VITAL STATISTICS OF THE UNITED STATES

VITAL STATISTICS OF THE UNITED STATES

BIRTHS, LIFE EXPECTANCY, DEATHS, AND SELECTED HEALTH DATA

SIXTH EDITION, 2014

Edited by Shana Hertz-Hattis

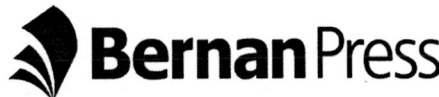
Bernan Press

Lanham • Boulder • New York • London

Published by Bernan Press
An imprint of The Rowman & Littlefield Publishing Group, Inc.
4501 Forbes Boulevard, Suite 200, Lanham, Maryland 20706
www.rowman.com
800-865-3457; info@bernan.com

16 Carlisle Street, London W1D 3BT, United Kingdom

ISBN-13: 978-1-59888-704-4

eISBN: 978-1-59888-705-1

ISSN: 1549-8603

∞™ The paper used in this publication meets the minimum requirements of American
National Standard for Information Sciences Permanence of Paper for Printed Library
Materials, ANSI/NISO Z39.48-1992.

Printed in the United States of America

CONTENTS

INTRODUCTION

Bernan Press is pleased to present a comprehensive collection of birth, mortality, health, and marriage data in the sixth edition of *Vital Statistics of the United States: Births, Life Expectancy, Deaths, and Selected Health Data.* This volume provides valuable information compiled by various government agencies including the Centers for Disease Control (CDC) and its National Center for Health Statistics (NCHS) and National Vital Statistics System (NVSS), the U.S. Census Bureau, and the Bureau of Labor Statistics (BLS).

Until 1993, the federal government published *Vital Statistics of the United States* in several thick-bound volumes. However, between the last publication of the federal volume and the first *Vital Statistics* edition from Bernan Press, nothing comparable was offered. During this time, the CDC continued to compile its information as periodical reports and news releases, and Bernan took this opportunity to streamline this information into a cohesive, inclusive volume.

The sixth edition builds upon the groundwork laid by the previous edition in the areas of birth, mortality, and health, and also includes a new chapter on marriages. Each part is preceded by highlights of salient data and contains a diverse array of information in its tables and figures. Notes and definitions and source information are also provided for all four parts.

The Birth section provides final data through 2011, as well as preliminary data for 2012. This section covers many aspects of natality, including birth and fertility rates, number of children, births to unmarried women, maternal health, methods of delivery, demographic characteristics of mothers, medical visits by pregnant women, and infant health status.

The Mortality section focuses on deaths and death rates, generally through 2010, as told through various medical, demographic, and social characteristics. Especially detailed are the tables on causes of death, which are shown by leading causes of death, age, sex, Hispanic origin, race, and (to a lesser extent) state of residence. Death rates are also given by marital status and level of educational attainment, and special tables are provided for infant mortality.

The Health section, the largest in the book, offers a collection of statistics concerning health and disease. While health is not a traditional component of vital statistics, its importance to this volume cannot be overstated. Health data provides the user with an even deeper picture of births and deaths in the United States. For example, a user interested in cancer deaths may glean useful information from tables about cancer incidence and survival rates. This chapter shows selected data on several topics, including determinants and measures of health, use of addictive substances, ambulatory care, inpatient care, health personnel, health expenditures, and health insurance.

The Marriage section, new to this edition, provides marriage and divorce rates by state and demographic characteristics. This chapter also provides statistics on multiple marriages, marriages ending in widowhood, and number of marriages for U.S. residents.

About the Editor

Shana Hertz-Hattis is an editor with over a decade of experience in statistical and government research publications. Past titles include *State Profiles: The Population and Economy of Each U.S. State, Housing Statistics of the United States,* and *The United States Government Internet Directory.* She earned her bachelor of science in journalism and master of science in education degrees from Northwestern University.

PART A

BIRTHS

CHAPTER 1: BIRTHS

Figure 1-1. Live Births and Fertility Rates, 1930–Preliminary 2012

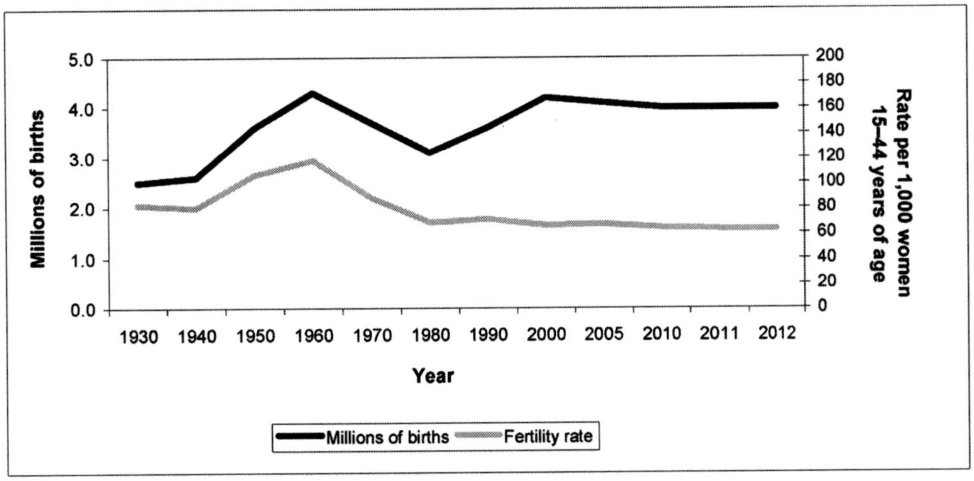

HIGHLIGHTS

- According to preliminary results, there were 3,952,937 births in the United States in 2012, down only slightly from 3,953,590 in 2011. Births increased for two racial groups: 7.5 percent for Asian or Other Pacific Islanders and 0.1 percent for non-Hispanic Blacks. Births declined 0.7 percent for American Indian and Alaska Natives and 0.6 percent for non-Hispanic Whites. Births also declined 1.2 percent for mothers of Hispanic ethnicity. (Table 1-1)

- The preliminary birth rate for teenagers age 15 to 19 years fell to 29.4 births per 1,000 females. From 1991 to 2012, this rate has declined 52.4 percent, and from 2011 to 2012, it declined 6.1 percent. (Table 1-6)

- In 2011, 40.7 percent of all births were to unmarried women, down from 41.0 percent in 2009. The numbers varied significantly by state. Utah had the lowest number of births to unmarried woman at 18.7 percent, followed by Colorado at 23.7 percent. Mississippi had the highest percentage of births to unmarried women of any state at 54.4 percent. The Virgin Islands had the highest percentage of births to unmarried women of any state or territory at 73.2 percent. (Table 1-46)

- In the 36 reporting states in 2011, South Carolina had the highest percentage of prepregnancy obesity (BMI of 30.0 or above) at 28.6 percent, while Utah had the lowest rate at 18.0 percent. In all of the states reporting, 47.3 percent of women had a normal prepregnancy BMI (18.5 to 24.9). (Table 1-70)

Table 1-1. Selected Characteristics, by Race and Hispanic Origin of Mother, Final 2011 and Preliminary 2012

(Number, rate, percent.)

Race and Hispanic origin of mother	Number		Birth rate		Fertility rate		Total fertility rate		Percent of births to unmarried women	
	2011	2012	2011	2012	2011	2012	2011	2012	2011	2012
All Races and Origins [1]	3,953,590	3,952,937	12.7	12.6	63.2	63.0	1,894.5	1,880.5	40.7	40.7
Non-Hispanic White [2]	2,146,566	2,133,115	10.8	10.7	58.7	58.7	1,773.5	1,761.5	29.0	29.4
Non-Hispanic Black [2]	582,345	583,060	14.7	14.6	65.4	65.0	1,919.5	1,898.5	72.3	72.2
American Indian or Alaska Native total [2,3]	46,419	46,093	10.7	10.5	47.7	47.0	1,373.5	1,350.0	66.2	66.9
Asian or Pacific Islander total [2,3]	253,915	272,949	14.5	15.1	59.9	62.2	1,706.5	1,770.0	17.2	17.1
Hispanic [4]	918,129	907,405	17.6	17.1	76.2	74.4	2,240.0	2,188.5	53.3	53.5

[1]Includes births to White Hispanic and Black Hispanic women and births with origin not stated, not shown separately.   [2]Race and Hispanic origin are reported separately on birth certificates. Persons of Hispanic origin may be of any race. Multiple-race data, when reported, were bridged to single-race categories in order to maintain comparability among all reported areas.   [3]Includes persons of Hispanic origin, and origin not stated, according to the mother's reported race.   [4]Persons of Hispanic origin may be of any race.

Table 1-2. Births and Birth Rates, by Race and Hispanic Origin of Mother, Final 2000–2011

(Number; rate. Birth rates are live births per 1,000 population in specified group. Fertility rates are live births per 1,000 women aged 15–44 years in specified group.)

Year and characteristic	All races and origins[1]	Non-Hispanic White[2]	Non-Hispanic Black[2]	American Indian or Alaska Native[2,3]	Asian or Pacific Islander[2,3]	Hispanic[4]
Number						
2000	4,058,814	2,362,968	604,346	41,668	200,543	815,868
2001	4,025,933	2,326,578	589,917	41,872	200,279	851,851
2002	4,021,726	2,298,156	578,335	42,368	210,907	876,642
2003	4,089,950	2,321,904	576,033	43,052	221,203	912,329
2004	4,112,052	2,296,683	578,772	43,927	229,123	946,349
2005	4,138,349	2,279,768	583,759	44,813	231,108	985,505
2006	4,265,555	2,308,640	617,247	47,721	241,045	1,039,077
2007	4,316,233	2,310,333	627,191	49,443	254,488	1,062,779
2008	4,247,694	2,267,817	623,029	49,537	253,185	1,041,239
2009	4,130,665	2,212,552	609,584	48,665	251,089	999,548
2010	3,999,386	2,162,406	589,808	46,760	246,886	945,180
2011	3,953,590	2,146,566	582,345	46,419	253,915	918,129
Birth Rate						
2000	14.4	12.2	17.3	14.0	17.1	23.1
2001	14.1	11.9	16.6	13.5	16.1	22.9
2002	14.0	11.7	16.1	13.2	16.3	22.7
2003	14.1	11.8	15.9	13.0	16.4	22.8
2004	14.0	11.7	15.8	12.8	16.4	22.8
2005	14.0	11.6	15.8	12.6	15.9	22.9
2006	14.3	11.7	16.5	12.9	16.0	23.3
2007	14.3	11.7	16.6	12.9	16.4	23.0
2008	14.0	11.5	16.3	12.4	15.7	21.8
2009	13.5	11.2	15.7	11.8	15.1	20.3
2010	13.0	10.9	15.1	11.0	14.5	18.7
2011	12.7	10.8	14.7	10.7	14.5	17.6
Fertility Rate						
2000	65.9	58.5	71.4	58.7	65.8	95.9
2001	65.1	57.7	69.1	57.0	62.5	95.4
2002	65.0	57.6	67.5	55.8	63.4	94.7
2003	66.1	58.9	67.1	55.0	64.2	95.2
2004	66.4	58.9	67.1	54.3	64.5	95.7
2005	66.7	59.0	67.2	53.6	63.0	96.4
2006	68.6	60.3	70.7	55.4	63.6	98.3
2007	69.3	61.0	71.4	55.6	65.3	97.4
2008	68.1	60.5	70.8	54.1	63.3	92.7
2009	66.2	59.6	68.9	51.7	61.3	86.5
2010	64.1	58.7	66.6	48.6	59.2	80.2
2011	63.2	58.7	65.4	47.7	59.9	76.2

[1]Includes births to race and origin groups not shown separately, such as White Hispanic and Black Hispanic women, and births with origin not stated.   [2]Race and Hispanic origin are reported separately on birth certificates. Persons of Hispanic origin may be of any race. Multiple-race data, when reported, were bridged to single-race categories in order to maintain comparability among all reported areas.   [3]Includes persons of Hispanic origin, and origin not stated, according to the mother's reported race.   [4]Persons of Hispanic origin may be of any race.

Table 1-3. Births and Birth Rates, by Age, Race, and Hispanic Origin of Mother, Final 2011 and Preliminary 2012

(Number, rates per 1,000 women in specified age group.)

Age, race, and Hispanic origin of mother	2011 Number	2011 Rate	2012 Number	2012 Rate
All Races and Origins [1]				
Total[2]	3,953,590	63.2	3,952,937	63.0
10 to 14 years	3,974	0.4	3,674	0.4
15 to 19 years	329,772	31.3	305,420	29.4
15 to 17 years	95,538	15.4	86,440	14.1
18 to 19 years	234,234	54.1	218,980	51.4
20 to 24 years	925,200	85.3	916,868	83.1
25 to 29 years	1,127,583	107.2	1,124,010	106.5
30 to 34 years	986,682	96.5	1,013,473	97.3
35 to 39 years	463,849	47.2	472,206	48.3
40 to 44 years	108,920	10.3	109,535	10.4
45 to 54 years[3]	7,610	0.7	7,750	0.7
Non-Hispanic White [4]				
Total[2]	2,146,566	58.7	2,133,115	58.7
10 to 14 years	869	0.2	866	0.2
15 to 19 years	129,329	21.7	119,777	20.5
15 to 17 years	31,461	9.0	29,008	8.4
18 to 19 years	97,868	39.9	90,769	37.9
20 to 24 years	451,939	71.8	444,371	70.2
25 to 29 years	647,520	105.2	641,353	104.4
30 to 34 years	591,266	100.1	602,549	100.5
35 to 39 years	260,596	45.8	261,509	46.8
40 to 44 years	60,724	9.3	58,515	9.1
45 to 54 years[3]	4,323	0.6	4,174	0.6
Non-Hispanic Black [4]				
Total[2]	582,345	65.4	583,080	65.0
10 to 14 years	1,378	0.9	1,263	0.8
15 to 19 years	78,558	47.3	71,271	43.9
15 to 17 years	23,659	24.6	20,553	21.9
18 to 19 years	54,899	78.8	50,719	74.1
20 to 24 years	186,229	112.3	187,386	109.0
25 to 29 years	147,708	101.7	149,548	101.7
30 to 34 years	104,274	73.9	107,768	75.1
35 to 39 years	50,245	37.8	51,461	38.9
40 to 44 years	12,952	9.3	13,360	9.6
45 to 54 years[3]	1,001	0.7	1,022	0.7
American Indian or Alaska Native Total [4,5]				
Total[2]	48,419	47.7	46,093	47.0
10 to 14 years	95	0.5	89	0.5
15 to 19 years	6,802	36.1	6,478	34.9
15 to 17 years	2,014	18.2	1,856	17.0
18 to 19 years	4,788	61.6	4,621	60.6
20 to 24 years	15,569	86.6	15,168	81.7
25 to 29 years	12,477	75.4	12,290	73.9
30 to 34 years	7,380	47.3	7,871	49.7
35 to 39 years	3,292	23.1	3,355	22.3
40 to 44 years	772	5.5	778	5.5
45 to 54 years[3]	32	0.2	64	0.5
Asian or Pacific Islander Total [4,5]				
Total[2]	253,915	59.9	272,949	62.2
10 to 14 years	65	0.1	62	0.1
15 to 19 years	5,708	10.2	5,544	9.7
15 to 17 years	1,532	4.6	1,414	4.2
18 to 19 years	4,176	18.1	4,131	17.8
20 to 24 years	27,783	41.9	28,580	41.4
25 to 29 years	70,461	93.7	74,254	95.8
30 to 34 years	88,660	114.9	97,986	121.4
35 to 39 years	49,474	64.1	53,392	68.1
40 to 44 years	10,963	15.2	12,196	16.1
45 to 54 years[3]	801	1.2	935	1.4
Hispanic [6]				
Total[2]	918,129	76.2	907,405	74.4
10 to 14 years	1,576	0.7	1,397	0.6
15 to 19 years	109,660	49.6	102,698	46.3
15 to 17 years	36,979	28.0	33,756	25.5
18 to 19 years	72,681	81.5	68,942	77.2
20 to 24 years	243,724	116.0	241,049	111.4
25 to 29 years	248,269	121.3	244,403	119.6
30 to 34 years	192,517	95.2	193,106	94.3
35 to 39 years	98,340	51.3	99,820	51.5
40 to 44 years	22,807	13.1	23,657	13.2
45 to 54 years[3]	1,236	0.8	1,275	0.8

[1]Includes births to race and origin groups not shown separately, such as White Hispanic and Black Hispanic women, and births with origin not stated.   [2]Includes births to women of all ages. The rate shown for all ages is the fertility rate, which is defined as the total number of births (regardless of the age of the mother) per 1,000 women age 15 to 44 years.   [3]The birth rate for women age 45 to 49 years is computed by relating the number of births to women age 45 and over to women age 45 to 49 years, as most of the births are to women age 45 to 49 years.   [4]Race and Hispanic origin are reported separately on birth certificates. Persons of Hispanic origin may be of any race. Multiple-race data, when reported, were bridged to single-race categories in order to maintain comparability among all reported areas.   [5]Includes persons of Hispanic origin, and origin not stated, according to the mother's reported race.   [6]Includes all persons of Hispanic origin of any race.

Table 1-4. Live Births, by Age of Mother, Live-Birth Order, and Race and Hispanic Origin of Mother, Preliminary 2012

(Number.)

Live-birth order and race and Hispanic origin of mother	All ages	Under 15 years	15 to 19 years	20 to 24 years	25 to 29 years	30 to 34 years	35 to 39 years	40 to 44 years	45 to 54 years
All Races and Origins [1]	3,952,937	3,674	305,420	916,868	1,124,010	1,013,473	472,206	109,535	7,750
1st child	1,569,943	3,580	250,985	461,445	421,522	299,379	106,715	24,208	2,109
2nd child	1,244,555	60	45,522	298,047	369,862	346,482	151,769	30,851	1,960
3rd child	650,242	8	6,380	111,071	202,018	201,814	105,269	22,471	1,211
4th child and over	465,373	8	865	41,077	124,590	160,074	105,457	31,219	2,383
Not stated	22,524	18	1,668	5,229	6,017	5,723	2,996	786	87
Non-Hispanic White [2]	2,133,115	866	119,777	444,371	641,353	602,549	261,509	58,515	4,174
1st child	894,666	841	102,656	242,556	271,221	195,337	65,928	14,857	1,270
2nd child	696,630	16	14,894	140,806	214,683	217,794	89,648	17,657	1,132
3rd child	328,230	2	1,624	45,605	100,746	111,875	56,268	11,476	634
4th child and over	205,299	2	174	13,655	52,321	75,210	48,585	14,243	1,110
Not stated	8,289	5	428	1,750	2,382	2,334	1,079	282	29
Non-Hispanic Black [2]	583,080	1,263	71,271	187,386	149,548	107,768	51,461	13,360	1,022
1st child	222,583	1,224	56,747	86,698	41,729	23,818	9,581	2,537	247
2nd child	165,147	26	11,498	59,390	46,090	31,087	13,546	3,281	228
3rd child	99,070	3	1,956	36,470	31,949	23,986	11,762	2,780	164
4th child and over	90,059	1	304	12,844	28,283	27,692	15,950	4,618	367
Not stated	6,222	9	767	1,984	1,497	1,186	620	144	15
American Indian or Alaska Native [2,3]	46,093	89	6,478	15,168	12,290	7,871	3,355	778	64
1st child	15,959	88	5,203	6,225	2,698	1,229	428	84	3
2nd child	12,417	1	1,062	5,152	3,531	1,880	644	129	17
3rd child	8,269	-	162	2,497	2,947	1,795	725	135	7
4th child and over	9,175	-	24	1,205	3,041	2,920	1,526	424	34
Not stated	274	-	26	90	72	46	31	6	3
Asian or Pacific Islander [2,3]	272,949	62	5,544	28,580	74,254	97,986	53,392	12,196	935
1st child	122,656	61	4,591	17,236	41,112	40,721	15,361	3,284	291
2nd child	97,554	1	818	7,885	22,055	39,290	22,708	4,512	284
3rd child	33,589	-	101	2,450	7,066	11,600	9,794	2,430	150
4th child and over	17,850	-	11	880	3,649	5,932	5,264	1,910	204
Not stated	1,300	-	22	130	373	443	265	60	6
Hispanic [4]	907,485	1,397	102,698	241,049	244,403	193,106	99,820	23,657	1,275
1st child	310,139	1,367	82,119	108,456	63,681	36,556	14,561	3,149	250
2nd child	270,546	17	17,349	84,965	83,094	55,389	24,499	4,982	250
3rd child	180,492	3	2,539	34,155	59,355	52,308	26,406	5,520	207
4th child and over	142,489	5	353	12,556	37,228	48,019	33,889	9,880	559
Not stated	3,739	4	338	917	1,045	834	466	126	9

- = Quantity zero.   [1]Includes births to race and origin groups not shown separately, such as White Hispanic and Black Hispanic women, and births with origin not stated.   [2]Race and Hispanic origin are reported separately on birth certificates. Persons of Hispanic origin may be of any race. Multiple-race data, when reported, were bridged to single-race categories in order to maintain comparability among all reported areas.   [3]Includes persons of Hispanic origin, and origin not stated, according to the mother's reported race.   [4]Persons of Hispanic origin may be of any race.

Table 1-5. Birth Rates, by Age of Mother, Live-Birth Order, and Race and Hispanic Origin of Mother, Preliminary 2012

(Rates per 1,000 women in specified age groups.)

Live-birth order, race, and Hispanic origin of mother	15 to 44 years[1]	10 to 14 years	15 to 19 years	20 to 24 years	25 to 29 years	30 to 34 years	35 to 39 years	40 to 44 years	45 to 49 years[2]
All Races and Origins[3]	63.0	0.4	29.4	83.1	106.5	97.3	48.3	10.4	0.7
1st child	25.2	0.4	24.3	42.1	40.2	28.9	11.0	2.3	0.2
2nd child	19.9	0.0	4.4	27.2	35.2	33.4	15.6	2.9	0.2
3rd child	10.4	*	0.6	10.1	19.2	19.5	10.8	2.1	0.1
4th child and over	7.5	*	0.1	3.7	11.9	15.5	10.9	3.0	0.2
Non-Hispanic White[4]	58.7	0.2	20.5	70.2	104.4	100.5	46.8	9.1	0.6
1st child	24.7	0.3	17.6	38.5	44.3	32.8	11.9	2.3	0.2
2nd child	19.2	*	2.6	22.3	35.1	36.4	16.1	2.8	0.2
3rd child	9.1	*	0.3	7.2	16.5	18.7	10.1	1.8	0.1
4th child and over	5.7	*	0.0	2.2	8.6	12.6	8.7	2.2	0.2
Non-Hispanic Black[4]	65.0	0.8	43.9	109.0	101.7	75.1	38.9	9.6	0.7
1st child	25.1	0.8	35.3	51.0	28.7	16.9	7.4	1.9	0.2
2nd child	18.6	0.0	7.2	34.9	31.7	21.9	10.4	2.4	0.2
3rd child	11.2	*	1.2	15.6	21.9	16.9	9.0	2.0	0.1
4th child and over	10.1	*	0.2	7.5	19.4	19.5	12.2	3.3	0.3
American Indian or Alaska Native Total[4,5]	47.0	0.5	34.9	81.7	73.9	49.7	23.3	5.5	0.5
1st child	16.4	0.5	28.2	33.7	16.3	7.8	3.0	0.6	*
2nd child	12.7	*	5.7	27.9	21.4	11.9	4.5	0.9	*
3rd child	8.5	*	0.9	13.5	17.8	11.4	5.1	1.0	*
4th child and over	9.4	*	0.1	6.5	18.4	18.5	10.7	3.0	0.3
Asian or Pacific Islander Total[4,5]	62.2	0.1	9.7	41.4	95.8	121.4	68.1	16.1	1.4
1st child	28.1	0.1	8.0	25.1	53.3	50.7	19.7	4.3	0.4
2nd child	22.3	*	1.4	11.5	28.6	48.9	29.1	6.0	0.4
3rd child	7.7	*	0.2	3.6	9.2	14.4	12.6	3.2	0.2
4th child and over	4.1	*	*	1.3	4.7	7.4	6.7	2.5	0.3
Hispanic[6]	74.4	0.6	46.3	111.4	119.6	94.3	51.5	13.2	0.8
1st child	25.5	0.6	37.1	50.3	31.3	17.9	7.6	1.8	0.2
2nd child	22.3	0.0	7.8	39.4	40.8	27.2	12.7	2.8	0.2
3rd child	14.9	*	1.1	15.8	29.2	25.6	13.7	3.1	0.1
4th child and over	11.7	*	0.2	5.8	18.3	23.5	17.6	5.5	0.4

* = Figure does not meet standards of reliability or precision.   0.0 = Quantity more than zero but less than 0.05.   [1]The rate shown is the fertility rate, which is defined as the total number of births (regardless of the age of the mother) per 1,000 women age 15 to 44 years.   [2]The birth rate for women age 45 to 49 years is computed by relating the number of births to women age 45 and over to women age 45 to 49 years, as most of the births are to women age 45 to 49 years.   [3]Includes births to race and origin groups not shown separately, such as White Hispanic and Black Hispanic women, and births with origin not stated.   [4]Race and Hispanic origin are reported separately on birth certificates. Persons of Hispanic origin may be of any race. Multiple-race data, when reported, were bridged to single-race categories in order to maintain comparability among all reported areas.   [5]Includes persons of Hispanic origin, and origin not stated, according to the mother's reported race.   [6]Includes all persons of Hispanic origin of any race.

Table 1-6. Birth Rates for Women Under 20 Years of Age, by Age and Race and Hispanic Origin of Mother, Selected Years, 1991–Preliminary 2012

(Rates per 1,000 women in specified group.)

Age, race, and Hispanic origin of mother	Year					Percent change		
	1991	2007	2010	2011	2012 (preliminary)	1991–2012	2007–2012	2011–2012
10 to 14 Years								
All races and origins[1]	1.4	0.6	0.4	0.4	0.4	-71.4	-33.3	†
Non-Hispanic White[2]	0.5	0.2	0.2	0.2	0.2	-60.0	†	†
Non-Hispanic Black[2]	4.9	1.4	1.0	0.9	0.8	-83.7	-42.9	-11.1
American Indian or Alaska Native total[2,3]	1.6	0.7	0.5	0.5	0.5	-68.8	-28.6	†
Asian or Pacific Islander total[2,3]	0.8	0.2	0.1	0.1	0.1	-87.5	-50.0	†
Hispanic[4]	2.4	1.2	0.8	0.8	0.7	-75.0	-50.0	-14.3
15 to 19 Years								
All races and origins[1]	61.8	41.5	34.2	31.3	29.4	-52.4	-29.2	-6.1
Non-Hispanic White[2]	43.4	27.2	23.5	21.7	20.5	-52.8	-24.6	-5.5
Non-Hispanic Black[2]	118.2	62.0	51.5	47.3	43.9	-62.9	-29.2	-7.2
American Indian or Alaska Native total[2,3]	84.1	49.3	38.7	36.1	34.9	-58.5	-29.2	-3.3
Asian or Pacific Islander total[2,3]	27.3	14.8	10.9	10.2	9.7	-64.5	-34.5	-4.9
Hispanic[4]	104.6	75.3	55.7	49.6	46.3	-55.7	-38.5	-6.7
15 to 17 Years								
All races and origins[1]	38.6	21.7	17.3	15.4	14.1	-63.5	-35.0	-8.4
Non-Hispanic White[2]	23.6	11.9	10.0	9.0	8.4	-64.4	-29.4	-6.7
Non-Hispanic Black[2]	86.1	34.6	27.4	24.6	21.9	-74.6	-36.7	-11.0
American Indian or Alaska Native total[2,3]	51.9	26.1	20.1	18.2	17.0	-67.2	-34.9	-6.6
Asian or Pacific Islander total[2,3]	16.3	7.4	5.1	4.6	4.2	-74.2	-43.2	-8.7
Hispanic[4]	69.2	44.4	32.3	28.0	25.5	-63.2	-42.6	-8.9
18 to 19 Years								
All races and origins[1]	94.0	71.7	58.2	54.1	51.4	-45.3	-28.3	-5.0
Non-Hispanic White[2]	70.6	50.4	42.5	39.9	37.9	-46.3	-24.8	-5.0
Non-Hispanic Black[2]	162.2	105.2	85.6	78.8	74.1	-54.3	-29.6	-6.0
American Indian or Alaska Native total[2,3]	134.2	86.3	66.1	61.6	60.6	-54.8	-29.8	†
Asian or Pacific Islander total[2,3]	42.2	24.9	18.7	18.1	17.8	-57.8	-28.5	†
Hispanic[4]	155.5	124.7	90.7	81.5	77.2	-50.4	-38.1	-5.3

† = Difference not statistically significant.   [1]Includes births to race and origin groups not shown separately, such as White Hispanic and Black Hispanic women, and births with origin not stated.   [2]Race and Hispanic origin are reported separately on birth certificates. Persons of Hispanic origin may be of any race. Multiple-race data, when reported, were bridged to single-race categories in order to maintain comparability among all reported areas.   [3]Includes persons of Hispanic origin, and origin not stated, according to the mother's reported race.   [4]Includes all persons of Hispanic origin of any race.

Table 1-7. Birth Rate for Teenagers Age 15 to 19 Years, by State and Territory, 2010 and 2011

(Rate per 1,000 female population age 15 to 19 years.)

State	2010	2011	Percent change
United States [1]	34.2	31.3	-8.5
Alabama	43.6	40.5	-7.1
Alaska	38.3	36.2	†
Arizona	41.9	38.5	-8.1
Arkansas	52.5	50.7	†
California	31.5	28.7	-8.9
Colorado	33.4	28.9	-13.5
Connecticut	18.7	16.4	-12.3
Delaware	30.5	29.3	†
District of Columbia	45.4	42.8	†
Florida	32.0	29.5	-7.8
Georgia	41.4	38.2	-7.7
Hawaii	32.5	30.0	-7.7
Idaho	33.0	27.7	-16.1
Illinois	33.0	29.5	-10.6
Indiana	37.3	34.8	-6.7
Iowa	28.6	25.3	-11.5
Kansas	39.3	35.4	-9.9
Kentucky	46.2	43.5	-5.8
Louisiana	47.7	45.1	-5.5
Maine	21.4	20.8	†
Maryland	27.3	24.7	-9.5
Massachusetts	17.2	15.4	-10.5
Michigan	30.1	27.8	-7.6
Minnesota	22.5	19.3	-14.2
Mississippi	55.0	50.2	-8.7
Missouri	37.1	34.5	-7.0
Montana	35.0	29.2	-16.6
Nebraska	31.1	27.2	-12.5
Nevada	38.6	36.1	-6.5
New Hampshire	15.7	13.7	-12.7
New Jersey	20.1	18.7	-7.0
New Mexico	53.0	48.8	-7.9
New York	22.7	21.2	-6.6
North Carolina	38.3	34.9	-8.9
North Dakota	28.8	28.2	†
Ohio	34.1	31.5	-7.6
Oklahoma	50.4	47.8	-5.2
Oregon	28.2	25.8	-8.5
Pennsylvania	27.0	24.9	-7.8
Rhode Island	22.3	21.3	†
South Carolina	42.6	39.1	-8.2
South Dakota	34.9	34.3	†
Tennessee	43.2	40.8	-5.6
Texas	52.2	46.9	-10.2
Utah	27.9	23.1	-17.2
Vermont	17.9	16.8	†
Virginia	27.4	24.5	-10.6
Washington	26.7	25.4	-4.9
West Virginia	44.4	43.5	†
Wisconsin	26.2	23.2	-11.5
Wyoming	39.0	35.2	-9.7
Puerto Rico	51.4	51.7	†
Virgin Islands	50.5	59.3	†
Guam	60.1	62.1	†
American Samoa	34.1	38.4	†
Northern Marianas	53.4	47.2	†

† = Difference not statistically significant.   [1] Excludes data for the territories.

Figure 1-2. Percent of Births, by Race and Hispanic Origin, Preliminary 2012

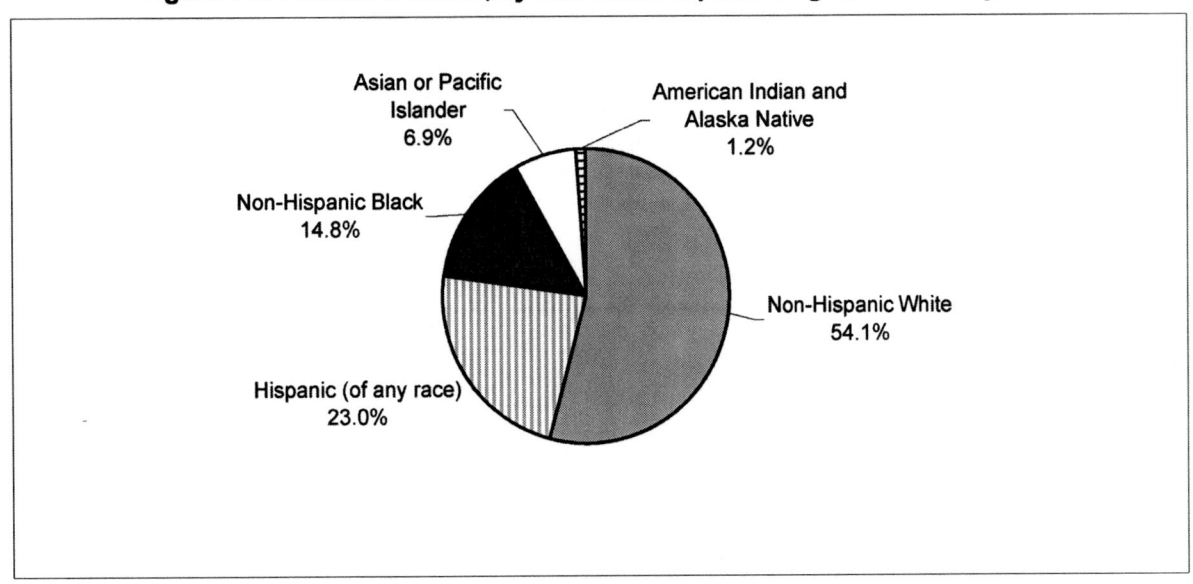

Figure 1-3. Percent of Births to Unmarried Women, by Race and Hispanic Origin, 2011

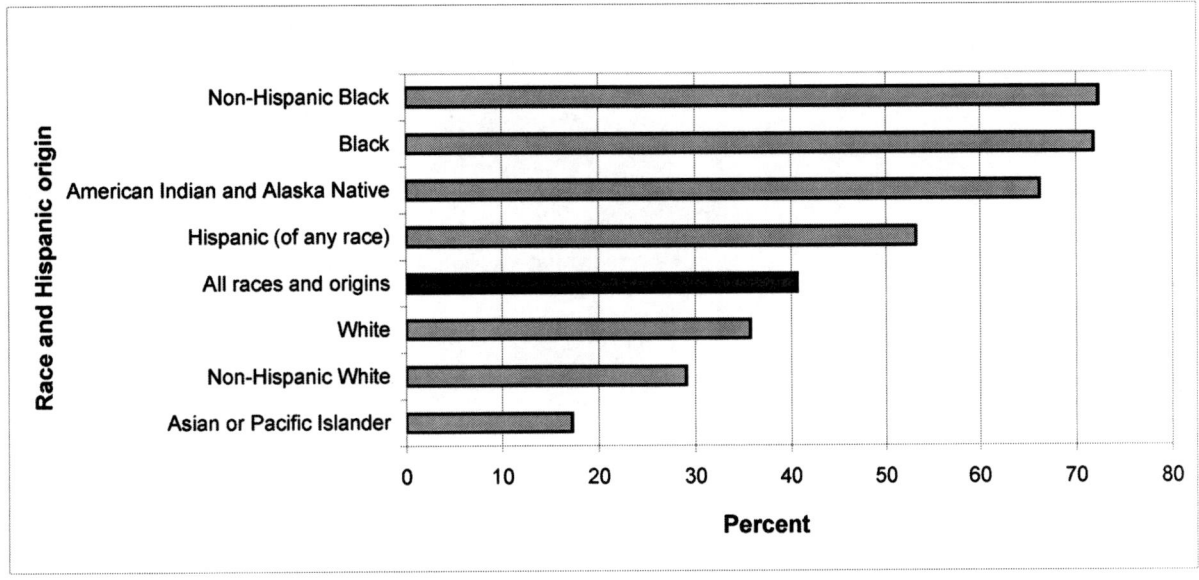

Table 1-8. Number, Percent, and Rate of Births to Unmarried Women, by Age, 2011

(Number, percent, rate per 1,000 unmarried women.)

Age of mother	Number	Percent	Rate
Total	1,607,773	40.7	NA
Under 20 years	295,675	18.4	NA
Under 15 years	3,939	99.1	NA
15 to 19 years	291,736	88.5	28.4
20 to 24 years	592,544	64.0	66.7
25 to 29 years	387,354	34.4	67.8
30 to 34 years	212,974	21.6	56.2
35 to 39 years	93,155	20.1	29.9
40 years and over	26,061	22.4	8.2

NA = Not available.

Table 1-9. Live Births, by Race and Hispanic Origin of Mother, and Birth and Fertility Rates, by State and Territory, 2011

(Birth rates are total births per 1,000 women; fertility rates are total births per 1,000 women age 15-44 years.)

State and territory	All races and origins[1]	Non-Hispanic White[2]	Non-Hispanic Black[2]	American Indian or Alaskan Native[2,3]	Asian or Pacific Islander[2,3]	Hispanic[4]	Birth rate for all races	Fertility rate for all races
United States [5]	3,953,590	2,146,566	582,345	46,419	253,915	918,129	12.7	63.2
Alabama	59,534	35,684	17,987	197	1,016	4,481	12.4	61.8
Alaska	11,456	6,082	437	2,842	1,040	757	15.9	78.5
Arizona	85,543	38,988	4,083	5,989	3,553	33,254	13.2	67.3
Arkansas	38,715	26,408	7,231	280	755	3,958	13.2	67.8
California	502,120	144,584	29,902	3,461	70,419	250,030	13.3	63.4
Colorado	65,055	40,439	3,054	675	2,546	18,077	12.7	62.7
Connecticut	37,281	21,538	4,476	255	2,289	8,393	10.4	54.3
Delaware	11,257	6,222	3,031	23	553	1,416	12.4	62.9
District of Columbia	9,295	2,626	4,809	20	554	1,371	15.0	56.0
Florida	213,414	97,304	49,084	435	7,286	58,739	11.2	59.6
Georgia	132,409	60,622	44,649	336	6,198	18,664	13.5	63.8
Hawaii	18,956	4,860	508	80	12,247	3,038	13.8	71.9
Idaho	22,305	17,869	192	414	440	3,475	14.1	72.3
Illinois	161,312	87,952	27,183	218	9,727	35,765	12.5	61.5
Indiana	83,701	64,482	9,825	157	2,025	7,180	12.8	65.0
Iowa	38,214	31,927	1,844	266	1,208	3,114	12.5	66.1
Kansas	39,642	28,814	2,934	380	1,342	6,294	13.8	71.2
Kentucky	55,370	46,190	5,204	86	1,185	2,782	12.7	64.7
Louisiana	61,888	33,112	23,608	381	1,340	3,607	13.5	66.4
Maine	12,704	11,747	395	111	211	208	9.6	53.1
Maryland	73,093	33,265	23,846	205	5,716	10,330	12.5	61.3
Massachusetts	73,166	46,570	7,161	165	6,278	12,573	11.1	54.3
Michigan	114,008	79,607	21,775	793	3,991	7,628	11.5	59.9
Minnesota	68,409	50,297	6,471	1,540	5,115	4,629	12.8	65.5
Mississippi	39,860	20,500	17,304	282	427	1,320	13.4	66.0
Missouri	76,117	57,815	11,433	395	2,006	4,113	12.7	64.8
Montana	12,069	9,934	75	1,486	143	449	12.1	66.7
Nebraska	25,720	19,301	1,708	514	723	3,646	14.0	72.0
Nevada	35,296	15,259	3,695	468	2,981	13,049	13.0	64.2
New Hampshire	12,851	11,392	234	22	521	540	9.7	51.9
New Jersey	105,883	49,661	16,047	182	11,852	28,013	12.0	61.3
New Mexico	27,289	7,719	473	3,617	525	15,061	13.1	68.2
New York	241,312	117,201	39,157	1,182	24,794	56,703	12.4	59.8
North Carolina	120,389	67,688	28,597	1,982	5,165	18,219	12.5	61.5
North Dakota	9,527	7,759	218	1,036	172	307	13.9	72.4
Ohio	137,918	104,506	22,835	273	3,509	6,337	11.9	62.1
Oklahoma	52,272	33,358	4,815	6,187	1,474	6,684	13.8	70.4
Oregon	45,155	31,768	1,168	873	2,687	8,742	11.7	59.4
Pennsylvania	143,178	100,790	21,027	383	6,289	14,178	11.2	58.8
Rhode Island	10,960	6,755	959	148	597	2,424	10.4	51.5
South Carolina	57,393	32,977	18,288	241	1,206	4,748	12.3	61.8
South Dakota	11,846	8,859	266	2,094	230	505	14.4	77.1
Tennessee	79,588	54,131	16,557	234	1,933	7,022	12.4	62.3
Texas	377,445	133,894	43,212	1,107	17,289	182,503	14.7	69.8
Utah	51,223	40,860	568	770	1,683	7,686	18.2	83.6
Vermont	6,078	5,727	89	17	158	72	9.7	51.8
Virginia	102,652	60,370	21,945	121	7,645	12,473	12.7	62.9
Washington	86,976	55,084	4,303	2,234	9,444	15,976	12.7	63.7
West Virginia	20,717	19,497	726	19	185	207	11.2	60.7
Wisconsin	67,810	50,500	6,592	975	3,141	6,525	11.9	62.0
Wyoming	7,399	6,072	65	268	102	864	13.0	69.1
Puerto Rico	41,080	1,175	133	NA	NA	39,706	11.1	53.6
Virgin Islands	1,491	111	1,017	4	22	320	14.1	72.2
Guam	3,294	194	33	6	3,022	52	20.6	95.9
American Samoa	1,256	NA	NA	-	1,252	NA	22.8	95.3
Northern Marianas	1,033	10	2	-	1,021	NA	19.8	74.0

NA = Not available. - = Quantity zero   [1]Includes births to race and origin groups not shown separately, such as White Hispanic and Black Hispanic women, and births with origin not stated.   [2]Race and Hispanic origin are reported separately on birth certificates.   [3]Includes persons of Hispanic origin according to the mother's reported race.   [4]Includes all persons of Hispanic origin of any race.   [5]Excludes data for the territories.

Table 1-10. Selected Characteristics of Births, by Race and Hispanic Origin of Mother, Final 2011 and Preliminary 2012

(Number, rate.)

Race and Hispanic origin of mother	Number		Cesarean rate[1]		Preterm				Low birthweight			
					Total[2]		Late[3]		Total[4]		Very low birthweight[5]	
	2011	2012	2011	2012	2011	2012	2011	2012	2011	2012	2011	2012
All Races and Origins [6]	3,953,590	3,952,937	32.8	32.8	11.7	11.5	8.3	8.1	8.1	8.0	1.4	1.4
Non-Hispanic White[7]	2,146,566	2,133,115	32.4	32.3	10.5	10.3	7.6	7.4	7.1	7.0	1.1	1.1
Non-Hispanic Black[7]	582,345	583,080	35.5	35.8	16.8	16.5	10.7	10.6	13.3	13.1	3.0	3.0
American Indian or Alaska Native total[7,8]	46,419	46,093	28.4	28.6	13.5	13.3	9.6	9.3	7.6	7.6	1.3	1.3
Asian or Pacific Islander total[7,8]	253,915	272,949	33.2	33.2	10.4	10.2	7.6	7.5	8.4	8.2	1.2	1.1
Hispanic[9]	918,129	907,405	32.0	32.2	11.7	11.6	8.4	8.3	7.0	7.0	1.2	1.2

[1]All births by cesarean delivery per 100 live births.   [2]Born prior to 37 completed weeks of gestation.   [3]Born between 34 and 36 completed weeks of gestation.   [4]Birthweight of less than 2,500 grams (5 lb 8 oz).   [5]Birthweight of less than 1,500 grams (3 lb 4 oz).   [6]Includes births to White Hispanic and Black Hispanic women and births with origin not stated, not shown separately.   [7]Race and Hispanic origin are reported separately on birth certificates. Persons of Hispanic origin may be of any race. Multiple-race data, when reported, were bridged to single-race categories in order to maintain comparability among all reported areas.   [8]Includes persons of Hispanic and non-Hispanic origin and origin not stated, according to the mother's reported race.   [9]Persons of Hispanic origin may be of any race.

Table 1-11. Low Birthweight Births, by State and Territory of Residence, Final 2011 and Preliminary 2012

(Percent.)

State and territory	2011	2012
United States [1]	8.1	8.0
Alabama	9.9	10.0
Alaska	6.0	5.6
Arizona	7.0	6.9
Arkansas	9.1	8.7
California	6.8	6.7
Colorado	8.7	8.8
Connecticut	7.7	7.9
Delaware	8.4	8.3
District of Columbia	10.4	9.6
Florida	8.7	8.6
Georgia	9.4	9.3
Hawaii	8.2	8.1
Idaho	6.1	6.4
Illinois	8.2	8.1
Indiana	8.1	7.9
Iowa	6.5	6.7
Kansas	7.2	7.1
Kentucky	9.1	8.6
Louisiana	10.9	10.8
Maine	6.7	6.6
Maryland	8.9	8.8
Massachusetts	7.6	7.5
Michigan	8.3	8.4
Minnesota	6.4	6.6
Mississippi	11.8	11.6
Missouri	7.9	7.7
Montana	7.2	7.4
Nebraska	6.6	6.7
Nevada	8.2	8.0
New Hampshire	7.1	7.3
New Jersey	8.5	8.2
New Mexico	8.8	8.8
New York	8.1	7.9
North Carolina	9.0	8.8
North Dakota	6.7	6.2
Ohio	8.6	8.6
Oklahoma	8.5	8.0
Oregon	6.1	6.1
Pennsylvania	8.2	8.1
Rhode Island	7.4	8.0
South Carolina	9.9	9.6
South Dakota	6.3	6.2
Tennessee	9.0	9.2
Texas	8.5	8.3
Utah	6.9	6.8
Vermont	6.7	6.2
Virginia	8.0	8.1
Washington	6.1	6.1
West Virginia	9.6	9.2
Wisconsin	7.2	7.1
Wyoming	8.1	8.5
Puerto Rico	12.5	11.6
Virgin Islands	10.4	NA
Guam	9.0	*
American Samoa	4.3	5.2
Northern Marianas	7.3	NA

* = Figure does not meet standards of reliability or precision.   NA = Not available.   [1]Excludes data for the territories.

Table 1-12. Preterm Births, Selected Years, 1990–2011 and Preliminary 2012

(Percent.)

Year	Total preterm[1]	Late preterm[2]	Early preterm (less than 34 weeks)		
			Total	32–33 weeks	Less than 32 weeks
1990	10.6	7.3	3.3	1.4	1.9
2006	12.8	9.1	3.7	1.6	2.0
2010	12.0	8.5	3.5	1.5	2.0
2011	11.7	8.3	3.4	1.5	2.0
2012 (preliminary)	11.5	8.1	3.4	1.5	1.9

[1]Preterm is less than 37 completed weeks of gestation.   [2]Late preterm is 34 to 36 completed weeks of gestation.

Table 1-13. Preterm and Late Term Births, by State and Territory of Residence, Final 2011 and Preliminary 2012

(Percent.)

Area	2011		2012	
	Late preterm[1]	Preterm[2]	Late preterm[1]	Preterm[2]
United States [3]	8.3	11.7	8.1	11.5
Alabama	10.3	14.9	10.0	14.6
Alaska	7.5	10.4	6.8	9.2
Arizona	9.2	12.1	8.3	11.6
Arkansas	9.6	13.2	9.8	13.3
California	7.1	9.8	6.9	9.6
Colorado	7.3	10.3	7.5	10.4
Connecticut	6.9	10.1	6.9	9.7
Delaware	7.4	11.2	8.1	12.3
District of Columbia	9.1	13.7	8.1	12.8
Florida	9.1	13.0	9.7	13.7
Georgia	9.3	13.2	8.8	12.7
Hawaii	8.7	12.3	9.0	12.2
Idaho	7.6	10.2	7.8	10.3
Illinois	8.4	12.1	8.3	12.0
Indiana	8.2	11.6	7.8	10.9
Iowa	8.0	11.1	8.2	11.5
Kansas	8.2	11.2	7.9	11.0
Kentucky	9.6	13.4	8.9	12.7
Louisiana	10.6	15.6	10.5	15.3
Maine	6.8	9.6	6.3	9.2
Maryland	8.6	12.5	8.4	12.2
Massachusetts	7.3	10.5	7.1	10.0
Michigan	8.3	12.0	8.1	11.8
Minnesota	7.1	9.9	7.1	10.2
Mississippi	11.9	16.9	11.9	17.1
Missouri	8.3	11.6	8.2	11.7
Montana	7.9	10.8	8.1	11.2
Nebraska	7.7	10.6	8.1	11.1
Nevada	9.7	13.2	9.4	13.0
New Hampshire	6.7	9.5	6.8	9.3
New Jersey	7.9	11.7	7.7	11.2
New Mexico	8.8	11.8	8.4	11.5
New York	7.7	10.9	7.6	10.7
North Carolina	8.4	12.6	8.0	12.0
North Dakota	7.0	9.9	7.1	9.9
Ohio	8.2	12.1	8.1	12.1
Oklahoma	9.4	13.2	9.4	13.0
Oregon	6.7	9.1	6.8	9.1
Pennsylvania	7.7	11.1	7.4	10.8
Rhode Island	7.2	10.4	7.3	11.0
South Carolina	9.5	14.1	9.3	13.7
South Dakota	8.2	11.2	7.5	10.7
Tennessee	9.1	12.8	8.8	12.5
Texas	9.2	12.8	8.8	12.4
Utah	8.2	10.9	7.7	10.2
Vermont	6.1	8.8	6.2	8.7
Virginia	7.8	11.2	7.8	11.3
Washington	8.0	9.8	7.2	9.9
West Virginia	8.9	12.8	8.7	12.4
Wisconsin	7.5	10.4	7.5	10.5
Wyoming	7.7	10.2	7.9	10.8
Puerto Rico	12.6	17.6	12.2	16.9
Virgin Islands	8.7	13.5	NA	NA
Guam	10.3	14.8	*	*
American Samoa	NA	NA	NA	NA
Northern Marianas	5.1	7.3	NA	NA

* = Figure does not meet standards of reliability or precision.   NA = Not available.   [1]Late preterm is 34 to 36 completed weeks of gestation.   [2]Preterm is less than 37 completed weeks of gestation.   [3]Excludes data for the territories.

Table 1-14. Births, by Cesarean Delivery and by State and Territory of Residence, Final 2011 and Preliminary 2012

(Percent.)

State and territory	2011	2012
United States [1]	32.8	32.8
Alabama	35.1	35.5
Alaska	22.4	23.4
Arizona	27.6	27.2
Arkansas	34.3	34.9
California	33.2	33.2
Colorado	25.3	25.9
Connecticut	35.8	34.8
Delaware	32.5	33.1
District of Columbia	33.9	33.5
Florida	38.1	38.1
Georgia	33.6	33.8
Hawaii	26.0	25.1
Idaho	24.5	24.9
Illinois	31.7	31.9
Indiana	30.6	30.7
Iowa	30.5	30.8
Kansas	30.2	30.2
Kentucky	36.3	36.2
Louisiana	39.9	40.2
Maine	30.9	30.5
Maryland	34.8	35.0
Massachusetts	32.5	31.6
Michigan	32.8	32.6
Minnesota	26.8	27.0
Mississippi	38.0	38.1
Missouri	31.4	31.8
Montana	29.5	31.2
Nebraska	30.8	31.5
Nevada	33.8	35.0
New Hampshire	30.8	30.8
New Jersey	39.1	38.7
New Mexico	23.0	23.9
New York	34.3	34.2
North Carolina	30.4	30.6
North Dakota	28.7	28.5
Ohio	31.2	30.9
Oklahoma	34.2	33.8
Oregon	28.9	28.3
Pennsylvania	31.4	31.5
Rhode Island	32.8	31.7
South Carolina	35.2	35.4
South Dakota	25.3	25.4
Tennessee	33.5	33.8
Texas	35.3	35.3
Utah	22.7	22.6
Vermont	27.8	27.1
Virginia	34.1	34.3
Washington	28.8	29.0
West Virginia	36.8	35.9
Wisconsin	25.8	26.3
Wyoming	26.9	29.2
Puerto Rico	46.7	48.5
Virgin Islands	27.8	NA
Guam	24.1	*
American Samoa	NA	NA
Northern Marianas	NA	NA

* = Figure does not meet standards of reliability or precision.   NA = Data not available.   [1]Excludes data for the territories.

Table 1-15. Birth Rates, by Age and Race and Hispanic Origin of Mother, 2000–2011

(Total fertility rates are sums of birth rates for 5-year age groups multiplied by 5; percent.)

Race, origin, and year	Total fertility rate	10 to 14 years	15 to 19 years Total	15 to 17 years	18 to 19 years	20 to 24 years	25 to 29 years	30 to 34 years	35 to 39 years	40 to 44 years	45 to 49 years[1]
All Races and Origins[2]											
2000	2,056.0	0.9	47.7	26.9	78.1	109.7	113.5	91.2	39.7	8.0	0.5
2001	2,030.5	0.8	45.0	24.5	75.5	105.6	113.8	91.8	40.5	8.1	0.5
2002	2,020.5	0.7	42.6	23.1	72.2	103.1	114.7	92.6	41.6	8.3	0.5
2003	2,047.5	0.6	41.1	22.2	69.6	102.3	116.7	95.7	43.9	8.7	0.5
2004	2,051.5	0.6	40.5	21.8	68.7	101.5	116.5	96.2	45.5	9.0	0.5
2005	2,057.0	0.6	39.7	21.1	68.4	101.8	116.5	96.7	46.4	9.1	0.6
2006	2,108.0	0.6	41.1	21.6	71.2	105.5	118.0	98.9	47.5	9.4	0.6
2007	2,120.0	0.6	41.5	21.7	71.7	105.4	118.1	100.6	47.6	9.6	0.6
2008	2,072.0	0.6	40.2	21.1	68.2	101.8	115.0	99.4	46.8	9.9	0.7
2009	2,002.0	0.5	37.9	19.6	64.0	96.2	111.5	97.5	46.1	10.0	0.7
2010	1,931.0	0.4	34.2	17.3	58.2	90.0	108.3	96.5	45.9	10.2	0.7
2011	1,894.5	0.4	31.3	15.4	54.1	85.3	107.2	96.5	47.2	10.3	0.7
Non-Hispanic White[3]											
2000	1,866.0	0.3	32.6	15.8	57.5	91.2	109.4	93.2	38.8	7.3	0.4
2001	1,846.0	0.3	30.3	14.0	54.7	87.0	109.6	94.3	39.8	7.5	0.4
2002	1,840.0	0.2	28.6	13.1	52.0	84.7	110.4	95.0	40.9	7.7	0.5
2003	1,874.5	0.2	27.4	12.4	50.0	84.1	112.7	98.4	43.5	8.1	0.5
2004	1,871.0	0.2	26.7	12.0	48.6	83.0	112.2	98.3	45.1	8.3	0.5
2005	1,869.0	0.2	26.0	11.5	48.0	82.7	111.7	98.4	46.0	8.3	0.5
2006	1,900.5	0.2	26.7	11.8	49.4	85.1	112.2	100.0	46.8	8.5	0.6
2007	1,908.0	0.2	27.2	11.9	50.4	85.1	112.0	101.5	46.3	8.7	0.6
2008	1,874.5	0.2	26.7	11.6	48.6	82.8	109.7	100.8	45.2	8.9	0.6
2009	1,830.0	0.2	25.7	11.0	46.2	79.2	107.1	99.7	44.4	9.1	0.6
2010	1,791.0	0.2	23.5	10.0	42.5	74.9	105.8	99.9	44.1	9.2	0.6
2011	1,773.5	0.2	21.7	9.0	39.9	71.8	105.2	100.1	45.8	9.3	0.6
Non-Hispanic Black[3]											
2000	2,178.5	2.4	79.2	50.1	121.9	145.4	102.8	66.5	31.8	7.2	0.4
2001	2,106.5	2.1	73.1	44.8	115.8	137.3	102.8	66.4	32.0	7.3	0.4
2002	2,053.0	1.9	67.7	40.6	109.5	131.4	103.1	66.5	32.1	7.5	0.4
2003	2,037.5	1.6	63.8	38.2	103.4	128.8	104.0	67.7	33.4	7.7	0.5
2004	2,030.5	1.6	61.9	36.4	101.6	127.9	105.0	67.8	33.6	7.8	0.5
2005	2,030.5	1.6	59.4	34.1	100.2	127.9	105.5	68.8	34.2	8.2	0.5
2006	2,128.5	1.5	61.9	35.2	105.0	134.4	110.0	73.2	35.9	8.3	0.5
2007	2,142.0	1.4	62.0	34.6	105.2	134.5	110.5	74.7	36.2	8.5	0.6
2008	2,115.0	1.4	60.4	33.6	100.0	131.5	108.8	75.3	36.3	8.7	0.6
2009	2,046.5	1.1	56.8	31.0	93.5	125.9	106.0	73.9	36.1	8.9	0.6
2010	1,971.5	1.0	51.5	27.4	85.6	119.4	102.5	73.6	36.4	9.2	0.7
2011	1,919.5	0.9	47.3	24.6	78.8	112.3	101.7	73.9	37.8	9.3	0.7
American Indian or Alaska Native[3,4]											
2000	1,772.5	1.1	58.3	34.1	97.1	117.2	91.8	55.5	24.6	5.7	0.3
2001	1,712.5	0.9	54.5	30.2	92.7	113.8	89.2	54.2	24.0	5.6	0.3
2002	1,675.5	0.8	50.9	28.8	85.3	110.7	88.9	53.7	24.1	5.7	0.3
2003	1,629.5	0.9	49.0	27.9	82.1	107.0	89.3	52.8	23.3	5.2	0.4
2004	1,610.5	0.8	47.2	26.7	79.9	105.4	87.1	51.9	23.9	5.6	0.2
2005	1,584.0	0.8	46.0	26.3	78.0	102.9	86.3	51.8	23.3	5.4	0.3
2006	1,625.0	0.7	46.9	25.9	80.8	106.8	89.0	52.0	23.9	5.4	0.3
2007	1,621.5	0.7	49.3	26.1	86.3	105.8	86.2	52.5	24.3	5.2	0.3
2008	1,569.0	0.7	47.3	25.8	80.2	102.7	83.2	51.2	23.1	5.3	0.3
2009	1,494.0	0.6	43.7	23.6	73.5	96.3	79.3	50.7	22.6	5.3	0.3
2010	1,404.0	0.5	38.7	20.1	66.1	91.0	74.4	48.4	22.3	5.2	0.3
2011	1,373.5	0.5	36.1	18.2	61.6	86.6	75.4	47.3	23.1	5.5	0.2
Asian or Pacific Islander[3,4]											
2000	1,892.0	0.3	20.5	11.6	32.6	60.3	108.4	116.5	59.0	12.6	0.8
2001	1,785.5	0.2	19.3	10.1	32.0	56.0	102.3	109.9	56.2	12.2	0.9
2002	1,798.5	0.3	17.7	8.8	29.9	55.5	102.4	112.5	57.8	12.6	0.9
2003	1,819.0	0.2	16.4	8.5	27.3	54.3	102.7	115.9	60.0	13.4	0.9
2004	1,825.0	0.2	16.0	8.4	26.6	53.3	100.4	118.3	62.2	13.6	1.0
2005	1,784.5	0.2	15.4	7.7	26.4	52.9	96.6	115.3	61.8	13.7	1.0
2006	1,803.0	0.1	15.3	8.2	25.4	53.8	95.7	117.3	63.4	14.0	1.0
2007	1,850.5	0.2	14.8	7.4	24.9	53.2	99.2	121.6	65.8	14.2	1.1
2008	1,797.5	0.2	13.8	7.0	23.0	50.4	96.6	117.6	64.9	14.7	1.2
2009	1,743.0	0.1	12.6	6.3	20.9	46.4	94.6	115.1	63.8	14.9	1.1
2010	1,689.0	0.1	10.9	5.1	18.7	42.6	91.5	113.6	62.8	15.1	1.2
2011	1,706.5	0.1	10.2	4.6	18.1	41.9	93.7	114.9	64.1	15.2	1.2
Hispanic[5]											
2000	2,730.0	1.7	87.3	55.5	132.6	161.3	139.9	97.1	46.6	11.5	0.6
2001	2,726.0	1.5	84.4	51.9	131.3	160.5	140.8	97.8	47.9	11.6	0.7
2002	2,711.0	1.4	80.6	49.3	127.1	159.0	141.6	98.3	48.8	11.7	0.8
2003	2,736.0	1.3	78.4	47.6	124.8	159.1	144.0	101.5	50.1	12.1	0.7
2004	2,759.0	1.2	78.1	47.3	124.8	159.2	144.7	103.4	52.2	12.3	0.7
2005	2,792.0	1.3	76.5	45.8	124.4	161.1	147.0	105.6	53.3	12.8	0.8
2006	2,856.0	1.2	77.4	45.1	128.7	166.7	149.9	107.5	54.6	13.1	0.8
2007	2,840.0	1.2	75.3	44.4	124.7	164.6	149.5	108.5	55.0	13.1	0.8
2008	2,706.0	1.1	70.3	42.2	114.0	154.1	142.3	105.3	54.0	13.3	0.8
2009	2,531.5	1.0	63.6	37.3	103.3	140.1	134.3	100.8	52.5	13.2	0.8
2010	2,350.0	0.8	55.7	32.3	90.7	126.1	125.3	96.6	51.7	13.0	0.8
2011	2,240.0	0.7	49.6	28.0	81.5	116.0	121.3	95.2	51.3	13.1	0.8

[1]Rates are computed by relating births to women age 45 years and over to women age 45 to 49. [2]Includes births to race and origin groups not shown separately, such as White Hispanic and Black Hispanic women, and births with origin not stated. [3]Race and Hispanic origin are reported separately on birth certificates. Persons of Hispanic origin may be of any race. Multiple-race data, when reported, were bridged to single-race categories in order to maintain comparability among all reported areas. [4]Includes persons of Hispanic origin, and origin not stated, according to the mother's reported race. [5]Includes all persons of Hispanic origin of any race.

Table 1-16. Birth Rates, by Live-Birth Order and by Race and Hispanic Origin of Mother, 2000–2011

(Rates are live births per 1,000 women age 15 to 44 years.)

Year, race, and Hispanic origin of mother	Fertility rate	Live-birth order			
		1st child	2nd child	3rd child	4th child and over
All Races and Origins[1,2]					
2000	65.9	26.5	21.4	11.0	7.0
2001	65.1	25.9	21.3	11.0	7.0
2002	65.0	25.8	21.2	10.9	7.0
2003	66.1	26.5	21.4	11.1	7.1
2004	66.4	26.4	21.4	11.2	7.3
2005	66.7	26.5	21.5	11.3	7.4
2006	68.6	27.4	21.9	11.6	7.7
2007	69.3	27.8	22.0	11.7	7.8
2008	68.1	27.5	21.5	11.4	7.8
2009	66.2	26.8	20.8	11.0	7.6
2010	64.1	25.9	20.2	10.6	7.5
2011	63.2	25.4	20.0	10.4	7.4
Non-Hispanic White[2,3]					
2000	58.5	24.2	19.8	9.4	5.1
2001	57.7	23.6	19.7	9.4	5.1
2002	57.6	23.6	19.6	9.3	5.1
2003	58.9	24.5	19.8	9.4	5.2
2004	58.9	24.4	19.8	9.5	5.3
2005	59.0	24.4	19.8	9.5	5.3
2006	60.3	25.1	20.0	9.6	5.5
2007	61.0	25.6	20.1	9.7	5.6
2008	60.5	25.5	19.8	9.5	5.6
2009	59.6	25.3	19.5	9.2	5.6
2010	58.7	25.0	19.2	9.1	5.5
2011	58.7	24.9	19.2	9.0	5.6
Non-Hispanic Black[2,3]					
2000	71.4	26.7	21.2	12.8	10.8
2001	69.1	25.9	20.4	12.4	10.5
2002	67.5	25.4	19.7	12.1	10.4
2003	67.1	25.4	19.6	11.9	10.3
2004	67.1	25.5	19.4	11.9	10.3
2005	67.2	25.8	19.3	11.8	10.3
2006	70.7	27.5	20.3	12.3	10.6
2007	71.4	27.9	20.4	12.3	10.8
2008	70.8	28.1	20.0	12.1	10.7
2009	68.9	27.3	19.4	11.7	10.5
2010	66.6	26.3	18.9	11.3	10.1
2011	65.4	25.6	18.5	11.1	10.1
Hispanic[4]					
2000	95.9	35.8	29.2	18.0	12.9
2001	95.4	35.2	29.3	18.0	12.9
2002	94.7	34.7	29.1	18.0	12.9
2003	95.2	34.5	29.4	18.3	13.0
2004	95.7	34.4	29.3	18.7	13.4
2005	96.4	34.4	29.6	19.0	13.5
2006	98.3	35.1	29.9	19.3	14.0
2007	97.4	34.7	29.4	19.3	14.1
2008	92.7	33.0	27.8	18.3	13.6
2009	86.5	30.6	25.9	17.0	13.0
2010	80.2	28.0	24.0	15.9	12.4
2011	76.2	26.3	22.9	15.2	11.8

[1]Includes births to race and origin groups not shown separately, such as White Hispanic and Black Hispanic women, and births with origin not stated.   [2]Includes origin not stated.   [3]Race and Hispanic origin are reported separately on birth certificates. Persons of Hispanic origin may be of any race. Multiple-race data, when reported, were bridged to single-race categories in order to maintain comparability among all reported areas.   [4]Includes all persons of Hispanic origin of any race.

Table 1-17. Births to Unmarried Mothers, by State and Territory of Residence, Final 2011 and Preliminary 2012

(Percent.)

State and territory	2011	2012
United States [1]	40.7	40.7
Alabama	42.1	42.6
Alaska	36.8	37.4
Arizona	44.7	45.5
Arkansas	44.9	45.2
California	40.4	40.1
Colorado	23.7	23.0
Connecticut	38.0	37.9
Delaware	48.6	47.5
District of Columbia	53.6	51.0
Florida	47.6	47.9
Georgia	45.4	45.2
Hawaii	37.5	37.3
Idaho	26.8	27.4
Illinois	40.0	40.4
Indiana	42.7	43.2
Iowa	33.8	34.8
Kansas	37.3	36.7
Kentucky	41.5	41.2
Louisiana	52.9	53.2
Maine	41.8	41.6
Maryland	41.2	40.7
Massachusetts	34.7	34.5
Michigan	42.3	42.3
Minnesota	32.7	33.1
Mississippi	54.4	54.7
Missouri	40.1	40.2
Montana	36.5	36.0
Nebraska	33.2	33.3
Nevada	44.2	45.2
New Hampshire	34.5	34.5
New Jersey	35.9	36.1
New Mexico	51.3	52.1
New York	41.1	40.9
North Carolina	40.9	41.0
North Dakota	33.4	32.4
Ohio	43.4	43.8
Oklahoma	41.8	42.3
Oregon	35.7	35.5
Pennsylvania	41.7	41.9
Rhode Island	44.5	46.4
South Carolina	47.1	47.9
South Dakota	38.9	38.6
Tennessee	44.1	44.1
Texas	42.0	42.1
Utah	18.7	18.7
Vermont	39.5	40.6
Virginia	35.5	35.2
Washington	32.8	32.5
West Virginia	43.9	44.8
Wisconsin	36.9	37.3
Wyoming	34.5	33.8
Puerto Rico	66.1	NA
Virgin Islands	73.2	NA
Guam	62.1	*
American Samoa	40.4	40.7
Northern Marianas	56.7	NA

NA = Not available.   * = Figure does not meet standards of reliability or precision.   [1] Excludes data for the territories.

Table 1-18. Total Count of Records and Completeness of Preliminary File of Live Births, by State and Territory, Preliminary 2012

(Number, percent.)

State and territory	Live births	
	Count of records	Percent complete
United States [1]	3,939,188	99.96
Alabama	56,941	100.00
Alaska	11,052	100.00
Arizona	87,207	100.00
Arkansas	37,326	100.00
California	504,634	100.00
Colorado	65,643	100.00
Connecticut	37,292	99.98
Delaware	11,376	100.00
District of Columbia	13,906	99.51
Florida	213,402	100.00
Georgia	131,861	99.85
Hawaii	18,974	100.00
Idaho	22,482	100.00
Illinois	155,814	100.00
Indiana	84,204	100.00
Iowa	38,427	100.00
Kansas	41,173	100.00
Kentucky	53,360	100.00
Louisiana	62,567	100.00
Maine	12,594	100.00
Maryland	70,415	100.00
Massachusetts	71,563	98.16
Michigan	112,154	100.00
Minnesota	68,054	100.00
Mississippi	37,787	100.00
Missouri	76,412	100.00
Montana	12,071	100.00
Nebraska	26,282	100.00
Nevada	34,625	100.00
New Hampshire	12,578	100.00
New Jersey	101,611	99.94
New Mexico	26,147	100.00
New York	242,217	100.00
New York excluding New York City	118,986	100.00
New York City	123,231	100.00
North Carolina	121,132	100.00
North Dakota	11,507	100.00
Ohio	139,066	100.00
Oklahoma	51,753	99.97
Oregon	45,557	99.98
Pennsylvania	141,981	100.00
Rhode Island	11,652	100.00
South Carolina	54,259	100.00
South Dakota	12,713	100.00
Tennessee	85,600	100.00
Texas	389,985	100.00
Utah	52,514	99.99
Vermont	5,686	100.00
Virginia	101,400	100.00
Washington	87,345	100.00
West Virginia	21,146	99.93
Wisconsin	66,975	100.00
Wyoming	6,856	99.99
Puerto Rico	38,903	99.60
Virgin Islands	NA	NA
Guam	2,396	66.48
American Samoa	1,163	100.00
Northern Marianas	NA	NA

NA = Not available.   [1] Excludes data for the territories.

Figure 1-4. Birth Rates for Teenagers (Age 15 to 19 Years), by Race and Hispanic Origin, 1991 and 2011

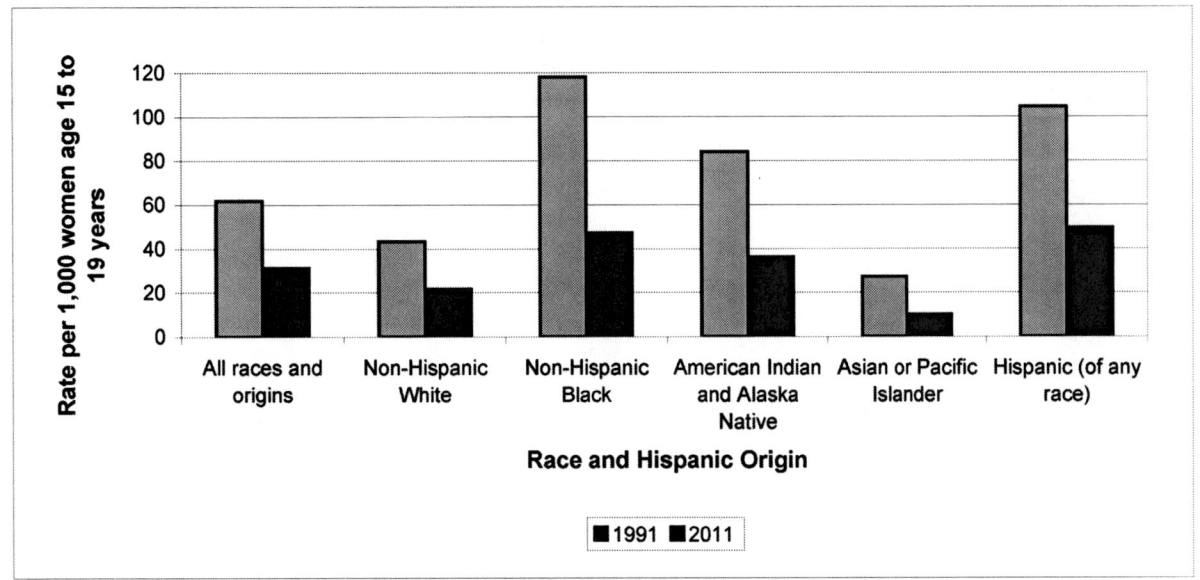

Figure 1-5. Highest and Lowest Birth Rates for Teenagers (Age 15 to 19 Years), by State, 2011

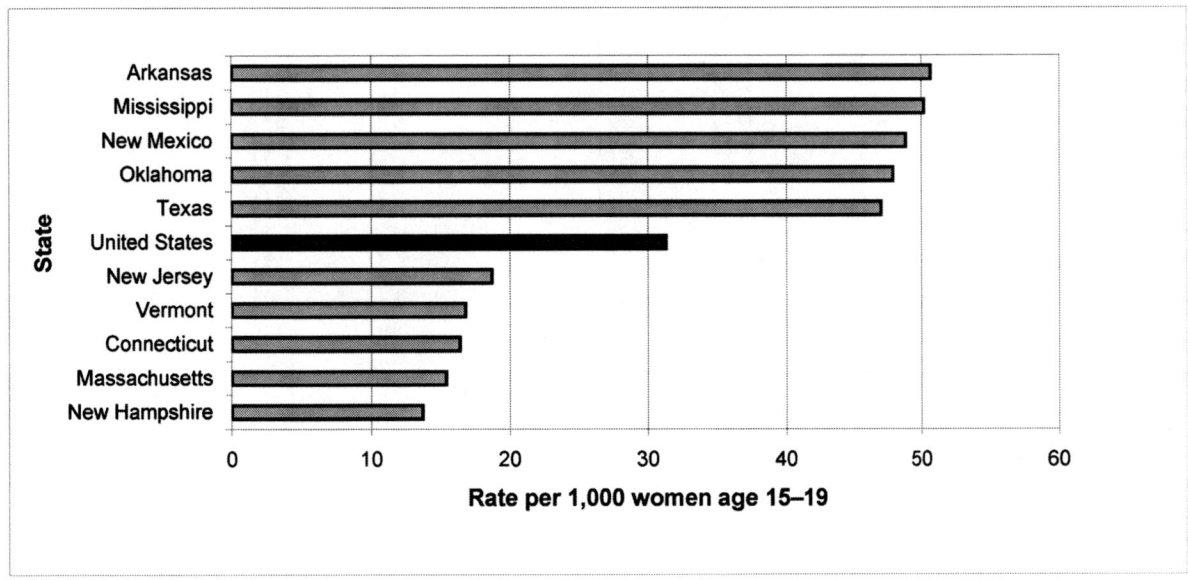

Table 1-19. Birth Rates for Teenagers Age 15 to 19 Years, by State and Territory of Residence, Selected Years, 1991–2011

(Birth rates per 1,000 estimated female population age 15 to 19 years in each area, percent.)

State and territory	1991	2005	2009	2010	2011	Percent change, 1991–2011	Percent change, 2005–2011	Percent change, 2009–2011	Percent change, 2010–2011
United States [1]	61.8	40.5	39.1	34.2	31.3	-49.4	-22.7	-19.9	-8.5
Alabama	73.6	49.7	50.7	43.6	40.5	-45.0	-18.5	-20.1	-7.1
Alaska	66.0	37.3	44.5	38.3	36.2	-45.2	-2.9	-18.7	-5.5
Arizona	79.7	58.2	50.6	41.9	38.5	-51.7	-33.8	-23.9	-8.1
Arkansas	79.5	59.1	59.2	52.5	50.7	-36.2	-14.2	-14.4	-3.4
California	73.8	38.8	36.6	31.5	28.7	-61.1	-26.0	-21.6	-8.9
Colorado	58.3	42.6	38.5	33.4	28.9	-50.4	-32.2	-24.9	-13.5
Connecticut	40.1	23.3	21.0	18.7	16.4	-59.1	-29.6	-21.9	-12.3
Delaware	60.4	44.0	35.3	30.5	29.3	-51.5	-33.4	-17.0	-3.9
District of Columbia	109.6	63.4	47.7	45.4	42.8	-60.9	-32.5	-10.3	-5.7
Florida	67.9	42.4	39.0	32.0	29.5	-56.6	-30.4	-24.4	-7.8
Georgia	76.0	52.7	47.7	41.4	38.2	-49.7	-27.5	-19.9	-7.7
Hawaii	59.2	36.2	40.9	32.5	30.0	-49.3	-17.1	-26.7	-7.7
Idaho	53.9	37.7	35.9	33.0	27.7	-48.6	-26.5	-22.8	-16.1
Illinois	64.5	38.6	36.1	33.0	29.5	-54.3	-23.6	-18.3	-10.6
Indiana	60.4	43.2	42.5	37.3	34.8	-42.4	-19.4	-18.1	-6.7
Iowa	42.5	32.6	32.1	28.6	25.3	-40.5	-22.4	-21.2	-11.5
Kansas	55.4	41.4	43.8	39.3	35.4	-36.1	-14.5	-19.2	-9.9
Kentucky	68.8	49.1	51.3	46.2	43.5	-36.8	-11.4	-15.2	-5.8
Louisiana	76.0	49.1	52.7	47.7	45.1	-40.7	-8.1	-14.4	-5.5
Maine	43.5	24.4	24.4	21.4	20.8	-52.2	-14.8	-14.8	-2.8
Maryland	54.1	31.8	31.3	27.3	24.7	-54.3	-22.3	-21.1	-9.5
Massachusetts	37.5	21.8	19.6	17.2	15.4	-58.9	-29.4	-21.4	-10.5
Michigan	58.9	32.5	32.7	30.1	27.8	-52.8	-14.5	-15.0	-7.6
Minnesota	37.3	26.1	24.3	22.5	19.3	-48.3	-26.1	-20.6	-14.2
Mississippi	85.3	60.5	64.2	55.0	50.2	-41.1	-17.0	-21.8	-8.7
Missouri	64.4	42.5	41.6	37.1	34.5	-46.4	-18.8	-17.1	-7.0
Montana	46.8	35.2	38.5	35.0	29.2	-37.6	-17.0	-24.2	-16.6
Nebraska	42.4	34.2	34.6	31.1	27.2	-35.8	-20.5	-21.4	-12.5
Nevada	74.5	50.1	47.4	38.6	36.1	-51.5	-27.9	-23.8	-6.5
New Hampshire	33.1	17.9	16.4	15.7	13.7	-58.6	-23.5	-16.5	-12.7
New Jersey	41.3	23.4	22.7	20.1	18.7	-54.7	-20.1	-17.6	-7.0
New Mexico	79.5	61.6	63.9	53.0	48.8	-38.6	-20.8	-23.6	-7.9
New York	45.5	26.5	24.4	22.7	21.2	-53.4	-20.0	-13.1	-6.6
North Carolina	70.0	48.5	44.9	38.3	34.9	-50.1	-28.0	-22.3	-8.9
North Dakota	35.5	29.7	27.9	28.8	28.2	-20.6	-5.1	1.1	-2.1
Ohio	60.5	38.9	38.9	34.1	31.5	-47.9	-19.0	-19.0	-7.6
Oklahoma	72.1	54.2	60.1	50.4	47.8	-33.7	-11.8	-20.5	-5.2
Oregon	54.8	33.0	33.1	28.2	25.8	-52.9	-21.8	-22.1	-8.5
Pennsylvania	46.7	30.4	29.3	27.0	24.9	-46.7	-18.1	-15.0	-7.8
Rhode Island	44.7	31.4	26.8	22.3	21.3	-52.3	-32.2	-20.5	-4.5
South Carolina	72.5	51.0	49.1	42.6	39.1	-46.1	-23.3	-20.4	-8.2
South Dakota	47.6	37.5	38.4	34.9	34.3	-27.9	-8.5	-10.7	-1.7
Tennessee	74.8	54.9	50.6	43.2	40.8	-45.5	-25.7	-19.4	-5.6
Texas	78.4	61.6	60.7	52.2	46.9	-40.2	-23.9	-22.7	-10.2
Utah	48.0	33.4	30.7	27.9	23.1	-51.9	-30.8	-24.8	-17.2
Vermont	39.2	18.6	17.4	17.9	16.8	-57.1	-9.7	-3.4	-6.1
Virginia	53.4	34.4	31.0	27.4	24.5	-54.1	-28.8	-21.0	-10.6
Washington	53.7	31.1	31.9	26.7	25.4	-52.7	-18.3	-20.4	-4.9
West Virginia	58.0	43.4	49.8	44.8	43.5	-25.0	0.2	-12.7	-2.9
Wisconsin	43.7	30.3	29.4	26.2	23.2	-46.9	-23.4	-21.1	-11.5
Wyoming	54.3	43.2	45.0	39.0	35.2	-35.2	-18.5	-21.8	-9.7
Puerto Rico	72.4	61.2	54.7	51.4	51.7	-28.6	-15.5	-5.5	0.6
Virgin Islands	77.9	50.0	51.5	50.5	59.3	-23.9	18.6	15.1	17.4
Guam	95.7	59.2	50.8	60.1	62.1	-35.1	4.9	22.2	3.3
America Samoa	NA	34.2	35.2	34.1	38.4	NA	12.3	9.1	12.6
Northern Marinas	NA	30.4	50.2	53.4	47.2	NA	55.3	-6.0	-11.6

[1] Excludes data for the territories.

Table 1-20. Probability of a First Birth, Age 15 to 20 Years, and for Females Age 15 to 24 Years, 2002 and 2006–2010

(Percent.)

Characteristic	Probability of a first birth by age					
	15	16	17	18	19	20
2002, Total	0.01	0.02	0.04	0.09	0.13	0.18
2006–2010[1], Total	0.00	0.01	0.04	0.08	0.13	0.18
2006–2010						
Hispanic Origin and Race						
Hispanic or Latina	0.01	0.03	0.09	0.16	0.23	0.30
Non-Hispanic White	0.00	0.01	0.03	0.05	0.09	0.14
Non-Hispanic Black	0.00	0.01	0.04	0.10	0.17	0.26
Contraceptive Use at First Sex						
Used contraception at first sex	0.00	0.01	0.03	0.09	0.13	0.20
Used more than one method at first sex	0.00	0.00	0.01	0.02	0.06	0.07
Did not use contraception at first sex	0.02	0.05	0.12	0.18	0.32	0.37
Mother's Age at First Birth						
Under 20 years	0.01	0.02	0.07	0.14	0.22	0.29
20 years or over	0.00	0.01	0.02	0.05	0.09	0.14
Mother's Education						
No high school diploma or GED[2]	0.01	0.04	0.11	0.18	0.28	0.37
High school diploma or GED	0.00	0.01	0.04	0.09	0.14	0.19
Some college or higher	0.00	0.01	0.01	0.04	0.07	0.12
Family Structure at Age 14						
Both biological or adoptive parents	0.00	0.01	0.02	0.04	0.07	0.11
Biological mother and stepfather	0.01	0.02	0.06	0.14	0.23	0.30
Other[3]	0.01	0.02	0.06	0.13	0.23	0.29

0.0 = Quantity more than zero but less than 0.01.   [1]Includes persons of other or unknown origin and race groups, those with a mother figure who had no births, and those who reported no mother-figure, not shown separately.   [2]GED is General Educational Development high school equivalency diploma.   [3]Refers to anything other than two biological or adoptive parents or biological mother and stepfather, including one biological parent and no other parents(s)/parent figures or no parent(s)/parent figures.

Table 1-21. Responses to the Statement, "If You Got Pregnant Now or Got a Female Pregnant Now, How Would You Feel?" for Never-Married Females and Males Age 15 to 19 Years, 2002 and 2006–2010

(Numbers in thousands, percent.)

Characteristic	Number of respondents	Percent surveyed[1]	Very upset		A little upset		A little pleased		Very pleased	
			Percent	Standard error	Percent	Standard error	Percent	Standard error	Percent	Standard error
2002, Total	9,598	100.0	60.2	1.8	26.7	1.6	8.0	0.9	4.7	0.8
2006–2010[2], Total	10,361	100.0	57.5	1.5	29.1	1.3	8.2	0.8	4.8	0.7
2006–2010										
Hispanic Origin and Race										
Hispanic or Latina	1,849	100.0	47.7	3.0	32.5	3.0	13.2	2.5	6.0	1.3
Non-Hispanic White	6,150	100.0	63.1	2.0	28.2	1.9	5.4	1.0	3.2	0.8
Non-Hispanic Black	1,691	100.0	48.9	3.0	30.6	2.4	9.9	1.6	9.5	1.7
Age										
15–17 years	5,820	100.0	63.3	1.9	28.6	1.6	5.7	1.0	2.2	0.5
18–19 years	4,541	100.0	50.0	2.3	29.7	2.1	11.5	1.1	8.3	1.4
Ever Had Sex										
Yes	4,417	100.0	44.2	2.1	33.9	1.9	12.7	1.4	8.6	1.4
No	5,944	100.0	67.3	2.0	25.5	1.8	4.9	0.9	2.1	0.6
Family Structure at Age 14										
Both biological or adoptive parents	6,317	100.0	63.7	2.0	25.2	1.8	7.1	1.0	3.8	0.8
Other[2]	4,044	100.0	47.7	2.1	35.2	1.8	10.1	1.3	6.6	1.1
Male										
Total 2002	10,139	100.0	51.4	2.0	33.4	1.8	11.0	1.4	3.7	0.6
Total 2006–2010	10,766	100.0	46.4	1.8	34.0	1.5	14.3	1.2	4.3	0.5
Male, 2006–2010										
Hispanic origin and race:										
Hispanic or Latino	2,000	100.0	26.6	2.9	37.8	2.6	23.3	3.2	11.7	2.2
Non-Hispanic White	6,405	100.0	56.0	2.1	32.1	2.0	9.7	1.2	1.5	0.5
Non-Hispanic Black	1,673	100.0	29.9	3.3	40.0	3.3	22.4	2.4	6.5	1.3
Age										
15–17 years	6,623	100.0	53.1	2.2	32.3	2.0	11.1	1.4	2.8	0.5
18–19 years	4,143	100.0	35.8	2.4	36.9	2.0	19.2	1.9	6.8	1.1
Ever Had Sex										
Yes	4,501	100.0	32.8	2.0	37.5	1.8	21.1	2.2	6.9	1.0
No	6,266	100.0	56.2	2.2	31.5	2.1	9.3	1.1	2.5	0.6
Family Structure at Age 14										
Both biological or adoptive parents	6,737	100.0	52.0	2.1	32.5	1.6	11.5	1.3	3.3	0.6
Other[3]	4,029	100.0	37.1	2.0	36.7	2.3	18.9	1.8	6.0	0.8

[1]Percentages may not add to 100 because responses of "would not care" (coded only if respondent insisted) are not shown separately. [2]Includes persons of other or unknown origin and race groups, not shown separately. [3]Refers to anything other than two biological or adoptive parents or biological mother and stepfather, including one biological parent and no other parents(s)/parent figures or no parent(s)/parent figures.

Table 1-22. Birth Rates for Women Age 10 to 19 Years, by Age, Race, and Hispanic Origin of Mother, Selected Years, 1991–2011

(Rates per 1,000 women in specified age, race, and Hispanic origin groups.)

Age, race, and Hispanic origin of mother	1991	2005	2007	2009	2010	2011	Percent change, 1991–2011	Percent change, 2005–2011	Percent change, 2007–2011	Percent change, 2010–2011
10 to 14 Years										
All races and origins[1]	1.4	0.6	0.6	0.6	0.4	0.4	-71.4	-33.3	-33.3	0.0
Non-Hispanic White[2]	0.5	0.2	0.2	0.2	0.2	0.2	-60.0	0.0	†	†
Non-Hispanic Black[2]	4.9	1.6	1.4	1.4	1.0	0.9	-81.6	-43.8	-35.7	-10.0
American Indian or Alaska Native total[2,3]	1.6	0.8	0.7	0.6	0.5	0.5	-68.8	-37.5	-28.6	†
Asian or Pacific Islander total[2,3]	0.8	0.2	0.2	0.1	0.1	0.1	-87.5	-50.0	-50.0	†
Hispanic[4]	2.4	1.3	1.2	1.1	0.8	0.7	-70.8	-46.2	-41.7	-12.5
15 to 19 Years										
All races and origins[1]	61.8	39.7	41.5	40.2	34.2	31.3	-49.4	-21.2	-24.6	-8.5
Non-Hispanic White[2]	43.4	26.0	27.2	26.7	23.5	21.7	-50.0	-16.5	-20.2	-7.7
Non-Hispanic Black[2]	118.2	59.4	62.0	60.4	51.5	47.3	-60.0	-20.4	-23.7	-8.2
American Indian or Alaska Native total[2,3]	84.1	46.0	49.3	43.7	38.7	36.1	-57.1	-21.5	-26.8	-6.7
Asian or Pacific Islander total[2,3]	27.3	15.4	14.8	12.6	10.9	10.2	-62.6	-33.8	-31.1	-6.4
Hispanic[4]	104.6	76.5	75.3	70.3	55.7	49.6	-52.6	-35.2	-34.1	-11.0
15 to 17 Years										
All races and origins[1]	38.6	21.1	21.7	21.1	17.3	15.4	-60.1	-27.0	-29.0	-11.0
Non-Hispanic White[2]	23.6	11.5	11.9	11.6	10.0	9.0	-61.9	-21.7	-24.4	-10.0
Non-Hispanic Black[2]	86.1	34.1	34.6	33.6	27.4	24.6	-71.4	-27.9	-28.9	-10.2
American Indian or Alaska Native total[2,3]	51.9	26.3	26.1	23.6	20.1	18.2	-64.9	-30.8	-30.3	-9.5
Asian or Pacific Islander total[2,3]	16.3	7.7	7.4	6.3	5.1	4.6	-71.8	-40.3	-37.8	-9.8
Hispanic[4]	69.2	45.8	44.4	42.2	32.3	28.0	-59.5	-38.9	-36.9	-13.3
18 to 19 Years										
All races and origins[1]	94.0	68.4	71.7	68.2	58.2	54.1	-42.4	-20.9	-24.5	-7.0
Non-Hispanic White[2]	70.6	48.0	50.4	48.6	42.5	39.9	-43.5	-16.9	-20.8	-6.1
Non-Hispanic Black[2]	162.2	100.2	105.2	100.0	85.6	78.8	-51.4	-21.4	-25.1	-7.9
American Indian or Alaska Native total[2,3]	134.2	78.0	86.3	73.5	66.1	61.6	-54.1	-21.0	-28.6	-6.8
Asian or Pacific Islander total[2,3]	42.2	26.4	24.9	20.9	18.7	18.1	-57.1	-31.4	-27.3	-3.2
Hispanic[4]	155.5	124.4	124.7	114.0	90.7	81.5	-47.6	-34.5	-34.6	-10.1

† = Difference not statistically significant.   [1]Includes births to race and origin groups not shown separately, such as White Hispanic and Black Hispanic women, and births with origin not stated.   [2]Race and Hispanic origin are reported separately on birth certificates. Persons of Hispanic origin may be of any race. Multiple-race data, when reported, were bridged to single-race categories in order to maintain comparability among all reported areas.   [3]Includes persons of Hispanic origin, and origin not stated, according to the mother's reported race.   [4]Includes all persons of Hispanic origin of any race.

Table 1-23. Mean Age of Mother, by Live-Birth Order and Race and Hispanic Origin of Mother, Selected Years, 1980–2011

(Arithmetic average of the age of mothers at the times of births.)

Year, race, and, Hispanic origin of mother	Total	Live-birth order							
		1	2	3	4	5	6 and 7	8 and over	Unknown or not stated
All Races [1]									
1980[2]	25.0	22.7	25.4	27.3	29.0	30.6	32.7	36.0	23.9
1985	25.8	23.7	26.3	27.9	29.3	30.6	32.5	35.7	26.1
1990	26.4	24.2	26.9	28.3	29.4	30.6	32.1	35.1	27.4
1995	26.9	24.5	27.5	29.1	30.1	31.2	32.6	35.4	27.1
2000	27.2	24.9	27.7	29.2	30.3	31.4	32.9	35.8	27.4
2001	27.3	25.0	27.8	29.2	30.3	31.4	32.9	35.9	27.0
2002	27.3	25.1	27.9	29.2	30.3	31.4	32.9	35.9	27.7
2003	27.4	25.2	28.0	29.3	30.4	31.4	33.0	35.8	27.9
2004	27.5	25.2	28.0	29.4	30.4	31.4	32.9	35.9	27.6
2005	27.4	25.2	28.0	29.4	30.4	31.4	32.9	35.9	28.0
2006	27.4	25.0	27.9	29.3	30.4	31.4	33.0	35.8	28.0
2007	27.4	25.0	27.9	29.3	30.4	31.5	32.9	35.7	27.9
2008	27.4	25.1	27.9	29.4	30.5	31.5	32.9	35.7	27.7
2009	27.5	25.2	28.0	29.5	30.6	31.6	32.9	35.7	27.6
2010	27.7	25.4	28.2	29.6	30.7	31.7	33.0	35.7	27.7
2011	27.9	25.6	28.3	29.7	30.8	31.8	33.1	35.5	28.2
Non-Hispanic White [3]									
1990[4]	27.1	25.0	27.6	29.1	30.3	31.6	33.2	36.2	28.5
1995	27.6	25.4	28.3	29.9	31.2	32.4	33.9	36.7	28.5
2000	28.0	25.9	28.6	30.0	31.3	32.4	34.0	37.0	28.9
2001	28.1	26.0	28.6	30.1	31.3	32.4	33.9	37.0	28.2
2002	28.2	26.1	28.7	30.1	31.2	32.3	33.9	37.1	28.6
2003	28.2	26.2	28.8	30.1	31.2	32.3	33.9	37.0	28.8
2004	28.2	26.2	28.8	30.2	31.2	32.2	33.8	36.9	28.7
2005	28.2	26.2	28.8	30.1	31.2	32.2	33.8	36.9	29.1
2006	28.1	26.0	28.8	30.1	31.1	32.1	33.7	36.7	29.1
2007	28.1	26.0	28.7	30.0	31.1	32.1	33.7	36.7	28.8
2008	28.1	26.0	28.7	30.1	31.1	32.1	33.6	36.7	28.7
2009	28.1	26.1	28.8	30.1	31.1	32.1	33.6	36.7	28.6
2010	28.3	26.3	28.9	30.2	31.1	32.2	33.6	36.6	28.7
2011	28.4	26.5	29.0	30.2	31.2	32.2	33.7	36.4	19.0
Non-Hispanic Black [3]									
1990[4]	24.4	21.7	24.6	26.3	27.4	28.7	30.3	33.3	26.0
1995	24.8	21.9	25.3	27.0	28.0	29.3	30.8	33.2	25.4
2000	25.2	22.3	25.5	27.1	28.2	29.5	31.0	33.9	26.0
2001	25.3	22.4	25.7	27.2	28.3	29.6	31.2	34.1	26.4
2002	25.4	22.6	25.8	27.3	28.5	29.6	31.2	34.1	26.5
2003	25.6	22.7	25.9	27.5	28.6	29.7	31.3	34.0	26.3
2004	25.6	22.7	25.9	27.5	28.6	29.8	31.2	34.1	25.7
2005	25.6	22.7	26.0	27.6	28.8	29.8	31.3	34.2	25.8
2006	25.6	22.7	26.0	27.7	28.8	29.9	31.4	34.1	25.9
2007	25.6	22.7	26.0	27.7	28.9	30.0	31.4	34.2	26.1
2008	25.6	22.8	26.0	27.8	29.0	30.0	31.5	34.2	26.2
2009	25.7	22.9	26.1	27.9	29.1	30.2	31.5	34.3	26.2
2010	25.9	23.1	26.3	28.0	29.3	30.3	31.7	34.2	26.5
2011	26.1	23.4	26.4	28.2	29.4	30.5	31.8	34.2	26.6
Hispanic [5]									
1990[4]	25.3	22.4	25.2	27.4	29.1	30.6	32.3	35.3	26.1
1995	25.4	22.4	25.5	27.8	29.6	31.1	32.8	35.5	24.2
2000	25.7	22.7	25.8	28.1	29.8	31.3	33.0	35.5	24.2
2001	25.9	22.8	25.9	28.2	29.9	31.4	33.1	35.7	24.4
2002	26.0	23.0	26.0	28.3	29.9	31.4	33.1	35.7	25.7
2003	26.1	23.1	26.1	28.4	30.0	31.4	33.1	35.4	25.8
2004	26.2	23.1	26.2	28.5	30.1	31.5	33.1	35.5	25.8
2005	26.2	23.1	26.2	28.5	30.1	31.4	33.2	35.6	26.5
2006	26.2	23.1	26.2	28.6	30.2	31.5	33.2	35.5	26.6
2007	26.3	23.1	26.3	28.6	30.3	31.6	33.1	35.3	26.7
2008	26.4	23.1	26.4	28.7	30.4	31.6	33.2	35.3	26.7
2009	26.5	23.3	26.5	28.9	30.5	31.8	33.1	35.3	26.8
2010	26.8	23.4	26.7	29.0	30.7	32.0	33.3	35.3	27.2
2011	27.0	23.7	26.9	29.2	30.9	32.1	33.3	35.0	28.0

[1]Includes races other than White and Black and origin not stated.   [2]Based on 100 percent of births in selected states and on a 50-percent sample of births in all other states.   [3]Race and Hispanic origin are reported separately on birth certificates. Persons of Hispanic origin may be of any race. Multiple-race data, when reported, were bridged to single-race categories in order to maintain comparability among all reported areas.   [4]Excludes data for New Hampshire and Oklahoma, which did not report Hispanic origin.   [5]Includes all persons of Hispanic origin of any race.

Table 1-24. Live Births, Birth Rates, and Fertility Rates, by Race, Selected Years, 1940–2011

(Number, rate per 1,000 population in specified group.)

Characteristic and year	Number					Birth rate					Fertility rate				
	All races[1]	White	Black	American Indian or Alaska Native	Asian or Pacific Islander	All races[1]	White	Black	American Indian or Alaska Native	Asian or Pacific Islander	All races[1]	White	Black	American Indian or Alaska Native	Asian or Pacific Islander
Race of Mother															
1980[2]	3,612,258	2,936,351	568,080	29,389	74,355	15.9	15.1	21.3	20.7	19.9	68.4	65.6	84.7	82.7	73.2
1981[2]	3,629,238	2,947,679	564,955	29,688	84,553	15.8	15.0	20.8	20.0	20.1	67.3	64.8	82.0	79.6	73.7
1982[2]	3,680,537	2,984,817	568,506	32,436	93,193	15.9	15.1	20.7	21.1	20.3	67.3	64.8	80.9	83.6	74.8
1983[2]	3,638,933	2,946,468	562,624	32,881	95,713	15.6	14.8	20.2	20.6	19.5	65.7	63.4	78.7	81.8	71.7
1984[2]	3,669,141	2,967,100	568,138	33,256	98,926	15.6	14.8	20.1	20.1	18.8	65.5	63.2	78.2	79.8	69.2
1985	3,760,561	3,037,913	581,824	34,037	104,606	15.8	15.0	20.4	19.8	18.7	66.3	64.1	78.8	78.6	68.4
1986	3,756,547	3,019,175	592,910	34,169	107,797	15.6	14.8	20.5	19.2	18.0	65.4	63.1	78.9	75.9	66.0
1987	3,809,394	3,043,828	611,173	35,322	116,560	15.7	14.9	20.8	19.1	18.4	65.8	63.3	80.1	75.6	67.1
1988	3,909,510	3,102,083	638,562	37,088	129,035	16.0	15.0	21.5	19.3	19.2	67.3	64.5	82.6	76.8	70.2
1989	4,040,958	3,192,355	673,124	39,478	133,075	16.4	15.4	22.3	19.7	18.7	69.2	66.4	86.2	79.0	68.2
1990	4,158,212	3,290,273	684,336	39,051	141,635	16.7	15.8	22.4	18.9	19.0	70.9	68.3	86.8	76.2	69.6
1991	4,110,907	3,241,273	682,602	38,841	145,372	16.2	15.3	21.8	18.3	18.3	69.3	66.7	84.8	73.9	67.1
1992	4,065,014	3,201,678	673,633	39,453	150,250	15.8	15.0	21.1	17.9	17.9	68.4	66.1	82.4	73.1	66.1
1993	4,000,240	3,149,833	658,875	38,732	152,800	15.4	14.6	20.2	17.0	17.3	67.0	64.9	79.6	69.7	64.3
1994	3,952,767	3,121,004	636,391	37,740	157,632	15.0	14.3	19.1	16.0	17.1	65.9	64.2	75.9	65.8	63.9
1995	3,899,589	3,098,885	603,139	37,278	160,287	14.6	14.1	17.8	15.3	16.7	64.6	63.6	71.0	63.0	62.6
1996	3,891,494	3,093,057	594,781	37,880	165,776	14.4	13.9	17.3	14.9	16.5	64.1	63.3	69.2	61.8	62.3
1997	3,880,894	3,072,640	599,913	38,572	169,769	14.2	13.7	17.1	14.7	16.2	63.6	62.8	69.0	60.8	61.3
1998	3,941,553	3,118,727	609,902	40,272	172,652	14.3	13.8	17.1	14.8	15.9	64.3	63.6	69.4	61.3	60.1
1999	3,959,417	3,132,501	605,970	40,170	180,776	14.2	13.7	16.8	14.2	15.9	64.4	64.0	68.5	59.0	60.9
2000	4,058,814	3,194,005	622,598	41,668	200,543	14.4	13.9	17.0	14.0	17.1	65.9	65.3	70.0	58.7	65.8
2001	4,025,933	3,177,626	606,156	41,872	200,279	14.1	13.7	16.3	13.5	16.1	65.1	65.0	67.5	56.8	62.5
2002	4,021,726	3,174,760	593,691	42,368	210,907	14.0	13.6	15.7	13.2	16.3	65.0	65.1	65.7	55.7	63.3
2003	4,089,950	3,225,848	599,847	43,052	221,203	14.1	13.7	15.7	13.0	16.4	66.1	66.4	66.0	54.8	64.2
2004	4,112,052	3,222,928	616,074	43,927	229,123	14.0	13.6	15.9	12.8	16.4	66.4	66.5	67.2	54.2	64.5
2005	4,138,349	3,229,294	633,134	44,813	231,108	14.0	13.6	16.1	12.6	15.9	66.7	66.8	68.5	53.6	63.0
2006	4,265,555	3,310,308	666,481	47,721	241,045	14.3	13.8	16.7	12.9	16.0	68.6	68.7	71.4	55.3	63.7
2007	4,316,233	3,336,626	675,676	49,443	254,488	14.3	13.8	16.7	12.9	16.4	69.3	69.4	71.7	55.5	65.3
2008	4,247,694	3,274,163	670,809	49,537	253,185	14.0	13.5	16.3	12.4	15.7	68.1	68.3	70.6	54.0	63.3
2009	4,130,665	3,173,293	657,618	48,665	251,089	13.5	13.0	15.8	11.8	15.1	66.2	66.4	68.8	51.6	61.3
2010	3,999,386	3,069,315	636,425	46,760	246,886	13.0	12.5	15.1	11.0	14.5	64.1	64.4	66.3	48.6	59.2
2011	3,953,590	3,020,355	632,901	46,419	253,915	12.7	12.2	14.8	10.7	14.5	63.2	63.4	65.5	47.7	59.9
Race of Child															
1960[3]	4,257,850	3,600,744	602,264	21,114	NA	23.7	22.7	31.9	NA	NA	118.0	113.2	153.5	NA	NA
1961[3]	4,268,326	3,600,864	611,072	21,464	NA	23.3	22.2	NA	NA	NA	117.1	112.3	NA	NA	NA
1962[3,4]	4,167,362	3,394,068	584,610	21,968	NA	22.4	21.4	NA	NA	NA	112.0	107.5	NA	NA	NA
1963[3,4]	4,098,020	3,326,344	580,658	22,358	NA	21.7	20.7	NA	NA	NA	108.3	103.6	NA	NA	NA
1964[3]	4,027,490	3,369,160	607,556	24,382	NA	21.1	20.0	29.5	NA	NA	104.7	99.8	142.6	NA	NA
1965[3]	3,760,358	3,123,860	581,126	24,066	NA	19.4	18.3	27.7	NA	NA	96.3	91.3	133.2	NA	NA
1966[3]	3,606,274	2,993,230	558,244	23,014	NA	18.4	17.4	26.2	NA	NA	90.8	86.2	124.7	NA	NA
1967[5]	3,520,959	2,922,502	543,976	22,665	NA	17.8	16.8	25.1	NA	NA	87.2	82.8	118.5	NA	NA
1968[3]	3,501,564	2,912,224	531,152	24,156	NA	17.6	16.6	24.2	NA	NA	85.2	81.3	112.7	NA	NA
1969[3]	3,600,206	2,993,614	543,132	24,008	NA	17.9	16.9	24.4	NA	NA	86.1	82.2	112.1	NA	NA
1970[3]	3,731,386	3,091,264	572,362	25,864	NA	18.4	17.4	25.3	NA	NA	87.9	84.1	115.4	NA	NA
1971[3]	3,555,970	2,919,746	564,960	27,148	NA	17.2	16.1	24.4	NA	NA	81.6	77.3	109.7	NA	NA
1972[2]	3,258,411	2,655,558	531,329	27,368	NA	15.6	14.5	22.5	NA	NA	73.1	68.9	99.9	NA	NA
1973[2]	3,136,965	2,551,030	512,597	26,464	NA	14.8	13.8	21.4	NA	NA	68.8	64.9	93.6	NA	NA
1974[2]	3,159,958	2,575,792	507,162	26,631	NA	14.8	13.9	20.8	NA	NA	67.8	64.2	89.7	NA	NA
1975[2]	3,144,198	2,551,996	511,581	27,546	NA	14.6	13.6	20.7	NA	NA	66.0	62.5	87.9	NA	NA
1976[2]	3,167,788	2,567,614	514,479	29,009	NA	14.6	13.6	20.5	NA	NA	65.0	61.5	85.8	NA	NA
1977[2]	3,326,632	2,691,070	544,221	30,500	NA	15.1	14.1	21.4	NA	NA	66.8	63.2	88.1	NA	NA
1978[2]	3,333,279	2,681,116	551,540	33,160	NA	15.0	14.0	21.3	NA	NA	65.5	61.7	86.7	NA	NA
1979[2]	3,494,398	2,808,420	577,855	34,269	NA	15.6	14.5	22.0	NA	NA	67.2	63.4	88.3	NA	NA
1980[2]	3,612,258	2,898,732	589,616	36,797	NA	15.9	14.9	22.1	NA	NA	68.4	64.7	88.1	NA	NA
Births adjusted for underregistration															
Race of Child															
1940	2,559,000	2,199,000	NA	NA	NA	19.4	18.6	NA	NA	NA	79.9	77.1	NA	NA	NA
1945	2,858,000	2,471,000	NA	NA	NA	20.4	19.7	NA	NA	NA	85.9	83.4	NA	NA	NA
1950	3,632,000	3,108,000	NA	NA	NA	24.1	23.0	NA	NA	NA	106.2	102.3	NA	NA	NA
1955	4,097,000	3,485,000	NA	NA	NA	25.0	23.8	NA	NA	NA	118.3	113.7	NA	NA	NA

NA = Not available. [1]Data for 1960–1991 includes births to races not shown separately. For 1992 and later years, unknown race of mother is imputed. [2]Based on 100 percent of births in selected states and on a 50 percent sample of births in all other states. [3]Based on a 50 percent sample of births. [4]Figures by race exclude New Jersey. [5]Based on a 20 to 50 percent sample of births.

Table 1-25. Births and Birth Rates, by Hispanic Origin of Mother and by Race for Mothers of Non-Hispanic Origin, 1989–2011

(Birth rates are live births per 1,000 population in specified group; fertility rates are live births per 1,000 women age 15 to 44 years in specified group.)

Measure and year	All origins[1]	Hispanic (may be of any race)						Non-Hispanic		
		Total	Mexican	Puerto Rican	Cuban	Central and South American	Other and unknown Hispanic	Total[2]	White	Black
Number										
1989[3]	3,903,012	532,249	327,233	56,229	10,842	72,443	65,502	3,297,493	2,526,367	611,269
1990[4]	4,092,994	595,073	385,640	58,807	11,311	83,008	56,307	3,457,417	2,626,500	661,701
1991[5]	4,094,566	623,085	411,233	59,833	11,058	86,908	54,053	3,434,464	2,589,878	666,758
1992[5]	4,049,024	643,271	432,047	59,569	11,472	89,031	51,152	3,365,862	2,527,207	657,450
1993	4,000,240	654,418	443,733	58,102	11,916	92,371	48,296	3,295,345	2,472,031	641,273
1994	3,952,767	665,026	454,536	57,240	11,889	93,485	47,876	3,245,115	2,438,855	619,198
1995	3,899,589	679,768	469,615	54,824	12,473	94,996	47,860	3,160,495	2,382,638	587,781
1996	3,891,494	701,339	489,666	54,863	12,613	97,888	46,309	3,133,484	2,358,989	578,099
1997	3,880,894	709,767	499,024	55,450	12,887	97,405	45,001	3,115,174	2,333,363	581,431
1998	3,941,553	734,661	516,011	57,349	13,226	98,226	49,849	3,158,975	2,361,462	593,127
1999	3,959,417	764,339	540,674	57,138	13,088	103,307	50,132	3,147,580	2,346,450	588,981
2000	4,058,814	815,868	581,915	58,124	13,429	113,344	49,056	3,199,994	2,362,968	604,346
2001	4,025,933	851,851	611,000	57,568	14,017	121,365	47,901	3,149,572	2,326,578	589,917
2002	4,021,726	876,642	627,505	57,465	14,232	125,981	51,459	3,119,944	2,298,156	578,335
2003	4,089,950	912,329	654,504	58,400	14,867	135,586	48,972	3,149,034	2,321,904	576,033
2004	4,112,052	946,349	677,621	61,221	14,943	143,520	49,044	3,133,125	2,296,683	578,772
2005	4,138,349	985,505	693,197	63,340	16,064	151,201	61,703	3,123,005	2,279,768	583,759
2006	4,265,555	1,039,077	718,146	66,932	16,936	165,321	71,742	3,196,082	2,308,640	617,247
2007	4,316,233	1,062,779	722,055	68,488	16,981	169,851	85,404	3,222,460	2,310,333	627,191
2008	4,247,694	1,041,239	684,883	69,015	16,718	155,578	115,045	3,173,629	2,267,817	623,029
2009	4,130,665	999,548	645,297	68,486	16,641	148,647	120,477	3,101,330	2,212,552	609,584
2010	3,999,396	945,180	598,317	66,368	16,882	142,692	120,921	3,026,314	2,162,406	589,808
2011	3,953,590	918,129	566,699	67,018	17,131	136,221	131,060	3,008,200	2,146,566	582,345
Birth Rate										
1989[3,6]	16.3	26.2	25.7	23.7	10.0	28.3	(6)	15.4	14.2	22.8
1990[4,6]	16.7	26.7	28.7	21.6	10.9	27.5	(6)	15.7	14.4	23.0
1991[5,6]	16.2	26.5	27.6	23.3	9.8	28.3	(6)	15.2	13.9	22.4
1992[5,6]	15.8	26.1	27.4	22.9	10.1	27.5	(6)	14.8	13.4	21.6
1993[6]	15.4	25.4	26.8	21.5	10.5	26.3	(6)	14.3	13.1	20.7
1994[6]	15.0	24.7	26.1	20.8	10.7	24.9	(6)	13.9	12.8	19.5
1995[6]	14.6	24.1	25.8	19.0	10.8	24.2	(6)	13.5	12.5	18.2
1996[6]	14.4	23.8	26.2	17.2	10.6	22.5	(6)	13.3	12.3	17.6
1997[6]	14.2	23.0	25.3	17.2	10.0	21.3	(6)	13.1	12.2	17.4
1998[6]	14.3	22.7	24.6	17.9	9.7	21.7	(6)	13.2	12.2	17.5
1999[6]	14.2	22.5	24.2	18.0	9.4	21.7	(6)	13.0	12.1	17.1
2000[6]	14.4	23.1	25.0	18.1	9.7	21.8	(6)	13.2	12.2	17.3
2001[6]	14.1	22.9	24.7	17.7	10.3	21.7	(6)	12.8	11.9	16.6
2002[6]	14.0	22.7	24.3	16.5	10.1	22.5	(6)	12.6	11.7	16.1
2003[6]	14.1	22.8	24.6	15.0	10.0	23.0	(6)	12.7	11.8	15.9
2004[6]	14.0	22.8	24.8	16.0	9.3	22.1	(6)	12.6	11.7	15.8
2005[6]	14.0	22.9	24.5	17.0	10.2	22.7	(6)	12.5	11.6	15.8
2006[6]	14.3	23.3	24.6	17.5	10.4	23.8	(6)	12.7	11.7	16.5
2007[6]	14.3	23.0	23.9	17.1	10.2	24.6	(6)	12.8	11.7	16.6
2008[6]	14.0	21.8	21.7	16.4	10.1	26.1	(6)	12.5	11.5	16.3
2009[6]	13.5	20.3	19.8	15.5	9.5	25.5	(6)	12.2	11.2	15.7
2010[6]	13.0	18.7	18.2	14.1	9.0	23.4	(6)	11.8	10.9	15.1
2011[6]	12.7	17.6	16.9	13.7	9.1	23.0	(6)	11.7	10.8	14.7
Fertility Rate										
1989[3,6]	69.2	104.9	106.6	86.6	49.8	95.8	(6)	65.7	60.5	84.8
1990[4,6]	71.0	107.7	118.9	82.9	52.6	102.7	(6)	67.1	62.8	89.0
1991[5,6]	69.3	106.9	114.9	87.9	47.6	105.5	(6)	65.2	60.9	87.0
1992[5,6]	68.4	106.1	113.3	87.9	49.4	104.7	(6)	64.2	60.0	84.5
1993[6]	67.0	103.3	110.9	79.8	53.9	101.5	(6)	62.7	58.9	81.5
1994[6]	65.9	100.7	109.9	78.2	53.6	93.2	(6)	61.6	58.2	77.5
1995[6]	64.6	98.8	109.9	71.3	52.2	89.1	(6)	60.2	57.5	72.8
1996[6]	64.1	97.5	110.7	66.5	55.1	84.2	(6)	59.6	57.1	70.7
1997[6]	63.6	94.2	106.6	65.8	53.1	80.6	(6)	59.3	56.8	70.3
1998[6]	64.3	93.2	103.2	69.7	46.5	83.5		60.0	57.6	70.9
1999[6]	64.4	93.0	101.5	71.1	47.0	84.8	(6)	60.0	57.7	69.9
2000[6]	65.9	95.9	105.1	73.5	49.3	85.1	(6)	61.1	58.5	71.4
2001[6]	65.1	95.4	105.0	71.7	56.4	82.2	(6)	60.0	57.7	69.1
2002[6]	65.0	94.7	103.0	65.6	59.3	86.5	(6)	59.8	57.6	67.5
2003[6]	66.1	95.2	103.7	60.6	60.8	89.7	(6)	60.7	58.9	67.1
2004[6]	66.4	95.7	104.5	66.8	52.2	87.4	(6)	60.8	58.9	67.1
2005[6]	66.7	96.4	104.5	69.8	49.1	90.5	(6)	60.8	59.0	67.2
2006[6]	68.6	98.3	105.6	71.6	47.9	95.6	(6)	62.5	60.3	70.7
2007[6]	69.3	97.4	102.8	70.3	47.6	100.1	(6)	63.3	61.0	71.4
2008[6]	68.1	92.7	92.6	67.0	50.1	109.1	(6)	62.7	60.5	70.8
2009[6]	66.2	86.5	84.8	63.7	46.0	107.5	(6)	61.6	59.6	68.9
2010[6]	64.1	80.2	78.2	59.7	46.4	97.1	(6)	60.4	58.7	66.6
2011[6]	63.2	76.2	73.0	59.6	46.1	96.3	(6)	60.1	58.7	65.4

[1]Includes origin not stated. [2]Includes races other than White and Black. [3]Excludes data for Louisiana, New Hampshire, and Oklahoma, which did not report Hispanic origin. [4]Excludes data for New Hampshire and Oklahoma, which did not report Hispanic origin. [5]Excludes data for New Hampshire, which did not report Hispanic origin. [6]Rates for the Central and South American population includes other and unknown Hispanic.

Table 1-26. Live Births, by Age of Mother, Live-Birth Order, and Race of Mother, 2011

(Number of children born alive to mother.)

Live birth order and race of mother	All ages	Under 15 years	Total	15 to 19 years					20 to 24 years	25 to 29 years	30 to 34 years	35 to 39 years	40 to 44 years	45 to 49 years	50 to 54 years
				15 years	16 years	17 years	18 years	19 years							
All Races	3,953,590	3,974	329,772	11,739	29,072	54,727	92,625	141,609	925,200	1,127,583	986,682	463,849	108,920	7,025	585
1st child	1,578,184	3,874	269,908	11,335	27,253	48,506	76,038	105,966	463,240	423,325	287,855	104,481	24,246	1,894	171
2nd child	1,239,690	64	50,349	314	1,555	5,386	14,079	29,015	300,457	369,858	337,298	149,282	30,463	1,771	148
3rd child	648,351	8	7,234	17	71	434	1,697	5,015	113,431	198,493	198,493	104,025	22,615	1,193	94
4th child	272,058	2	762	1	4	27	156	574	31,731	90,414	90,414	53,341	13,459	710	59
5th child	104,355	-	93	-	3	8	16	66	7,539	36,614	36,614	24,001	7,177	464	59
6th child	43,121	-	16	-	-	3	3	10	1,668	15,755	15,755	11,588	3,920	294	18
7th child	19,464	-	8	-	-	-	4	4	359	7,269	7,269	6,027	2,192	186	10
8th child and over	19,945	-	6	-	-	1	1	4	349	5,815	5,815	7,523	3,914	423	16
Not stated	28,422	26	2,206	72	186	362	631	955	6,426	7,169	7,169	3,581	934	90	10
White	3,020,355	2,339	232,122	7,710	20,116	38,369	65,259	100,668	680,525	883,545	776,706	356,327	83,084	5,311	396
1st child	1,203,508	2,296	191,452	7,487	18,978	34,298	54,166	76,523	347,466	336,977	225,615	79,454	18,706	1,432	110
2nd child	959,521	30	34,655	190	998	3,611	9,648	20,208	224,294	295,543	267,202	113,364	22,982	1,355	96
3rd child	502,388	3	4,515	9	52	276	1,061	3,117	79,753	157,648	160,656	81,725	17,144	874	70
4th child	205,546	1	439	-	3	16	86	334	20,137	60,160	71,476	42,281	10,465	542	45
5th child	75,552	-	52	-	3	4	10	35	4,316	19,217	27,503	18,610	5,473	338	43
6th child	30,035	-	7	-	-	-	2	5	864	6,014	11,160	8,736	3,012	228	14
7th child	13,139	-	6	-	-	-	3	3	179	1,861	4,902	4,371	1,673	141	6
8th child and over	13,608	-	3	-	-	1	1	1	220	1,045	3,536	5,449	3,010	341	4
Not stated	17,058	9	993	24	82	163	282	442	3,296	5,080	4,656	2,337	619	60	8
Black	632,901	1,475	85,140	3,590	7,899	14,308	23,829	35,514	201,323	161,100	113,936	54,756	14,101	972	98
1st child	244,236	1,424	67,459	3,421	7,280	12,402	18,943	25,413	92,585	44,826	24,852	10,279	2,555	229	27
2nd child	177,501	28	13,751	114	496	1,563	3,908	7,670	63,414	49,660	32,585	14,387	3,447	200	29
3rd child	106,328	5	2,430	7	18	139	574	1,692	28,593	34,127	25,492	12,497	2,987	187	10
4th child	51,635	1	286	1	1	9	60	215	10,062	17,342	14,315	7,587	1,931	103	8
5th child	22,826	-	36	-	-	4	5	27	2,795	7,494	7,166	4,017	1,213	97	8
6th child	10,455	-	7	-	-	2	1	4	694	38,182	3,750	2,128	650	42	2
7th child	5,115	-	2	-	-	-	1	1	160	1,319	1,948	1,275	376	32	3
8th child and over	5,179	-	3	-	-	-	-	3	114	744	1,904	1,644	702	59	9
Not stated	9,626	17	1,166	47	104	189	337	489	2,906	2,406	1,924	942	240	23	2
American Indian or Alaska Native	46,419	95	6,802	258	624	1,132	1,904	2,884	15,569	12,477	7,380	3,292	772	30	2
1st child	16,537	92	5,475	255	591	993	1,563	2,073	6,402	2,808	1,221	436	96	6	1
2nd child	12,427	3	1,107	3	33	118	302	651	5,194	3,609	1,715	651	140	8	-
3rd child	8,208	-	172	-	-	15	30	127	2,679	2,850	1,691	677	135	3	1
4th child	4,603	-	23	-	-	-	7	16	907	1,750	1,266	534	122	1	-
5th child	2,322	-	4	-	-	-	-	4	258	858	721	387	91	3	-
6th child	1,076	-	1	-	-	1	-	-	56	341	361	243	70	4	-
7th child	545	-	-	-	-	-	-	-	12	139	190	164	38	2	-
8th child and over	486	-	-	-	-	-	-	-	7	55	171	180	71	2	-
Not stated	215	-	20	-	-	5	2	13	54	67	44	20	9	1	-
Asian or Pacific Islander	253,915	65	5,708	181	433	918	1,633	2,543	27,783	70,461	88,660	49,474	10,963	712	89
1st child	113,903	62	4,712	172	404	813	1,366	1,957	16,787	38,714	36,167	14,312	2,889	227	33
2nd child	90,241	3	836	7	28	94	221	486	7,555	21,046	35,796	20,880	3,894	208	23
3rd child	31,427	-	117	1	1	4	32	79	2,406	6,633	10,654	9,126	2,349	129	13
4th child	10,274	-	14	-	-	2	3	9	625	2,328	3,357	2,939	941	64	6
5th child	3,655	-	1	-	-	-	1	-	170	839	1,224	987	400	26	8
6th child	1,555	-	1	-	-	-	-	1	54	325	484	481	188	20	2
7th child	665	-	-	-	-	-	-	-	8	94	229	229	105	11	1
8th child and over	672	-	-	-	-	-	-	-	8	55	204	204	131	21	3
Not stated	1,523	-	27	1	-	5	10	11	170	427	545	545	66	6	-

– = Quantity zero.

Table 1-27. Live Births, by Age of Mother, Live-Birth Order, and Hispanic Origin, 2011

(Number of children born alive to mother; includes births with stated origin of mother only.)

Live-birth order and origin of mother	All ages	Under 15 years	Total	15 years	16 years	17 years	18 years	19 years	20 to 24 years	25 to 29 years	30 to 34 years	35 to 39 years	40 to 44 years	45 to 49 years	50 to 54 years
Hispanic[1], Total	918,129	1,576	109,660	4,758	11,779	20,442	30,667	42,014	243,724	248,269	192,517	98,340	22,807	1,184	52
1st child	315,396	1,542	86,852	4,596	10,961	17,689	23,994	29,612	108,318	64,725	36,054	14,504	3,207	183	11
2nd child	274,887	24	19,240	143	737	2,438	5,746	10,176	86,771	84,296	55,256	24,266	4,783	239	12
3rd child	181,812	3	2,828	6	41	216	729	1,836	35,045	59,744	52,455	26,108	5,386	231	12
4th child	86,111	-	292	-	2	14	63	213	9,619	25,564	28,712	17,579	4,156	183	6
5th child	33,558	-	31	-	2	1	6	22	2,277	8,510	11,532	8,559	2,511	141	6
6th child	12,873	-	2	-	-	-	1	1	464	2,785	4,466	3,746	1,325	81	4
7th child	5,133	-	3	-	-	-	1	2	100	900	1,794	1,649	651	35	1
8th child and over	3,744	-	1	-	-	-	-	1	82	469	1,118	1,372	641	76	-
Not stated	4,615	7	411	13	36	84	84	151	1,048	1,276	1,139	572	147	15	-
Mexican	566,699	1,019	71,672	3,191	7,933	13,624	20,034	26,890	152,375	153,360	115,157	59,076	13,383	643	14
1st child	181,607	1,002	56,221	3,077	7,374	11,741	15,516	18,513	63,700	35,236	17,273	6,651	1,453	66	5
2nd child	164,672	13	13,097	100	509	1,692	3,905	6,891	56,210	51,187	29,677	12,229	2,162	93	4
3rd child	119,962	1	1,914	6	30	141	494	1,243	23,626	40,229	34,372	16,531	3,161	127	1
4th child	59,927	-	194	-	1	7	42	144	6,444	17,593	20,290	12,456	2,830	120	-
5th child	23,441	-	23	-	2	1	4	16	1,494	5,753	8,052	6,175	1,852	90	2
6th child	8,935	-	2	-	-	-	1	1	311	1,889	3,042	2,689	941	60	1
7th child	3,494	-	1	-	-	-	-	1	74	595	1,187	1,152	458	26	1
8th child and over	2,517	-	1	-	-	-	-	1	54	290	737	923	457	55	-
Not stated	2,144	3	219	8	17	42	72	80	462	588	527	270	69	6	-
Puerto Rican	67,018	118	9,283	313	873	1,653	2,698	3,746	21,116	17,244	12,130	5,743	1,299	83	14
1st child	26,878	114	7,565	303	820	1,456	2,159	2,827	9,978	4,915	2,878	1,175	234	19	5
2nd child	20,151	3	1,447	7	44	165	459	772	7,027	5,801	3,799	1,671	379	24	4
3rd child	11,268	1	214	-	5	20	63	126	2,880	3,770	2,764	1,350	273	16	1
4th child	4,935	-	15	-	-	-	8	7	867	1,665	1,414	766	200	7	-
5th child	1,970	-	4	-	-	-	1	3	210	651	649	353	94	9	2
6th child	833	-	-	-	-	-	-	-	36	233	309	194	56	4	1
7th child	358	-	-	-	-	-	-	-	7	83	143	105	20	-	1
8th child and over	287	-	-	-	-	-	-	-	6	47	95	101	35	3	-
Not stated	338	-	38	3	4	12	8	11	105	79	79	28	9	1	-
Cuban	17,131	5	956	33	69	138	277	439	3,837	5,022	4,068	2,572	633	34	4
1st child	7,988	5	848	33	68	128	253	366	2,436	2,366	1,495	673	157	8	-
2nd child	6,163	-	91	-	1	9	20	61	1,068	1,819	1,724	1,187	258	14	2
3rd child	1,995	-	9	-	-	-	4	5	229	561	589	465	134	7	1
4th child	607	-	4	-	-	-	-	4	59	180	166	150	45	3	-
5th child	179	-	-	-	-	-	-	-	17	46	44	53	17	1	1
6th child	62	-	-	-	-	-	-	-	5	13	23	13	8	-	-
7th child	20	-	-	-	-	-	-	-	-	2	6	7	5	-	-
8th child and over	28	-	-	-	-	-	-	-	-	3	11	7	6	1	-
Not stated	89	-	4	-	-	1	-	3	23	32	10	17	3	-	-
Central and South American	136,221	154	8,759	374	913	1,529	2,369	3,574	27,777	38,249	36,610	19,487	4,867	292	26
1st child	46,665	145	7,068	363	838	1,331	1,869	2,667	13,945	11,900	8,809	3,856	878	58	6
2nd child	44,629	7	1,416	10	69	163	429	745	9,541	13,990	12,306	5,963	1,326	75	5
3rd child	26,060	1	179	-	-	17	39	123	3,097	7,876	8,839	4,828	1,183	49	8
4th child	10,670	-	21	-	1	4	3	13	727	2,905	3,886	2,493	680	44	4
5th child	4,144	-	1	-	-	-	1	-	161	843	1,537	1,213	354	34	1
6th child	1,540	-	-	-	-	-	-	-	23	235	556	515	198	11	2
7th child	637	-	-	-	-	-	-	-	4	60	194	260	113	6	-
8th child and over	443	-	-	-	-	-	-	-	6	44	111	178	90	11	-
Not stated	1,343	1	74	1	5	14	28	26	273	396	369	181	45	4	-
Other and Unknown Hispanic	131,060	280	18,990	847	1,991	3,498	5,289	7,365	38,619	34,394	24,552	11,462	2,625	132	6
1st child	52,258	276	15,150	820	1,861	3,033	4,197	5,239	18,259	10,308	5,599	2,149	485	32	-
2nd child	39,272	1	3,189	26	114	409	933	1,707	12,925	11,499	7,750	3,216	658	33	1
3rd child	22,527	-	512	-	6	38	129	339	5,213	7,308	5,891	2,934	635	32	2
4th child	9,882	-	58	-	-	3	10	45	1,522	3,221	2,956	1,714	401	9	1
5th child	3,824	-	3	-	-	-	-	3	395	1,217	1,241	765	194	7	2
6th child	1,503	-	-	-	-	-	-	-	89	415	536	335	122	6	-
7th child	624	-	2	-	-	-	1	1	15	160	264	125	55	3	-
8th child and over	469	-	-	-	-	-	-	-	16	85	161	148	53	6	-
Not stated	701	3	76	-	10	15	19	31	185	181	154	76	22	4	-

– = Quantity zero.   [1]Includes all persons of Hispanic origin of any race.

Table 1-28. Live Births, by Race of Mother, by State and Territory, 2011

(Number.)

State and territory	All races	White	Black	American Indian or Alaska Native	Asian or Pacific Islander
United States [1]	3,953,590	3,020,355	632,901	46,419	253,915
Alabama	59,354	40,066	18,075	197	1,016
Alaska	11,456	7,053	521	2,842	1,040
Arizona	85,543	71,526	4,475	5,989	3,553
Arkansas	38,715	30,370	7,310	280	755
California	502,120	395,419	32,821	3,461	70,419
Colorado	65,055	58,382	3,452	675	2,546
Connecticut	37,281	29,491	5,426	255	2,289
Delaware	11,257	7,571	3,110	23	553
District of Columbia	9,295	3,492	5,229	20	554
Florida	213,414	152,835	52,858	435	7,286
Georgia	132,409	77,416	48,459	336	6,198
Hawaii	18,956	5,978	651	80	12,247
Idaho	22,305	21,221	230	414	440
Illinois	161,312	123,442	27,925	218	9,727
Indiana	83,071	71,292	10,227	157	2,025
Iowa	38,214	34,790	1,950	266	1,208
Kansas	39,642	34,804	3,116	380	1,342
Kentucky	55,370	48,647	5,452	86	1,185
Louisiana	61,888	35,806	24,361	381	1,340
Maine	12,704	11,974	408	111	211
Maryland	73,093	42,024	25,148	205	5,716
Massachusetts	73,166	57,261	9,462	165	6,278
Michigan	114,008	86,838	22,386	793	3,991
Minnesota	68,409	54,963	6,791	1,540	5,115
Mississippi	39,860	21,819	17,332	282	427
Missouri	76,117	61,895	11,821	395	2,006
Montana	12,069	10,344	96	1,486	143
Nebraska	25,720	22,635	1,848	514	723
Nevada	35,296	27,916	3,931	468	2,981
New Hampshire	12,851	12,022	286	22	521
New Jersey	105,833	74,496	19,353	182	11,852
New Mexico	27,289	22,517	630	3,617	525
New York	241,312	165,598	49,738	1,182	24,794
North Carolina	120,389	81,604	31,638	1,982	5,165
North Dakota	9,527	8,074	245	1,036	172
Ohio	137,918	110,001	24,135	273	3,509
Oklahoma	52,272	39,589	5,022	6,187	1,474
Oregon	45,155	40,326	1,269	873	2,687
Pennsylvania	143,178	111,053	25,453	383	6,289
Rhode Island	10,960	8,797	1,418	148	597
South Carolina	57,393	36,916	19,030	241	1,206
South Dakota	11,846	9,240	282	2,094	230
Tennessee	79,588	60,052	17,369	234	1,933
Texas	377,445	312,247	46,102	1,107	17,289
Utah	51,223	47,977	793	770	1,683
Vermont	6,078	5,812	91	17	158
Virginia	102,652	72,333	22,553	121	7,645
Washington	86,976	70,156	5,142	2,234	9,444
West Virginia	20,717	19,777	736	19	185
Wisconsin	67,810	56,858	6,836	975	3,141
Wyoming	7,399	6,940	89	268	102
Puerto Rico	41,080	36,940	4,584	NA	NA
Virgin Islands	1,491	357	1,108	4	22
Guam	3,294	226	40	6	3,022
American Samoa	1,256	4	-	-	1,252
Northern Marianas	1,033	10	2	-	1,021

NA = Not available.   - = Quantity zero.   [1] Excludes data for the territories.

Table 1-29. Live Births, by Hispanic Origin of Mother and by Race for Mothers of Non-Hispanic Origin, by State and Territory, 2011

(Number.)

State and territory	All origins	Hispanic (may be of any race)						Non-Hispanic			Not stated
		Total	Mexican	Puerto Rican	Cuban	Central and South American	Other and unknown Hispanic	Total[1]	White	Black	
United States [2]	3,953,590	918,129	566,699	67,018	17,131	136,221	131,060	3,008,200	2,146,566	582,345	27,261
Alabama	59,354	4,481	2,958	178	41	1,221	83	54,862	35,684	17,987	11
Alaska	11,456	757	345	96	14	117	185	10,231	6,082	437	468
Arizona	85,543	33,254	31,044	403	106	944	757	51,992	38,988	4,083	297
Arkansas	38,715	3,958	3,030	59	14	701	154	34,661	26,408	7,231	96
California	502,120	250,030	195,099	2,030	685	21,324	30,892	243,306	144,584	29,902	8,784
Colorado	65,055	18,077	12,102	350	85	1,008	4,532	46,353	40,439	3,054	625
Connecticut	37,281	8,393	953	4,490	81	2,735	134	28,805	21,538	4,776	83
Delaware	11,257	1,416	676	293	9	361	77	9,821	6,222	3,031	20
District of Columbia	9,295	1,371	158	32	13	1,009	159	7,834	2,626	4,809	90
Florida	213,414	58,739	12,626	11,590	11,658	18,681	4,184	153,587	97,304	49,084	1,088
Georgia	132,409	18,664	11,285	1,052	263	3,955	2,109	111,017	60,622	44,649	2,728
Hawaii	18,956	3,038	720	898	28	184	1,208	15,890	4,860	508	28
Idaho	22,305	3,475	2,858	40	12	166	399	18,785	17,869	192	45
Illinois	161,312	35,765	29,843	2,452	185	2,361	924	124,916	87,952	27,183	631
Indiana	83,701	7,180	5,699	299	38	659	485	76,345	64,482	9,825	176
Iowa	38,214	3,114	2,336	74	15	516	173	35,094	31,927	1,844	6
Kansas	39,642	6,294	4,564	122	25	553	1,030	33,306	28,814	2,934	42
Kentucky	55,370	2,782	1,743	176	135	460	268	52,530	46,190	5,204	58
Louisiana	61,888	3,607	1,583	166	125	1,388	345	58,280	33,112	23,608	1
Maine	12,704	208	26	31	13	48	90	12,453	11,747	395	43
Maryland	73,093	10,330	1,901	630	85	6,717	997	62,574	33,265	23,846	189
Massachusetts	73,166	12,573	420	4,070	107	3,601	4,375	60,027	46,570	7,161	566
Michigan	114,008	7,628	4,893	502	93	724	1,416	105,990	79,607	21,775	390
Minnesota	68,409	4,629	3,241	137	47	837	367	63,087	50,297	6,471	693
Mississippi	39,860	1,320	601	42	8	307	362	38,512	20,500	17,304	28
Missouri	76,117	4,113	2,731	158	75	670	479	71,479	57,815	11,433	525
Montana	12,069	449	261	24	6	30	128	11,521	9,934	75	99
Nebraska	25,720	3,646	2,598	54	48	668	278	22,052	19,301	1,708	22
Nevada	35,296	13,049	10,226	264	256	1,226	1,077	22,163	15,259	3,695	84
New Hampshire	12,851	540	79	136	12	97	216	12,154	11,392	234	157
New Jersey	105,883	28,013	5,771	6,754	695	12,765	2,028	77,554	49,661	16,047	316
New Mexico	27,289	15,061	5,248	88	28	108	9,589	11,936	7,719	473	292
New York	241,312	56,703	10,396	13,807	545	16,929	15,026	181,086	117,201	39,157	3,523
North Carolina	120,389	18,219	11,752	1,236	208	3,900	1,123	102,112	67,688	28,597	58
North Dakota	9,527	307	203	28	5	31	40	9,103	7,759	218	117
Ohio	137,918	6,337	3,074	1,398	72	1,029	764	130,939	104,506	22,835	642
Oklahoma	52,272	6,684	5,219	178	28	619	640	45,496	33,358	4,815	92
Oregon	45,155	8,742	7,558	116	47	535	486	36,197	31,768	1,168	216
Pennsylvania	143,178	14,178	2,759	7,143	201	1,624	2,451	127,816	100,790	21,027	1,184
Rhode Island	10,960	2,424	140	641	16	756	871	8,311	6,755	959	225
South Carolina	57,393	4,748	2,893	404	53	999	399	52,481	32,977	18,288	164
South Dakota	11,846	505	285	46	2	111	61	11,328	8,859	266	13
Tennessee	79,588	7,022	4,588	318	100	1,450	566	72,511	54,131	16,557	55
Texas	377,445	182,503	133,750	1,716	534	11,742	34,761	194,578	133,894	43,212	364
Utah	51,223	7,686	5,546	108	28	1,075	929	43,533	40,860	568	4
Vermont	6,078	72	19	12	4	20	17	5,991	5,727	89	15
Virginia	102,652	12,473	2,963	964	132	7,723	691	89,967	60,370	21,945	212
Washington	86,976	15,976	12,305	407	103	1,038	2,123	69,715	55,084	4,303	1,285
West Virginia	20,717	207	82	33	1	49	42	20,424	19,497	726	86
Wisconsin	67,810	6,525	4,991	752	45	398	339	61,030	50,500	6,592	255
Wyoming	7,399	864	558	21	2	52	231	6,465	6,072	65	70
Puerto Rico	41,080	39,706	30	38,529	21	209	917	1,314	1,175	133	60
Virgin Islands	1,491	320	-	74	1	110	135	1,153	111	1,017	18
Guam	3,294	52	19	11	2	8	12	3,195	194	33	47
American Samoa	1,256	NA	NA	NA	NA	NA	NA	NA	NA	NA	1,256
Northern Marianas	1,033	NA	NA	NA	NA	NA	NA	1,030	10	2	3

NA = Not available.   - = Quantity zero.   [1]Includes races other than White and Black.   [2]Excludes data for the territories.

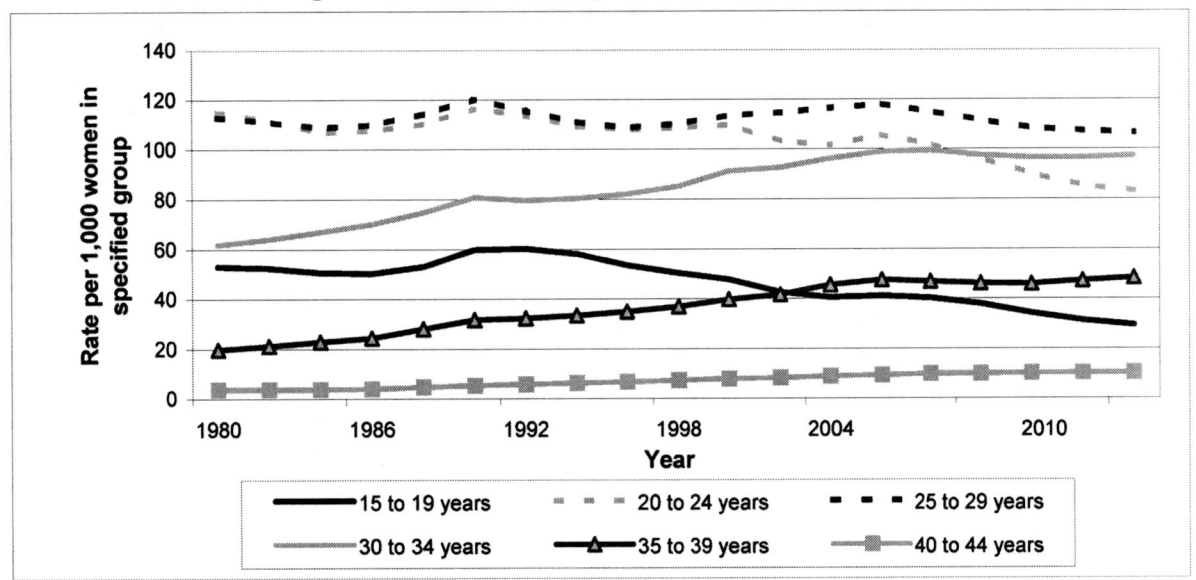

Figure 1-6. Birth Rates, by Age of Mother, 1980–2011

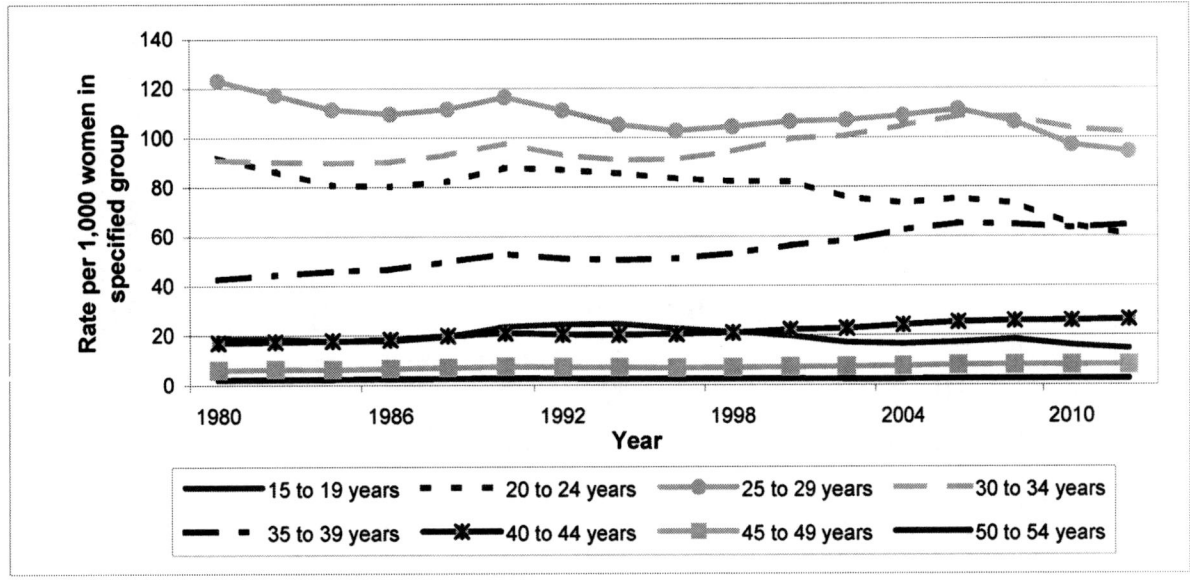

Figure 1-7. Birth Rates, by Age of Father, 1980–2011

Table 1-30. Birth Rates, by Age of Mother, State, and Territory, 2011

(Fertility rates are births per 1,000 women age 15 to 44 years estimated in each area; total fertility rates are sums of birth rates for 5-year age groups multiplied by 5; birth rates by age are births per 1,000 women in specified age group estimated in each area.)

State and territory	Birth rate	Fertility rate	Total fertility rate	10 to 14 years	15 to 19 years			20 to 24 years	25 to 29 years	30 to 34 years	35 to 39 years	40 to 44 years	45 to 49 years[1]
					Total	15 to 17 years	18 to 19 years						
United States [2]	12.7	63.2	1,894.5	0.4	31.3	15.4	54.1	85.3	107.2	96.5	47.2	10.3	0.7
Alabama	12.4	61.8	1,836.5	0.6	40.5	20.7	68.8	101.0	111.4	77.1	30.4	6.0	0.3
Alaska	15.9	78.5	2,277.0	*	36.2	13.3	73.9	125.8	127.0	102.2	51.9	11.5	*
Arizona	13.2	67.3	1,999.5	0.5	38.5	18.7	68.4	98.3	113.6	92.9	45.5	10.0	0.6
Arkansas	13.2	67.8	1,995.5	0.6	50.7	23.2	91.0	119.4	118.1	75.4	28.8	5.8	0.3
California	13.3	63.4	1,900.0	0.3	28.7	14.8	49.5	74.9	100.1	102.1	58.2	14.5	1.2
Colorado	12.7	62.7	1,854.5	0.4	28.9	14.4	49.7	78.7	100.2	99.8	50.8	11.3	0.8
Connecticut	10.4	54.3	1,708.0	0.2	16.4	7.3	29.4	57.8	90.7	109.1	55.0	11.6	0.8
Delaware	12.4	62.9	1,904.5	*	29.3	14.3	48.8	82.0	113.3	98.5	48.0	8.9	*
District of Columbia	15.0	56.0	1,636.5	2.3	42.8	33.6	49.1	55.6	47.5	85.0	71.0	21.1	2.0
Florida	11.2	59.6	1,799.0	0.3	29.5	13.7	52.7	82.9	101.9	89.6	44.9	10.1	0.6
Georgia	13.5	63.8	1,927.0	0.5	38.2	19.0	66.0	99.2	107.7	88.5	41.3	9.3	0.7
Hawaii	13.8	71.9	2,114.0	*	30.0	12.0	58.9	98.8	110.7	104.8	61.5	15.7	1.0
Idaho	14.1	72.3	2,145.5	*	27.7	11.5	50.7	113.3	138.8	98.9	40.8	8.9	0.4
Illinois	12.5	61.5	1,838.5	0.3	29.5	15.4	50.6	75.0	98.9	101.9	50.7	10.7	0.7
Indiana	12.8	65.0	1,951.5	0.4	34.8	16.0	61.2	97.0	124.1	90.2	36.2	7.3	0.3
Iowa	12.5	66.1	1,972.5	0.2	25.3	11.8	43.0	84.4	134.9	103.4	38.8	7.2	0.3
Kansas	13.8	71.2	2,091.0	0.5	35.4	15.5	63.3	102.8	129.8	99.3	41.8	8.2	0.4
Kentucky	12.7	64.7	1,939.0	0.4	43.5	19.6	78.1	108.8	116.2	80.3	32.0	6.2	0.4
Louisiana	13.5	66.4	1,910.0	0.7	45.1	20.7	79.8	107.2	111.3	78.7	32.4	6.4	0.2
Maine	9.6	53.1	1,665.0	*	20.8	9.3	36.9	79.2	104.3	86.3	35.1	6.8	0.4
Maryland	12.5	61.3	1,854.0	0.4	24.7	12.1	43.1	72.0	99.6	104.7	56.3	12.2	0.9
Massachusetts	11.1	54.3	1,666.0	0.2	15.4	7.9	24.4	46.7	80.0	114.0	63.0	13.0	0.9
Michigan	11.5	59.9	1,843.5	0.3	27.8	12.6	49.3	80.9	115.3	95.9	39.9	8.1	0.5
Minnesota	12.8	65.5	1,947.0	0.2	19.3	8.8	34.3	70.9	120.2	116.0	51.9	10.2	0.7
Mississippi	13.4	66.0	1,940.0	1.0	50.2	26.1	83.8	120.2	114.6	69.9	26.5	5.3	0.3
Missouri	12.7	64.8	1,915.0	0.3	34.5	15.8	60.8	96.5	115.4	91.2	37.5	7.2	0.4
Montana	12.1	66.7	1,961.5	*	29.2	12.4	52.5	96.7	120.5	96.5	40.3	8.5	*
Nebraska	14.0	72.0	2,112.0	*	27.2	12.6	46.9	91.8	136.7	111.1	45.8	9.0	0.6
Nevada	13.0	64.2	1,911.5	0.4	36.1	18.4	66.3	93.6	106.9	88.6	45.7	10.4	0.6
New Hampshire	9.7	51.9	1,671.5	*	13.7	5.4	24.5	61.9	102.3	103.5	44.2	8.2	0.4
New Jersey	12.0	61.3	1,884.0	0.2	18.7	8.8	34.9	65.9	98.8	116.9	62.0	13.2	1.1
New Mexico	13.1	68.2	2,001.5	0.6	48.8	26.3	82.1	110.2	112.0	80.6	38.3	9.3	0.5
New York	12.4	59.8	1,786.0	0.3	21.2	10.1	36.7	65.2	91.4	102.6	61.0	14.4	1.1
North Carolina	12.5	61.5	1,860.0	0.5	34.9	16.6	60.0	94.1	105.6	88.3	40.0	8.1	0.5
North Dakota	13.9	72.4	2,080.0	*	28.2	10.7	47.9	80.7	142.2	110.0	45.3	8.3	*
Ohio	11.9	62.1	1,881.5	0.4	31.5	14.4	56.4	90.8	113.9	92.8	39.0	7.4	0.5
Oklahoma	13.8	70.4	2,039.5	0.5	47.8	22.9	82.7	117.1	121.5	79.9	33.9	6.9	0.3
Oregon	11.7	59.4	1,756.5	0.2	25.8	11.9	45.7	76.5	101.2	90.3	46.8	9.9	0.6
Pennsylvania	11.2	58.8	1,800.0	0.4	24.9	12.9	40.5	72.4	105.0	101.7	46.3	8.7	0.6
Rhode Island	10.4	51.5	1,602.5	*	21.3	12.6	30.4	53.4	92.0	96.4	47.3	9.4	0.5
South Carolina	12.3	61.8	1,839.5	0.5	39.1	19.2	65.3	95.4	106.9	83.0	35.5	7.3	0.2
South Dakota	14.4	77.1	2,253.0	*	34.3	15.2	59.9	102.4	150.5	108.3	44.8	9.4	*
Tennessee	12.4	62.3	1,866.0	0.5	40.8	18.5	73.8	102.9	109.1	79.8	33.1	6.6	0.4
Texas	14.7	69.8	2,074.5	0.6	46.9	25.6	79.0	106.0	113.6	93.2	44.1	9.9	0.6
Utah	18.2	83.6	2,377.5	0.2	23.1	11.1	39.2	102.3	163.6	121.8	53.2	10.7	0.6
Vermont	9.7	51.8	1,627.0	*	16.8	8.2	26.1	64.1	96.6	93.6	45.1	8.3	*
Virginia	12.7	61.9	1,853.0	0.2	24.5	11.2	42.7	78.0	102.3	101.2	52.3	11.3	0.8
Washington	12.7	63.7	1,886.0	0.2	25.4	11.7	46.0	79.8	108.6	100.0	51.1	11.3	0.8
West Virginia	11.2	60.7	1,842.5	0.5	43.5	20.5	74.7	107.1	114.2	71.3	26.2	5.3	0.4
Wisconsin	11.9	62.0	1,873.0	0.3	23.2	10.6	40.5	75.9	118.8	104.6	43.4	8.0	0.4
Wyoming	13.0	69.1	1,976.0	*	35.2	14.7	63.7	106.8	124.2	86.9	35.1	6.5	*
Puerto Rico	11.1	53.6	1,596.5	0.7	51.7	31.8	81.1	102.5	82.3	54.2	22.8	4.8	0.3
Virgin Islands	14.1	72.2	2,344.0	*	59.3	25.1	111.5	150.4	128.7	84.2	36.4	8.1	*
Guam	20.6	95.9	2,875.5	*	62.1	34.3	105.1	145.6	155.6	127.1	63.9	17.4	*
American Samoa	22.8	95.3	3,095.0	*	38.4	19.2	67.2	150.8	165.5	154.5	91.8	16.6	*
Northern Marianas	19.8	74.0	2,169.0	*	47.2	28.1	71.8	102.4	81.6	81.1	91.3	27.1	*

* = Figure does not meet standards of reliability or percision; birth rates based on fewer than 20 births.   [1]Birth rates computed by relating births to women age 45 years and over to women age 45 to 49 years.   [2]Excludes data for the territories.

Table 1-31. Birth Rates, by Age of Mother, Live-Birth Order, and Race of Mother, 2011

(Live births per 1,000 women in specified age and racial group.)

Live-birth order and race of mother	15 to 44 years	10 to 14 years	15 to 19 years			20 to 24 years	25 to 29 years	30 to 34 years	35 to 39 years	40 to 44 years	45 to 49 years[1]
			Total	15 to 17 years	18 to 19 years						
All Races	63.2	0.4	31.3	15.4	54.1	85.3	107.2	96.5	47.2	10.3	0.7
1st child	25.4	0.4	25.7	14.1	42.4	43.0	40.5	28.3	10.7	2.3	0.2
2nd child	20.0	0.0	4.8	1.2	10.0	27.9	35.4	33.2	15.3	2.9	0.2
3rd child	10.4	*	0.7	0.1	1.6	10.5	19.3	19.5	10.7	2.2	0.1
4th child	4.4	*	0.1	0.0	0.2	2.9	7.8	8.9	5.5	1.3	0.1
5th child	1.7	*	0.0	*	0.0	0.7	2.7	3.6	2.5	0.7	0.0
6th and 7th child	1.0	*	0.0	*	0.0	0.2	1.3	2.3	1.8	0.6	0.0
8th child and over	0.3	*	*	*	*	0.0	0.2	0.6	0.8	0.4	0.0
White	63.4	0.3	29.1	14.1	50.8	83.0	110.2	100.1	47.6	10.1	0.6
1st child	25.4	0.3	24.1	13.0	40.2	42.6	42.3	29.2	10.7	2.3	0.2
2nd child	20.3	0.0	4.4	1.0	9.2	27.5	37.1	34.6	15.3	2.8	0.2
3rd child	10.6	*	0.6	0.1	1.3	9.8	19.8	20.8	11.0	2.1	0.1
4th child	4.3	*	0.1	*	0.1	2.5	7.5	9.3	5.7	1.3	0.1
5th child	1.6	*	0.0	*	0.0	0.5	2.4	3.6	2.5	0.7	0.0
6th and 7th child	0.9	*	*	*	*	0.1	1.0	2.1	1.8	0.6	0.0
8th child and over	0.3	*	*	*	*	0.0	0.1	0.5	0.7	0.4	0.0
Black	65.5	0.9	47.3	24.7	78.8	111.9	101.7	74.1	38.0	9.4	0.7
1st child	25.7	0.9	38.0	22.4	59.7	52.2	28.7	16.4	7.3	1.7	0.2
2nd child	18.7	0.0	7.8	2.1	15.6	35.8	31.8	21.5	10.2	2.3	0.2
3rd child	11.2	*	1.4	0.2	3.1	16.1	21.9	16.9	8.8	2.0	0.1
4th child	5.4	*	0.2	*	0.4	5.7	11.1	9.5	5.4	1.3	0.1
5th child	2.4	*	0.0	*	0.0	1.6	4.8	4.7	2.8	0.8	0.1
6th and 7th child	1.6	*	*	*	*	0.5	2.9	3.8	2.4	0.7	0.1
8th child and over	0.5	*	*	*	*	0.1	0.5	1.3	1.2	0.5	0.0
American Indian or Alaska Native	47.7	0.5	36.1	18.2	61.6	86.6	75.4	47.3	23.1	5.5	0.2
1st child	17.1	0.5	29.1	16.7	46.9	35.7	17.1	7.9	3.1	0.7	*
2nd child	12.8	*	5.9	1.4	12.3	29.0	21.9	11.1	4.6	1.0	*
3rd child	8.5	*	0.9	*	2.0	15.0	17.3	10.9	4.8	1.0	*
4th child	4.8	*	0.1	*	0.3	5.1	10.6	8.2	3.8	0.9	*
5th child	2.4	*	*	*	*	1.4	5.2	4.6	2.7	0.7	*
6th and 7th child	1.7	*	*	*	*	0.4	2.9	3.6	2.9	0.8	*
8th child and over	0.5	*	*	*	*	*	0.3	1.1	1.3	0.5	*
Asian or Pacific Islander	59.9	0.1	10.2	4.6	18.1	41.9	93.7	114.9	64.1	15.2	1.2
1st child	27.0	*	8.4	4.2	14.5	25.4	51.8	47.2	18.7	4.0	0.4
2nd child	21.4	*	1.5	0.4	3.1	11.5	28.2	46.7	27.2	5.4	0.4
3rd child	7.5	*	0.2	*	0.5	3.6	8.9	13.9	11.9	3.3	0.2
4th child	2.4	*	*	*	*	0.9	3.1	4.4	3.8	1.3	0.1
5th child	0.9	*	*	*	*	0.3	1.1	1.6	1.3	0.6	0.1
6th and 7th child	0.5	*	*	*	*	0.1	0.6	0.9	0.9	0.4	0.1
8th child and over	0.2	*	*	*	*	*	0.1	0.3	0.3	0.2	0.0

* = Figure does not meet standards of reliability or precision.   0.0 = Quantity more than zero but less than 0.05.   [1]Birth rates computed by relating births to women age 45 years and over to women age 45 to 49 years.

Table 1-32. Birth Rates, by Age and Selected Race of Father, 1980–2011

(Rates are births per 1,000 men in specified group.)

Year and race of father	Total, 15 to 54 years[1]	Age of father								
		15 to 19 years[2]	20 to 24 years	25 to 29 years	30 to 34 years	35 to 39 years	40 to 44 years	45 to 49 years	50 to 54 years	55 years and over
All Races[3]										
1980[4]	57.0	18.8	92.0	123.1	91.0	42.8	17.1	6.1	2.2	0.3
1981[4]	56.3	18.4	88.4	119.1	88.7	43.3	17.0	6.2	2.3	0.4
1982[4]	56.4	18.6	86.5	117.3	90.3	44.5	17.5	6.4	2.3	0.4
1983[4]	55.1	18.2	82.6	113.0	89.1	45.2	17.4	6.4	2.3	0.4
1984[4]	55.0	17.8	80.7	111.4	89.9	46.0	17.8	6.3	2.4	0.4
1985	55.6	18.0	81.2	112.3	91.1	47.3	18.1	6.6	2.5	0.4
1986	54.8	17.9	80.3	109.6	90.3	46.8	18.3	6.7	2.6	0.4
1987	55.0	18.3	80.5	109.9	91.2	48.6	19.0	6.9	2.6	0.4
1988	55.8	19.6	82.4	111.6	93.2	49.9	19.9	7.1	2.7	0.4
1989	57.2	21.9	85.4	114.3	94.8	51.3	20.4	7.4	2.7	0.6
1990	58.4	23.5	88.0	116.4	97.8	53.0	21.0	7.5	2.8	0.4
1991	56.8	24.7	87.9	113.5	94.3	51.6	20.2	7.4	2.7	0.4
1992	55.3	24.4	87.1	111.1	93.0	51.1	20.4	7.3	2.7	0.4
1993	53.7	24.4	86.0	108.1	91.7	50.7	20.2	7.3	2.7	0.4
1994	52.4	24.6	85.6	105.3	91.1	50.5	20.3	7.2	2.6	0.3
1995	51.0	23.9	83.9	103.2	90.7	50.4	20.3	7.0	2.5	0.3
1996	50.2	22.7	83.4	102.8	91.3	51.1	20.5	6.9	2.5	0.3
1997	49.4	21.9	82.1	102.6	92.0	51.5	20.7	7.0	2.5	0.3
1998	49.6	21.3	82.3	104.4	94.4	53.1	21.0	7.1	2.5	0.3
1999	49.2	20.6	81.1	105.3	95.9	53.9	21.1	7.0	2.4	0.3
2000	50.0	19.8	82.1	106.5	99.5	56.3	22.2	7.3	2.5	0.3
2001	48.9	18.3	78.3	106.7	99.9	57.1	22.3	7.3	2.4	0.3
2002	48.7	17.2	75.7	107.1	100.7	58.3	22.7	7.4	2.4	0.3
2003	49.3	16.6	74.7	109.1	104.0	60.9	23.6	7.6	2.5	0.3
2004	49.3	16.6	73.4	108.9	104.7	62.5	24.1	7.7	2.4	0.3
2005	49.3	16.4	72.7	109.4	105.9	63.4	24.5	7.9	2.5	0.2
2006	50.4	17.3	75.3	111.4	108.6	65.2	25.3	8.1	2.6	0.2
2007	50.8	18.2	75.6	110.4	110.3	65.6	25.7	8.2	2.6	0.3
2008	49.8	18.4	73.2	106.4	108.3	64.8	25.8	8.3	2.6	0.3
2009	48.3	17.7	69.5	101.5	105.5	63.8	25.9	8.2	2.6	0.3
2010	46.8	16.1	64.6	97.1	103.6	63.4	25.9	8.2	2.6	0.3
2011	46.1	14.7	60.5	94.4	102.2	64.6	26.4	8.3	2.6	0.3
White										
1980[4]	53.4	15.4	84.9	119.4	87.8	39.7	15.0	5.1	1.8	0.3
1981[4]	52.9	15.0	81.7	115.8	85.8	40.3	15.0	5.2	1.8	0.3
1982[4]	53.1	14.9	80.1	114.2	87.5	41.7	15.6	5.3	1.9	0.3
1983[4]	52.0	14.4	76.3	110.2	86.8	42.6	15.5	5.3	1.8	0.3
1984[4]	51.8	14.0	74.3	108.8	87.9	43.5	16.0	5.3	1.9	0.3
1985	52.6	14.0	74.7	109.9	89.5	44.8	16.3	5.6	1.9	0.3
1986	51.7	13.8	73.3	107.0	88.7	44.4	16.6	5.7	2.0	0.3
1987	51.6	13.9	72.8	107.0	89.5	46.2	17.3	5.9	2.0	0.3
1988	52.2	14.8	73.7	108.3	91.2	47.6	18.1	6.1	2.1	0.3
1989	53.3	16.7	75.9	110.8	93.0	49.1	18.7	6.3	2.1	0.4
1990	54.6	18.1	78.3	113.2	96.1	50.9	19.2	6.5	2.2	0.3
1991	53.1	19.0	78.4	110.2	92.8	49.6	18.5	6.5	2.2	0.3
1992	51.8	18.8	77.8	108.2	91.9	49.1	18.8	6.4	2.2	0.3
1993	50.3	18.9	77.2	105.5	90.7	48.9	18.7	6.4	2.2	0.2
1994	49.3	19.5	77.4	103.1	90.4	48.9	18.9	6.3	2.2	0.3
1995	48.4	19.4	77.0	101.7	90.4	49.1	19.1	6.2	2.1	0.2
1996	47.7	18.7	76.7	101.4	91.1	49.9	19.2	6.1	2.1	0.2
1997	46.8	18.0	75.3	100.9	91.7	50.2	19.3	6.2	2.1	0.3
1998	47.1	17.7	75.6	102.7	94.3	51.9	19.6	6.3	2.1	0.3
1999	46.9	17.3	74.7	104.1	96.2	52.7	19.8	6.3	2.1	0.3
2000	47.6	16.6	75.8	105.4	99.5	54.7	20.7	6.5	2.1	0.3
2001	46.9	15.4	73.1	106.6	100.3	55.8	20.8	6.5	2.0	0.3
2002	46.8	14.7	71.4	107.5	101.2	57.0	21.2	6.6	2.1	0.3
2003	47.5	14.1	70.7	109.9	104.5	59.6	22.0	6.8	2.1	0.3
2004	47.4	14.1	69.1	109.6	105.0	61.1	22.5	6.9	2.0	0.2
2005	47.3	14.0	68.2	110.0	106.2	61.9	22.8	6.9	2.1	0.2
2006	48.3	14.6	70.5	112.0	108.8	63.4	23.5	7.1	2.1	0.1
2007	48.6	15.5	70.6	111.1	110.5	63.5	23.8	7.1	2.1	0.3
2008	47.7	15.7	68.1	107.0	108.8	62.6	23.9	7.2	2.1	0.3
2009	46.3	15.2	64.3	102.0	106.2	61.7	24.0	7.1	2.1	0.3
2010	44.8	13.9	59.6	97.5	104.6	61.3	24.0	7.1	2.0	0.2
2011	44.1	12.8	55.5	94.5	103.0	62.5	24.3	7.1	2.0	0.2
Black										
1980[4]	83.0	40.1	145.3	152.8	109.6	62.0	31.2	13.6	5.9	1.1
1981[4]	80.4	38.9	138.4	145.6	104.3	61.3	29.7	13.3	5.7	1.2
1982[4]	79.5	40.3	133.4	141.2	103.6	61.1	29.6	13.9	6.0	1.2
1983[4]	77.2	40.7	129.1	134.4	99.0	59.6	29.6	13.5	6.0	1.2
1984[4]	76.7	40.9	128.0	132.2	98.3	58.4	29.3	13.3	6.1	1.2
1985	77.2	41.8	129.5	132.7	97.3	59.4	29.5	13.3	6.5	1.2
1986	77.2	42.6	131.4	131.6	97.4	58.0	29.1	13.5	6.7	1.3
1987	78.3	44.6	136.1	133.9	97.4	58.0	30.0	13.8	6.6	1.3
1988	80.7	48.1	144.1	137.9	100.0	58.0	30.6	14.3	6.9	1.4
1989	84.1	52.9	153.4	143.5	101.4	59.9	31.1	14.9	6.9	2.7
1990	84.9	55.2	158.2	144.9	103.2	60.4	31.1	15.0	7.1	1.4
1991	83.0	57.8	158.5	142.0	99.2	58.5	29.4	14.1	6.7	1.4
1992	80.4	57.0	157.1	138.6	95.8	56.7	28.4	13.7	6.1	1.4
1993	77.6	56.2	152.7	134.2	94.0	56.3	27.7	13.4	6.3	1.3
1994	74.0	54.1	149.1	129.6	91.4	53.8	26.4	12.8	5.8	1.1
1995	69.1	49.9	139.2	123.9	87.7	52.0	25.7	11.9	5.4	1.1
1996	67.2	46.7	137.6	123.9	87.0	51.8	25.7	11.3	5.3	1.1
1997	66.7	45.1	136.3	126.3	88.8	52.6	26.1	11.4	5.2	1.0
1998	66.8	42.8	137.0	130.3	90.9	54.0	26.7	11.6	5.0	1.0
1999	65.4	41.0	133.8	129.6	91.6	54.3	26.5	11.2	4.9	1.0

Table 1-32. Birth Rates, by Age and Selected Race of Father, 1980–2011—*Continued*

(Rates are births per 1,000 men in specified group.)

Year and race of father	Total, 15 to 54 years[1]	Age of father								
		15 to 19 years[2]	20 to 24 years	25 to 29 years	30 to 34 years	35 to 39 years	40 to 44 years	45 to 49 years	50 to 54 years	55 years and over
2000	66.2	39.6	135.5	131.0	95.2	56.9	28.4	11.7	5.0	1.0
2001	63.3	36.2	124.9	127.6	96.1	57.1	28.2	11.8	4.6	1.0
2002	61.2	32.8	117.3	126.4	95.1	58.0	28.4	11.9	4.7	0.9
2003	61.2	31.8	114.4	127.7	97.6	60.1	29.3	12.3	4.7	0.9
2004	61.7	31.8	113.9	129.0	100.2	62.0	30.2	12.5	4.8	0.7
2005	62.5	31.1	114.7	131.5	102.8	64.2	31.2	13.3	5.0	0.7
2006	64.8	32.9	119.8	135.1	107.1	67.5	32.4	13.7	5.3	0.6
2007	63.8	33.9	118.5	128.1	105.1	67.7	33.2	13.9	5.4	1.0
2008	64.4	35.8	115.8	119.0	103.5	68.3	34.0	14.4	5.7	1.0
2009	61.9	32.2	114.4	122.3	102.1	66.0	33.3	13.9	5.5	1.0
2010	59.6	29.0	107.0	117.0	98.9	65.7	33.9	13.8	5.8	1.0
2011	58.7	26.6	99.4	114.6	98.3	66.7	34.5	14.2	5.7	1.0

NOTE: Race and Hispanic origin are reported separately on birth certificates.

[1]Rates computed by relating total births, regardless of age of father, to men age 15 to 54 years.   [2]Rates computed by relating births to fathers under 20 years of age to men age 15 to 19 years.   [3]Includes races other than White and Black.   [4]Based on 100 percent of births in selected states and on a 50-percent sample of births in all other states.

Table 1-33. Total Fertility Rates and Birth Rates by Age of Mother and by Age and Race of Mother, 1980–2011

(Live births per 1,000 women in specified group.)

Year and race	Total fertility rate	10 to 14 years	15 to 19 years Total	15 to 17 years	18 to 19 years	20 to 24 years	25 to 29 years	30 to 34 years	35 to 39 years	40 to 44 years	45 to 49 years[1]
All Races [2]											
1980[3]	1,839.5	1.1	53.0	32.5	82.1	115.1	112.9	61.9	19.8	3.9	0.2
1981[3]	1,812.0	1.1	52.2	32.0	80.0	112.2	111.5	61.4	20.0	3.8	0.2
1982[3]	1,827.5	1.1	52.4	32.3	79.4	111.6	111.0	64.1	21.2	3.9	0.2
1983[3]	1,799.0	1.1	51.4	31.8	77.4	107.8	108.5	64.9	22.0	3.9	0.2
1984[3]	1,806.5	1.2	50.6	31.0	77.4	106.8	108.7	67.0	22.9	3.9	0.2
1985	1,844.0	1.2	51.0	31.0	79.6	108.3	111.0	69.1	24.0	4.0	0.2
1986	1,837.5	1.3	50.2	30.5	79.6	107.4	109.8	70.1	24.4	4.1	0.2
1987	1,872.0	1.3	50.6	31.7	78.5	107.9	111.6	72.1	26.3	4.4	0.2
1988	1,934.0	1.3	53.0	33.6	79.9	110.2	114.4	74.8	28.1	4.8	0.2
1989	2,014.0	1.4	57.3	36.4	84.2	113.8	117.6	77.4	29.9	5.2	0.2
1990	2,081.0	1.4	59.9	37.5	88.6	116.5	120.2	80.8	31.7	5.5	0.2
1991	2,062.5	1.4	61.8	38.6	94.0	115.3	117.2	79.2	31.9	5.5	0.2
1992	2,046.0	1.4	60.3	37.6	93.6	113.7	115.7	79.6	32.3	5.9	0.3
1993	2,019.5	1.4	59.0	37.5	91.1	111.3	113.2	79.9	32.7	6.1	0.3
1994	2,001.5	1.4	58.2	37.2	90.2	109.2	111.0	80.4	33.4	6.4	0.3
1995	1,978.0	1.3	56.0	35.5	87.7	107.5	108.8	81.1	34.0	6.6	0.3
1996	1,976.0	1.2	53.5	33.3	84.7	107.8	108.6	82.1	34.9	6.8	0.3
1997	1,971.0	1.1	51.3	31.4	82.1	107.3	108.3	83.0	35.7	7.1	0.4
1998	1,999.0	1.0	50.3	29.9	80.9	108.4	110.2	85.2	36.9	7.4	0.4
1999	2,007.5	0.9	48.8	28.2	79.1	107.9	111.2	87.1	37.8	7.4	0.4
2000	2,056.0	0.9	47.7	26.9	78.1	109.7	113.5	91.2	39.7	8.0	0.5
2001	2,030.5	0.8	45.0	24.5	75.5	105.6	113.8	91.8	40.5	8.1	0.5
2002	2,020.5	0.7	42.6	23.1	72.2	103.1	114.7	92.6	41.6	8.3	0.5
2003	2,047.5	0.6	41.1	22.2	69.6	102.3	116.7	95.7	43.9	8.7	0.5
2004	2,051.5	0.6	40.5	21.8	68.7	101.5	116.5	96.2	45.5	9.0	0.5
2005	2,057.0	0.6	39.7	21.1	68.4	101.8	116.5	96.7	46.4	9.1	0.6
2006	2,108.0	0.6	41.1	21.6	71.2	105.5	118.0	98.9	47.5	9.4	0.6
2007	2,120.0	0.6	41.5	21.7	71.7	105.4	118.1	100.6	47.6	9.6	0.6
2008	2,072.0	0.6	40.2	21.1	68.2	101.8	115.0	99.4	46.8	9.9	0.7
2009	2,002.0	0.5	37.9	19.6	64.0	96.2	111.5	97.5	46.1	10.0	0.7
2010	1,931.0	0.4	34.2	17.3	58.2	90.0	108.3	96.5	45.9	10.2	0.7
2011	1,894.5	0.4	31.3	15.4	54.1	85.3	107.2	96.5	47.2	10.3	0.7
White											
1980[3]	1,773.0	0.6	45.4	25.5	73.2	111.1	113.8	61.2	18.8	3.5	0.2
1981[3]	1,748.0	0.5	44.9	25.4	71.5	108.3	112.3	61.0	19.0	3.4	0.2
1982[3]	1,767.0	0.6	45.0	25.5	70.8	107.7	111.9	64.0	20.4	3.6	0.2
1983[3]	1,740.5	0.6	43.9	25.0	68.8	103.8	109.4	65.3	21.3	3.6	0.2
1984[3]	1,748.5	0.6	42.9	24.3	68.4	102.7	109.8	67.7	22.2	3.6	0.2
1985	1,787.0	0.6	43.3	24.4	70.4	104.1	112.3	69.9	23.3	3.7	0.2
1986	1,776.0	0.6	42.3	23.8	70.1	102.7	110.8	70.9	23.9	3.8	0.2
1987	1,804.5	0.6	42.5	24.6	68.9	102.3	112.3	73.0	25.9	4.1	0.2
1988	1,856.5	0.6	44.4	26.0	69.6	103.7	114.8	75.4	27.7	4.5	0.2
1989	1,931.0	0.7	47.9	28.1	72.9	106.9	117.8	78.1	29.7	4.9	0.2
1990	2,003.0	0.7	50.8	29.5	78.0	109.8	120.7	81.7	31.5	5.2	0.2
1991	1,988.0	0.8	52.6	30.5	83.3	108.8	118.0	80.2	31.8	5.2	0.2
1992	1,978.0	0.8	51.4	29.9	83.2	107.7	116.9	80.8	32.1	5.7	0.2
1993	1,961.5	0.8	50.6	30.0	81.5	106.1	114.7	81.3	32.6	5.9	0.3
1994	1,957.5	0.8	50.5	30.4	81.2	105.0	113.0	82.2	33.5	6.2	0.3
1995	1,954.5	0.8	49.5	29.6	80.2	104.7	111.7	83.3	34.2	6.4	0.3
1996	1,960.5	0.7	47.5	28.0	77.6	105.3	111.7	84.6	35.3	6.7	0.3
1997	1,955.0	0.7	45.5	26.6	75.0	104.5	111.3	85.7	36.1	6.9	0.3
1998	1,991.0	0.6	44.9	25.6	74.1	105.4	113.6	88.5	37.5	7.3	0.4
1999	2,007.5	0.6	44.0	24.4	73.0	105.0	114.9	90.7	38.5	7.4	0.4
2000	2,051.0	0.6	43.2	23.3	72.3	106.6	116.7	94.6	40.2	7.9	0.4
2001	2,042.5	0.5	41.0	21.4	70.4	103.4	117.8	95.9	41.4	8.0	0.5
2002	2,041.5	0.5	39.2	20.4	67.7	101.6	119.0	96.7	42.6	8.2	0.5
2003	2,075.0	0.5	38.0	19.6	65.6	100.9	121.3	100.1	45.0	8.7	0.5
2004	2,074.5	0.5	37.4	19.4	64.4	99.8	120.8	100.3	46.7	8.9	0.5
2005	2,078.5	0.5	36.7	18.8	64.0	99.9	120.7	100.7	47.6	9.0	0.6
2006	2,125.0	0.5	37.9	19.2	66.7	103.4	122.0	102.7	48.6	9.3	0.6
2007	2,137.0	0.5	38.4	19.5	67.2	103.5	122.0	104.4	48.5	9.5	0.6
2008	2,087.0	0.4	37.3	19.1	64.0	99.8	118.8	103.3	47.5	9.7	0.6
2009	2,016.5	0.4	35.3	17.8	60.2	94.1	114.9	101.3	46.7	9.9	0.7
2010	1,947.5	0.3	31.9	15.8	54.8	87.9	111.9	100.5	46.4	10.0	0.6
2011	1,905.0	0.3	29.1	14.1	50.8	83.0	110.2	100.1	47.6	10.1	0.6
Black											
1980[3]	2,176.5	4.3	97.8	72.5	135.1	140.0	103.9	59.9	23.5	5.6	0.3
1981[3]	2,117.5	4.0	94.5	69.3	131.0	136.5	102.3	57.4	23.1	5.4	0.3
1982[3]	2,106.5	4.0	94.3	69.7	128.9	135.4	101.3	57.5	23.3	5.1	0.4
1983[3]	2,066.0	4.1	93.9	69.6	127.1	131.9	98.4	56.2	23.3	5.1	0.3
1984[3]	2,070.5	4.4	94.1	69.2	128.1	132.2	98.4	56.7	23.3	4.8	0.2
1985	2,109.0	4.5	95.4	69.3	132.4	135.0	100.2	57.9	23.9	4.6	0.3
1986	2,135.5	4.7	95.8	69.3	135.1	137.3	101.1	59.3	23.8	4.8	0.3
1987	2,198.0	4.8	97.6	72.1	135.8	142.7	104.3	60.6	24.6	4.8	0.2
1988	2,298.0	4.9	102.7	75.7	142.7	149.7	108.2	63.1	25.6	5.1	0.3
1989	2,432.5	5.1	111.5	81.9	151.9	156.8	114.4	66.3	26.7	5.4	0.3

Table 1-33. Total Fertility Rates and Birth Rates by Age of Mother and by Age and Race of Mother, 1980–2011—*Continued*

(Live births per 1,000 women in specified group.)

Year and race	Total fertility rate	10 to 14 years	15 to 19 years			20 to 24 years	25 to 29 years	30 to 34 years	35 to 39 years	40 to 44 years	45 to 49 years[1]
			Total	15 to 17 years	18 to 19 years						
1990	2,480.0	4.9	112.8	82.3	152.9	160.2	115.5	68.7	28.1	5.5	0.3
1991	2,462.0	4.7	114.8	83.5	157.6	159.7	112.0	67.3	28.2	5.5	0.2
1992	2,416.0	4.6	111.3	80.5	156.3	156.2	109.7	67.0	28.6	5.6	0.2
1993	2,351.0	4.5	107.3	78.9	150.2	150.2	106.4	66.6	29.0	5.9	0.3
1994	2,258.5	4.5	102.9	75.1	146.2	142.9	101.5	65.0	28.7	5.9	0.3
1995	2,127.5	4.1	94.4	68.5	135.0	133.7	95.6	63.0	28.4	6.0	0.3
1996	2,088.5	3.5	89.6	63.3	130.5	133.2	94.3	62.0	28.7	6.1	0.3
1997	2,091.5	3.1	86.3	59.3	127.7	135.2	95.0	62.6	29.3	6.5	0.3
1998	2,111.5	2.8	83.5	55.4	124.8	138.4	97.5	63.2	30.0	6.6	0.3
1999	2,082.5	2.5	79.1	50.5	120.6	137.9	97.3	62.7	30.2	6.5	0.3
2000	2,129.0	2.3	77.4	49.0	118.8	141.3	100.3	65.4	31.5	7.2	0.4
2001	2,049.5	2.0	71.3	43.7	112.9	132.9	99.6	64.9	31.6	7.2	0.4
2002	1,990.0	1.8	65.8	39.5	106.3	126.9	99.4	64.7	31.6	7.4	0.4
2003	1,994.5	1.5	62.5	37.5	101.3	125.9	101.4	66.4	33.1	7.6	0.5
2004	2,026.0	1.6	61.7	36.3	101.3	127.5	104.4	67.8	33.8	7.9	0.5
2005	2,062.0	1.6	60.1	34.5	101.2	129.5	107.0	70.2	35.1	8.4	0.5
2006	2,143.0	1.5	62.2	35.3	105.6	135.2	110.6	73.8	36.3	8.5	0.5
2007	2,145.5	1.4	62.1	34.7	105.2	134.6	110.4	74.9	36.4	8.7	0.6
2008	2,102.5	1.3	60.1	33.5	99.5	130.6	107.9	74.8	36.4	8.8	0.6
2009	2,036.0	1.1	56.5	30.9	92.9	125.1	105.3	73.5	36.2	8.9	0.6
2010	1,957.0	1.0	51.1	27.3	84.8	118.1	101.8	73.0	36.4	9.3	0.7
2011	1,920.0	0.9	47.3	24.7	78.8	111.9	101.7	74.1	38.0	9.4	0.7
American Indian or Alaska Native											
1980[3]	2,165.0	1.9	82.2	51.5	129.5	143.7	106.6	61.8	28.1	8.2	*
1981[3]	2,092.5	2.1	78.4	49.7	121.5	141.2	105.6	58.9	25.2	6.6	*
1982[3]	2,215.0	1.4	83.5	52.6	127.6	148.1	115.8	60.9	26.9	6.0	*
1983[3]	2,182.0	1.9	84.2	55.2	121.4	145.5	113.7	58.9	25.5	6.4	*
1984[3]	2,137.5	1.7	81.5	50.7	124.7	142.4	109.2	60.5	26.3	5.6	*
1985	2,129.5	1.7	79.2	47.7	124.1	139.1	109.6	62.6	27.4	6.0	*
1986	2,083.0	1.8	78.1	48.7	125.3	138.8	107.9	60.7	23.8	5.3	*
1987	2,100.5	1.7	77.2	48.8	122.2	140.0	107.9	63.0	24.4	5.6	*
1988	2,155.0	1.7	77.5	49.7	121.1	145.2	110.9	64.5	25.6	5.3	*
1989	2,248.5	1.5	82.7	51.6	128.9	152.4	114.2	64.8	27.4	6.4	*
1990	2,184.5	1.6	81.1	48.5	129.3	148.7	110.3	61.5	27.5	5.9	*
1991	2,142.5	1.6	84.1	51.9	134.2	143.8	105.6	60.8	26.4	5.8	0.4
1992	2,135.5	1.6	82.4	52.3	130.5	142.3	107.0	61.0	26.7	5.9	*
1993	2,048.5	1.4	79.8	51.5	126.3	134.2	103.5	59.5	25.5	5.6	*
1994	1,950.0	1.8	76.4	48.4	123.7	126.5	98.2	56.6	24.8	5.4	0.3
1995	1,878.5	1.6	72.9	44.6	122.2	123.1	91.6	56.5	24.3	5.5	*
1996	1,855.0	1.6	68.2	42.7	113.3	123.5	91.1	56.5	24.4	5.5	*
1997	1,834.5	1.5	65.2	41.0	107.1	122.5	91.6	56.0	24.4	5.4	0.3
1998	1,851.0	1.5	64.7	39.7	106.9	125.1	92.0	56.8	24.6	5.3	*
1999	1,783.5	1.4	59.9	36.5	98.0	120.7	90.6	53.8	24.3	5.7	0.3
2000	1,772.5	1.1	58.3	34.1	97.1	117.2	91.8	55.5	24.6	5.7	0.3
2001	1,675.5	0.8	50.9	28.8	85.3	110.7	88.9	53.7	24.1	5.7	0.3
2002	1,639.5	0.9	49.0	27.9	82.1	107.0	89.3	52.8	23.3	5.2	0.4
2003	1,610.5	0.8	47.2	26.7	79.9	105.4	87.1	51.9	23.9	5.6	0.2
2004	1,584.0	0.8	46.0	26.3	78.0	102.9	86.3	51.8	23.3	5.4	0.3
2005	1,625.0	0.7	46.9	25.9	80.8	106.8	89.0	52.0	23.9	5.4	0.3
2006	1,621.5	0.7	49.3	26.1	86.3	105.8	86.2	52.5	24.3	5.2	0.3
2007	1,569.0	0.7	47.3	25.8	80.2	102.7	83.2	51.2	23.1	5.3	0.3
2008	1,569.0	0.7	47.3	25.8	80.2	102.7	83.2	51.2	23.1	5.3	0.3
2009	1,494.0	0.6	43.7	23.6	73.5	96.3	79.3	50.7	22.6	5.3	0.3
2010	1,404.0	0.5	38.7	20.1	66.1	91.0	74.4	48.4	22.3	5.2	0.3
2011	1,373.5	0.5	36.1	18.2	61.6	86.6	75.4	47.3	23.1	5.5	0.2

Table 1-33. Total Fertility Rates and Birth Rates by Age of Mother and by Age and Race of Mother, 1980–2011—*Continued*

(Live births per 1,000 women in specified group.)

Year and race	Total fertility rate	10 to 14 years	15 to 19 years			20 to 24 years	25 to 29 years	30 to 34 years	35 to 39 years	40 to 44 years	45 to 49 years[1]
			Total	15 to 17 years	18 to 19 years						
Asian or Other Pacific Islander											
1980[3]	1,953.5	0.3	26.2	12.0	46.2	93.3	127.4	96.0	38.3	8.5	0.7
1981[3]	1,976.0	0.3	28.5	13.4	49.5	96.4	129.1	93.4	38.0	8.6	0.9
1982[3]	2,015.5	0.4	29.4	14.0	50.8	98.9	130.9	94.4	39.2	8.8	1.1
1983[3]	1,943.5	0.5	26.1	12.9	44.5	94.0	126.2	93.3	39.4	8.2	1.0
1984[3]	1,892.0	0.5	24.2	12.6	40.7	86.7	124.3	92.4	40.6	8.7	1.0
1985	1,885.0	0.4	23.8	12.5	40.8	83.6	123.0	93.6	42.7	8.7	1.2
1986	1,836.0	0.5	22.8	12.1	38.8	79.2	119.9	92.6	41.9	9.3	1.0
1987	1,886.0	0.6	22.4	12.6	37.0	79.7	122.7	97.0	44.2	9.5	1.1
1988	1,983.5	0.6	24.2	13.6	39.6	80.7	128.0	104.4	47.5	10.3	1.0
1989	1,947.5	0.6	25.6	15.0	40.4	78.8	124.0	102.3	47.0	10.2	1.0
1990	2,002.5	0.7	26.4	16.0	40.2	79.2	126.3	106.5	49.6	10.7	1.1
1991	1,928.0	0.8	27.3	16.3	42.2	73.8	118.9	103.3	49.2	11.2	1.1
1992	1,894.5	0.7	26.5	15.4	41.9	71.7	114.6	102.7	50.7	11.1	0.9
1993	1,841.5	0.7	26.5	16.1	41.2	68.1	110.3	101.2	49.4	11.2	0.9
1994	1,834.0	0.7	26.6	16.3	41.3	66.4	108.0	102.2	50.4	11.5	1.0
1995	1,795.5	0.7	25.5	15.6	40.1	64.2	103.7	102.3	50.1	11.8	0.8
1996	1,787.0	0.6	23.5	14.7	36.8	63.5	102.8	104.1	50.2	11.9	0.8
1997	1,757.5	0.5	22.3	14.0	34.9	61.2	101.6	102.5	51.0	11.5	0.9
1998	1,731.5	0.5	22.2	13.8	34.5	59.2	98.7	101.6	51.4	11.8	0.9
1999	1,754.5	0.4	21.4	12.4	33.9	58.9	100.8	104.3	52.9	11.3	0.9
2000	1,892.0	0.3	20.5	11.6	32.6	60.3	108.4	116.5	59.0	12.6	0.8
2001	1,785.0	0.2	19.3	10.1	32.0	56.0	102.3	109.9	56.2	12.2	0.9
2002	1,798.5	0.3	17.7	8.8	29.9	55.5	102.4	112.5	57.8	12.6	0.9
2003	1,819.0	0.2	16.4	8.5	27.3	54.3	102.7	115.9	60.0	13.4	0.9
2004	1,825.0	0.2	16.0	8.4	26.6	53.3	100.4	118.3	62.2	13.6	1.0
2005	1,784.5	0.2	15.4	7.7	26.4	52.9	96.6	115.3	61.8	13.7	1.0
2006	1,803.0	0.1	15.3	8.2	25.4	53.8	95.7	117.3	63.4	14.0	1.0
2007	1,850.5	0.2	14.8	7.4	24.9	53.2	99.2	121.6	65.8	14.2	1.1
2008	1,797.5	0.2	13.8	7.0	23.0	50.4	96.6	117.7	64.9	14.7	1.2
2009	1,743.0	0.1	12.6	6.3	20.9	46.4	94.6	115.1	63.8	14.9	1.1
2010	1,689.0	0.1	10.9	5.1	18.7	42.6	91.5	113.6	62.8	15.1	1.2
2011	1,706.5	0.1	10.2	4.6	18.1	41.9	93.7	114.9	64.1	15.2	1.2

* = Figure does not meet standards of reliability or precision.   [1]Beginning in 1997, rates computed by relating births to women age 45 years and over to women age 45 to 49 years.   [2]For 1970 to 1991 includes births to races not shown separately. For 1992 and later years, unknown race of mother is imputed.   [3]Based on 100 percent of births in selected states and on a 50 percent sample of births in all other states.

Table 1-34. Fertility Rates and Birth Rates, by Age, Live-Birth Order, Specified Hispanic Origin, and Race of Mother, 2011

(Live births per 1,000 women in specified age and race groups.)

Live-birth order and race of mother	15 to 44 years[1]	10 to 14 years	15 to 19 years Total	15 to 17 years	18 to 19 years	20 to 24 years	25 to 29 years	30 to 34 years	35 to 39 years	40 to 44 years	45 to 49 years[2]
HISPANIC [3]											
Total	76.2	0.7	49.6	28.0	81.5	116.0	121.3	95.2	51.3	13.1	0.8
1st child	26.3	0.7	39.4	25.3	60.4	51.8	31.8	17.9	7.6	1.8	0.1
2nd child	22.9	0.0	8.7	2.5	17.9	41.5	41.4	27.5	12.7	2.8	0.2
3rd child	15.2	*	1.3	0.2	2.9	16.7	29.3	26.1	13.7	3.1	0.2
4th child	7.2	*	0.1	*	0.3	4.6	12.6	14.3	9.2	2.4	0.1
5th child	2.8	*	0.0	*	0.0	1.1	4.2	5.7	4.5	1.4	0.1
6th and 7th child	1.5	*	*	*	*	0.3	1.8	3.1	2.8	1.1	0.1
8th child and over	0.3	*	*	*	*	0.0	0.2	0.6	0.7	0.4	0.0
Mexican	73.0	0.6	47.9	27.7	77.6	111.6	118.2	89.3	47.9	12.4	0.7
1st child	23.5	0.6	37.7	24.9	56.4	46.8	27.3	13.5	5.4	1.4	0.1
2nd child	21.3	*	8.8	2.6	17.9	41.3	39.6	23.1	10.0	2.0	0.1
3rd child	15.5	*	1.3	0.2	2.9	17.4	31.1	26.8	13.5	2.9	0.1
4th child	7.7	*	0.1	*	0.3	4.7	13.6	15.8	10.1	2.6	0.1
5th child	3.0	*	0.0	*	0.0	1.1	4.5	6.3	5.0	1.7	0.1
6th and 7th child	1.6	*	*	*	*	0.3	1.9	3.3	3.1	1.3	0.1
8th child and over	0.3	*	*	*	*	0.0	0.2	0.6	0.8	0.4	0.1
Puerto Rican	59.6	0.5	42.8	22.9	69.5	106.0	93.8	64.9	33.2	7.8	0.5
1st child	24.0	0.5	35.1	20.9	53.9	50.3	26.9	15.5	6.8	1.4	*
2nd child	18.0	*	6.7	1.8	13.3	35.4	31.7	20.5	9.7	2.3	0.1
3rd child	10.1	*	1.0	0.2	2.0	14.5	20.6	14.9	7.9	1.7	*
4th child	4.4	*	*	*	*	4.4	9.1	7.6	4.5	1.2	*
5th child	1.8	*	*	*	*	1.1	3.6	3.5	2.1	0.6	*
6th and 7th child	1.1	*	*	*	*	0.2	1.7	2.4	1.7	0.5	*
8th child and over	0.3	*	*	*	*	*	0.3	0.5	0.6	0.2	*
Cuban	46.1	*	15.8	6.7	29.0	54.7	86.1	78.4	42.0	9.1	0.5
1st child	21.6	*	14.1	6.4	25.2	34.9	40.8	28.9	11.0	2.3	*
2nd child	16.7	*	1.5	*	3.3	15.3	31.4	33.3	19.5	3.7	*
3rd child	5.4	*	*	*	*	3.3	9.7	11.4	7.6	1.9	*
4th child	1.6	*	*	*	*	0.8	3.1	3.2	2.5	0.6	*
5th child	0.5	*	*	*	*	*	0.8	0.8	0.9	*	*
6th and 7th child	0.2	*	*	*	*	*	*	0.6	0.3	*	*
8th child and over	0.1	*	*	*	*	*	*	*	*	*	*
Other Hispanic [3]	96.3	1.1	62.1	35.1	99.9	142.3	150.3	127.3	68.6	16.7	1.1
1st child	35.9	1.0	50.0	31.8	75.5	69.5	46.3	30.2	13.4	3.1	0.2
2nd child	30.5	*	10.4	3.1	20.6	48.5	53.1	42.1	20.5	4.5	0.3
3rd child	17.6	*	1.6	0.2	3.4	17.9	31.7	30.9	17.4	4.1	0.2
4th child	7.5	*	0.2	*	0.4	4.9	12.8	14.4	9.4	2.4	0.1
5th child	2.9	*	*	*	*	1.2	4.3	5.8	4.4	1.2	0.1
6th and 7th child	1.6	*	*	*	*	0.3	1.8	3.3	2.8	1.1	0.1
8th child and over	0.3	*	*	*	*	0.0	0.3	0.6	0.7	0.3	*
NON-HISPANIC [4]											
Total [5]	60.1	0.3	26.5	12.0	47.0	78.0	103.8	96.8	46.2	9.8	0.7
1st child	25.2	0.3	22.1	11.1	37.7	40.9	42.7	30.9	11.5	2.4	0.2
2nd child	19.3	0.0	3.8	0.8	8.0	24.6	34.0	34.6	15.9	2.9	0.2
3rd child	9.3	*	0.5	0.1	1.2	9.0	16.8	17.9	9.9	2.0	0.1
4th child	3.7	*	0.1	*	0.1	2.6	6.7	7.6	4.6	1.1	0.1
5th child	1.4	*	0.0	*	0.0	0.6	2.4	3.1	2.0	0.5	0.0
6th and 7th child	0.9	*	*	*	*	0.2	1.1	2.1	1.6	0.5	0.0
8th child and over	0.3	*	*	*	*	0.0	0.2	0.6	0.8	0.4	0.0
White	58.7	0.2	21.7	9.0	39.9	71.8	105.2	100.1	45.8	9.3	0.6
1st child	24.9	0.2	18.6	8.5	33.0	39.3	44.9	32.4	11.5	2.4	0.2
2nd child	19.2	*	2.8	0.5	6.1	22.8	35.2	36.4	15.9	2.8	0.2
3rd child	9.0	*	0.3	0.0	0.7	7.5	16.5	18.8	10.0	1.8	0.1
4th child	3.4	*	0.0	*	0.1	1.8	5.9	7.5	4.5	1.0	0.1
5th child	1.2	*	0.0	*	0.0	0.4	1.8	2.8	1.8	0.5	0.0
6th and 7th child	0.7	*	*	*	*	0.1	0.7	1.7	1.4	0.4	0.0
8th child and over	0.3	*	*	*	*	0.0	0.1	0.4	0.7	0.4	0.0
Black	65.4	0.9	47.3	24.6	78.8	112.3	101.7	73.9	37.8	9.3	0.7
1st child	25.6	0.9	38.0	22.3	59.6	52.2	28.8	16.5	7.3	1.8	0.2
2nd child	18.5	0.0	7.8	2.1	15.7	35.8	31.5	21.4	10.1	2.3	0.2
3rd child	11.1	*	1.4	0.2	3.1	16.3	21.8	16.6	8.7	2.0	0.1
4th child	5.4	*	0.2	*	0.4	5.8	11.2	9.4	5.3	1.3	0.1
5th child	2.4	*	0.0	*	0.0	1.6	4.9	4.8	2.8	0.8	0.1
6th and 7th child	1.7	*	*	*	*	0.5	3.0	3.9	2.4	0.7	0.1
8th child and over	0.6	*	*	*	*	0.1	0.5	1.3	1.2	0.5	0.0

* = Figure does not meet standards of reliability or precision.   0.0 = Quantity more than zero but less than 0.05.   [1]Fertility rates computed by relating total births, regardless of age of mother, to women age 15 to 44 years.   [2]Birth rates computed by relating births to women age 45 years and over to women age 45 to 49 years.   [3]Includes Central and South American and other and unknown Hispanic. Includes all persons of Hispanic origin of any race.   [4]Includes origin not stated.   [5]Includes races other than White and Black.

Table 1-35. Total Fertility Rates, Fertility Rates, and Birth Rates, by Age and Hispanic Origin of Mother and by Race for Mothers of Non-Hispanic Origin, 1989–2011

(Total fertility rates are sums of birth rates for 5-year age groups multiplied by 5; fertility rates are live births per 1,000 women age 15 to 44 years in specified racial group; birth rates are live births per 1,000 women in specified age group.)

Year, origin, and race of mother	Total fertility rate	Fertility rate[1]	10–14 years	15–19 years Total	15–17 years	18–19 years	20–24 years	25–29 years	30–34 years	35–39 years	40–44 years	45–49 years[2]
ALL ORIGINS												
1989	2,014.0	69.2	1.4	57.3	36.4	84.2	113.8	117.6	77.4	29.9	5.2	0.2
1990	2,081.0	70.9	1.4	59.9	37.5	88.6	116.5	120.2	80.8	31.7	5.5	0.2
1991	2,062.5	69.3	1.4	61.8	38.6	94.0	115.3	117.2	79.2	31.9	5.5	0.2
1992	2,046.0	68.4	1.4	60.3	37.6	93.6	113.7	115.7	79.6	32.3	5.9	0.3
1993	2,019.5	67.0	1.4	59.0	37.5	91.1	111.3	113.2	79.9	32.7	6.1	0.3
1994	2,001.5	65.9	1.4	58.2	37.2	90.2	109.2	111.0	80.4	33.4	6.4	0.3
1995	1,978.0	64.6	1.3	56.0	35.5	87.7	107.5	108.8	81.1	34.0	6.6	0.3
1996	1,976.0	64.1	1.2	53.5	33.3	84.7	107.8	108.6	82.1	34.9	6.8	0.3
1997	1,971.0	63.6	1.1	51.3	31.4	82.1	107.3	108.3	83.0	35.7	7.1	0.4
1998	1,999.0	64.3	1.0	50.3	29.9	80.9	108.4	110.2	85.2	36.9	7.4	0.4
1999	2,007.5	64.4	0.9	48.8	28.2	79.1	107.9	111.2	87.1	37.8	7.4	0.4
2000	2,056.0	65.9	0.9	47.7	26.9	78.1	109.7	113.5	91.2	39.7	8.0	0.5
2001	2,030.5	65.1	0.8	45.0	24.5	75.5	105.6	113.8	91.8	40.5	8.1	0.5
2002	2,020.5	65.0	0.7	42.6	23.1	72.2	103.1	114.7	92.6	41.6	8.3	0.5
2003	2,047.5	66.1	0.6	41.1	22.2	69.6	102.3	116.7	95.7	43.9	8.7	0.5
2004	2,051.5	66.4	0.6	40.5	21.8	68.7	101.5	116.5	96.2	45.5	9.0	0.5
2005	2,057.0	66.7	0.6	39.7	21.1	68.4	101.8	116.5	96.7	46.4	9.1	0.6
2006	2,108.0	68.6	0.6	41.1	21.6	71.2	105.5	118.0	98.9	47.5	9.4	0.6
2007	2,120.0	69.3	0.6	41.5	21.7	71.7	105.4	118.1	100.6	47.6	9.6	0.6
2008	2,072.0	68.1	0.6	40.2	21.1	68.2	101.8	115.0	99.4	46.8	9.9	0.7
2009	2,002.0	66.2	0.5	37.9	19.6	64.0	96.2	111.5	97.5	46.1	10.0	0.7
2010	1,931.0	64.1	0.4	34.2	17.3	58.2	90.0	108.3	96.5	45.9	10.2	0.7
2011	1,894.5	63.2	0.4	31.3	15.4	54.1	85.3	107.2	96.5	47.2	10.3	0.7
HISPANIC [3]												
Total												
1989 [4]	2,903.5	104.9	2.3	100.8	NA	NA	184.4	146.6	92.1	43.5	10.4	0.6
1990 [5]	2,959.5	107.7	2.4	100.3	65.9	147.7	181.0	153.0	98.3	45.3	10.9	0.7
1991 [6]	2,963.5	106.9	2.4	104.6	69.2	155.5	184.6	150.0	95.1	44.7	10.7	0.6
1992 [6]	2,957.5	106.1	2.5	103.3	68.9	153.9	185.2	148.8	94.8	45.3	11.0	0.6
1993	2,894.5	103.3	2.6	101.8	68.5	151.1	180.0	146.0	93.2	44.1	10.6	0.6
1994	2,839.0	100.7	2.6	101.3	69.9	147.5	175.7	142.4	91.1	43.4	10.7	0.6
1995	2,798.5	98.8	2.6	99.3	68.3	145.4	171.9	140.4	90.5	43.7	10.7	0.6
1996	2,772.0	97.5	2.4	94.6	64.2	140.0	170.2	140.7	91.3	43.9	10.7	0.6
1997	2,680.5	94.2	2.1	89.6	61.1	132.4	162.6	137.5	89.6	43.4	10.7	0.6
1998	2,652.5	93.2	1.9	87.9	58.5	131.5	159.3	136.1	90.5	43.4	10.8	0.6
1999	2,649.0	93.0	1.9	86.8	56.9	129.5	157.3	135.8	92.3	44.5	10.6	0.6
2000	2,730.0	95.9	1.7	87.3	55.5	132.6	161.3	139.9	97.1	46.6	11.5	0.6
2001	2,030.5	65.1	0.8	45.0	24.5	75.5	105.6	113.8	91.8	40.5	8.1	0.5
2002	2,020.5	65.0	0.7	42.6	23.1	72.2	103.1	114.7	92.6	41.6	8.3	0.5
2003	2,047.5	66.1	0.6	41.1	22.2	69.6	102.3	116.7	95.7	43.9	8.7	0.5
2004	2,051.5	66.4	0.6	40.5	21.8	68.7	101.5	116.5	96.2	45.5	9.0	0.5
2005	2,057.0	66.7	0.6	39.7	21.1	68.4	101.8	116.5	96.7	46.4	9.1	0.6
2006	2,108.0	68.6	0.6	41.1	21.6	71.2	105.5	118.0	98.9	47.5	9.4	0.6
2007	2,120.0	69.3	0.6	41.5	21.7	71.7	105.4	118.1	100.6	47.6	9.6	0.6
2008	2,072.0	68.1	0.6	40.2	21.1	68.2	101.8	115.0	99.4	46.8	9.9	0.7
2009	2,002.0	66.2	0.5	37.9	19.6	64.0	96.2	111.5	97.5	46.1	10.0	0.7
2010	1,931.0	64.1	0.4	34.2	17.3	58.2	90.0	108.3	96.5	45.9	10.2	0.7
2011	1,894.5	63.2	0.4	31.3	15.4	54.1	85.3	107.2	96.5	47.2	10.3	0.7
Mexican												
1989 [4]	2,916.5	106.6	2.0	94.5	NA	NA	184.3	153.7	96.1	41.0	11.1	0.6
1990 [5]	3,214.0	118.9	2.5	108.0	69.7	162.2	200.3	165.3	104.4	49.1	12.4	0.8
1991 [6]	3,103.5	114.9	2.5	108.3	70.0	164.7	192.4	156.1	99.7	49.1	11.9	0.7
1992 [6]	3,107.0	113.3	2.4	105.1	NA	NA	196.6	160.2	97.1	47.4	11.8	0.8
1993	3,041.5	110.9	2.5	103.6	68.4	156.6	187.9	159.5	97.2	45.5	11.3	0.8
1994	3,024.0	109.9	2.7	109.2	73.6	163.3	189.1	153.6	92.5	45.3	11.7	0.7
1995	3,033.5	109.9	2.7	115.9	79.1	170.7	190.4	146.6	93.0	45.5	11.9	0.7
1996	3,052.0	110.7	2.6	112.2	77.7	161.6	185.3	154.7	96.5	46.4	12.0	0.7
1997	2,957.0	106.6	2.3	103.4	71.3	151.6	180.9	150.0	95.3	47.4	11.5	0.6
1998	2,878.0	103.2	2.1	96.4	62.9	149.2	176.5	147.4	94.9	46.9	10.8	0.6
1999	2,823.0	101.5	2.1	94.3	60.8	145.6	170.8	141.4	97.4	47.2	10.7	0.7
2000	2,906.5	105.1	1.9	95.4	60.6	146.7	174.9	144.7	102.3	49.2	12.2	0.7
2001	2,905.0	105.0	1.7	93.2	58.2	142.5	173.8	146.8	102.1	50.1	12.6	0.7
2002	2,869.0	103.0	1.5	91.4	57.0	141.0	171.2	146.8	101.1	48.5	12.5	0.8
2003	2,903.0	103.7	1.4	88.8	54.4	140.7	172.2	151.0	104.2	49.6	12.7	0.7
2004	2,948.5	104.5	1.4	90.3	55.6	142.5	173.4	152.5	105.5	53.5	12.4	0.7
2005	2,954.5	104.5	1.4	87.5	52.3	144.5	173.5	152.1	107.1	55.3	13.2	0.8
2006	2,997.0	105.6	1.3	86.6	50.7	145.4	180.3	152.3	109.0	55.5	13.6	0.8
2007	2,944.5	102.8	1.2	81.7	49.9	130.6	176.0	150.2	110.1	55.4	13.5	0.8
2008	2,663.5	92.6	1.1	71.4	44.4	111.7	154.3	138.4	101.9	51.4	13.4	0.8
2009	2,442.0	84.8	1.0	62.9	37.8	100.5	135.2	129.0	96.0	50.6	13.0	0.7
2010	2,276.5	78.2	0.8	55.3	32.6	89.9	123.3	122.9	91.5	48.1	12.7	0.7
2011	2,143.0	73.0	0.6	47.9	27.7	77.6	111.6	118.2	89.3	47.9	12.4	0.7
Puerto Rican												
1989 [4]	2,421.0	86.6	3.8	112.7	NA	NA	171.0	98.0	65.2	26.9	6.3	*
1990 [5]	2,301.0	82.9	2.9	101.6	71.6	141.6	150.1	109.9	62.8	26.2	6.2	0.5
1991 [6]	2,573.5	87.9	2.7	111.0	*	*	193.3	108.9	68.1	23.9	6.5	*
1992 [6]	2,568.5	87.9	3.4	106.5	NA	NA	199.1	102.6	65.3	29.9	6.6	*
1993	2,416.0	79.8	3.1	104.9	70.1	*	184.6	102.8	54.4	26.7	6.2	*
1994	2,341.5	78.2	3.1	99.6	68.8	*	169.0	103.8	59.5	27.5	5.6	0.2
1995	2,078.0	71.3	2.9	82.8	57.3	*	138.1	97.9	61.2	26.9	5.5	0.3
1996	1,965.0	66.5	1.9	76.5	48.6	*	133.7	95.6	54.3	25.2	5.6	*
1997	1,931.5	65.8	1.7	68.9	45.0	*	136.0	92.9	54.1	26.1	6.2	0.4
1998	2,043.5	69.7	1.8	76.2	51.7	*	146.7	88.7	61.9	25.8	7.2	0.4

Table 1-35. Total Fertility Rates, Fertility Rates, and Birth Rates, by Age and Hispanic Origin of Mother and by Race for Mothers of Non-Hispanic Origin, 1989–2011—Continued

(Total fertility rates are sums of birth rates for 5-year age groups multiplied by 5; fertility rates are live births per 1,000 women age 15 to 44 years in specified racial group; birth rates are live births per 1,000 women in specified age group.)

Year, origin, and race of mother	Total fertility rate	Fertility rate[1]	10–14 years	15–19 years Total	15–19 years 15–17 years	15–19 years 18–19 years	20–24 years	25–29 years	30–34 years	35–39 years	40–44 years	45–49 years[2]
1999	2,104.5	71.1	1.6	74.0	49.4	*	146.0	106.5	58.0	27.3	7.2	0.3
2000	2,178.5	73.5	1.7	82.9	54.7	120.4	149.5	101.6	61.1	32.0	6.6	0.3
2001	2,144.5	71.7	1.7	80.3	*	*	144.5	93.9	70.6	30.8	6.7	0.4
2002	1,937.0	65.6	1.3	59.3	38.6	*	132.2	92.1	63.6	32.0	6.4	0.5
2003	1,805.0	60.6	1.0	57.9	34.4	*	124.5	86.3	55.4	29.2	6.3	0.4
2004	2,005.0	66.8	0.9	59.1	37.0	*	133.9	101.5	66.0	32.4	6.7	0.5
2005	2,065.5	69.8	0.9	59.2	35.1	*	124.1	108.8	76.6	35.3	7.8	0.4
2006	2,088.5	71.6	1.0	64.7	35.8	*	130.7	100.7	72.3	39.2	8.5	0.6
2007	2,101.0	70.3	0.8	61.8	32.8	*	139.2	105.9	65.0	39.8	7.3	0.4
2008	2,004.0	67.0	0.7	56.0	28.8	*	119.3	114.3	65.9	37.3	6.9	0.4
2009	1,922.5	63.7	0.7	50.8	28.2	82.4	118.9	106.6	66.9	32.6	7.4	0.6
2010	1,747.5	59.7	0.6	45.4	25.0	73.4	105.7	90.7	66.0	32.6	7.9	0.6
2011	1,747.5	59.6	0.5	42.8	22.9	69.5	106.0	93.8	64.9	33.2	7.8	0.5
Cuban												
1989 [4]	1,479.0	49.8	*	*	NA	NA	*	*	*	*	*	*
1990 [5]	1,459.5	52.6	*	30.3	18.2	46.1	64.6	95.4	67.6	28.2	4.9	*
1991 [6]	1,352.5	47.6	*	*	*	*	*	*	*	*	*	*
1992 [6]	1,453.5	49.4	*	*	NA	NA	*	*	*	*	*	*
1993	1,570.0	53.9	*	*	*	*	*	*	*	*	*	*
1994	1,587.0	53.6	*	*	*	*	*	*	*	*	*	*
1995	1,584.0	52.2	*	*	*	*	*	*	*	*	*	*
1996	1,617.0	55.1	*	*	*	*	*	*	*	*	*	*
1997	1,619.5	53.1	*	*	*	*	*	*	*	*	*	*
1998	1,402.5	46.5	*	*	*	*	*	*	*	*	*	*
1999	1,388.5	47.0	*	*	*	*	*	*	*	*	*	*
2000	1,528.0	49.3	*	23.5	14.2	43.4	64.2	104.0	68.1	37.3	7.9	*
2001	1,786.0	56.4	*	*	*	*	*	*	*	*	*	*
2002	1,958.5	59.3	*	*	*	*	*	*	*	*	*	*
2003	2,032.5	60.8	*	*	*	*	*	*	*	*	*	*
2004	1,699.5	52.2	*	*	*	*	*	*	*	*	*	*
2005	1,540.5	49.1	*	*	*	*	*	*	*	*	*	*
2006	1,556.5	47.9	*	*	*	*	*	*	*	*	6.8	*
2007	1,542.5	47.6	*	*	*	*	*	*	*	*	6.4	*
2008	1,536.5	50.1	*	*	*	*	*	*	*	*	*	*
2009	1,352.0	46.0	*	*	*	*	*	*	*	*	*	*
2010	1,452.5	46.4	*	17.8	8.0	29.7	61.6	80.6	82.8	39.1	8.0	0.5
2011	1,433.5	46.1	*	15.8	6.7	29.0	54.7	86.1	78.4	42.0	9.1	0.5
Other Hispanic [7]												
1989 [4]	2,683.0	95.8	1.7	66.4	NA	NA	159.2	150.4	85.1	60.3	12.7	0.8
1990 [5]	2,877.0	102.7	2.1	86.0	57.2	123.8	162.9	155.8	106.9	49.4	11.6	0.7
1991 [6]	3,064.5	105.5	2.2	100.7	67.3	145.6	184.1	164.5	100.2	49.2	11.4	0.6
1992 [6]	2,989.0	104.7	2.4	108.2	NA	NA	168.0	151.9	104.4	49.9	12.5	0.5
1993	2,914.5	101.5	2.6	102.0	74.7	134.6	167.5	139.4	106.7	51.7	12.5	0.5
1994	2,693.0	93.2	2.5	82.6	62.7	105.0	151.2	137.0	104.4	48.4	11.9	0.6
1995	2,629.5	89.1	2.3	72.1	51.3	99.4	144.3	147.7	97.9	49.4	11.6	0.6
1996	2,516.5	84.2	2.2	64.8	43.4	95.6	149.6	127.9	98.0	49.1	11.0	0.7
1997	2,376.5	80.6	1.8	66.4	44.5	98.0	129.3	125.8	95.6	43.9	11.8	0.7
1998	2,448.5	83.5	1.8	75.0	53.3	100.3	122.7	133.6	97.8	45.4	12.8	0.6
1999	2,517.0	84.8	1.5	75.5	53.1	100.5	130.2	138.4	98.3	46.5	12.3	0.7
2000	2,563.5	85.1	1.2	69.9	44.4	102.0	133.2	143.9	103.6	47.7	12.5	0.7
2001	2,503.5	82.2	1.1	63.8	35.0	111.6	133.6	143.7	95.6	50.4	11.6	0.9
2002	2,612.0	86.5	1.1	60.9	33.7	105.4	138.8	149.5	101.7	57.3	12.3	0.8
2003	2,690.0	89.7	1.0	57.5	34.9	88.0	138.4	152.3	111.8	62.4	13.8	0.8
2004	2,594.0	87.4	1.1	54.6	31.1	90.2	131.1	143.5	113.5	59.2	15.0	0.8
2005	2,737.0	90.5	1.1	58.2	35.0	90.2	148.1	152.3	115.0	57.6	14.3	0.8
2006	2,918.0	95.6	1.1	62.5	36.3	99.7	154.3	172.7	118.0	59.3	14.7	1.0
2007	2,995.0	100.1	1.2	68.1	38.8	113.4	154.5	173.4	124.1	60.7	15.9	1.1
2008	3,278.0	109.1	1.4	80.5	47.9	129.3	180.5	171.1	135.9	69.1	16.0	1.1
2009	3,248.5	107.5	1.3	78.4	44.2	131.3	181.3	169.4	133.5	68.3	16.3	1.2
2010	2,870.0	97.1	1.0	67.4	39.6	105.2	146.6	154.2	120.5	67.0	16.2	1.1
2011	2,847.5	96.3	1.1	62.1	35.1	99.9	142.3	150.3	127.3	68.6	16.7	1.1
NON-HISPANIC [8]												
Total [9]												
1989 [4]	1,921.0	65.7	1.3	53.4	---	---	107.8	113.4	74.7	28.6	4.8	0.2
1990 [5]	1,979.5	67.1	1.3	54.8	33.8	81.4	108.1	116.5	79.2	30.7	5.1	0.2
1991 [6]	1,953.0	65.2	1.3	56.1	34.4	86.1	106.5	113.1	77.5	30.8	5.1	0.2
1992 [6]	1,929.0	64.2	1.2	54.3	33.2	85.3	104.3	111.4	77.9	31.1	5.4	0.2
1993	1,901.5	62.7	1.2	52.7	32.9	82.3	101.7	108.7	78.4	31.6	5.7	0.3
1994	1,883.5	61.6	1.2	51.7	32.3	81.4	99.5	106.5	79.1	32.4	6.0	0.3
1995	1,856.5	60.2	1.1	49.3	30.5	78.6	97.4	104.1	79.9	33.0	6.2	0.3
1996	1,852.0	59.6	1.0	47.0	28.4	75.8	97.3	103.6	80.8	33.9	6.5	0.3
1997	1,853.0	59.3	0.9	45.0	26.7	73.7	97.4	103.5	82.0	34.8	6.7	0.3
1998	1,887.5	60.0	0.8	44.0	25.2	72.4	98.9	105.8	84.4	36.2	7.0	0.4
1999	1,894.0	60.0	0.8	42.2	23.3	70.2	98.4	106.7	86.2	37.0	7.1	0.4
2000	1,931.5	61.1	0.7	40.7	21.9	68.2	99.5	108.4	90.2	38.8	7.6	0.4
2001	1,898.0	60.0	0.6	37.8	19.6	65.0	94.6	108.1	90.8	39.5	7.7	0.5
2002	1,885.0	59.8	0.6	35.4	18.2	61.6	91.8	108.7	91.6	40.5	7.9	0.5
2003	1,909.0	60.7	0.5	33.9	17.2	58.9	90.6	110.6	94.6	42.8	8.3	0.5
2004	1,906.0	60.8	0.5	33.1	16.7	57.6	89.5	110.1	94.7	44.3	8.5	0.5
2005	1,902.0	60.8	0.5	32.1	15.9	56.9	89.2	109.5	94.7	45.2	8.6	0.6
2006	1,946.0	62.5	0.5	33.2	16.5	59.0	92.3	110.7	96.9	46.2	8.8	0.6
2007	1,959.5	63.3	0.5	33.8	16.4	60.1	92.3	110.9	98.7	46.1	9.0	0.6
2008	1,926.0	62.7	0.4	33.1	16.0	57.8	90.0	108.6	97.9	45.3	9.3	0.6
2009	1,877.5	61.6	0.4	31.6	15.1	54.7	86.0	106.0	96.7	44.7	9.4	0.7
2010	1,831.0	60.4	0.3	28.8	13.4	50.3	81.5	104.2	96.5	44.5	9.7	0.7
2011	1,810.5	60.1	0.3	26.5	12.0	47.0	78.0	103.8	96.8	46.2	9.8	0.7

Table 1-35. Total Fertility Rates, Fertility Rates, and Birth Rates, by Age and Hispanic Origin of Mother and by Race for Mothers of Non-Hispanic Origin, 1989–2011—*Continued*

(Total fertility rates are sums of birth rates for 5-year age groups multiplied by 5; fertility rates are live births per 1,000 women age 15 to 44 years in specified racial group; birth rates are live births per 1,000 women in specified age group.)

Year, origin, and race of mother	Total fertility rate	Fertility rate[1]	10–14 years	15–19 years Total	15–17 years	18–19 years	20–24 years	25–29 years	30–34 years	35–39 years	40–44 years	45–49 years[2]
White												
1989[4]	1,770.0	60.5	0.4	39.9	NA	NA	94.7	111.7	75.0	27.8	4.3	0.2
1990[5]	1,850.5	62.8	0.5	42.5	23.2	66.6	97.5	115.3	79.4	30.0	4.7	0.2
1991[6]	1,822.5	60.9	0.5	43.4	23.6	70.6	95.7	112.1	77.7	30.2	4.7	0.2
1992[6]	1,803.5	60.0	0.5	41.7	22.7	69.8	93.9	110.6	78.3	30.4	5.1	0.2
1993	1,786.0	58.9	0.5	40.7	22.7	67.7	92.2	108.2	79.0	31.0	5.4	0.2
1994	1,782.5	58.2	0.5	40.4	22.7	67.6	90.9	106.6	80.2	32.0	5.7	0.2
1995	1,777.5	57.5	0.4	39.3	22.0	66.2	90.2	105.1	81.5	32.8	5.9	0.3
1996	1,781.0	57.1	0.4	37.6	20.6	64.0	90.1	104.9	82.8	33.9	6.2	0.3
1997	1,785.5	56.8	0.4	36.0	19.3	62.1	90.0	104.8	84.3	34.8	6.5	0.3
1998	1,825.0	57.6	0.3	35.3	18.3	60.9	91.2	107.4	87.2	36.4	6.8	0.4
1999	1,838.5	57.7	0.3	34.1	17.1	59.4	90.6	108.6	89.5	37.3	6.9	0.4
2000	1,866.0	58.5	0.3	32.6	15.8	57.5	91.2	109.4	93.2	38.8	7.3	0.4
2001	1,846.0	57.7	0.3	30.3	14.0	54.7	87.0	109.6	94.3	39.8	7.5	0.4
2002	1,840.0	57.6	0.2	28.6	13.1	52.0	84.7	110.4	95.0	40.9	7.7	0.5
2003	1,874.5	58.9	0.2	27.4	12.4	50.0	84.1	112.7	98.4	43.5	8.1	0.5
2004	1,871.0	58.9	0.2	26.7	12.0	48.6	83.0	112.1	98.3	45.1	8.3	0.5
2005	1,869.0	59.0	0.2	26.0	11.5	48.0	82.7	111.7	98.4	46.0	8.3	0.5
2006	1,900.5	60.3	0.2	26.7	11.8	49.4	85.1	112.2	100.0	46.8	8.5	0.6
2007	1,908.0	61.0	0.2	27.2	11.9	50.4	85.1	112.0	101.5	46.3	8.7	0.6
2008	1,874.5	60.5	0.2	26.7	11.6	48.6	82.8	109.7	100.8	45.2	8.9	0.6
2009	1,830.0	59.6	0.2	25.7	11.0	46.2	79.2	107.1	99.7	44.4	9.1	0.6
2010	1,791.0	58.7	0.2	23.5	10.0	42.5	74.9	105.8	99.9	44.1	9.2	0.6
2011	1,773.5	58.7	0.2	21.7	9.0	39.9	71.8	105.2	100.1	45.8	9.3	0.6
Black												
1989[4]	2,424.0	84.8	5.2	111.9	NA	NA	156.3	113.8	65.7	26.3	5.3	0.3
1990[5]	2,547.5	89.0	5.0	116.2	84.9	157.5	165.1	118.4	70.2	28.7	5.6	0.3
1991[6]	2,532.0	87.0	4.9	118.2	86.1	162.2	164.8	115.1	68.9	28.7	5.6	0.2
1992[6]	2,482.5	84.5	4.8	114.7	82.9	161.1	160.8	112.8	68.4	29.1	5.7	0.2
1993	2,412.5	81.5	4.6	110.5	81.1	154.6	154.5	109.2	68.1	29.4	5.9	0.3
1994	2,314.5	77.5	4.6	105.7	77.0	150.4	146.8	104.1	66.3	29.1	6.0	0.3
1995	2,186.5	72.8	4.2	97.2	70.4	139.2	137.8	98.5	64.4	28.8	6.1	0.3
1996	2,140.0	70.7	3.6	91.9	64.8	134.1	137.0	96.7	63.2	29.1	6.2	0.3
1997	2,137.5	70.3	3.2	88.3	60.7	131.0	138.8	97.2	63.6	29.6	6.5	0.3
1998	2,164.0	70.9	2.9	85.7	56.8	128.2	142.5	99.9	64.4	30.4	6.7	0.3
1999	2,134.0	69.9	2.6	81.0	51.7	123.9	142.1	99.8	63.9	30.6	6.5	0.3
2000	2,178.5	71.4	2.4	79.2	50.1	121.9	145.4	102.8	66.5	31.8	7.2	0.4
2001	2,107.0	69.1	2.1	73.1	44.8	115.9	137.3	102.8	66.4	32.0	7.3	0.4
2002	2,053.0	67.5	1.9	67.7	40.6	109.5	131.4	103.1	66.5	32.1	7.5	0.4
2003	2,037.5	67.1	1.6	63.8	38.2	103.4	128.8	104.0	67.7	33.4	7.7	0.5
2004	2,030.5	67.1	1.6	61.9	36.4	101.6	127.9	105.0	67.8	33.6	7.8	0.5
2005	2,030.5	67.2	1.6	59.4	34.1	100.2	127.9	105.5	68.8	34.2	8.2	0.5
2006	2,128.5	70.7	1.5	61.9	35.2	105.1	134.4	110.0	73.2	35.9	8.3	0.5
2007	2,142.0	71.4	1.4	62.0	34.6	105.2	134.5	110.5	74.7	36.2	8.5	0.6
2008	2,115.5	70.8	1.4	60.4	33.6	100.0	131.6	108.8	75.3	36.3	8.7	0.6
2009	2,046.5	68.9	1.1	56.8	31.0	93.5	125.9	106.0	73.9	36.1	8.9	0.6
2010	1,971.5	66.6	1.0	51.5	27.4	85.6	119.4	102.5	73.6	36.4	9.2	0.7
2011	1,919.5	65.4	0.9	47.3	24.6	78.8	112.3	101.7	73.9	37.8	9.3	0.7

NA = Not available.   * = Figure does not meet standards of reliability or precision.   [1]Fertility rates computed by relating total births, regardless of age of mother, to women age 15 to 44 years.   [2]Beginning in 1997, rates computed by relating births to women age 45 to 54 years to women age 45 to 49 years.   [3]Includes all persons of Hispanic origin of any race.   [4]Excludes data for Louisiana, New Hampshire, and Oklahoma, which did not report Hispanic origin.   [5]Excludes data for New Hampshire and Oklahoma, which did not report Hispanic origin.   [6]Excludes data for New Hampshire, which did not report Hispanic origin.   [7]Includes Central and South American and other and unknown Hispanic.   [8]Includes origin not stated.   [9]Includes races other than White and Black.

Table 1-36. Fertility Rates and Birth Rates, by Live-Birth Order and by Race and Hispanic Origin of Mother, 1980–2011

(Births per 1,000 women age 15 to 44 years.)

Year, race, and Hispanic origin of mother	Fertility rate	Live-birth order						
		1	2	3	4	5	6 and 7	8 and over
All Races [1,2]								
1980 [3]	68.4	29.5	21.8	10.3	3.9	1.5	1.0	0.4
1981 [3]	67.3	29.0	21.6	10.1	3.8	1.5	0.9	0.4
1982 [3]	67.3	28.6	22.0	10.2	3.8	1.4	0.9	0.3
1983 [3]	65.7	27.8	21.5	10.1	3.7	1.4	0.9	0.3
1984 [3]	65.5	27.4	21.7	10.1	3.7	1.4	0.9	0.3
1985	66.3	27.6	22.0	10.4	3.8	1.4	0.8	0.3
1986	65.4	27.2	21.6	10.3	3.8	1.4	0.8	0.3
1987	65.8	27.2	21.6	10.5	3.9	1.4	0.8	0.3
1988	67.3	27.6	22.0	10.9	4.1	1.5	0.9	0.3
1989	69.2	28.4	22.4	11.3	4.3	1.6	0.9	0.3
1990	70.9	29.0	22.8	11.7	4.5	1.7	1.0	0.3
1991	69.3	28.2	22.3	11.4	4.4	1.7	1.0	0.3
1992	68.4	27.6	22.2	11.2	4.4	1.7	1.0	0.3
1993	67.0	27.3	21.7	10.9	4.3	1.6	1.0	0.3
1994	65.9	27.1	21.2	10.6	4.1	1.6	0.9	0.3
1995	64.6	26.9	20.7	10.3	4.0	1.5	0.9	0.3
1996	64.1	26.3	20.7	10.4	4.0	1.5	0.9	0.3
1997	63.6	25.9	20.7	10.4	4.0	1.5	0.9	0.3
1998	64.3	25.9	21.0	10.6	4.1	1.5	0.9	0.3
1999	64.4	26.0	21.0	10.7	4.1	1.5	0.9	0.3
2000	65.9	26.5	21.4	11.0	4.2	1.6	0.9	0.3
2001	65.1	25.9	21.3	11.0	4.3	1.6	0.9	0.3
2002	65.0	25.8	21.2	10.9	4.3	1.6	0.9	0.3
2003	66.1	26.5	21.4	11.1	4.3	1.6	0.9	0.3
2004	66.4	26.4	21.4	11.2	4.4	1.6	0.9	0.3
2005	66.7	26.5	21.5	11.3	4.5	1.6	0.9	0.3
2006	68.6	27.4	21.9	11.6	4.7	1.7	1.0	0.3
2007	69.3	27.8	22.0	11.7	4.7	1.8	1.0	0.3
2008	68.1	27.5	21.5	11.4	4.7	1.7	1.0	0.3
2009	66.2	26.8	20.8	11.0	4.6	1.7	1.0	0.3
2010	64.1	25.9	20.2	10.6	4.4	1.7	1.0	0.3
2011	63.2	25.4	20.0	10.4	4.4	1.7	1.0	0.3
Non-Hispanic White [2,4]								
1990 [5]	62.8	26.7	21.2	9.9	3.3	1.1	0.5	0.2
1991 [6]	60.9	25.8	20.6	9.6	3.2	1.0	0.5	0.2
1992 [6]	60.0	25.1	20.5	9.5	3.2	1.0	0.5	0.2
1993	58.9	24.8	20.1	9.2	3.1	1.0	0.5	0.2
1994	58.2	24.6	19.7	9.1	3.1	1.0	0.5	0.2
1995	57.5	24.5	19.3	8.9	3.0	1.0	0.5	0.2
1996	57.1	24.1	19.3	8.9	3.0	1.0	0.5	0.2
1997	56.8	23.8	19.3	8.9	3.0	1.0	0.5	0.2
1998	57.6	23.8	19.7	9.2	3.1	1.0	0.6	0.2
1999	57.7	24.0	19.6	9.2	3.2	1.0	0.6	0.2
2000	58.5	24.2	19.8	9.4	3.3	1.1	0.6	0.2
2001	57.7	23.6	19.7	9.4	3.3	1.1	0.6	0.2
2002	57.6	23.6	19.6	9.3	3.3	1.1	0.6	0.2
2003	58.9	24.5	19.8	9.4	3.3	1.1	0.6	0.2
2004	58.9	24.4	19.8	9.5	3.3	1.1	0.6	0.2
2005	59.0	24.4	19.8	9.5	3.4	1.1	0.6	0.2
2006	60.3	25.1	20.0	9.6	3.5	1.1	0.6	0.2
2007	61.0	25.6	20.1	9.7	3.5	1.2	0.7	0.2
2008	60.5	25.5	19.8	9.5	3.5	1.2	0.7	0.2
2009	59.6	25.3	19.5	9.2	3.4	1.2	0.7	0.3
2010	58.7	25.0	19.2	9.1	3.4	1.2	0.7	0.3
2011	58.7	24.9	19.2	9.0	3.4	1.2	0.7	0.3
Non-Hispanic Black [2,4]								
1990 [5]	89.0	33.2	26.3	16.0	7.6	3.3	2.0	0.6
1991 [6]	87.0	32.1	25.5	15.7	7.5	3.4	2.2	0.6
1992 [6]	84.5	31.1	24.8	15.2	7.3	3.4	2.2	0.6
1993	81.5	30.5	23.6	14.3	7.0	3.2	2.2	0.7
1994	77.5	30.0	22.4	13.2	6.3	2.9	2.0	0.6
1995	72.8	28.9	20.9	12.1	5.8	2.7	1.9	0.6
1996	70.7	27.6	20.5	12.0	5.6	2.6	1.8	0.6
1997	70.3	27.2	20.6	12.0	5.7	2.5	1.8	0.6
1998	70.9	27.0	21.0	12.3	5.7	2.6	1.8	0.6
1999	69.9	26.4	20.8	12.3	5.7	2.5	1.7	0.6
2000	71.4	26.7	21.2	12.8	5.9	2.6	1.8	0.6
2001	69.1	25.9	20.4	12.4	5.8	2.5	1.7	0.6
2002	67.5	25.4	19.7	12.1	5.7	2.5	1.7	0.6
2003	67.1	25.4	19.6	11.9	5.6	2.5	1.6	0.5
2004	67.1	25.5	19.4	11.9	5.6	2.5	1.7	0.5
2005	67.2	25.8	19.3	11.8	5.6	2.5	1.7	0.5
2006	70.7	27.5	20.3	12.3	5.8	2.5	1.7	0.5
2007	71.4	27.9	20.4	12.3	5.9	2.6	1.7	0.5
2008	70.8	28.1	20.0	12.1	5.8	2.6	1.7	0.5
2009	68.9	27.3	19.4	11.7	5.7	2.5	1.7	0.6
2010	66.6	26.3	18.9	11.3	5.4	2.5	1.7	0.5
2011	65.4	25.6	18.5	11.1	5.4	2.4	1.7	0.6

Table 1-36. Fertility Rates and Birth Rates, by Live-Birth Order and by Race and Hispanic Origin of Mother, 1980–2011—*Continued*

(Births per 1,000 women age 15 to 44 years.)

Year, race, and Hispanic origin of mother	Fertility rate	Live-birth order						
		1	2	3	4	5	6 and 7	8 and over
Hispanic [7]								
1990 [5]	107.7	40.7	30.9	19.5	9.3	4.0	2.6	0.8
1991 [6]	106.9	40.8	30.6	19.2	9.2	3.9	2.5	0.7
1992 [6]	106.1	40.1	30.9	19.0	9.1	3.9	2.5	0.7
1993	103.3	39.3	30.4	18.3	8.6	3.7	2.3	0.6
1994	100.7	39.0	29.7	17.6	8.2	3.4	2.1	0.6
1995	98.8	38.4	29.3	17.4	7.8	3.3	2.0	0.6
1996	97.5	37.2	29.4	17.4	7.8	3.2	1.9	0.5
1997	94.2	35.6	28.6	17.1	7.6	3.0	1.8	0.5
1998	93.2	34.8	28.5	17.2	7.6	3.0	1.7	0.4
1999	93.0	34.6	28.5	17.3	7.5	2.9	1.7	0.4
2000	95.9	35.8	29.2	18.0	7.7	3.0	1.7	0.4
2001	95.4	35.2	29.3	18.0	7.9	3.0	1.7	0.4
2002	94.7	34.7	29.1	18.0	7.9	3.0	1.6	0.4
2003	95.2	34.5	29.4	18.3	8.0	3.0	1.6	0.4
2004	95.7	34.4	29.3	18.7	8.2	3.1	1.6	0.4
2005	96.4	34.4	29.6	19.0	8.4	3.1	1.6	0.4
2006	98.3	35.1	29.9	19.3	8.7	3.3	1.7	0.4
2007	97.4	34.7	29.4	19.3	8.7	3.3	1.7	0.4
2008	92.7	33.0	27.8	18.3	8.4	3.2	1.7	0.3
2009	86.5	30.6	25.9	17.0	8.0	3.0	1.6	0.3
2010	80.2	28.0	24.0	15.9	7.5	2.9	1.5	0.3
2011	76.2	26.3	22.9	15.2	7.2	2.8	1.5	0.3

[1] Includes races other than White and Black.   [2] Includes origin not stated.   [3] Based on 100 percent of births in selected states and on a 50 percent sample of births in all other states.   [4] Race and Hispanic origin are reported separately on birth certificates. Persons of Hispanic origin may be of any race. Multiple-race data, when reported, were bridged to single-race categories in order to maintain comparability among all reported areas. Persons of Hispanic origin may be of any race.   [5] Excludes data for New Hampshire and Oklahoma, which did not report Hispanic origin.   [6] Excludes data for New Hampshire, which did not report Hispanic origin.   [7] Includes all persons of Hispanic origin of any race.

Table 1-37. Selected Demographic Characteristics of Births, by Race of Mother, 2011

(Number; rates are live births per 1,000 population; percent.)

Characteristic	All Races	White	Black	American Indian or Alaska Native	Asian or Pacific Islander
Number					
Births	3,953,590	3,020,355	632,901	46,419	253,915
Rate					
Birth rate	12.7	12.2	14.8	10.7	14.5
Fertility rate	63.2	63.4	65.5	47.7	59.9
Total fertility rate	1,894.5	1,905.0	1,920.0	1,373.5	1,706.5
Sex ratio[1]	1,049	1,051	1,034	1,046	1,061
Percent, All Births					
Births to mothers under 20 years	8.4	7.8	13.7	14.9	2.3
4th and higher-order births[2]	11.7	11.3	15.3	19.5	6.7
Births to unmarried mothers	40.7	35.7	71.8	66.2	17.2
Mothers born in the 50 states and DC	77.1	80.1	83.7	93.5	21.9
Mean					
Age of mother at first birth	25.6	25.8	23.4	22.4	29.1

[1] Male live births per 1,000 female live births.   [2] Based on live-birth order.

Table 1-38. Live Births, by Day of Week and Index of Occurrence, by Method of Delivery, 2011

(Number, ratio.)

Day of the week	Average number of births	Index of occurrence[1]		
		Total[2]	Method of delivery	
			Vaginal	Cesarean
Total, All Days	10,832	100.0	100.0	100.0
Sunday	7,045	65.0	73.8	47.0
Monday	11,402	105.3	101.0	114.0
Tuesday	12,657	116.8	112.7	125.4
Wednesday	12,385	114.3	112.0	119.2
Thursday	12,327	113.8	111.5	118.6
Friday	12,048	111.2	106.4	121.1
Saturday	8,012	74.0	82.9	55.6

[1] Index is the ratio of the average number of births by a specified method of delivery on a given day of the week to the average daily number of births by a specified method of delivery for the year, multiplied by 100.   [2] Includes method of delivery not stated.

Table 1-39. Live Births and Observed and Seasonally Adjusted Birth and Fertility Rates, by Month, 2011

(Rates on an annual basis per 1,000 population for specified month; birth rates are live births per 1,000 total population; fertility rates are births per 1,000 women age 15 to 44 years.)

Month	Number	Observed		Seasonally adjusted[1]	
		Birth rate	Fertility rate	Birth rate	Fertility rate
Total, All Months	3,953,590	12.7	63.2	X	X
January	320,477	12.2	60.4	13.9	66.6
February	297,961	12.5	62.2	13.9	66.6
March	330,151	12.5	62.2	13.8	66.4
April	313,275	12.3	61.0	13.7	66.1
May	326,647	12.4	61.6	13.8	66.5
June	337,280	13.2	65.7	13.8	66.4
July	345,560	13.1	65.1	13.8	66.5
August	359,404	13.6	67.7	13.8	66.6
September	345,548	13.5	67.2	13.7	66.2
October	328,488	12.4	61.8	13.7	66.4
November	321,479	12.5	62.5	13.6	65.8
December	327,320	12.3	61.6	13.7	66.3

X = Not applicable.   [1] Method of seasonal adjustment developed by the U.S. Census Bureau. For more information, see: http://www.census.gov/ts/papers/ShiskinYoungMusgrave1967.pdf

Figure 1-8. Percent of Births to Unmarried Women Within Age Group, by Age, 2011

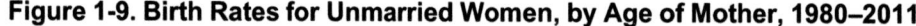

Figure 1-9. Birth Rates for Unmarried Women, by Age of Mother, 1980–2011

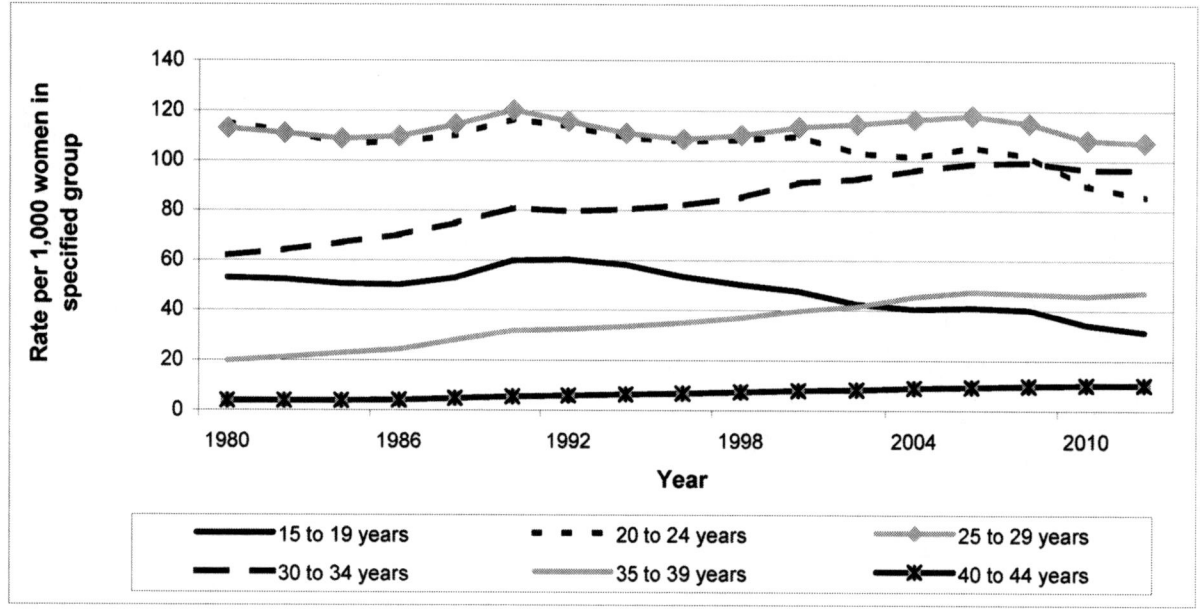

Table 1-40. Number, Rate, and Percent of Births to Unmarried Women and Birth Rate for Married Women, Selected Years, 1980–2011

(Number, rate per 1,000 women age 15 to 44 years; percent.)

Year	Births to unmarried women			Birth rate for married women[3]
	Number	Rate[1]	Percent[2]	
1980	665,747	29.4	18.4	97.0
1985	828,174	32.8	22.0	93.3
1990	1,165,384	43.8	28.0	93.2
1995	1,253,976	44.3	32.2	82.6
2000	1,347,043	44.1	33.2	87.4
2001	1,349,249	43.7	33.5	86.6
2002	1,365,966	43.6	34.0	86.9
2003	1,415,995	44.7	34.6	88.4
2004	1,470,189	46.0	35.8	88.1
2005	1,527,034	47.2	36.9	87.9
2006	1,641,946	50.3	38.5	88.7
2007	1,715,047	51.8	39.7	89.1
2008	1,726,566	51.8	40.6	86.9
2009	1,693,658	49.9	41.0	85.6
2010	1,633,471	47.5	40.8	84.3
2011	1,607,773	46.0	40.7	85.1

[1] Births to unmarried women per 1,000 unmarried women age 15 to 44 years.   [2] Percentage of all births to unmarried women.   [3] Births to married women per 1,000 married women age 15 to 44 years.

Table 1-41. Birth Rates for Unmarried Women, by Age, Race, and Hispanic Origin of Mother, Selected Years, 1970–2011

(Births to unmarried women per 1,000 unmarried women.)

Characteristic	15 to 44 years[1]	15 to 19 years Total	15 to 17 years	18 to 19 years	20 to 24 years	25 to 29 years	30 to 34 years	35 to 39 years	40 to 44 years[2]
All Races[3]									
1970[4,5]	26.4	22.4	17.1	32.9	38.4	37.0	27.1	13.6	3.5
1975[5,6]	24.5	23.9	19.3	32.5	31.2	27.5	17.9	9.1	2.6
1980[5,6]	29.4	27.6	20.6	39.0	40.9	34.0	21.1	9.7	2.6
1980[6,7]	28.4	27.5	20.7	38.7	39.7	31.4	18.5	8.4	2.3
1981[6,7]	29.5	27.9	20.9	39.0	41.1	34.5	20.8	9.8	2.6
1982[6,7]	30.0	28.7	21.5	39.6	41.5	35.1	21.9	10.0	2.7
1983[6,7]	30.3	29.5	22.0	40.7	41.8	35.5	22.4	10.2	2.6
1984[6,7]	31.0	30.0	21.9	42.5	43.0	37.1	23.3	10.9	2.5
1985[7]	32.8	31.4	22.4	45.9	46.5	39.9	25.2	11.6	2.5
1986[7]	34.2	32.3	22.8	48.0	49.3	42.2	27.2	12.2	2.7
1987[7]	36.0	33.8	24.5	48.9	52.6	44.5	29.6	13.5	2.9
1988[7]	38.5	36.4	26.4	51.5	56.0	48.5	32.0	15.0	3.2
1989[7]	41.6	40.1	28.7	56.0	61.2	52.8	34.9	16.0	3.4
1990[7]	43.8	42.5	29.6	60.7	65.1	56.0	37.6	17.3	3.6
1991[7]	45.0	44.6	30.8	65.4	67.8	56.0	37.9	17.9	3.8
1992[7]	44.9	44.2	30.2	66.7	67.9	55.6	37.6	18.8	4.1
1993[7]	44.8	44.0	30.3	66.2	68.5	55.9	38.0	18.9	4.4
1994[7]	46.2	45.8	31.7	69.1	70.9	57.4	39.6	19.7	4.7
1995[7]	44.3	43.8	30.1	66.5	68.7	54.3	38.9	19.3	4.7
1996[7]	43.8	42.2	28.5	64.9	68.9	54.5	40.2	19.9	4.8
1997[7]	42.9	41.4	27.7	63.9	68.9	53.4	37.9	18.7	4.6
1998[7]	43.3	40.9	26.5	63.6	70.4	55.4	38.1	18.7	4.6
1999[7]	43.3	39.7	25.0	62.3	70.8	56.9	38.1	19.0	4.6
2000[7]	44.1	39.0	23.9	62.2	72.2	58.5	39.3	19.7	5.0
2001[7]	43.7	36.8	21.8	60.2	70.8	59.6	40.3	20.4	5.3
2002[7]	43.6	35.1	20.7	58.1	70.0	62.0	41.3	20.9	5.4
2003[7]	44.7	34.3	20.1	56.6	71.0	66.2	44.2	22.3	5.8
2004[7]	46.0	34.2	19.9	56.6	72.3	69.1	47.3	23.5	6.0
2005[7]	47.2	33.9	19.4	57.0	74.5	71.5	50.4	24.5	6.2
2006[7]	50.3	35.5	20.1	60.3	79.1	75.4	55.3	26.8	6.5
2007[7]	51.8	36.5	20.4	61.9	79.8	76.9	58.0	28.7	6.8
2008[7]	51.8	35.9	20.1	59.7	78.1	75.7	58.8	30.2	7.5
2009[7]	49.9	34.0	18.8	56.3	74.4	73.0	57.1	29.7	7.8
2010[7]	47.5	31.1	16.8	52.0	70.0	69.2	56.3	29.6	8.0
2011[7]	46.0	28.4	14.9	48.2	66.7	67.8	56.2	29.9	8.2
White									
1980[6,7]	18.1	16.5	12.0	24.1	25.1	21.5	14.1	7.1	1.8
1981[6,7]	18.6	17.2	12.6	24.6	25.8	22.3	14.2	7.2	1.9
1982[6,7]	19.3	18.0	13.1	25.3	26.5	23.1	15.3	7.4	2.1
1983[6,7]	19.8	18.7	13.6	26.4	27.1	23.8	15.9	7.8	2.0
1984[6,7]	20.6	19.3	13.7	27.9	28.5	25.5	16.8	8.4	2.0
1985[7]	22.5	20.8	14.5	31.2	31.7	28.5	18.4	9.0	2.0
1986[7]	23.9	21.8	14.9	33.5	34.2	30.5	20.1	9.7	2.2
1987[7]	25.3	23.2	16.2	34.5	36.6	32.0	22.3	10.7	2.4
1988[7]	27.4	25.3	17.6	36.8	39.2	35.4	24.2	12.1	2.7
1989[7]	30.2	28.0	19.3	40.2	43.8	39.1	26.8	13.1	2.9
1990[7]	32.9	30.6	20.4	44.9	48.2	43.0	29.9	14.5	3.2
1991[7]	34.5	32.7	21.7	49.4	51.4	44.3	30.9	15.2	3.2
1992[7]	35.0	32.7	21.4	51.2	52.4	44.8	31.3	16.1	3.6
1993[7]	35.6	33.3	21.9	52.0	53.8	46.0	31.9	16.3	3.9
1994[7]	37.8	35.8	23.9	55.8	57.5	48.6	33.8	17.2	4.3
1995[7]	37.0	35.0	23.3	54.7	57.2	47.4	33.7	16.8	4.2
1996[7]	37.0	34.0	22.3	53.5	57.9	48.1	35.4	17.7	4.3
1997[7]	36.3	33.6	22.0	52.9	57.9	47.0	33.6	16.6	3.9
1998[7]	36.9	33.6	21.5	53.1	59.5	48.6	34.1	16.9	4.1
1999[7]	37.4	33.2	20.6	52.9	60.2	50.8	34.9	17.4	4.1
2000[7]	38.2	32.7	19.7	53.1	61.7	52.9	35.9	17.9	4.5
2001[7]	38.4	31.2	18.1	51.9	61.5	54.9	37.2	18.6	4.9
2002[7]	39.0	30.3	17.5	50.8	61.6	57.5	38.8	19.5	5.1
2003[7]	40.5	29.9	17.1	50.0	63.2	61.7	42.3	21.3	5.5
2004[7]	41.8	29.9	17.0	49.9	64.5	65.0	46.2	22.8	5.6
2005[7]	43.2	29.7	16.7	50.3	67.0	67.7	49.8	23.9	5.9
2006[7]	46.4	31.1	17.3	53.3	71.7	72.4	55.5	26.6	6.3
2007[7]	48.3	32.3	17.9	55.1	72.6	74.3	59.5	29.1	6.5
2008[7]	48.4	31.9	17.8	53.3	70.9	73.1	60.0	31.1	7.3
2009[7]	46.6	30.4	16.7	50.5	67.3	69.7	57.7	30.6	7.8
2010[7]	44.5	27.9	15.1	46.9	63.4	65.8	56.8	30.7	8.1
2011[7]	42.7	25.5	13.4	43.4	60.1	63.8	56.2	30.6	8.3
Non-Hispanic White									
1990[7,8]	24.4	25.0	16.2	37.0	36.4	30.3	20.5	6.1	NA
1991[7]	NA	NA	NA	NA	NA	NA	NA	NA	NA
1992[7]	NA	NA	NA	NA	NA	NA	NA	NA	NA
1993[7]	NA	NA	NA	NA	NA	NA	NA	NA	NA
1994[7]	28.4	28.1	17.9	45.0	43.8	34.7	24.6	12.8	3.1
1995[7]	28.1	27.7	17.6	44.6	43.9	34.4	25.1	12.9	3.2
1996[7]	28.2	27.0	16.9	43.9	44.5	35.0	26.4	13.8	3.3
1997[7]	27.5	26.4	16.2	43.3	44.8	34.4	24.9	12.7	2.9
1998[7]	27.9	26.2	15.5	43.1	46.3	35.4	25.0	13.1	3.1
1999[7]	27.9	25.6	14.6	42.7	46.3	36.2	24.8	13.0	3.1
2000[7]	28.0	24.7	13.6	42.1	47.0	36.9	24.8	12.9	3.3
2001[7]	27.8	23.1	12.1	40.3	46.4	37.8	25.4	13.2	3.6
2002[7]	27.9	22.1	11.4	38.8	46.3	38.9	26.2	13.6	3.7
2003[7]	28.8	21.5	11.0	37.8	47.6	41.5	28.0	14.8	4.1
2004[7]	29.6	21.3	10.7	37.4	48.6	44.2	30.0	15.7	4.2

Table 1-41. Birth Rates for Unmarried Women, by Age, Race, and Hispanic Origin of Mother, Selected Years, 1970–2011—*Continued*

(Births to unmarried women per 1,000 unmarried women.)

Characteristic	15 to 44 years[1]	15 to 19 years			20 to 24 years	25 to 29 years	30 to 34 years	35 to 39 years	40 to 44 years[2]
		Total	15 to 17 years	18 to 19 years					
2005[7]	30.4	20.9	10.3	37.4	49.9	46.0	31.7	16.2	4.3
2006[7]	32.4	21.6	10.7	38.9	52.6	49.1	35.1	17.9	4.5
2007[7]	33.8	22.6	10.9	40.7	53.4	50.7	37.2	19.2	4.6
2008[7]	34.3	22.5	10.8	39.7	52.9	50.8	38.4	20.4	5.2
2009[7]	33.6	21.8	10.4	38.1	51.4	49.3	37.9	20.0	5.5
2010[7]	32.9	20.3	9.5	36.0	49.5	48.0	38.7	20.2	5.8
2011[7]	32.3	18.8	8.6	33.6	47.8	47.8	39.2	20.7	6.0
Black									
1980[6,7]	81.1	87.9	68.8	118.2	112.3	81.4	46.7	19.0	5.5
1981[6,7]	79.4	85.0	65.9	114.2	110.7	83.1	45.5	19.6	5.6
1982[6,7]	77.9	85.1	66.3	112.7	109.3	82.7	44.1	19.5	5.2
1983[6,7]	76.2	85.5	66.8	111.9	107.2	79.7	43.8	19.4	4.8
1984[6,7]	75.2	86.1	66.5	113.6	107.9	77.8	43.8	19.4	4.3
1985[7]	77.0	87.6	66.8	117.9	113.1	79.3	47.5	20.4	4.3
1986[7]	79.0	88.5	67.0	121.1	118.0	84.6	50.0	20.6	4.4
1987[7]	82.6	90.9	69.9	123.0	126.1	91.6	53.1	22.4	4.7
1988[7]	86.5	96.1	73.5	130.5	133.6	97.2	57.4	24.1	5.0
1989[7]	90.7	104.5	78.9	140.9	142.4	102.9	60.5	24.9	5.0
1990[7]	90.5	106.0	78.8	143.7	144.8	105.3	61.5	25.5	5.1
1991[7]	89.0	107.8	79.9	147.7	146.4	100.0	59.8	25.5	5.4
1992[7]	85.7	104.8	77.2	146.4	142.6	96.8	57.3	25.6	5.4
1993[7]	83.0	101.2	75.9	140.0	139.9	92.8	56.7	25.7	5.8
1994[7]	80.8	99.3	73.9	139.6	135.2	91.3	56.5	26.0	5.9
1995[7]	74.5	91.2	67.4	129.2	124.6	82.3	53.3	25.3	6.0
1996[7]	72.8	87.5	62.6	127.2	122.6	81.2	53.4	25.2	6.1
1997[7]	71.5	84.5	59.0	124.8	124.2	81.4	51.0	24.3	6.5
1998[7]	71.6	81.5	55.0	121.5	127.8	86.5	50.5	24.3	6.0
1999[7]	69.7	76.5	50.0	115.8	126.8	85.5	49.0	24.2	5.8
2000[7]	70.5	75.0	48.3	115.0	129.0	85.9	50.2	25.4	6.3
2001[7]	68.0	69.4	43.5	109.1	122.5	84.4	51.2	25.4	6.3
2002[7]	66.1	64.0	39.4	102.8	119.0	86.3	50.2	24.9	6.3
2003[7]	65.9	61.0	37.4	98.0	117.8	91.3	51.2	25.2	6.5
2004[7]	66.8	60.1	36.1	98.0	119.6	92.5	52.0	25.7	6.8
2005[7]	67.2	58.7	34.4	97.9	120.4	94.7	53.9	25.9	7.1
2006[7]	70.7	61.1	35.4	103.3	125.5	98.0	58.4	27.3	7.2
2007[7]	71.4	61.3	34.8	103.6	125.3	99.1	59.9	28.0	7.4
2008[7]	71.0	59.7	33.9	98.4	124.0	97.0	61.1	28.5	7.6
2009[7]	68.7	55.9	31.1	91.3	119.5	95.6	60.3	28.4	7.6
2010[7]	65.3	50.8	27.6	83.6	112.6	92.5	58.6	27.8	7.8
2011[7]	63.7	46.7	24.7	77.4	106.9	92.4	59.1	28.9	7.8
Asian or Pacific Islander									
2000[7]	20.9	15.2	9.6	23.2	24.2	25.4	29.7	18.4	6.9
2001[7]	20.5	14.2	8.5	22.4	23.9	25.7	28.7	19.5	6.3
2002[7]	20.6	13.0	7.3	21.0	24.4	26.7	29.4	19.1	6.9
2003[7]	21.1	12.3	7.1	19.6	24.2	29.0	31.8	19.8	7.9
2004[7]	22.1	12.3	7.3	19.4	24.8	30.7	35.8	20.7	8.6
2005[7]	22.8	11.9	6.8	19.3	25.8	31.4	36.8	24.6	9.3
2006[7]	23.4	12.0	7.3	18.9	26.8	30.5	37.6	29.7	9.4
2007[7]	23.9	11.9	6.7	19.2	27.1	32.3	36.9	28.8	9.9
2008[7]	23.9	11.4	6.3	18.4	26.4	33.5	37.9	30.3	10.8
2009[7]	23.6	10.6	5.9	17.1	25.3	36.2	39.2	27.3	9.9
2010[7]	22.3	9.2	4.8	15.4	23.2	35.0	40.0	26.6	9.9
2011[7]	22.4	8.6	4.4	14.8	22.3	35.1	42.3	27.0	9.9
Hispanic[9]									
1990[7,8]	89.6	65.9	45.9	98.9	129.8	131.7	88.1	50.8	13.7
1991[7]	92.5	71.0	49.5	107.5	134.2	135.1	88.2	47.6	14.1
1992[7]	92.8	70.3	49.2	106.6	138.2	133.4	89.9	47.8	14.6
1993[7]	91.4	71.1	49.6	108.8	134.3	130.4	87.8	47.1	14.1
1994[7]	95.8	77.7	55.7	115.4	144.5	131.7	91.2	47.4	13.9
1995[7]	88.8	73.2	52.8	108.6	135.8	122.3	84.1	42.2	12.1
1996[7]	86.2	69.3	49.7	102.3	131.6	122.0	84.6	41.2	12.3
1997[7]	83.2	69.2	50.7	100.6	122.8	114.8	78.8	40.5	12.1
1998[7]	82.8	69.3	49.8	101.2	120.6	115.9	78.2	38.8	12.0
1999[7]	84.9	68.6	48.7	99.9	126.1	119.6	84.2	42.4	11.2
2000[7]	87.2	68.5	47.0	102.2	130.5	121.6	89.4	46.1	12.2
2001[7]	86.8	65.5	43.4	101.1	129.8	121.0	91.4	49.6	12.2
2002[7]	87.0	63.9	41.9	100.7	127.2	125.1	91.0	52.4	12.8
2003[7]	89.9	63.5	41.1	101.2	130.2	135.6	98.7	54.0	13.2
2004[7]	92.7	64.2	41.2	102.9	133.4	142.5	108.8	56.0	13.7
2005[7]	96.2	63.7	40.3	103.9	142.5	151.2	116.7	58.1	14.1
2006[7]	101.5	65.9	40.5	110.2	155.1	160.7	122.9	61.3	14.8
2007[7]	102.1	65.4	40.6	109.2	153.8	161.1	127.0	64.9	14.9
2008[7]	97.3	62.4	39.4	101.1	141.0	151.1	121.6	66.9	16.2
2009[7]	89.4	56.7	35.3	90.9	125.4	139.4	112.4	63.7	17.1
2010[7]	80.6	50.0	30.8	79.8	110.5	123.9	105.8	61.7	16.3
2011[7]	75.1	44.7	27.0	71.7	100.6	116.2	106.0	58.0	16.2

NA = Not available.   [1] Rates computed by relating total births to unmarried mothers, regardless of age of mother, to unmarried women age 15 to 44 years.   [2] Beginning in 1997, birth rates computed by relating births to unmarried mothers age 40 years and over to unmarried women age 40 to 44 years.   [3] Includes races other than White, Black, and Asian or Other Pacific Islander.   [4] Births to unmarried women are estimated for the United States from data for registration areas in which marital status of mother was reported.   [5] Based on a 50 percent sample of births.   [6] Based on 100 percent of births in selected states and on a 50 percent sample of births in all other states.   [7] Data for states in which marital status was not reported have been inferred and included with data from the remaining states.   [8] Rates based on data for 48 states and the District of Columbia that reported Hispanic origin on the birth certificate. Rate for age group 35–39 years are based on births to unmarried women aged 35–44 years.   [9] Persons of Hispanic origin may be of any race.

Table 1-42. Births and Birth Rates for Unmarried Women, by Age, Race, and Hispanic Origin of Mother, 2011

(Number, rate, percent.)

Measure and age of mother	All races[1]	White		Black		American Indian or Alaska Native[2]	Asian or Pacific Islander[2]	Hispanic[3]
		Total[2]	Non-Hispanic	Total[2]	Non-Hispanic			
Number								
All ages	1,607,773	1,079,091	622,972	454,403	420,879	30,713	43,566	489,667
Under 15 years	3,939	2,309	859.0	1,472	1,375	93.0	65.0	1,558
15 to 19 years	291,736	197,922	109,016	82,904	76,797	6,267	4,643	95,246
15 years	11,586	7,574	3,226	3,581	3,278	257.0	174.0	4,670
16 years	28,012	19,151	8,632	7,855	7,192	612.0	394.0	11,207
17 years	51,455	35,395	17,668	14,157	13,054	1,076	827.0	18,880
18 years	82,590	56,176	31,478	23,289	21,508	1,771	1,354	26,572
19 years	118,093	79,626	48,012	34,022	31,765	2,551	1,894	33,917
20 to 24 years	592,554	392,501	243,305	175,823	164,015	11,779	12,451	161,244
25 to 29 years	387,354	260,370	150,801	107,181	99,047	7,156	12,647	117,671
30 to 34 years	212,974	143,534	75,974	57,871	53,079	3,612	7,957	72,252
35 to 39 years	93,155	64,110	32,632	23,115	21,094	1,467	4,463	33,372
40 years and over	26,061	18,345	10,385	6,037	5,472	339	1,340	8,324
Rate per 1,000 Unmarried Women in Specified Group								
15 to 44 years[4]	46.0	42.7	32.3	63.7	NA	NA	22.4	75.1
15 to 19 years	28.4	25.5	18.8	46.7	NA	NA	8.6	44.7
15 to 17 years	14.9	13.4	8.6	24.7	NA	NA	4.4	27.0
18 to 19 years	48.2	43.4	33.6	77.4	NA	NA	14.8	71.7
20 to 24 years	66.7	60.1	47.8	106.9	NA	NA	22.3	100.6
25 to 29 years	67.8	63.8	47.8	92.4	NA	NA	35.1	116.2
30 to 34 years	56.2	56.2	39.2	59.1	NA	NA	42.3	106.0
35 to 39 years	29.9	30.6	20.7	28.9	NA	NA	27.0	58.0
40 to 44 years[5]	8.2	8.3	6.0	7.8	NA	NA	9.9	16.2
Percent of Births to Unmarried Women								
All ages	40.7	35.7	29.0	71.8	72.3	66.2	17.2	53.3
Under 15 years	99.1	98.7	98.8	99.8	99.8	97.9	100.0	98.9
15 to 19 years	88.5	85.3	84.3	97.4	97.8	92.1	81.3	86.9
15 years	98.7	98.2	98.4	99.7	99.9	99.6	96.1	98.2
16 years	96.4	95.2	95.4	99.4	99.7	98.1	91.0	95.1
17 years	94.0	92.2	92.3	98.9	99.2	95.1	90.1	92.4
18 years	89.2	86.1	86.0	97.7	98.1	93.0	82.9	86.6
19 years	83.4	79.1	78.4	95.8	96.3	88.5	74.5	80.7
20 to 24 years	64.0	57.7	53.8	87.3	88.1	75.7	44.8	66.2
25 to 29 years	34.4	29.5	23.3	66.5	67.1	57.4	17.9	47.4
30 to 34 years	21.6	18.5	12.8	50.8	50.9	48.9	9.0	37.5
35 to 39 years	20.1	18.0	12.5	42.2	42.0	44.6	9.0	33.9
40 years and over	22.4	20.7	16.0	39.8	39.2	42.2	11.4	34.6

NA = Not available.   [1] Includes races other than White and Black and origin not stated.   [2] Race and Hispanic origin are reported separately on birth certificates. Persons of Hispanic origin may be of any race. Multiple-race data, when reported, were bridged to single-race categories in order to maintain comparability among all reported areas.   [3] Persons of Hispanic origin may be of any race.   [4] Birth rates computed by relating total births to unmarried mothers, regardless of age of mother, to unmarried women age 15 to 44 years.   [5] Birth rates computed by relating births to unmarried mothers age 40 years and over to unmarried women age 40 to 44 years.

Table 1-43. Selected Demographic Characteristics of Births, by Hispanic Origin of Mother and by Race for Mothers of Non-Hispanic Origin, 2011

(Birth rates are births per 1,000 population; fertility rates are computed by relating total births, regardless of age of mother, to women age 15 to 44 years; total fertility rates are sums of birth rates for 5-year age groups multiplied by 5.)

Characteristic	All origins[1]	Hispanic[2]						Non-Hispanic		
		Total	Mexican	Puerto Rican	Cuban	Central and South American	Other and unknown Hispanic	Total[3]	White	Black
Number										
Births	3,953,590	918,129	566,699	67,018	17,131	136,221	131,060	3,008,200	2,146,566	582,345
Rate										
Birth rate[4]	12.7	17.6	16.9	13.7	9.1	23.0	(4)	11.7	10.8	14.7
Fertility rate[4]	63.2	76.2	73.0	59.6	46.1	96.3	(4)	60.1	58.7	65.4
Total fertility rate[4]	1,894.5	2,240.0	2,143.0	1,747.5	1,433.5	2,847.5	(4)	1,810.5	1,773.5	1,919.5
Sex ratio[5]	1,049	1,040	1,043	1,046	1,053	1,030	1,033	1,052	1,055	1,033
Percent										
Births to mothers under 20 years	8.4	12.1	12.8	14.0	5.6	6.5	14.7	7.3	6.1	13.7
4th and higher-order births[6]	11.7	15.5	17.4	12.6	5.3	13.0	12.5	10.5	9.5	15.4
Births to unmarried mothers	40.7	53.3	52.0	65.0	48.2	51.2	55.9	36.8	29.0	72.3
Mothers born in the 50 states and D.C.	77.1	46.0	44.1	72.9	48.5	16.0	71.9	86.6	92.9	86.3
Mean										
Age of mother at first birth	25.6	23.7	23.1	23.4	26.5	26.0	23.4	26.1	26.5	23.4

[1] Includes origin not stated.   [2] Persons of Hispanic origin may be of any race.   [3] Includes races other than White and Black.   [4] Rates for Central and South American include other and unknown Hispanic.
[5] Male births per 1,000 female births.   [6] Based on live-birth order.

Table 1-44. Percent of Births with Selected Medical or Health Characteristics, by Race of Mother, 2011

(Percent, rate.)

Characteristic	All races	White	Black	American or Alaska Indian Native	Asian or Pacific Islander
ALL BIRTHS					
Mother					
Diabetes during pregnancy	5.5	5.3	5.0	7.5	9.2
Weight gain of less than 11 lbs	8.5	7.7	12.9	11.9	6.0
Weight gain of more than 40 lbs	21.2	21.7	21.1	21.4	15.2
Induction of labor	23.2	24.1	21.9	21.9	17.2
CNM delivery[1]	7.8	7.9	7.4	16.7	6.5
Cesarean delivery	32.8	32.3	35.2	28.4	33.2
Infant					
Gestational age					
Preterm[2]	11.7	10.8	16.5	13.5	10.4
Early preterm[3]	3.4	3.0	5.9	3.9	2.8
Late preterm[4]	8.3	7.8	10.6	9.6	7.6
Birthweight					
Very low birthweight[5]	1.4	1.2	2.9	1.3	1.2
Low birthweight[6]	8.1	7.1	13.0	7.5	8.4
4,000 grams or more[7]	7.8	8.7	4.4	9.8	4.8
Low 5-minute Apgar[8]	1.9	1.6	3.1	2.3	1.2
Twin birth[9] (rate)	33.2	32.8	36.4	23.4	31.2
Triplet or higher-order multiple birth[10] (rate)	137.0	145.5	110.3	43.1	119.7

[1] Births delivered by certified nurse midwives.   [2] Born prior to 37 completed weeks of gestation.   [3] Born prior to 34 completed weeks of gestation.   [4] Born between 34 and 36 completed weeks of gestation.
[5] Birthweight of less than 1,500 grams (3 lb 4 oz).   [6] Birthweight of less than 2,500 grams (5 lb 8 oz).   [7] Equivalent to 8 lb 14 oz.   [8] Score of less than 7 on a 10-point scale.   [9] Live births in twin deliveries per 1,000 live births.   [10] Live births in triplet and other higher-order multiple deliveries per 100,000 live births.

Table 1-45. Percent of Births with Selected Medical or Health Characteristics, by Hispanic Origin of Mother and by Race for Mothers of Non-Hispanic Origin, 2011

(Percent, rate.)

Characteristic	All origins[1]	Origin of mother								
		Hispanic						Non-Hispanic		
		Total	Mexican	Puerto Rican	Cuban	Central and South American	Other and un-known Hispanic	Total[2]	White	Black
ALL BIRTHS										
Mother										
Diabetes during pregnancy	5.5	5.8	6.2	6.1	5.1	5.5	4.6	5.4	5.1	4.9
Weight gain of less than 11 lbs	8.5	9.4	9.8	8.8	5.1	8.7	8.8	8.2	7.1	13.1
Weight gain of more than 40 lbs	21.2	16.7	15.5	22.7	27.1	15.3	19.3	22.6	23.8	21.2
Induction of labor	23.2	18.0	17.4	21.2	20.5	16.5	19.7	24.9	26.6	22.0
CNM delivery[3]	7.8	8.0	7.5	10.3	4.6	9.4	7.8	7.8	7.9	7.1
Cesarean delivery	32.8	32.0	30.8	34.5	47.9	32.8	33.5	33.0	32.4	35.5
Infant										
Gestational age										
Preterm[4]	11.7	11.7	11.3	13.2	12.4	11.8	12.3	11.7	10.5	16.8
Early preterm[5]	3.4	3.3	3.1	4.0	3.4	3.3	3.5	3.5	2.9	6.0
Late preterm[6]	8.3	8.4	8.2	9.2	9.0	8.5	8.8	8.2	7.6	10.7
Birthweight										
Very low birthweight[7]	1.4	1.2	1.1	1.8	1.3	1.2	1.4	1.5	1.1	3.0
Low birthweight[8]	8.1	7.0	6.5	9.7	7.1	6.7	8.0	8.4	7.1	13.3
4,000 grams or more[9]	7.8	7.2	7.6	5.8	7.3	7.0	6.1	8.0	9.3	4.2
Low 5-minute Apgar[10]	1.9	1.4	1.3	1.7	1.4	1.3	1.6	2.0	1.8	3.2
Twin birth[11] (rate)	33.2	23.1	20.9	32.0	29.4	25.2	25.3	36.1	36.6	37.2
Triplet or higher-order multiple birth[12] (rate)	137.0	78.7	60.7	114.9	181.0	105.7	96.9	153.2	171.0	108.9

[1] Includes origin not stated.   [2] Includes races other than White and Black.   [3] Births delivered by certified nurse midwives.   [4] Born prior to 37 completed weeks of gestation.   [5] Born prior to 34 completed weeks of gestation.   [6] Born between 34 and 36 completed weeks of gestation.   [7] Birthweight of less than 1,500 grams (3 lb 4 oz).   [8] Birthweight of less than 2,500 grams (5 lb 8 oz).   [9] Equivalent to 8 lb 14 oz.   [10] Score of less than 7 on a 10 point scale.   [11] Live births in twin deliveries per 1,000 live births.   [12] Live births in triplet and other higher-order multiple deliveries per 100,000 live births.

Table 1-46. Births to Unmarried Women, by Race and Hispanic Origin of Mother, by State and Territory of Residence, 2011

(Number, percent.)

State and territory	Births to unmarried women				Percent unmarried			
	All races[1]	Non-Hispanic		Hispanic[3]	All races[1]	Non-Hispanic		Hispanic[3]
		White[2]	Black[2]			White[2]	Black[2]	
United States [4]	1,607,773	622,972	420,879	489,667	40.7	29.0	72.3	53.3
Alabama	25,012	10,015	13,578	1,200	42.1	28.1	75.5	26.8
Alaska	4,217	1,377	200	242	36.8	22.6	45.8	32.0
Arizona	38,227	11,690	2,586	18,867	44.7	30.0	63.3	56.7
Arkansas	17,370	9,272	5,780	2,001	44.9	35.1	79.9	50.6
California	202,689	35,035	20,371	132,435	40.4	24.2	68.1	53.0
Colorado	15,403	7,072	1,301	6,413	23.7	17.5	42.6	35.5
Connecticut	14,177	5,137	3,259	5,533	38.0	23.9	68.2	65.9
Delaware	5,469	2,282	2,185	942	48.6	36.7	72.1	66.5
District of Columbia	4,979	155	3,781	924	53.6	5.9	78.6	67.4
Florida	101,545	35,384	34,608	29,762	47.6	36.4	70.5	50.7
Georgia	60,169	16,525	31,597	9,857	45.4	27.3	70.8	52.8
Hawaii	7,104	1,195	140	1,472	37.5	24.6	27.6	48.5
Idaho	5,968	4,102	80	1,515	26.8	23.0	41.7	43.6
Illinois	64,501	22,564	21,777	18,939	40.0	25.7	80.1	53.0
Indiana	35,774	23,912	7,852	3,641	42.7	37.1	79.9	50.7
Iowa	12,923	9,682	1,336	1,562	33.8	30.3	72.5	50.2
Kansas	14,791	8,884	2,162	3,364	37.3	30.8	73.7	53.4
Kentucky	22,970	17,378	3,966	1,435	41.5	37.6	76.2	51.6
Louisiana	32,763	11,415	18,917	1,996	52.9	34.5	80.1	55.3
Maine	5,309	4,948	132	89	41.8	42.1	33.4	42.8
Maryland	30,091	8,569	15,075	5,798	41.2	25.8	63.2	56.1
Massachusetts	25,359	12,168	4,042	8,004	34.7	26.1	56.4	63.7
Michigan	48,238	25,760	17,551	3,992	42.3	32.4	80.6	52.3
Minnesota	22,395	12,861	3,768	2,662	32.7	25.6	58.2	57.5
Mississippi	21,703	6,513	14,151	730	54.4	31.8	81.8	55.3
Missouri	30,508	18,715	8,943	2,090	40.1	32.4	78.2	50.8
Montana	4,405	3,043	35	217	36.5	30.6	46.7	48.3
Nebraska	8,548	5,175	1,171	1,809	33.2	26.8	68.6	49.6
Nevada	15,597	4,923	2,684	6,925	44.2	32.3	72.6	53.1
New Hampshire	4,440	3,964	81	289	34.5	34.8	34.6	53.5
New Jersey	37,967	9,190	11,102	17,012	35.9	18.5	69.2	60.7
New Mexico	13,994	2,404	254	8,542	51.3	31.1	53.7	56.7
New York	99,288	29,854	27,205	37,156	41.1	25.5	69.5	65.5
North Carolina	49,237	17,693	20,557	9,378	40.9	26.1	71.9	51.5
North Dakota	3,183	2,104	87	139	33.4	27.1	39.9	45.3
Ohio	59,860	37,122	18,004	3,844	43.4	35.5	78.8	60.7
Oklahoma	21,846	11,603	3,585	3,178	41.8	34.8	74.5	47.5
Oregon	16,124	10,061	707	4,345	35.7	31.7	60.5	49.7
Pennsylvania	59,761	32,018	16,613	9,498	41.7	31.8	79.0	67.0
Rhode Island	4,875	2,403	634	1,535	44.5	35.6	66.1	63.3
South Carolina	27,018	10,199	14,209	2,261	47.1	30.9	77.7	47.6
South Dakota	4,604	2,462	125	288	38.9	27.8	47.0	57.0
Tennessee	35,086	18,153	13,027	3,570	44.1	33.5	78.7	50.8
Texas	158,708	36,108	28,440	92,159	42.0	27.0	65.8	50.5
Utah	9,564	5,412	235	3,292	18.7	13.2	41.4	42.8
Vermont	2,399	2,291	38	30	39.5	40.0	42.7	41.7
Virginia	36,412	14,606	14,611	6,467	35.5	24.2	66.6	51.8
Washington	28,555	15,032	2,198	8,109	32.8	27.3	51.1	50.8
West Virginia	9,093	8,363	559	86	43.9	42.9	77.0	41.5
Wisconsin	25,001	14,350	5,548	3,616	36.9	28.4	84.2	55.4
Wyoming	2,554	1,829	32	457	34.5	30.1	49.2	52.9
Puerto Rico	27,156	743	83	26,271	66.1	63.2	62.4	66.2
Virgin Islands	1,092	37	797	240	73.2	33.3	78.4	75.0
Guam	2,044	28	8	12	62.1	14.4	*	*
American Samoa	508	NA	NA	NA	40.4	NA	NA	NA
Northern Marianas	586	3	1	—	56.7	*	*	*

NA = Not available.   - = Quantity zero.   * = Figure does not meet standards of reliability or precision.   [1] Includes races other than White and Black and origin not stated.   [2] Race and Hispanic origin are reported separately on birth certificates. Persons of Hispanic origin may be of any race. Multiple-race data, when reported, were bridged to single-race categories in order to maintain comparability among all reported areas.   [3] Includes all persons of Hispanic origin of any race.   [4] Excludes data for the territories.

Table 1-47. Births, by Weight Gain of Mother During Pregnancy, by Plurality, Gestational Age, and Race and Hispanic Origin of Mother, 2011

(Number, percent distribution.)

Period of gestation[1], race, and Hispanic origin of mother	All births	Less than 11 pounds	11 to 20 pounds	21 to 30 pounds	31 to 40 pounds	41 to 98 pounds	Not stated
NUMBER							
All Pluralities							
All Gestational Ages [2]							
All races[3]	3,953,590	317,512	612,561	1,075,375	953,797	796,496	197,849
Non-Hispanic White[4]	2,146,566	145,241	279,492	576,188	566,081	489,141	90,423
Non-Hispanic Black[4]	582,345	70,683	102,328	139,096	113,420	114,445	42,373
Hispanic[5]	918,129	81,724	181,781	266,118	197,669	145,997	44,840
Under 37 Weeks							
All races[3]	463,163	54,421	90,222	120,321	88,832	78,863	30,504
Non-Hispanic White[4]	225,150	21,817	38,124	58,822	48,117	45,280	12,990
Non-Hispanic Black[4]	97,543	15,894	20,399	22,490	15,300	14,998	8,462
Hispanic[5]	106,884	13,364	24,756	29,374	18,882	14,179	6,329
37 Weeks and Over							
All races[3]	3,485,581	262,614	521,998	954,646	864,580	717,309	164,434
Non-Hispanic White[4]	1,919,036	123,221	241,194	517,138	517,730	443,680	76,073
Non-Hispanic Black[4]	483,974	54,627	81,846	116,531	98,051	99,376	33,543
Hispanic[5]	810,465	68,277	156,960	236,666	178,723	131,764	38,075
Live Births in Singleton Deliveries							
All Gestational Ages [2]							
All races[3]	3,816,904	305,063	624,006	1,121,227	959,049	759,357	218,406
Non-Hispanic White[4]	2,064,258	133,891	280,558	594,932	563,989	462,497	90,274
Non-Hispanic Black[4]	560,030	68,773	103,319	146,566	115,388	108,905	42,830
Hispanic[5]	896,170	84,089	193,002	286,223	205,025	143,993	63,900
Under 37 Weeks							
All races[3]	383,027	50,051	87,173	114,732	77,790	56,633	29,356
Non-Hispanic White[4]	177,069	18,755	35,714	54,620	40,049	29,884	10,390
Non-Hispanic Black[4]	83,787	15,133	19,840	22,095	14,239	11,838	7,992
Hispanic[5]	94,271	13,198	25,472	29,191	17,954	11,760	8,212
37 Weeks and Over							
All races[3]	3,429,172	254,504	536,425	1,005,954	880,863	702,348	186,178
Non-Hispanic White[4]	1,884,879	114,900	244,654	540,049	523,721	432,401	78,757
Non-Hispanic Black[4]	475,444	53,510	83,395	124,376	101,092	97,001	34,441
Hispanic[5]	801,139	70,793	167,426	256,900	186,990	132,167	54,999
PERCENT DISTRIBUTION							
All Pluralities							
All Gestational Ages [2]							
All races[3]	100.0	8.5	16.3	28.6	25.4	21.2	X
Non-Hispanic White[4]	100.0	7.1	13.6	28.0	27.5	23.8	X
Non-Hispanic Black[4]	100.0	13.1	19.0	25.8	21.0	21.2	X
Hispanic[5]	100.0	9.4	20.8	30.5	22.6	16.7	X
Under 37 Weeks							
All races[3]	100.0	12.6	20.9	27.8	20.5	18.2	X
Non-Hispanic White[4]	100.0	10.3	18.0	27.7	22.7	21.3	X
Non-Hispanic Black[4]	100.0	17.8	22.9	25.2	17.2	16.8	X
Hispanic[5]	100.0	13.3	24.6	29.2	18.8	14.1	X
37 Weeks and Over							
All races[3]	100.0	7.9	15.7	28.7	26.0	21.6	X
Non-Hispanic White[4]	100.0	6.7	13.1	28.1	28.1	24.1	X
Non-Hispanic Black[4]	100.0	12.1	18.2	25.9	21.8	22.1	X
Hispanic[5]	100.0	8.8	20.3	30.6	23.1	17.1	X
Live Births in Singleton Deliveries							
All Gestational Ages [2]							
All races[3]	100.0	8.5	16.5	28.9	25.4	20.6	X
Non-Hispanic White[4]	100.0	7.1	13.8	28.4	27.6	23.0	X
Non-Hispanic Black[4]	100.0	13.1	19.1	26.0	21.0	20.7	X
Hispanic[5]	100.0	9.4	21.0	30.7	22.6	16.4	X
Under 37 Weeks							
All races[3]	100.0	13.6	22.6	29.1	19.9	14.9	X
Non-Hispanic White[4]	100.0	11.4	20.0	29.7	22.1	16.8	X
Non-Hispanic Black[4]	100.0	18.5	23.9	25.9	16.8	14.9	X
Hispanic[5]	100.0	14.0	25.8	29.8	18.2	12.2	X
37 Weeks and Over							
All races[3]	100.0	8.0	15.8	28.9	26.1	21.2	X
Non-Hispanic White[4]	100.0	6.7	13.2	28.3	28.2	23.6	X
Non-Hispanic Black[4]	100.0	12.2	18.3	26.0	21.8	21.8	X
Hispanic[5]	100.0	8.9	20.4	30.8	23.1	16.8	X

NOTE: Excludes data for California, which did not require reporting of weight gain during pregnancy.

X = Not applicable. [1]Expressed in completed weeks. [2]Includes births with period of gestation not stated. [3]Includes races other than White and Black and origin not stated. [4]Race and Hispanic origin are reported separately on birth certificates. Persons of Hispanic origin may be of any race. Multiple-race data, when reported, were bridged to single-race categories in order to maintain comparability among all reported areas. [5]Includes all persons of Hispanic origin of any race.

Table 1-48. Selected Risk Factors, Obstetric Procedures, Characteristics of Labor and Delivery, and Congenital Anomalies, by Age, Race, and Hispanic Origin of Mother, 2011

(Rates are number of live births with specified risk factors, procedures, or anomaly per 1,000 live births in specified group; congenital anomalies are per 100,000 live births.)

Risk factor, procedure, characteristic, and anomaly	All births[1]	Factor reported	All ages	Under 20 years	20 to 24 years	25 to 29 years	30 to 34 years	35 to 39 years	40 to 54 years	Not stated[2]
ALL RACES[3]										
Risk Factors in This Pregnancy										
Diabetes	3,953,590	217,367	55.2	18.1	31.3	50.6	69.0	95.6	119.4	18,169
Hypertension, pregnancy-associated	3,953,590	173,694	44.1	46.5	43.0	43.3	42.6	46.2	59.1	18,169
Hypertension, chronic	3,953,590	56,562	14.4	5.0	8.3	12.5	17.2	25.6	39.2	18,169
Obstetric Procedures and Characteristics of Labor or Delivery										
Induction of labor	3,953,590	916,043	232.5	262.1	249.5	238.0	218.0	201.9	203.5	13,539
Tocolysis[4]	3,903,618	37,765	9.7	10.7	10.2	9.5	9.3	9.4	10.0	20,302
Meconium, moderate/heavy[5]	3,942,333	193,816	49.3	54.7	50.4	48.9	48.3	47.2	46.6	13,757
Breech/malpresentation	3,953,590	216,383	55.8	44.2	46.9	52.7	60.8	71.0	88.9	78,739
Precipitous labor[5]	3,942,333	97,402	24.8	16.9	22.3	25.3	27.4	28.3	26.9	18,759
Congenital Anomalies[4]										
Anencephaly	3,953,590	410	10.5	14.8	11.9	9.3	10.9	8.3	*	32,884
Meningomyelocele/Spina Bifida	3,953,590	586	14.9	17.8	15.4	15.4	12.6	15.2	18.2	32,884
Congenital diaphragmatic hernia	3,953,590	667	17.0	19.3	18.9	16.0	15.5	15.7	23.4	32,884
Omphalocele/Gastroschisis	3,953,590	1,515	38.6	110.5	63.9	28.0	14.2	17.6	26.0	32,884
Cleft lip/palate	3,953,590	2,693	68.7	69.5	74.9	68.5	63.4	64.6	80.6	32,884
Down syndrome	3,953,590	1,873	47.8	28.7	22.3	27.7	38.7	105.3	346.7	32,884
NON-HISPANIC WHITE[6]										
Risk Factors in This Pregnancy										
Diabetes	2,146,566	109,025	51.0	21.4	32.6	46.6	58.7	79.3	99.3	9,493
Hypertension, pregnancy-associated	2,146,566	102,516	48.0	50.6	48.2	48.4	45.2	48.1	61.8	9,493
Hypertension, chronic	2,146,566	29,151	13.6	5.0	8.1	12.0	15.6	22.3	32.9	9,493
Obstetric Procedures and Characteristics of Labor or Delivery										
Induction of labor	2,146,566	569,403	266.2	326.9	297.5	273.1	243.7	225.5	225.1	7,365
Tocolysis4	2,113,936	23,067	11.0	13.3	12.0	10.7	10.3	10.4	10.6	10,131
Meconium, moderate/heavy[5]	2,140,344	93,844	44.0	46.1	43.6	44.0	44.3	43.2	43.5	7,461
Breech/malpresentation	2,146,566	117,250	55.4	42.5	44.9	52.1	60.4	69.5	87.0	31,948
Precipitous labor[5]	2,140,344	53,320	25.0	15.2	21.3	24.7	28.1	29.4	28.1	9,717
Congenital Anomalies[4]										
Anencephaly	2,146,566	245	11.5	23.2	12.0	10.6	12.6	*	*	17,663
Meningomyelocele/Spina Bifida	2,146,566	372	17.5	20.9	17.6	18.7	13.6	19.4	*	17,663
Congenital diaphragmatic hernia	2,146,566	440	20.7	28.6	24.3	19.8	18.6	15.9	*	17,663
Omphalocele/Gastroschisis	2,146,566	924	43.4	149.3	79.8	33.9	15.4	17.4	31.1	17,663
Cleft lip/palate	2,146,566	1,716	80.6	95.9	95.9	80.1	70.5	71.3	77.7	17,663
Down syndrome	2,146,566	1,132	53.2	44.1	27.0	32.2	42.3	105.0	354.3	17,663
NON-HISPANIC BLACK[6]										
Risk Factors in This Pregnancy										
Diabetes	582,345	28,425	49.2	15.8	27.8	51.1	74.6	102.9	123.9	5,082
Hypertension, pregnancy-associated	582,345	31,696	54.9	55.8	49.8	53.7	58.9	63.0	71.9	5,082
Hypertension, chronic	582,345	16,988	29.4	8.2	14.5	28.7	45.7	67.0	99.5	5,082
Obstetric Procedures and Characteristics of Labor or Delivery										
Induction of labor	582,345	127,368	220.1	247.4	224.6	216.7	209.7	197.5	196.8	3,561
Tocolysis[4]	572,083	6,647	11.7	12.7	12.1	11.3	11.1	11.4	12.8	6,141
Meconium, moderate/heavy[5]	579,314	35,373	61.4	65.0	60.1	59.3	63.0	63.9	61.5	3,590
Breech/malpresentation	582,345	31,133	54.6	42.2	48.3	54.0	62.0	73.8	93.5	12,300
Precipitous labor[5]	579,314	15,542	27.1	21.7	26.0	28.9	29.4	29.5	27.5	5,132
Congenital Anomalies										
Anencephaly	582,345	55	9.6	*	12.5	*	*	*	*	7,875
Meningomyelocele/Spina Bifida	582,345	60	10.4	*	*	*	*	*	*	7,875
Congenital diaphragmatic hernia	582,345	72	12.5	*	12.0	*	*	*	*	7,875
Omphalocele/Gastroschisis	582,345	188	32.7	74.8	35.4	22.6	*	*	*	7,875
Cleft lip/palate	582,345	227	39.5	44.4	39.2	34.3	43.7	*	*	7,875
Down syndrome	582,345	196	34.1	*	15.8	20.6	31.1	92.9	356.4	7,875
HISPANIC[7]										
Risk Factors in This Pregnancy										
Diabetes	918,129	53,486	58.4	15.3	29.7	53.1	83.3	119.1	154.1	1,773
Hypertension, pregnancy-associated	918,129	30,435	33.2	35.7	30.2	29.5	34.1	40.7	52.7	1,773
Hypertension, chronic	918,129	7,288	8.0	3.0	4.4	6.1	10.3	17.6	27.2	1,773
Obstetric Procedures and Characteristics of Labor or Delivery										
Induction of labor	918,129	164,634	179.6	203.1	190.0	175.4	167.4	163.8	170.3	1,272
Tocolysis[4]	912,755	5,841	6.4	6.6	6.0	6.4	6.5	7.0	7.3	2,058
Meconium, moderate/heavy[5]	916,713	48,858	53.4	57.1	54.4	53.3	51.8	50.7	49.6	1,323
Breech/malpresentation	918,129	51,165	57.4	48.7	49.9	54.5	62.9	74.6	88.8	26,741
Precipitous labor[5]	916,713	20,600	22.5	15.1	20.5	24.9	25.2	24.4	23.4	1,956
Congenital Anomalies										
Anencephaly	918,129	88	9.6	*	9.9	9.3	*	*	*	3,792
Meningomyelocele/Spina Bifida	918,129	132	14.4	*	16.5	12.5	14.1	*	*	3,792
Congenital diaphragmatic hernia	918,129	92	10.1	*	8.6	9.7	11.5	*	*	3,792
Omphalocele/Gastroschisis	918,129	322	35.2	91.1	53.5	18.2	12.5	*	*	3,792
Cleft lip/palate	918,129	526	57.5	52.3	58.9	56.6	50.1	66.4	100.4	3,792
Down syndrome	918,129	416	45.5	21.7	18.5	23.9	31.8	134.8	397.2	3,792

* = Figure does not meet standards of reliability or precision; precision; based on fewer than 20 births in the numerator.   [1]Total number of births to residents of areas reporting risk factors, procedure or anomaly. [2]No response reported for specific item. [3]Includes races not shown. [4]Data on tocolysis for Arkansas and Delaware are excluded. [5]Excludes data for Delaware. [6]Race and Hispanic origin are reported separately on birth certificates. Persons of Hispanic origin may be of any race. Multiple-race data, when reported, were bridged to single-race categories in order to maintain comparability among all reported areas. [7]Includes all persons of Hispanic origin of any race.

Table 1-49. Pregnancy Risk Factors, by Age and Race and Hispanic Origin of Mother, 27 Reporting States, 2008

(Number; rates are number of live births with specified risk factor per 1,000 live births in specified group.)

Risk factor and race and Hispanic origin of mother	All birth[1]	Factor reported	All ages	Under 20 years	20 to 24 years	25 to 29 years	30–34 years	35–39 years	40–54 years	Not stated[2]
All Races [3]										
Diabetes										
Prepregnancy (diagnosis prior to this pregnancy)	2,748,302	17,688	6.5	2.3	4.2	6.1	8.3	11.3	14.9	38,770
Gestational (diagnosis in this pregnancy)	2,748,302	110,140	40.6	12.7	23.7	38.5	54.2	70.6	88.6	38,770
Hypertension										
Prepregnancy (chronic)	2,748,302	29,989	11.1	4.5	6.8	10.0	13.6	19.4	30.6	38,770
Gestational (PIH, preeclampsia)[4]	2,748,302	104,850	38.7	41.3	38.0	37.8	37.0	40.7	50.2	38,770
Eclampsia[5]	2,128,437	3,818	1.8	2.6	1.9	1.6	1.6	1.8	2.2	30,752
Previous preterm birth	2,748,302	50,575	18.7	6.4	17.1	20.6	21.0	23.0	23.5	38,770
Other previous poor pregnancy outcome	2,748,302	50,811	18.8	6.7	15.1	19.2	22.1	27.0	32.5	38,770
Mother had a previous cesarean delivery[6]	1,782,194	346,180	196.4	117.8	163.4	184.0	214.8	247.5	254.7	19,811
White [7]										
Diabetes										
Prepregnancy (diagnosis prior to this pregnancy)	1,366,527	7,979	5.9	2.3	4.3	5.6	6.9	8.5	10.4	8,697
Gestational (diagnosis in this pregnancy)	1,366,527	53,107	39.1	15.0	25.3	36.6	47.3	60.7	74.6	8,697
Hypertension										
Prepregnancy (chronic)	1,366,527	15,902	11.7	5.1	7.5	10.7	13.8	18.3	27.0	8,697
Gestational (PIH, preeclampsia)[4]	1,366,527	59,692	44.0	47.2	45.0	44.6	40.7	43.2	52.5	8,697
Eclampsia[5]	947,743	1,905	2.0	2.7	2.2	1.9	1.8	2.0	2.4	6,995
Previous preterm birth	1,366,527	28,742	21.2	7.0	19.2	22.3	23.1	25.6	26.6	8,697
Other previous poor pregnancy outcome	1,366,527	31,636	23.3	8.5	18.4	22.6	26.3	32.9	40.5	8,697
Mother had a previous cesarean delivery[6]	871,960	165,349	190.4	105.2	153.0	172.2	206.3	242.8	252.6	3,396
Black [7]										
Diabetes										
Prepregnancy (diagnosis prior to this pregnancy)	349,243	3,139	9.2	2.8	5.5	9.2	14.0	21.9	26.4	8,702
Gestational (diagnosis in this pregnancy)	349,243	11,892	34.9	11.5	20.9	37.7	54.9	72.2	88.1	8,702
Hypertension										
Prepregnancy (chronic)	349,243	7,749	22.8	7.5	11.8	22.2	36.0	54.2	81.3	8,702
Gestational (PIH, preeclampsia)[4]	349,243	16,738	49.2	48.9	44.7	47.5	54.1	57.5	64.9	8,702
Eclampsia[5]	259,004	761	3.0	3.9	2.9	2.6	2.8	3.5	3.8	8,292
Previous preterm birth	349,243	9,599	28.2	9.0	24.7	35.2	36.6	39.4	35.4	8,702
Other previous poor pregnancy outcome	349,243	8,064	23.7	9.0	20.6	27.8	31.5	33.6	35.2	8,702
Mother had a previous cesarean delivery[6]	228,425	44,549	198.1	125.4	176.4	198.8	219.0	249.6	248.8	3,523
Hispanic [8]										
Diabetes										
Prepregnancy (diagnosis prior to this pregnancy)	787,484	5,003	6.4	1.8	3.3	5.7	10.0	14.0	20.4	5,195
Gestational (diagnosis in this pregnancy)	787,484	31,442	40.2	11.1	22.0	38.6	61.4	84.1	110.2	5,195
Hypertension										
Prepregnancy (chronic)	787,484	4,588	5.9	2.6	3.6	4.9	8.1	12.0	22.2	5,195
Gestational (PIH, preeclampsia)[4]	787,484	22,350	28.6	32.3	26.5	24.9	28.7	34.9	46.2	5,195
Eclampsia[5]	721,835	942	1.3	2.0	1.3	1.0	1.2	1.5	1.5	4,736
Previous preterm birth	787,484	9,136	11.7	4.4	10.7	13.4	14.3	14.8	15.4	5,195
Other previous poor pregnancy outcome	787,484	7,933	10.1	3.7	8.1	11.0	13.0	16.1	17.4	5,195
Mother had a previous cesarean delivery[6]	533,199	109,848	207.0	127.0	174.2	201.2	233.6	260.7	266.2	2,618

[1]Refers to total number of births to residents of areas reporting specified pregnancy risk factor.   [2]No response reported for pregnancy risk factor; includes births to residents of states using the 2003 U.S. Standard Certificate of Live Birth occurring in states using the 1989 U.S. Standard Certificate of Live Birth.   [3]Includes other races not shown and origin not stated.   [4]PIH is pregnancy-induced hypertension. Includes California, Colorado, Delaware, Florida, Georgia, Idaho, Indiana, Iowa, Kansas, Kentucky, Michigan, Montana, Nebraska, New Hampshire, New Mexico, New York, North Dakota, Ohio, Oregon, Pennsylvania, South Carolina, South Dakota, Tennessee, Texas, Vermont, Washington, and Wyoming. Births to residents of states using the 2003 U.S. Standard Certificate of Live Birth occurring in states using the 1989 Standard Certificate of Live Birth (0.6 percent) are included in the "not stated" category.   [5]Excludes data for Idaho, Kentucky, Michigan, Nebraska, New York City, Pennsylvania, South Carolina, Tennessee, and Washington, which did not report eclampsia.   [6]Excludes women who have not had a previous pregnancy and for whom total birth order is unknown.   [7]Race and Hispanic origin are reported separately on the birth certificate.   [8]Persons of Hispanic origin may be of any race.

Table 1-50. Births Delivered by Forceps or Vacuum Extraction, Selected Years, 1990–2011

(Percent.)

Year and type of birth	Forceps	Vacuum extraction	Forceps or vacuum
All Births			
1990[1]	5.1	3.9	9.0
1995	3.5	5.9	9.4
2000	2.1	4.9	7.0
1005	0.9	3.9	4.8
2007	0.8	3.5	4.2
2008	0.7	3.2	3.9
2009	0.7	3.0	3.7
2010	0.7	3.0	3.6
2011	0.7	2.9	3.5

[1]Excludes data for Oklahoma, which did not require reporting method of delivery.

Table 1-51. Births, by Method of Delivery and Race and Hispanic Origin of Mother, 1989–2011

(Number, rate.)

Year	All births	Vaginal				Cesarean							
		Number				Number				Percentage of all live births by cesarean delivery			
		Total[1]	Non-Hispanic White[2]	Non-Hispanic Black[2]	Hispanic[3]	Total[1]	Non-Hispanic White[2]	Non-Hispanic Black[2]	Hispanic[3]	Total[1]	Non-Hispanic White[2]	Non-Hispanic Black[2]	Hispanic[3]
1989 [4]	3,798,734	2,793,463	1,806,753	440,310	385,462	826,955	556,585	125,290	105,268	22.8	23.6	22.2	21.5
1990 [5]	4,110,563	3,111,421	1,972,754	503,720	458,242	914,096	603,467	142,838	122,969	22.7	23.4	22.1	21.2
1991 [6]	4,110,907	3,100,891	1,941,726	507,522	472,126	905,077	587,802	142,417	129,752	22.6	23.2	21.9	21.6
1992 [6]	4,065,014	3,100,710	1,916,414	502,669	494,338	888,622	566,788	143,153	133,369	22.3	22.8	22.2	21.2
1993	4,000,240	3,098,796	1,902,433	496,333	514,493	861,987	542,013	139,702	136,279	21.8	22.2	22.0	20.9
1994	3,952,767	3,087,576	1,896,609	480,551	525,928	830,517	518,021	134,526	135,569	21.2	21.5	21.9	20.5
1995	3,899,589	3,063,724	1,867,024	457,104	539,731	806,722	496,103	127,171	136,640	20.8	21.0	21.8	20.2
1996	3,891,494	3,061,092	1,851,058	449,544	558,105	797,119	485,530	124,836	139,554	20.7	20.8	21.7	20.0
1997	3,880,894	3,046,621	1,829,213	451,744	563,114	799,033	481,982	126,138	142,907	20.8	20.9	21.8	20.2
1998	3,941,553	3,078,537	1,842,420	457,186	580,143	825,870	495,550	131,999	150,317	21.2	21.2	22.4	20.6
1999	3,959,417	3,063,870	1,810,682	449,580	599,118	862,086	514,051	135,508	161,035	22.0	22.1	23.2	21.2
2000	4,058,814	3,108,188	1,804,550	454,736	633,220	923,991	540,794	146,042	179,583	22.9	23.1	24.3	22.1
2001	4,025,933	3,027,993	1,746,551	435,455	648,821	978,411	567,488	151,908	199,874	24.4	24.5	25.9	23.6
2002	4,021,726	2,958,423	1,687,144	416,516	653,516	1,043,846	598,682	159,297	219,777	26.1	26.2	27.7	25.2
2003	4,089,950	2,949,853	1,671,414	405,671	667,656	1,119,388	637,482	167,506	241,159	27.5	27.6	29.2	26.5
2004	4,112,052	2,903,341	1,617,994	397,877	679,118	1,190,210	667,836	178,461	263,454	29.1	29.2	31.0	28.0
2005	4,138,349	2,873,918	1,579,613	392,064	698,089	1,248,815	690,260	189,287	285,376	30.3	30.4	32.6	29.0
2006	4,265,555	2,929,590	1,580,794	411,097	728,854	1,321,054	718,960	203,723	307,981	31.1	31.3	33.1	29.7
2007	4,316,233	2,933,056	1,565,555	413,088	737,478	1,367,340	735,744	211,615	322,554	31.8	32.0	33.9	30.4
2008	4,247,694	2,864,343	1,527,340	406,379	716,811	1,369,273	732,641	214,416	321,859	32.3	32.4	34.5	31.0
2009	4,130,665	2,764,285	1,481,660	392,715	682,512	1,353,572	723,687	214,810	315,025	32.9	32.8	35.4	31.6
2010	3,999,386	2,680,947	1,454,861	379,617	643,682	1,309,182	702,548	208,520	300,138	32.8	32.6	35.5	31.8
2011	3,953,590	2,651,428	1,447,969	374,978	623,010	1,293,267	693,591	206,009	293,816	32.8	32.4	35.5	32.0

[1]Includes races other than White and Black and origin not stated.   [2]Race and Hispanic origin are reported separately on birth certificates. Persons of Hispanic origin may be of any race. Multiple-race data, when reported, were bridged to single-race categories in order to maintain comparability among all reported areas.   [3]Includes all persons of Hispanic origin of any race.   [4]Excludes data for Louisiana, Maryland, Nebraska, Nevada, and Oklahoma, which did not report method of delivery on the birth certificate; data by Hispanic origin also excludes New Hampshire, which did not report Hispanic origin.   [5]Excludes data for New Hampshire and Oklahoma, which did not report data by Hispanic origin. Oklahoma did not report method of delivery.   [6]Excludes data for New Hampshire, which did not report Hispanic origin.

Table 1-52. Births, by Method of Delivery and Age, Race, and Hispanic Origin of Mother, 2011

(Number; rate of cesarean delivery.)

Age, race, and Hispanic origin of mother	Number				Cesarean delivery rate[1]
	All births	Vaginal	Cesarean	Not stated	
All Races [2]	3,953,590	2,651,428	1,293,267	8,895	32.8
Under 20 years	333,746	258,683	74,508	555	22.4
20 to 24 years	925,200	664,885	258,298	2,017	28.0
25 to 29 years	1,127,583	770,437	354,571	2,575	31.5
30 to 34 years	986,682	631,051	353,369	2,262	35.9
35 to 39 years	463,849	267,302	195,410	1,137	42.2
40 years and over	116,530	59,070	57,111	349	49.2
Non-Hispanic White [3]	2,146,566	1,447,969	693,591	5,006	32.4
Under 20 years	130,198	100,701	29,247	250	22.5
20 to 24 years	451,939	327,599	123,269	1,071	27.3
25 to 29 years	647,520	448,462	197,585	1,473	30.6
30 to 34 years	591,266	384,477	205,447	1,342	34.8
35 to 39 years	260,596	153,110	106,810	676	41.1
40 years and over	65,047	33,620	31,233	194	48.2
Non-Hispanic Black [3]	582,345	374,978	206,009	1,358	35.5
Under 20 years	79,936	60,061	19,726	149	24.7
20 to 24 years	186,229	127,147	58,690	392	31.6
25 to 29 years	147,708	93,839	53,526	343	36.3
30 to 34 years	104,274	61,070	42,901	303	41.3
35 to 39 years	50,245	26,438	23,677	130	47.2
40 years and over	13,953	6,423	7,489	41	53.8
Hispanic [4]	918,129	623,010	293,816	1,303	32.0
Under 20 years	111,236	87,718	23,397	121	21.1
20 to 24 years	243,724	177,357	66,031	336	27.1
25 to 29 years	248,269	168,953	78,945	371	31.8
30 to 34 years	192,517	121,120	71,118	279	37.0
35 to 39 years	98,340	55,671	42,517	152	43.3
40 years and over	24,043	12,191	11,808	44	49.2

[1]Percentage of all live births by cesarean delivery.   [2]Includes races other than White and Black and origin not stated.   [3]Race and Hispanic origin are reported separately on birth certificates. Persons of Hispanic origin may be of any race. Multiple-race data, when reported, were bridged to single-race categories in order to maintain comparability among all reported areas.   [4]Includes all persons of Hispanic origin of any race.

Figure 1-10. Cesarean Deliveries, by Age of Mother, 2011 and Preliminary 2012

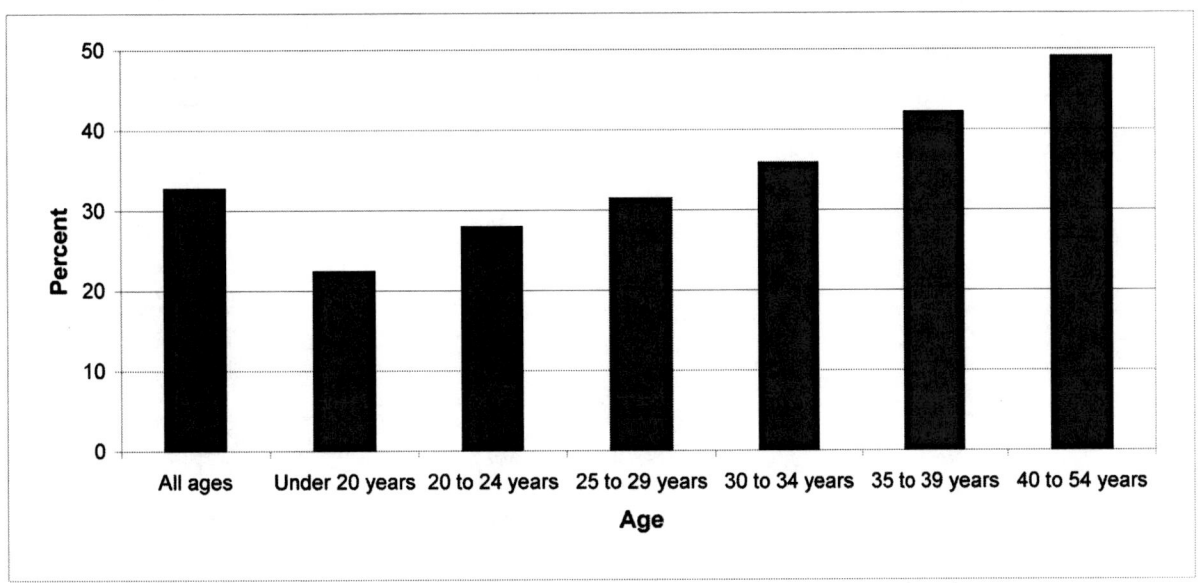

Figure 1-11. Percent of Births with Low and Very Low Birthweights, Selected Years, 1986–2011

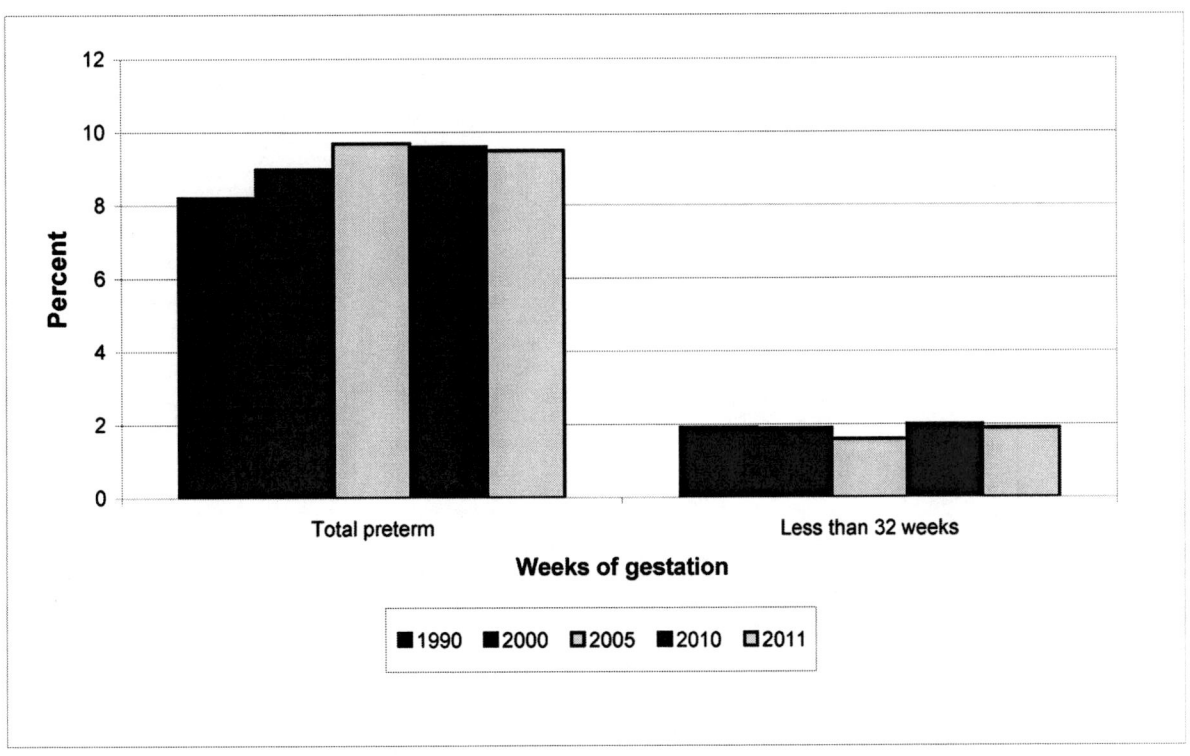

Table 1-53. Cesarean Deliveries, by Race and Hispanic Origin of Mother, by State and Territory of Residence, 2011

(Percent.)

| State and territory | Total cesarean delivery rate[1] | | | |
| | All races[2] | Non-Hispanic | | Hispanic[4] |
		White[3]	Black[3]	
United States [5]	32.8	32.4	35.5	32.0
Alabama	35.1	35.4	37.1	25.2
Alaska	22.4	25.0	29.5	28.0
Arizona	27.6	29.0	31.3	25.7
Arkansas	34.3	34.6	35.1	30.5
California	33.2	32.7	37.7	32.9
Colorado	25.3	26.2	26.8	22.3
Connecticut	35.8	36.0	38.6	33.4
Delaware	32.5	33.0	33.3	29.1
District of Columbia	33.9	33.3	35.7	28.8
Florida	38.1	36.1	37.8	41.5
Georgia	33.6	33.8	35.7	27.7
Hawaii	26.0	24.2	31.0	26.4
Idaho	24.5	23.7	30.4	27.3
Illinois	31.7	32.5	31.6	28.8
Indiana	30.6	30.5	32.7	28.5
Iowa	30.5	30.2	32.0	31.7
Kansas	30.2	30.8	32.1	26.7
Kentucky	36.3	36.6	36.8	32.5
Louisiana	39.9	41.1	39.2	35.3
Maine	30.9	30.8	30.7	34.3
Maryland	34.8	33.2	38.2	31.1
Massachusetts	32.5	33.0	33.5	31.2
Michigan	32.8	32.8	32.9	30.6
Minnesota	26.8	27.3	29.0	25.0
Mississippi	38.0	38.7	38.3	28.2
Missouri	31.4	31.6	31.4	28.5
Montana	29.5	28.6	32.4	34.7
Nebraska	30.8	31.4	30.7	28.5
Nevada	33.8	34.3	40.4	30.8
New Hampshire	30.8	30.6	33.8	31.5
New Jersey	39.1	38.9	40.5	37.7
New Mexico	23.0	24.3	27.9	23.0
New York	34.3	33.8	37.8	33.5
North Carolina	30.4	31.3	32.4	24.3
North Dakota	28.7	28.4	22.0	28.7
Ohio	31.2	31.2	31.8	29.3
Oklahoma	34.2	34.7	35.7	29.9
Oregon	28.9	28.8	31.2	27.0
Pennsylvania	31.4	31.5	31.2	30.6
Rhode Island	32.8	35.0	32.3	28.8
South Carolina	35.2	35.2	36.5	29.5
South Dakota	25.3	24.8	24.1	25.7
Tennessee	33.5	34.0	34.0	28.4
Texas	35.3	35.6	37.9	34.5
Utah	22.7	22.2	30.5	23.5
Vermont	27.8	27.8	25.8	31.9
Virginia	34.1	33.4	35.5	31.3
Washington	28.8	28.1	32.4	27.4
West Virginia	36.8	36.9	38.5	31.2
Wisconsin	25.8	26.6	23.8	24.3
Wyoming	26.9	26.6	*	27.9
Puerto Rico	46.7	43.1	55.6	46.8
Virgin Islands	27.8	22.9	27.8	30.8
Guam	24.1	19.2	*	
American Samoa	NA	NA	NA	NA
Northern Marianas	NA	NA	NA	NA

NA = Not available.   * = Figure does not meet standards of reliability or precision.   [1]Percent of all live births by cesarean delivery.   [2]Includes races other than White and Black and origin not stated.   [3]Race and Hispanic origin are reported separately on birth certificates. Persons of Hispanic origin may be of any race. Multiple-race data, when reported, were bridged to single-race categories in order to maintain comparability among all reported areas   [4]Includes all persons of Hispanic origin of any race.   [5]Excludes data for the territories.

Table 1-54. Births, by Birthweight, Gestational Age, and Race and Hispanic Origin of Mother, 2011

(Number, percent.)

| Birthweight[1], race, and Hispanic origin of mother | All births | Period of gestation[2] | | | | | | | | | Postterm | Not stated |
| | | Preterm | | | | | Term | | | | | |
		Total under 37 weeks	Under 28 weeks	28 to 31 weeks	32 to 33 weeks	34 to 36 weeks	Total, 37 to 41 weeks	37 to 38 weeks	39 weeks	40 to 41 weeks	42 weeks and over	
ALL RACES [3]												
Total	3,953,590	463,163	28,762	47,437	59,831	327,133	3,265,736	1,021,205	1,152,661	1,091,870	219,845	4,846
Less than 500 grams	5,942	5,886	5,664	203	7	12	19	9	7	3	3	34
500 to 999 grams	21,289	21,073	15,767	4,850	305	151	149	66	51	32	18	49
1,000 to 1,499 grams	29,523	27,688	3,872	16,024	4,989	2,803	1,537	743	371	423	256	42
1,500 to 1,999 grams	62,504	52,633	781	11,519	18,545	21,788	9,001	6,013	1,600	1,388	796	74
2,000 to 2,499 grams	200,453	102,427	609	3,609	16,619	81,590	93,054	60,841	18,908	13,305	4,746	226
2,500 to 2,999 grams	728,201	123,043	1,102	3,943	8,185	109,813	573,268	272,293	177,375	123,600	31,191	699
3,000 to 3,499 grams	1,545,355	87,840	–	4,698	7,117	76,025	1,368,985	428,553	505,148	435,284	87,387	1,143
3,500 to 3,999 grams	1,048,902	33,718	–	2,481	3,276	27,961	943,592	204,471	351,612	387,509	70,934	658
4,000 to 4,499 grams	265,040	6,231	–	–	585	5,646	237,789	40,897	84,346	112,546	20,831	189
4,500 to 4,999 grams	37,475	1,027	–	–	88	939	33,190	5,902	11,456	15,832	3,224	34
5,000 grams or more	4,357	190	–	–	17	173	3,800	983	1,332	1,485	356	11
Not stated	4,549	1,407	967	110	98	232	1,352	434	455	463	103	1,687
Percent												
Very low birthweight[4]	1.1	10.5	90.8	44.5	8.7	0.9	0.0	0.1	0.0	0.0	0.1	3.2
Low birthweight[5]	7.1	45.0	96.0	77.8	71.6	32.6	2.7	6.0	1.5	1.1	2.3	11.4
NON-HISPANIC WHITE [6]												
Total	2,146,566	225,150	11,225	21,884	28,645	163,396	1,796,185	528,419	644,131	623,635	122,851	2,380
Less than 500 grams	2,190	2,161	2,055	96	6	4	13	6	5	2	3	13
500 to 999 grams	8,629	8,521	6,169	2,139	141	72	80	32	30	18	13	15
1,000 to 1,499 grams	13,642	12,817	1,641	7,485	2,333	1,358	697	320	180	197	109	19
1,500 to 1,999 grams	30,532	25,880	300	5,676	9,336	10,568	4,237	2,784	779	674	388	27
2,000 to 2,499 grams	97,054	51,708	262	1,580	8,645	41,221	42,978	28,371	8,569	6,038	2,272	96
2,500 to 2,999 grams	344,184	61,138	432	1,539	3,422	55,745	267,855	127,708	82,836	57,311	14,886	305
3,000 to 3,499 grams	816,932	41,955	–	2,042	2,827	37,086	728,129	222,147	271,373	234,609	46,325	523
3,500 to 3,999 grams	631,614	16,550	–	1,269	1,522	13,759	571,918	118,359	216,035	237,524	42,803	343
4,000 to 4,499 grams	172,430	3,189	–	–	305	2,884	155,501	24,498	55,675	75,328	13,619	121
4,500 to 4,999 grams	24,456	523	–	–	50	473	21,752	3,442	7,585	10,725	2,158	23
5,000 grams or more	2,559	87	–	–	7	80	2,245	511	795	939	223	4
Not stated	2,344	621	366	58	51	146	780	241	269	270	52	891
Percent												
Very low birthweight[4]	1.2	10.3	91.1	44.4	8.7	0.8	0.0	0.1	0.0	0.0	0.1	3.1
Low birthweight[5]	7.2	44.2	96	78.1	71.4	31.8	2.7	5.5	1.5	1.2	2.3	12.2
NON-HISPANIC BLACK [6]												
Total	582,345	97,543	9,879	11,966	13,245	62,453	454,302	162,978	154,675	136,649	29,672	828
Less than 500 grams	2,222	2,206	2,137	62	1	6	4	3	–	1	–	12
500 to 999 grams	7,100	7,044	5,414	1,507	76	47	35	19	8	8	2	19
1,000 to 1,499 grams	8,039	7,511	1,190	4,318	1,331	672	442	226	87	129	75	11
1,500 to 1,999 grams	14,850	12,401	270	2,551	4,295	5,285	2,241	1,479	418	344	186	22
2,000 to 2,499 grams	45,307	21,760	183	909	3,207	17,461	22,300	14,409	4,682	3,209	1,181	66
2,500 to 2,999 grams	147,180	24,368	344	1,140	2,048	20,836	116,127	55,364	35,752	25,011	6,491	194
3,000 to 3,499 grams	225,648	15,829	–	1,057	1,652	13,120	196,738	64,418	71,885	60,435	12,813	268
3,500 to 3,999 grams	106,629	4,997	–	398	522	4,077	94,447	22,379	34,262	37,806	7,092	93
4,000 to 4,499 grams	21,216	845	–	–	76	769	18,806	3,854	6,520	8,432	1,547	18
4,500 to 4,999 grams	2,884	122	–	–	11	111	2,530	613	845	1,072	230	2
5,000 grams or more	393	25	–	–	3	22	336	102	116	118	29	3
Not stated	877	435	341	24	23	47	296	112	100	84	26	120
Percent												
Very low birthweight[4]	3.0	17.3	91.6	49.3	10.6	1.2	0.1	0.2	0.1	0.1	0.3	5.9
Low birthweight[5]	13.3	52.4	96.4	78.3	67.4	37.6	5.5	9.9	3.4	2.7	4.9	18.4
HISPANIC [7]												
Total	918,129	106,884	5,824	10,330	13,705	77,025	758,222	247,458	263,232	247,532	52,243	780
Less than 500 grams	1,115	1,106	1,068	36	–	2	2	–	2	–	–	7
500 to 999 grams	4,195	4,161	3,210	863	66	22	25	6	13	6	1	8
1,000 to 1,499 grams	5,712	5,361	819	3,076	929	537	293	144	78	71	54	4
1,500 to 1,999 grams	12,281	10,310	162	2,523	3,554	4,071	1,787	1,214	288	285	172	12
2,000 to 2,499 grams	41,146	21,066	134	902	3,612	16,418	19,092	12,229	3,923	2,940	953	35
2,500 to 2,999 grams	168,690	28,375	256	990	2,135	24,994	132,887	63,263	40,581	29,043	7,307	121
3,000 to 3,499 grams	376,835	24,012	–	1,260	2,180	20,572	330,750	107,686	119,925	103,139	21,843	230
3,500 to 3,999 grams	241,873	10,088	–	669	1,026	8,393	214,916	50,844	78,007	86,065	16,731	138
4,000 to 4,499 grams	56,503	1,812	–	–	167	1,645	50,255	10,212	17,595	22,448	4,408	28
4,500 to 4,999 grams	8,074	312	–	–	20	292	7,083	1,512	2,431	3,140	674	5
5,000 grams or more	1,105	58	–	–	4	54	959	300	334	325	84	4
Not stated	600	223	175	11	12	25	173	48	55	70	16	188
Percent												
Very low birthweight[4]	1.2	10.0	90.2	38.5	7.3	0.7	0.0	0.1	0.0	0.0	0.1	*
Low birthweight[5]	7.0	39.4	95.5	71.7	59.6	27.3	2.8	5.5	1.6	1.3	2.3	11.1

* = Figure does not meet the standards for reliability or precision.   – = Quantity zero.   0.0 = Quantity more than zero but less than 0.05.   [1]Equivalents of the gram weights in pounds and ounces are shown in Notes.   [2]Expressed in completed weeks.   [3]Includes races other than White and Black and origin not stated.   [4]Birthweight of less than 1,500 grams (3 lb 4 oz).   [5]Birthweight of less than 2,500 grams (5 lb 8 oz).   [6]Race and Hispanic origin are reported separately on birth certificates. Persons of Hispanic origin may be of any race. Multiple-race data, when reported, were bridged to single-race categories in order to maintain comparability among all reported areas   [7]Includes all persons of Hispanic origin of any race.

Table 1-55A. Very Preterm and Preterm Births, by Race and Hispanic Origin of Mother, 1981–2011

(Percent.)

Year	Very preterm[1]				Preterm[2]			
	All races[3]	Non-Hispanic		Hispanic[5]	All races[3]	Non-Hispanic		Hispanic[5]
		White[4]	Black[4]			White[4]	Black[4]	
1981	1.81	---	---	---	9.44	---	---	---
1982	1.84	---	---	---	9.50	---	---	---
1983	1.86	---	---	---	9.61	---	---	---
1984	1.83	---	---	---	9.40	---	---	---
1985	1.88	---	---	---	9.76	---	---	---
1986	1.90	---	---	---	9.97	---	---	---
1987	1.96	---	---	---	10.20	---	---	---
1988	1.96	---	---	---	10.22	---	---	---
1989[6]	1.95	1.34	4.68	1.76	10.58	8.40	19.05	11.10
1990[7]	1.92	1.33	4.63	1.69	10.62	8.50	18.89	10.96
1991[8]	1.94	1.35	4.65	1.65	10.82	8.73	19.00	10.96
1992[8]	1.91	1.33	4.50	1.64	10.69	8.72	18.49	10.75
1993	1.93	1.39	4.45	1.67	10.99	9.08	18.58	10.98
1994	1.91	1.39	4.36	1.67	11.02	9.27	18.18	10.94
1995	1.89	1.41	4.29	1.66	10.99	9.40	17.77	10.91
1996	1.89	1.43	4.17	1.66	10.99	9.50	17.51	10.89
1997	1.94	1.49	4.19	1.68	11.36	9.94	17.61	11.20
1998	1.96	1.52	4.15	1.72	11.69	10.24	17.60	11.43
1999	1.96	1.54	4.18	1.68	11.77	10.52	17.63	11.43
2000	1.93	1.51	4.09	1.69	11.64	10.43	17.41	11.24
2001	1.95	1.55	4.05	1.69	11.95	10.81	17.63	11.45
2002	1.96	1.56	4.04	1.72	12.08	10.98	17.66	11.61
2003	1.97	1.60	3.99	1.73	12.33	11.30	17.83	11.87
2004	2.01	1.63	4.05	1.77	12.49	11.50	17.91	12.00
2005	2.03	1.64	4.17	1.79	12.73	11.69	18.43	12.13
2006	2.04	1.66	4.08	1.80	12.80	11.70	18.46	12.25
2007	2.04	1.64	4.08	1.82	12.68	11.50	18.29	12.29
2008	1.99	1.60	3.84	1.80	12.33	11.14	17.54	12.10
2009	1.97	1.57	3.87	1.77	12.18	10.92	17.47	11.97
2010	1.96	1.58	3.79	1.78	11.99	10.77	17.12	11.79
2011	1.93	1.54	3.76	1.76	11.73	10.50	16.77	11.65

NA = Not available.   [1]Births of less than 32 completed weeks of gestation.   [2]Births of less than 37 completed weeks of gestation.   [3]Includes races other than White and Black and origin not stated.   [4]Race and Hispanic origin are reported separately on birth certificates. Persons of Hispanic origin may be of any race. Multiple-race data, when reported, were bridged to single-race categories in order to maintain comparability among all reported areas.   [5]Includes all persons of Hispanic origin of any race.   [6]Data by Hispanic origin exclude New Hampshire, Oklahoma, and Louisiana, which did not report Hispanic origin.   [7]Data by Hispanic origin exclude New Hampshire and Oklahoma, which did not report Hispanic origin.   [8]Data by Hispanic origin exclude New Hampshire, which did not report Hispanic origin.

Table 1-55B. Very Low Birthweight and Low Birthweight Births, by Race and Hispanic Origin of Mother, 1981–2011

(Percent.)

Year	Very low birthweight[1]				Low birthweight[2]			
	All races[3]	Non-Hispanic		Hispanic[5]	All races[3]	Non-Hispanic		Hispanic[5]
		White[4]	Black[4]			White[4]	Black[4]	
1981	1.16	---	---	---	6.81	---	---	---
1982	1.18	---	---	---	6.75	---	---	---
1983	1.19	---	---	---	6.82	---	---	---
1984	1.19	---	---	---	6.72	---	---	---
1985	1.21	---	---	---	6.75	---	---	---
1986	1.21	---	---	---	6.81	---	---	---
1987	1.24	---	---	---	6.90	---	---	---
1988	1.24	---	---	---	6.93	---	---	---
1989[6]	1.28	0.93	2.97	1.05	7.05	5.62	13.61	6.18
1990[7]	1.27	0.93	2.93	1.03	6.97	5.61	13.32	6.06
1991[8]	1.29	0.94	2.97	1.02	7.12	5.72	13.62	6.15
1992[8]	1.29	0.94	2.97	1.04	7.08	5.73	13.40	6.10
1993	1.33	1.00	2.99	1.06	7.22	5.92	13.43	6.24
1994	1.33	1.01	2.99	1.08	7.28	6.06	13.34	6.25
1995	1.35	1.04	2.98	1.11	7.32	6.20	13.21	6.29
1996	1.37	1.08	3.02	1.12	7.39	6.36	13.12	6.28
1997	1.42	1.12	3.05	1.13	7.51	6.47	13.11	6.42
1998	1.45	1.15	3.11	1.15	7.57	6.55	13.17	6.44
1999	1.45	1.15	3.18	1.14	7.62	6.64	13.23	6.38
2000	1.43	1.14	3.10	1.14	7.57	6.60	13.13	6.41
2001	1.44	1.17	3.08	1.14	7.68	6.76	13.07	6.47
2002	1.46	1.17	3.15	1.17	7.82	6.91	13.39	6.55
2003	1.45	1.18	3.12	1.16	7.93	7.04	13.55	6.69
2004	1.48	1.20	3.15	1.20	8.08	7.20	13.74	6.79
2005	1.49	1.21	3.27	1.20	8.19	7.29	14.02	6.88
2006	1.49	1.20	3.15	1.19	8.26	7.32	13.97	6.99
2007	1.49	1.19	3.20	1.21	8.22	7.28	13.90	6.93
2008	1.46	1.18	3.01	1.20	8.18	7.22	13.71	6.96
2009	1.45	1.16	3.06	1.19	8.16	7.19	13.61	6.94
2010	1.45	1.16	2.98	1.20	8.15	7.14	13.53	6.97
2011	1.44	1.14	2.99	1.20	8.10	7.09	13.33	7.02

NA = Not available. [1]Less than 1,500 grams (3 lb. 4 oz.). [2]Less than 2,500 grams (5 lb. 8 oz.). [3]Includes races other than White and Black and origin not stated. [4]Race and Hispanic origin are reported separately on birth certificates. Persons of Hispanic origin may be of any race. Multiple-race data, when reported, were bridged to single-race categories in order to maintain comparability among all reported areas. [5]Includes all persons of Hispanic origin of any race. [6]Data by Hispanic origin exclude New Hampshire, Oklahoma, and Louisiana, which did not report Hispanic origin. [7]Data by Hispanic origin exclude New Hampshire and Oklahoma, which did not report Hispanic origin. [8]Data by Hispanic origin exclude New Hampshire, which did not report Hispanic origin.

Table 1-56. Birthweight Distribution in 500-Gram Intervals, Selected Years, 1990–2011

(Percent.)

Weight	All births					Percent change		
	1990	2006	2008	2009	2011	1990–2009	1990–2011	2009–2011
Less than 1,000 grams	0.63	0.72	0.70	0.70	0.69	11.1	9.7	-1.3
1,000–1,499 grams	0.65	0.76	0.75	0.75	0.75	15.4	14.9	-0.4
1,500–1,999 grams	1.33	1.63	1.58	1.59	1.58	19.5	18.9	-0.6
2,000–2,499 grams	4.37	5.15	5.14	5.12	5.07	17.2	16.0	-1.0
2,500–2,999 grams	16.03	18.44	18.57	18.59	18.42	16.0	14.9	-0.9
3,000–3,499 grams	36.71	38.87	39.20	39.22	39.09	6.8	6.5	-0.3
3,500–3,999 grams	29.40	26.61	26.41	26.43	26.53	-10.1	-9.8	0.4
4,000–4,499 grams	9.10	6.75	6.60	6.57	6.70	-27.8	-26.3	2.0
4,500–4,999 grams	1.59	0.96	0.92	0.92	0.95	-42.1	-40.4	3.0
5,000 grams or more	0.19	0.11	0.10	0.10	0.11	-47.4	-39.6	14.8

Table 1-57. Preterm and Low Birthweight Births, by Age and Race and Hispanic Origin of Mother, 2011

(Percent, number.)

Age, race, and Hispanic origin of mother	Preterm[1]							Low birthweight[2]						
	Percent			Number				Percent			Number			
	Total	Early[3]	Late[4]	Total	Early[3]	Late[4]	Unknown	Total	Very[5]	Moder-ately[6]	Total	Very[5]	Moder-ately[6]	Unknown
All Races[7]														
All ages	11.7	3.4	8.3	463,163	136,030	327,133	4,846	8.1	1.4	6.7	319,711	56,754	262,957	4,549
Under 15 years	21.1	7.9	13.2	835	314	521	21	11.7	2.7	9.0	463	108	355	9
15 to 19 years	13.5	4.4	9.1	44,507	14,496	30,011	438	9.6	1.7	7.9	31,584	5,615	25,969	325
15 years	16.5	6.0	10.6	1,933	696	1,237	39	10.5	2.2	8.3	1,228	256	972	13
16 years	15.4	5.4	10.0	4,468	1,574	2,894	47	9.8	1.9	7.9	2,853	564	2,289	26
17 years	14.2	4.8	9.5	7,779	2,595	5,184	75	9.9	1.7	8.2	5,411	941	4,470	55
18 years	13.5	4.4	9.1	12,480	4,059	8,421	113	9.7	1.7	8.0	8,941	1,564	7,377	95
19 years	12.6	3.9	8.7	17,847	5,572	12,275	164	9.3	1.6	7.7	13,151	2,290	10,861	136
20 to 24 years	11.7	3.5	8.2	107,858	31,916	75,942	1,127	8.3	1.4	6.9	76,840	13,255	63,585	986
25 to 29 years	10.7	3.0	7.7	120,486	34,218	86,268	1,449	7.3	1.3	6.1	82,356	14,241	68,115	1,331
30 to 34 years	11.1	3.2	7.9	109,509	31,303	78,206	1,108	7.5	1.4	6.2	74,256	13,387	60,869	1,131
35 to 39 years	13.2	3.9	9.3	60,980	17,894	43,086	539	8.8	1.6	7.2	40,821	7,590	33,231	602
40 to 44 years	15.6	4.8	10.8	16,913	5,167	11,746	153	10.8	2.1	8.8	11,764	2,242	9,522	152
45 to 54 years	27.3	9.5	17.8	2,075	722	1,353	11	21.4	4.2	17.3	1,627	316	1,311	13
Non-Hispanic White[8]														
All ages	10.5	2.9	7.6	225,150	61,754	163,396	2,380	7.1	1.1	6.0	152,047	24,461	10.5	2.9
Under 15 years	17.8	5.8	12.0	154	50	104	4	10.1	2.5	7.5	87	22	17.8	5.8
15 to 19 years	11.9	3.7	8.2	15,371	4,773	10,598	162	8.4	1.4	7.0	10,845	1,850	11.9	3.7
15 years	14.7	4.9	9.8	481	160	321	8	9.4	1.8	7.6	307	59	14.7	4.9
16 years	13.8	5.1	8.7	1,246	457	789	17	9.1	1.9	7.2	821	173	13.8	5.1
17 years	12.5	4.1	8.4	2,388	788	1,600	24	8.7	1.7	7.0	1,659	319	12.5	4.1
18 years	11.9	3.7	8.2	4,336	1,337	2,999	45	8.5	1.4	7.1	3,109	505	11.9	3.7
19 years	11.3	3.3	8.0	6,920	2,031	4,889	68	8.1	1.3	6.8	4,949	794	11.3	3.3
20 to 24 years	10.3	2.9	7.5	46,696	12,932	33,764	489	7.2	1.1	6.1	32,613	5,139	10.3	2.9
25 to 29 years	9.7	2.6	7.1	62,688	16,869	45,819	730	6.5	1.0	5.5	41,943	6,676	9.7	2.6
30 to 34 years	10.1	2.7	7.4	59,393	15,863	43,530	602	6.6	1.1	5.6	39,229	6,306	10.1	2.7
35 to 39 years	12.0	3.2	8.8	31,229	8,441	22,788	311	7.9	1.3	6.6	20,508	3,297	12.0	3.2
40 to 44 years	14.0	4.1	10.0	8,514	2,457	6,057	76	9.9	1.7	8.2	5,980	1,028	14.0	4.1
45 to 54 years	25.6	8.6	17.1	1,105	369	736	6	19.5	3.3	16.2	842	143	25.6	8.6
Non-Hispanic Black[8]														
All ages	16.8	6.0	10.7	97,543	35,090	62,453	828	13.3	3.0	10.4	77,518	17,361	60,157	877
Under 15 years	25.5	11.0	14.5	349	151	198	8	14.6	3.4	11.2	200	46	154	3
15 to 19 years	17.3	6.4	10.8	13,536	5,032	8,504	137	13.7	2.8	11.0	10,775	2,162	8,613	103
15 years	20.9	8.0	12.8	681	262	419	18	14.0	3.3	10.7	460	108	352	5
16 years	18.8	7.4	11.4	1,354	530	824	7	13.4	2.9	10.5	966	211	755	3
17 years	18.4	6.9	11.5	2,413	901	1,512	29	13.9	2.6	11.3	1,831	342	1,489	20
18 years	17.3	6.4	10.9	3,778	1,401	2,377	26	13.7	2.7	11.1	3,007	587	2,420	27
19 years	16.1	5.9	10.2	5,310	1,938	3,372	57	13.7	2.8	10.9	4,511	914	3,597	48
20 to 24 years	16.0	5.6	10.4	29,692	10,359	19,333	271	13.2	2.7	10.5	24,497	5,024	19,473	275
25 to 29 years	15.9	5.6	10.3	23,391	8,234	15,157	193	12.6	2.8	9.8	18,545	4,138	14,407	215
30 to 34 years	17.1	6.2	10.9	17,826	6,477	11,349	147	13.3	3.3	9.9	13,789	3,470	10,319	169
35 to 39 years	19.2	7.3	11.9	9,655	3,664	5,991	57	14.7	3.8	10.8	7,348	1,913	5,435	92
40 to 44 years	21.6	8.1	13.5	2,790	1,042	1,748	14	16.3	4.2	12.1	2,111	545	1,566	19
45 to 54 years	30.4	13.1	17.3	304	131	173	1	25.3	6.3	19.0	253	63	190	1
Hispanic[9]														
All ages	11.7	3.3	8.4	106,884	29,859	77,025	780	7.0	1.2	5.8	64,449	11,022	53,427	600
Under 15 years	18.6	6.2	12.4	291	97	194	8	10.2	2.3	7.9	160	36	124	1
15 to 19 years	12.7	3.8	8.9	13,860	4,117	9,743	101	8.1	1.3	6.8	8,832	1,410	7,422	82
15 years	14.9	5.3	9.6	706	249	457	12	8.9	1.8	7.1	422	84	338	1
16 years	14.4	4.5	10.0	1,694	523	1,171	15	8.1	1.3	6.9	955	148	807	7
17 years	13.1	3.9	9.1	2,669	802	1,867	16	8.4	1.2	7.2	1,721	251	1,470	12
18 years	12.7	3.9	8.8	3,883	1,180	2,703	31	8.3	1.4	6.9	2,533	425	2,108	34
19 years	11.7	3.3	8.4	4,908	1,363	3,545	27	7.6	1.2	6.4	3,201	502	2,699	28
20 to 24 years	10.8	3.0	7.9	26,365	7,212	19,153	217	6.7	1.1	5.6	16,224	2,568	13,656	142
25 to 29 years	10.5	2.8	7.8	26,150	6,908	19,242	216	6.2	1.0	5.2	15,470	2,523	12,947	180
30 to 34 years	11.8	3.3	8.4	22,631	6,404	16,227	154	6.9	1.3	5.7	13,360	2,449	10,911	118
35 to 39 years	13.8	4.0	9.8	13,593	3,926	9,667	60	8.1	1.6	6.5	7,909	1,528	6,381	57
40 to 44 years	16.1	4.8	11.3	3,668	1,093	2,575	24	9.9	2.0	7.9	2,246	458	1,788	18
45 to 54 years	26.4	8.3	18.1	326	102	224	0	20.1	4.1	16.1	248	50	198	2

[1]Less than 37 completed weeks of gestation.   [2]Less than 2,500 grams.   [3]Less than 34 completed weeks of gestation.   [4]Includes 34 to 36 completed weeks of gestation.   [5]Less than 1,500 grams.   [6]Includes 1,500–2,499 grams.   [7]Includes races other than White and Black and origin not stated.   [8]Race and Hispanic origin are reported separately on birth certificates. Persons of Hispanic origin may be of any race. Multiple-race data, when reported, were bridged to single-race categories in order to maintain comparability among all reported areas.   [9]Includes all persons of Hispanic origin of any race.

Table 1-58. Births of Very Low Birthweight, by Race and Hispanic Origin of Mother and by State and Territory of Residence, 2011

(Number, percent.)

State and territory	Number				Percent			
	All races[1]	Non-Hispanic White[2]	Non-Hispanic Black[2]	Hispanic[3]	All races[1]	Non-Hispanic White[2]	Non-Hispanic Black[2]	Hispanic[3]
United States [4]	56,754	24,461	17,361	11,022	1.4	1.1	3.0	1.2
Alabama	1,138	461	612	52	1.9	1.3	3.4	1.2
Alaska	108	42	8	7	0.9	0.7	*	*
Arizona	994	436	104	349	1.2	1.1	2.5	1.0
Arkansas	632	321	258	39	1.6	1.2	3.6	1.0
California	5,717	1,412	757	2,593	1.1	1.0	2.5	1.0
Colorado	810	468	63	220	1.2	1.2	2.1	1.2
Connecticut	573	254	153	129	1.5	1.2	3.2	1.5
Delaware	206	67	104	28	1.8	1.1	3.4	2.0
District of Columbia	199	24	138	29	2.1	0.9	2.9	2.1
Florida	3,388	1,035	1,467	766	1.6	1.1	3.0	1.3
Georgia	2,338	695	1,314	213	1.8	1.2	3.0	1.1
Hawaii	232	44	9	43	1.2	0.9	*	1.4
Idaho	215	168	6	30	1.0	0.9	*	0.9
Illinois	2,498	1,048	844	451	1.5	1.2	3.1	1.3
Indiana	1,227	811	286	103	1.5	1.3	2.9	1.4
Iowa	428	339	46	24	1.1	1.1	2.5	0.8
Kansas	509	333	84	76	1.3	1.2	2.9	1.2
Kentucky	861	642	164	40	1.6	1.4	3.2	1.4
Louisiana	1,272	446	763	47	2.1	1.3	3.2	1.3
Maine	136	127	6	2	1.1	1.1	*	*
Maryland	1,280	338	720	137	1.8	1.0	3.0	1.3
Massachusetts	960	519	162	189	1.3	1.1	2.3	1.5
Michigan	1,764	922	697	95	1.5	1.2	3.2	1.2
Minnesota	712	449	145	46	1.0	0.9	2.2	1.0
Mississippi	872	286	561	16	2.2	1.4	3.2	*
Missouri	1,026	581	353	54	1.4	1.0	3.1	1.3
Montana	118	96	-	5	1.0	1.0	*	*
Nebraska	279	196	35	40	1.1	1.0	2.1	1.1
Nevada	471	176	102	152	1.3	1.2	2.8	1.2
New Hampshire	160	146	2	8	1.2	1.3	*	*
New Jersey	1,686	584	525	406	1.6	1.2	3.3	1.5
New Mexico	359	84	14	213	1.3	1.1	*	1.4
New York	3,533	1,320	1,118	780	1.5	1.1	2.9	1.4
North Carolina	2,084	849	904	240	1.7	1.3	3.2	1.3
North Dakota	105	82	1	5	1.1	1.1	*	*
Ohio	2,298	1,419	728	89	1.7	1.4	3.2	1.4
Oklahoma	750	422	157	81	1.4	1.3	3.3	1.2
Oregon	443	295	21	95	1.0	0.9	1.8	1.1
Pennsylvania	2,151	1,125	696	188	1.5	1.1	3.3	1.3
Rhode Island	155	79	20	40	1.4	1.2	2.1	1.7
South Carolina	1,054	420	563	49	1.8	1.3	3.1	1.0
South Dakota	127	85	8	2	1.1	1.0	*	*
Tennessee	1,187	621	472	73	1.5	1.1	2.9	1.0
Texas	5,340	1,593	1,211	2,293	1.4	1.2	2.8	1.3
Utah	548	419	18	84	1.1	1.0	*	1.1
Vermont	74	66	5	-	1.2	1.2	*	*
Virginia	1,597	707	625	159	1.6	1.2	2.9	1.3
Washington	841	470	94	157	1.0	0.9	2.2	1.0
West Virginia	333	311	19	1	1.6	1.6	*	*
Wisconsin	885	564	197	77	1.3	1.1	3.0	1.2
Wyoming	81	64	2	7	1.1	1.1	*	*
Puerto Rico	572	16	3	522	1.4	*	*	1.4
Virgin Islands	38	6	26	6	2.6	*	2.6	*
Guam	36	1	1	1	1.1	*	*	*
American Samoa	9	NA	NA	NA	*	NA	NA	NA
Northern Marianas	10	-	-	-	*	*	*	NA

NA = Not available.   – = Quantity zero.   * = Figure does not meet standards of reliability or precision.   [1]Includes races other than White and Black and origin not stated.   [2]Race and Hispanic origin are reported separately on birth certificates. Persons of Hispanic origin may be of any race. Multiple-race data, when reported, were bridged to single-race categories in order to maintain comparability among all reported areas.   [3]Includes all persons of Hispanic origin of any race.   [4]Excludes data for the territories.

Table 1-59. Preterm Births (Less Than 37 Completed Weeks of Gestation), by Race and Hispanic Origin of Mother, by State and Territory of Residence, 2011

(Number, percent.)

State and territory	Number				Percent			
	All races[1]	Non-Hispanic		Hispanic[3]	All races[1]	Non-Hispanic		Hispanic[3]
		White[2]	Black[2]			White[2]	Black[2]	
United States [4]	463,163	225,150	97,543	106,884	11.7	10.5	16.8	11.7
Alabama	8,817	4,511	3,558	621	14.9	12.6	19.8	13.9
Alaska	1,188	516	59	83	10.4	8.5	13.6	11.0
Arizona	10,356	4,332	657	4,067	12.1	11.1	16.1	12.2
Arkansas	5,096	3,158	1,321	465	13.2	12.0	18.3	11.8
California	48,942	12,647	4,034	24,824	9.8	8.8	13.5	9.9
Colorado	6,712	3,951	423	1,948	10.3	9.8	13.9	10.8
Connecticut	3,760	1,933	670	893	10.1	9.0	14.1	10.6
Delaware	1,264	577	442	176	11.2	9.3	14.6	12.4
District of Columbia	1,270	219	832	154	13.7	8.3	17.3	11.2
Florida	27,829	10,789	8,563	7,528	13.0	11.1	17.5	12.8
Georgia	17,492	6,583	7,606	2,206	13.2	10.9	17.1	11.9
Hawaii	2,338	448	66	386	12.3	9.2	13.0	12.7
Idaho	2,264	1,727	31	399	10.2	9.7	16.1	11.5
Illinois	19,580	9,486	4,625	4,300	12.1	10.8	17.0	12.0
Indiana	9,664	7,070	1,564	798	11.6	11.0	15.9	11.1
Iowa	4,226	3,417	323	338	11.1	10.7	17.5	10.9
Kansas	4,455	3,016	497	760	11.2	10.5	17.0	12.1
Kentucky	7,413	6,014	902	358	13.4	13.0	17.3	12.9
Louisiana	9,673	4,261	4,733	486	15.6	12.9	20.1	13.5
Maine	1,220	1,121	50	17	9.6	9.6	12.7	*
Maryland	9,160	3,358	3,877	1,338	12.5	10.1	16.3	13.0
Massachusetts	7,564	4,545	935	1,384	10.5	9.9	13.2	11.1
Michigan	13,710	8,346	3,867	947	12.0	10.5	17.8	12.4
Minnesota	6,779	4,741	823	486	9.9	9.4	12.7	10.5
Mississippi	6,730	2,844	3,604	183	16.9	13.9	20.9	13.9
Missouri	8,834	6,090	1,980	476	11.6	10.6	17.4	11.6
Montana	1,301	1,020	13	48	10.8	10.3	*	10.7
Nebraska	2,722	1,908	244	479	10.6	9.9	14.3	13.1
Nevada	4,654	1,762	652	1,762	13.2	11.6	17.7	13.5
New Hampshire	1,222	1,068	33	68	9.5	9.4	14.1	12.6
New Jersey	12,340	5,192	2,523	3,427	11.7	10.5	15.7	12.2
New Mexico	3,214	784	77	1,831	11.8	10.2	16.3	12.2
New York	26,302	11,067	5,936	6,568	10.9	9.4	15.2	11.6
North Carolina	15,111	7,245	4,893	2,241	12.6	10.7	17.1	12.3
North Dakota	946	735	26	25	9.9	9.5	11.9	8.1
Ohio	16,689	11,477	3,940	777	12.1	11.0	17.3	12.3
Oklahoma	6,878	4,087	923	894	13.2	12.3	19.2	13.4
Oregon	4,093	2,742	140	856	9.1	8.6	12.0	9.8
Pennsylvania	15,778	10,038	3,336	1,652	11.1	10.0	15.9	11.7
Rhode Island	1,135	641	125	278	10.4	9.5	13.1	11.5
South Carolina	8,066	3,990	3,343	550	14.1	12.1	18.3	11.6
South Dakota	1,323	862	35	57	11.2	9.7	13.2	11.3
Tennessee	10,141	6,222	2,883	832	12.8	11.5	17.5	11.9
Texas	48,336	15,058	7,259	23,985	12.8	11.2	16.8	13.1
Utah	5,580	4,233	132	905	10.9	10.4	23.3	11.8
Vermont	533	503	10	7	8.8	8.8	*	*
Virginia	11,484	5,896	3,282	1,499	11.2	9.8	15.0	12.0
Washington	8,524	4,970	530	1,736	9.8	9.0	12.3	10.9
West Virginia	2,640	2,482	105	24	12.8	12.7	14.5	11.6
Wisconsin	7,060	4,870	1,051	666	10.4	9.6	16.0	10.2
Wyoming	755	598	10	96	10.2	9.8	*	11.1
Puerto Rico	7,220	182	26	7,006	17.6	15.5	19.5	17.7
Virgin Islands	199	17	134	43	13.5	*	13.3	13.7
Guam	484	14	1	6	14.8	*	*	*
American Samoa	NA	NA	NA	NA	NA	NA	NA	NA
Northern Marianas	75	–	–	–	7.3	*	*	*

NA = Not available.   – = Quantity zero.   * = Figure does not meet standards of reliability or precision.   [1]Includes races other than White and Black and origin not stated.   [2]Race and Hispanic origin are reported separately on birth certificates. Persons of Hispanic origin may be of any race. Multiple-race data, when reported, were bridged to single-race categories in order to maintain comparability among all reported areas.   [3]Includes all persons of Hispanic origin of any race.   [4]Excludes data for the territories.

Table 1-60. Low Birthweight Births (Less Than 2,500 Grams or 5 Lbs 8 Oz), by Race and Hispanic Origin of Mother, by State and Territory of Residence, 2011

(Number, percent.)

State and territory	Number				Percent			
	All races[1]	Non-Hispanic		Hispanic[3]	All races[1]	Non-Hispanic		Hispanic[3]
		White[2]	Black[2]			White[2]	Black[2]	
United States [4]	319,711	152,047	77,518	64,449	8.1	7.1	13.3	7.0
Alabama	5,896	2,812	2,696	287	9.9	7.9	15.0	6.4
Alaska	690	305	42	53	6.0	5.0	9.6	7.0
Arizona	5,988	2,631	523	2,147	7.0	6.7	12.8	6.5
Arkansas	3,516	2,056	1,119	244	9.1	7.8	15.5	6.2
California	33,946	8,813	3,422	15,487	6.8	6.1	11.4	6.2
Colorado	5,640	3,405	388	1,481	8.7	8.4	12.7	8.2
Connecticut	2,883	1,427	565	659	7.7	6.6	11.8	7.9
Delaware	942	404	388	96	8.4	6.5	12.8	6.8
District of Columbia	970	160	648	111	10.4	6.1	13.5	8.1
Florida	18,527	7,056	6,437	4,293	8.7	7.3	13.1	7.3
Georgia	12,333	4,449	5,906	1,192	9.4	7.4	13.3	6.4
Hawaii	1,557	304	50	261	8.2	6.3	9.8	8.6
Idaho	1,352	1,057	14	229	6.1	5.9	7.3	6.6
Illinois	13,232	6,215	3,665	2,381	8.2	7.1	13.5	6.7
Indiana	6,786	4,821	1,305	481	8.1	7.5	13.3	6.7
Iowa	2,495	2,017	219	170	6.5	6.3	11.9	5.5
Kansas	2,854	1,934	374	417	7.2	6.7	12.8	6.6
Kentucky	5,040	4,004	716	208	9.1	8.7	13.8	7.5
Louisiana	6,773	2,771	3,612	255	10.9	8.4	15.3	7.1
Maine	846	774	36	13	6.7	6.6	9.2	6.3
Maryland	6,466	2,236	2,990	750	8.9	6.7	12.6	7.3
Massachusetts	5,481	3,179	737	1,006	7.6	7.0	10.4	8.1
Michigan	9,508	5,483	3,052	523	8.3	6.9	14.0	6.9
Minnesota	4,384	2,924	660	267	6.4	5.8	10.2	5.8
Mississippi	4,710	1,846	2,747	58	11.8	9.0	15.9	4.4
Missouri	5,995	3,889	1,617	262	7.9	6.8	14.2	6.4
Montana	867	703	8	32	7.2	7.1	10.7	7.1
Nebraska	1,702	1,154	215	265	6.6	6.0	12.6	7.3
Nevada	2,906	1,204	477	911	8.2	7.9	12.9	7.0
New Hampshire	911	811	20	41	7.1	7.1	8.5	7.6
New Jersey	9,005	3,765	1,988	2,145	8.5	7.6	12.4	7.7
New Mexico	2,385	627	59	1,363	8.8	8.1	12.5	9.1
New York	19,557	8,086	4,886	4,282	8.1	6.9	12.5	7.6
North Carolina	10,839	5,038	4,008	1,252	9.0	7.4	14.0	6.9
North Dakota	637	514	14	23	6.7	6.6	6.4	7.5
Ohio	11,901	7,929	3,096	498	8.6	7.6	13.6	7.9
Oklahoma	4,431	2,687	724	478	8.5	8.1	15.1	7.2
Oregon	2,764	1,839	115	549	6.1	5.8	9.8	6.3
Pennsylvania	11,662	7,060	2,753	1,214	8.2	7.0	13.2	8.6
Rhode Island	813	464	106	166	7.4	6.9	11.1	6.9
South Carolina	5,650	2,555	2,693	271	9.9	7.8	14.7	5.7
South Dakota	744	520	29	33	6.3	5.9	10.9	6.5
Tennessee	7,176	4,279	2,294	457	9.0	7.9	13.9	6.5
Texas	32,018	10,167	5,891	14,283	8.5	7.6	13.6	7.8
Utah	3,544	2,705	84	568	6.9	6.6	14.8	7.4
Vermont	404	382	9	3	6.7	6.7	10.1	4.2
Virginia	8,184	3,992	2,713	777	8.0	6.6	12.4	6.2
Washington	5,340	3,036	403	997	6.1	5.5	9.4	6.2
West Virginia	1,985	1,866	87	11	9.6	9.6	12.0	5.3
Wisconsin	4,876	3,211	911	425	7.2	6.4	13.8	6.5
Wyoming	600	481	7	74	8.1	7.9	10.8	8.6
Puerto Rico	5,119	127	18	4,962	12.5	10.8	*	12.5
Virgin Islands	152	13	99	37	10.4	*	9.9	11.8
Guam	294	9	3	5	9.0	*	*	*
American Samoa	54	NA	NA	NA	4.3	NA	NA	NA
Northern Marianas	75	-	-	NA	7.3	*	*	NA

NA = Not available.   – = Quantity zero.   * = Figure does not meet standards of reliability or precision.   [1]Includes races other than White and Black and origin not stated.   [2]Race and Hispanic origin are reported separately on birth certificates. Persons of Hispanic origin may be of any race. Multiple-race data, when reported, were bridged to single-race categories in order to maintain comparability among all reported areas   [3]Includes all persons of Hispanic origin of any race.   [4]Excludes data for the territories.

Table 1-61. Births, by Plurality, Age, and Race and Hispanic Origin of Mother, 2011

(Number, rate as stated.)

Plurality, race, and Hispanic origin of mother	All ages	Under 15 years	15 to 19 years			20 to 24 years	25 to 29 years	30 to 34 years	35 to 39 years	40 to 44 years	45 to 54 years
			Total	15 to 17 years	18 to 19 years						
NUMBER											
All Live Births											
All races[1]	3,953,590	3,974	329,772	95,538	234,234	925,200	1,127,583	986,682	463,849	108,920	7,610
Non-Hispanic White[2]	2,146,566	869	129,329	31,461	97,868	451,939	647,520	591,266	260,596	60,724	4,323
Non-Hispanic Black[2]	582,345	1,378	78,558	23,659	54,899	186,229	147,708	104,274	50,245	12,952	1,001
Hispanic[3]	918,129	1,576	109,660	36,979	72,681	243,724	248,269	192,517	98,340	22,807	1,236
Live Births in Single Deliveries											
All races[1]	3,816,904	3,927	324,557	94,238	230,319	903,329	1,092,096	944,983	439,941	102,176	5,895
Non-Hispanic White[2]	2,064,258	860	127,357	31,000	96,357	441,810	626,004	563,617	245,120	56,203	3,287
Non-Hispanic Black[2]	560,030	1,354	76,948	23,272	53,676	179,854	141,582	99,402	47,727	12,327	836
Hispanic[3]	896,170	1,564	108,173	36,566	71,607	239,238	242,453	186,753	94,973	21,979	1,037
Live Births in Twin Deliveries											
All races[1]	131,269	44	5,142	1,291	3,851	21,475	34,229	39,692	22,654	6,408	1,625
Non-Hispanic White[2]	78,638	9	1,944	457	1,487	9,929	20,637	26,227	14,598	4,289	1,005
Non-Hispanic Black[2]	21,681	21	1,586	385	1,201	6,257	5,975	4,689	2,409	594	150
Hispanic[3]	21,236	12	1,466	410	1,056	4,435	5,647	5,488	3,208	799	181
Live Births in Triplet and Higher-Order Multiple Births [4]											
All races[1]	5,417	3	73	9	64	396	1,258	2,007	1,254	336	90
Non-Hispanic White[2]	3,670	–	28	4	24	200	879	1,422	878	232	31
Non-Hispanic Black[2]	634	3	24	2	22	118	151	183	109	31	15
Hispanic[3]	723	–	21	3	18	51	169	276	159	29	18
RATE PER 1,000 LIVE BIRTHS											
All Multiple Births											
All races[1]	34.6	11.8	15.8	13.6	16.7	23.6	31.5	42.3	51.5	61.9	225.4
Non-Hispanic White[2]	38.3	*	15.2	14.7	15.4	22.4	33.2	46.8	59.4	74.5	239.6
Non-Hispanic Black[2]	38.3	17.4	20.5	16.4	22.3	34.2	41.5	46.7	50.1	48.3	164.8
Hispanic[3]	23.9	*	13.6	11.2	14.8	18.4	23.4	29.9	34.2	36.3	161.0
Twin Births											
All races[1]	33.2	11.1	15.6	13.5	16.4	23.2	30.4	40.2	48.8	58.8	213.5
Non-Hispanic White[2]	36.6	*	15.0	14.5	15.2	22.0	31.9	44.4	56.0	70.6	232.5
Non-Hispanic Black[2]	37.2	15.2	20.2	16.3	21.9	33.6	40.5	45.0	47.9	45.9	149.9
Hispanic[3]	23.1	*	13.4	11.1	14.5	18.2	22.7	28.5	32.6	35.0	146.4
RATE PER 100,000 LIVE BIRTHS											
Triplet and Higher-Order Multiple Births [4]											
All races[1]	137.0	*	22.1	*	27.3	42.8	111.6	203.4	270.3	308.5	1,182.7
Non-Hispanic White[2]	171.0	*	21.7	*	24.5	44.3	135.7	240.5	336.9	382.1	717.1
Non-Hispanic Black[2]	108.9	*	30.6	*	40.1	63.4	102.2	175.5	216.9	239.3	*
Hispanic[3]	78.7	*	19.2	*	*	20.9	68.1	143.4	161.7	127.2	*

– = Quantity zero.   * = Figure does not meet standards of reliability or precision.   [1]Includes races other than White and Black and origin not stated.   [2]Race and Hispanic origin are reported separately on birth certificates. Persons of Hispanic origin may be of any race. Multiple-race data, when reported, were bridged to single-race categories in order to maintain comparability among all reported areas.   [3]Includes all persons of Hispanic origin of any race.   [4]Triplet, quadruplet, quintuplet, and higher-order multiple deliveries.

Table 1-62. Numbers and Rates of Twin and Triplet and Higher-Order Multiple Births, by Race and Hispanic Origin of Mother, 1980–2011

(Number, rate per 1,000 live births; rate per 100,000 live births, as stated.)

Year, race, and Hispanic origin of mother	Total births	Twin births	Triplet and higher-order births	Multiple birth rate[1]	Twin birth rate[2]	Triplet or higher-order birth rate[3]
All Races [4]						
1980	3,612,258	68,339	1,337	19.3	18.9	37.0
1981	3,629,238	70,049	1,385	19.7	19.3	38.2
1982	3,680,537	71,631	1,484	19.9	19.5	40.3
1983	3,638,933	72,287	1,575	20.3	19.9	43.3
1984	3,669,141	72,949	1,653	20.3	19.9	45.1
1985	3,760,561	77,102	1,925	21.0	20.5	51.2
1986	3,756,547	79,485	1,814	21.6	21.2	48.3
1987	3,809,394	81,778	2,139	22.0	21.5	56.2
1988	3,909,510	85,315	2,385	22.4	21.8	61.0
1989	4,040,958	90,118	2,798	23.0	22.3	69.2
1990	4,158,212	93,865	3,028	23.3	22.6	72.8
1991	4,110,907	94,779	3,346	23.9	23.1	81.4
1992	4,065,014	95,372	3,883	24.4	23.5	95.5
1993	4,000,240	96,445	4,168	25.2	24.1	104.2
1994	3,952,767	97,064	4,594	25.7	24.6	116.2
1995	3,899,589	96,736	4,973	26.1	24.8	127.5
1996	3,891,494	100,750	5,939	27.4	25.9	152.6
1997	3,880,894	104,137	6,737	28.6	26.8	173.6
1998	3,941,553	110,670	7,625	30.0	28.1	193.5
1999	3,959,417	114,307	7,321	30.7	28.9	184.9
2000	4,058,814	118,916	7,325	31.1	29.3	180.5
2001	4,025,933	121,246	7,471	32.0	30.1	185.6
2002	4,021,726	125,134	7,401	33.0	31.1	184.0
2003	4,089,950	128,665	7,663	33.3	31.5	187.4
2004	4,112,052	132,219	7,275	33.9	32.2	176.9
2005	4,138,349	133,122	6,694	33.8	32.2	161.8
2006	4,265,555	137,085	6,540	33.7	32.1	153.3
2007	4,316,233	138,961	6,427	33.7	32.2	148.9
2008	4,247,694	138,660	6,268	34.1	32.6	147.6
2009	4,130,665	137,217	6,340	34.8	33.2	153.5
2010	3,999,386	132,562	5,503	34.5	33.1	137.6
2011	3,953,590	131,269	5,417	34.6	33.2	137.0
Non-Hispanic White [5]						
1990 [6]	2,626,500	60,210	2,358	23.8	22.9	89.8
1991 [7]	2,589,878	60,904	2,612	24.5	23.5	100.9
1992 [7]	2,527,207	60,640	3,115	25.2	24.0	123.3
1993	2,472,031	61,525	3,360	26.2	24.9	135.9
1994	2,438,855	62,476	3,721	27.1	25.6	152.6
1995	2,382,638	62,370	4,050	27.9	26.2	170.0
1996	2,358,989	65,523	4,885	29.8	27.8	207.1
1997	2,333,363	67,191	5,386	31.1	28.8	230.8
1998	2,283,986	71,270	6,206	32.8	30.2	262.8
1999	2,346,450	73,964	5,909	34.0	31.5	251.8
2000	2,362,968	76,018	5,821	34.6	32.2	246.3
2001	2,326,578	77,882	5,894	36.0	33.5	253.3
2002	2,298,156	79,949	5,754	37.3	34.8	250.4
2003	2,321,904	81,691	5,922	37.7	35.2	255.0
2004	2,296,683	83,346	5,590	38.7	36.3	243.4
2005	2,279,768	82,223	4,966	38.2	36.1	217.8
2006	2,308,640	83,108	4,805	38.1	36.0	208.1
2007	2,310,333	83,632	4,559	38.2	36.2	197.3
2008	2,267,817	82,903	4,493	38.5	36.6	198.1
2009	2,212,552	81,954	4,457	39.1	37.0	201.4
2010	2,162,406	79,728	3,842	38.6	36.9	177.7
2011	2,146,566	78,638	3,670	38.3	36.6	171.0
Non-Hispanic Black [5]						
1990 [6]	661,701	17,646	306	27.1	26.7	46.2
1991 [7]	666,758	18,243	367	27.9	27.4	55.0
1992 [7]	657,450	18,294	346	28.4	27.8	52.6
1993	641,273	18,115	314	28.7	28.2	49.0
1994	619,198	17,934	357	29.5	29.0	57.7
1995	587,781	16,622	340	28.9	28.3	57.8
1996	578,099	16,873	425	29.9	29.2	73.5
1997	581,431	17,472	523	30.9	30.0	90.0
1998	593,127	18,589	518	32.2	31.3	87.3
1999	588,981	18,920	561	33.1	32.1	95.2
2000	604,346	20,173	506	34.2	33.4	83.7
2001	589,917	19,974	531	34.8	33.9	90.0
2002	578,335	20,064	591	35.7	34.7	102.2
2003	576,033	20,010	631	35.8	34.7	109.5
2004	578,772	20,605	577	36.6	35.6	99.7
2005	583,759	21,254	616	37.5	36.4	105.5
2006	617,247	22,702	580	37.7	36.8	94.0
2007	627,191	23,101	612	37.8	36.8	97.6
2008	623,029	22,924	569	37.7	36.8	91.3
2009	609,584	23,159	644	39.0	38.0	105.6
2010	589,808	21,804	574	37.9	37.0	97.3
2011	582,345	21,681	634	38.3	37.2	108.9

Table 1-62. Numbers and Rates of Twin and Triplet and Higher-Order Multiple Births, by Race and Hispanic Origin of Mother, 1980–2011—*Continued*

(Number, rate per 1,000 live births; rate per 100,000 live births, as stated.)

Year, race, and Hispanic origin of mother	Total births	Twin births	Triplet and higher-order births	Multiple birth rate[1]	Twin birth rate[2]	Triplet or higher-order birth rate[3]
Hispanic [8]						
1990 [6]	595,073	10,713	235	18.4	18.0	39.5
1991 [7]	623,085	11,356	235	18.6	18.2	37.7
1992 [7]	643,271	11,932	239	18.9	18.5	37.2
1993	654,418	12,294	321	19.3	18.8	49.1
1994	665,026	12,206	348	18.9	18.4	52.3
1995	679,768	12,685	355	19.2	18.7	52.2
1996	701,339	13,014	409	19.1	18.6	58.3
1997	709,767	13,821	516	20.2	19.5	72.7
1998	734,661	15,015	553	21.2	20.4	75.3
1999	764,339	15,388	583	20.9	20.1	76.3
2000	815,868	16,470	659	21.0	20.2	80.8
2001	851,851	17,257	710	21.1	20.3	83.3
2002	876,642	18,128	737	21.5	20.7	84.1
2003	912,329	19,472	784	22.2	21.3	85.9
2004	946,349	20,351	723	22.3	21.5	76.4
2005	985,505	21,723	761	22.8	22.0	77.2
2006	1,039,077	22,698	787	22.6	21.8	75.7
2007	1,062,779	23,405	857	22.8	22.0	80.6
2008	1,041,239	23,266	834	23.1	22.3	80.1
2009	999,548	22,481	835	23.3	22.5	83.5
2010	945,180	21,359	721	23.4	22.6	76.3
2011	918,129	21,236	723	23.9	23.1	78.7

[1]The number of live births in all multiple deliveries per 1,000 live births.   [2]The number of live births in twin deliveries per 1,000 live births.   [3]The number of live births in triplet and other higher-order deliveries per 100,000 live births.   [4]Includes races other than White and Black and origin not stated.   [5]Race and Hispanic origin are reported separately on birth certificates. Persons of Hispanic origin may be of any race. Multiple-race data, when reported, were bridged to single-race categories in order to maintain comparability among all reported areas.   [6]Excludes data for New Hampshire and Oklahoma, which did not report Hispanic origin.   [7]Excludes data for New Hampshire, which did not report Hispanic origin.   [8]Includes all persons of Hispanic origin of any race.

Table 1-63. Twin, Triplet, and Higher-Order Multiple Births, by State, 2009–2011

(Number, rate per 1,000 births.)

State	Twin		Triplet or higher order[1]	
	Number	Rate per 1,000 live births	Number	Rate per 100,000 live births
United States	401,048	33.2	17,260	142.8
Alabama	6,080	33.4	274	150.6
Alaska	1,011	29.5	25	73.0
Arizona	7,252	27.3	287	108.0
Arkansas	3,454	29.5	84	71.8
California	46,896	30.5	1,889	122.7
Colorado	6,357	31.8	270	135.0
Connecticut	4,981	43.7	224	196.7
Delaware	1,145	33.5	39	114.1
District of Columbia	1,069	38.9	40	145.5
Florida	20,233	31.2	846	130.3
Georgia	13,723	33.7	485	119.0
Hawaii	1,742	30.7	69	121.4
Idaho	2,016	29.1	92	132.9
Illinois	18,323	36.8	848	170.4
Indiana	7,973	31.4	438	172.2
Iowa	3,949	33.9	193	165.5
Kansas	3,718	30.6	130	106.8
Kentucky	5,340	31.7	196	116.2
Louisiana	6,044	31.9	290	153.2
Maine	1,215	31.0	33	84.3
Maryland	8,342	37.6	279	125.7
Massachusetts	9,755	44.1	364	164.7
Michigan	12,104	35.0	608	175.8
Minnesota	7,195	34.6	305	146.9
Mississippi	4,199	34.2	134	109.1
Missouri	7,821	33.7	423	182.5
Montana	1,081	29.7	20	55.0
Nebraska	2,572	32.7	167	212.5
Nevada	3,197	29.4	152	139.7
New Hampshire	1,538	39.3	65	166.2
New Jersey	14,391	44.5	691	213.8
New Mexico	2,074	24.6	62	73.7
New York	27,744	37.8	1,444	196.8
North Carolina	12,378	33.5	578	156.4
North Dakota	847	30.7	57	206.3
Ohio	14,264	33.8	760	180.1
Oklahoma	4,729	29.5	198	123.7
Oregon	4,374	31.7	147	106.7
Pennsylvania	15,255	35.2	662	152.9
Rhode Island	1,201	35.8	39	116.1
South Carolina	5,851	33.2	235	133.3
South Dakota	988	27.8	38	106.8
Tennessee	7,383	30.6	254	105.3
Texas	35,363	30.3	1,654	141.9
Utah	4,874	31.0	203	129.0
Vermont	547	29.7	15	*
Virginia	11,032	35.5	379	122.0
Washington	8,273	31.5	222	84.5
West Virginia	1,897	30.4	47	75.3
Wisconsin	6,609	31.9	282	136.1
Wyoming	649	28.4	24	105.1

* = Figure does not meet standards of reliability or precision.   [1]Includes triplet, quadruplet, and other higher-order multiple births.

Figure 1-12. Percent of Preterm Births, by Completed Weeks of Gestation, Selected Years, 1990–2011

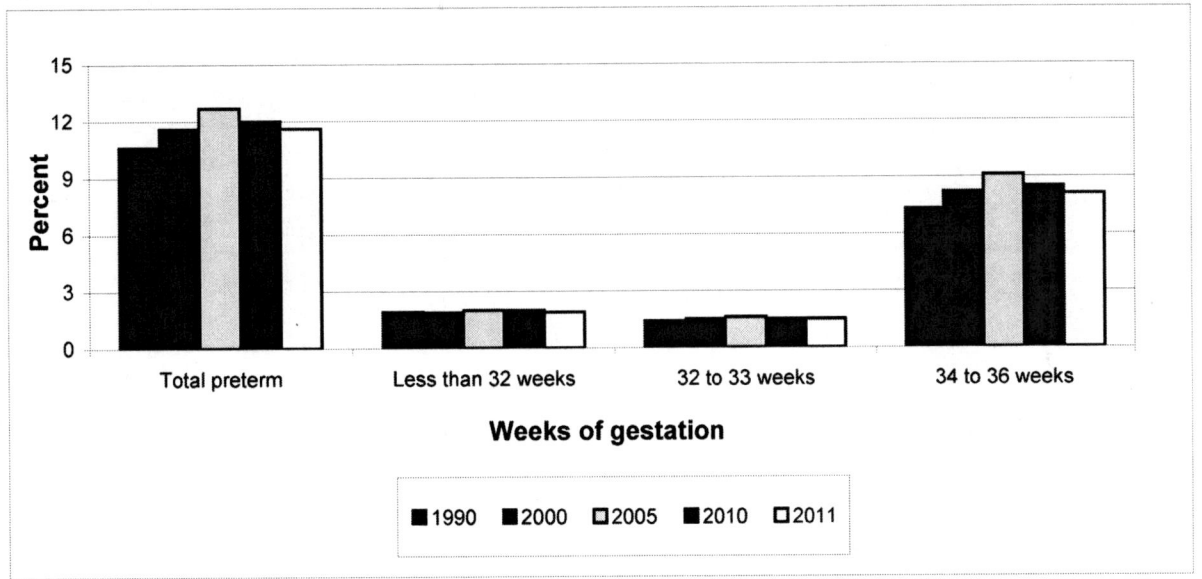

Figure 1-13. Twin, Triplet, and Higher Order Birth Rates, Selected Years, 1980–2011

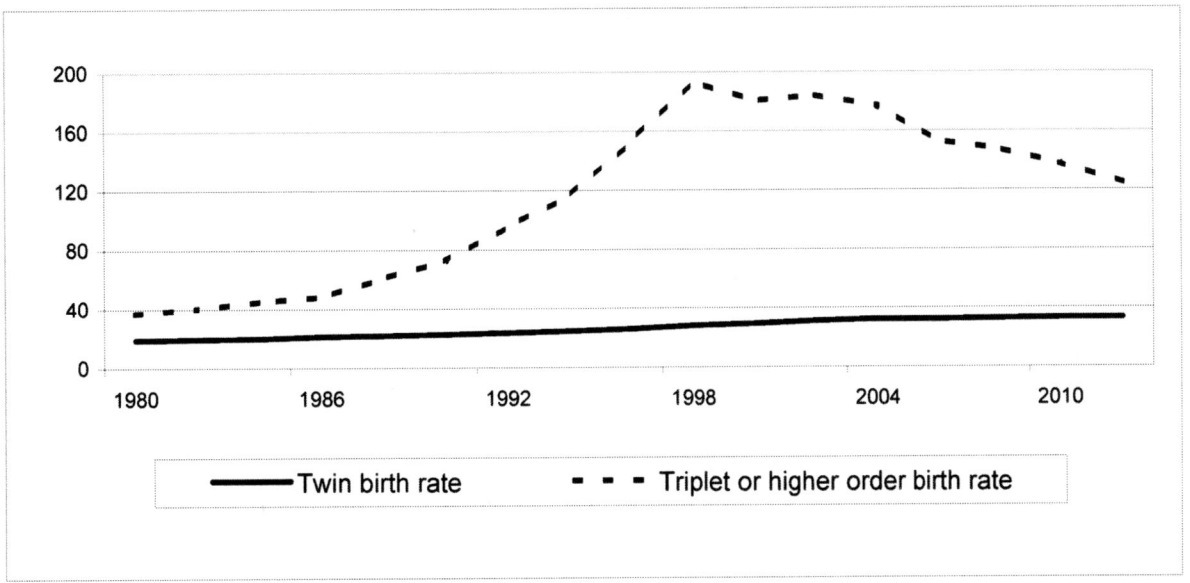

Table 1-64. Gestational Age and Birthweight Characteristics, by Plurality, 2011

(Number, percent.)

Characteristic	All births	Singletons	Twins	Triplets	Quadruplets	Quintuplets and higher-order multiples[1]
Number of Births	3,953,590	3,816,904	131,269	5,137	239	41
Percent, very preterm[2]	1.9	1.6	11.3	36.5	67.4	73.2
Percent, preterm[3]	11.7	10.0	57.3	93.4	92.8	100.0
Percent, very low birthweight[4]	1.4	1.1	9.8	35.3	68.9	100.0
Percent, low birthweight[5]	8.1	6.3	56.3	94.4	97.9	100.0

[1]Quintuplets, sextuplets, and higher-order multiple births are not differentiated in the national data set.   [2]Very preterm is less than 32 completed weeks of gestation.   [3]Preterm is less than 37 completed weeks of gestation.   [4]Very low birthweight is less than 1,500 grams. [5]Low birthweight is less than 2,500 grams.

Table 1-65A. Distribution of Births, by Gestational Age for All Births, Selected Years, 1990–2011

(Percent.)

Gestational age	All births					
	1990	2000	2005	2006	2010	2011
Under 28 weeks	0.7	0.7	0.8	0.8	0.7	0.7
28 to 31 weeks	1.2	1.2	1.3	1.3	1.2	1.2
32 to 33 weeks	1.4	1.5	1.6	1.6	1.5	1.5
Total under 34 weeks	3.3	3.4	3.6	3.7	3.5	3.4
34 to 36 weeks	7.3	8.2	9.1	9.2	8.5	8.3
Total under 37 weeks	10.6	11.6	12.7	12.8	12.0	11.7
37 to 38 weeks	19.7	24.5	28.3	28.9	26.9	25.9
39 weeks	21.7	24.3	25.3	25.4	28.3	29.2
40 weeks	22.6	21.3	19.2	18.9	19.1	19.3
41 weeks	14.1	11.0	8.7	8.3	8.2	8.4
42 weeks or more	11.3	7.3	5.8	5.7	5.5	5.6

Table 1-65B. Distribution of Births, by Gestational Age for Singleton Births Only, Selected Years, 1990–2011

(Percent.)

Gestational age	Singleton births					
	1990	2000	2005	2006	2010	2011
Under 28 weeks	0.6	0.6	0.6	0.6	0.6	0.6
28 to 31 weeks	1.1	1.0	1.0	1.0	1.0	1.0
32 to 33 weeks	1.2	1.2	1.3	1.3	1.2	1.2
Total under 34 weeks	2.9	2.8	2.9	3.0	2.8	2.8
34 to 36 weeks	6.8	7.3	8.1	8.1	7.5	7.3
Total under 37 weeks	9.7	10.1	11.0	11.1	10.3	10.1
37 to 38 weeks	19.4	24.4	28.3	28.9	26.7	25.7
39 weeks	22.0	24.9	26.0	26.2	29.1	30.1
40 weeks	23.0	21.9	19.8	19.4	19.7	19.9
41 weeks	14.4	11.3	8.9	8.6	8.5	8.6
42 weeks or more	11.5	7.5	6.0	5.8	5.6	5.7

Table 1-66. Quitting Smoking Prior to Pregnancy, by Race, Hispanic Origin, Age of Mother, and Reporting Area, 36 States, 2011

(Percent.)

Reporting area	Race and Hispanic Origin				Age of mother in years					
	Total	Non-Hispanic White	Non-Hispanic Black	Hispanic	Under 20 years	20 to 24 years	25 to 29 years	30 to 35 years	35 to 39 years	40 to 54 years
Total	23.8	22.4	23.1	39.2	22.6	22.3	24.6	26.7	24.3	20.0
California	34.6	31.2	25.2	45.4	33.4	34.7	34.3	36.4	35.3	24.3
Colorado	21.3	20.3	17.7	25.6	22.7	21.1	20.9	23.5	19.0	*
Delaware	14.3	13.5	13.5	*	*	15.0	13.4	17.6	*	*
District of Columbia	36.8	*	35.4	*	*	41.3	40.7	23.0	*	*
Florida	17.5	15.6	16.9	33.6	19.6	16.7	17.7	17.7	17.9	15.1
Georgia	12.8	12.1	12.5	28.3	10.5	12.9	12.7	14.4	12.9	*
Idaho	26.2	24.9	*	35.3	22.5	25.1	29.7	25.4	24.1	*
Illinois	16.1	16.1	12.0	29.1	17.3	14.4	17.2	18.1	13.9	12.3
Indiana	19.6	18.8	23.0	34.2	20.8	18.7	19.8	20.8	18.8	17.4
Iowa	25.8	25.5	22.4	38.9	25.3	23.8	28.5	27.5	23.3	*
Kansas	15.7	15.8	6.4	26.4	16.7	15.1	16.3	15.3	18.2	*
Kentucky	12.9	12.3	18.2	31.8	12.5	11.7	13.7	15.1	13.1	14.5
Louisiana	18.0	18.3	16.0	30.9	17.0	17.0	18.5	19.5	20.1	*
Maryland	35.8	34.3	35.1	58.2	30.3	33.8	37.4	39.5	36.5	30.8
Missouri	26.8	26.8	25.3	35.8	25.6	24.0	27.9	33.2	25.2	16.4
Montana	15.2	15.9	*	*	16.7	12.9	15.5	17.3	19.7	*
Nebraska	28.4	28.1	18.7	39.1	25.4	28.0	29.3	30.0	25.9	*
Nevada	15.4	13.4	15.1	22.7	14.0	18.4	15.5	14.1	11.3	*
New Hampshire	14.2	14.2	*	*	11.8	12.3	14.9	17.1	16.7	*
New Mexico	39.9	31.8	*	44.7	45.7	41.8	39.6	35.5	32.6	*
New York	28.1	26.0	28.0	41.8	23.8	24.1	28.7	34.4	31.7	28.0
North Carolina	25.2	23.5	28.0	43.1	25.9	25.6	24.5	26.1	23.1	18.6
North Dakota	26.0	27.2	*	45.3	22.7	22.6	30.4	28.3	27.4	*
Ohio	23.9	23.3	26.0	32.7	20.9	21.9	24.9	28.4	26.4	22.1
Oklahoma	18.5	18.2	15.3	31.4	19.3	18.3	18.8	19.1	15.3	*
Oregon	16.3	15.6	*	26.3	16.8	15.0	16.6	17.6	18.5	*
Pennsylvania	26.5	26.4	22.9	33.7	22.5	23.5	28.2	30.7	28.4	25.2
South Carolina	25.1	23.2	29.4	45.7	22.7	25.2	25.3	26.7	26.4	*
South Dakota	32.6	30.9	*	29.8	36.9	31.0	33.1	35.0	23.1	*
Tennessee	22.5	21.8	23.5	43.8	22.4	20.7	23.1	26.6	21.3	22.4
Texas	32.4	28.4	30.3	49.6	31.7	31.2	33.2	34.5	32.5	24.9
Utah	26.2	25.5	*	32.3	29.1	27.5	26.2	22.7	23.9	*
Vermont	17.7	17.4	*	*	21.7	13.7	16.8	28.4	*	*
Washington	19.6	18.9	15.0	28.7	18.3	19.8	20.0	19.4	19.9	19.4
Wisconsin	24.9	25.7	16.4	32.4	22.1	23.0	25.9	28.3	25.6	18.9
Wyoming	25.3	24.2	*	33.6	24.3	25.5	26.1	26.3	*	*

* = Figure does not meet standards of reliability or precision.

Table 1-67. Use of Contraception Among Sexually Experienced Males and Females Age 15 to 19 Years, by Method of Contraception, Selected Years, 1995–2010

(Number in thousands, percent.)

Method	Females		
	1995	2002	2006–2010
Percent Who Ever Used Method of Birth Control			
Any method	96.2	97.7	98.9
Pill	51.6	61.4	55.6
Injectable	9.7	20.7	20.3
Emergency contraception	*	8.1	13.7
Contraceptive patch	NA	1.5	10.3
Contraceptive ring	NA	NA	5.2
Condom	93.5	93.7	95.9
Female condom	1.1	1.7	1.5
Periodic abstinence-calendar	13.2	10.8	15
Withdrawal	42.3	55.0	57.3
Other methods	14.5	9.9	7.1

NA = Not available.   * = Figure does not meet standards of reliability or precision.

Table 1-68. Use of Contraception at First Sex Among Females and Males Age 15 to 19 Years, by Method Used, Selected Years, 1988–2010

(Number in thousands, percent.)

Characteristic	Number	Any method	No method	Pill (at all)[1]	Other hormonal[1,2]	Condom (at all)[1]	All other methods[3]	Dual methods (hormonal and condom)
Females								
1988	4,410	66.9	33.1	8.0	X	50.4	10.0	1.8
2002	4,598	74.5	25.5	16.5	2.1	66.4	2.6	13.1
2006–2010[4]	4,532	78.3	21.7	15.7	6.1	68.0	3.4	14.8
Females, 2006–2010								
Hispanic Origin and Race								
Hispanic or Latina	833	74.0	26.0	7.2	5.8	65.4	1.3	5.7
Non-Hispanic White	2,633	82.3	17.7	21.8	6.3	70.7	4.3	20.8
Non-Hispanic Black	785	71.1	28.9	8.9	6.6	64.1	*	9.5
Age at First Sex								
14 years or under	1,244	59.1	40.9	7.1	2.4	53.5	2.3	6.3
15 to 16 years	2,108	83.1	16.9	16.7	9.0	69.6	3.6	15.8
17 to 19 years	1,180	90.1	9.9	22.8	4.7	80.5	4.2	22.0
Age Difference Between Female and First Male Partner								
Male partner same age or younger	1,252	82.9	17.1	17.3	7.6	71.8	1.0	14.7
Male partner 1 year older	1,222	78.7	21.3	14.4	6.5	71.0	4.5	17.6
Male partner 2 to 3 years older	1,326	81.7	18.3	16.6	5.3	68.3	5.6	14.0
Male partner 4 or more years older	732	63.7	36.3	13.4	4.2	56.3	1.7	11.7
Males								
1988	5,379	71.4	28.6	9.5	X	55.0	10.6	2.6
1995	4,989	75.7	24.3	10.3	0.4	69.3	4.4	6.8
2002	4,697	82.0	18.0	14.9	2.1	70.9	4.7	10.4
2006–2010[4]	4,551	85.4	14.6	17.9	1.4	79.6	2.7	16.2
Males, 2006–2010								
Hispanic Origin and Race								
Hispanic or Latino	931	84.1	15.9	9.1	*	78.5	4.5	8.3
Non-Hispanic White	2,387	88.5	11.5	24.8	2.4	80.9	2.6	22.3
Non-Hispanic Black	977	81.7	18.3	11.7	*	79.6	*	11.1
Age at First Sex								
14 years or under	1,513	74.9	25.1	8.0	*	71.0	3.3	9.0
15 to 16 years	1,994	89.3	10.7	19.8	1.8	82.2	3.5	18.0
17 to 19 years	1,044	93.3	6.7	28.7	*	86.9	*	23.2
Age Difference Between Male and First Female Partner								
Female partner younger	723	88.3	11.7	14.5	*	79.6	5.0	15.1
Female partner same age	2,034	89.4	10.6	16.1	1.3	85.2	1.9	15.1
Female partner 1 year older	1,011	83.2	16.8	22.4	*	78.5	*	19.1
Female partner 2 or more years older	783	75.4	24.6	20.1	-	66.4	5.1	16.2

NOTE: Statistics not available for females in 1995 because of differences in the universe of respondents asked the questions.

X = Category not applicable.   - = Quantity zero.   * = Figure does not meet standards of reliability or precision.   [1]Statistics for condom "at all," pill "at all," and other hormonal reflect use of that method regardless of whether it was used alone or in combination with another method.   [2]Includes Lunelle injectable, emergency contraception, and contraceptive patch in 2002; adds contraceptive ring (Nuva-Ring) and Implanon implant in 2006–2010.   [3]Excludes condom and hormonal methods. Thus, if other method was combined with condom or hormonal method, it is not counted. Other methods include withdrawal, sterilization, IUD, female condom, diaphragm, cervical cap, spermicidal foam, jelly, cream or suppository, sponge, calendar rhythm method, and "other" methods.   [4]Includes persons of other or unknown origin and race groups.

Table 1-69. Use of Contraception at Last Sex in the Prior 3 Months Among Never-Married Females and Males Age 15 to 19 Years, by Method Used, Selected Years, 1988–2010

(Number in thousands, percent)

Characteristic	Number	Any method	No method	Pill (at all)	Other hormonal[1]	Condom (at all)	All other methods[2]	Dual methods (hormonal and condom)
FEMALE								
1988	3,521	79.9	20.1	42.7	X	31.3	9.3	3.3
1995	3,225	70.7	29.3	25.0	7.0	38.2	9.6	8.4
2002	3,304	83.2	16.8	34.2	9.1	54.3	5.1	19.5
Total, 2006–2010 [3]	3,175	85.6	14.4	30.5	12.2	52.0	11.0	20.1
Female, 2006–2010								
Hispanic Origin and Race								
Hispanic or Latina	539	79.5	20.5	17.2	18.0	47.7	10.6	14.0
Non-Hispanic White	1,873	89.3	10.7	38.6	10.5	52.4	12.3	24.4
Non-Hispanic Black	564	81.1	18.9	14.4	16.2	57.6	5.7	12.8
Age at First Sex								
14 years or under	835	73.0	27.0	18.0	11.6	38.3	16.7	11.7
15 to 16 years	1,528	88.7	11.3	33.5	12.9	50.1	10.9	18.7
17 to 19 years	812	92.8	7.2	37.9	11.3	69.6	5.5	31.4
MALE								
1988	3,847	84.2	15.8	37.4	...	53.3	13.6	15.2
1995	3,416	81.8	18.2	28.2	2.8	63.9	10.0	16.5
2002	3,165	90.7	9.3	31.0	6.3	70.7	2.0	23.9
Total, 2006–2010 [3]	2,970	92.5	7.5	39.0	9.3	74.7	3.4	33.9
Male, 2006–2010								
Hispanic Origin and Race								
Hispanic or Latino	593	86.2	13.8	29.4	6.8	65.5	4.3	19.6
Non-Hispanic White	1,567	96.8	3.2	49.6	11.0	76.8	2.9	43.4
Non-Hispanic Black	638	91.6	8.4	25.6	9.8	79.0	4.1	26.9
Age at First Sex								
14 years or under	1,009	85.3	14.7	31.1	11.1	68.0	5.0	29.7
15 to 16 years	1,363	95.3	4.7	41.3	10.1	74.4	3.6	34.2
17 to 19 years	598	98.1	*	47.2	4.5	86.3	*	40.2

NOTE: Statistics for condom "at all," pill "at all," and other hormonal reflect use of that method regardless of whether it was used alone or in combination with another method.

X = Not applicable.   * = Figure does not meet standards of reliability or precision.   [1]Includes Depo-Provera injectable and Norplant implants in 1995; adds Lunelle injectable, emergency contraception, and contraceptive patch in 2002; adds contraceptive ring (Nuva-Ring) and Implanon implant in 2006–2010.   [2]Excludes condom and hormonal methods. Thus, if other method was combined with condom or hormonal method, it is not counted. Other methods include withdrawal, sterilization, IUD, female condom, diaphragm, cervical cap, spermicidal foam, jelly, cream or suppository, sponge, calendar rhythm method, and "other" methods.   [3]Includes persons of other or unknown origin and race groups.

Table 1-70. Maternal Prepregnancy Body Mass Index, by Reporting Area, and Prepregnancy Obesity, by Race, Hispanic Origin, and Age of Mother, 36 States, the District of Columbia, and Puerto Rico, 2011

(Percent.)

Reporting Area	Total	BMI[1] Under-weight (BMI less than 18.5)	Normal (BMI 18.5 to 24.9)	Over-weight (BMI 25.0 to 29.9)	Obese (BMI greater than 30.0)	Race and Hispanic origin of mother Total	Non-Hispanic White[2]	Non-Hispanic Black[2]	Hispanic[3]	Age of mother in years Under 20 years	20 to 24 years	25 to 29 years	30 to 34 years	35 to 39 years	40 to 54 years
Total [4]	100.0	3.9	47.3	25.3	23.4	23.4	21.8	32.6	25.2	15.0	23.9	24.8	23.6	24.7	25.1
California	100.0	3.8	48.5	26.2	21.6	21.6	17.1	29.4	26.8	13.6	22.7	23.5	21.4	21.2	22.2
Colorado	100.0	4.1	52.3	24.8	18.8	18.8	16.6	24.2	24.5	11.6	19.9	20.3	18.1	19.3	19.4
Delaware	100.0	4.5	45.1	25.7	24.7	24.7	21.8	33.3	25.4	15.3	23.4	24.8	26.6	29.0	26.0
District of Columbia	100.0	4.3	52.7	22.7	20.3	20.3	4.8	30.0	20.6	17.0	26.7	27.9	16.2	14.2	13.7
Florida	100.0	4.8	48.3	25.1	21.8	21.8	19.3	30.5	20.2	13.7	21.8	23.0	22.1	23.1	23.8
Georgia	100.0	3.7	42.6	26.4	27.3	27.3	23.5	35.9	24.6	18.6	28.2	28.8	27.1	29.1	30.3
Idaho	100.0	3.3	50.1	24.8	21.7	21.7	20.7	19.2	27.2	13.9	20.4	22.2	23.0	26.0	28.0
Illinois	100.0	3.5	46.0	26.4	24.1	24.1	21.9	34.1	26.4	15.9	25.1	25.4	23.7	25.6	25.6
Indiana	100.0	4.2	45.0	25.2	25.7	25.7	24.9	33.9	26.0	15.9	25.6	26.4	27.4	28.3	30.9
Iowa	100.0	3.2	46.5	25.6	24.8	24.8	25.0	29.5	25.5	16.0	25.3	25.3	24.6	29.1	23.7
Kansas	100.0	3.5	46.8	26.0	23.7	23.7	23.4	28.8	25.8	14.2	24.2	24.8	24.5	25.7	28.2
Kentucky	100.0	4.6	43.7	24.3	27.4	27.4	27.1	36.1	23.8	18.3	28.0	28.4	28.4	31.1	31.8
Louisiana	100.0	4.4	43.8	24.6	27.2	27.2	23.2	34.7	22.0	17.2	26.2	29.3	29.4	31.3	33.7
Maryland	100.0	3.5	46.5	26.3	23.7	23.7	19.8	33.6	22.0	17.1	25.0	24.6	23.0	23.8	26.8
Michigan	100.0	3.5	45.1	25.5	25.9	25.9	24.4	34.5	27.7	17.1	26.2	26.7	26.1	29.1	28.9
Missouri	100.0	4.2	47.3	24.1	24.4	24.4	23.5	31.5	24.1	14.6	24.2	25.5	25.6	27.1	29.8
Montana	100.0	3.1	49.0	25.0	22.9	22.9	21.3	*	26.6	12.9	22.4	23.9	23.3	27.7	26.7
Nebraska	100.0	3.3	48.4	24.9	23.5	23.5	22.7	30.4	25.7	14.6	23.2	23.5	23.5	28.3	31.9
Nevada	100.0	4.7	48.8	25.4	21.1	21.1	19.5	24.2	23.7	11.0	20.8	22.5	22.4	22.7	24.4
New Hampshire	100.0	3.5	50.1	23.8	22.6	22.6	23.2	22.0	22.6	16.1	23.1	23.9	22.0	23.1	20.4
New Mexico	100.0	4.0	43.2	28.1	24.8	24.8	19.1	23.6	26.1	13.0	23.8	27.0	28.2	29.8	27.6
New York	100.0	4.2	50.0	25.4	20.4	20.4	19.5	30.3	21.9	15.4	20.6	21.7	19.8	20.5	21.1
North Carolina	100.0	4.2	46.4	25.0	24.4	24.4	21.1	35.4	22.6	16.1	25.2	25.5	24.0	26.6	28.0
North Dakota	100.0	2.6	41.0	27.9	28.5	28.5	27.2	22.9	31.9	16.6	27.6	27.7	30.2	39.6	29.0
Ohio	100.0	4.2	46.9	24.1	24.8	24.8	23.7	32.5	26.3	15.7	25.1	26.1	24.8	27.9	28.6
Oklahoma	100.0	4.5	45.2	24.8	25.4	25.4	24.3	30.8	26.0	15.1	25.1	26.7	27.9	30.6	30.8
Oregon	100.0	3.2	48.5	24.9	23.4	23.4	22.6	27.7	27.4	15.3	24.6	24.8	22.6	24.1	23.1
Pennsylvania	100.0	3.9	49.2	24.1	22.9	22.9	21.8	31.8	23.7	15.1	22.9	24.2	22.5	24.6	25.1
South Carolina	100.0	4.1	42.5	24.8	28.6	28.6	23.2	40.5	25.0	18.6	29.3	30.2	29.1	31.1	30.9
South Dakota	100.0	3.6	47.8	25.5	23.2	23.2	22.2	13.9	24.6	10.2	22.4	24.2	24.6	29.1	28.8
Tennessee	100.0	4.8	46.5	24.3	24.3	24.3	22.6	33.0	21.3	15.2	24.4	26.0	24.9	27.9	27.7
Texas	100.0	4.0	47.4	25.3	23.3	23.3	20.5	29.4	25.4	13.3	23.2	25.1	24.8	26.0	26.3
Utah	100.0	4.3	54.9	22.7	18.0	18.0	17.0	25.0	21.7	12.7	15.5	17.5	19.4	24.0	25.5
Vermont	100.0	3.1	49.4	24.3	23.2	23.2	23.7	*	*	20.9	25.8	25.1	21.8	20.6	15.6
Washington	100.0	2.9	46.4	25.9	24.7	24.7	24.1	30.9	29.8	16.6	26.5	25.5	24.0	25.1	27.0
Wisconsin	100.0	2.6	43.1	26.5	27.8	27.8	26.7	37.0	29.9	19.7	27.3	28.3	27.8	31.5	30.8
Wyoming	100.0	3.6	50.1	24.3	22.1	22.1	21.8		22.2	13.8	21.4	22.2	24.9	26.1	20.6
Puerto Rico	100.0	7.4	46.9	25.2	20.5	20.5	NA	NA	20.4	10.3	18.8	24.1	25.0	27.3	32.4

NA = Not available.   * = Figure does not meet standards of reliability or precision.   [1]BMI is Body Mass Index.   [2]Race and Hispanic origin are reported separately on birth certificates. Persons of Hispanic origin may be of any race. Multiple-race data, when reported, were bridged to single-race categories in order to maintain comparability among all reported areas.   [3]Includes all persons of Hispanic origin of any race.   [4]Excludes data for Puerto Rico.

Table 1-71. Number of Live Births by Attendant, Place of Delivery, Race, and Hispanic Origin of Mother, 2011

(Number.)

Place of delivery and race and Hispanic origin of mother	All births	Physician			Midwife			Other	Unspecified
		Total	Doctor of medicine	Doctor of osteopathy	Total	Certified nurse midwife	Other midwife		
ALL RACES [1]									
Total	3,953,590	3,588,203	3,359,909	228,294	335,525	309,514	26,011	25,782	4,080
In hospital [2]	3,903,569	3,585,862	3,357,836	228,026	300,072	294,684	5,388	14,433	3,202
Not in hospital	49,893	2,300	2,035	265	35,440	14,821	20,619	11,317	836
Freestanding birthing center	14,206	553	449	104	13,233	7,121	6,112	354	66
Clinic or doctor's office	408	185	142	43	178	152	26	42	3
Residence	33,043	1,121	1,025	96	21,569	7,396	14,173	9,702	651
Other	2,236	441	419	22	460	152	308	1,219	116
Not specified	128	41	38	3	13	9	4	32	42
NON-HISPANIC WHITE [3]									
Total	2,146,566	1,938,445	1,790,807	147,638	191,087	170,465	20,622	15,424	1,610
In hospital [2]	2,105,931	1,936,952	1,789,551	147,401	160,589	157,898	2,691	7,194	1,196
Not in hospital	40,580	1,465	1,231	234	30,486	12,559	17,927	8,218	411
Freestanding birthing center	11,839	503	400	103	10,975	5,875	5,100	312	49
Clinic or doctor's office	312	133	90	43	151	130	21	27	1
Residence	27,256	640	567	73	18,967	6,435	12,532	7,332	317
Other	1,173	189	174	15	393	119	274	547	44
Not specified	55	28	25	3	12	8	4	12	3
NON-HISPANIC BLACK [3]									
Total	582,345	534,765	510,641	24,124	42,543	41,508	1,035	3,847	1,190
In hospital [2]	579,556	534,314	510,210	24,104	41,540	40,965	575	2,661	1,041
Not in hospital	2,780	448	428	20	1,003	543	460	1,183	146
Freestanding birthing center	583	24	24	–	542	322	220	8	9
Clinic or doctor's office	18	10	10	–	6	5	1	2	–
Residence	1,783	280	264	16	433	202	231	955	115
Other	396	134	130	4	22	14	8	218	22
Not specified	9	3	3	–	–	–	–	3	3
HISPANIC [4]									
Total	918,129	836,577	791,936	44,641	76,218	73,218	3,000	4,493	841
In hospital [2]	914,123	836,321	791,687	44,634	73,683	72,139	1,544	3,446	673
Not in hospital	3,995	249	242	7	2,534	1,078	1,456	1,044	168
Freestanding birthing center	1,331	21	20	1	1,283	687	596	21	6
Clinic or doctor's office	24	7	7	–	16	12	4	1	–
Residence	2,302	154	149	5	1,213	366	847	798	137
Other	338	67	66	1	22	13	9	224	25
Not specified	11	7	7	–	1	1	–	3	–

– = Quantity zero.   [1]Includes races other than White and Black and origin not stated.   [2]Includes births occurring en route to or on arrival at hospital.   [3]Race and Hispanic origin are reported separately on birth certificates. Persons of Hispanic origin may be of any race. Multiple-race data, when reported, were bridged to single-race categories in order to maintain comparability among all reported areas.   [4]Includes all persons of Hispanic origin of any race.

Table 1-72. Educational Attainment of Mother, by Age and Hispanic Origin and Race of Mother: Total of 27 Reporting States, 2008

(Number, rates per 100,000 in specified group; age-adjusted rates per 100,000 U.S. standard population.)

Education level and sex	All ages	Under 20	20 to 24 years	25 to 29 years	30 to 34 years	35 to 39 years	40 to 54 years
All Races [1]	100.0	100.0	100.0	100.0	100.0	100.0	100.0
12 grade or less with no diploma	22.2	57.5	25.6	17.3	13.5	13.1	14.7
High school graduate [2]	27.0	33.7	39.5	25.6	17.8	16.7	17.8
Some college credit, but no degree	19.6	8.5	25.8	22.2	17.0	15.5	15.5
Associate's degree [3]	6.8	0.3	4.7	8.9	8.5	8.5	8.2
Bachelor's degree [4]	16.3	0.0	4.1	19.4	26.9	27.5	25.8
Master's degree [5]	6.4	*	0.3	5.6	12.8	13.9	12.6
Doctorate or professional degree [6]	1.8	*	0.0	1.0	3.5	4.8	5.3
All births	2,748,302	289,202	684,971	769,935	613,235	316,488	74,471
Not stated [7]	52,906	4,488	11,131	14,108	12,984	7,736	2,459
White [8]	100.0	100.0	100.0	100.0	100.0	100.0	100.0
12 grade or less with no diploma	11.3	50.0	17.2	7.2	3.7	3.2	3.7
High school graduate [2]	24.7	39.1	40.7	23.0	14.3	13.4	14.7
Some college credit, but no degree	21.4	10.5	29.5	23.9	17.5	16.1	16.4
Associate's degree [3]	8.7	0.4	6.4	11.2	10.0	9.6	9.3
Bachelor's degree [4]	22.5	*	5.7	26.1	34.0	34.0	32.7
Master's degree [5]	9.1	*	0.4	7.4	16.5	17.9	16.5
Doctorate or professional degree [6]	2.3	–	0.0	1.3	4.0	5.7	6.7
All births	1,366,527	103,622	313,625	404,436	333,446	171,589	39,809
Not stated [7]	9,276	707	1,851	2,443	2,358	1,446	471
Black [8]	100.0	100.0	100.0	100.0	100.0	100.0	100.0
12 grade or less with no diploma	22.7	55.4	20.5	15.3	12.0	11.4	13.9
High school graduate [2]	34.7	34.9	42.9	32.5	27.4	25.7	27.1
Some college credit, but no degree	24.6	9.4	29.7	28.9	25.5	22.4	20.8
Associate's degree [3]	5.9	0.2	3.7	8.0	9.6	10.2	10.0
Bachelor's degree [4]	8.4	*	3.0	11.7	16.3	18.4	16.7
Master's degree [5]	3.1	*	0.2	3.1	7.5	9.5	9.2
Doctorate or professional degree [6]	0.6	*	0.0	0.5	1.6	2.4	2.4
All births	349,243	58,110	109,188	88,153	56,649	29,446	7,697
Not stated [7]	4,175	627	1,136	1,035	787	456	134
Hispanic [9]	100.0	100.0	100.0	100.0	100.0	100.0	100.0
12 grade or less with no diploma	43.7	65.9	40.8	39.4	39.2	40.1	43.3
High school graduate [2]	29.2	27.9	36.2	29.0	24.1	22.4	21.9
Some college credit, but no degree	14.9	6.0	18.2	17.2	14.7	13.2	12.8
Associate's degree [3]	3.8	0.2	2.8	5.1	5.5	5.4	5.0
Bachelor's degree [4]	6.1	0.0	1.8	7.5	11.5	12.5	11.0
Master's degree [5]	1.7	*	0.1	1.5	3.9	4.9	4.3
Doctorate or professional degree [6]	0.5	*	0.0	0.3	1.1	1.6	1.8
All births	787,484	112,705	221,920	210,785	150,512	74,250	17,312
Not stated [7]	12,437	1,555	3,260	3,366	2,549	1,331	376

NOTE: Includes California, Colorado, Delaware, Florida, Georgia, Idaho, Indiana, Iowa, Kansas, Kentucky, Michigan, Montana, Nebraska, New Hampshire, New Mexico, New York, North Dakota, Ohio, Oregon, Pennsylvania, South Carolina, South Dakota, Tennessee, Texas, Vermont, Washington, and Wyoming.

– = Quantity zero.   * = Figure does not meet standards of reliability or precision.   0.0 = Quantity more than zero but less than 0.5.   [1]Includes other races not shown and origin not stated.   [2]Includes General Educational Development (GED).   [3]Includes Associate in Arts and Associate in Science.   [4]Includes Bachelor of Arts and Bachelor of Science.   [5]Includes Master of Arts and Master of Science.   [6]Includes Doctor of Philosophy, Doctor of Education, Doctor of Medicine, Doctor of Dental Surgery, Doctor of Veterinary Medicine, Doctor of Laws, and Juris Doctor.   [7]No response reported for education attainment of mother item; includes births to residents of states using the 2003 U.S. Standard Certificate of Live Birth occurring in states using the 1989 U.S. Standard Certificate of Live Birth.   [8]Race and Hispanic origin are reported separately on birth certificates. Persons of Hispanic origin may be of any race. Multiple-race data, when reported, were bridged to single-race categories in order to maintain comparability among all reported areas.   [9]Includes all persons of Hispanic origin of any race.

Table 1-73. Mother Received WIC Food During This Pregnancy, by Race and Hispanic Origin, and Age of Mother, 36 States, the District of Columbia, and Puerto Rico, 2011

(Percent.)

Reporting area	Race and Hispanic origin of mother				Age of mother in years					
	Total	Non-Hispanic White[1]	Non-Hispanic Black[1]	Hispanic[2]	Under 20 years	20 to 24 years	25 to 29 years	30 to 34 years	35 to 39 years	40 to 54 years
Total [3]	47.8	33.0	67.9	71.4	81.2	68.8	43.9	31.1	29.7	29.7
California	54.3	26.1	69.6	76.2	87.7	77.7	55.0	38.9	35.6	34.3
Colorado	33.0	19.8	53.1	60.2	71.7	53.8	30.3	18.9	17.4	16.9
Delaware	35.7	25.4	45.5	67.6	61.6	52.7	33.8	22.4	20.2	19.5
District of Columbia	44.5	2.4	59.2	77.5	76.9	67.4	54.3	27.9	21.3	14.5
Florida	54.0	39.9	73.0	64.5	83.7	73.8	50.9	38.3	37.0	36.8
Georgia	51.5	38.1	66.4	64.9	81.9	71.1	47.4	33.6	30.4	28.1
Idaho	44.2	38.0	69.5	73.1	80.6	60.4	39.7	27.1	28.8	28.3
Illinois	41.6	26.6	66.4	66.3	77.7	68.0	39.0	24.9	23.5	23.4
Indiana	46.9	40.0	73.0	75.1	81.3	67.6	38.6	28.0	28.2	28.8
Iowa	37.6	31.5	72.2	75.7	80.5	60.4	29.9	20.9	22.9	23.3
Kansas	39.0	29.8	63.3	70.0	71.8	57.8	31.6	22.8	22.3	22.6
Kentucky	49.5	46.9	65.4	69.5	81.0	68.1	41.1	28.3	28.1	28.0
Louisiana	55.2	42.5	72.6	61.8	81.8	70.4	47.8	36.5	35.0	34.2
Maryland	41.9	24.1	59.5	69.6	83.2	69.3	41.1	26.5	22.7	22.3
Michigan	46.7	38.9	70.3	69.7	80.6	70.7	42.3	26.7	27.0	26.2
Missouri	46.6	40.0	71.6	70.3	84.6	69.1	38.4	25.9	25.7	24.9
Montana	35.8	30.8	48.0	47.5	67.5	54.2	30.1	19.8	20.3	19.8
Nebraska	36.3	25.5	70.9	72.1	75.1	58.3	29.6	20.9	23.4	26.1
Nevada	40.7	23.0	53.5	61.3	68.8	53.7	35.7	30.2	30.1	28.5
New Hampshire	28.1	26.4	51.0	57.1	73.6	54.3	26.6	13.5	11.5	11.3
New Mexico	55.9	34.2	54.9	66.1	77.8	66.7	48.8	43.0	43.0	42.6
New York	48.0	30.1	69.7	68.9	81.0	72.4	51.2	33.8	30.4	30.2
North Carolina	49.1	34.8	69.3	73.5	83.0	69.9	43.9	31.1	27.1	29.1
North Dakota	31.6	23.8	74.2	46.8	73.1	50.5	24.6	15.1	21.4	20.9
Ohio	42.8	35.9	69.5	64.9	79.7	65.6	36.4	23.3	21.2	21.7
Oklahoma	53.9	45.2	69.6	75.5	83.1	69.6	44.0	35.5	34.8	35.6
Oregon	45.7	37.2	61.2	77.3	82.0	67.9	43.3	30.1	28.8	28.8
Pennsylvania	39.9	29.2	68.0	73.4	78.4	64.3	36.3	22.6	20.9	22.6
South Carolina	53.9	39.9	76.7	68.4	84.7	73.3	47.3	33.5	32.0	30.7
South Dakota	40.0	28.5	60.1	62.5	78.2	62.1	31.5	23.1	23.2	26.1
Tennessee	49.2	43.3	62.0	68.7	79.7	66.3	42.3	30.1	28.1	28.5
Texas	53.5	29.5	62.8	71.8	80.8	69.6	48.2	37.5	36.5	36.5
Utah	28.3	21.5	57.0	58.2	65.2	40.2	24.1	19.4	19.8	20.4
Vermont	42.9	42.7	73.2	38.0	82.6	71.9	42.7	24.5	18.3	19.7
Washington	41.5	32.2	56.8	73.8	79.5	63.9	39.3	26.8	24.5	23.9
Wisconsin	37.2	26.6	75.2	71.2	79.9	62.8	31.9	20.8	20.7	21.2
Wyoming	34.4	30.0	52.5	55.1	69.4	47.8	27.1	20.8	17.7	19.1
Puerto Rico	87.1	NA	NA	87.5	95.1	93.3	87.3	75.6	68.9	69.0

NA = Not available.   [1]Race and Hispanic origin are reported separately on birth certificates. Persons of Hispanic origin may be of any race. Multiple-race data, when reported, were bridged to single-race categories in order to maintain comparability among all reported areas.   [2]Includes all persons of Hispanic origin of any race. [3]Excludes data for Puerto Rico.

Table 1-74. Pregnancy Resulted from Infertility Therapy, by Race and Hispanic Origin, and Age of Mother, 36 States, the District of Columbia, and Puerto Rico, 2011

(Percent.)

Reporting area	Race and Hispanic origin of mother				Age of mother in years					
	Total	Non-Hispanic White[1]	Non-Hispanic Black[1]	Hispanic[2]	Under 20 years	20 to 24 years	25 to 29 years	30 tos 34 years	35 to 39 years	40 to 54 years
Total [3]	1.4	2.0	0.4	0.4	0.0	0.2	0.9	1.9	3.2	6.8
California	1.0	1.9	0.4	0.3	*	0.1	0.4	1.1	2.2	6.4
Colorado	1.8	2.4	*	0.5	*	0.2	1.0	2.3	3.9	10.9
Delaware	2.2	3.1	*	*	*	0.1	1.5	3.8	4.7	9.3
District of Columbia	2.7	7.9	*	*	*	*	*	2.4	6.6	17.1
Florida	0.6	1.0	0.2	0.4	*	0.1	0.3	1.0	1.6	3.3
Georgia	1.0	1.7	0.3	0.4	*	0.1	0.6	1.6	2.9	6.0
Idaho	1.2	1.4	*	*	*	0.3	1.1	1.8	2.7	7.5
Illinois	2.5	3.7	0.5	0.7	*	0.2	1.5	3.4	5.7	11.5
Indiana	0.9	1.1	0.2	*	*	0.2	0.8	1.6	2.1	2.9
Iowa	2.5	2.8	*	0.7	*	0.3	2.3	4.0	5.0	9.7
Kansas	1.2	1.5	*	0.3	*	*	1.1	2.1	3.0	3.9
Kentucky	0.8	0.9	*	*	*	0.1	0.8	1.3	1.9	4.5
Louisiana	0.5	0.9	0.2	*	*	*	0.5	1.2	1.3	3.5
Maryland	3.7	5.4	1.8	1.3	*	0.6	2.2	4.7	8.0	13.8
Michigan	1.1	1.3	0.2	0.5	*	0.1	0.9	1.6	2.5	4.4
Missouri	1.1	1.3	0.2	*	*	0.2	0.9	1.9	2.8	4.2
Montana	1.1	1.2	*	*	*	*	0.6	2.0	2.6	*
Nebraska	1.2	1.6	*	*	*	*	1.1	1.9	2.7	*
Nevada	1.5	2.4	*	0.6	*	0.3	1.0	2.0	3.8	*
New Hampshire	2.2	2.2	*	*	*	*	1.1	2.9	4.9	*
New Mexico	0.3	0.6	*	*	*	*	0.2	0.6	*	*
New York	1.6	3.3	0.8	0.6	*	0.3	1.1	2.6	4.2	8.8
North Carolina	0.9	1.3	0.3	0.3	*	0.1	0.6	1.4	2.1	4.6
North Dakota	1.5	1.8	*	*	*	*	1.1	2.7	3.4	*
Ohio	1.7	2.0	0.4	0.7	*	0.2	1.4	2.8	4.2	7.6
Oklahoma	0.8	1.1	*	*	*	*	0.8	1.4	2.2	4.3
Oregon	1.9	2.3	*	0.6	*	*	1.2	2.6	4.5	9.5
Pennsylvania	1.8	2.3	0.4	0.6	*	0.2	1.2	2.6	4.3	8.0
South Carolina	0.7	1.1	0.2	*	*	*	0.5	1.3	2.2	3.7
South Dakota	1.4	1.8	*	*	*	0.5	1.4	2.1	2.6	*
Tennessee	0.8	1.1	0.1	*	*	0.1	0.7	1.5	2.2	4.3
Texas	0.8	1.5	0.3	0.3	*	0.1	0.5	1.3	2.0	4.9
Utah	4.9	5.6	*	2.1	*	2.5	5.4	6.0	7.4	10.4
Vermont	2.0	2.1	*	*	*	*	1.0	2.3	5.4	*
Washington	1.2	1.4	0.4	0.5	*	0.1	0.7	1.6	2.8	7.4
Wisconsin	2.0	2.4	0.4	0.7	*	0.2	1.6	3.0	4.3	6.9
Wyoming	1.0	1.2	*	*	*	*	0.9	1.7	*	*
Puerto Rico	0.4	NA	NA	*	*	*	0.2	0.7	2.1	*

NA = Not available.   * = Figure does not meet standards of reliability or precision.   0.0 = Quantity more than zero but less than 0.05.   [1]Race and Hispanic origin are reported separately on birth certificates. Persons of Hispanic origin may be of any race. Multiple-race data, when reported, were bridged to single-race categories in order to maintain comparability among all reported areas.   [2]Includes all persons of Hispanic origin of any race.   [3]Excludes data for Puerto Rico.

94 VITAL STATISTICS OF THE UNITED STATES (BERNAN PRESS)

Table 1-75. Abnormal Conditions of the Newborn, by Age and Race and Hispanic Origin of Mother, 27 Reporting States, 2008

(Number; rate per 1,000 live births in specified group.)

Abnormal condition and race and Hispanic origin of mother	All births[1]	Condition reported	All ages	Under 20 years	20 to 24 years	25 to 29 years	30 to 34 years	35 to 39 years	40 to 54 years	Not stated[2]
All Races [3]										
Assisted ventilation required immediately following delivery	2,748,302	110,715	41.0	44.2	40.1	39.2	40.5	43.1	49.1	45,689
Assisted ventilation required for more than 6 hours	2,748,302	23,697	8.8	9.8	8.5	8.3	8.5	9.2	11.9	45,689
NICU admission	2,748,302	180,274	66.7	68.4	62.6	62.6	66.1	77.3	100.1	45,689
Surfactant replacement therapy given to newborn	2,748,302	9,139	3.4	3.7	3.2	3.2	3.3	3.6	4.8	45,689
Antibiotics received by newborn for suspected neonatal sepsis	2,748,302	46,874	17.3	21.0	18.2	16.4	15.9	16.7	19.9	45,689
Seizure or serious neurologic dysfunction	2,748,302	754	0.3	0.3	0.3	0.2	0.3	0.3	0.4	45,689
Significant birth injury	2,748,302	1,881	0.7	0.7	0.7	0.7	0.6	0.7	1.0	45,689
White [4]										
Assisted ventilation required immediately following delivery	1,366,527	61,396	45.3	49.7	44.3	43.7	44.8	47.4	54.0	12,072
Assisted ventilation required for more than 6 hours	1,366,527	13,479	10.0	11.7	9.9	9.6	9.5	10.0	13.1	12,072
NICU admission	1,366,527	89,207	65.9	66.1	61.5	62.4	65.0	75.7	99.3	12,072
Surfactant replacement therapy given to newborn	1,366,527	5,606	4.1	5.0	4.0	4.0	3.9	4.3	5.5	12,072
Antibiotics received by newborn for suspected neonatal sepsis	1,366,527	25,987	19.2	24.1	20.8	18.5	17.2	18.1	22.2	12,072
Seizure or serious neurologic dysfunction	1,366,527	481	0.4	0.4	0.4	0.3	0.3	0.3	*	12,072
Significant birth injury	1,366,527	998	0.7	0.9	0.8	0.7	0.6	0.6	1.0	12,072
Black [4]										
Assisted ventilation required immediately following delivery	349,243	17,584	51.9	52.2	49.2	50.3	54.2	58.3	62.8	10,184
Assisted ventilation required for more than 6 hours	349,243	4,071	12.0	12.0	11.3	11.3	13.0	13.8	16.9	10,184
NICU admission	349,243	31,483	92.9	87.2	85.5	87.6	100.9	120.7	133.8	10,184
Surfactant replacement therapy given to newborn	349,243	1,576	4.6	4.7	4.3	4.2	5.1	6.1	5.6	10,184
Antibiotics received by newborn for suspected neonatal sepsis	349,243	6,887	20.3	21.9	20.6	18.0	20.8	22.1	20.9	10,184
Seizure or serious neurologic dysfunction	349,243	77	0.2	0.4	*	*	0.4	*	*	10,184
Significant birth injury	349,243	160	0.5	0.6	0.4	0.4	0.6	*	*	10,184
Hispanic [5]										
Assisted ventilation required immediately following delivery	787,484	24,601	31.5	35.3	30.8	28.9	31.4	33.9	38.5	6,835
Assisted ventilation required for more than 6 hours	787,484	4,674	6.0	7.1	5.6	5.4	5.8	7.0	8.2	6,835
NICU admission	787,484	44,993	57.6	60.3	53.1	53.2	59.2	69.3	88.4	6,835
Surfactant replacement therapy given to newborn	787,484	1,397	1.8	2.0	1.8	1.5	1.8	1.9	3.6	6,835
Antibiotics received by newborn for suspected neonatal sepsis	787,484	10,476	13.4	17.4	13.6	12.0	12.2	13.0	15.6	6,835
Seizure or serious neurologic dysfunction	787,484	144	0.2	0.2	0.2	0.2	0.2	*	*	6,835
Significant birth injury	787,484	471	0.6	0.6	0.6	0.6	0.6	0.6	*	6,835

NOTE: Includes California, Colorado, Delaware, Florida, Georgia, Idaho, Indiana, Iowa, Kansas, Kentucky, Michigan, Montana, Nebraska, New Hampshire, New Mexico, New York, North Dakota, Ohio, Oregon, Pennsylvania, South Carolina, South Dakota, Tennessee, Texas, Vermont, Washington, and Wyoming.

* = Figure does not meet standards of reliability or precision.   [1]Refers to total number of births to residents of areas reporting specified abnormal condition.   [2]No response reported for abnormal conditions of the newborn item; includes births to residents of states using the 2003 U.S. Standard Certificate of Live Birth occurring in states using the 1989 U.S. Standard Certificate of Live Birth.   [3]Includes other races not shown and origin not stated.   [4]Race and Hispanic origin are reported separately on birth certificates. Persons of Hispanic origin may be of any race. Multiple-race data, when reported, were bridged to single-race categories in order to maintain comparability among all reported areas.   [5]Includes all persons of Hispanic origin of any race.

Table 1-76. Congenital Anomaly of the Newborn, by Age and Race and Hispanic Origin of Mother, 27 Reporting States, 2008

(Number; rate per 1,000 live births in specified group.)

Congenital anomaly	All births[1]	Condition reported	All ages	Under 20 years	20 to 24 years	25 to 29 years	30 to 34 years	35 to 39 years	40 to 54 years	Not stated[2]
Anencephaly	2,748,302	372	13.8	16.5	13.2	17.1	10.6	11.6	*	50,501
Menigomyelocele or spina bifida	2,748,302	402	14.9	16.5	14.9	14.8	15.3	12.6	*	50,501
Cyanotic congenital heart disease	2,748,302	1,225	45.4	38.0	38.5	42.9	45.5	60.3	100.1	50,501
Congenital diaphragmatic hernia	2,748,302	293	10.9	10.6	11.0	12.0	9.8	10.6	*	50,501
Omphalocele	2,748,302	193	7.2	7.7	6.8	5.7	5.8	11.0	*	50,501
Gastroschisis	2,748,302	790	29.3	95.0	52.2	15.5	5.3	*	*	50,501
Limb reduction defect	2,748,302	438	16.2	18.3	20.2	16.5	12.5	13.5	*	50,501
Cleft lip with or without cleft palate	2,748,302	1,396	51.7	59.1	55.0	52.8	44.2	52.2	42.5	50,501
Cleft palate alone	2,748,302	596	22.1	23.6	25.1	20.8	18.3	23.8	*	50,501
Down syndrome	2,748,302	1,298	48.1	28.2	22.0	22.8	44.2	119.2	359.3	50,501
Suspected chromosomal disorder	2,748,302	1,093	40.5	36.6	37.6	31.8	37.4	51.2	153.6	50,501
Hypospadias[3]	2,748,302	1,434	53.2	46.1	52.6	56.1	54.5	54.8	37.0	50,501
Males only[4]	1,406,875	1,434	103.8	89.8	103.0	109.6	106.3	106.9	72.2	25,868

NOTE: Includes California, Colorado, Delaware, Florida, Georgia, Idaho, Indiana, Iowa, Kansas, Kentucky, Michigan, Montana, Nebraska, New Hampshire, New Mexico, New York, North Dakota, Ohio, Oregon, Pennsylvania, South Carolina, South Dakota, Tennessee, Texas, Vermont, Washington, and Wyoming.

* = Figure does not meet standards of reliability or precision; based on fewer than 20 births in the numerator.   [1]Refers to total number of births to residents of areas reporting specified abnormal condition.   [2]No response reported for congenital anomaly of the newborn item; includes births to residents of states using the 2003 U.S. Standard Certificate of Live Birth occurring in states using the 1989 U.S. Standard Certificate of Live Birth.   [3]Denominator includes both male and female births.   [4]Denominator includes male only.

Table 1-77. Principal Source of Payment for the Delivery, 36 States, the District of Columbia, and Puerto Rico, 2011

(Percent.)

Reporting area	All births	Medicaid	Private insurance	Self-pay[1]	Other
Total [2]	100.0	44.9	46.1	4.2	4.8
California	100.0	46.9	46.5	2.1	4.5
Colorado	100.0	35.9	52.8	3.5	7.8
Delaware	100.0	49.2	46.5	1.4	2.9
District of Columbia	100.0	46.1	41.8	0.6	11.6
Florida	100.0	49.8	38.9	8.6	2.6
Georgia	100.0	47.3	35.1	5.1	12.6
Idaho	100.0	39.3	48.0	8.2	4.5
Illinois	100.0	49.0	48.8	1.0	1.2
Indiana	100.0	46.0	48.0	4.5	1.5
Iowa	100.0	38.6	57.2	3.0	1.2
Kansas	100.0	33.8	50.8	7.2	8.2
Kentucky	100.0	43.7	43.9	2.8	9.5
Louisiana	100.0	64.2	32.3	0.9	2.7
Maryland	100.0	30.6	59.6	3.7	6.0
Michigan	100.0	45.0	53.1	1.3	0.5
Missouri	100.0	45.0	49.8	3.1	2.1
Montana	100.0	35.4	46.6	7.1	10.9
Nebraska	100.0	30.7	58.9	6.8	3.6
Nevada	100.0	32.7	47.6	14.5	5.2
New Hampshire	100.0	31.1	63.7	2.1	3.0
New Mexico	100.0	58.2	23.9	6.9	11.1
New York	100.0	45.6	48.8	1.6	4.0
North Carolina	100.0	45.8	44.7	6.9	2.6
North Dakota	100.0	28.8	56.6	3.1	11.6
Ohio	100.0	40.5	49.8	4.9	4.7
Oklahoma	100.0	54.8	33.9	2.2	9.1
Oregon	100.0	45.5	50.8	2.2	1.5
Pennsylvania	100.0	32.7	59.5	5.1	2.8
South Carolina	100.0	51.0	38.6	5.1	5.3
South Dakota	100.0	35.4	56.0	2.2	6.4
Tennessee	100.0	53.8	41.8	1.8	2.6
Texas	100.0	47.9	36.6	7.8	7.7
Utah	100.0	29.4	60.8	6.0	3.8
Vermont	100.0	45.9	49.4	1.7	3.0
Washington	100.0	39.7	49.2	1.2	9.9
Wisconsin	100.0	38.9	54.1	2.9	4.1
Wyoming	100.0	37.6	51.9	5.8	4.7
Puerto Rico	100.0	73.4	25.5	1.1	*

* = Figure does not meet standards of reliability or precision; based on fewer than 20 births in the numerator.   [1]No third-party payer listed; uninsured.   [2]Excludes data for Puerto Rico.

Table 1-78. Births Insured by Medicaid, by Race and Hispanic Origin, and Age of Mother, 36 States, the District of Columbia, and Puerto Rico, 2011

(Percent.)

Reporting area	Race and Hispanic origin or mother				Age of mother in years					
	Total	Non-Hispanic White[1]	Non-Hispanic Black[1]	Hispanic[2]	Under 20 years	20 to 24 years	25 to 29 years	30 to 34 years	35 to 39 years	40 to 54 years
Total[3]	44.9	32.7	66.8	61.4	76.1	66.4	41.8	28.0	26.1	26.6
California	46.9	23.5	56.4	66.0	75.9	68.0	47.8	33.0	30.5	29.7
Colorado	35.9	22.5	57.9	63.1	72.2	58.1	33.6	21.4	19.1	20.9
Delaware	49.2	35.8	67.2	80.7	79.1	72.9	47.3	30.5	29.1	29.0
District of Columbia	46.1	1.7	72.4	44.2	79.9	75.2	56.3	26.4	19.6	17.4
Florida	49.8	41.7	68.8	50.0	80.2	71.7	47.9	32.3	29.9	29.9
Georgia	47.3	36.5	65.2	42.6	76.7	67.8	43.4	28.4	25.5	24.6
Idaho	39.3	36.1	60.6	52.3	77.3	56.6	33.5	22.7	23.0	21.5
Illinois	49.0	30.9	78.3	77.0	85.7	78.4	47.4	30.4	28.4	28.6
Indiana	46.0	38.4	76.3	73.6	76.2	67.4	38.9	26.8	25.6	28.7
Iowa	38.6	33.9	81.2	59.8	79.6	64.6	31.3	20.3	20.4	23.8
Kansas	33.8	29.5	67.6	39.1	66.7	53.4	27.3	16.8	14.7	15.6
Kentucky	43.7	42.7	56.1	43.0	70.4	61.4	36.8	23.7	22.9	24.9
Louisiana	64.2	47.6	85.4	79.8	93.0	82.8	56.7	41.8	39.0	36.7
Maryland	30.6	18.7	45.1	42.6	63.0	51.9	30.4	18.3	15.6	15.5
Michigan	45.0	39.2	58.4	71.3	72.2	67.8	42.4	26.0	26.1	25.7
Missouri	45.0	37.7	77.2	58.8	81.5	68.1	37.4	24.2	23.1	22.6
Montana	35.4	30.7	36.0	51.0	65.9	54.9	29.9	19.8	15.9	15.6
Nebraska	30.7	24.4	68.3	40.9	64.4	52.8	25.5	15.3	16.4	17.6
Nevada	32.7	25.2	55.9	37.6	62.2	49.2	28.7	20.4	16.9	20.6
New Hampshire	31.1	30.6	48.5	43.6	60.1	57.9	31.4	17.6	13.4	14.7
New Mexico	58.2	42.9	54.2	59.7	75.2	69.6	53.6	43.0	40.5	43.3
New York	45.6	25.9	63.3	70.9	71.3	68.1	50.0	32.4	29.3	28.1
North Carolina	45.8	35.3	70.6	47.1	80.4	66.4	40.7	27.1	24.0	26.5
North Dakota	28.8	21.1	60.8	41.2	59.8	47.3	23.9	13.6	16.7	15.4
Ohio	40.5	33.9	71.4	45.2	71.8	64.1	35.7	20.9	18.1	19.8
Oklahoma	54.8	46.2	74.2	78.8	81.9	70.4	46.3	35.5	35.7	36.3
Oregon	45.5	37.4	66.5	74.3	77.1	68.0	43.8	30.5	27.9	30.1
Pennsylvania	32.7	24.2	58.5	56.3	63.4	55.3	30.1	17.2	15.3	16.3
South Carolina	51.0	40.3	72.5	46.7	81.5	71.1	44.6	30.3	26.9	27.8
South Dakota	35.4	24.0	62.2	47.2	65.8	56.9	28.6	18.9	19.7	19.6
Tennessee	53.8	45.5	76.9	69.2	83.3	73.1	46.9	32.6	30.0	32.5
Texas	47.9	33.2	62.6	57.5	76.7	66.9	42.9	29.5	26.7	27.4
Utah	29.4	23.1	63.9	59.2	70.9	44.4	24.6	19.2	19.3	23.4
Vermont	45.9	45.8	72.2	35.7	78.0	75.2	47.2	27.6	22.7	17.5
Washington	39.7	29.9	56.7	71.8	72.0	57.5	38.8	27.1	25.4	25.8
Wisconsin	38.9	28.6	78.9	73.2	74.4	65.1	35.0	22.3	22.3	25.1
Wyoming	37.6	32.8	47.5	56.3	67.8	52.9	29.9	23.8	20.3	22.9
Puerto Rico	73.4	NA	NA	73.5	95.2	89.7	67.2	45.0	38.2	41.1

NA = Not available.   [1]Race and Hispanic origin are reported separately on birth certificates. Persons of Hispanic origin may be of any race. Multiple-race data, when reported, were bridged to single-race categories in order to maintain comparability among all reported areas.   [2]Includes all persons of Hispanic origin of any race.   [3]Excludes data for Puerto Rico.

Table 1-79. Maternal Morbidity, 35 States, the District of Columbia, and Puerto Rico, 2011

(Number, rate per 100,000 births.)

Reporting area	Rate per 100,000 births					
	Maternal transfusion	3rd or 4th degree perineal laceration	Ruptured Uterus	Unplanned hysterectomy	Admission to ICU	Unplanned operating room procedure
Total[1]	271.6	867.0	26.2	37.4	149.9	275.0
California	135.5	645.6	12.2	25.1	97.4	95.8
Colorado	209.1	661.2	*	61.5	67.7	201.4
District of Columbia	*	877.0	*	*	*	*
Florida	124.5	472.9	17.9	28.8	166.4	75.9
Georgia	154.7	608.3	47.6	23.0	113.4	135.6
Idaho	462.3	1,238.7	*	*	*	206.5
Illinois	373.1	791.1	34.3	54.8	204.3	238.6
Indiana	249.7	835.3	28.7	40.6	130.2	234.2
Iowa	366.8	1,412.2	*	*	138.9	332.7
Kansas	265.0	903.4	*	*	128.7	194.3
Kentucky	243.5	679.7	*	*	105.4	516.1
Louisiana	294.8	511.5	39.1	39.1	231.3	104.2
Maryland	195.8	2,114.9	*	*	84.7	895.7
Michigan	277.8	882.4	36.5	30.3	124.7	255.6
Missouri	360.9	1,035.2	39.5	43.5	122.5	234.4
Montana	456.7	664.3	*	*	*	307.2
Nebraska	230.2	4,550.2	*	*	82.0	796.1
Nevada	229.9	933.7	90.8	*	122.0	153.2
New Hampshire	404.9	1,077.0	*	*	*	542.6
New Mexico	217.0	742.9	*	*	327.3	125.0
New York	436.6	1,010.8	24.1	52.8	132.6	247.0
North Carolina	224.6	808.9	33.4	39.2	224.6	218.7
North Dakota	326.7	1,380.4	*	*	*	274.0
Ohio	289.6	1,152.5	31.2	52.0	148.5	1,861.0
Oklahoma	239.2	741.0	38.9	*	103.1	134.2
Oregon	483.0	1,209.7	*	*	161.7	587.1
Pennsylvania	362.1	732.0	19.7	43.7	128.2	217.7
South Carolina	170.9	915.4	*	*	108.1	108.1
South Dakota	414.5	1,345.1	*	*	*	245.3
Tennessee	193.1	979.4	30.3	35.3	73.2	116.1
Texas	202.2	569.3	22.0	31.8	284.9	102.6
Utah	1,244.5	1,314.8	*	58.6	125.0	207.1
Vermont	396.6	1,801.4	*	*	*	710.6
Washington	391.6	1,210.6	26.6	52.0	100.5	259.9
Wisconsin	446.5	1,401.7	41.5	53.4	157.2	384.2
Wyoming	594.9	797.7	*	*	*	378.6
Puerto Rico	185.0	447.9	17.0	31.6	68.2	150.9
Total[1]	8,774	28,005	847	1,209	4,842	8,883
California	680	3,240	61	126	489	481
Colorado	136	430	8	40	44	131
District of Columbia	10	71	1	1	3	3
Florida	264	1,003	38	61	353	161
Georgia	195	767	60	29	143	171
Idaho	103	276	5	6	17	46
Illinois	599	1,270	55	88	328	383
Indiana	209	699	24	34	109	196
Iowa	140	539	13	18	53	127
Kansas	105	358	13	14	51	77
Kentucky	134	374	19	19	58	284
Louisiana	181	314	24	24	142	64
Maryland	141	1,523	16	18	61	645
Michigan	312	991	41	34	140	287
Missouri	274	786	30	33	93	178
Montana	55	80	6	5	12	37
Nebraska	59	1,166	6	6	21	204
Nevada	81	329	32	15	43	54
New Hampshire	50	133	5	10	15	67
New Mexico	59	202	2	7	89	34
New York	1,034	2,394	57	125	314	585
North Carolina	269	969	40	47	269	262
North Dakota	31	131	2	3	13	26
Ohio	390	1,552	42	70	200	2,506
Oklahoma	123	381	20	14	53	69
Oregon	218	546	6	14	73	265
Pennsylvania	514	1,039	28	62	182	309
South Carolina	98	525	14	14	62	62
South Dakota	49	159	4	2	9	29
Tennessee	153	776	24	28	58	92
Texas	763	2,148	83	120	1,075	387
Utah	637	673	10	30	64	106
Vermont	24	109	2	5	5	43
Washington	339	1,048	23	45	87	225
Wisconsin	301	945	28	36	106	259
Wyoming	44	59	5	6	8	28
Puerto Rico	76	184	7	13	28	62

NOTE: Excludes Delaware. ICU is intensive care unit.

* = Figure does not meet standards of reliability or precision; based on fewer than 20 births in the numerator.   [1]Excludes data for Puerto Rico.

NOTES AND DEFINITIONS

SOURCES OF DATA

All of the tables in Part 1 are from the National Center for Health Statistics (NCHS), a component of the Centers for Disease Control and Prevention (CDC). Five different publications were used to obtain the data.

Most of the tables found in Part 1 were obtained from: Martin JA, Hamilton BE, Ventura SJ, et al. *Births: Final Data for 2011*. National Vital Statistics Reports: Volume 62, No 1. Hyattsville, MD: National Center for Health Statistics. 2013.

Data for Tables 1-1 (partial), 1-3 through 1-6, 1-8, 1-10 through 1-14, and 1-17 through 1-18 were obtained from were derived from Hamilton BE, Martin JA, Ventura SJ. *Births: Preliminary Data for 2012*. National Vital Statistics Reports: Volume 62, No 3. Hyattsville, MD: National Center for Health Statistics. 2013.

Data for Tables 1-66, 1-70, 1-73 through 1-74, and 1-77 through 1-79 were obtained from Osterman MJK, Martin JA, Curtin, SC, et al. *Newly Released Data from the Revised U.S. Birth Certificate, 2011*. National Vital Statistics Reports: Volume 62, No 4. Hyattsville, MD: National Center for Health Statistics, 2013.

Data for Tables 1-49, 1-72, and 1-75 through 1-76 were obtained from Osterman MJK, Martin JA, Mathews TJ, Hamilton BE. *Expanded Data From The New Birth Certificate, 2008*. National Vital Statistics Reports: Volume 59, No 7. Hyattsville, MD: National Center for Health Statistics. July 2011.

Data for Tables 1-20, 1-21, and 1-67 through 1-69 were derived from Martinez G, Copen, CE, Abma, JC. *Teenagers in the United States: Sexual Activity, Contraceptive Use, and Childbearing, 2006–2010 National Survey of Family Growth*. National Center for Health Statistics. Vital Health Stat 23 (31). 2011.

NOTES ON THE DATA

The preliminary 2012 findings are based on nearly 100 percent of registered vital records from calendar year 2012; these were received and processed by NCHS as of April 24, 2013. Final data are based on 100 percent of the birth certificates filed in all states and the District of Columbia.

Race and Hispanic origin are noted separately on birth certificates. Some rates for 2001 through 2009 have been revised using new population estimates that are based on the 2010 census; thus, these rates may differ from those previously published. Population estimates are generally for July 1 of the year shown.

CONCEPTS AND DEFINITIONS

Anencephaly—A congenital anomaly that consists of a partial or complete absence of the brain and skull.

Apgar score—This has been employed for over 50 years to assess the physical condition and short term prognosis of newborns. Historically, the score has been measured at 1 minute, 5 minutes, and if needed, at additional 5-minute intervals after delivery. Information on the 5 minute score is included in national birth certificate data. The Apgar score measures five easily identifiable characteristics of newborns. A 5-minute score of 0 to 3 indicates an infant in immediate need of resuscitation; 4 to 6 is considered intermediate, and 7 to 10 is considered normal. The Apgar score is a useful clinical indicator for reporting overall status of the neonate and need for, and response to resuscitation efforts.

Birth cohort—Consists of all persons born within a given period of time, such as a calendar year.

Birthweight—The first weight of the newborn obtained after birth. Low birthweight is defined as less than 2,500 grams or 5 pounds 8 ounces. Very low birthweight is defined as less than 1,500 grams or 3 pounds 4 ounces. Before 1979, low birthweight was defined as weighing 2,500 grams or less, and very low birthweight was defined as 1,500 grams or less. Equivalents of the gram weights in terms of pounds and ounces are as follows:

Less than 500 grams = 1 lb 1 oz or less

500–999 grams = 1 lb 2 oz–2 lb 3 oz

3 oz 1,000–1,499 grams = 2 lb 4 oz–3 lb 4 oz

1,500–1,999 grams = 3 lb 5 oz–4 lb 6 oz

2,000–2,499 grams = 4 lb 7 oz–5 lb 8 oz

2,500–2,999 grams = 5 lb 9 oz–6 lb 9 oz

3,000–3,499 grams = 6 lb 10 oz–7 lb 11 oz

3,500–3,999 grams = 7 lb 12 oz–8 lb 13 oz

4,000–4,499 grams = 8 lb 14 oz–9 lb 14 oz

4,500–4,999 grams = 9 lb 15 oz–11 lb 0 oz

5,000 grams or more = 11lb 1oz or more

Birth rate—Calculated by dividing the number of live births in a population in a year by the midyear resident population.

Birth rates are expressed as the number of live births per 1,000 population. The rate may be restricted to births to women of specific age, race, marital status, or geographic location (specific rate), or it may be related to the entire population (crude rate).

Breech/malpresentation—Presenting part of the fetus listed as breech, complete breech, frank breech, footling breech.

Cervical cerclage—Circumferential banding or suture of the cervix to prevent or treat early dilation of the cervix (e.g., incompetent cervix) in an attempt to avoid premature delivery.

Cleft lip/palate—Incomplete closure of the lip. May be unilateral, bilateral, or median. Cleft palate is incomplete fusion of the palatal shelves. May be limited to the soft palate, or may extend into the hard palate.

Contraception—The National Survey of Family Growth collects information on contraceptive use reported by women 15–44 years old. For current contraceptive use, women were asked about contraceptive use during the month of interview. Women were classified by whether they reported using any of the 19 methods of contraception at any time in the month of interview.

Cyanotic heart disease—Congenital heart defects resulting in lack of oxygen that cause cyanosis.

Down syndrome—The most common chromosomal defect (trisomy 21).

Fertility rate—Total number of live births per 1,000 women of reproductive age (defined as women age 15 to 44 years).

Gestation—The time period between the first day of the last normal menstrual period and the day of birth or day of termination of pregnancy according to the National Vital Statistics System and the CDC's Abortion Surveillance.

Hispanic origin—Includes persons of Mexican, Puerto Rican, Cuban, Central and South American, and other or unknown Latin American or Spanish origins. Persons of Hispanic origin may be of any race.

Hypertension, chronic—Diagnosis prior to the onset of this pregnancy of elevated blood pressure above normal for age, gender, and physiological condition.

Hypertension, pregnancy-associated—Diagnosis in pregnancy of elevated blood pressure above normal for age, gender, and physiological condition.

Induction of labor—Initiation of uterine contractions by medical and/or surgical means for the purpose of delivery before the spontaneous onset of labor.

Maternal morbidities—Information on six maternal morbidities is collected on the 2003 revised birth certificate: maternal transfusion, third-or fourth-degree perineal laceration, ruptured uterus, unplanned hysterectomy, admission to intensive care unit, and unplanned operating room procedure. More than one morbidity may be reported. Maternal morbidity data are not available for Delaware for 2011 because of concerns with data quality.

Meconium, moderate/heavy—Staining of the amniotic fluid caused by passage of fetal bowel contents during labor and/or at delivery that is more than enough to cause a greenish color change of an otherwise clear fluid.

Meningomyecele/Spina bifida—Meningomyelocele is herniation of meninges and spinal cord tissue. Meningocele (herniation of meninges without spinal cord tissue) should also be included in this category. Both open and closed (covered with skin) lesions should be included. Spina bifida is herniation of the meninges and/or spinal cord tissue through a bony defect of spine closure.

Nonvertex presentation—Includes any nonvertex fetal presentation, that is, presentation of a part of the infant's body other than the upper and back part of the infant's head.

Omphalocele/Gastroschisis—Omphalocele is a defect in the anterior abdominal wall, accompanied by herniation of some abdominal organs through a widened umbilical ring into the umbilical stalk. Gastroschisis is an abnormality of the anterior abdominal wall, lateral to the umbilicus, resulting in herniation of the abdominal contents directly into the amniotic cavity

Precipitous labor—Labor lasting less than 3 hours.

Prenatal care—Medical care provided to a pregnant woman to prevent complications and decrease the incidence of maternal and prenatal mortality. Information on when pregnancy care began is recorded on the birth certificate. Between 1970 and 1980, the reporting area for prenatal care expanded. In 1970, 39 states and the District of Columbia (D.C.) reported prenatal care on the birth certificate. Data were not available from Alabama, Alaska, Arkansas, Connecticut, Delaware, Georgia, Idaho, Massachusetts, New Mexico, Pennsylvania, and Virginia. In 1975, these data were available from three additional states—Connecticut, Delaware, and Georgia—increasing the number of states reporting prenatal care to 42 and D.C. During 1980–2002, prenatal care information was available for the entire United States.

Prepregnancy BMI—The 2003 Standard Certificate of Live Birth includes the components needed to compute both prepregnancy BMI and maternal weight gain (i.e., maternal height, prepregnancy weight, and weight at delivery). BMI is calculated as weight in kilograms divided by height in meters squared (kg/m^2)(4).

Suspected chromosomal disorder—Includes any constellation of congenital malformations resulting from, or compatible with, known syndromes caused by detectable defects in chromosome structure.

Tocolysis—Administration of any agent with the intent to inhibit preterm uterine contractions to extend the length of the pregnancy.

WIC Program—The WIC program is run by the U.S. Department of Agriculture. It is intended to help low-income pregnant women, infants, and children through age 5 years receive proper nutrition by providing vouchers for food, nutrition counseling, health care screenings, and referrals.

PART B

MORTALITY

CHAPTER 2: MORTALITY

Figure 2-1. Age-Adjusted Death Rates, 1940–2010

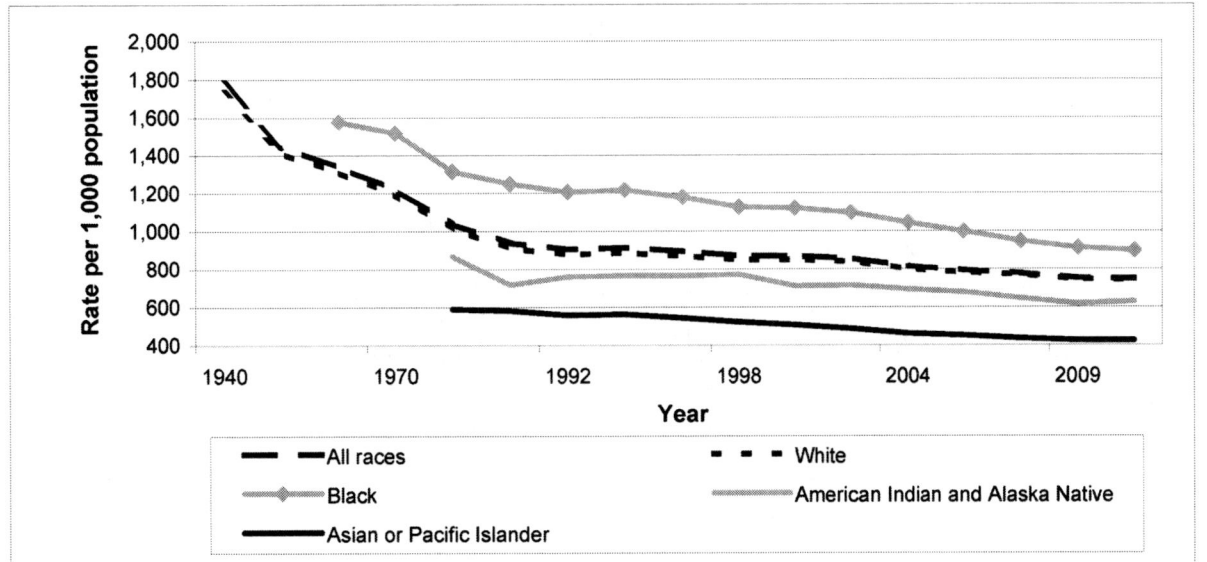

HIGHLIGHTS

- In 2010, 2,468,435 deaths were registered in the United States. The age-adjusted death rate declined to a low of 747.0 per 100,000 standard population. Among all states, Mississippi had the highest age-adjusted death rate at 962.0, while Hawaii had the lowest age-adjusted death rate at 589.6. (Tables 2-1 and 2-31)

- Hispanics had the highest life expectancy of all races and ethnic origins at 83.8 years in 2010. Life expectancy increased for the entire population from 78.2 years in 2008 to 78.7 years in 2010. (Table 2-7)

- While age-adjusted death rates declined for 9 of the 15 leading causes of deaths in 2010, including heart disease, cancer, and cerebrovascular disease, death rates increased for accidents (unintentional injuries); Alzheimer's disease; nephritis, nephrotic syndrome and nephrosis; intentional self-harm (suicide); essential hypertension and hypertensive renal disease; and Parkinson's disease. (Table 2-10)

- The infant mortality rate declined to a record-low in 2010—dropping to 6.2 deaths per 1,000 live births, down from rates of 6.6 in 2008 and 6.4 in 2009. The neonatal mortality rate also declined, falling from 4.3 in 2008 to 4.1 in 2010. The postneonatal mortality rate, however, increased from 2.1 in 2009 to 2.2 in 2010; both rates were lower than the rate of 2.3 in 2008. (Table 2-45)

- The leading cause of infant deaths in 2010 was congenital malformations, deformations, and chromosomal abnormalities, followed by disorders related to length of gestation and fetal malnutrition. (Table 2-46)

Table 2-1. Number of Deaths, Death Rates, and Age-Adjusted Death Rates, by Race and Sex, Selected Years, 1940–2010

(Number, rate per 100,000 population.)

Year	All races[1]			White[2]			Black[2]			American Indian or Alaska Native[2,3]			Asian or Pacific Islander[2,4]		
	Both sexes	Male	Female	Both sexes	Male	Female	Both sexes	Male	Female	Both sexes	Male	Female	Both sexes	Male	Female
Number															
1940	1,417,269	791,003	626,266	1,231,223	690,901	540,322	178,743	95,517	83,226	4,791	2,527	2,264	NA	NA	NA
1950	1,452,454	827,749	624,705	1,276,085	731,366	544,719	169,606	92,004	77,602	4,440	2,497	1,943	NA	NA	NA
1960	1,711,982	975,648	736,334	1,505,335	860,857	644,478	196,010	107,701	88,309	4,528	2,658	1,870	NA	NA	NA
1970	1,921,031	1,078,478	842,553	1,682,096	942,437	739,659	225,647	127,540	98,107	5,675	3,391	2,284	NA	NA	NA
1980	1,989,841	1,075,078	914,763	1,738,607	933,878	804,729	233,135	130,138	102,997	6,923	4,193	2,730	11,071	6,809	4,262
1981	1,977,981	1,063,772	914,209	1,731,233	925,490	805,743	228,560	127,296	101,264	6,608	4,016	2,592	11,475	6,908	4,567
1982	1,974,797	1,056,440	918,357	1,729,085	919,239	809,846	226,513	125,610	100,903	6,679	3,974	2,705	12,430	7,564	4,866
1983	2,019,201	1,071,923	947,278	1,765,582	931,779	833,803	233,124	127,911	105,213	6,839	4,064	2,775	13,554	8,126	5,428
1984	2,039,369	1,076,514	962,855	1,781,897	934,529	847,368	235,884	129,147	106,737	6,949	4,117	2,832	14,483	8,627	5,856
1985	2,086,440	1,097,758	988,682	1,819,054	950,455	868,599	244,207	133,610	110,597	7,154	4,181	2,973	15,887	9,441	6,446
1986	2,105,361	1,104,005	1,001,356	1,831,083	952,554	878,529	250,326	137,214	113,112	7,301	4,365	2,936	16,514	9,795	6,719
1987	2,123,323	1,107,958	1,015,365	1,843,067	953,382	889,685	254,814	139,551	115,263	7,602	4,432	3,170	17,689	10,496	7,193
1988	2,167,999	1,125,540	1,042,459	1,876,906	965,419	911,487	264,019	144,228	119,791	7,917	4,617	3,300	18,963	11,155	7,808
1989	2,150,466	1,114,190	1,036,276	1,853,841	950,852	902,989	267,642	146,393	121,249	8,614	5,066	3,548	20,042	11,688	8,354
1990	2,148,463	1,113,417	1,035,046	1,853,254	950,812	902,442	265,498	145,359	120,139	8,316	4,877	3,439	21,127	12,211	8,916
1991	2,169,518	1,121,665	1,047,853	1,868,904	956,497	912,407	269,525	147,331	122,194	8,621	4,948	3,673	22,173	12,727	9,446
1992	2,175,613	1,122,336	1,053,277	1,873,781	956,957	916,824	269,219	146,630	122,589	8,953	5,181	3,772	23,660	13,568	10,092
1993	2,268,553	1,161,797	1,106,756	1,951,437	988,329	963,108	282,151	153,502	128,649	9,579	5,434	4,145	25,386	14,532	10,854
1994	2,278,994	1,162,747	1,116,247	1,959,875	988,823	971,052	282,379	153,019	129,360	9,637	5,497	4,140	27,103	15,408	11,695
1995	2,312,132	1,172,959	1,139,173	1,987,437	997,277	990,160	286,401	154,175	132,226	9,997	5,574	4,423	28,297	15,933	12,364
1996	2,314,690	1,163,569	1,151,121	1,992,966	991,984	1,000,982	282,089	149,472	132,617	10,127	5,563	4,564	29,508	16,550	12,958
1997	2,314,245	1,154,039	1,160,206	1,996,393	986,884	1,009,509	276,520	144,110	132,410	10,576	5,985	4,591	30,756	17,060	13,696
1998	2,337,256	1,157,260	1,179,996	2,015,984	990,190	1,025,794	278,440	143,417	135,023	10,845	5,994	4,851	31,987	17,659	14,328
1999	2,391,399	1,175,460	1,215,939	2,061,348	1,005,335	1,056,013	285,064	145,703	139,361	11,312	6,092	5,220	33,675	18,330	15,345
2000	2,403,351	1,177,578	1,225,773	2,071,287	1,007,191	1,064,096	285,826	145,184	140,642	11,363	6,185	5,178	34,875	19,018	15,857
2001	2,416,425	1,183,421	1,233,004	2,079,691	1,011,218	1,068,473	287,709	145,908	141,801	11,977	6,466	5,511	37,048	19,829	17,219
2002	2,443,387	1,199,264	1,244,123	2,102,589	1,025,196	1,077,393	290,051	146,835	143,216	12,415	6,750	5,665	38,332	20,483	17,849
2003	2,448,288	1,201,964	1,246,324	2,103,714	1,025,650	1,078,064	291,300	148,022	143,278	13,147	7,106	6,041	40,127	21,186	18,941
2004	2,397,615	1,181,668	1,215,947	2,056,643	1,007,266	1,049,377	287,315	145,970	141,345	13,124	7,134	5,990	40,533	21,298	19,235
2005	2,448,017	1,207,675	1,240,342	2,098,097	1,028,152	1,069,945	292,808	149,108	143,700	13,918	7,607	6,311	43194	22808	20386
2006	2,426,264	1,201,942	1,224,322	2,077,549	1,022,328	1,055,221	289,971	148,602	141,369	14,037	7,630	6,407	44707	23382	21325
2007	2,423,712	1,203,968	1,219,744	2,074,151	1,023,951	1,050,200	289,585	148,309	141,276	14,367	7,885	6,482	45609	23823	21786
2008	2,471,984	1,226,197	1,245,787	2,120,233	1,046,183	1,074,050	289,072	147,143	141,929	14,776	8,163	6,613	47903	24708	23195
2009	2,437,163	1,217,379	1,219,784	2,086,355	1,037,475	1,048,880	286,623	146,239	140,384	14,960	8,105	6,855	49,225	25,560	23,665
2010	2,468,435	1,232,432	1,236,003	2,114,749	1,051,514	1,063,235	286,959	145,802	141,157	15,565	8,516	7,049	51,162	26,600	24,562
Death Rate															
1940	1,076.4	1,197.4	954.6	1,041.5	1,162.2	919.4	NA	NA	NA	NA	NA	NA	NA	NA	NA
1950	963.8	1,106.1	823.5	945.7	1,089.5	803.3	NA	NA	NA	NA	NA	NA	NA	NA	NA
1960	954.7	1,104.5	809.2	947.8	1,098.5	800.9	1,038.6	1,181.7	905.0	NA	NA	NA	NA	NA	NA
1970	945.3	1,090.3	807.8	946.3	1,086.7	812.6	999.3	1,186.6	829.2	NA	NA	NA	NA	NA	NA
1980	878.3	976.9	785.3	892.5	983.3	806.1	875.4	1,034.1	733.3	487.4	597.1	380.1	296.9	375.3	222.5
1981	862.0	954.0	775.0	880.4	965.2	799.8	842.4	992.6	707.7	445.6	547.9	345.6	272.3	336.2	211.5
1982	852.4	938.4	771.2	873.1	951.8	798.2	823.4	966.2	695.5	434.5	522.9	348.1	271.3	338.3	207.4
1983	863.7	943.2	788.4	885.4	957.7	816.4	836.6	971.2	715.9	428.5	515.1	343.9	276.1	339.1	216.1
1984	864.8	938.8	794.7	887.8	954.1	824.6	836.1	968.5	717.4	419.6	502.7	338.4	275.9	336.5	218.1
1985	876.9	948.6	809.1	900.4	963.6	840.1	854.8	989.3	734.2	416.4	492.5	342.5	283.4	344.6	224.9
1986	876.7	944.7	812.3	900.1	958.6	844.3	864.9	1,002.6	741.5	409.5	494.9	325.9	276.2	335.1	219.9
1987	876.4	939.3	816.7	900.1	952.7	849.8	868.9	1,006.2	745.7	410.7	483.8	339.0	278.9	338.3	222.0
1988	886.7	945.1	831.2	910.5	957.9	865.3	888.3	1,026.1	764.6	411.7	485.0	339.9	282.0	339.0	227.4
1989	871.3	926.3	818.9	893.2	936.5	851.8	887.9	1,026.7	763.2	430.5	510.7	351.3	280.9	334.5	229.4
1990	863.8	918.4	812.0	888.0	930.9	846.9	871.0	1,008.0	747.9	402.8	476.4	330.4	283.3	334.3	234.3
1991	857.6	908.8	808.7	883.2	922.7	845.2	861.4	994.8	741.4	405.3	468.9	342.7	278.7	326.9	232.4
1992	848.1	896.1	802.4	875.8	912.2	840.8	841.8	967.6	728.6	406.6	474.1	340.0	282.1	331.1	235.3
1993	872.8	915.0	832.5	902.7	931.8	874.6	864.6	992.2	749.6	419.8	479.6	360.7	288.0	338.1	240.3
1994	866.1	904.2	829.7	897.8	922.6	873.8	849.0	970.2	739.7	408.2	468.8	348.3	294.6	344.0	247.7
1995	868.3	900.8	837.2	901.8	921.0	883.2	846.2	960.2	743.2	409.4	459.4	360.1	294.6	341.4	250.4
1996	859.2	882.8	836.7	896.0	907.1	885.3	819.7	915.3	733.3	399.5	441.5	358.0	294.4	340.2	251.1
1997	848.8	864.6	833.6	889.1	893.3	885.0	789.9	867.1	720.1	402.7	458.2	347.7	294.1	336.8	253.9
1998	847.3	856.4	838.5	889.5	887.3	891.6	782.3	848.2	722.6	397.8	441.9	354.2	293.8	335.4	254.9
1999	857.0	859.2	854.9	901.4	892.1	910.4	788.1	847.4	734.3	399.3	431.8	367.1	296.8	333.2	262.5
2000	854.0	853.0	855.0	900.2	887.8	912.3	781.1	834.1	733.0	380.8	415.6	346.1	296.6	332.9	262.3
2001 [5]	848.0	846.0	849.9	895.7	882.5	908.5	772.4	822.7	726.6	386.7	418.5	355.1	298.1	328.9	269.1
2002 [5]	849.5	849.2	849.8	899.6	888.5	910.4	768.4	816.8	724.4	387.7	422.4	353.1	295.9	326.5	267.2
2003 [5]	843.9	843.9	843.9	894.7	883.6	905.6	762.4	813.6	715.8	396.9	429.9	364.1	298.1	325.6	272.3
2004 [5]	818.8	821.6	816.2	869.0	861.6	876.3	741.7	790.7	697.1	382.7	416.5	348.9	290.2	315.9	266.2
2005 [5]	828.4	831.7	825.1	880.9	873.5	888.1	745.4	796.1	699.2	391.6	428.4	354.8	298.0	326.6	271.4
2006 [5]	813.1	819.6	806.9	866.3	862.3	870.3	727.5	781.4	678.3	380.6	413.7	347.6	297.5	323.4	273.4
2007 [5]	804.6	813.1	796.4	859.3	857.8	860.6	715.9	768.1	668.2	375.1	411.1	339.0	293.1	318.7	269.5
2008 [5]	812.9	820.3	805.8	872.6	870.6	874.6	704.2	750.6	661.8	370.9	408.7	332.9	297.6	320.0	277.0
2009 [5]	794.5	807.2	782.1	853.7	858.2	849.3	688.5	735.3	645.6	361.2	389.9	332.4	296.4	321.2	273.5
2010	799.5	812.0	787.4	861.7	866.1	857.3	682.2	725.4	642.7	365.1	397.5	332.4	301.1	327.0	277.3
Age-Adjusted Death Rate [6]															
1940	1,785.0	1,976.0	1,599.4	1,735.3	1,925.2	1,550.4	NA	NA	NA	NA	NA	NA	NA	NA	NA
1950	1,446.0	1,674.2	1,236.0	1,410.8	1,642.5	1,198.0	NA	NA	NA	NA	NA	NA	NA	NA	NA
1960	1,339.2	1,609.0	1,105.3	1,311.3	1,586.0	1,074.4	1,577.5	1,811.1	1,369.7	NA	NA	NA	NA	NA	NA
1970	1,222.6	1,542.1	971.4	1,193.3	1,513.7	944.0	1,518.1	1,873.9	1,228.7	NA	NA	NA	NA	NA	NA
1980	1,039.1	1,348.1	817.9	1,012.7	1,317.6	796.1	1,314.8	1,697.8	1,033.3	867.0	1,111.5	662.4	589.9	786.5	425.9
1981	1,007.1	1,308.2	792.7	984.0	1,282.2	773.6	1,258.4	1,626.6	986.6	784.6	1,030.2	588.0	544.7	710.3	405.3
1982	985.0	1,279.9	776.6	963.6	1,255.9	758.7	1,221.3	1,580.4	960.1	757.0	940.1	604.4	550.4	738.2	410.3
1983	990.0	1,284.5	783.3	967.3	1,259.4	763.9	1,240.5	1,600.7	980.7	757.3	945.0	605.5	565.1	718.8	428.8
1984	982.5	1,271.4	779.8	959.7	1,245.9	760.7	1,236.7	1,600.8	976.9	761.7	946.0	567.9	574.4	724.7	443.1

Table 2-1. Number of Deaths, Death Rates, and Age-Adjusted Death Rates, by Race and Sex, Selected Years, 1940–2010—*Continued*

(Number, rate per 100,000 population.)

Year	All races[1]			White[2]			Black[2]			American Indian or Alaska Native[2,3]			Asian or Pacific Islander[2,4]		
	Both sexes	Male	Female	Both sexes	Male	Female	Both sexes	Male	Female	Both sexes	Male	Female	Both sexes	Male	Female
1985	988.1	1,278.1	784.5	963.6	1,249.8	764.3	1,261.2	1,634.5	994.4	731.7	926.1	577.2	586.5	755.4	456.7
1986	978.6	1,261.7	778.7	952.8	1,230.5	758.1	1,266.7	1,650.1	994.4	720.8	926.7	549.3	576.4	730.5	445.4
1987	970.0	1,246.1	774.2	943.4	1,213.4	753.3	1,263.1	1,650.3	989.7	719.8	899.3	583.7	577.3	732.4	448.1
1988	975.7	1,250.7	781.0	947.6	1,215.9	759.1	1,284.3	1,677.6	1,006.8	718.6	917.4	563.6	584.2	732.0	451.0
1989	950.5	1,215.0	761.8	920.2	1,176.6	738.8	1,275.5	1,670.1	998.1	761.6	999.8	586.3	581.3	729.6	458.4
1990	938.7	1,202.8	750.9	909.8	1,165.9	728.8	1,250.3	1,644.5	975.1	716.3	916.2	561.8	582.0	716.4	469.3
1991	922.3	1,180.5	738.2	893.2	1,143.1	716.1	1,235.4	1,626.1	963.3	763.9	970.6	608.3	566.2	703.4	453.2
1992	905.6	1,158.3	725.5	877.7	1,122.4	704.1	1,206.7	1,587.8	942.5	759.0	970.4	599.4	558.5	697.3	445.8
1993	926.1	1,177.3	745.9	897.0	1,138.9	724.1	1,241.2	1,632.2	969.5	796.4	1,006.3	641.6	565.8	709.9	450.4
1994	913.5	1,155.5	738.6	885.6	1,118.7	717.5	1,216.9	1,592.8	954.6	764.8	953.3	618.8	562.7	702.5	452.1
1995	909.8	1,143.9	739.4	882.3	1,107.5	718.7	1,213.9	1,585.7	955.9	771.2	932.0	643.9	554.8	693.4	446.7
1996	894.1	1,115.7	733.0	869.0	1,082.9	713.6	1,178.4	1,524.2	940.3	763.6	924.8	641.7	543.2	676.1	439.6
1997	878.1	1,088.1	725.6	855.7	1,059.1	707.8	1,139.8	1,458.8	922.1	774.0	974.8	625.3	531.8	660.2	432.6
1998	870.6	1,069.4	724.7	849.3	1,042.0	707.3	1,127.8	1,430.5	921.6	770.4	943.9	640.5	522.4	646.9	426.7
1999	875.6	1,067.0	734.0	854.6	1,040.0	716.6	1,135.7	1,432.6	933.6	780.9	925.9	668.2	519.7	641.2	427.5
2000	869.0	1,053.8	731.4	849.8	1,029.4	715.3	1,121.4	1,403.5	927.6	709.3	841.5	604.5	506.4	624.2	416.8
2001[5]	858.8	1,035.4	725.6	840.7	1,012.1	710.4	1,106.2	1,380.5	917.9	714.1	834.4	617.1	495.4	603.7	413.9
2002[5]	855.9	1,030.6	723.6	839.0	1,009.0	709.3	1,097.3	1,364.8	913.5	713.0	841.3	611.1	486.5	595.3	405.5
2003[5]	843.5	1,010.3	715.2	827.1	988.8	701.6	1,080.5	1,343.5	898.3	726.3	850.6	628.1	480.5	583.6	404.2
2004[5]	813.7	973.3	690.5	798.5	953.2	677.7	1,043.8	1,296.8	869.8	691.8	811.4	594.9	460.7	557.4	389.1
2005[5]	815.0	971.9	692.3	801.1	952.9	680.9	1,035.1	1,281.3	862.7	701.1	824.5	601.8	459.6	560.6	385.2
2006[5]	791.8	943.5	672.2	779.3	925.8	662.3	997.9	1,239.5	828.4	676.6	780.8	589.0	450.7	544.9	381.2
2007[5]	775.3	922.9	658.1	764.3	907.1	649.4	972.0	1,204.8	808.1	661.3	780.3	565.2	436.2	525.9	369.2
2008[5]	774.9	918.8	659.9	767.2	907.1	653.7	947.7	1,168.0	792.0	644.0	757.2	548.7	435.1	518.5	372.4
2009[5]	749.6	890.9	636.8	742.8	880.5	631.3	912.8	1,123.1	763.3	616.0	709.0	536.4	424.6	509.2	361.1
2010	747.0	887.1	634.9	741.8	878.5	630.8	898.2	1,104.0	752.5	628.3	730.2	541.7	424.3	512.1	359.0

NA= Not available.   [1]For 1940–1991, data includes deaths among races not shown separately; beginning in 1992, records coded as "other races" and records for which race was unknown, not stated, or not classifiable were assigned to the race of previous record.   [2]Multiple-race data were reported by 37 states and the District of Columbia in 2010, 34 states and the District of Columbia in 2008, by 27 states and the District of Columbia in 2007, by 25 states and the District of Columbia in 2006, by 21 states and the District of Columbia in 2005, by 15 states in 2004, and by 7 states in 2003. The multiple-race data for these reporting areas were bridged to the single-race categories of the 1977 OMB standards for comparability with other reporting areas.   [3]Includes Aleuts and Eskimos.   [4]Includes Chinese, Filipinos, Hawaiians, Japanese, and other Asian or Pacific Islander persons.   [5]Rates are revised using updated intercensal population estimates and may differ from rates previously published.   [6]For method of computation, see chapter notes.

Table 2-2. Number of Deaths, Death Rates, and Age-Adjusted Death Rates, by Hispanic Origin, Race for Non-Hispanic Population, and Sex, 1997–2010

(Number, rate per 100,000 population in specified group.)

Year	All origins[1]			Hispanic			Non-Hispanic[2]			Non-Hispanic White[3]			Non-Hispanic Black[3]		
	Both sexes	Male	Female	Both sexes	Male	Female	Both sexes	Male	Female	Both sexes	Male	Female	Both sexes	Male	Female
Number															
1997	2,314,245	1,154,039	1,160,206	95,460	54,348	41,112	2,209,450	1,094,541	1,114,909	1,895,461	929,703	965,758	273,381	142,241	131,140
1998	2,337,256	1,157,260	1,179,996	98,406	55,821	42,585	2,230,127	1,096,677	1,133,450	1,912,802	931,844	980,958	275,264	141,627	133,637
1999	2,391,399	1,175,460	1,215,939	103,740	57,991	45,749	2,279,325	1,112,718	1,166,607	1,953,197	944,913	1,008,284	281,979	143,883	138,096
2000	2,403,351	1,177,578	1,225,773	107,254	60,172	47,082	2,287,846	1,112,704	1,175,142	1,959,919	944,781	1,015,138	282,676	143,297	139,379
2001	2,416,425	1,183,421	1,233,004	113,413	63,317	50,096	2,295,244	1,115,683	1,179,561	1,962,810	945,967	1,016,843	284,343	143,971	140,372
2002	2,443,387	1,199,264	1,244,123	117,135	65,703	51,432	2,318,269	1,129,090	1,189,179	1,981,973	957,645	1,024,328	286,573	144,802	141,771
2003	2,448,288	1,201,964	1,246,324	122,026	68,119	53,907	2,319,476	1,129,927	1,189,549	1,979,465	956,194	1,023,271	287,968	146,136	141,832
2004	2,397,615	1,181,668	1,215,947	122,416	68,544	53,872	2,269,583	1,109,848	1,159,735	1,933,382	938,143	995,239	283,859	144,022	139,837
2005	2,448,017	1,207,675	1,240,342	131,161	73,788	57,373	2,312,028	1,131,013	1,181,015	1,967,142	954,402	1,012,740	289,163	147,010	142,153
2006	2,426,264	1,201,942	1,224,322	133,004	74,250	58,754	2,288,424	1,124,813	1,163,611	1,944,617	947,966	996,651	286,581	146,729	139,852
2007	2,423,712	1,203,968	1,219,744	135,519	75,708	59,811	2,284,446	1,125,974	1,158,472	1,939,606	948,662	990,944	286,366	146,474	139,892
2008	2,471,984	1,226,197	1,245,787	139,241	76,861	62,380	2,327,636	1,146,394	1,181,242	1,981,034	969,288	1,011,746	285,522	145,168	140,354
2009	2,437,163	1,217,379	1,219,784	141,576	78,157	63,419	2,289,999	1,135,852	1,154,147	1,944,606	959,014	985,592	282,982	144,197	138,785
2010	2,468,435	1,232,432	1,236,003	144,490	79,622	64,868	2,318,218	1,149,438	1,168,780	1,969,916	971,604	998,312	283,438	143,824	139,614
Death Rate															
1997	848.8	864.6	833.6	309	343.2	272.9	913.9	930.4	898.3	967.4	970.6	964.3	813.5	892.9	741.9
1998	847.3	856.4	838.5	303.9	336.0	270.0	916.0	925.3	907.1	972.9	969.2	976.5	805.6	873.7	744.1
1999	857.0	859.2	854.9	305.7	332.6	277.2	929.9	932.2	927.8	990.7	979.6	1001.3	812.1	872.8	757.3
2000	854.0	853.0	855.0	303.8	331.3	274.6	929.6	928.1	931.0	993.2	978.5	1,007.3	805.5	859.5	756.7
2001 [4]	848.0	846.0	849.9	305.3	331.8	277.4	926.2	923.5	928.7	992.1	976.3	1,007.2	797.9	849.6	751.0
2002 [4]	849.5	849.2	849.8	303.3	331.5	273.6	931.0	930.0	932.0	1,000.5	986.7	1,013.8	794.9	844.5	750.0
2003 [4]	843.9	843.9	843.9	304.7	332.0	276.0	927.6	926.8	928.3	998.3	984.1	1,011.8	790.6	843.7	742.5
2004 [4]	818.8	821.6	816.2	295.0	322.8	265.8	903.1	905.3	901.0	973.4	963.2	983.2	770.3	821.2	724.1
2005 [4]	828.4	831.7	825.1	304.9	335.6	272.7	915.7	918.0	913.5	989.1	978.1	999.7	775.8	828.4	728.1
2006 [4]	813.1	819.6	806.9	298.2	326.1	269.0	901.8	908.0	895.8	976.2	969.4	982.8	759.8	816.5	708.1
2007 [4]	804.6	813.1	796.4	293.4	321.6	264.0	895.7	904.2	887.6	972.3	968.3	976.1	749.9	804.9	699.9
2008 [4]	812.9	820.3	805.8	291.3	316.0	265.8	908.2	915.9	900.8	991.6	987.5	995.6	738.7	787.8	694.0
2009 [4]	794.5	807.2	782.1	287.0	311.8	261.4	889.5	903.3	876.3	972.3	975.7	969.1	723.7	773.2	678.5
2010	799.5	812.0	787.4	286.2	310.8	260.9	897.6	911.1	884.7	984.3	987.5	981.2	718.7	764.5	676.9
Age-Adjusted Death Rate [5]															
1997	878.1	1088.1	725.6	669.3	840.5	538.8	885.3	1096.4	732.6	859.7	1063.2	712.5	1154.3	1476.7	934.2
1998	870.6	1,069.40	724.7	665.4	833.6	536.9	878.4	1,078.20	732.4	854.1	1,046.70	712.8	1,141.80	1,448.20	932.9
1999	875.6	1067.0	734.0	676.4	830.5	555.9	883.9	1076.4	741.9	859.8	1045.5	722.3	1150.1	1449.4	946.0
2000	869.0	1053.8	731.4	665.7	818.1	546.0	877.9	1063.8	740.0	855.5	1035.4	721.5	1137.0	1422.0	941.2
2001 [4]	858.8	1,035.4	725.6	662.6	808.6	547.0	868.4	1,046.1	734.9	847.1	1,018.8	717.3	1,122.3	1,400.4	931.5
2002 [4]	855.9	1,030.6	723.6	652.2	799.9	535.9	866.4	1,042.1	733.8	846.4	1,016.5	717.1	1,114.1	1,385.1	927.9
2003 [4]	843.5	1,010.3	715.2	645.3	784.0	534.2	854.6	1,022.6	725.8	834.9	996.7	709.8	1,099.0	1,366.8	913.6
2004 [4]	813.7	973.3	690.5	616.8	750.1	509.5	825.9	986.7	702.2	807.6	962.5	687.2	1,062.8	1,320.9	885.4
2005 [4]	815.0	971.9	692.3	627.6	771.2	513.8	827.3	985.0	704.4	810.1	961.5	690.7	1,055.1	1,306.1	879.4
2006 [4]	791.8	943.5	672.2	604.0	732.3	500.2	804.9	958.0	684.6	789.1	935.7	672.4	1,019.3	1,267.0	845.6
2007 [4]	775.3	922.9	658.1	586.1	711.4	484.4	789.5	938.7	671.4	775.3	918.4	660.6	994.4	1,233.2	826.4
2008 [4]	774.9	918.8	659.9	579.8	695.3	484.7	790.0	935.9	673.7	779.4	920.2	665.4	969.2	1,195.4	809.6
2009 [4]	749.6	890.9	636.8	559.7	675.5	466.1	764.7	908.0	650.5	755.1	893.7	643.1	934.4	1,150.5	781.0
2010	747.0	887.1	634.9	558.6	677.7	463.4	762.6	904.6	649.2	755.0	892.5	643.3	920.4	1,131.7	770.8

[1]Figures for origin not stated are included in "All origins" but are not distributed among specified origins.   [2]Includes races other than White and Black.   [3]Multiple-race data were reported by 37 states and the District of Columbia in 2010, 34 states and the District of Columbia in 2008, by 27 states and the District of Columbia in 2007, by 25 states and the District of Columbia in 2006, by 21 states and the District of Columbia in 2005, by 15 states in 2004, and by 7 states in 2003. The multiple-race data for these reporting areas were bridged to the single-race categories of the 1977 OMB standards for comparability with other reporting areas.   [4]Rates are revised using updated intercensal population estimates and may differ from rates previously published.   [5]For method of computation, see chapter notes.

Table 2-3. Number of Deaths and Death Rates, by Age, Race, and Sex, 2010

(Number, rate per 100,000 population in specified group.)

Age	All races			White[1]			Black[1]			American Indian or Alaska Native[1,2]			Asian or Pacific Islander[1,3]		
	Both sexes	Male	Female	Both sexes	Male	Female	Both sexes	Male	Female	Both sexes	Male	Female	Both sexes	Male	Female
Number															
All ages	2,468,435	1,232,432	1,236,003	2,114,749	1,051,514	1,063,235	286,959	145,802	141,157	15,565	8,516	7,049	51,162	26,600	24,562
Under 1 year	24,586	13,702	10,884	15,954	8,871	7,083	7,401	4,116	3,285	354	213	141	877	502	375
1 to 4 years	4,316	2,460	1,856	3,015	1,718	1,297	1,041	595	446	93	55	38	167	92	75
5 to 9 years	2,330	1,325	1,005	1,691	957	734	494	283	211	46	29	17	99	56	43
10 to 14 years	2,949	1,729	1,220	2,150	1,265	885	651	384	267	62	40	22	86	40	46
15 to 19 years	10,887	7,866	3,021	7,847	5,549	2,298	2,531	1,965	566	242	176	66	267	176	91
20 to 24 years	18,664	13,924	4,740	13,662	10,112	3,550	4,144	3,164	980	373	280	93	485	368	117
25 to 29 years	20,263	14,429	5,834	15,097	10,817	4,280	4,246	2,997	1,249	376	246	130	544	369	175
30 to 34 years	21,996	14,763	7,233	16,328	11,066	5,262	4,674	3,074	1,600	419	279	140	575	344	231
35 to 39 years	28,012	17,614	10,398	20,935	13,391	7,544	5,810	3,440	2,370	513	321	192	754	462	292
40 to 44 years	42,021	25,820	16,201	32,125	20,095	12,030	8,206	4,675	3,531	650	428	222	1,040	622	418
45 to 49 years	73,569	44,946	28,623	57,398	35,738	21,660	13,581	7,665	5,916	990	607	383	1,600	936	664
50 to 54 years	109,638	67,072	42,566	85,651	53,279	32,372	20,512	11,728	8,784	1,213	704	509	2,262	1,361	901
55 to 59 years	139,961	86,775	53,186	110,343	69,195	41,148	25,246	14,939	10,307	1,380	837	543	2,992	1,804	1,188
60 to 64 years	170,841	102,520	68,321	139,240	84,101	55,139	26,570	15,519	11,051	1,324	753	571	3,707	2,147	1,560
65 to 69 years	189,962	109,519	80,443	158,882	92,184	66,698	25,781	14,289	11,492	1,349	738	611	3,950	2,308	1,642
70 to 74 years	217,189	120,185	97,004	184,095	102,609	81,486	26,710	14,106	12,604	1,454	769	685	4,930	2,701	2,229
75 to 79 years	273,348	143,006	130,342	237,879	125,427	112,452	28,238	13,898	14,340	1,388	705	683	5,843	2,976	2,867
80 to 84 years	352,303	168,824	183,479	314,629	152,116	162,513	29,305	12,704	16,601	1,297	593	704	7,072	3,411	3,661
85 years and over	765,474	275,866	489,608	697,733	252,958	444,775	51,795	16,243	35,552	2,042	743	1,299	13,904	5,922	7,982
Not stated	126	87	39	95	66	29	23	18	5	-	-	-	8	3	5
Rate															
All ages[4]	799.5	812.0	787.4	861.7	866.1	857.3	682.2	725.4	642.7	365.1	397.5	332.4	301.1	327.0	277.3
Under 1 year[5]	623.4	680.2	564.0	537.2	584.3	488.0	1,102.1	1,206.5	994.4	455.3	542.5	366.4	389.3	434.4	341.8
1 to 4 years	26.5	29.6	23.3	24.6	27.4	21.6	38.1	42.9	33.2	29.4	34.3	24.4	17.9	19.3	16.3
5 to 9 years	11.5	12.8	10.1	10.9	12.1	9.7	15.0	16.9	13.0	12.2	15.2	*	8.5	9.6	7.4
10 to 14 years	14.3	16.3	12.1	13.6	15.6	11.5	19.1	22.2	16.0	16.6	21.1	12.0	7.8	7.2	8.5
15 to 19 years	49.4	69.6	28.1	47.0	64.7	28.3	67.0	102.5	30.5	61.5	87.1	34.5	22.8	29.3	15.9
20 to 24 years	86.5	126.4	44.8	82.7	119.2	44.2	122.4	189.1	57.3	102.8	147.5	53.7	36.9	55.3	18.0
25 to 29 years	96.0	135.7	55.7	92.6	130.0	53.6	140.3	206.0	79.5	110.4	139.6	79.1	37.9	53.7	23.4
30 to 34 years	110.2	147.7	72.6	106.1	141.5	69.5	164.6	228.4	107.1	134.7	174.5	92.6	40.5	51.4	30.8
35 to 39 years	138.8	175.4	102.6	133.8	169.5	97.3	208.7	263.0	160.5	175.4	216.1	133.5	51.9	67.2	38.1
40 to 44 years	201.1	248.4	154.3	194.7	241.8	146.9	291.4	351.2	237.7	232.1	302.3	160.4	80.3	101.8	61.1
45 to 49 years	324.0	401.0	248.9	314.4	392.5	236.7	458.8	549.8	377.8	348.7	431.2	267.6	132.6	164.8	104.0
50 to 54 years	491.7	613.5	374.5	471.9	592.7	353.5	731.5	893.0	589.3	477.8	570.0	390.5	207.2	268.6	154.0
55 to 59 years	711.7	911.2	524.5	678.9	869.4	496.1	1,104.8	1,425.7	833.0	699.4	878.5	532.2	322.1	427.8	234.2
60 to 64 years	1,015.8	1,269.2	781.7	982.4	1,222.1	756.2	1,523.4	1,977.9	1,151.8	892.0	1,047.5	745.9	492.9	632.2	378.1
65 to 69 years	1,527.6	1,871.3	1,222.0	1,495.8	1,825.2	1,197.3	2,148.8	2,745.1	1,691.9	1,377.8	1,591.5	1,185.6	765.6	982.5	584.3
70 to 74 years	2,340.9	2,831.9	1,926.9	2,315.5	2,792.1	1,905.9	3,041.6	3,862.0	2,457.3	2,202.4	2,555.9	1,906.4	1,285.7	1,555.4	1,062.5
75 to 79 years	3,735.4	4,493.7	3,151.9	3,734.9	4,472.1	3,154.8	4,450.5	5,677.3	3,679.8	3,221.2	3,840.9	2,761.3	2,155.2	2,598.0	1,831.3
80 to 84 years	6,134.1	7,358.2	5,319.8	6,171.5	7,379.2	5,351.7	6,710.4	8,414.7	5,809.8	4,811.0	5,489.7	4,357.2	3,895.1	4,791.6	3,316.8
85 years and over	13,934.3	15,414.3	13,219.2	14,147.6	15,640.3	13,419.3	13,187.2	14,715.3	12,589.9	9,615.3	10,268.1	9,277.9	9,418.1	10,824.5	8,590.1

- = Quantity zero.   * = Figure does not meet standards of reliability or precision.   [1]Race categories are consistent with the 1977 Office of Management and Budget (OMB) standards. In 2010, multiple-race data were reported by 37 states and the District of Columbia. The multiple-race data for these reporting areas were bridged to the single-race categories of the 1977 OMB standards for comparability with other reporting areas.   [2]Includes Aleuts and Eskimos.   [3]Includes Chinese, Filipinos, Hawaiians, Japanese, and other Asian or Pacific Islander persons.   [4]Figures for age not stated are included in "All ages" but not distributed among age groups.   [5]Death rates for "Under 1 year" (based on population estimates) differ from infant mortality rates (based on live births); for more information, see chapter notes.

Table 2-4. Number of Deaths and Death Rates, by Hispanic Origin, Race for Non-Hispanic Population, Age, and Sex, 2010

(Number, rate per 100,000 population in specified group.)

Age	All origins[1]			Hispanic			Non-Hispanic[2]			Non-Hispanic White[3]			Non-Hispanic Black[3]		
	Both sexes	Male	Female	Both sexes	Male	Female	Both sexes	Male	Female	Both sexes	Male	Female	Both sexes	Male	Female
Number															
All ages	2,468,435	1,232,432	1,236,003	144,490	79,622	64,868	2,318,218	1,149,438	1,168,780	1,969,916	971,604	998,312	283,438	143,824	139,614
Under 1 year	24,586	13,702	10,884	5,170	2,870	2,300	19,189	10,709	8,480	11,025	6,144	4,881	7,071	3,931	3,140
1–4 years	4,316	2,460	1,856	930	524	406	3,373	1,931	1,442	2,139	1,219	920	993	570	423
5–9 years	2,330	1,325	1,005	423	245	178	1,901	1,077	824	1,283	722	561	481	275	206
10–14 years	2,949	1,729	1,220	528	298	230	2,406	1,420	986	1,627	969	658	637	374	263
15–19 years	10,887	7,866	3,021	1,883	1,436	447	8,964	6,400	2,564	6,013	4,152	1,861	2,482	1,929	553
20–24 years	18,664	13,924	4,740	2,912	2,253	659	15,696	11,629	4,067	10,834	7,927	2,907	4,064	3,104	960
25–29 years	20,263	14,429	5,834	2,940	2,217	723	17,255	12,156	5,099	12,207	8,637	3,570	4,172	2,940	1,232
30–34 years	21,996	14,763	7,233	3,082	2,244	838	18,845	12,470	6,375	13,279	8,846	4,433	4,614	3,031	1,583
35–39 years	28,012	17,614	10,398	3,497	2,399	1,098	24,435	15,160	9,275	17,508	11,045	6,463	5,710	3,368	2,342
40–44 years	42,021	25,820	16,201	4,645	3,061	1,584	37,213	22,649	14,564	27,491	17,025	10,466	8,097	4,607	3,490
45–49 years	73,569	44,946	28,623	6,640	4,310	2,330	66,657	40,459	26,198	50,736	31,406	19,330	13,423	7,568	5,855
50–54 years	109,638	67,072	42,566	8,275	5,317	2,958	100,918	61,448	39,470	77,298	47,889	29,409	20,275	11,578	8,697
55–59 years	139,961	86,775	53,186	9,504	6,100	3,404	129,931	80,304	49,627	100,742	62,997	37,745	24,964	14,768	10,196
60–64 years	170,841	102,520	68,321	10,562	6,409	4,153	159,734	95,733	64,001	128,523	77,555	50,968	26,324	15,370	10,954
65–69 years	189,962	109,519	80,443	10,765	6,223	4,542	178,654	102,928	75,726	148,016	85,858	62,158	25,491	14,113	11,378
70–74 years	217,189	120,185	97,004	12,197	6,817	5,380	204,474	113,049	91,425	171,789	95,709	76,080	26,439	13,947	12,492
75–79 years	273,348	143,006	130,342	14,654	7,664	6,990	258,146	135,025	123,121	223,128	117,699	105,429	27,956	13,738	14,218
80–84 years	352,303	168,824	183,479	16,710	8,059	8,651	335,038	160,476	174,562	297,855	144,024	153,831	28,986	12,543	16,443
85 years and over	765,474	275,866	489,608	29,166	11,171	17,995	735,305	264,358	470,947	668,361	241,741	426,620	51,242	16,055	35,187
Not stated	126	87	39	7	5	2	84	57	27	62	40	22	17	15	2
Rate															
All ages[4]	799.5	812.0	787.4	286.2	310.8	260.9	897.6	911.1	884.7	984.3	987.5	981.2	718.7	764.5	676.9
Under 1 year[5]	623.4	680.2	564.0	510.7	556.8	462.9	654.5	714.5	591.8	529.3	575.9	480.4	1,170.4	1,281.5	1,055.7
1–4 years	26.5	29.6	23.3	22.7	25.0	20.2	27.7	31.1	24.3	24.7	27.5	21.8	40.2	45.4	34.8
5–9 years	11.5	12.8	10.1	8.8	10.0	7.6	12.2	13.6	10.8	11.4	12.5	10.2	15.9	17.9	13.9
10–14 years	14.3	16.3	12.1	11.7	12.9	10.4	14.9	17.2	12.5	13.8	16.0	11.5	20.2	23.4	17.0
15–19 years	49.4	69.6	28.1	41.5	61.2	20.4	51.2	71.4	30.0	47.5	63.9	30.1	70.6	108.0	31.9
20–24 years	86.5	126.4	44.8	67.4	97.9	32.6	90.9	133.5	47.6	85.4	123.2	46.5	129.5	200.2	60.5
25–29 years	96.0	135.7	55.7	68.2	97.4	35.5	102.8	145.4	60.5	98.0	137.6	57.8	149.2	219.0	84.7
30–34 years	110.2	147.7	72.6	74.7	104.7	42.3	119.0	158.8	79.8	113.6	150.1	76.5	175.4	243.4	114.3
35–39 years	138.8	175.4	102.6	90.7	121.7	58.2	149.7	187.8	112.4	144.0	180.8	106.9	218.7	274.7	169.2
40–44 years	201.1	248.4	154.3	134.9	173.6	94.4	213.3	262.4	165.2	205.5	253.9	156.9	304.2	366.4	248.5
45–49 years	324.0	401.0	248.9	219.7	282.6	155.6	338.6	417.8	261.9	327.0	406.9	247.9	475.4	569.2	392.0
50–54 years	491.7	613.5	374.5	338.9	439.1	240.4	508.2	632.0	389.5	485.2	607.1	365.7	753.0	918.4	607.4
55–59 years	711.7	911.2	524.5	516.1	686.1	357.5	729.0	930.0	540.1	691.4	881.6	508.4	1,132.8	1,462.7	853.9
60–64 years	1,015.8	1,269.2	781.7	769.6	992.8	571.4	1,034.2	1,288.1	798.7	995.3	1,233.3	769.4	1,561.9	2,027.9	1,181.1
65–69 years	1,527.6	1,871.3	1,222.0	1,134.9	1,450.9	874.0	1,555.3	1,897.8	1,249.0	1,518.9	1,844.8	1,221.1	2,195.3	2,802.4	1,730.3
70–74 years	2,340.9	2,831.9	1,926.9	1,742.1	2,229.5	1,364.2	2,383.7	2,870.6	1,970.4	2,353.0	2,822.4	1,945.9	3,110.7	3,947.8	2,515.2
75–79 years	3,735.4	4,493.7	3,151.9	2,868.8	3,592.4	2,349.8	3,792.4	4,547.8	3,208.0	3,786.8	4,518.2	3,207.2	4,542.9	5,789.4	3,760.6
80–84 years	6,134.1	7,358.2	5,319.8	4,754.1	5,795.9	4,072.2	6,213.8	7,445.5	5,393.5	6,246.1	7,459.8	5,420.4	6,834.3	8,566.4	5,921.1
85 years and over	13,934.3	15,414.3	13,219.2	10,777.9	11,779.8	10,237.3	14,078.7	15,597.8	13,348.9	14,286.1	15,816.6	13,543.5	13,385.7	14,974.2	12,767.7

- = Quantity zero.   [1]Figures for origin not stated are included in "All origins" but not distributed among specified origins.   [2]Includes races other than White and Black.   [3]Race categories are consistent with the 1977 Office of Management and Budget (OMB) standards. In 2010, multiple-race data were reported by 37 states and the District of Columbia. The multiple-race data for these reporting areas were bridged to the single-race categories of the 1977 OMB standards for comparability with other reporting areas.   [4]Figures for age not stated are included in "All ages" but not distributed among age groups.   [5]Death rates for "Under 1 year" (based on population estimates) differ from infant mortality rates (based on live births); for more information, see chapter notes.

Table 2-5. Number of Deaths and Death Rates, by Age, and Age-Adjusted Death Rates, by Specified Hispanic Origin, Race for Non-Hispanic Population, and Sex, 2010

(Number, rate per 100,000 population in specified group.)

Origin, race, and sex	All ages	Under 1 year[1]	1 to 4 years	5 to 14 years	15 to 24 years	25 to 34 years	35 to 44 years	45 to 54 years	55 to 64 years	65 to 74 years	75 to 84 years	85 years and over	Age not stated	Age-adjusted rate[2]
NUMBER														
All Origins	2,468,435	24,586	4,316	5,279	29,551	42,259	70,033	183,207	310,802	407,151	625,651	765,474	126	X
Male	1,232,432	13,702	2,460	3,054	21,790	29,192	43,434	112,018	189,295	229,704	311,830	275,866	87	X
Female	1,236,003	10,884	1,856	2,225	7,761	13,067	26,599	71,189	121,507	177,447	313,821	489,608	39	X
Hispanic (of any race)	144,490	5,170	930	951	4,795	6,022	8,142	14,915	20,066	22,962	31,364	29,166	7	X
Male	79,622	2,870	524	543	3,689	4,461	5,460	9,627	12,509	13,040	15,723	11,171	5	X
Female	64,868	2,300	406	408	1,106	1,561	2,682	5,288	7,557	9,922	15,641	17,995	2	X
Mexican	80,578	3,488	664	661	3,243	3,835	5,022	8,800	11,479	12,503	16,700	14,179	4	X
Male	45,633	1,921	381	370	2,515	2,858	3,384	5,778	7,148	7,086	8,372	5,817	3	X
Female	34,945	1,567	283	291	728	977	1,638	3,022	4,331	5,417	8,328	8,362	1	X
Puerto Rican	18,681	503	76	92	402	630	1,033	2,110	3,050	3,428	3,960	3,395	2	X
Male	10,283	299	42	61	299	453	648	1,312	1,957	1,992	1,971	1,248	1	X
Female	8,398	204	34	31	103	177	385	798	1,093	1,436	1,989	2,147	1	X
Cuban	14,085	83	9	13	91	115	242	720	1,154	2,229	4,232	5,197	-	X
Male	7,275	47	3	12	71	85	175	492	773	1,350	2,321	1,946	-	X
Female	6,810	36	6	1	20	30	67	228	381	879	1,911	3,251	-	X
Central and South American	13,406	486	87	84	537	807	982	1,458	1,822	2,072	2,597	2,474	-	X
Male	6,923	255	49	44	428	627	684	899	1,041	1,059	1,113	724	-	X
Female	6,483	231	38	40	109	180	298	559	781	1,013	1,484	1,750	-	X
Other and unknown Hispanic	17,740	610	94	101	522	635	863	1,827	2,561	2,730	3,875	3,921	1	X
Male	9,508	348	49	56	376	438	569	1,146	1,590	1,553	1,946	1,436	1	X
Female	8,232	262	45	45	146	197	294	681	971	1,177	1,929	2,485	-	X
Non-Hispanic[3]	2,318,218	19,189	3,373	4,307	24,660	36,100	61,648	167,575	289,665	383,128	593,184	735,305	84	X
Male	1,149,438	10,709	1,931	2,497	18,029	24,626	37,809	101,907	176,037	215,977	295,501	264,358	57	X
Female	1,168,780	8,480	1,442	1,810	6,631	11,474	23,839	65,668	113,628	167,151	297,683	470,947	27	X
White[4]	1,969,916	11,025	2,139	2,910	16,847	25,486	44,999	128,034	229,265	319,805	520,983	668,361	62	X
Male	971,604	6,144	1,219	1,691	12,079	17,483	28,070	79,295	140,552	181,567	261,723	241,741	40	X
Female	998,312	4,881	920	1,219	4,768	8,003	16,929	48,739	88,713	138,238	259,260	426,620	22	X
Black[4]	283,438	7,071	993	1,118	6,546	8,786	13,807	33,698	51,288	51,930	56,942	51,242	17	X
Male	143,824	3,931	570	649	5,033	5,971	7,975	19,146	30,138	28,060	26,281	16,055	15	X
Female	139,614	3,140	423	469	1,513	2,815	5,832	14,552	21,150	23,870	30,661	35,187	2	X
Origin Not Stated[5]	5,727	227	13	21	96	137	243	717	1,071	1,061	1,103	1,003	35	X
Male	3,372	123	5	14	72	105	165	484	749	687	606	337	25	X
Female	2,355	104	8	7	24	32	78	233	322	374	497	666	10	X
RATE[6]														
All Origins[7]	799.5	623.4	26.5	12.9	67.7	102.9	170.5	407.1	851.9	1,875.1	4,790.2	13,934.3	X	747.0
Male	812.0	680.2	29.6	14.6	97.6	141.5	212.5	505.9	1,075.5	2,275.1	5,693.7	15,414.3	X	887.1
Female	787.4	564.0	23.3	11.1	36.4	64.0	128.9	311.4	643.5	1,527.5	4,137.7	13,219.2	X	634.9
Hispanic	286.2	510.7	22.7	10.2	54.2	71.4	111.6	273.0	624.4	1,392.7	3,637.3	10,777.9	X	558.6
Male	310.8	556.8	25.0	11.4	79.4	100.9	146.2	351.9	815.1	1,775.0	4,461.9	11,779.8	X	677.7
Female	260.9	462.9	20.2	8.9	26.3	38.9	75.2	193.9	450.1	1,085.5	3,067.4	10,237.3	X	463.4
Mexican	244.7	547.3	22.4	10.0	54.6	69.8	106.6	272.8	624.5	1,408.0	3,748.1	9,599.5	X	545.8
Male	269.8	597.0	25.2	10.9	80.0	98.8	138.0	348.6	789.3	1,745.4	4,441.6	10,858.7	X	656.9
Female	218.2	496.6	19.5	8.9	26.1	37.6	72.6	192.8	464.5	1,123.8	3,239.6	8,883.0	X	453.5
Puerto Rican	398.2	610.3	20.9	10.8	47.9	88.6	163.1	389.0	865.0	1,773.0	4,438.2	11,160.4	X	673.4
Male	447.3	740.7	22.0	13.9	70.9	129.9	214.1	498.5	1,218.1	2,274.5	5,438.0	12,650.8	X	839.5
Female	350.9	485.1	19.7	7.5	24.6	48.8	116.4	285.8	569.4	1,357.8	3,754.2	10,445.1	X	546.0
Cuban	751.8	416.7	*	*	37.2	52.6	84.3	248.2	610.7	1,437.4	3,553.3	12,950.4	X	575.0
Male	769.2	463.3	*	*	57.6	76.4	115.7	313.3	830.6	1,957.7	4,434.0	14,631.6	X	715.1
Female	733.9	368.3	*	*	16.5	28.0	49.3	171.4	397.3	1,020.8	2,862.7	12,117.0	X	461.6
Central and South American	179.1	422.8	16.7	7.9	43.7	55.4	80.1	153.0	344.5	838.0	2,318.3	8,163.7	X	371.1
Male	184.4	455.8	18.5	8.2	64.4	80.4	110.2	199.0	438.1	1,083.2	2,963.7	9,850.3	X	468.5
Female	173.9	391.4	14.9	7.5	19.3	26.6	49.2	111.5	268.1	677.7	1,992.9	7,623.6	X	312.4
Other and unknown Hispanic	471.7	1,082.4	36.4	16.4	78.1	118.9	171.1	378.5	776.9	1,522.1	4,060.1	11,066.9	X	647.1
Male	523.2	1,270.5	37.7	17.1	110.2	166.3	246.0	517.2	1,080.7	1,981.5	4,980.8	12,591.0	X	813.4
Female	423.5	904.5	35.0	15.5	44.6	72.7	107.7	260.8	532.1	1,165.5	3,422.0	10,343.4	X	522.7
Non-Hispanic	897.6	654.5	27.7	13.6	70.9	110.6	182.5	423.8	870.7	1,909.5	4,862.6	14,078.7	X	762.6
Male	911.1	714.5	31.1	15.4	102.0	151.9	226.4	525.1	1,095.7	2,307.0	5,766.6	15,597.8	X	904.6
Female	884.7	591.8	24.3	11.7	38.8	69.9	139.7	326.1	660.5	1,561.7	4,207.9	13,348.9	X	649.2
White	984.3	529.3	24.7	12.6	66.4	105.6	176.2	407.2	834.2	1,876.2	4,886.8	14,286.1	X	755.0
Male	987.5	575.9	27.5	14.3	93.4	143.6	219.1	508.1	1,046.2	2,256.9	5,770.3	15,816.6	X	892.5
Female	981.2	480.4	21.8	10.9	38.4	66.8	133.1	307.7	631.5	1,535.9	4,232.6	13,543.5	X	643.3
Black	718.7	1,170.4	40.2	18.1	98.3	161.9	261.9	610.9	1,318.8	2,582.2	5,477.8	13,385.7	X	920.4
Male	764.5	1,281.5	45.4	20.7	150.8	230.8	321.1	739.1	1,705.0	3,274.7	6,849.1	14,974.2	X	1,131.7
Female	676.9	1,055.7	34.8	15.5	45.6	99.1	209.1	497.4	996.9	2,068.1	4,675.5	12,767.7	X	770.8

X = Not applicable.   - = Quantity zero.   * = Figure does not meet standards of reliability or precision.   [1]Death rates for "Under 1 year" (based on population estimates) differ from infant mortality rates (based on live births); see chapter notes for more information.   [2]For method of computation, see chapter notes.   [3]Includes races other than White and Black.   [4]Race categories are consistent with the 1977 Office of Management and Budget (OMB) standards. In 2010, multiple-race data were reported by 37 states and the District of Columbia. The multiple-race data for these reporting areas were bridged to the single-race categories of the 1977 OMB standards for comparability with other reporting areas.   [5]Includes deaths for which Hispanic origin was not reported on the death certificate.   [6]Figures for age not stated are included in "All ages" but not distributed among age groups.   [7]Figures for origin not stated are included in "All origins" but not distributed among specified origins.

Table 2-6. Abridged Life Table for the Total Population, 2010

(Number.)

Age	Probability of dying between ages x to x + n	Number surviving to age x	Number dying between ages x to x + n	Person-years lived between ages x to x + n	Total number of person-years lived above age x	Expectancy of life at age x
	$n q x$	$l x$	$n d x$	$n L x$	$T x$	$e x$
0 to 1 years	0.006123	100,000	612	99,465	7,866,031	78.7
1 to 5 years	0.001071	99,388	106	397,294	7,766,566	78.1
5 to 10 years	0.000573	99,281	57	496,250	7,369,272	74.2
10 to 15 years	0.000708	99,224	70	495,989	6,873,022	69.3
15 to 20 years	0.002463	99,154	244	495,240	6,377,033	64.3
20 to 25 years	0.004317	98,910	427	493,529	5,881,793	59.5
25 to 30 years	0.004791	98,483	472	491,249	5,388,265	54.7
30 to 35 years	0.005500	98,011	539	488,743	4,897,016	50.0
35 to 40 years	0.006913	97,472	674	485,752	4,408,273	45.2
40 to 45 years	0.009979	96,798	966	481,756	3,922,521	40.5
45 to 50 years	0.016044	95,832	1,538	475,582	3,440,766	35.9
50 to 55 years	0.024343	94,295	2,295	466,064	2,965,184	31.4
55 to 60 years	0.035106	91,999	3,230	452,346	2,499,119	27.2
60 to 65 years	0.049847	88,770	4,425	433,346	2,046,773	23.1
65 to 70 years	0.074412	84,345	6,276	406,910	1,613,427	19.1
70 to 75 years	0.112312	78,068	8,768	369,609	1,206,518	15.5
75 to 80 years	0.174772	69,300	12,112	317,693	836,909	12.1
80 to 85 years	0.274365	57,189	15,691	248,042	519,216	9.1
85 to 90 years	0.430887	41,498	17,881	162,716	271,174	6.5
90 to 95 years	0.615150	23,617	14,528	79,221	108,458	4.6
95 to 100 years	0.783137	9,089	7,118	24,685	29,237	3.2
100 years and over	1.000000	1,971	1,971	4,552	4,552	2.3

Figure 2-2. Life Expectancy at Selected Ages, by Sex, 2010

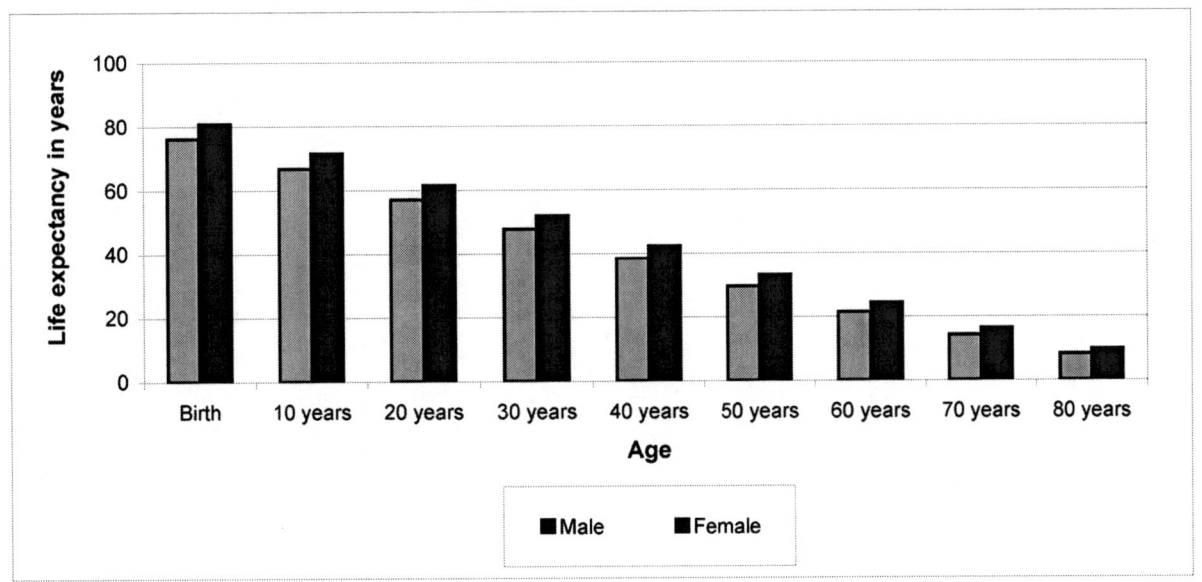

Figure 2-3. Life Expectancy at Selected Ages, by Race, 2010

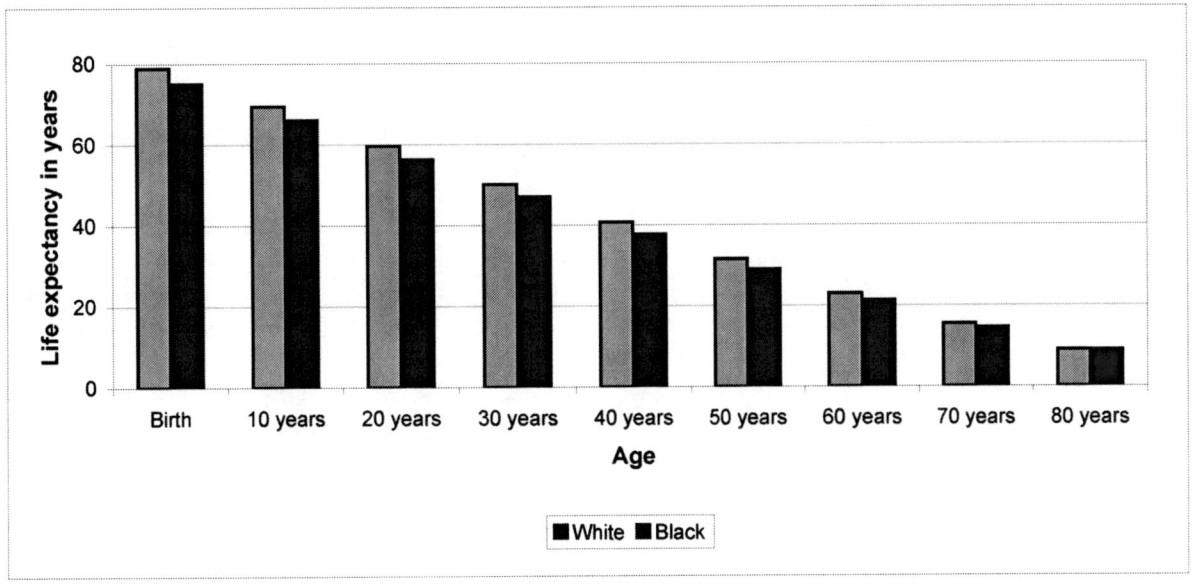

Table 2-7. Life Expectancy at Birth by Race and Sex, Selected Years, 1940–2010

(Number.)

Year	All races and origins[1]			White[2]			Black[2]			Hispanic[3]			Non-Hispanic White			Non-Hispanic Black		
	Both sexes	Male	Female	Both sexes	Male	Female	Both sexes	Male	Female	Both sexes	Male	Female	Both sexes	Male	Female	Both sexes	Male	Female
1940	62.9	60.8	65.2	64.2	62.1	66.6	NA	NA	NA	NA	NA	NA	NA	NA	NA	NA	NA	NA
1950	68.2	65.6	71.1	69.1	66.5	72.2	NA	NA	NA	NA	NA	NA	NA	NA	NA	NA	NA	NA
1960	69.7	66.6	73.1	70.6	67.4	74.1	NA	NA	NA	NA	NA	NA	NA	NA	NA	NA	NA	NA
1970	70.8	67.1	74.7	71.7	68.0	75.6	64.1	60.0	68.3	NA	NA	NA	NA	NA	NA	NA	NA	NA
1975	72.6	68.8	76.6	73.4	69.5	77.3	66.8	62.4	71.3	NA	NA	NA	NA	NA	NA	NA	NA	NA
1976	72.9	69.1	76.8	73.6	69.9	77.5	67.2	62.9	71.6	NA	NA	NA	NA	NA	NA	NA	NA	NA
1977	73.3	69.5	77.2	74.0	70.2	77.9	67.7	63.4	72.0	NA	NA	NA	NA	NA	NA	NA	NA	NA
1978	73.5	69.6	77.3	74.1	70.4	78.0	68.1	63.7	72.4	NA	NA	NA	NA	NA	NA	NA	NA	NA
1979	73.9	70.0	77.8	74.6	70.8	78.4	68.5	64.0	72.9	NA	NA	NA	NA	NA	NA	NA	NA	NA
1980	73.7	70.0	77.4	74.4	70.7	78.1	68.1	63.8	72.5	NA	NA	NA	NA	NA	NA	NA	NA	NA
1981	74.1	70.4	77.8	74.8	71.1	78.4	68.9	64.5	73.2	NA	NA	NA	NA	NA	NA	NA	NA	NA
1982	74.5	70.8	78.1	75.1	71.5	78.7	69.4	65.1	73.6	NA	NA	NA	NA	NA	NA	NA	NA	NA
1983	74.6	71.0	78.1	75.2	71.6	78.7	69.4	65.2	73.5	NA	NA	NA	NA	NA	NA	NA	NA	NA
1984	74.7	71.1	78.2	75.3	71.8	78.7	69.5	65.3	73.6	NA	NA	NA	NA	NA	NA	NA	NA	NA
1985	74.7	71.1	78.2	75.3	71.8	78.7	69.3	65.0	73.4	NA	NA	NA	NA	NA	NA	NA	NA	NA
1986	74.7	71.2	78.2	75.4	71.9	78.8	69.1	64.8	73.4	NA	NA	NA	NA	NA	NA	NA	NA	NA
1987	74.9	71.4	78.3	75.6	72.1	78.9	69.1	64.7	73.4	NA	NA	NA	NA	NA	NA	NA	NA	NA
1988	74.9	71.4	78.3	75.6	72.2	78.9	68.9	64.4	73.2	NA	NA	NA	NA	NA	NA	NA	NA	NA
1989	75.1	71.7	78.5	75.9	72.5	79.2	68.8	64.3	73.3	NA	NA	NA	NA	NA	NA	NA	NA	NA
1990	75.4	71.8	78.8	76.1	72.7	79.4	69.1	64.5	73.6	NA	NA	NA	NA	NA	NA	NA	NA	NA
1991	75.5	72.0	78.9	76.3	72.9	79.6	69.3	64.6	73.8	NA	NA	NA	NA	NA	NA	NA	NA	NA
1992	75.8	72.3	79.1	76.5	73.2	79.8	69.6	65.0	73.9	NA	NA	NA	NA	NA	NA	NA	NA	NA
1993	75.5	72.2	78.8	76.3	73.1	79.5	69.2	64.6	73.7	NA	NA	NA	NA	NA	NA	NA	NA	NA
1994	75.7	72.4	79.0	76.5	73.3	79.6	69.5	64.9	73.9	NA	NA	NA	NA	NA	NA	NA	NA	NA
1995	75.8	72.5	78.9	76.5	73.4	79.6	69.6	65.2	73.9	NA	NA	NA	NA	NA	NA	NA	NA	NA
1996	76.1	73.1	79.1	76.8	73.9	79.7	70.2	66.1	74.2	NA	NA	NA	NA	NA	NA	NA	NA	NA
1997	76.5	73.6	79.4	77.1	74.3	79.9	71.1	67.2	74.7	NA	NA	NA	NA	NA	NA	NA	NA	NA
1998	76.7	73.8	79.5	77.3	74.5	80.0	71.3	67.6	74.8	NA	NA	NA	NA	NA	NA	NA	NA	NA
1999	76.7	73.9	79.4	77.3	74.6	79.9	71.4	67.8	74.7	NA	NA	NA	NA	NA	NA	NA	NA	NA
2000	76.8	74.1	79.3	77.3	74.7	79.9	71.8	68.2	75.1	NA	NA	NA	NA	NA	NA	NA	NA	NA
2001[4,5]	77.0	74.3	79.5	77.5	74.9	80.0	72.0	68.5	75.3	NA	NA	NA	NA	NA	NA	NA	NA	NA
2002[4,5]	77.0	74.4	79.6	77.5	74.9	80.1	72.2	68.7	75.4	NA	NA	NA	NA	NA	NA	NA	NA	NA
2003[4,5,6]	77.2	74.5	79.7	77.7	75.1	80.2	72.4	68.9	75.7	NA	NA	NA	NA	NA	NA	NA	NA	NA
2004[4,5,6]	77.6	75.0	80.1	78.1	75.5	80.5	72.9	69.4	76.1	NA	NA	NA	NA	NA	NA	NA	NA	NA
2005[4,5,6]	77.6	75.0	80.1	78.0	75.5	80.5	73.0	69.5	76.2	NA	NA	NA	NA	NA	NA	NA	NA	NA
2006[4,5,6]	77.8	75.2	80.3	78.3	75.8	80.7	73.4	69.9	76.7	80.3	77.5	82.9	78.2	75.7	80.6	73.1	69.5	76.4
2007[4,5,6]	78.1	75.5	80.6	78.5	76.0	80.9	73.8	70.3	77.0	80.7	77.8	83.2	78.4	75.9	80.8	73.5	69.9	76.7
2008[4,5,6]	78.2	75.6	80.6	78.5	76.1	80.9	74.3	70.9	77.3	80.8	78.0	83.3	78.4	76.0	80.7	73.9	70.5	77.0
2009[4,5,6]	78.5	76.0	80.9	78.8	76.4	81.2	74.7	71.4	77.7	81.1	78.4	83.5	78.7	76.3	81.1	74.3	70.9	77.4
2010[4,6]	78.7	76.2	81.0	78.9	76.5	81.3	75.1	71.8	78.0	81.2	78.5	83.8	78.8	76.4	81.1	74.7	71.4	77.7

NA = Not available.   [1]Includes races other than White and Black.   [2]Includes Hispanic and non-Hispanic persons.   [3]Life expectancies for the Hispanic population are based on death rates adjusted for misclassification; please see chapter notes.   [4]Life table data for 2001–2010 are based on revised life table methodology.   [5]Life table data for 2001–2009 have been re-estimated using new 2001–2009 intercensal population estimates and may differ from data previously published.   [6]Race categories are consistent with the 1977 Office of Management and Budget (OMB) standards. Multiple-race data were reported by 37 states and the District of Columbia in 2010, by 34 states and the District of Columbia in 2009 and 2008, by 27 states and the District of Columbia in 2007, by 25 states and the District of Columbia in 2006, by 21 states and the District of Columbia in 2005, by 15 states in 2004, and by 7 states in 2003. The multiple-race data for these reporting areas were bridged to the single-race categories of the 1977 OMB standards for comparability with other reporting areas.

Table 2-8. Life Expectancy at Selected Ages by Race, Hispanic Origin, Race for Non-Hispanic Population, and Sex, 2010

(Number.)

Exact age in years	All races and origins[1]			White[2]			Black[2]			Hispanic[3]			Non-Hispanic White[2]			Non-Hispanic Black[2]		
	Both sexes	Male	Female	Both sexes	Male	Female	Both sexes	Male	Female	Both sexes	Male	Female	Both sexes	Male	Female	Both sexes	Male	Female
0 years	78.7	76.2	81.0	78.9	76.5	81.3	75.1	71.8	78.0	81.2	78.5	83.8	78.8	76.4	81.1	74.7	71.4	77.7
1 year	78.1	75.7	80.5	78.4	76.0	80.7	75.0	71.8	77.8	80.7	78.0	83.2	78.2	75.8	80.5	74.6	71.3	77.5
5 years	74.2	71.8	76.6	74.4	72.1	76.7	71.1	67.9	73.9	76.7	74.0	79.2	74.3	71.9	76.6	70.7	67.5	73.6
10 years	69.3	66.8	71.6	69.5	67.1	71.8	66.1	62.9	69.0	71.8	69.1	74.3	69.3	67.0	71.6	65.8	62.5	68.7
15 years	64.3	61.9	66.6	64.5	62.1	66.8	61.2	58.0	64.0	66.8	64.1	69.3	64.4	62.0	66.6	60.8	57.6	63.7
20 years	59.5	57.1	61.7	59.7	57.3	61.9	56.4	53.3	59.1	62.0	59.3	64.4	59.5	57.2	61.7	56.0	52.9	58.8
25 years	54.7	52.4	56.9	54.9	52.7	57.0	51.7	48.8	54.3	57.1	54.6	59.5	54.7	52.5	56.9	51.4	48.4	54.0
30 years	50.0	47.8	52.0	50.1	48.0	52.2	47.1	44.3	49.5	52.3	49.8	54.6	50.0	47.9	52.0	46.7	43.9	49.2
35 years	45.2	43.1	47.2	45.4	43.3	47.4	42.4	39.7	44.7	47.5	45.1	49.7	45.3	43.2	47.2	42.1	39.4	44.5
40 years	40.5	38.5	42.4	40.7	38.7	42.6	37.8	35.2	40.1	42.7	40.4	44.8	40.6	38.6	42.5	37.6	34.9	39.8
45 years	35.9	33.9	37.7	36.0	34.1	37.9	33.4	30.8	35.5	38.0	35.7	40.0	36.0	34.0	37.8	33.1	30.5	35.3
50 years	31.4	29.6	33.2	31.6	29.7	33.3	29.1	26.6	31.1	33.5	31.2	35.3	31.5	29.7	33.2	28.8	26.3	31.0
55 years	27.2	25.4	28.8	27.3	25.5	28.8	25.1	22.7	27.0	29.0	26.9	30.8	27.2	25.5	28.8	24.9	22.5	26.8
60 years	23.1	21.5	24.5	23.1	21.6	24.5	21.3	19.2	23.0	24.7	22.8	26.3	23.1	21.5	24.4	21.2	19.0	22.9
65 years	19.1	17.7	20.3	19.2	17.8	20.3	17.8	15.9	19.3	20.6	18.8	22.0	19.1	17.7	20.3	17.7	15.8	19.1
70 years	15.5	14.2	16.5	15.5	14.2	16.4	14.6	12.9	15.8	16.8	15.1	18.0	15.4	14.2	16.4	14.5	12.8	15.7
75 years	12.1	11.0	12.9	12.1	11.0	12.8	11.6	10.2	12.5	13.2	11.7	14.1	12.0	11.0	12.8	11.6	10.1	12.5
80 years	9.1	8.2	9.7	9.0	8.2	9.6	9.0	7.8	9.6	9.9	8.7	10.7	9.0	8.1	9.6	8.9	7.8	9.6
85 years	6.5	5.8	6.9	6.5	5.8	6.9	6.8	5.9	7.1	7.1	6.1	7.7	6.5	5.8	6.9	6.7	5.9	7.1
90 years	4.6	4.1	4.8	4.5	4.0	4.8	5.0	4.4	5.2	5.0	4.2	5.4	4.5	4.0	4.8	5.0	4.4	5.2
95 years	3.2	2.9	3.3	3.2	2.8	3.3	3.7	3.3	3.8	3.5	2.9	3.7	3.2	2.8	3.3	3.8	3.3	3.8
100 years	2.3	2.1	2.3	2.3	2.0	2.3	2.8	2.5	2.8	2.4	2.1	2.6	2.3	2.1	2.3	2.9	2.6	2.8

[1]Includes races other than White and Black.   [2]Race categories are consistent with the 1977 Office of Management and Budget (OMB) standards. Multiple-race data were reported by 37 states and the District of Columbia in 2010; see Technical Notes. The multiple-race data for these reporting areas were bridged to the single-race categories of the 1977 OMB standards for comparability with other reporting areas.   [3]Life expectancies for the Hispanic population are based on death rates adjusted for misclassification; please see chapter notes.

Table 2-9A. Life Expectancy at Birth, at 65 Years of Age, and at 75 Years of Age, by Race and Sex, Selected Years, 1900–2009

(Number.)

Specified age and year	All races			White			Black or African American[1]		
	Both sexes	Male	Female	Both sexes	Male	Female	Both sexes	Male	Female
	Remaining life expectancy in years								
At Birth									
1900 [2,3]	47.3	46.3	48.3	47.6	46.6	48.7	33.0	32.5	33.5
1950 [3]	68.2	65.6	71.1	69.1	66.5	72.2	60.8	59.1	62.9
1960 [3]	69.7	66.6	73.1	70.6	67.4	74.1	63.6	61.1	66.3
1970	70.8	67.1	74.7	71.7	68.0	75.6	64.1	60.0	68.3
1975	72.6	68.8	76.6	73.4	69.5	77.3	66.8	62.4	71.3
1980	73.7	70.0	77.4	74.4	70.7	78.1	68.1	63.8	72.5
1981	74.1	70.4	77.8	74.8	71.1	78.4	68.9	64.5	73.2
1982	74.5	70.8	78.1	75.1	71.5	78.7	69.4	65.1	73.6
1983	74.6	71.0	78.1	75.2	71.6	78.7	69.4	65.2	73.5
1984	74.7	71.1	78.2	75.3	71.8	78.7	69.5	65.3	73.6
1985	74.7	71.1	78.2	75.3	71.8	78.7	69.3	65.0	73.4
1986	74.7	71.2	78.2	75.4	71.9	78.8	69.1	64.8	73.4
1987	74.9	71.4	78.3	75.6	72.1	78.9	69.1	64.7	73.4
1988	74.9	71.4	78.3	75.6	72.2	78.9	68.9	64.4	73.2
1989	75.1	71.7	78.5	75.9	72.5	79.2	68.8	64.3	73.3
1990	75.4	71.8	78.8	76.1	72.7	79.4	69.1	64.5	73.6
1991	75.5	72.0	78.9	76.3	72.9	79.6	69.3	64.6	73.8
1992	75.8	72.3	79.1	76.5	73.2	79.8	69.6	65.0	73.9
1993	75.5	72.2	78.8	76.3	73.1	79.5	69.2	64.6	73.7
1994	75.7	72.4	79.0	76.5	73.3	79.6	69.5	64.9	73.9
1995	75.8	72.5	78.9	76.5	73.4	79.6	69.6	65.2	73.9
1996	76.1	73.1	79.1	76.8	73.9	79.7	70.2	66.1	74.2
1997	76.5	73.6	79.4	77.1	74.3	79.9	71.1	67.2	74.7
1998	76.7	73.8	79.5	77.3	74.5	80.0	71.3	67.6	74.8
1999	76.7	73.9	79.4	77.3	74.6	79.9	71.4	67.8	74.7
2000	76.8	74.1	79.3	77.3	74.7	79.9	71.8	68.2	75.1
2001	76.9	74.2	79.4	77.4	74.8	79.9	72.0	68.4	75.2
2002	76.9	74.3	79.5	77.4	74.9	79.9	72.1	68.6	75.4
2003	77.1	74.5	79.6	77.6	75.0	80.0	72.3	68.8	75.6
2004	77.5	74.9	79.9	77.9	75.4	80.4	72.8	69.3	76.0
2005	77.4	74.9	79.9	77.9	75.4	80.4	72.8	69.3	76.1
2006	77.7	75.1	80.2	78.2	75.7	80.6	73.2	69.7	76.5
2007	77.9	75.4	80.4	78.4	75.9	80.8	73.6	70.0	76.8
2008	78.1	75.6	80.6	78.5	76.1	80.9	74.0	70.6	77.2
2009	78.5	76.0	80.9	78.8	76.4	81.2	74.5	71.1	77.6
At 65 Years									
1950 [3]	13.9	12.8	15.0	14.1	12.8	15.1	13.9	12.9	14.9
1960 [3]	14.3	12.8	15.8	14.4	12.9	15.9	13.9	12.7	15.1
1970	15.2	13.1	17.0	15.2	13.1	17.1	14.2	12.5	15.7
1975	16.1	13.8	18.1	16.1	13.8	18.2	15.0	13.1	16.7
1980	16.4	14.1	18.3	16.5	14.2	18.4	15.1	13.0	16.8
1981	16.6	14.3	18.6	16.7	14.4	18.7	15.5	13.4	17.2
1982	16.8	14.5	18.7	16.9	14.5	18.8	15.7	13.5	17.5
1983	16.7	14.4	18.6	16.8	14.5	18.7	15.4	13.2	17.2
1984	16.8	14.5	18.6	16.8	14.6	18.7	15.4	13.2	17.2
1985	16.7	14.5	18.5	16.8	14.5	18.7	15.2	13.0	16.9
1986	16.8	14.6	18.6	16.9	14.7	18.7	15.2	13.0	17.0
1987	16.9	14.7	18.7	17.0	14.8	18.8	15.2	13.0	17.0
1988	16.9	14.7	18.6	17.0	14.8	18.7	15.1	12.9	16.9
1989	17.1	15.0	18.8	17.2	15.1	18.9	15.2	13.0	16.9
1990	17.2	15.1	18.9	17.3	15.2	19.1	15.4	13.2	17.2
1991	17.4	15.3	19.1	17.5	15.4	19.2	15.5	13.4	17.2
1992	17.5	15.4	19.2	17.6	15.5	19.3	15.7	13.5	17.4
1993	17.3	15.3	18.9	17.4	15.4	19.0	15.5	13.4	17.1
1994	17.4	15.5	19.0	17.5	15.6	19.1	15.7	13.6	17.2
1995	17.4	15.6	18.9	17.6	15.7	19.1	15.6	13.6	17.1
1996	17.5	15.7	19.0	17.6	15.8	19.1	15.8	13.9	17.2
1997	17.7	15.9	19.2	17.8	16.0	19.3	16.1	14.2	17.6
1998	17.8	16.0	19.2	17.8	16.1	19.3	16.1	14.3	17.4
1999	17.7	16.1	19.1	17.8	16.1	19.2	16.0	14.3	17.3
2000	17.6	16.0	19.0	17.7	16.1	19.1	16.1	14.1	17.5
2001	17.7	16.2	19.0	17.8	16.3	19.1	16.2	14.2	17.6
2002	17.8	16.2	19.1	17.9	16.3	19.2	16.3	14.4	17.7
2003	17.9	16.4	19.2	18.0	16.5	19.3	16.4	14.5	17.9
2004	18.2	16.7	19.5	18.3	16.8	19.5	16.7	14.8	18.2
2005	18.2	16.8	19.5	18.3	16.9	19.5	16.8	14.9	18.2
2006	18.5	17.0	19.7	18.6	17.1	19.8	17.1	15.1	18.6
2007	18.6	17.2	19.9	18.7	17.3	19.9	17.2	15.2	18.7
2008	18.8	17.3	20.0	18.8	17.4	20.0	17.4	15.4	18.9
2009	19.2	17.6	20.3	19.1	17.7	20.4	17.8	15.8	19.3
At 75 Years									
1980	10.4	8.8	11.5	10.4	8.8	11.5	9.7	8.3	10.7
1981	10.6	9.0	11.7	10.6	9.0	11.7	10.4	9.0	11.4
1982	10.7	9.1	11.9	10.7	9.0	11.9	10.6	9.1	11.6
1983	10.6	9.0	11.7	10.6	8.9	11.7	10.3	8.9	11.4
1984	10.7	9.0	11.8	10.7	9.0	11.8	10.3	8.9	11.4
1985	10.6	9.0	11.7	10.6	9.0	11.7	10.1	8.7	11.1
1986	10.7	9.1	11.7	10.7	9.1	11.8	10.1	8.6	11.1
1987	10.7	9.1	11.8	10.7	9.1	11.8	10.1	8.6	11.1
1988	10.6	9.1	11.7	10.7	9.1	11.7	10.0	8.5	11.0
1989	10.9	9.3	11.9	10.9	9.3	11.9	10.1	8.6	11.0
1990	10.9	9.4	12.0	11.0	9.4	12.0	10.2	8.6	11.2
1991	11.1	9.5	12.1	11.1	9.5	12.1	10.2	8.7	11.2
1992	11.2	9.6	12.2	11.2	9.6	12.2	10.4	8.9	11.4
1993	10.9	9.5	11.9	11.0	9.5	12.0	10.2	8.7	11.1
1994	11.0	9.6	12.0	11.1	9.6	12.0	10.3	8.9	11.2

Table 2-9A. Life Expectancy at Birth, at 65 Years of Age, and at 75 Years of Age, by Race and Sex, Selected Years, 1900–2009—*Continued*

(Number.)

Specified age and year	All races			White			Black or African American[1]		
	Both sexes	Male	Female	Both sexes	Male	Female	Both sexes	Male	Female
	Remaining life expectancy in years								
1995	11.0	9.7	11.9	11.1	9.7	12.0	10.2	8.8	11.1
1996	11.1	9.8	12.0	11.1	9.8	12.0	10.3	9.0	11.2
1997	11.2	9.9	12.1	11.2	9.9	12.1	10.7	9.3	11.5
1998	11.3	10.0	12.2	11.3	10.0	12.2	10.5	9.2	11.3
1999	11.2	10.0	12.1	11.2	10.0	12.1	10.4	9.2	11.1
2000	11.0	9.8	11.8	11.0	9.8	11.9	10.4	9.0	11.3
2001	11.1	9.9	11.9	11.1	9.9	11.9	10.5	9.1	11.4
2002	11.0	9.9	11.9	11.1	9.9	11.9	10.5	9.2	11.4
2003	11.1	10.0	11.9	11.1	10.0	11.9	10.6	9.3	11.5
2004	11.4	10.3	12.2	11.4	10.3	12.2	10.8	9.5	11.7
2005	11.3	10.2	12.1	11.4	10.3	12.1	10.8	9.5	11.7
2006	11.6	10.5	12.3	11.5	10.5	12.3	11.1	9.8	12.0
2007	11.7	10.6	12.5	11.7	10.6	12.4	11.2	9.9	12.1
2008	11.8	10.7	12.6	11.8	10.7	12.6	11.3	9.9	12.3
2009	12.2	11.0	12.9	12.1	11.0	12.9	11.7	10.3	12.6

[1]Data shown for 1900-1960 are for the Non-White population.   [2]Death registration area only. The death registration area increased from 10 states and the District of Columbia (D.C.) in 1900 to the coterminous United States in 1933.   [3]Includes deaths of persons who were not residents of the 50 states and D.C.

Table 2-9B. Life Expectancy at Birth, at 65 Years of Age, and at 75 Years of Age, by Hispanic Origin and Sex, Selected Years, 2006–2009

(Number.)

Specified age and year	Hispanic[1]			Non-Hispanic White			Non-Hispanic Black		
	Both sexes	Male	Female	Both sexes	Male	Female	Both sexes	Male	Female
	Remaining life expectancy in years								
At Birth									
2006	78.1	75.6	80.4	72.9	69.2	76.2	80.6	77.9	83.1
2007	78.2	75.8	80.6	73.2	69.6	76.5	80.9	78.2	83.4
2008	78.4	75.9	80.8	73.7	70.2	76.9	81.0	78.4	83.3
2009	78.7	76.3	81.1	74.2	70.7	77.3	81.2	78.7	83.5
At 65 Years									
2006	18.5	17.1	19.7	17.0	15.0	18.4	20.6	19.0	21.7
2007	18.7	17.2	19.8	17.1	15.1	18.5	20.8	19.2	21.9
2008	18.8	17.3	20.0	17.3	15.3	18.8	20.7	19.1	21.8
2009	19.1	17.6	20.3	17.7	15.7	19.1	20.9	19.4	22.0
At 75 Years									
2006	11.5	10.4	12.3	11.0	9.7	11.9	13.3	12.1	14.1
2007	11.6	10.6	12.4	11.1	9.8	12.0	13.5	12.3	14.1
2008	11.8	10.7	12.6	11.3	9.8	12.2	13.4	12.2	14.0
2009	12.1	11.0	12.9	11.7	10.2	12.5	13.6	12.4	14.3

[1]Hispanic origin was added to the U.S. standard death certificate in 1989 and was adopted by every state in 1997. To estimate life expectancy, age-specific death rates were corrected to address racial and ethnic misclassification, which underestimates deaths in the Hispanic population. To address the effects of age misstatement at the oldest ages, the probability of death for Hispanic persons older than 80 years is estimated as a function of non-Hispanic white mortality with the use of the Brass relational logit model.

Table 2-10. Death Rates by Age and Age-Adjusted Death Rates for the 15 Leading Causes of Death, 1999–2010

(Rate per 100,000 population in specified group; age-adjusted rates per 100,000 U.S. standard population.)

Cause of death (based on ICD-10, 2004) and year	All ages[1]	Age												Age-adjusted rate[3]
		Under 1 year[2]	1 to 4 years	5 to 14 years	15 to 24 years	25 to 34 years	35 to 44 years	45 to 54 years	55 to 64 years	65 to 74 years	75 to 84 years	85 years and over	
All Causes													
1999	857.0	736.0	34.2	18.6	79.3	102.2	198.0	418.2	1,005.0	2,457.3	5,714.5	15,554.6	875.6
2000	854.0	736.7	32.4	18.0	79.9	101.4	198.9	425.6	992.2	2,399.1	5,666.5	15,524.4	869.0
2001 [4]	848.0	687.0	33.4	17.2	80.2	105.6	203.5	426.7	972.5	2,344.2	5,573.7	15,432.6	858.8
2002 [4]	849.5	709.5	31.4	17.4	80.9	105.1	204.2	431.0	948.7	2,300.3	5,543.8	15,589.5	855.9
2003 [4]	843.9	704.9	31.8	16.9	81.1	105.2	202.6	433.1	937.3	2,235.0	5,451.3	15,401.4	843.5
2004 [4]	818.8	695.9	30.3	16.7	79.7	104.1	194.9	426.8	903.2	2,141.0	5,267.4	14,777.6	813.7
2005 [4]	828.4	710.2	29.9	16.3	80.7	106.8	194.9	431.9	898.5	2,109.7	5,251.8	14,982.4	815.0
2006 [4]	813.1	705.8	29.1	15.2	81.4	109.0	192.0	427.5	881.3	2,031.4	5,096.1	14,426.7	791.8
2007 [4]	804.6	702.5	29.4	15.2	78.8	107.2	186.0	420.3	866.7	1,976.0	4,987.1	14,160.9	775.3
2008 [4]	812.9	678.9	29.3	13.9	74.2	105.1	181.0	419.6	867.1	1,958.4	4,998.1	14,332.4	774.9
2009 [4]	794.5	659.7	27.4	13.8	69.8	104.4	180.0	418.1	856.7	1,888.7	4,820.2	13,660.1	749.6
2010 [4]	799.5	623.4	26.5	12.9	67.7	102.9	170.5	407.1	851.9	1,875.1	4,790.2	13,934.3	747.0
Diseases of Heart (I00–I09, I11, I13, I20–I51)													
1999	259.9	13.8	1.2	0.7	2.8	7.6	30.2	95.7	269.9	701.7	1,849.9	6,063.0	266.5
2000	252.6	13.0	1.2	0.7	2.6	7.4	29.2	94.2	261.2	665.6	1,780.3	5,926.1	257.6
2001 [4]	245.7	11.9	1.5	0.7	2.5	8.0	29.6	92.4	248.9	632.6	1,723.0	5,784.1	249.5
2002 [4]	242.3	12.7	1.1	0.6	2.5	8.0	30.7	93.9	240.5	612.0	1,673.2	5,726.3	244.6
2003 [4]	236.1	11.0	1.2	0.6	2.7	8.3	30.8	92.4	232.3	579.8	1,607.7	5,570.7	236.3
2004 [4]	222.8	10.5	1.2	0.6	2.5	8.1	29.5	90.2	217.1	535.7	1,504.1	5,233.8	221.6
2005 [4]	220.7	8.9	0.9	0.6	2.6	8.3	29.2	89.7	212.8	512.3	1,458.5	5,188.3	216.8
2006 [4]	211.7	8.6	1.0	0.6	2.5	8.4	28.5	88.0	205.1	483.0	1,378.0	4,877.6	205.5
2007 [4]	204.5	10.2	1.1	0.6	2.5	8.1	27.7	85.2	197.8	454.8	1,308.6	4,668.1	196.1
2008 [4]	202.8	9.6	1.2	0.6	2.5	8.1	26.9	85.2	195.3	441.4	1,271.7	4,598.4	192.1
2009 [4]	195.4	9.6	0.9	0.5	2.4	7.8	26.7	82.3	190.0	422.8	1,210.8	4,316.9	182.8
2010 [4]	193.6	8.3	1.0	0.5	2.4	7.8	25.8	81.6	186.6	409.2	1,172.0	4,285.2	179.1
Malignant Neoplasms (C00–C97)													
1999	197.0	1.8	2.7	2.5	4.5	10.0	37.1	127.6	374.6	827.1	1,331.5	1,805.8	200.8
2000	196.5	2.4	2.7	2.5	4.4	9.8	36.6	127.5	366.7	816.3	1,335.6	1,819.4	199.6
2001 [4]	194.3	1.6	2.7	2.4	4.2	10.1	36.8	125.8	359.4	799.7	1,313.7	1,802.9	196.5
2002 [4]	193.7	1.9	2.6	2.6	4.2	9.8	36.0	124.1	349.7	787.2	1,308.8	1,812.4	194.3
2003 [4]	192.0	1.9	2.5	2.6	4.0	9.5	35.1	122.1	341.6	763.5	1,299.7	1,792.3	190.9
2004 [4]	189.2	1.8	2.5	2.5	4.1	9.3	33.6	119.0	330.8	746.8	1,278.6	1,767.4	186.8
2005 [4]	189.3	1.9	2.4	2.5	4.0	9.2	33.5	118.6	323.9	733.2	1,272.8	1,778.2	185.1
2006 [4]	187.6	1.9	2.4	2.2	3.8	9.3	32.2	116.3	317.7	716.3	1,259.2	1,748.3	181.8
2007 [4]	186.9	1.7	2.3	2.4	3.8	8.7	31.0	114.2	311.4	702.9	1,250.1	1,739.4	179.3
2008 [4]	186.0	1.7	2.4	2.2	3.8	8.8	30.1	113.4	304.7	688.4	1,230.9	1,724.6	176.4
2009 [4]	185.0	1.8	2.2	2.2	3.8	9.0	30.2	112.8	301.7	668.2	1,213.0	1,699.3	173.5
2010 [4]	186.2	1.6	2.1	2.2	3.7	8.8	28.8	111.6	300.1	666.1	1,202.2	1,729.5	172.8
Chronic Lower Respiratory Disease (J40–J47)													
1999	44.5	0.9	0.4	0.3	0.5	0.8	2.0	8.5	47.5	177.2	397.8	646.0	45.4
2000	43.4	0.9	0.3	0.3	0.5	0.7	2.1	8.6	44.2	169.4	386.1	648.6	44.2
2001 [4]	43.2	1.0	0.3	0.3	0.4	0.7	2.2	8.4	44.5	167.3	379.3	658.3	43.9
2002 [4]	43.4	1.0	0.4	0.3	0.5	0.8	2.3	8.7	42.2	162.0	385.8	670.3	43.9
2003 [4]	43.6	0.8	0.4	0.3	0.5	0.7	2.2	8.7	43.1	161.7	382.2	670.2	43.7
2004 [4]	41.7	0.9	0.3	0.3	0.4	0.6	2.0	8.4	40.1	152.1	366.2	643.2	41.6
2005 [4]	44.3	0.8	0.4	0.3	0.3	0.7	2.0	9.4	41.6	158.4	385.0	691.9	43.9
2006 [4]	41.8	0.7	0.3	0.3	0.4	0.6	1.9	9.1	38.8	147.0	362.0	641.3	41.0
2007 [4]	42.5	1.0	0.4	0.3	0.3	0.7	1.9	9.5	38.6	145.5	367.1	652.0	41.4
2008 [4]	46.4	0.8	0.3	0.3	0.4	0.6	1.9	9.9	41.1	155.9	395.4	722.7	44.7
2009 [4]	44.8	0.7	0.4	0.3	0.4	0.7	1.8	10.4	40.0	147.5	376.4	684.9	42.7
2010 [4]	44.7	0.9	0.3	0.3	0.3	0.7	1.7	9.9	39.0	146.3	369.9	690.7	42.2
Cerebrovascular Diseases (I60–I69)													
1999	60.0	2.7	0.3	0.2	0.5	1.4	5.7	15.2	40.6	130.8	469.8	1,614.8	61.6
2000	59.6	3.3	0.3	0.2	0.5	1.5	5.8	16.0	41.0	128.6	461.3	1,589.2	60.9
2001 [4]	57.4	2.7	0.4	0.2	0.5	1.5	5.5	15.0	38.3	122.9	443.3	1,532.0	58.4
2002 [4]	56.6	3.0	0.3	0.2	0.4	1.4	5.4	15.1	37.1	119.6	430.0	1,520.1	57.2
2003 [4]	54.4	2.5	0.3	0.2	0.5	1.5	5.6	15.0	35.5	111.9	409.8	1,446.0	54.6
2004 [4]	51.3	3.2	0.3	0.2	0.5	1.4	5.4	14.8	34.0	106.6	385.6	1,331.9	51.2
2005 [4]	48.6	3.1	0.4	0.2	0.5	1.4	5.2	15.0	32.7	99.8	358.4	1,239.7	48.0
2006 [4]	46.0	3.5	0.3	0.2	0.5	1.3	5.1	14.6	32.9	94.9	333.9	1,131.7	44.8
2007 [4]	45.1	3.2	0.3	0.2	0.5	1.3	5.0	14.5	31.7	91.4	320.8	1,110.7	43.5
2008 [4]	44.1	3.4	0.4	0.2	0.4	1.3	4.8	13.7	30.6	87.3	313.3	1,071.0	42.1
2009 [4]	42.0	3.7	0.3	0.2	0.4	1.3	4.6	13.7	29.7	82.8	294.9	992.2	39.6
2010 [4]	41.9	3.3	0.3	0.2	0.4	1.3	4.6	13.1	29.3	81.7	288.3	993.8	39.1
Accidents (Unintentional Injuries) (V01–X59, Y85–Y86)													
1999	35.1	22.3	12.4	7.6	35.3	29.6	33.8	31.8	30.6	44.6	100.5	282.4	35.3
2000	34.8	23.1	11.9	7.3	36.0	29.5	34.1	32.6	30.9	41.9	95.1	273.5	34.9
2001 [4]	35.6	24.3	11.2	6.9	35.8	30.0	35.4	33.9	30.5	42.6	100.7	282.2	35.7
2002 [4]	37.1	23.9	10.6	6.6	37.7	31.9	37.4	36.7	31.3	44.0	101.1	289.6	37.1
2003 [4]	37.7	23.8	11.0	6.4	36.9	32.0	38.0	38.8	32.7	43.7	101.6	294.3	37.6
2004 [4]	38.3	26.2	10.4	6.5	36.8	33.2	37.6	40.7	32.9	43.5	103.6	295.8	38.1
2005 [4]	39.9	27.0	10.5	5.9	37.1	35.7	38.9	43.2	35.4	45.7	106.0	303.5	39.5
2006 [4]	40.8	28.4	10.1	5.6	37.9	38.0	40.5	45.5	35.8	43.8	104.7	299.2	40.2
2007 [4]	41.1	31.0	9.9	5.4	36.8	37.7	39.6	46.2	36.8	44.4	105.0	313.6	40.4
2008 [4]	40.1	31.8	9.1	4.6	32.5	36.3	38.1	45.8	37.4	43.9	105.7	318.3	39.2
2009 [4]	38.5	29.5	9.0	4.1	28.6	34.5	36.4	44.5	36.5	42.1	103.5	310.9	37.5
2010 [4]	39.1	28.1	8.6	4.0	28.3	35.5	36.0	43.7	38.4	43.3	106.1	328.4	38.0

Table 2-10. Death Rates by Age and Age-Adjusted Death Rates for the 15 Leading Causes of Death, 1999–2010—*Continued*

(Rate per 100,000 population in specified group; age-adjusted rates per 100,000 U.S. standard population.)

Cause of death (based on ICD–10, 2004) and year	All ages[1]	Under 1 year[2]	1 to 4 years	5 to 14 years	15 to 24 years	25 to 34 years	35 to 44 years	45 to 54 years	55 to 64 years	65 to 74 years	75 to 84 years	85 years and over	Age-adjusted rate[3]
Alzheimer's Disease (G30)													
1999	16.0	*	*	*	*	*	*	0.2	1.9	17.4	129.5	601.3	16.5
2000	17.6	*	*	*	*	*	*	0.2	2.0	18.7	139.6	667.7	18.1
2001 [4]	18.9	*	*	*	*	*	*	0.2	2.1	18.6	147.2	725.4	19.3
2002 [4]	20.5	*	*	*	*	*	*	0.1	1.9	19.6	157.7	790.9	20.8
2003 [4]	21.9	*	*	*	*	*	*	0.2	2.0	20.7	164.1	846.8	22.1
2004 [4]	22.5	*	*	*	*	*	*	0.2	1.8	19.5	168.5	875.3	22.6
2005 [4]	24.2	*	*	*	*	*	*	0.2	2.1	20.2	177.0	935.5	24.0
2006 [4]	24.3	*	*	*	*	*	*	0.2	2.1	19.9	175.0	923.4	23.7
2007 [4]	24.8	*	*	*	*	*	*	0.2	2.2	20.2	175.8	928.7	23.8
2008 [4]	27.1	*	*	*	*	*	*	0.2	2.2	21.1	192.5	1,002.2	25.8
2009 [4]	25.8	*	*	*	*	*	*	0.2	2.0	19.4	179.1	945.3	24.2
2010 [4]	27.0	*	*	*	*	*	*	0.3	2.1	19.8	184.5	987.1	25.1
Diabetes Mellitus (E10–E14)													
1999	24.5	*	*	0.1	0.4	1.4	4.3	12.9	38.3	91.8	178.0	317.2	25.0
2000	24.6	*	*	0.1	0.4	1.6	4.3	13.1	37.8	90.7	179.5	319.7	25.0
2001 [4]	25.0	*	*	0.1	0.4	1.5	4.3	13.6	38.1	91.0	181.1	328.6	25.4
2002 [4]	25.5	*	*	0.1	0.4	1.6	4.8	13.7	37.5	90.9	182.4	337.0	25.6
2003 [4]	25.6	*	*	0.1	0.4	1.7	4.6	13.9	38.3	90.0	180.7	335.1	25.5
2004 [4]	25.0	*	*	0.1	0.4	1.5	4.6	13.4	36.8	86.2	176.6	328.2	24.7
2005 [4]	25.4	*	*	0.1	0.5	1.6	4.7	13.4	36.9	85.7	177.0	338.8	24.9
2006 [4]	24.3	*	*	0.1	0.4	1.7	4.8	13.1	35.8	80.6	166.2	310.4	23.6
2007 [4]	23.7	*	*	0.1	0.4	1.5	4.6	13.1	34.1	76.7	161.9	302.2	22.8
2008 [4]	23.2	*	*	0.1	0.5	1.4	4.4	12.6	33.3	74.7	153.2	298.9	22.0
2009 [4]	22.4	*	*	0.1	0.4	1.5	4.5	12.8	32.1	69.6	145.8	282.6	21.0
2010 [4]	22.4	*	*	0.1	0.4	1.5	4.4	12.5	32.0	67.6	144.1	285.5	20.8
Nephritis, Nephrotic Syndrome and Nephrosis (N00–N07, N17–N19, N25–N27)													
1999	12.7	4.4	*	0.1	0.2	0.6	1.6	4.0	12.0	37.1	97.6	268.9	13.0
2000	13.2	4.3	*	0.1	0.2	0.6	1.6	4.4	12.8	38.0	100.8	277.8	13.5
2001 [4]	13.9	3.3	*	*	0.2	0.6	1.7	4.6	13.1	40.0	104.0	293.8	14.1
2002 [4]	14.2	4.4	*	0.1	0.2	0.7	1.7	4.7	12.9	39.0	108.9	303.4	14.4
2003 [4]	14.6	4.6	*	0.1	0.2	0.7	1.8	4.9	13.6	39.7	109.3	309.3	14.7
2004 [4]	14.5	4.3	*	0.1	0.2	0.6	1.8	5.0	13.5	38.1	108.2	306.4	14.5
2005 [4]	14.9	4.0	*	0.1	0.2	0.7	1.7	4.8	13.5	38.8	110.2	313.1	14.7
2006 [4]	15.2	4.0	*	*	0.2	0.7	1.8	5.2	13.7	38.8	111.0	316.2	14.8
2007 [4]	15.4	3.5	0.1	0.1	0.2	0.7	1.8	5.1	13.4	39.4	112.4	317.9	14.9
2008 [4]	15.9	3.5	*	*	0.2	0.6	1.8	5.0	14.1	39.9	113.3	325.6	15.1
2009 [4]	16.0	2.8	*	*	0.2	0.7	2.0	5.2	13.5	38.7	115.1	321.4	15.1
2010 [4]	16.3	2.7	*	0.1	0.2	0.6	1.8	4.9	13.9	39.3	115.7	333.8	15.3
Influenza and Pneumonia (J09–J18)													
1999	22.8	8.4	0.8	0.2	0.5	0.8	2.4	4.6	11.0	37.2	157.0	751.8	23.5
2000	23.2	7.6	0.7	0.2	0.5	0.9	2.4	4.7	11.9	39.1	160.3	744.1	23.7
2001 [4]	21.8	7.5	0.7	0.2	0.5	0.9	2.2	4.6	10.8	36.2	148.3	700.1	22.2
2002 [4]	22.8	6.7	0.7	0.2	0.4	0.9	2.2	4.8	11.2	37.2	156.6	732.4	23.2
2003 [4]	22.5	8.1	1.0	0.4	0.5	1.0	2.2	5.2	11.2	36.9	150.8	703.0	22.6
2004 [4]	20.4	6.8	0.8	0.2	0.4	0.8	2.0	4.6	10.8	34.2	139.1	622.8	20.4
2005 [4]	21.3	6.6	0.7	0.3	0.4	0.9	2.1	5.1	11.2	35.1	142.0	644.9	21.0
2006 [4]	18.9	6.5	0.8	0.2	0.4	0.9	1.9	4.6	9.9	31.6	127.3	547.0	18.4
2007 [4]	17.5	5.4	0.7	0.3	0.4	0.8	1.8	4.3	9.5	28.2	113.5	506.7	16.8
2008 [4]	18.5	5.5	0.9	0.2	0.5	0.9	2.1	5.1	10.9	30.5	118.6	512.3	17.6
2009 [4]	17.5	6.3	0.9	0.6	1.0	2.0	3.2	6.5	11.7	29.5	107.0	433.8	16.5
2010 [4]	16.2	4.9	0.6	0.2	0.4	0.9	1.9	4.3	9.9	27.9	102.4	426.2	15.1
Intentional Self-Harm (Suicide) (*U03, X60–X84, Y87.0)													
1999	10.5	NA	NA	0.6	10.1	12.7	14.3	13.9	12.2	13.4	18.1	19.3	10.5
2000	10.4	NA	NA	0.7	10.2	12.0	14.5	14.4	12.1	12.5	17.6	19.6	10.4
2001 [4,5]	10.7	NA	NA	0.7	9.9	12.8	14.7	15.1	13.2	13.2	17.4	17.8	10.7
2002 [4]	11.0	NA	NA	0.6	9.8	12.8	15.3	15.8	13.5	13.4	17.7	18.9	10.9
2003 [4]	10.9	NA	NA	0.6	9.6	12.9	15.0	15.9	13.7	12.6	16.4	17.9	10.8
2004 [4]	11.1	NA	NA	0.7	10.3	12.9	15.2	16.6	13.7	12.2	16.3	17.6	11.0
2005 [4]	11.0	NA	NA	0.7	9.9	12.7	15.1	16.5	13.7	12.4	16.8	18.3	10.9
2006 [4]	11.2	NA	NA	0.5	9.8	12.7	15.2	17.2	14.4	12.4	15.8	17.3	11.0
2007 [4]	11.5	NA	NA	0.5	9.6	13.3	15.7	17.7	15.3	12.4	16.2	17.0	11.3
2008 [4]	11.8	NA	NA	0.5	9.9	13.2	15.9	18.6	16.0	13.6	16.1	16.4	11.6
2009 [4]	12.0	NA	NA	0.6	10.0	13.1	16.1	19.2	16.4	13.7	15.8	16.4	11.8
2010 [4]	12.4	NA	NA	0.7	10.5	14.0	16.0	19.6	17.5	13.7	15.7	17.6	12.1
Septicemia (A40–A41)													
1999	11.0	7.5	0.6	0.2	0.3	0.7	1.8	4.6	11.4	31.2	79.4	220.7	11.3
2000	11.1	7.2	0.6	0.2	0.3	0.7	1.9	4.9	11.9	31.0	80.4	215.7	11.3
2001 [4]	11.3	7.8	0.7	0.2	0.3	0.7	1.8	5.0	12.4	32.6	82.2	210.3	11.5
2002 [4]	11.8	7.5	0.5	0.2	0.3	0.8	1.9	5.2	12.6	34.5	86.3	213.4	11.9
2003 [4]	11.7	7.0	0.5	0.2	0.4	0.8	2.1	5.3	13.0	32.3	84.8	213.7	11.8
2004 [4]	11.4	6.8	0.5	0.2	0.3	0.8	1.9	5.4	12.8	32.1	81.5	199.6	11.3
2005 [4]	11.6	7.5	0.5	0.2	0.3	0.8	1.9	5.2	12.8	32.2	81.3	203.4	11.4
2006 [4]	11.5	6.7	0.6	0.2	0.3	0.7	2.0	5.2	12.6	31.6	82.1	193.0	11.2
2007 [4]	11.6	6.8	0.5	0.2	0.4	0.7	2.1	5.5	12.8	32.2	79.5	190.8	11.2
2008 [4]	11.8	7.0	0.6	0.2	0.3	0.9	2.1	5.7	13.3	31.4	82.0	189.8	11.3
2009 [4]	11.6	5.5	0.4	0.2	0.3	0.9	2.2	5.4	13.1	31.4	79.2	182.4	11.0
2010 [4]	11.3	5.5	0.4	0.2	0.3	0.8	1.9	5.2	12.6	30.1	76.0	179.0	10.6

Table 2-10. Death Rates by Age and Age-Adjusted Death Rates for the 15 Leading Causes of Death, 1999–2010—*Continued*

(Rate per 100,000 population in specified group; age-adjusted rates per 100,000 U.S. standard population.)

Cause of death (based on ICD–10, 2004) and year	All ages[1]	Under 1 year[2]	1 to 4 years	5 to 14 years	15 to 24 years	25 to 34 years	35 to 44 years	45 to 54 years	55 to 64 years	65 to 74 years	75 to 84 years	85 years and over	Age-adjusted rate[3]
Chronic Liver Disease and Cirrhosis (K70, K73–K74)													
1999	9.4	*	*	*	0.1	1.0	7.3	17.4	23.7	30.6	31.9	23.2	9.6
2000	9.4	*	*	*	0.1	1.0	7.5	17.7	23.8	29.8	31.0	23.1	9.5
2001 [4]	9.5	*	*	*	0.1	1.0	7.4	18.4	22.9	29.8	30.2	22.7	9.5
2002 [4]	9.5	*	*	*	0.1	1.0	7.1	18.0	22.8	29.3	31.3	22.5	9.4
2003 [4]	9.5	*	*	*	*	0.9	6.8	18.3	22.9	29.2	29.9	21.2	9.3
2004 [4]	9.2	*	*	*	*	0.8	6.4	18.0	22.4	27.4	28.7	21.1	9.0
2005 [4]	9.3	*	*	*	0.1	0.8	6.2	17.7	23.3	26.8	28.9	21.3	8.9
2006 [4]	9.2	*	*	*	0.1	0.8	5.9	17.8	22.6	25.6	28.9	21.1	8.8
2007 [4]	9.7	*	*	*	0.1	1.0	6.0	18.7	24.2	26.2	28.2	21.7	9.1
2008 [4]	9.9	*	*	*	0.1	1.1	6.1	18.5	25.0	26.3	28.0	21.9	9.2
2009 [4]	10.0	*	*	*	0.1	1.1	6.0	18.7	25.9	25.4	27.2	21.1	9.1
2010 [4]	10.3	*	*	*	0.1	1.2	5.9	19.2	26.8	26.3	27.7	21.8	9.4
Essential Hypertension and Hypertensive Renal Disease (I10, I12, I15)													
1999	6.1	*	*	*	*	0.2	0.7	2.2	5.5	15.2	43.6	152.1	6.2
2000	6.4	*	*	*	*	0.2	0.8	2.3	5.9	15.1	45.5	162.9	6.5
2001 [4]	6.8	*	*	*	0.1	0.3	0.7	2.4	5.8	15.4	47.6	175.6	6.9
2002 [4]	7.0	*	*	*	0.1	0.2	0.8	2.3	5.7	15.9	48.1	189.6	7.1
2003 [4]	7.6	*	*	*	0.1	0.2	0.8	2.5	6.3	16.8	51.6	199.4	7.6
2004 [4]	7.9	*	*	*	0.1	0.3	0.8	2.7	6.3	16.9	52.5	212.2	7.9
2005 [4]	8.4	*	*	*	0.1	0.2	0.9	2.7	6.4	17.5	55.5	228.0	8.3
2006 [4]	8.0	*	*	*	0.0	0.3	0.9	3.0	6.8	16.5	50.8	206.1	7.7
2007 [4]	8.0	*	*	*	0.1	0.2	0.9	2.8	6.4	15.9	49.2	209.1	7.6
2008 [4]	8.5	*	*	*	0.1	0.3	1.0	3.0	7.2	16.5	51.9	215.3	8.0
2009 [4]	8.4	*	*	*	0.1	0.3	1.0	3.1	7.1	16.3	51.0	208.0	7.8
2010 [4]	8.6	*	*	*	0.0	0.3	1.0	3.1	7.3	16.7	51.8	212.0	8.0
Parkinson's Disease (G20–G21)													
1999	5.2	*	*	*	*	*	*	0.1	1.0	11.0	58.2	124.4	5.4
2000	5.6	*	*	*	*	*	*	0.1	1.1	11.5	61.9	131.9	5.7
2001 [4]	5.8	*	*	*	*	*	*	0.1	1.2	11.7	64.5	137.0	5.9
2002 [4]	5.9	*	*	*	*	*	*	0.1	1.2	12.1	63.8	142.2	6.0
2003 [4]	6.2	*	*	*	*	*	*	0.2	1.3	12.6	67.6	145.8	6.3
2004 [4]	6.1	*	*	*	*	*	*	0.2	1.2	11.9	67.4	145.1	6.2
2005 [4]	6.6	*	*	*	*	*	*	0.2	1.4	12.8	71.1	156.0	6.6
2006 [4]	6.6	*	*	*	*	*	*	0.2	1.2	12.0	69.5	157.6	6.5
2007 [4]	6.7	*	*	*	*	*	*	0.1	1.2	11.7	71.5	157.0	6.5
2008 [4]	6.7	*	*	*	*	*	*	0.2	1.2	12.3	71.2	157.4	6.6
2009 [4]	6.7	*	*	*	*	*	*	0.2	1.3	11.2	70.8	157.0	6.5
2010 [4]	7.1	*	*	*	*	*	*	0.2	1.3	11.8	74.8	165.9	6.8
Pneumonitis due to solids and liquids (J69)													
1999	5.5	*	*	*	0.1	0.2	0.4	0.8	2.5	9.5	41.1	175.6	5.6
2000	5.9	*	*	*	0.1	0.2	0.4	1.0	2.5	10.3	44.5	187.6	6.1
2001 [4]	6.1	*	*	*	0.1	0.2	0.4	1.0	2.6	10.0	45.7	193.4	6.2
2002 [4]	6.1	*	*	*	0.1	0.2	0.4	0.9	2.5	9.8	46.2	195.5	6.2
2003 [4]	6.0	*	*	*	0.1	0.2	0.4	1.0	2.8	9.5	44.9	186.0	6.0
2004 [4]	5.7	*	*	*	0.1	0.2	0.4	0.9	2.5	9.5	42.8	176.3	5.7
2005 [4]	5.8	*	*	*	0.1	0.2	0.4	1.1	2.7	9.2	42.5	178.0	5.8
2006 [4]	5.7	*	*	*	0.1	0.2	0.4	1.0	2.7	9.1	40.4	169.6	5.5
2007 [4]	5.6	*	*	*	0.1	0.2	0.4	1.0	2.7	8.8	39.6	167.7	5.4
2008 [4]	5.5	*	*	*	0.1	0.2	0.4	1.1	2.7	8.2	38.5	157.8	5.2
2009 [4]	5.2	*	*	*	0.1	0.2	0.4	1.1	2.8	7.7	35.7	146.7	4.9
2010 [4]	5.5	*	*	*	0.1	0.2	0.3	1.1	2.8	8.6	38.2	152.3	5.1

NA = Not applicable.   * = Figure does not meet standards of reliability or precision.   [1]Figures for age not stated included in "All ages" but not distributed among age groups.   [2]Death rates for "Under 1 year" (based on population estimates) differ from infant mortality rates (based on live births); please see chapter notes for more information.   [3]For method of computation, please see chapter notes.   [4]Rates are revised using updated intercensal population estimates and may differ from rates previously published.   [5]Figures include September 11, 2001 related deaths for which death certificates were filed as of October 24, 2002.

Table 2-11. Number of Deaths from Selected Causes, by Age, 2010

(Number.)

Causes of death (based on ICD-10, 2004)	All ages	Under 1 year	1 to 4 years	5 to 14 years	15 to 24 years	25 to 34 years	35 to 44 years	45 to 54 years	55 to 64 years	65 to 74 years	75 to 84 years	85 years and over	Not stated
All Causes	2,468,435	24,586	4,316	5,279	29,551	42,259	70,033	183,207	310,802	407,151	625,651	765,474	126
Salmonella infections	28	1	-	-	-	-	1	4	4	3	10	5	-
Shigellosis and amebiasis	3	-	-	-	1	1	-	-	-	-	-	1	-
Certain other intestinal infections	10,276	322	20	12	16	26	61	264	635	1,400	3,267	4,253	-
Tuberculosis	569	-	1	3	6	14	26	66	107	111	126	108	1
Respiratory tuberculosis	423	-	-	2	5	10	16	47	80	83	92	88	1
Other tuberculosis	146	-	1	1	1	4	10	19	27	28	34	20	1
Whooping cough	26	25	-	-	-	-	-	-	1	-	-	-	-
Scarlet fever and erysipelas	3	-	-	-	1	-	-	-	1	-	-	1	-
Meningococcal infection	79	11	10	4	16	6	8	9	7	1	4	3	-
Septicemia	34,812	215	62	67	141	312	767	2,333	4,604	6,545	9,931	9,834	1
Syphilis	28	2	-	-	-	-	1	-	7	8	6	4	-
Acute poliomyelitis	-	-	-	-	-	-	-	-	-	-	-	-	-
Arthropod-borne viral encephalitis	9	-	1	1	-	-	-	3	1	2	-	1	-
Measles	2	-	-	-	-	1	-	1	-	-	-	-	-
Viral hepatitis	7,564	1	-	1	8	51	342	2,376	3,218	879	510	178	-
Human immunodeficiency virus (HIV) disease	8,369	-	2	3	147	741	1,898	3,123	1,822	486	124	23	-
Malaria	10	-	-	-	-	3	-	-	4	2	1	-	-
Other and unspecified infectious and parasitic diseases and their sequelae	5,805	119	67	48	69	115	216	460	956	1,149	1,444	1,162	-
Malignant Neoplasms	574,743	62	346	916	1,604	3,619	11,809	50,211	109,501	144,635	157,025	95,010	5
Lip, oral cavity and pharynx	8,474	-	1	1	31	43	231	1,157	2,214	2,007	1,721	1,068	-
Esophagus	14,490	-	-	-	2	32	222	1,483	3,683	3,953	3,517	1,598	-
Stomach	11,390	-	-	1	22	136	433	1,180	2,075	2,590	2,901	2,052	-
Colon, rectum and anus	52,622	-	-	4	54	312	1,345	5,052	9,453	11,459	13,846	11,096	1
Liver and intrahepatic bile ducts	20,305	4	19	20	31	90	315	2,493	5,819	4,814	4,569	2,130	1
Pancreas	36,888	-	-	3	8	64	468	2,869	7,382	9,658	10,452	5,984	-
Larynx	3,691	-	-	-	1	6	41	413	955	1,068	855	352	-
Trachea, bronchus and lung	158,318	-	-	7	31	162	1,351	12,093	31,147	48,606	46,658	18,262	1
Skin	9,154	-	-	2	40	169	447	1,115	1,911	2,063	2,165	1,242	-
Breast	41,435	-	-	1	8	323	2,045	5,915	9,104	8,710	8,385	6,945	-
Cervix uteri	3,939	-	-	-	12	191	531	989	916	606	438	256	-
Corpus uteri and uterus, part unspecified	8,402	-	-	-	3	31	166	679	1,892	2,323	2,035	1,273	-
Ovary	14,572	-	-	2	22	97	345	1,510	3,104	3,724	3,722	2,046	-
Prostate	28,561	-	-	-	2	1	20	493	2,555	5,866	10,135	9,488	1
Kidney and renal pelvis	13,219	-	16	30	30	41	246	1,262	2,778	3,418	3,348	2,050	-
Bladder	14,731	-	-	-	-	17	90	602	1,731	3,019	5,027	4,244	1
Meninges, brain and other parts of central nervous system	14,164	13	101	296	206	366	782	1,987	3,347	3,305	2,711	1,050	-
Lymphoid, hematopoietic and related tissue	55,590	28	115	286	533	771	1,261	3,439	8,002	12,789	17,069	11,297	-
Hodgkin's disease	1,231	-	-	3	48	119	122	124	203	220	259	133	-
Non-Hodgkin's lymphoma	20,294	2	3	30	103	204	429	1,316	2,912	4,621	6,223	4,451	-
Leukemia	22,569	25	112	253	376	439	608	1,377	2,973	4,914	6,883	4,609	-
Multiple myeloma and immuno-proliferative neoplasms	11,428	-	-	-	4	8	101	619	1,898	3,027	3,686	2,085	-
Other and unspecified malignant neoplasms of lymphoid, hematopoietic and related tissue	68	1	-	-	2	1	1	3	16	7	18	19	-
All other and unspecified malignant neoplasms	64,798	17	94	263	569	767	1,470	5,480	11,433	14,657	17,471	12,577	-
In situ neoplasms, benign neoplasms and neoplasms of uncertain or unknown behavior	14,917	48	59	82	93	163	279	751	1,438	2,580	4,710	4,714	-
Anemias	4,852	15	29	26	109	142	178	264	369	524	1,091	2,104	1
Diabetes mellitus	69,071	3	4	26	165	606	1,789	5,610	11,677	14,687	18,822	15,682	-
Nutritional deficiencies	2,948	3	6	2	7	18	37	106	240	380	803	1,346	-
Malnutrition	2,790	2	3	-	7	17	36	98	231	366	772	1,258	-
Other nutritional deficiencies	158	1	3	2	-	1	1	8	9	14	31	88	-
Meningitis	608	58	22	11	22	33	53	97	115	67	83	47	-
Parkinson's disease	22,032	-	-	-	3	5	7	80	489	2,567	9,769	9,112	-
Alzheimer's disease	83,494	-	-	-	-	-	7	121	750	4,291	24,099	54,226	-

Table 2-11. Number of Deaths from Selected Causes, by Age, 2010—*Continued*

(Number.)

Causes of death (based on ICD-10, 2004)	All ages	Under 1 year	1 to 4 years	5 to 14 years	15 to 24 years	25 to 34 years	35 to 44 years	45 to 54 years	55 to 64 years	65 to 74 years	75 to 84 years	85 years and over	Not stated
Major cardiovascular diseases	780,213	468	213	282	1,286	4,012	13,313	45,149	83,886	114,483	205,180	311,910	31
Diseases of heart	597,689	329	159	185	1,028	3,222	10,594	36,729	68,077	88,851	153,080	235,407	28
Acute rheumatic fever and chronic rheumatic heart diseases	2,987	1	2	3	12	25	56	163	342	534	852	997	-
Hypertensive heart disease	33,678	-	-	2	47	371	1,358	4,097	5,369	4,567	6,330	11,529	8
Hypertensive heart and renal disease	2,807	-	-	-	1	19	84	193	311	330	702	1,167	-
Ischemic heart diseases	379,559	20	5	9	113	1,023	5,330	23,008	46,291	60,934	100,056	142,754	16
Acute myocardial infarction	122,071	14	2	4	61	353	2,053	8,862	17,680	22,219	32,058	38,763	2
Other acute ischemic heart diseases	4,170	2	-	-	4	21	94	383	657	709	995	1,305	-
Other forms of chronic ischemic heart disease	253,318	4	3	5	48	649	3,183	13,763	27,954	38,006	67,003	102,686	14
Atherosclerotic cardiovascular disease, so described	57,438	-	-	-	12	257	1,345	5,949	10,711	9,917	12,458	16,781	8
All other forms of chronic ischemic heart disease	195,880	4	3	5	36	392	1,838	7,814	17,243	28,089	54,545	85,905	6
Other heart diseases	178,658	308	152	171	855	1,784	3,766	9,268	15,764	22,486	45,140	78,960	4
Acute and subacute endocarditis	1,103	1	2	-	15	37	61	149	217	235	256	130	-
Diseases of pericardium and acute myocarditis	776	25	18	7	36	48	58	95	120	97	147	125	-
Heart failure	57,757	26	13	9	42	107	298	1,116	2,912	5,864	15,094	32,274	2
All other forms of heart disease	119,022	256	119	155	762	1,592	3,349	7,908	12,515	16,290	29,643	46,431	2
Essential hypertension and hypertensive renal disease	26,634	3	1	2	21	110	394	1,384	2,672	3,636	6,763	11,648	-
Cerebrovascular diseases	129,476	130	50	90	190	517	1,904	5,910	10,693	17,736	37,659	54,595	2
Atherosclerosis	7,230	2	-	-	2	6	23	126	366	741	1,802	4,162	-
Other diseases of circulatory system	19,184	4	3	5	45	157	398	1,000	2,078	3,519	5,876	6,098	1
Aortic aneurysm and dissection	10,431	-	-	3	38	110	311	621	1,219	2,049	3,390	2,690	-
Other diseases of arteries, arterioles and capillaries	8,753	4	3	2	7	47	87	379	859	1,470	2,486	3,408	1
Other disorders of circulatory system	4,241	39	3	2	48	140	327	634	687	600	822	938	1
Influenza and pneumonia	50,097	195	91	71	181	385	773	1,926	3,627	6,066	13,369	23,411	2
Influenza	500	16	13	12	31	44	53	103	84	39	44	61	-
Pneumonia	49,597	179	78	59	150	341	720	1,823	3,543	6,027	13,325	23,350	2
Other acute lower respiratory infections	213	28	12	4	3	2	10	21	17	14	31	71	-
Acute bronchitis and bronchiolitis	177	27	12	4	3	2	10	19	15	12	21	52	-
Other and unspecified acute lower respiratory infections	36	1	-	-	-	-	-	2	2	2	10	19	-
Chronic lower respiratory diseases	138,080	37	51	133	149	272	709	4,452	14,242	31,777	48,309	37,945	4
Bronchitis, chronic and unspecified	620	25	16	5	6	8	8	22	52	92	127	259	-
Emphysema	10,034	1	-	1	2	9	44	411	1,264	2,650	3,556	2,095	1
Asthma	3,404	6	31	119	132	210	303	571	513	374	498	647	-
Other chronic lower respiratory diseases	124,022	5	4	8	9	45	354	3,448	12,413	28,661	44,128	34,944	3
Pneumoconioses and chemical effects	845	-	1	-	-	1	2	19	47	155	364	256	-
Pneumonitis due to solids and liquids	17,011	18	13	9	42	69	142	487	1,005	1,869	4,990	8,367	-
Other diseases of respiratory system	31,187	296	114	68	134	239	468	1,455	3,268	6,267	10,067	8,811	-
Peptic ulcer	2,977	-	-	1	4	23	58	241	420	495	809	925	1
Diseases of appendix	415	7	2	6	9	8	13	35	57	68	101	109	-
Hernia	1,832	27	5	3	7	4	30	112	191	274	496	683	-
Chronic liver disease and cirrhosis	31,903	3	2	3	34	487	2,423	8,651	9,764	5,720	3,620	1,195	1
Alcoholic liver disease	15,990	-	-	-	24	378	1,769	5,465	5,257	2,209	762	125	1
Other chronic liver disease and cirrhosis	15,913	3	2	3	10	109	654	3,186	4,507	3,511	2,858	1,070	-
Cholelithiasis and other disorders of gallbladder	3,332	-	-	-	7	15	51	102	288	505	942	1,421	1
Nephritis, nephrotic syndrome and nephrosis	50,476	105	13	22	68	243	726	2,222	5,082	8,541	15,118	18,335	1
Acute and rapidly progressive nephritic and nephrotic syndrome	203	5	3	2	-	5	8	10	13	32	67	58	-
Chronic glomerulonephritis, nephritis and nephropathy not specified as acute or chronic, and renal sclerosis unspecified	5,894	-	-	4	3	17	48	154	367	681	1,652	2,968	-
Renal failure	44,362	100	10	16	65	220	668	2,057	4,698	7,824	13,395	15,308	1
Other disorders of kidney	17	-	-	-	-	1	2	1	4	4	4	1	-

Table 2-11. Number of Deaths from Selected Causes, by Age, 2010—*Continued*

(Number.)

Causes of death (based on ICD-10, 2004)	All ages	Under 1 year	1 to 4 years	5 to 14 years	15 to 24 years	25 to 34 years	35 to 44 years	45 to 54 years	55 to 64 years	65 to 74 years	75 to 84 years	85 years and over	Not stated
Infections of kidney	608	7	2	2	9	6	20	60	63	97	145	197	-
Hyperplasia of prostate	489	-	-	-	-	-	1	3	13	44	140	288	-
Inflammatory diseases of female pelvic organs	137	-	-	-	3	2	6	10	17	26	40	33	-
Pregnancy, childbirth and the puerperium	825	X	X	1	163	367	223	64	6	1	-	-	-
Pregnancy with abortive outcome	37	X	X	-	7	16	13	1	-	-	-	-	-
Other complications of pregnancy, childbirth and the puerperium	788	X	X	1	156	351	210	63	6	1	-	-	-
Certain conditions originating in the perinatal period	12,128	12,008	52	25	13	9	11	4	2	2	1	-	1
Congenital malformations, deformations and chromosomal abnormalities	9,673	5,107	507	298	412	397	449	680	774	396	351	302	-
Symptoms, signs and abnormal clinical and laboratory findings, not elsewhere classified	38,360	3,052	243	100	510	888	1,225	2,204	2,548	3,105	6,827	17,631	27
All other diseases (Residual)	269,844	753	482	779	1,872	3,297	6,576	16,727	26,186	32,793	65,182	115,192	5
Accidents (unintentional injuries)	120,859	1,110	1,394	1,643	12,341	14,573	14,792	19,667	14,023	9,407	13,853	18,040	16
Transport accidents	37,961	81	469	956	7,549	6,090	5,124	5,955	4,806	2,942	2,620	1,366	3
Motor vehicle accidents	35,332	79	449	890	7,250	5,746	4,745	5,392	4,335	2,676	2,458	1,309	3
Other land transport accidents	1,029	2	17	30	154	134	149	208	156	89	63	27	-
Water, air and space, and other and unspecified transport accidents and their sequelae	1,600	-	3	36	145	210	230	355	315	177	99	30	-
Nontransport accidents	82,898	1,029	925	687	4,792	8,483	9,668	13,712	9,217	6,465	11,233	16,674	13
Falls	26,009	10	24	28	211	299	493	1,283	2,011	2,988	7,249	11,412	1
Accidental discharge of firearms	606	-	25	37	145	107	91	89	50	38	19	5	-
Accidental drowning and submersion	3,782	39	436	251	656	476	409	578	417	276	171	70	3
Accidental exposure to smoke, fire and flames	2,782	21	147	135	127	155	231	446	468	398	400	253	1
Accidental poisoning and exposure to noxious substances	33,041	6	34	54	3,183	6,767	7,476	9,662	4,451	837	338	227	6
Other and unspecified nontransport accidents and their sequelae	16,678	953	259	182	470	679	968	1,654	1,820	1,928	3,056	4,707	2
Intentional Self-Harm (Suicide)	38,364	X	X	274	4,600	5,735	6,571	8,799	6,384	2,974	2,052	968	7
By discharge of firearms	19,392	X	X	81	2,046	2,594	2,914	4,092	3,387	2,053	1,544	679	2
By other and unspecified means and their sequelae	18,972	X	X	193	2,554	3,141	3,657	4,707	2,997	921	508	289	5
Assault (Homicide)	16,259	311	385	261	4,678	4,258	2,473	1,997	1,065	452	250	112	17
By discharge of firearms	11,078	11	43	165	3,889	3,331	1,673	1,097	533	207	90	34	5
By other and unspecified means and their sequelae	5,181	300	342	96	789	927	800	900	532	245	160	78	12
Legal intervention	412	-	1	1	74	102	108	70	46	9	1	-	-
Events of undetermined intent	4,908	108	82	67	456	806	932	1,295	726	195	136	102	3
Discharge of firearms, undetermined intent	252	-	3	14	53	54	26	44	33	10	10	5	-
Other and unspecified events of undetermined intent and their sequelae	4,656	108	79	53	403	752	906	1,251	693	185	126	97	3
Operations of war and their sequelae	9	-	-	-	-	2	-	-	4	-	-	3	-
Complications of medical and surgical care	2,490	22	19	22	40	61	122	242	418	499	629	416	-
Enterocolitis due to Clostridium difficile[1]	7,298	2	-	4	6	6	27	149	426	1,063	2,462	3,153	-
Drug-induced deaths[2,3]	40,393	23	43	63	3,667	7,864	8,923	11,935	5,911	1,137	520	303	4
Alcohol-induced deaths[2,4]	25,692	1	-	-	152	899	3,076	8,612	7,986	3,420	1,250	291	5
Injury by firearms[2,5]	31,672	11	71	298	6,201	6,172	4,790	5,380	4,039	2,316	1,664	723	7

X = Not applicable. - = Quantity zero. [1]Included in "Certain other intestinal infections (A04, A07–A09)" shown above. Beginning with data year 2006, Enterocolitis due to Clostridium difficile (A04.7) is shown separately at the bottom of the table and is included in the list of rankable causes. [2]Included in selected categories above. [3]Includes ICD–10 codes D52.1, D59.0, D59.2, D61.1, D64.2, E06.4, E16.0, E23.1, E24.2, E27.3, E66.1, F11.1–F11.5, F11.7–F11.9, F12.1–F12.5, F12.7–F12.9, F13.1–F13.5, F13.7–F13.9, F14.1–F14.5, F14.7–F14.9, F15.1–F15.5, F15.7–F15.9, F16.1–F16.5, F16.7–F16.9, F17.3–F17.5, F17.7–F17.9, F18.1–F18.5, F18.7–F18.9, F19.1–F19.5, F19.7–F19.9, G21.1, G24.0, G25.1, G25.4, G25.6, G44.4, G62.0, G72.0, I95.2, J70.2–J70.4, K85.3, L10.5, L27.0–L27.1, M10.2, M32.0, M80.4, M81.4, M83.5, M87.1, R50.2, R78.1–R78.5, X40–X44, X60–X64, X85, and Y10–Y14. Trend data for drug-induced deaths, previously shown in this report, can be found at http://www.cdc.gov/nchs/deaths.htm. [4]Includes ICD–10 codes E24.4, F10, G31.2, G62.1, G72.1, I42.6, K29.2, K70, K85.2, K86.0, R78.0, X45, X65, and Y15. Trend data for alcohol-induced deaths, previously shown in this report, can be found at http://www.cdc.gov/nchs/deaths.htm. [5]Includes ICD–10 codes *U01.4, W32–W34, X72–X74, X93–X95, Y22–Y24, and Y35.0. Trend data for Injury by firearms, previously shown in this report, can be found at http://www.cdc.gov/nchs/deaths.htm.

Table 2-12. Death Rates for Selected Causes, by Age, 2010

(Number.)

Cause of death (based on ICD-10, 2004)	All ages[1]	Under 1 year[2]	1 to 4 years	5 to 14 years	15 to 24 years	25 to 34 years	35 to 44 years	45 to 54 years	55 to 64 years	65 to 74 years	75 to 84 years	85 years and over
All Causes	799.5	623.4	26.5	12.9	67.7	102.9	170.5	407.1	851.9	1,875.1	4,790.2	13,934.3
Salmonella infections	0.0	*	*	*	*	*	*	*	*	*	*	*
Shigellosis and amebiasis	*	*	*	*	*	*	*	*	*	*	*	*
Certain other intestinal infections	3.3	8.2	0.1			0.1	0.1	0.6	1.7	6.4	25.0	77.4
Tuberculosis	0.2	*				*	0.1	0.1	0.3	0.5	1.0	2.0
Respiratory tuberculosis	0.1	*				*	*	0.1	0.2	0.4	0.7	1.6
Other tuberculosis	0.0	*							0.1	0.1	0.3	0.4
Whooping cough	0.0	0.6	*	*	*	*	*	*	*	*	*	*
Scarlet fever and erysipelas	*	*	*	*	*	*	*	*	*	*	*	*
Meningococcal infection	0.0	*	*	*	*	*	*	*	*	*	*	*
Septicemia	11.3	5.5	0.4	0.2	0.3	0.8	1.9	5.2	12.6	30.1	76.0	179.0
Syphilis	0.0	*	*	*	*	*	*	*	*	*	*	*
Acute poliomyelitis	*	*	*	*	*	*	*	*	*	*	*	*
Arthropod-borne viral encephalitis	*	*	*	*	*	*	*	*	*	*	*	*
Measles	*	*	*	*	*	*	*	*	*	*	*	*
Viral hepatitis	2.4	*	*	*	*	0.1	0.8	5.3	8.8	4.0	3.9	3.2
Human immunodeficiency virus (HIV) disease	2.7	*	*	*	0.3	1.8	4.6	6.9	5.0	2.2	0.9	0.4
Malaria	*	*	*	*	*	*	*	*	*	*	*	*
Other and unspecified infectious and parasitic diseases and their sequelae	1.9	3.0	0.4	0.1	0.2	0.3	0.5	1.0	2.6	5.3	11.1	21.2
Malignant Neoplasms	186.2	1.6	2.1	2.2	3.7	8.8	28.8	111.6	300.1	666.1	1,202.2	1,729.5
Lip, oral cavity and pharynx	2.7	*	*	*	0.1	0.1	0.6	2.6	6.1	9.2	13.2	19.4
Esophagus	4.7	*	*	*	*	0.1	0.5	3.3	10.1	18.2	26.9	29.1
Stomach	3.7	*	*	*	0.1	0.3	1.1	2.6	5.7	11.9	22.2	37.4
Colon, rectum and anus	17.0	*	*	*	0.1	0.8	3.3	11.2	25.9	52.8	106.0	202.0
Liver and intrahepatic bile ducts	6.6	*	*	0.0	0.1	0.2	0.8	5.5	16.0	22.2	35.0	38.8
Pancreas	11.9	*	*	*	*	0.2	1.1	6.4	20.2	44.5	80.0	108.9
Larynx	1.2	*	*	*	*	*	0.1	0.9	2.6	4.9	6.5	6.4
Trachea, bronchus and lung	51.3	*	*	*	0.1	0.4	3.3	26.9	85.4	223.9	357.2	332.4
Melanoma of skin	3.0	*	*	*	0.1	0.4	1.1	2.5	5.2	9.5	16.6	22.6
Breast	13.4	*	*	*	*	0.8	5.0	13.1	25.0	40.1	64.2	126.4
Cervix uteri	1.3	*	*	*	*	0.5	1.3	2.2	2.5	2.8	3.4	4.7
Corpus uteri and uterus, part unspecified	2.7	*	*	*	*	0.1	0.4	1.5	5.2	10.7	15.6	23.2
Ovary	4.7	*	*	*	0.1	0.2	0.8	3.4	8.5	17.2	28.5	37.2
Prostate	9.3	*	*	*	*	*	*	0.0	1.1	7.0	27.0	77.6	172.7
Kidney and renal pelvis	4.3	*	*	0.1	0.1	0.1	0.6	2.8	7.6	15.7	25.6	37.3
Bladder	4.8	*	*	*	*	*	0.2	1.3	4.7	13.9	38.5	77.3
Meninges, brain and other parts of central nervous system	4.6	*	0.6	0.7	0.5	0.9	1.9	4.4	9.2	15.2	20.8	19.1
Lymphoid, hematopoietic and related tissue	18.0	0.7	0.7	0.7	1.2	1.9	3.1	7.6	21.9	58.9	130.7	205.6
Hodgkin's disease	0.4	*	*	*	0.1	0.3	0.3	0.3	0.6	1.0	2.0	2.4
Non-Hodgkin's lymphoma	6.6	*	*	0.1	0.2	0.5	1.0	2.9	8.0	21.3	47.6	81.0
Leukemia	7.3	0.6	0.7	0.6	0.9	1.1	1.5	3.1	8.1	22.6	52.7	83.9
Multiple myeloma and immunoproliferative neoplasms	3.7	*	*	*	*	*	0.2	1.4	5.2	13.9	28.2	38.0
Other and unspecified malignant neoplasms of lymphoid, hematopoietic and related tissue	0.0	*	*	*	*	*	*	*	*	*	*	*
All other and unspecified malignant neoplasms	21.0	*	0.6	0.6	1.3	1.9	3.6	12.2	31.3	67.5	133.8	228.9
In situ neoplasms, benign neoplasms and neoplasms of uncertain or unknown behavior	4.8	1.2	0.4	0.2	0.2	0.4	0.7	1.7	3.9	11.9	36.1	85.8
Anemias	1.6	*	0.2	0.1	0.2	0.3	0.4	0.6	1.0	2.4	8.4	38.3
Diabetes mellitus	22.4	*	*	0.1	0.4	1.5	4.4	12.5	32.0	67.6	144.1	285.5
Nutritional deficiencies	1.0	*	*	*	*	*	0.1	0.2	0.7	1.8	6.1	24.5
Malnutrition	0.9	*	*	*	*	*	0.1	0.2	0.6	1.7	5.9	22.9
Other nutritional deficiencies	0.1	*	*	*	*	*	*	*	*	*	0.2	1.6
Meningitis	0.2	1.5	0.1	*	0.1	0.1	0.1	0.2	0.3	0.3	0.6	0.9
Parkinson's disease	7.1	*	*	*	*	*	*	0.2	1.3	11.8	74.8	165.9
Alzheimer's disease	27.0	*	*	*	*	*	*	0.3	2.1	19.8	184.5	987.1

Table 2-12. Death Rates for Selected Causes, by Age, 2010—*Continued*

(Number.)

Cause of death (based on ICD-10, 2004)	All ages[1]	Under 1 year[2]	1 to 4 years	5 to 14 years	15 to 24 years	25 to 34 years	35 to 44 years	45 to 54 years	55 to 64 years	65 to 74 years	75 to 84 years	85 years and over
Major cardiovascular diseases	252.7	11.9	1.3	0.7	2.9	9.8	32.4	100.3	229.9	527.2	1,570.9	5,677.9
Diseases of heart	193.6	8.3	1.0	0.5	2.4	7.8	25.8	81.6	186.6	409.2	1,172.0	4,285.2
Acute rheumatic fever and chronic rheumatic heart diseases	1.0	*	*	*	*	0.1	0.1	0.4	0.9	2.5	6.5	18.1
Hypertensive heart disease	10.9	*	*	*	0.1	0.9	3.3	9.1	14.7	21.0	48.5	209.9
Hypertensive heart and renal disease	0.9	*	*	*	*	*	0.2	0.4	0.9	1.5	5.4	21.2
Ischemic heart diseases	122.9	0.5	*	*	0.3	2.5	13.0	51.1	126.9	280.6	766.1	2,598.6
Acute myocardial infarction	39.5	*	*	*	0.1	0.9	5.0	19.7	48.5	102.3	245.4	705.6
Other acute ischemic heart diseases	1.4	*	*	*	*	0.1	0.2	0.9	1.8	3.3	7.6	23.8
Other forms of chronic ischemic heart disease	82.0	*	*	*	0.1	1.6	7.8	30.6	76.6	175.0	513.0	1,869.3
Atherosclerotic cardiovascular disease, so described	18.6	*	*	*	*	0.6	3.3	13.2	29.4	45.7	95.4	305.5
All other forms of chronic ischemic heart disease	63.4	*	*	*	0.1	1.0	4.5	17.4	47.3	129.4	417.6	1,563.8
Other heart diseases	57.9	7.8	0.9	0.4	2.0	4.3	9.2	20.6	43.2	103.6	345.6	1,437.4
Acute and subacute endocarditis	0.4	*	*	*	*	0.1	0.1	0.3	0.6	1.1	2.0	2.4
Diseases of pericardium and acute myocarditis	0.3	0.6	*	*	0.1	0.1	0.1	0.2	0.3	0.4	1.1	2.3
Heart failure	18.7	0.7	*	*	0.1	0.3	0.7	2.5	8.0	27.0	115.6	587.5
All other forms of heart disease	38.6	6.5	0.7	0.4	1.7	3.9	8.2	17.6	34.3	75.0	227.0	845.2
Essential hypertension and hypertensive renal disease	8.6	*	*	*	0.0	0.3	1.0	3.1	7.3	16.7	51.8	212.0
Cerebrovascular diseases	41.9	3.3	0.3	0.2	0.4	1.3	4.6	13.1	29.3	81.7	288.3	993.8
Atherosclerosis	2.3	*	*	*	*	*	0.1	0.3	1.0	3.4	13.8	75.8
Other diseases of circulatory system	6.2	*	*	*	0.1	0.4	1.0	2.2	5.7	16.2	45.0	111.0
Aortic aneurysm and dissection	3.4	*	*	*	0.1	0.3	0.8	1.4	3.3	9.4	26.0	49.0
Other diseases of arteries, arterioles and capillaries	2.8	*	*	*	*	0.1	0.2	0.8	2.4	6.8	19.0	62.0
Other disorders of circulatory system	1.4	1.0	*	*	0.1	0.3	0.8	1.4	1.9	2.8	6.3	17.1
Influenza and pneumonia	16.2	4.9	0.6	0.2	0.4	0.9	1.9	4.3	9.9	27.9	102.4	426.2
Influenza	0.2	*	*	*	0.1	0.1	0.1	0.2	0.2	0.2	0.3	1.1
Pneumonia	16.1	4.5	0.5	0.1	0.3	0.8	1.8	4.1	9.7	27.8	102.0	425.1
Other acute lower respiratory infections	0.1	0.7	*	*	*	*	*	*	0.0	*	0.2	1.3
Acute bronchitis and bronchiolitis	0.1	0.7	*	*	*	*	*	*	*	*	0.2	0.9
Other and unspecified acute lower respiratory infections	0.0	*	*	*	*	*	*	*	*	*	*	*
Chronic lower respiratory diseases	44.7	0.9	0.3	0.3	0.3	0.7	1.7	9.9	39.0	146.3	369.9	690.7
Bronchitis, chronic and unspecified	0.2	0.6	*	*	*	*	*	0.0	0.1	0.4	1.0	4.7
Emphysema	3.2	*	*	*	*	*	0.1	0.9	3.5	12.2	27.2	38.1
Asthma	1.1	*	0.2	0.3	0.3	0.5	0.7	1.3	1.4	1.7	3.8	11.8
Other chronic lower respiratory diseases	40.2	*	*	*	*	0.1	0.9	7.7	34.0	132.0	337.9	636.1
Pneumoconioses and chemical effects	0.3	*	*	*	*	*	*	*	0.1	0.7	2.8	4.7
Pneumonitis due to solids and liquids	5.5	*	*	*	0.1	0.2	0.3	1.1	2.8	8.6	38.2	152.3
Other diseases of respiratory system	10.1	7.5	0.7	0.2	0.3	0.6	1.1	3.2	9.0	28.9	77.1	160.4
Peptic ulcer	1.0	*	*	*	*	0.1	0.1	0.5	1.2	2.3	6.2	16.8
Diseases of appendix	0.1	*	*	*	*	*	*	0.1	0.2	0.3	0.8	2.0
Hernia	0.6	0.7	*	*	*	*	0.1	0.2	0.5	1.3	3.8	12.4
Chronic liver disease and cirrhosis	10.3	*	*	*	0.1	1.2	5.9	19.2	26.8	26.3	27.7	21.8
Alcoholic liver disease	5.2	*	*	*	0.1	0.9	4.3	12.1	14.4	10.2	5.8	2.3
Other chronic liver disease and cirrhosis	5.2	*	*	*	*	0.3	1.6	7.1	12.4	16.2	21.9	19.5
Cholelithiasis and other disorders of gallbladder	1.1	*	*	*	*	*	0.1	0.2	0.8	2.3	7.2	25.9
Nephritis, nephrotic syndrome and nephrosis	16.3	2.7	*	0.1	0.2	0.6	1.8	4.9	13.9	39.3	115.7	333.8
Acute and rapidly progressive nephritic and nephrotic syndrome	0.1	*	*	*	*	*	*	*	*	0.1	0.5	1.1
Chronic glomerulonephritis, nephritis and nephropathy not specified as acute or chronic, and renal sclerosis unspecified	1.9	*	*	*	*	*	0.1	0.3	1.0	3.1	12.6	54.0
Renal failure	14.4	2.5	*	*	0.1	0.5	1.6	4.6	12.9	36.0	102.6	278.7
Other disorders of kidney	*	*	*	*	*	*	*	*	*	*	*	*

Table 2-12. Death Rates for Selected Causes, by Age, 2010—*Continued*

(Number.)

Cause of death (based on ICD-10, 2004)	All ages[1]	Under 1 year[2]	1 to 4 years	5 to 14 years	15 to 24 years	25 to 34 years	35 to 44 years	45 to 54 years	55 to 64 years	65 to 74 years	75 to 84 years	85 years and over
Infections of kidney	0.2	*	*	*	*	*	0.0	0.1	0.2	0.4	1.1	3.6
Hyperplasia of prostate	0.2	*	*	*	*	*	*	*	*	0.2	1.1	5.2
Inflammatory diseases of female pelvic organs	0.0	*	*	*	*	*	*	*	*	0.1	0.3	0.6
Pregnancy, childbirth and the puerperium	0.3	X	X	*	0.4	0.9	0.5	0.1	*	*	*	*
Pregnancy with abortive outcome	0.0	X	X	*	*	*	*	*	*	*	*	*
Other complications of pregnancy, childbirth and the puerperium	0.3	X	X	*	0.4	0.9	0.5	0.1	*	*	*	*
Certain conditions originating in the perinatal period	3.9	304.5	0.3	0.1	*	*	*	*	*	*	*	*
Congenital malformations, deformations and chromosomal abnormalities	3.1	129.5	3.1	0.7	0.9	1.0	1.1	1.5	2.1	1.8	2.7	5.5
Symptoms, signs and abnormal clinical and laboratory findings, not elsewhere classified	12.4	77.4	1.5	0.2	1.2	2.2	3.0	4.9	7.0	14.3	52.3	320.9
All other diseases (Residual)	87.4	19.1	3.0	1.9	4.3	8.0	16.0	37.2	71.8	151.0	499.1	2,096.9
Accidents (unintentional injuries)	39.1	28.1	8.6	4.0	28.3	35.5	36.0	43.7	38.4	43.3	106.1	328.4
Transport accidents	12.3	2.1	2.9	2.3	17.3	14.8	12.5	13.2	13.2	13.5	20.1	24.9
Motor vehicle accidents	11.4	2.0	2.8	2.2	16.6	14.0	11.6	12.0	11.9	12.3	18.8	23.8
Other land transport accidents	0.3	*	*	0.1	0.4	0.3	0.4	0.5	0.4	0.4	0.5	0.5
Water, air and space, and other and unspecified transport accidents and their sequelae	0.5	*	*	0.1	0.3	0.5	0.6	0.8	0.9	0.8	0.8	0.5
Nontransport accidents	26.8	26.1	5.7	1.7	11.0	20.7	23.5	30.5	25.3	29.8	86.0	303.5
Falls	8.4	*	0.1	0.1	0.5	0.7	1.2	2.9	5.5	13.8	55.5	207.7
Accidental discharge of firearms	0.2	*	0.2	0.1	0.3	0.3	0.2	0.2	0.1	0.2	*	*
Accidental drowning and submersion	1.2	1.0	2.7	0.6	1.5	1.2	1.0	1.3	1.1	1.3	1.3	1.3
Accidental exposure to smoke, fire and flames	0.9	0.5	0.9	0.3	0.3	0.4	0.6	1.0	1.3	1.8	3.1	4.6
Accidental poisoning and exposure to noxious substances	10.7	*	0.2	0.1	7.3	16.5	18.2	21.5	12.2	3.9	2.6	4.1
Other and unspecified nontransport accidents and their sequelae	5.4	24.2	1.6	0.4	1.1	1.7	2.4	3.7	5.0	8.9	23.4	85.7
Intentional Self-Harm (Suicide)	12.4	X	X	0.7	10.5	14.0	16.0	19.6	17.5	13.7	15.7	17.6
By discharge of firearms	6.3	X	X	0.2	4.7	6.3	7.1	9.1	9.3	9.5	11.8	12.4
By other and unspecified means and their sequelae	6.1	X	X	0.5	5.9	7.6	8.9	10.5	8.2	4.2	3.9	5.3
Assault (Homicide)	5.3	7.9	2.4	0.6	10.7	10.4	6.0	4.4	2.9	2.1	1.9	2.0
By discharge of firearms	3.6	*	0.3	0.4	8.9	8.1	4.1	2.4	1.5	1.0	0.7	0.6
By other and unspecified means and their sequelae	1.7	7.6	2.1	0.2	1.8	2.3	1.9	2.0	1.5	1.1	1.2	1.4
Legal intervention	0.1	*	*	*	0.2	0.2	0.3	0.2	0.1	*	*	*
Events of undetermined intent	1.6	2.7	0.5	0.2	1.0	2.0	2.3	2.9	2.0	0.9	1.0	1.9
Discharge of firearms, undetermined intent	0.1	*	*	*	0.1	0.1	0.1	0.1	0.1	*	*	*
Other and unspecified events of undetermined intent and their sequelae	1.5	2.7	0.5	0.1	0.9	1.8	2.2	2.8	1.9	0.9	1.0	1.8
Operations of war and their sequelae	*	*	*	*	*	*	*	*	*	*	*	*
Complications of medical and surgical care	0.8	0.6	*	0.1	0.1	0.1	0.3	0.5	1.1	2.3	4.8	7.6
Enterocolitis due to Clostridium difficile[3]	2.4	*	*	*	*	*	0.1	0.3	1.2	4.9	18.8	57.4
Drug-induced deaths[4,5]	13.1	0.6	0.3	0.2	8.4	19.2	21.7	26.5	16.2	5.2	4.0	5.5
Alcohol-induced deaths[4,6]	8.3	*	*	*	0.3	2.2	7.5	19.1	21.9	15.8	9.6	5.3
Injury by firearms[4,7]	10.3	*	0.4	0.7	14.2	15.0	11.7	12.0	11.1	10.7	12.7	13.2

X = Not applicable.   * = Figure does not meet standards of reliability or precision.   0.0 = Quantity more than zero but less than 0.05.   [1]Figures for age not stated included in "All ages" but not distributed among age groups.   [2]Death rates for "Under 1 year" (based on population estimates) differ from infant mortality rates (based on live births); for more information, see chapter notes.   [3]Included in "Certain other intestinal infections (A04, A07–A09)" shown above. Beginning with data year 2006, Enterocolitis due to Clostridium difficile (A04.7) is shown separately at the bottom of the tables and is included in the list of rankable causes.   [4]Included in selected categories above.   [5]Includes ICD–10 codes D52.1, D59.0, D59.2, D61.1, D64.2, E06.4, E16.0, E23.1, E24.2, E27.3, E66.1, F11.1–F11.5, F11.7–F11.9, F12.1–F12.5, F12.7–F12.9, F13.1–F13.5, F13.7–F13.9, F14.1–F14.5, F14.7–F14.9, F15.1–F15.5, F15.7–F15.9, F16.1–F16.5, F16.7–F16.9, F17.3–F17.5, F17.7–F17.9, F18.1–F18.5, F18.7–F18.9, F19.1–F19.5, F19.7–F19.9, G21.1, G24.0, G25.1, G25.4, G25.6, G44.4, G62.0, G72.0, I95.2, J70.2–J70.4, K85.3, L10.5, L27.0–L27.1, M10.2, M32.0, M80.4, M81.4, M83.5, M87.1, R50.2, R78.1–R78.5, X40–X44, X60–X64, X85, and Y10–Y14. Trend data for drug-induced deaths, previously shown in this report, can be found at http://www.cdc.gov/nchs/deaths.htm available from http://www.cdc.gov/nchs/deaths.htm   [6]Includes ICD–10 codes E24.4, F10, G31.2, G62.1, G72.1, I42.6, K29.2, K70, K85.2, K86.0, R78.0, X45, X65, and Y15. Trend data for alcohol-induced deaths, previously shown in this report, can be found at http://www.cdc.gov/nchs/deaths.htm.   [7]Includes ICD–10 codes *U01.4, W32–W34, X72–X74, X93–X95, Y22–Y24, and Y35.0. Trend data for Injury by firearms, previously shown in this report, can be found through a link from the online version of this report, available at http://www.cdc.gov/nchs/deaths.htm.

Table 2-13A. Number of Deaths from Selected Causes, by Race and Sex, 2010

(Number.)

Cause of death (based on ICD-10, 2004)	All races			White[1]			Black[1]		
	Both sexes	Male	Female	Both sexes	Male	Female	Both sexes	Male	Female
All Causes	2,468,435	1,232,432	1,236,003	2,114,749	1,051,514	1,063,235	286,959	145,802	141,157
Salmonella infections	28	17	11	19	14	5	5	1	4
Shigellosis and amebiasis	3	1	2	1	1	-	1	-	1
Certain other intestinal infections	10,276	4,046	6,230	9,248	3,582	5,666	827	370	457
Tuberculosis	569	351	218	338	200	138	120	86	34
Respiratory tuberculosis	423	276	147	239	146	93	94	74	20
Other tuberculosis	146	75	71	99	54	45	26	12	14
Whooping cough	26	13	13	24	11	13	2	2	-
Scarlet fever and erysipelas	3	1	2	2	1	1	-	-	-
Meningococcal infection	79	40	39	67	34	33	9	5	4
Septicemia	34,812	16,069	18,743	27,985	12,976	15,009	6,001	2,691	3,310
Syphilis	28	20	8	15	12	3	12	8	4
Acute poliomyelitis	-	-	-	-	-	-	-	-	-
Arthropod-borne viral encephalitis	9	4	5	8	3	5	-	-	-
Measles	2	1	1	1	1	-	-	-	-
Viral hepatitis	7,564	5,038	2,526	6,061	4,097	1,964	1,101	707	394
Human immunodeficiency virus (HIV) disease	8,369	6,099	2,270	3,575	2,951	624	4,662	3,047	1,615
Malaria	10	7	3	2	1	1	6	5	1
Other and unspecified infectious and parasitic diseases and their sequelae	5,805	2,970	2,835	4,802	2,439	2,363	777	407	370
Malignant Neoplasms	574,743	301,037	273,706	491,686	258,272	233,414	65,930	33,967	31,963
Lip, oral cavity and pharynx	8,474	5,815	2,659	7,151	4,885	2,266	1,006	727	279
Esophagus	14,490	11,416	3,074	12,761	10,148	2,613	1,437	1,044	393
Stomach	11,390	6,703	4,687	8,524	5,023	3,501	2,000	1,180	820
Colon, rectum and anus	52,622	27,284	25,338	43,854	22,765	21,089	7,005	3,618	3,387
Liver and intrahepatic bile ducts	20,305	13,658	6,647	15,949	10,627	5,322	2,826	1,986	840
Pancreas	36,888	18,699	18,189	31,413	16,064	15,349	4,327	2,096	2,231
Larynx	3,691	2,951	740	3,007	2,410	597	613	480	133
Trachea, bronchus and lung	158,318	87,740	70,578	137,698	75,675	62,023	16,688	9,793	6,895
Melanoma of skin	9,154	6,002	3,152	8,944	5,905	3,039	135	62	73
Breast	41,435	439	40,996	34,183	349	33,834	6,109	78	6,031
Cervix uteri	3,939	X	3,939	2,970	X	2,970	790	X	790
Corpus uteri and uterus, part unspecified	8,402	X	8,402	6,688	X	6,688	1,437	X	1,437
Ovary	14,572	X	14,572	12,841	X	12,841	1,279	X	1,279
Prostate	28,561	28,561	X	23,172	23,172	X	4,854	4,854	X
Kidney and renal pelvis	13,219	8,436	4,783	11,659	7,474	4,185	1,185	708	477
Bladder	14,731	10,429	4,302	13,404	9,647	3,757	1,073	615	458
Meninges, brain and other parts of central nervous system	14,164	7,977	6,187	12,876	7,305	5,571	896	466	430
Lymphoid, hematopoietic and related tissue	55,590	30,777	24,813	48,584	27,084	21,500	5,450	2,824	2,626
Hodgkin's disease	1,231	714	517	1,087	633	454	114	60	54
Non-Hodgkin's lymphoma	20,294	11,047	9,247	18,198	9,907	8,291	1,509	825	684
Leukemia	22,569	12,851	9,718	20,088	11,524	8,564	1,816	957	859
Multiple myeloma and immunoproliferative neoplasms	11,428	6,117	5,311	9,154	4,979	4,175	2,003	978	1,025
Other and unspecified malignant neoplasms of lymphoid, hematopoietic and related tissue	68	48	20	57	41	16	8	4	4
All other and unspecified malignant neoplasms	64,798	34,150	30,648	56,008	29,739	26,269	6,820	3,436	3,384
In situ neoplasms, benign neoplasms and neoplasms of uncertain or unknown behavior	14,917	7,721	7,196	13,287	6,966	6,321	1,220	550	670
Anemias	4,852	2,017	2,835	3,741	1,525	2,216	1,007	446	561
Diabetes mellitus	69,071	35,490	33,581	54,250	28,486	25,764	12,126	5,640	6,486
Nutritional deficiencies	2,948	1,141	1,807	2,503	974	1,529	367	134	233
Malnutrition	2,790	1,079	1,711	2,358	919	1,439	357	129	228
Other nutritional deficiencies	158	62	96	145	55	90	10	5	5
Meningitis	608	303	305	442	221	221	138	64	74
Parkinson's disease	22,032	12,871	9,161	20,792	12,173	8,619	804	452	352
Alzheimer's disease	83,494	25,364	58,130	76,928	23,442	53,486	5,220	1,488	3,732
Major cardiovascular diseases	780,213	383,547	396,666	667,081	327,381	339,700	92,898	45,572	47,326
Diseases of heart	597,689	307,384	290,305	514,323	264,425	249,898	69,083	35,089	33,994
Acute rheumatic fever and chronic rheumatic heart diseases	2,987	996	1,991	2,644	885	1,759	232	79	153
Hypertensive heart disease	33,678	16,242	17,436	25,097	11,726	13,371	7,729	4,075	3,654
Hypertensive heart and renal disease	2,807	1,285	1,522	1,960	864	1,096	748	377	371
Ischemic heart diseases	379,559	207,580	171,979	330,277	181,386	148,891	39,630	20,615	19,015
Acute myocardial infarction	122,071	67,435	54,636	106,204	59,181	47,023	12,743	6,445	6,298
Other acute ischemic heart diseases	4,170	2,156	2,014	3,519	1,798	1,721	557	303	254
Other forms of chronic ischemic heart disease	253,318	137,989	115,329	220,554	120,407	100,147	26,330	13,867	12,463
Atherosclerotic cardiovascular disease, so described	57,438	33,703	23,735	47,470	27,790	19,680	8,361	4,930	3,431
All other forms of chronic ischemic heart disease	195,880	104,286	91,594	173,084	92,617	80,467	17,969	8,937	9,032
Other heart diseases	178,658	81,281	97,377	154,345	69,564	84,781	20,744	9,943	10,801
Acute and subacute endocarditis	1,103	627	476	889	507	382	183	100	83
Diseases of pericardium and acute myocarditis	776	405	371	617	320	297	126	64	62
Heart failure	57,757	24,385	33,372	51,290	21,540	29,750	5,528	2,444	3,084
All other forms of heart disease	119,022	55,864	63,158	101,549	47,197	54,352	14,907	7,335	7,572
Essential hypertension and hypertensive renal disease	26,634	10,846	15,788	20,560	8,229	12,331	5,116	2,218	2,898
Cerebrovascular diseases	129,476	52,367	77,109	109,119	43,424	65,695	15,965	6,938	9,027
Atherosclerosis	7,230	2,933	4,297	6,513	2,618	3,895	594	254	340
Other diseases of circulatory system	19,184	10,017	9,167	16,566	8,685	7,881	2,140	1,073	1,067
Aortic aneurysm and dissection	10,431	6,096	4,335	9,134	5,359	3,775	972	552	420
Other diseases of arteries, arterioles and capillaries	8,753	3,921	4,832	7,432	3,326	4,106	1,168	521	647

Table 2-13A. Number of Deaths from Selected Causes, by Race and Sex, 2010—*Continued*

(Number.)

Cause of death (based on ICD-10, 2004)	All races			White[1]			Black[1]		
	Both sexes	Male	Female	Both sexes	Male	Female	Both sexes	Male	Female
Other disorders of circulatory system	4,241	2,053	2,188	3,377	1,616	1,761	763	383	380
Influenza and pneumonia	50,097	23,615	26,482	43,296	20,238	23,058	4,936	2,380	2,556
Influenza	500	250	250	409	205	204	68	32	36
Pneumonia	49,597	23,365	26,232	42,887	20,033	22,854	4,868	2,348	2,520
Other acute lower respiratory infections	213	94	119	182	80	102	22	10	12
Acute bronchitis and bronchiolitis	177	74	103	147	61	86	21	9	12
Other and unspecified acute lower respiratory infections	36	20	16	35	19	16	1	1	-
Chronic lower respiratory diseases	138,080	65,423	72,657	127,176	59,632	67,544	8,715	4,532	4,183
Bronchitis, chronic and unspecified	620	267	353	557	232	325	48	26	22
Emphysema	10,034	5,227	4,807	9,294	4,764	4,530	596	363	233
Asthma	3,404	1,283	2,121	2,366	790	1,576	879	408	471
Other chronic lower respiratory diseases	124,022	58,646	65,376	114,959	53,846	61,113	7,192	3,735	3,457
Pneumoconioses and chemical effects	845	812	33	803	773	30	36	33	3
Pneumonitis due to solids and liquids	17,011	9,208	7,803	15,235	8,264	6,971	1,380	724	656
Other diseases of respiratory system	31,187	15,791	15,396	27,376	13,968	13,408	2,926	1,378	1,548
Peptic ulcer	2,977	1,460	1,517	2,572	1,233	1,339	296	172	124
Diseases of appendix	415	258	157	355	216	139	44	30	14
Hernia	1,832	814	1,018	1,635	714	921	166	82	84
Chronic liver disease and cirrhosis	31,903	20,798	11,105	28,014	18,352	9,662	2,635	1,715	920
Alcoholic liver disease	15,990	11,441	4,549	13,997	10,125	3,872	1,226	822	404
Other chronic liver disease and cirrhosis	15,913	9,357	6,556	14,017	8,227	5,790	1,409	893	516
Cholelithiasis and other disorders of gallbladder	3,332	1,552	1,780	2,912	1,368	1,544	300	121	179
Nephritis, nephritic syndrome and nephrosis	50,476	24,865	25,611	40,205	20,172	20,033	8,841	4,016	4,825
Acute and rapidly progressive nephritic and nephritic syndrome	203	97	106	161	75	86	32	18	14
Chronic glomerulonephritis, nephritis and nephropathy not specified as acute or chronic, and renal sclerosis unspecified	5,894	2,775	3,119	4,770	2,270	2,500	948	432	516
Renal failure	44,362	21,989	22,373	35,261	17,824	17,437	7,857	3,565	4,292
Other disorders of kidney	17	4	13	13	3	10	4	1	3
Infections of kidney	608	187	421	526	158	368	65	26	39
Hyperplasia of prostate	489	489	X	444	444	X	37	37	X
Inflammatory diseases of female pelvic organs	137	X	137	113	X	113	21	X	21
Pregnancy, childbirth and the puerperium	825	X	825	504	X	504	264	X	264
Pregnancy with abortive outcome	37	X	37	19	X	19	18	X	18
Other complications of pregnancy, childbirth and the puerperium	788	X	788	485	X	485	246	X	246
Certain conditions originating in the perinatal period	12,128	6,803	5,325	7,513	4,233	3,280	4,031	2,216	1,815
Congenital malformations, deformations and chromosomal abnormalities	9,673	4,960	4,713	7,566	3,860	3,706	1,656	872	784
Symptoms, signs and abnormal clinical and laboratory findings, not elsewhere classified	38,360	16,057	22,303	32,668	13,321	19,347	4,935	2,351	2,584
All other diseases (Residual)	269,844	109,547	160,297	235,449	94,966	140,483	28,532	11,902	16,630
Accidents (unintentional injuries)	120,859	75,921	44,938	104,945	65,360	39,585	12,069	8,074	3,995
Transport accidents	37,961	26,783	11,178	31,637	22,348	9,289	4,751	3,421	1,330
Motor vehicle accidents	35,332	24,723	10,609	29,392	20,589	8,803	4,477	3,206	1,271
Other land transport accidents	1,029	794	235	840	647	193	136	106	30
Water, air and space, and other and unspecified transport accidents and their sequelae	1,600	1,266	334	1,405	1,112	293	138	109	29
Nontransport accidents	82,898	49,138	33,760	73,308	43,012	30,296	7,318	4,653	2,665
Falls	26,009	13,049	12,960	24,133	11,967	12,166	1,164	669	495
Accidental discharge of firearms	606	515	91	474	396	78	113	101	12
Accidental drowning and submersion	3,782	2,936	846	2,970	2,267	703	571	478	93
Accidental exposure to smoke, fire and flames	2,782	1,624	1,158	2,135	1,251	884	577	335	242
Accidental poisoning and exposure to noxious substances	33,041	21,117	11,924	29,283	18,717	10,566	2,988	1,896	1,092
Other and unspecified nontransport accidents and their sequelae	16,678	9,897	6,781	14,313	8,414	5,899	1,905	1,174	731
Intentional Self-Harm (Suicide)	38,364	30,277	8,087	34,690	27,422	7,268	2,144	1,755	389
By discharge of firearms	19,392	16,962	2,430	17,909	15,648	2,261	1,079	965	114
By other and unspecified means and their sequelae	18,972	13,315	5,657	16,781	11,774	5,007	1,065	790	275
Assault (Homicide)	16,259	12,774	3,485	7,863	5,648	2,215	7,818	6,704	1,114
By discharge of firearms	11,078	9,340	1,738	4,647	3,555	1,092	6,151	5,553	598
By other and unspecified means and their sequelae	5,181	3,434	1,747	3,216	2,093	1,123	1,667	1,151	516
Legal intervention	412	399	13	295	287	8	98	96	2
Events of undetermined intent	4,908	2,930	1,978	4,147	2,448	1,699	594	381	213
Discharge of firearms, undetermined intent	252	203	49	210	171	39	32	25	7
Other and unspecified events of undetermined intent and their sequelae	4,656	2,727	1,929	3,937	2,277	1,660	562	356	206
Operations of war and their sequelae	9	9	-	7	7	-	1	1	-
Complications of medical and surgical care	2,490	1,167	1,323	2,023	971	1,052	401	169	232
Enterocolitis due to Clostridium difficile[2]	7,298	2,889	4,409	6,671	2,623	4,048	488	203	285
Drug-induced deaths[3,4]	40,393	24,376	16,017	36,020	21,697	14,323	3,561	2,210	1,351
Alcohol-induced deaths[3,5]	25,692	19,038	6,654	22,167	16,527	5,640	2,330	1,686	644
Injury by firearms[3,6]	31,672	27,356	4,316	23,490	20,014	3,476	7,454	6,721	733

X = Not applicable.   - = Quantity zero.   [1]Race categories are consistent with the 1977 Office of Management and Budget (OMB) standards. Multiple-race data were reported by 37 states and the District of Columbia in 2010. The multiple-race data for these reporting areas were bridged to the single-race categories of the 1977 OMB standards for comparability with other reporting areas.   [2]Included in certain other intestinal infections (A04, A07–A09). Beginning with data year 2006, Enterocolitis due to Clostridium difficile (A04.7) is shown separately at the bottom of the table and is included in the list of rankable causes.   [3]Included in selected categories above.   [4]Includes ICD–10 codes D52.1, D59.0, D59.2, D61.1, D64.2, E06.4, E16.0, E23.1, E24.2, E27.3, E66.1, F11.1–F11.5, F11.7–F11.9, F12.1–F12.5, F12.7–F12.9, F13.1–F13.5, F13.7–F13.9, F14.1–F14.5, F14.7–F14.9, F15.1–F15.5, F15.7–F15.9, F16.1–F16.5, F16.7–F16.9, F17.3–F17.5, F17.7–F17.9, F18.1–F18.5, F18.7–F18.9, F19.1–F19.5, F19.7–F19.9, G21.1, G24.0, G25.1, G25.4, G25.6, G44.4, G62.0, G72.0, I95.2, J70.2–J70.4, K85.3, L10.5, L27.0–L27.1, M10.2, M32.0, M80.4, M81.4, M83.5, M87.1, R50.2, R78.1–R78.5, X40–X44, X60–X64, X85, and Y10–Y14. Trend data for drug-induced deaths, previously shown in this report, can be found at http://www.cdc.gov/nchs/deaths.htm.   [5]Includes ICD–10 codes E24.4, F10, G31.2, G62.1, G72.1, I42.6, K29.2, K70, K85.2, K86.0, R78.0, X45, X65, and Y15. Trend data for alcohol-induced deaths, previously shown in this report, can be found at http://www.cdc.gov/nchs/deaths.htm.   [6]Includes ICD–10 codes *U01.4, W32–W34, X72–X74, X93–X95, Y22–Y24, and Y35.0. Trend data for Injury by firearms, previously shown in this report, can be found at http://www.cdc.gov/nchs/deaths.htm.

Table 2-13B. Number of Deaths from Selected Causes, by Race and Sex, 2010

(Number.)

Cause of death (based on ICD-10, 2004)	American Indian and Alaskan Native[1,2]			Asian or Pacific Islander[1,3]		
	Both sexes	Male	Female	Both sexes	Male	Female
All Causes	15,565	8,516	7,049	51,162	26,600	24,562
Salmonella infections	-	-	-	4	2	2
Shigellosis and amebiasis	-	-	-	1	-	1
Certain other intestinal infections	62	30	32	139	64	75
Tuberculosi	15	6	9	96	59	37
Respiratory tuberculosis	12	5	7	78	51	27
Other tuberculosis	3	1	2	18	8	10
Whooping cough	-	-	-	-	-	-
Scarlet fever and erysipelas	-	-	-	1	-	1
Meningococcal infection	-	-	-	3	1	2
Septicemia	244	106	138	582	296	286
Syphilis	-	-	-	1	-	1
Acute poliomyelitis	-	-	-	-	-	-
Arthropod-borne viral encephalitis	-	-	-	1	1	-
Measles	-	-	-	-	-	-
Viral hepatitis	1	1	-	-	-	-
Human immunodeficiency virus (HIV) disease	99	63	36	303	171	132
	61	48	13	71	53	18
Malaria	-	-	-	2	1	1
Other and unspecified infectious and parasitic diseases and their sequelae	53	28	25	173	96	77
Malignant Neoplasms	2,962	1,588	1,374	14,165	7,210	6,955
Lip, oral cavity and pharynx	41	25	16	276	178	98
Esophagus	63	49	14	229	175	54
Stomach	87	57	30	779	443	336
Colon, rectum and anus	287	152	135	1,476	749	727
Liver and intrahepatic bile ducts	196	143	53	1,334	902	432
Pancreas	177	97	80	971	442	529
Larynx	25	20	5	46	41	5
Trachea, bronchus and lung	785	445	340	3,147	1,827	1,320
Skin	22	12	10	53	23	30
Breast	172	2	170	971	10	961
Cervix uteri	36	X	36	143	X	143
Corpus uteri and uterus, part unspecified	36	X	36	241	X	241
Ovary	73	X	73	379	X	379
Prostate	117	117	X	418	418	X
Kidney and renal pelvis	110	74	36	265	180	85
Bladder	47	31	16	207	136	71
Meninges, brain and other parts of central nervous system	73	38	35	319	168	151
Lymphoid, hematopoietic and related tissue	230	129	101	1,326	740	586
Hodgkin's disease	5	3	2	25	18	7
Non-Hodgkin's lymphoma	70	41	29	517	274	243
Leukemi	107	59	48	558	311	247
Multiple myeloma and immunoproliferative neoplasms	48	26	22	223	134	89
Other and unspecified malignant neoplasms of lymphoid, hemato-poietic and related tissue	-	-	-	3	3	-
All other and unspecified malignant neoplasms	385	197	188	1,585	778	807
In situ neoplasms, benign neoplasms and neoplasms of uncertain or unknown behavior	60	33	27	350	172	178
Anemias	18	5	13	86	41	45
Diabetes mellitus	857	432	425	1,838	932	906
Nutritional deficiencies	29	9	20	49	24	25
Malnutrition	28	9	19	47	22	25
Other nutritional deficiencies	1	-	1	2	2	-
Meningitis	7	4	3	21	14	7
Parkinson's disease	62	40	22	374	206	168
Alzheimer's disease	264	89	175	1,082	345	737
Major cardiovascular diseases	3,603	1,972	1,631	16,631	8,622	8,009
Diseases of heart	2,793	1,608	1,185	11,490	6,262	5,228
Acute rheumatic fever and chronic rheumatic heart diseases	14	6	8	97	26	71
Hypertensive heart disease	169	100	69	683	341	342
Hypertensive heart and renal disease	18	10	8	81	34	47
Ischemic heart diseases	1,831	1,098	733	7,821	4,481	3,340
Acute myocardial infarction	594	367	227	2,530	1,442	1,088
Other acute ischemic heart diseases	39	24	15	55	31	24
Other forms of chronic ischemic heart disease	1,198	707	491	5,236	3,008	2,228
Atherosclerotic cardiovascular disease, so described	372	233	139	1,235	750	485
All other forms of chronic ischemic heart disease	826	474	352	4,001	2,258	1,743
Other heart diseases	761	394	367	2,808	1,380	1,428
Acute and subacute endocarditis	11	5	6	20	15	5
Diseases of pericardium and acute myocarditis	10	7	3	23	14	9
Heart failure	225	91	134	714	310	404
All other forms of heart disease	515	291	224	2,051	1,041	1,010
Essential hypertension and hypertensive renal disease	144	62	82	814	337	477
Cerebrovascular diseases	559	258	301	3,833	1,747	2,086
Atherosclerosis	19	5	14	104	56	48
Other diseases of circulatory system	88	39	49	390	220	170
Aortic aneurysm and dissection	48	26	22	277	159	118
Other diseases of arteries, arterioles and capillaries	40	13	27	113	61	52

Table 2-13B. Number of Deaths from Selected Causes, by Race and Sex, 2010—*Continued*

(Number.)

Cause of death (based on ICD-10, 2004)	American Indian and Alaskan Native[1,2]			Asian or Pacific Islander[1,3]		
	Both sexes	Male	Female	Both sexes	Male	Female
Other disorders of circulatory system	23	9	14	78	45	33
Influenza and pneumonia	326	172	154	1,539	825	714
Influenza	4	2	2	19	11	8
Pneumonia	322	170	152	1,520	814	706
Other acute lower respiratory infections	2	1	1	7	3	4
Acute bronchitis and bronchiolitis	2	1	1	7	3	4
Other and unspecified acute lower respiratory infections	-	-	-	-	-	-
Chronic lower respiratory diseases	702	349	353	1,487	910	577
Bronchitis, chronic and unspecified	4	4	-	11	5	6
Emphysema	44	21	23	100	79	21
Asthma	23	12	11	136	73	63
Other chronic lower respiratory diseases	631	312	319	1,240	753	487
Pneumoconioses and chemical effects	4	4	-	2	2	-
Pneumonitis due to solids and liquids	83	40	43	313	180	133
Other diseases of respiratory system	238	113	125	647	332	315
Peptic ulcer	22	8	14	87	47	40
Diseases of appendix	5	3	2	11	9	2
Hernia	14	8	6	17	10	7
Chronic liver disease and cirrhosis	787	429	358	467	302	165
Alcoholic liver disease	592	351	241	175	143	32
Other chronic liver disease and cirrhosis	195	78	117	292	159	133
Cholelithiasis and other disorders of gallbladder	20	11	9	100	52	48
Nephritis, nephritic syndrome and nephrosis	339	153	186	1,091	524	567
Acute and rapidly progressive nephritic and nephritic syndrome	1	-	1	9	4	5
Chronic glomerulonephritis, nephritis and nephropathy not specified as acute or chronic, and renal sclerosis unspecified	41	20	21	135	53	82
Renal failure	297	133	164	947	467	480
Other disorders of kidney	-	-	-	-	-	-
Infections of kidney	5	1	4	12	2	10
Hyperplasia of prostate	-	-	X	8	8	X
Inflammatory diseases of female pelvic organs	3	X	3	-	X	-
Pregnancy, childbirth and the puerperium	15	X	15	42	X	42
Pregnancy with abortive outcome	-	X	-	-	X	-
Other complications of pregnancy, childbirth and the puerperium	15	X	15	42	X	42
Certain conditions originating in the perinatal period	117	76	41	467	278	189
Congenital malformations, deformations and chromosomal abnormalities	130	71	59	321	157	164
Symptoms, signs and abnormal clinical and laboratory findings, not elsewhere classified	240	129	111	517	256	261
All other diseases (Residual)	1,549	725	824	4,314	1,954	2,360
Accidents (unintentional injuries)	1,701	1,150	551	2,144	1,337	807
Transport accidents	684	462	222	889	552	337
Motor vehicle accidents	638	425	213	825	503	322
Other land transport accidents	22	19	3	31	22	9
Water, air and space, and other and unspecified transport accidents and their sequelae	24	18	6	33	27	6
Nontransport accidents	1,017	688	329	1,255	785	470
Falls	161	97	64	551	316	235
Accidental discharge of firearms	14	14	-	5	4	1
Accidental drowning and submersion	68	60	8	173	131	42
Accidental exposure to smoke, fire and flames	45	26	19	25	12	13
Accidental poisoning and exposure to noxious substances	521	332	189	249	172	77
Other and unspecified nontransport accidents and their sequelae	208	159	49	252	150	102
Intentional Self-Harm (Suicide)	469	344	125	1,061	756	305
By discharge of firearms	178	146	32	226	203	23
By other and unspecified means and their sequelae	291	198	93	835	553	282
Assault (Homicide)	257	204	53	321	218	103
Assault (homicide) by discharge of firearms	113	98	15	167	134	33
Assault (homicide) by other and unspecified means and their sequelae	144	106	38	154	84	70
Legal intervention	9	6	3	10	10	-
Events of undetermined intent	87	46	41	80	55	25
Discharge of firearms, undetermined intent	7	4	3	3	3	-
Other and unspecified events of undetermined intent and their sequelae	80	42	38	77	52	25
Operations of war and their sequelae	-	-	-	1	1	-
Complications of medical and surgical care	21	10	11	45	17	28
Enterocolitis due to Clostridium difficile[4]	39	20	19	100	43	57
Drug-induced deaths[5,6]	458	250	208	354	219	135
Alcohol-induced deaths[5,7]	931	611	320	264	214	50
Injury by firearms[5,8]	317	267	50	411	354	57

X = Not applicable.   - = Quantity zero.   [1]Race categories are consistent with the 1977 Office of Management and Budget (OMB) standards. Multiple-race data were reported by 37 states and the District of Columbia in 2010. The multiple-race data for these reporting areas were bridged to the single-race categories of the 1977 OMB standards for comparability with other reporting areas.   [2]Includes Aleuts and Eskimos.   [3]Includes Chinese, Filipinos, Hawaiians, Japanese, and other Asian and Pacific Islander persons.   [4]Included in certain other intestinal infections (A04, A07–A09). Beginning with data year 2006, Enterocolitis due to Clostridium difficile (A04.7) is shown separately at the bottom of the table and is included in the list of rankable causes.   [5]Included in selected categories above.   [6]Includes ICD–10 codes D52.1, D59.0, D59.2, D61.1, D64.2, E06.4, E16.0, E23.1, E24.2, E27.3, E66.1, F11.1–F11.5, F11.7–F11.9, F12.1–F12.5, F12.7–F12.9, F13.1–F13.5, F13.7–F13.9, F14.1–F14.5, F14.7–F14.9, F15.1–F15.5, F15.7–F15.9, F16.1–F16.5, F16.7–F16.9, F17.3–F17.5, F17.7–F17.9, F18.1–F18.5, F18.7–F18.9, F19.1–F19.5, F19.7–F19.9, G21.1, G24.0, G25.1, G25.4, G25.6, G44.4, G62.0, G72.0, I95.2, J70.2–J70.4, K85.3, L10.5, L27.0–L27.1, M10.2, M32.0, M80.4, M81.4, M83.5, M87.1, R50.2, R78.1–R78.5, X40–X44, X60–X64, X85, and Y10–Y14. Trend data for drug-induced deaths, previously shown in this report, can be found at http://www.cdc.gov/nchs/deaths.htm.   [7]Includes ICD–10 codes E24.4, F10, G31.2, G62.1, G72.1, I42.6, K29.2, K70, K85.2, K86.0, R78.0, X45, X65, and Y15. Trend data for alcohol-induced deaths, previously shown in this report, can be found at http://www.cdc.gov/nchs/deaths.htm.   [8]Includes ICD–10 codes *U01.4, W32–W34, X72–X74, X93–X95, Y22–Y24, and Y35.0. Trend data for Injury by firearms, previously shown in this report, can be found at http://www.cdc.gov/nchs/deaths.htm.

Table 2-14A. Death Rates for Selected Causes, by Race and Sex, 2010

(Rates per 100,000 population in specified group.)

Cause of death (based on ICD-10, 2004)	All races			White[1]			Black[1]		
	Both sexes	Male	Female	Both sexes	Male	Female	Both sexes	Male	Female
All Causes	799.5	812.0	787.4	861.7	866.1	857.3	682.2	725.4	642.7
Salmonella infections	0.0	*	*	*	*	*	*	*	*
Shigellosis and amebiasis	*	*	*	*	*	*	*	*	*
Certain other intestinal infections	3.3	2.7	4.0	3.8	3.0	4.6	2.0	1.8	2.1
Tuberculosis	0.2	0.2	0.1	0.1	0.2	0.1	0.3	0.4	0.2
Respiratory tuberculosis	0.1	0.2	0.1	0.1	0.1	0.1	0.2	0.4	0.1
Other tuberculosis	0.0	0.0	0.0	0.0	0.0	0.0	0.1	*	*
Whooping cough	0.0	*	*	0.0	*	*	*	*	*
Scarlet fever and erysipelas	*	*	*	*	*	*	*	*	*
Meningococcal infection	0.0	0.0	0.0	0.0	0.0	0.0	*	*	*
Septicemia	11.3	10.6	11.9	11.4	10.7	12.1	14.3	13.4	15.1
Syphilis	0.0	0.0	*	0.0	*	*	*	*	*
Acute poliomyelitis	*	*	*	*	*	*	*	*	*
Arthropod-borne viral encephalitis	*	*	*	*	*	*	*	*	*
Measles	*	*	*	*	*	*	*	*	*
Viral hepatitis	2.4	3.3	1.6	2.5	3.4	1.6	2.6	3.5	1.8
Human immunodeficiency virus (HIV) disease	2.7	4.0	1.4	1.5	2.4	0.5	11.1	15.2	7.4
Malaria	*	*	*	*	*	*	*	*	*
Other and unspecified infectious and parasitic diseases and their sequelae	1.9	2.0	1.8	2.0	2.0	1.9	1.8	2.0	1.7
Malignant Neoplasms	186.2	198.3	174.4	200.3	212.7	188.2	156.7	169.0	145.5
Lip, oral cavity and pharynx	2.7	3.8	1.7	2.9	4.0	1.8	2.4	3.6	1.3
Esophagus	4.7	7.5	2.0	5.2	8.4	2.1	3.4	5.2	1.8
Stomach	3.7	4.4	3.0	3.5	4.1	2.8	4.8	5.9	3.7
Colon, rectum and anus	17.0	18.0	16.1	17.9	18.8	17.0	16.7	18.0	15.4
Liver and intrahepatic bile ducts	6.6	9.0	4.2	6.5	8.8	4.3	6.7	9.9	3.8
Pancreas	11.9	12.3	11.6	12.8	13.2	12.4	10.3	10.4	10.2
Larynx	1.2	1.9	0.5	1.2	2.0	0.5	1.5	2.4	0.6
Trachea, bronchus and lung	51.3	57.8	45.0	56.1	62.3	50.0	39.7	48.7	31.4
Melanoma of skin	3.0	4.0	2.0	3.6	4.9	2.5	0.3	0.3	0.3
Breast	13.4	0.3	26.1	13.9	0.3	27.3	14.5	0.4	27.5
Cervix uteri	1.3	X	2.5	1.2	X	2.4	1.9	X	3.6
Corpus uteri and uterus, part unspecified	2.7	X	5.4	2.7	X	5.4	3.4	X	6.5
Ovary	4.7	X	9.3	5.2	X	10.4	3.0	X	5.8
Prostate	9.3	18.8	X	9.4	19.1	X	11.5	24.1	X
Kidney and renal pelvis	4.3	5.6	3.0	4.8	6.2	3.4	2.8	3.5	2.2
Bladder	4.8	6.9	2.7	5.5	7.9	3.0	2.6	3.1	2.1
Meninges, brain and other parts of central nervous system	4.6	5.3	3.9	5.2	6.0	4.5	2.1	2.3	2.0
Lymphoid, hematopoietic and related tissue	18.0	20.3	15.8	19.8	22.3	17.3	13.0	14.0	12.0
Hodgkin's disease	0.4	0.5	0.3	0.4	0.5	0.4	0.3	0.3	0.2
Non-Hodgkin's lymphoma	6.6	7.3	5.9	7.4	8.2	6.7	3.6	4.1	3.1
Leukemia	7.3	8.5	6.2	8.2	9.5	6.9	4.3	4.8	3.9
Multiple myeloma and immunoproliferative neoplasms	3.7	4.0	3.4	3.7	4.1	3.4	4.8	4.9	4.7
Other and unspecified malignant neoplasms of lymphoid, hematopoietic and related tissue	0.0	0.0	0.0	0.0	0.0	*	*	*	*
All other and unspecified malignant neoplasms	21.0	22.5	19.5	22.8	24.5	21.2	16.2	17.1	15.4
In situ neoplasms, benign neoplasms and neoplasms of uncertain or unknown behavior	4.8	5.1	4.6	5.4	5.7	5.1	2.9	2.7	3.1
Anemias	1.6	1.3	1.8	1.5	1.3	1.8	2.4	2.2	2.6
Diabetes mellitus	22.4	23.4	21.4	22.1	23.5	20.8	28.8	28.1	29.5
Nutritional deficiencies	1.0	0.8	1.2	1.0	0.8	1.2	0.9	0.7	1.1
Malnutrition	0.9	0.7	1.1	1.0	0.8	1.2	0.8	0.6	1.0
Other nutritional deficiencies	0.1	0.0	0.1	0.1	0.0	0.1	*	*	*
Meningitis	0.2	0.2	0.2	0.2	0.2	0.2	0.3	0.3	0.3
Parkinson's disease	7.1	8.5	5.8	8.5	10.0	6.9	1.9	2.2	1.6
Alzheimer's disease	27.0	16.7	37.0	31.3	19.3	43.1	12.4	7.4	17.0
Major cardiovascular diseases	252.7	252.7	252.7	271.8	269.7	273.9	220.8	226.7	215.5
Diseases of heart	193.6	202.5	184.9	209.6	217.8	201.5	164.2	174.6	154.8
Acute rheumatic fever and chronic rheumatic heart diseases	1.0	0.7	1.3	1.1	0.7	1.4	0.6	0.4	0.7
Hypertensive heart disease	10.9	10.7	11.1	10.2	9.7	10.8	18.4	20.3	16.6
Hypertensive heart and renal disease	0.9	0.8	1.0	0.8	0.7	0.9	1.8	1.9	1.7
Ischemic heart diseases	122.9	136.8	109.6	134.6	149.4	120.1	94.2	102.6	86.6
Acute myocardial infarction	39.5	44.4	34.8	43.3	48.7	37.9	30.3	32.1	28.7
Other acute ischemic heart diseases	1.4	1.4	1.3	1.4	1.5	1.4	1.3	1.5	1.2
Other forms of chronic ischemic heart disease	82.0	90.9	73.5	89.9	99.2	80.8	62.6	69.0	56.7
Atherosclerotic cardiovascular disease, so described	18.6	22.2	15.1	19.3	22.9	15.9	19.9	24.5	15.6
All other forms of chronic ischemic heart disease	63.4	68.7	58.4	70.5	76.3	64.9	42.7	44.5	41.1
Other heart diseases	57.9	53.6	62.0	62.9	57.3	68.4	49.3	49.5	49.2
Acute and subacute endocarditis	0.4	0.4	0.3	0.4	0.4	0.3	0.4	0.5	0.4
Diseases of pericardium and acute myocarditis	0.3	0.3	0.2	0.3	0.3	0.2	0.3	0.3	0.3
Heart failure	18.7	16.1	21.3	20.9	17.7	24.0	13.1	12.2	14.0
All other forms of heart disease	38.6	36.8	40.2	41.4	38.9	43.8	35.4	36.5	34.5
Essential hypertension and hypertensive renal disease	8.6	7.1	10.1	8.4	6.8	9.9	12.2	11.0	13.2
Cerebrovascular diseases	41.9	34.5	49.1	44.5	35.8	53.0	38.0	34.5	41.1
Atherosclerosis	2.3	1.9	2.7	2.7	2.2	3.1	1.4	1.3	1.5
Other diseases of circulatory system	6.2	6.6	5.8	6.7	7.2	6.4	5.1	5.3	4.9
Aortic aneurysm and dissection	3.4	4.0	2.8	3.7	4.4	3.0	2.3	2.7	1.9
Other diseases of arteries, arterioles and capillaries	2.8	2.6	3.1	3.0	2.7	3.3	2.8	2.6	2.9
Other disorders of circulatory system	1.4	1.4	1.4	1.4	1.3	1.4	1.8	1.9	1.7
Influenza and pneumonia	16.2	15.6	16.9	17.6	16.7	18.6	11.7	11.8	11.6
Influenza	0.2	0.2	0.2	0.2	0.2	0.2	0.2	0.2	0.2
Pneumonia	16.1	15.4	16.7	17.5	16.5	18.4	11.6	11.7	11.5

Table 2-14A. Death Rates for Selected Causes, by Race and Sex, 2010—*Continued*

(Rates per 100,000 population in specified group.)

Cause of death (based on ICD-10, 2004)	All races Both sexes	All races Male	All races Female	White[1] Both sexes	White[1] Male	White[1] Female	Black[1] Both sexes	Black[1] Male	Black[1] Female
Other acute lower respiratory infections	0.1	0.1	0.1	0.1	0.1	0.1	0.1	*	*
Acute bronchitis and bronchiolitis	0.1	0.0	0.1	0.1	0.1	0.1	0.0	*	*
Other and unspecified acute lower respiratory infections	0.0	0.0	*	0.0	*	*	*	*	*
Chronic lower respiratory diseases	44.7	43.1	46.3	51.8	49.1	54.5	20.7	22.5	19.0
Bronchitis, chronic and unspecified	0.2	0.2	0.2	0.2	0.2	0.3	0.1	0.1	0.1
Emphysema	3.2	3.4	3.1	3.8	3.9	3.7	1.4	1.8	1.1
Asthma	1.1	0.8	1.4	1.0	0.7	1.3	2.1	2.0	2.1
Other chronic lower respiratory diseases	40.2	38.6	41.7	46.8	44.4	49.3	17.1	18.6	15.7
Pneumoconioses and chemical effects	0.3	0.5	0.0	0.3	0.6	0.0	0.1	0.2	*
Pneumonitis due to solids and liquids	5.5	6.1	5.0	6.2	6.8	5.6	3.3	3.6	3.0
Other diseases of respiratory system	10.1	10.4	9.8	11.2	11.5	10.8	7.0	6.9	7.0
Peptic ulcer	1.0	1.0	1.0	1.0	1.0	1.1	0.7	0.9	0.6
Diseases of appendix	0.1	0.2	0.1	0.1	0.2	0.1	0.1	0.1	*
Hernia	0.6	0.5	0.6	0.7	0.6	0.7	0.4	0.4	0.4
Chronic liver disease and cirrhosis	10.3	13.7	7.1	11.4	15.1	7.8	6.3	8.5	4.2
Alcoholic liver disease	5.2	7.5	2.9	5.7	8.3	3.1	2.9	4.1	1.8
Other chronic liver disease and cirrhosis	5.2	6.2	4.2	5.7	6.8	4.7	3.3	4.4	2.3
Cholelithiasis and other disorders of gallbladder	1.1	1.0	1.1	1.2	1.1	1.2	0.7	0.6	0.8
Nephritis, nephrotic syndrome and nephrosis	16.3	16.4	16.3	16.4	16.6	16.2	21.0	20.0	22.0
Acute and rapidly progressive nephritic and nephrotic syndrome	0.1	0.1	0.1	0.1	0.1	0.1	0.1	*	*
Chronic glomerulonephritis, nephritis and nephropathy not specified as acute or chronic, and renal sclerosis unspecified	1.9	1.8	2.0	1.9	1.9	2.0	2.3	2.1	2.3
Renal failure	14.4	14.5	14.3	14.4	14.7	14.1	18.7	17.7	19.5
Other disorders of kidney	*	*	*	*	*	*	*	*	*
Infections of kidney	0.2	0.1	0.3	0.2	0.1	0.3	0.2	0.1	0.2
Hyperplasia of prostate	0.2	0.3	X	0.2	0.4	X	0.1	0.2	X
Inflammatory diseases of female pelvic organs	0.0	X	0.1	0.0	X	0.1	0.0	X	0.1
Pregnancy, childbirth and the puerperium	0.3	X	0.5	0.2	X	0.4	0.6	X	1.2
Pregnancy with abortive outcome	0.0	X	0.0	*	X	*	*	X	*
Other complications of pregnancy, childbirth and the puerperium	0.3	X	0.5	0.2	X	0.4	0.6	X	1.1
Certain conditions originating in the perinatal period	3.9	4.5	3.4	3.1	3.5	2.6	9.6	11.0	8.3
Congenital malformations, deformations and chromosomal abnormalities	3.1	3.3	3.0	3.1	3.2	3.0	3.9	4.3	3.6
Symptoms, signs and abnormal clinical and laboratory findings, not elsewhere classified	12.4	10.6	14.2	13.3	11.0	15.6	11.7	11.7	11.8
All other diseases (Residual)	87.4	72.2	102.1	95.9	78.2	113.3	67.8	59.2	75.7
Accidents (unintentional injuries)	39.1	50.0	28.6	42.8	53.8	31.9	28.7	40.2	18.2
Transport accidents	12.3	17.6	7.1	12.9	18.4	7.5	11.3	17.0	6.1
Motor vehicle accidents	11.4	16.3	6.8	12.0	17.0	7.1	10.6	15.9	5.8
Other land transport accidents	0.3	0.5	0.1	0.3	0.5	0.2	0.3	0.5	0.1
Water, air and space, and other and unspecified transport accidents and their sequelae	0.5	0.8	0.2	0.6	0.9	0.2	0.3	0.5	0.1
Nontransport accidents	26.8	32.4	21.5	29.9	35.4	24.4	17.4	23.1	12.1
Falls	8.4	8.6	8.3	9.8	9.9	9.8	2.8	3.3	2.3
Accidental discharge of firearms	0.2	0.3	0.1	0.2	0.3	0.1	0.3	0.5	*
Accidental drowning and submersion	1.2	1.9	0.5	1.2	1.9	0.6	1.4	2.4	0.4
Accidental exposure to smoke, fire and flames	0.9	1.1	0.7	0.9	1.0	0.7	1.4	1.7	1.1
Accidental poisoning and exposure to noxious substances	10.7	13.9	7.6	11.9	15.4	8.5	7.1	9.4	5.0
Other and unspecified nontransport accidents and their sequelae	5.4	6.5	4.3	5.8	6.9	4.8	4.5	5.8	3.3
Intentional Self-Harm (Suicide)	12.4	19.9	5.2	14.1	22.6	5.9	5.1	8.7	1.8
By discharge of firearms	6.3	11.2	1.5	7.3	12.9	1.8	2.6	4.8	0.5
By other and unspecified means and their sequelae	6.1	8.8	3.6	6.8	9.7	4.0	2.5	3.9	1.3
Assault (Homicide)	5.3	8.4	2.2	3.2	4.7	1.8	18.6	33.4	5.1
By discharge of firearms	3.6	6.2	1.1	1.9	2.9	0.9	14.6	27.6	2.7
By other and unspecified means and their sequelae	1.7	2.3	1.1	1.3	1.7	0.9	4.0	5.7	2.3
Legal intervention	0.1	0.3	*	0.1	0.2	*	0.2	0.5	*
Events of undetermined intent	1.6	1.9	1.3	1.7	2.0	1.4	1.4	1.9	1.0
Discharge of firearms, undetermined intent	0.1	0.1	0.0	0.1	0.1	0.0	0.1	0.1	*
Other and unspecified events of undetermined intent and their sequelae	1.5	1.8	1.2	1.6	1.9	1.3	1.3	1.8	0.9
Operations of war and their sequelae	*	*	*	*	*	*	*	*	*
Complications of medical and surgical care	0.8	0.8	0.8	0.8	0.8	0.8	1.0	0.8	1.1
Enterocolitis due to Clostridium difficile[2]	2.4	1.9	2.8	2.7	2.2	3.3	1.2	1.0	1.3
Drug-induced deaths[3,4]	13.1	16.1	10.2	14.7	17.9	11.5	8.5	11.0	6.2
Alcohol-induced deaths[3,5]	8.3	12.5	4.2	9.0	13.6	4.5	5.5	8.4	2.9
Injury by firearms[3,6]	10.3	18.0	2.7	9.6	16.5	2.8	17.7	33.4	3.3

* = Figure does not meet standards of reliability or precision.   [1]Race categories are consistent with the 1977 Office of Management and Budget (OMB) standards. Multiple-race data were reported by 37 states and the District of Columbia in 2010. The multiple-race data for these reporting areas were bridged to the single-race categories of the 1977 OMB standards for comparability with other reporting areas.   [2]Included in certain other intestinal infections (A04, A07–A09). Beginning with data year 2006, Enterocolitis due to Clostridium difficile (A04.7) is shown separately at the bottom of the table and is included in the list of rankable causes.   [3]Included in selected categories above.   [4]Includes ICD–10 codes D52.1, D59.0, D59.2, D61.1, D64.2, E06.4, E16.0, E23.1, E24.2, E27.3, E66.1, F11.1–F11.5, F11.7–F11.9, F12.1–F12.5, F12.7–F12.9, F13.1–F13.5, F13.7–F13.9, F14.1–F14.5, F14.7–F14.9, F15.1–F15.5, F15.7–F15.9, F16.1–F16.5, F16.7–F16.9, F17.3–F17.5, F17.7–F17.9, F18.1–F18.5, F18.7–F18.9, F19.1–F19.5, F19.7–F19.9, G21.1, G24.0, G25.1, G25.4, G25.6, G44.4, G62.0, G72.0, I95.2, J70.2–J70.4, K85.3, L10.5, L27.0–L27.1, M10.2, M32.0, M80.4, M81.4, M83.5, M87.1, R50.2, R78.1–R78.5, X40–X44, X60–X64, X85, and Y10–Y14. Trend data for drug-induced deaths, previously shown in this report, can be found at http://www.cdc.gov/nchs/deaths.htm.   [5]Includes ICD–10 codes E24.4, F10, G31.2, G62.1, G72.1, I42.6, K29.2, K70, K85.2, K86.0, R78.0, X45, X65, and Y15. Trend data for alcohol-induced deaths, previously shown in this report, can be found at http://www.cdc.gov/nchs/deaths.htm.   [6]Includes ICD–10 codes *U01.4, W32–W34, X72–X74, X93–X95, Y22–Y24, and Y35.0. Trend data for Injury by firearms, previously shown in this report, can be found at http://www.cdc.gov/nchs/deaths.htm.

Table 2-14B. Death Rates for Selected Causes, by Race and Sex, 2010

(Rates per 100,000 population in specified group.)

Cause of death (based on ICD-10, 2004)	American Indian or Alaska Native[1]			Asian or Pacific Islander[2]		
	Both sexes	Male	Female	Both sexes	Male	Female
All Causes	365.1	397.5	332.4	301.1	327.0	277.3
Salmonella infections	*	*	*	*	*	*
Shigellosis and amebiasis	*	*	*	*	*	
Certain other intestinal infections	1.5	1.4	1.5	0.8	0.8	0.8
Tuberculosis	*	*	*	0.6	0.7	0.4
Respiratory tuberculosis	*	*	*	0.5	0.6	0.3
Other tuberculosis	*	*	*			
Whooping cough	*	*	*	*	*	*
Scarlet fever and erysipelas	*	*	*	*	*	*
Meningococcal infection	*	*	*	*	*	*
Septicemia	5.7	4.9	6.5	3.4	3.6	3.2
Syphilis	*	*	*	*	*	*
Acute poliomyelitis	*	*	*	*	*	*
Arthropod-borne viral encephalitis	*	*	*	*	*	*
Measles	*	*	*	*	*	*
Viral hepatitis	2.3	2.9	1.7	1.8	2.1	1.5
Human immunodeficiency virus (HIV) disease	1.4	2.2	*	0.4	0.7	*
Malaria	*	*		*	*	
Other and unspecified infectious and parasitic diseases and their sequelae	1.2	1.3	1.2	1.0	1.2	0.9
Malignant Neoplasms	69.5	74.1	64.8	83.4	88.6	78.5
Lip, oral cavity and pharynx	1.0	1.2	*	1.6	2.2	1.1
Esophagus	1.5	2.3	*	1.3	2.2	0.6
Stomach	2.0	2.7	1.4	4.6	5.4	3.8
Colon, rectum and anus	6.7	7.1	6.4	8.7	9.2	8.2
Liver and intrahepatic bile ducts	4.6	6.7	2.5	7.9	11.1	4.9
Pancreas	4.2	4.5	3.8	5.7	5.4	6.0
Larynx	0.6	0.9	*	0.3	0.5	*
Trachea, bronchus and lung	18.4	20.8	16.0	18.5	22.5	14.9
Melanoma of skin	0.5	*	*	0.3	0.3	0.3
Breast	4.0	*	8.0	5.7	*	10.8
Cervix uteri	0.8	X	1.7	0.8	X	1.6
Corpus uteri and uterus, part unspecified	0.8	X	1.7	1.4	X	2.7
Ovary	1.7	X	3.4	2.2	X	4.3
Prostate	2.7	5.5	X	2.5	5.1	X
Kidney and renal pelvis	2.6	3.5	1.7	1.6	2.2	1.0
Bladder	1.1	1.4	*	1.2	1.7	0.8
Meninges, brain and other parts of central nervous system	1.7	1.8	1.7	1.9	2.1	1.7
Lymphoid, hematopoietic and related tissue	5.4	6.0	4.8	7.8	9.1	6.6
Hodgkin's disease	*	*	*	0.1	*	*
Non-Hodgkin's lymphoma	1.6	1.9	1.4	3.0	3.4	2.7
Leukemia	2.5	2.8	2.3	3.3	3.8	2.8
Multiple myeloma and immunoproliferative neoplasms	1.1	1.2	1.0	1.3	1.6	1.0
Other and unspecified malignant neoplasms of lymphoid, hematopoietic and related tissue	*	*	*	*	*	*
All other and unspecified malignant neoplasms	9.0	9.2	8.9	9.3	9.6	9.1
In situ neoplasms, benign neoplasms and neoplasms of uncertain or unknown behavior	1.4	1.5	1.3	2.1	2.1	2.0
Anemias	*	*	*	0.5	0.5	0.5
Diabetes mellitus	20.1	20.2	20.0	10.8	11.5	10.2
Nutritional deficiencies	0.7	*	0.9	0.3	0.3	0.3
Malnutrition	0.7	*	*	0.3	0.3	0.3
Other nutritional deficiencies	*	*	*	*	*	*
Meningitis	*	*	*	0.1	*	*
Parkinson's disease	1.5	1.9	1.0	2.2	2.5	1.9
Alzheimer's disease	6.2	4.2	8.3	6.4	4.2	8.3
Major cardiovascular diseases	84.5	92.0	76.9	97.9	106.0	90.4
Diseases of heart	65.5	75.0	55.9	67.6	77.0	59.0
Acute rheumatic fever and chronic rheumatic heart diseases	*	*	*	0.6	0.3	0.8
Hypertensive heart disease	4.0	4.7	3.3	4.0	4.2	3.9
Hypertensive heart and renal disease	*	*	*	0.5	0.4	0.5
Ischemic heart diseases	42.9	51.2	34.6	46.0	55.1	37.7
Acute myocardial infarction	13.9	17.1	10.7	14.9	17.7	12.3
Other acute ischemic heart diseases	0.9	1.1	*	0.3	0.4	0.3
Other forms of chronic ischemic heart disease	28.1	33.0	23.2	30.8	37.0	25.2
Atherosclerotic cardiovascular disease, so described	8.7	10.9	6.6	7.3	9.2	5.5
All other forms of chronic ischemic heart disease	19.4	22.1	16.6	23.5	27.8	19.7
Other heart diseases	17.8	18.4	17.3	16.5	17.0	16.1
Acute and subacute endocarditis	*	*	*	0.1	*	*
Diseases of pericardium and acute myocarditis	*	*	*	0.1	*	*
Heart failure	5.3	4.2	6.3	4.2	3.8	4.6
All other forms of heart disease	12.1	13.6	10.6	12.1	12.8	11.4
Essential hypertension and hypertensive renal disease	3.4	2.9	3.9	4.8	4.1	5.4
Cerebrovascular diseases	13.1	12.0	14.2	22.6	21.5	23.5
Atherosclerosis	*	*	*	0.6	0.7	0.5
Other diseases of circulatory system	2.1	1.8	2.3	2.3	2.7	1.9
Aortic aneurysm and dissection	1.1	1.2	1.0	1.6	2.0	1.3
Other diseases of arteries, arterioles and capillaries	0.9	*	1.3	0.7	0.7	0.6
Other disorders of circulatory system	0.5	*	*	0.5	0.6	0.4
Influenza and pneumonia	7.6	8.0	7.3	9.1	10.1	8.1
Influenza	*	*	*	*	*	*
Pneumonia	7.6	7.9	7.2	8.9	10.0	8.0
Other acute lower respiratory infections	*	*	*	*	*	*
Acute bronchitis and bronchiolitis	*	*	*	*	*	*
Other and unspecified acute lower respiratory infections	*	*	*	*	*	*
Chronic lower respiratory diseases	16.5	16.3	16.6	8.8	11.2	6.5
Bronchitis, chronic and unspecified	*	*	*	*	*	*
Emphysema	1.0	1.0	1.1	0.6	1.0	0.2
Asthma	0.5	*	*	0.8	0.9	0.7
Other chronic lower respiratory diseases	14.8	14.6	15.0	7.3	9.3	5.5

Table 2-14B. Death Rates for Selected Causes, by Race and Sex, 2010—*Continued*

(Rates per 100,000 population in specified group.)

Cause of death (based on ICD-10, 2004)	American Indian or Alaska Native[1]			Asian or Pacific Islander[2]		
	Both sexes	Male	Female	Both sexes	Male	Female
Pneumoconioses and chemical effects	*	*	*	*	*	*
Pneumonitis due to solids and liquids	1.9	1.9	2.0	1.8	2.2	1.5
Other diseases of respiratory system	5.6	5.3	5.9	3.8	4.1	3.6
Peptic ulcer	0.5	*	*	0.5	0.6	0.5
Diseases of appendix	*	*	*	*	*	*
Hernia	*	*	*	*	*	*
Chronic liver disease and cirrhosis	18.5	20.0	16.9	2.7	3.7	1.9
Alcoholic liver disease	13.9	16.4	11.4	1.0	1.8	0.4
Other chronic liver disease and cirrhosis	4.6	3.6	5.5	1.7	2.0	1.5
Cholelithiasis and other disorders of gallbladder	0.5	*	*	0.6	0.6	0.5
Nephritis, nephrotic syndrome and nephrosis	8.0	7.1	8.8	6.4	6.4	6.4
Acute and rapidly progressive nephritic and nephrotic syndrome	*	*	*	*	*	*
Chronic glomerulonephritis, nephritis and nephropathy not specified as acute or chronic, and renal sclerosis unspecified	1.0	0.9	1.0	0.8	0.7	0.9
Renal failure	7.0	6.2	7.7	5.6	5.7	5.4
Other disorders of kidney	*	*	*	*	*	*
Infections of kidney	*	*	*	*	*	*
Hyperplasia of prostate	*	*	X	*	*	X
Inflammatory diseases of female pelvic organs	*	X	*	*	X	*
Pregnancy, childbirth and the puerperium	*	X	*	0.2	X	0.5
Pregnancy with abortive outcome	*	X	*	*	X	*
Other complications of pregnancy, childbirth and the puerperium	*	X	*	0.2	X	0.5
Certain conditions originating in the perinatal period	2.7	3.5	1.9	2.7	3.4	2.1
Congenital malformations, deformations and chromosomal abnormalities	3.0	3.3	2.8	1.9	1.9	1.9
Symptoms, signs and abnormal clinical and laboratory findings, not elsewhere classified	5.6	6.0	5.2	3.0	3.1	2.9
All other diseases (Residual)	36.3	33.8	38.9	25.4	24.0	26.6
Accidents (unintentional injuries)	39.9	53.7	26.0	12.6	16.4	9.1
Transport accidents	16.0	21.6	10.5	5.2	6.8	3.8
Motor vehicle accidents	15.0	19.8	10.0	4.9	6.2	3.6
Other land transport accidents	0.5	*	*	0.2	0.3	*
Water, air and space, and other and unspecified transport accidents and their sequelae	0.6	*	*	0.2	0.3	*
Nontransport accidents	23.9	32.1	15.5	7.4	9.7	5.3
Falls	3.8	4.5	3.0	3.2	3.9	2.7
Accidental discharge of firearms	*	*	*	*	*	*
Accidental drowning and submersion	1.6	2.8	*	1.0	1.6	0.5
Accidental exposure to smoke, fire and flames	1.1	1.2	*	0.1	*	*
Accidental poisoning and exposure to noxious substances	12.2	15.5	8.9	1.5	2.1	0.9
Other and unspecified nontransport accidents and their sequelae	4.9	7.4	2.3	1.5	1.8	1.2
Intentional Self-Harm (Suicide)	11.0	16.1	5.9	6.2	9.3	3.4
By discharge of firearms	4.2	6.8	1.5	1.3	2.5	0.3
By other and unspecified means and their sequelae	6.8	9.2	4.4	4.9	6.8	3.2
Assault (Homicide)	6.0	9.5	2.5	1.9	2.7	1.2
By discharge of firearms	2.7	4.6	*	1.0	1.6	0.4
By other and unspecified means and their sequelae	3.4	4.9	1.8	0.9	1.0	0.8
Legal intervention	*	*	*	*	*	*
Events of undetermined intent	2.0	2.1	1.9	0.5	0.7	0.3
Discharge of firearms, undetermined intent	*	*	*	*	*	*
Other and unspecified events of undetermined intent and their sequelae	1.9	2.0	1.8	0.5	0.6	0.3
Operations of war and their sequelae	*	*	*	*	*	*
Complications of medical and surgical care	0.5	*	*	0.3	*	0.3
Enterocolitis due to Clostridium difficile[3]	0.9	0.9	*	0.6	0.5	0.6
Drug-induced deaths[4,5]	10.7	11.7	9.8	2.1	2.7	1.5
Alcohol-induced deaths[4,6]	21.8	28.5	15.1	1.6	2.6	0.6
Injury by firearms[4,7]	7.4	12.5	2.4	2.4	4.4	0.6

X = Not applicable.   0.0 = Quantity more than zero but less than 0.05.   * = Figure does not meet standards of reliability or precision.   [1]Race categories are consistent with the 1977 Office of Management and Budget (OMB) standards. Multiple-race data were reported by 37 states and the District of Columbia in 2010. The multiple-race data for these reporting areas were bridged to the single-race categories of the 1977 OMB standards for comparability with other reporting areas.   [2]Includes Chinese, Filipino, Hawaiian, Japanese, and Other Asian and Pacific Islander.   [3]Included in certain other intestinal infections (A04, A07–A09). Beginning with data year 2006, Enterocolitis due to Clostridium difficile (A04.7) is shown separately at the bottom of the table and is included in the list of rankable causes.   [4]Included in selected categories above.   [5]Includes ICD–10 codes D52.1, D59.0, D59.2, D61.1, D64.2, E06.4, E16.0, E23.1, E24.2, E27.3, E66.1, F11.1–F11.5, F11.7–F11.9, F12.1–F12.5, F12.7–F12.9, F13.1–F13.5, F13.7–F13.9, F14.1–F14.5, F14.7–F14.9, F15.1–F15.5, F15.7–F15.9, F16.1–F16.5, F16.7–F16.9, F17.3–F17.5, F17.7–F17.9, F18.1–F18.5, F18.7–F18.9, F19.1–F19.5, F19.7–F19.9, G21.1, G24.0, G25.1, G25.4, G25.6, G44.4, G62.0, G72.0, I95.2, J70.2–J70.4, K85.3, L10.5, L27.0–L27.1, M10.2, M32.0, M80.4, M81.4, M83.5, M87.1, R50.2, R78.1–R78.5, X40–X44, X60–X64, X85, and Y10–Y14. Trend data for drug-induced deaths, previously shown in this report, can be found at http://www.cdc.gov/nchs/deaths.htm.   [6]Includes ICD–10 codes E24.4, F10, G31.2, G62.1, G72.1, I42.6, K29.2, K70, K85.2, K86.0, R78.0, X45, X65, and Y15. Trend data for alcohol-induced deaths, previously shown in this report, can be found at http://www.cdc.gov/nchs/deaths.htm.   [7]Includes ICD–10 codes *U01.4, W32–W34, X72–X74, X93–X95, Y22–Y24, and Y35.0. Trend data for Injury by firearms, previously shown in this report, can be found at http://www.cdc.gov/nchs/deaths.htm.

Table 2-15A. Number of Deaths from Selected Causes, by Hispanic Origin and Sex, 2010

(Number.)

Cause of death (based on ICD–10, 2004)	All origins			Hispanic[1]			Non–Hispanic[2]		
	Both sexes	Male	Female	Both sexes	Male	Female	Both sexes	Male	Female
All Causes	2,468,435	1,232,432	1,236,003	144,490	79,622	64,868	2,318,218	1,149,438	1,168,780
Salmonella infections	28	17	11	3	-	3	25	17	8
Shigellosis and amebiasis	3	1	2	-	-	-	3	1	2
Certain other intestinal infections	10,276	4,046	6,230	603	269	334	9,657	3,770	5,887
Tuberculosis	569	351	218	98	63	35	467	285	182
Respiratory tuberculosis	423	276	147	73	52	21	347	222	125
Other tuberculosis	146	75	71	25	11	14	120	63	57
Whooping cough	26	13	13	11	5	6	15	8	7
Scarlet fever and erysipelas	3	1	2	1	1	-	2	-	2
Meningococcal infection	79	40	39	22	10	12	57	30	27
Septicemia	34,812	16,069	18,743	2,035	1,012	1,023	32,716	15,028	17,688
Syphilis	28	20	8	3	3	-	25	17	8
Acute poliomyelitis	-	-	-	-	-	-	-	-	-
Arthropod-borne viral encephalitis	9	4	5	-	-	-	9	4	5
Measles	2	2	-	1	1	-	1	1	-
Viral hepatitis	7,564	5,038	2,526	1,118	766	352	6,414	4,248	2,166
Human immunodeficiency virus (HIV) disease	8,369	6,099	2,270	1,134	910	224	7,175	5,140	2,035
Malaria	10	7	3	-	-	-	10	7	3
Other and unspecified infectious and parasitic diseases and their sequelae	5,805	2,970	2,835	441	233	208	5,353	2,732	2,621
Malignant Neoplasms	574,543	301,037	273,706	31,119	16,450	14,669	542,481	284,018	258,263
Lip, oral cavity and pharynx	8,474	5,815	2,659	412	298	114	8,035	5,497	2,538
Esophagus	14,490	11,416	3,074	592	475	117	13,870	10,919	2,951
Stomach	11,390	6,703	4,687	1,554	873	681	9,814	5,815	3,999
Colon, rectum and anus	52,622	27,284	25,338	3,179	1,782	1,397	49,358	25,455	23,903
Liver and intrahepatic bile ducts	20,305	13,658	6,647	2,331	1,584	747	17,929	12,045	5,884
Pancreas	36,888	18,699	18,189	2,142	1,046	1,096	34,694	17,620	17,074
Larynx	3,691	2,951	740	211	188	23	3,469	2,753	716
Trachea, bronchus and lung	158,318	87,740	70,578	4,953	3,046	1,907	153,042	84,519	68,523
Skin	9,154	6,002	3,152	216	125	91	8,926	5,870	3,056
Breast	41,435	439	40,996	2,312	17	2,295	39,044	421	38,623
Cervix uteri	3,939	X	3,939	476	X	476	3,456	X	3,456
Corpus uteri and uterus, part unspecified	8,402	X	8,402	528	X	528	7,853	X	7,853
Ovary	14,572	X	14,572	848	X	848	13,691	X	13,691
Prostate	28,561	28,561	X	1,535	1,535	X	26,973	26,973	X
Kidney and renal pelvis	13,219	8,436	4,783	944	588	356	12,255	7,832	4,423
Bladder	14,731	10,429	4,302	519	352	167	14,187	10,063	4,124
Meninges, brain and other parts of central nervous system	14,164	7,977	6,187	884	514	370	13,269	7,456	5,813
Lymphoid, hematopoietic and related tissue	55,590	30,777	24,813	3,634	1,968	1,666	51,881	28,760	23,121
Hodgkin's disease	1,231	714	517	133	82	51	1,095	629	466
Non-Hodgkin's lymphoma	20,294	11,047	9,247	1,327	711	616	18,937	10,314	8,623
Leukemia	22,569	12,851	9,718	1,444	785	659	21,096	12,051	9,045
Multiple myeloma and immunoproliferative neoplasms	11,428	6,117	5,311	728	388	340	10,687	5,720	4,967
Other and unspecified malignant neoplasms of lymphoid, hematopoietic and related tissue	68	48	20	2	2	-	66	46	20
All other and unspecified malignant neoplasms	64,798	34,150	30,648	3,849	2,059	1,790	60,835	32,020	28,815
In situ neoplasms, benign neoplasms and neoplasms of uncertain or unknown behavior	14,917	7,721	7,196	784	404	380	14,107	7,302	6,805
Anemias	4,852	2,017	2,835	236	117	119	4,602	1,892	2,710
Diabetes mellitus	69,071	35,490	33,581	6,556	3,372	3,184	62,357	32,027	30,330
Nutritional deficiencies	2,948	1,141	1,807	175	81	94	2,768	1,057	1,711
Malnutrition	2,790	1,079	1,711	166	78	88	2,620	999	1,621
Other nutritional deficiencies	158	62	96	9	3	6	148	58	90
Meningitis	608	303	305	71	33	38	533	266	267
Parkinson's disease	22,032	12,871	9,161	982	555	427	21,035	12,308	8,727
Alzheimer's disease	83,494	25,364	58,130	3,427	1,171	2,256	79,984	24,169	55,815
Major cardiovascular diseases	780,213	383,547	396,666	40,154	21,220	18,934	738,164	361,226	376,938
Diseases of heart	597,689	307,384	290,305	30,006	16,421	13,585	566,098	290,006	276,092
Acute rheumatic fever and chronic rheumatic heart diseases	2,987	996	1,991	154	52	102	2,830	942	1,888
Hypertensive heart disease	33,678	16,242	17,436	2,094	1,169	925	31,406	14,967	16,439
Hypertensive heart and renal disease	2,807	1,285	1,522	215	108	107	2,586	1,174	1,412
Ischemic heart diseases	379,559	207,580	171,979	20,494	11,546	8,948	357,969	195,358	162,611
Acute myocardial infarction	122,071	67,435	54,636	6,554	3,726	2,828	115,254	63,543	51,711
Other acute ischemic heart diseases	4,170	2,156	2,014	134	60	74	4,029	2,090	1,939
Other forms of chronic ischemic heart disease	253,318	137,989	115,329	13,806	7,760	6,046	238,686	129,725	108,961
Atherosclerotic cardiovascular disease, so described	57,438	33,703	23,735	3,419	2,242	1,177	53,660	31,208	22,452
All other forms of chronic ischemic heart disease	195,880	104,286	91,594	10,387	5,518	4,869	185,026	98,517	86,509
Other heart diseases	178,658	81,281	97,377	7,049	3,546	3,503	171,307	77,565	93,742
Acute and subacute endocarditis	1,103	627	476	78	47	31	1,023	579	444
Diseases of pericardium and acute myocarditis	776	405	371	57	31	26	716	372	344
Heart failure	57,757	24,385	33,372	2,024	936	1,088	55,661	23,409	32,252
All other forms of heart disease	119,022	55,864	63,158	4,890	2,532	2,358	113,907	53,205	60,702

Table 2-15A. Number of Deaths from Selected Causes, by Hispanic Origin and Sex, 2010—Continued

(Number.)

Cause of death (based on ICD–10, 2004)	All origins			Hispanic[1]			Non–Hispanic[2]		
	Both sexes	Male	Female	Both sexes	Male	Female	Both sexes	Male	Female
Essential hypertension and hypertensive renal disease	26,634	10,846	15,788	1,712	764	948	24,872	10,058	14,814
Cerebrovascular diseases	129,476	52,367	77,109	7,274	3,382	3,892	122,000	48,894	73,106
Atherosclerosis	7,230	2,933	4,297	269	127	142	6,952	2,803	4,149
Other diseases of circulatory system	19,184	10,017	9,167	893	526	367	18,242	9,465	8,777
Aortic aneurysm and dissection	10,431	6,096	4,335	438	295	143	9,966	5,781	4,185
Other diseases of arteries, arterioles and capillaries	8,753	3,921	4,832	455	231	224	8,276	3,684	4,592
Other disorders of circulatory system	4,241	2,053	2,188	259	135	124	3,964	1,908	2,056
Influenza and pneumonia	50,097	23,615	26,482	3,025	1,565	1,460	46,937	21,981	24,956
Influenza	500	250	250	92	51	41	408	199	209
Pneumonia	49,597	23,365	26,232	2,933	1,514	1,419	46,529	21,782	24,747
Other acute lower respiratory infections	213	94	119	13	8	5	200	86	114
Acute bronchitis and bronchiolitis	177	74	103	12	7	5	165	67	98
Other and unspecified acute lower respiratory infections	36	20	16	1	1	-	35	19	16
Chronic lower respiratory diseases	138,080	65,423	72,657	4,172	2,174	1,998	133,638	63,100	70,538
Bronchitis, chronic and unspecified	620	267	353	45	21	24	574	245	329
Emphysema	10,034	5,227	4,807	250	152	98	9,749	5,051	4,698
Asthma	3,404	1,283	2,121	292	120	172	3,099	1,157	1,942
Other chronic lower respiratory diseases	124,022	58,646	65,376	3,585	1,881	1,704	120,216	56,647	63,569
Pneumoconioses and chemical effects	845	812	33	23	23	-	820	787	33
Pneumonitis due to solids and liquids	17,011	9,208	7,803	691	396	295	16,300	8,796	7,504
Other diseases of respiratory system	31,187	15,791	15,396	2,021	1,013	1,008	29,107	14,737	14,370
Peptic ulcer	2,977	1,460	1,517	140	76	64	2,826	1,376	1,450
Diseases of appendix	415	258	157	28	22	6	385	234	151
Hernia	1,832	814	1,018	120	44	76	1,707	766	941
Chronic liver disease and cirrhosis	31,903	20,798	11,105	4,348	3,067	1,281	27,455	17,657	9,798
Alcoholic liver disease	15,990	11,441	4,549	2,389	1,937	452	13,540	9,458	4,082
Other chronic liver disease and cirrhosis	15,913	9,357	6,556	1,959	1,130	829	13,915	8,199	5,716
Cholelithiasis and other disorders of gallbladder	3,332	1,552	1,780	247	130	117	3,075	1,419	1,656
Nephritis, nephrotic syndrome and nephrosis	50,476	24,865	25,611	3,252	1,670	1,582	47,120	23,140	23,980
Acute and rapidly progressive nephritic and nephrotic syndrome	203	97	106	12	6	6	191	91	100
Chronic glomerulonephritis, nephritis and nephropathy not specified as acute or chronic, and renal sclerosis unspecified	5,894	2,775	3,119	326	162	164	5,552	2,603	2,949
Renal failure	44,362	21,989	22,373	2,913	1,502	1,411	41,361	20,442	20,919
Other disorders of kidney	17	4	13	1	-	1	16	4	12
Infections of kidney	608	187	421	44	12	32	562	175	387
Hyperplasia of prostate	489	489	X	28	28	X	459	459	X
Inflammatory diseases of female pelvic organs	137	X	137	12	X	12	125	X	125
Pregnancy, childbirth and the puerperium	825	X	825	146	X	146	670	X	670
Pregnancy with abortive outcome	37	X	37	8	X	8	28	X	28
Other complications of pregnancy, childbirth and the puerperium	788	X	788	138	X	138	642	X	642
Certain conditions originating in the perinatal period	12,128	6,803	5,325	2,529	1,456	1,073	9,446	5,269	4,177
Congenital malformations, deformations and chromosomal abnormalities	9,673	4,960	4,713	1,786	903	883	7,845	4,032	3,813
Symptoms, signs and abnormal clinical and laboratory findings, not elsewhere classified	38,360	16,057	22,303	2,069	1,065	1,004	36,151	14,900	21,251
All other diseases (Residual)	269,844	109,547	160,297	13,964	6,565	7,399	255,372	102,717	152,655
Accidents (unintentional injuries)	120,859	75,921	44,938	10,476	7,594	2,882	109,968	68,032	41,936
Transport accidents	37,961	26,783	11,178	4,778	3,518	1,260	33,045	23,165	9,880
Motor vehicle accidents	35,332	24,723	10,609	4,509	3,291	1,218	30,700	21,345	9,355
Other land transport accidents	1,029	794	235	169	146	23	854	642	212
Water, air and space, and other and unspecified transport accidents and their sequelae	1,600	1,266	334	100	81	19	1,491	1,178	313
Nontransport accidents	82,898	49,138	33,760	5,698	4,076	1,622	76,923	44,867	32,056
Falls	26,009	13,049	12,960	1,275	791	484	24,683	12,234	12,449
Accidental discharge of firearms	606	515	91	37	34	3	568	480	88
Accidental drowning and submersion	3,782	2,936	846	527	447	80	3,241	2,476	765
Accidental exposure to smoke, fire and flames	2,782	1,624	1,158	171	113	58	2,595	1,499	1,096
Accidental poisoning and exposure to noxious substances	33,041	21,117	11,924	2,601	1,918	683	30,292	19,086	11,206
Other and unspecified nontransport accidents and their sequelae	16,678	9,897	6,781	1,087	773	314	15,544	9,092	6,452
Intentional Self-Harm (Suicide)	38,364	30,277	8,087	2,661	2,168	493	35,562	27,994	7,568
By discharge of firearms	19,392	16,962	2,430	962	868	94	18,365	16,036	2,329
By other and unspecified means and their sequelae	18,972	13,315	5,657	1,699	1,300	399	17,197	11,958	5,239
Assault (Homicide)	16,259	12,774	3,485	2,890	2,435	455	13,252	10,238	3,014
By discharge of firearms	11,078	9,340	1,738	1,919	1,706	213	9,082	7,565	1,517
By other and unspecified means and their sequelae	5,181	3,434	1,747	971	729	242	4,170	2,673	1,497
Legal intervention	412	399	13	75	75	-	335	322	13
Events of undetermined intent	4,908	2,930	1,978	349	242	107	4,531	2,667	1,864
Discharge of firearms, undetermined intent	252	203	49	25	21	4	227	182	45
Other and unspecified events of undetermined intent and their sequelae	4,656	2,727	1,929	324	221	103	4,304	2,485	1,819
Operations of war and their sequelae	9	9	-	-	-	-	9	9	-
Complications of medical and surgical care	2,490	1,167	1,323	148	80	68	2,337	1,084	1,253
Enterocolitis due to Clostridium difficile[3]	7,298	2,889	4,409	380	158	222	6,908	2,726	4,182
Drug-induced deaths[4,5]	40,393	24,376	16,017	2,788	1,944	844	37,420	22,303	15,117
Alcohol-induced deaths[4,6]	25,692	19,038	6,654	3,326	2,759	567	22,242	16,178	6,064
Injury by firearms[4,7]	31,672	27,356	4,316	3,008	2,694	314	28,519	24,532	3,987

X = Not applicable.   – = Quantity zero.   [1]Includes races other than White and Black.   [2]Race categories are consistent with the 1977 Office of Management and Budget (OMB) standards. Multiple-race data were reported by 37 states and the District of Columbia in 2010. The multiple-race data for these reporting areas were bridged to the single-race categories of the 1977 OMB standards for comparability with other reporting areas.   [3]Included in certain other intestinal infections (A04, A07–A09). Beginning with data year 2006, Enterocolitis due to Clostridium difficile (A04.7) is shown separately at the bottom of the table and is included in the list of rankable causes.   [4]Included in selected categories above.   [5]Includes ICD–10 codes D52.1, D59.0, D59.2, D61.1, D64.2, E06.4, E16.0, E23.1, E24.2, E27.3, E66.1, F11.1–F11.5, F11.7–F11.9, F12.1–F12.5, F12.7–F12.9, F13.1–F13.5, F13.7–F13.9, F14.1–F14.5, F14.7–F14.9, F15.1–F15.5, F15.7–F15.9, F16.1–F16.5, F16.7–F16.9, F17.3–F17.5, F17.7–F17.9, F18.1–F18.5, F18.7–F18.9, F19.1–F19.5, F19.7–F19.9, G21.1, G24.0, G25.1, G25.4, G25.6, G44.4, G62.0, G72.0, I95.2, J70.2–J70.4, K85.3, L10.5, L27.0–L27.1, M10.2, M32.0, M80.4, M81.4, M83.5, M87.1, R50.2, R78.1–R78.5, X40–X44, X60–X64, X85, and Y10–Y14. Trend data for drug-induced deaths, previously shown in this report, can be found at http://www.cdc.gov/nchs/deaths.htm.   [6]Includes ICD–10 codes E24.4, F10, G31.2, G62.1, G72.1, I42.6, K29.2, K70, K85.2, K86.0, R78.0, X45, X65, and Y15. Trend data for alcohol-induced deaths, previously shown in this report, can be found at http://www.cdc.gov/nchs/deaths.htm.   [7]Includes ICD–10 codes *U01.4, W32–W34, X72–X74, X93–X95, Y22–Y24, and Y35.0. Trend data for Injury by firearms, previously shown in this report, can be found at http://www.cdc.gov/nchs/deaths.htm.

Table 2-15B. Number of Deaths from Selected Causes, by Race for Non-Hispanic Population and Sex, 2010

(Number.)

Cause of death (based on ICD-10, 2004)	Non-Hispanic White[1]			Non-Hispanic Black[1]			Origin not stated[2]		
	Both sexes	Male	Female	Both sexes	Male	Female	Both sexes	Male	Female
All Causes	1,969,916	971,601	998,312	283,438	143,824	139,614	5,727	3,372	2,355
Salmonella infections	16	14	2	5	1	4	-	-	-
Shigellosis and amebiasis	1	1	-	1	-	1	-	-	-
Certain other intestinal infections	8,661	3,323	5,338	801	357	444	16	7	9
Tuberculosis	238	135	103	119	86	33	4	3	1
Respiratory tuberculosis	165	93	72	93	74	19	3	2	1
Other tuberculosis	73	42	31	26	12	14	1	1	-
Whooping cough	13	6	7	2	2	-	-	-	-
Scarlet fever and erysipelas	1	-	1	-	-	-	-	-	-
Meningococcal infection	46	25	21	8	4	4	-	-	-
Septicemia	25,951	11,963	13,988	5,958	2,673	3,285	61	29	32
Syphilis	12	9	3	12	8	4	-	-	-
Acute poliomyelitis	-	-	-	-	-	-	-	-	-
Arthropod-borne viral encephalitis	8	3	5	-	-	-	-	-	-
Measles	-	-	-	-	-	-	-	-	-
Viral hepatitis	4,942	3,331	1,611	1,089	697	392	32	24	8
Human immunodeficiency virus (HIV) disease	2,454	2,046	408	4,598	3,000	1,598	60	49	11
Malaria	2	1	1	6	5	1	-	-	-
Other and unspecified infectious and parasitic diseases and their sequelae	4,359	2,205	2,154	771	404	367	11	5	6
Malignant Neoplasms	460,567	241,816	218,751	65,276	33,607	31,669	1043	569	474
Lip, oral cavity and pharynx	6,728	4,580	2,148	996	719	277	27	20	7
Esophagus	12,161	9,665	2,496	1,424	1,037	387	28	22	6
Stomach	6,983	4,157	2,826	1,974	1,162	812	22	15	7
Colon, rectum and anus	40,686	20,990	19,696	6,946	3,584	3,362	85	47	38
Liver and intrahepatic bile ducts	13,643	9,069	4,574	2,788	1,958	830	45	29	16
Pancreas	29,278	15,013	14,265	4,292	2,079	2,213	52	33	19
Larynx	2,793	2,219	574	605	473	132	11	10	1
Trachea, bronchus and lung	132,658	72,584	60,074	16,536	9,711	6,825	323	175	148
Melanoma of skin	8,721	5,775	2,946	134	61	73	12	7	5
Breast	31,868	333	31,535	6,063	77	5,986	79	1	78
Cervix uteri	2,506	X	2,506	776	X	776	7	X	7
Corpus uteri and uterus, part unspecified	6,162	X	6,162	1,421	X	1,421	21	X	21
Ovary	11,984	X	11,984	1,264	X	1,264	33	X	33
Prostate	21,657	21,657	X	4,801	4,801	X	53	53	X
Kidney and renal pelvis	10,713	6,882	3,831	1,175	702	473	20	16	4
Bladder	12,877	9,289	3,588	1,065	610	455	25	14	11
Meninges, brain and other parts of central nervous system	12,002	6,801	5,201	881	453	428	11	7	4
Lymphoid, hematopoietic and related tissue	44,975	25,120	19,855	5,390	2,792	2,598	75	49	26
Hodgkin's disease	952	549	403	114	60	54	3	3	-
Non-Hodgkin's lymphoma	16,873	9,192	7,681	1,488	813	675	30	22	8
Leukemia	18,654	10,744	7,910	1,794	945	849	29	15	14
Multiple myeloma and immunoproliferative neoplasms	8,441	4,596	3,845	1,986	970	1,016	13	9	4
Other and unspecified malignant neoplasms of lymphoid, hematopoietic and related tissue	55	39	16	8	4	4	-	-	-
All other and unspecified malignant neoplasms	52,172	27,682	24,490	6,745	3,388	3,357	114	71	43
In situ neoplasms, benign neoplasms and neoplasms of uncertain or unknown behavior	12,494	6,557	5,937	1,211	543	668	26	15	11
Anemias	3,503	1,404	2,099	995	442	553	14	8	6
Diabetes mellitus	47,746	25,134	22,612	11,996	5,572	6,424	158	91	67
Nutritional deficiencies	2,325	891	1,434	366	134	232	5	3	2
Malnutrition	2,190	840	1,350	356	129	227	4	2	2
Other nutritional deficiencies	135	51	84	10	5	5	1	1	-
Meningitis	369	185	184	137	63	74	4	4	-
Parkinson's disease	19,818	11,627	8,191	795	445	350	15	8	7
Alzheimer's disease	73,502	22,278	51,224	5,169	1,471	3,698	83	24	59
Major cardiovascular diseases	626,610	305,928	320,682	91,807	44,993	46,814	1,895	1,101	794
Diseases of heart	483,973	247,765	236,208	68,215	34,597	33,618	1,585	957	628
Acute rheumatic fever and chronic rheumatic heart diseases	2,493	831	1,662	228	79	149	3	2	1
Hypertensive heart disease	22,966	10,533	12,433	7,611	4,007	3,604	178	106	72
Hypertensive heart and renal disease	1,744	757	987	747	377	370	6	3	3
Ischemic heart diseases	309,492	169,637	139,855	39,047	20,282	18,765	1,096	676	420
Acute myocardial infarction	99,600	55,411	44,189	12,597	6,366	6,231	263	166	97
Other acute ischemic heart diseases	3,388	1,739	1,649	549	298	251	7	6	1
Other forms of chronic ischemic heart disease	206,504	112,487	94,017	25,901	13,618	12,283	826	504	322
Atherosclerotic cardiovascular disease, so described	43,882	25,424	18,458	8,216	4,832	3,384	359	253	106
All other forms of chronic ischemic heart disease	162,622	87,063	75,559	17,685	8,786	8,899	467	251	216
Other heart diseases	147,278	66,007	81,271	20,582	9,852	10,730	302	170	132
Acute and subacute endocarditis	810	460	350	183	100	83	2	1	1
Diseases of pericardium and acute myocarditis	563	290	273	124	64	60	3	2	1
Heart failure	49,253	20,596	28,657	5,497	2,428	3,069	72	40	32
All other forms of heart disease	96,652	44,661	51,991	14,778	7,260	7,518	225	127	98

Table 2-15B. Number of Deaths from Selected Causes, by Race for Non-Hispanic Population and Sex, 2010—*Continued*

(Number.)

Cause of death (based on ICD-10, 2004)	Non-Hispanic White[1]			Non-Hispanic Black[1]			Origin not stated[2]		
	Both sexes	Male	Female	Both sexes	Male	Female	Both sexes	Male	Female
Essential hypertension and hypertensive renal disease	18,878	7,476	11,402	5,059	2,196	2,863	50	24	26
Cerebrovascular diseases	101,849	40,040	61,809	15,833	6,890	8,943	202	91	111
Atherosclerosis	6,242	2,490	3,752	588	252	336	9	3	6
Other diseases of circulatory system	15,668	8,157	7,511	2,112	1,058	1,054	49	26	23
Aortic aneurysm and dissection	8,697	5,063	3,634	956	541	415	27	20	7
Other diseases of arteries, arterioles and capillaries	6,971	3,094	3,877	1,156	517	639	22	6	16
Other disorders of circulatory system	3,118	1,483	1,635	749	374	375	18	10	8
Influenza and pneumonia	40,244	18,657	21,587	4,854	2,340	2,514	135	69	66
Influenza	319	155	164	66	31	35	-	-	-
Pneumonia	39,925	18,502	21,423	4,788	2,309	2,479	135	69	66
Other acute lower respiratory infections	169	72	97	22	10	12	-	-	-
Acute bronchitis and bronchiolitis	135	54	81	21	9	12	-	-	-
Other and unspecified acute lower respiratory infections	34	18	16	1	1	-	-	-	-
Chronic lower respiratory diseases	122,887	57,390	65,497	8,614	4,480	4,134	270	149	121
Bronchitis, chronic and unspecified	514	212	302	48	26	22	1	1	-
Emphysema	9,021	4,594	4,427	586	358	228	35	24	11
Asthma	2,082	676	1,406	862	399	463	13	6	7
Other chronic lower respiratory diseases	111,270	51,908	59,362	7,118	3,697	3,421	221	118	103
Pneumoconioses and chemical effects	778	748	30	36	33	3	2	2	-
Pneumonitis due to solids and liquids	14,539	7,862	6,677	1,369	716	653	20	16	4
Other diseases of respiratory system	25,350	12,949	12,401	2,900	1,360	1,540	59	41	18
Peptic ulcer	2,428	1,153	1,275	290	168	122	11	8	3
Diseases of appendix	328	195	133	42	28	14	2	2	-
Hernia	1,515	671	844	162	78	84	5	4	1
Chronic liver disease and cirrhosis	23,655	15,270	8,385	2,601	1,694	907	100	74	26
Alcoholic liver disease	11,607	8,185	3,422	1,206	808	398	61	46	15
Other chronic liver disease and cirrhosis	12,048	7,085	4,963	1,395	886	509	39	28	11
Cholelithiasis and other disorders of gallbladder	2,663	1,236	1,427	296	120	176	10	3	7
Nephritis, nephrotic syndrome and nephrosis	36,963	18,503	18,460	8,769	3,984	4,785	104	55	49
Acute and rapidly progressive nephritic and nephrotic syndrome	150	70	80	32	18	14	-	-	-
Chronic glomerulonephritis, nephritis and nephropathy not specified as acute or chronic, and renal sclerosis unspecified	4,445	2,108	2,337	937	427	510	16	10	6
Renal failure	32,356	16,322	16,034	7,796	3,538	4,258	88	45	43
Other disorders of kidney	12	3	9	4	1	3	-	-	-
Infections of kidney	481	147	334	65	26	39	2	-	2
Hyperplasia of prostate	416	416	X	35	35	X	2	2	X
Inflammatory diseases of female pelvic organs	101	X	101	21	X	21	-	X	-
Pregnancy, childbirth and the puerperium	357	X	357	261	X	261	9	X	9
Pregnancy with abortive outcome	11	X	11	17	X	17	1	X	1
Other complications of pregnancy, childbirth and the puerperium	346	X	346	244	X	244	8	X	8
Certain conditions originating in the perinatal period	5,065	2,830	2,235	3,846	2,116	1,730	153	78	75
Congenital malformations, deformations and chromosomal abnormalities	5,832	2,981	2,851	1,608	850	758	42	25	17
Symptoms, signs and abnormal clinical and laboratory findings, not elsewhere classified	30,602	12,246	18,356	4,840	2,293	2,547	140	92	48
All other diseases (Residual)	221,437	88,360	133,077	28,230	11,758	16,472	508	265	243
Accidents (unintentional injuries)	94,420	57,747	36,673	11,853	7,920	3,933	415	295	120
Transport accidents	26,868	18,845	8,023	4,668	3,358	1,310	138	100	38
Motor vehicle accidents	24,898	17,318	7,580	4,398	3,146	1,252	123	87	36
Other land transport accidents	669	499	170	135	105	30	6	6	-
Water, air and space, and other and unspecified transport accidents and their sequelae	1,301	1,028	273	135	107	28	9	7	2
Nontransport accidents	67,552	38,902	28,650	7,185	4,562	2,623	277	195	82
Falls	22,842	11,178	11,664	1,147	660	487	51	24	27
Accidental discharge of firearms	439	364	75	112	100	12	1	1	-
Accidental drowning and submersion	2,462	1,838	624	551	459	92	14	13	1
Accidental exposure to smoke, fire and flames	1,956	1,130	826	569	331	238	16	12	4
Accidental poisoning and exposure to noxious substances	26,620	16,746	9,874	2,938	1,861	1,077	148	113	35
Other and unspecified nontransport accidents and their sequelae	13,233	7,646	5,587	1,868	1,151	717	47	32	15
Intentional Self-Harm (Suicide)	32,010	25,238	6,772	2,091	1,712	379	141	115	26
By discharge of firearms	16,928	14,762	2,166	1,057	946	111	65	58	7
By other and unspecified means and their sequelae	15,082	10,476	4,606	1,034	766	268	76	57	19
Assault (Homicide)	5,035	3,267	1,768	7,679	6,580	1,099	117	101	16
By discharge of firearms	2,775	1,894	881	6,051	5,460	591	77	69	8
By other and unspecified means and their sequelae	2,260	1,373	887	1,628	1,120	508	40	32	8
Legal intervention	220	212	8	97	95	2	2	2	-
Events of undetermined intent	3,783	2,194	1,589	587	377	210	28	21	7
Discharge of firearms, undetermined intent	186	151	35	32	25	7	-	-	-
Other and unspecified events of undetermined intent and their sequelae	3,597	2,043	1,554	555	352	203	28	21	7
Operations of war and their sequelae	7	7	-	1	1	-	-	-	-
Complications of medical and surgical care	1,875	888	987	398	169	229	5	3	2
Enterocolitis due to Clostridium difficile[3]	6,298	2,471	3,827	476	196	280	10	5	5
Drug-induced deaths[4,5]	33,145	19,689	13,456	3,502	2,170	1,332	185	129	56
Alcohol-induced deaths[4,6]	18,806	13,735	5,071	2,296	1,661	635	124	101	23
Injury by firearms[4,7]	20,513	17,350	3,163	7,330	6,607	723	145	130	15

X = Not applicable.   – = Quantity zero.   [1]Race categories are consistent with the 1977 Office of Management and Budget (OMB) standards. Multiple-race data were reported by 37 states and the District of Columbia in 2010. The multiple-race data for these reporting areas were bridged to the single-race categories of the 1977 OMB standards for comparability with other reporting areas.   [2]Includes deaths for which Hispanic origin was not reported on the death certificate.   [3]Included in certain other intestinal infections (A04, A07–A09). Beginning with data year 2006, Enterocolitis due to Clostridium difficile (A04.7) is shown separately at the bottom of the table and is included in the list of rankable causes.   [4]Included in selected categories above.   [5]Includes ICD–10 codes D52.1, D59.0, D59.2, D61.1, D64.2, E06.4, E16.0, E23.1, E24.2, E27.3, E66.1, F11.1–F11.5, F11.7–F11.9, F12.1–F12.5, F12.7–F12.9, F13.1–F13.5, F13.7–F13.9, F14.1–F14.5, F14.7–F14.9, F15.1–F15.5, F15.7–F15.9, F16.1–F16.5, F16.7–F16.9, F17.3–F17.5, F17.7–F17.9, F18.1–F18.5, F18.7–F18.9, F19.1–F19.5, F19.7–F19.9, G21.1, G24.0, G25.1, G25.4, G25.6, G44.4, G62.0, G72.0, I95.2, J70.2–J70.4, K85.3, L10.5, L27.0–L27.1, M10.2, M32.0, M80.4, M81.4, M83.5, M87.1, R50.2, R78.1–R78.5, X40–X44, X60–X64, X85, and Y10–Y14. Trend data for drug-induced deaths, previously shown in this report, can be found at http://www.cdc.gov/nchs/deaths.htm.   [6]Includes ICD–10 codes E24.4, F10, G31.2, G62.1, G72.1, I42.6, K29.2, K70, K85.2, K86.0, R78.0, X45, X65, and Y15. Trend data for alcohol-induced deaths, previously shown in this report, can be found at http://www.cdc.gov/nchs/deaths.htm.   [7]Includes ICD–10 codes *U01.4, W32–W34, X72–X74, X93–X95, Y22–Y24, and Y35.0. Trend data for Injury by firearms, previously shown in this report, can be found at http://www.cdc.gov/nchs/deaths.htm.

Table 2-16A. Death Rates from Selected Causes, by Hispanic Origin and Sex, 2010

(Rates per 100,000 population in specified group.)

Cause of death (based on ICD-10, 2004)	All origins[1]			Hispanic[2]			Non-Hispanic		
	Both sexes	Male	Female	Both sexes	Male	Female	Both sexes	Male	Female
All Causes	799.5	812.0	787.4	286.2	310.8	260.9	897.6	911.1	884.7
Salmonella infections	0.0	*	*	*	*	*	0.0	*	*
Shigellosis and amebiasis	*	*	*	*	*	*	*	*	*
Certain other intestinal infections	3.3	2.7	4.0	1.2	1.1	1.3	3.7	3.0	4.5
Tuberculosis	0.2	0.2	0.1	0.2	0.2	0.1	0.2	0.2	0.1
Respiratory tuberculosis	0.1	0.2	0.1	0.1	0.2	0.1	0.1	0.2	0.1
Other tuberculosis	0.0	0.0	0.0	0.0	*	*	0.0	0.0	0.0
Whooping cough	0.0	*	*	*	*	*	*	*	*
Scarlet fever and erysipelas	*	*	*	*	*	*	*	*	*
Meningococcal infection	0.0	0.0	0.0	0.0	*	*	0.0	0.0	0.0
Septicemia	11.3	10.6	11.9	4.0	4.0	4.1	12.7	11.9	13.4
Syphilis	0.0	0.0	*	*	*	*	0.0	*	*
Acute poliomyelitis	*	*	*	*	*	*	*	*	*
Arthropod-borne viral encephalitis	*	*	*	*	*	*	*	*	*
Measles	*	*	*	*	*	*	*	*	*
Viral hepatitis	2.4	3.3	1.6	2.2	3.0	1.4	2.5	3.4	1.6
Human immunodeficiency virus (HIV) disease	2.7	4.0	1.4	2.2	3.6	0.9	2.8	4.1	1.5
Malaria	*	*	*	*	*	*	*	*	*
Other and unspecified infectious and parasitic diseases and their sequelae	1.9	2.0	1.8	0.9	0.9	0.8	2.1	2.2	2.0
Malignant Neoplasms	186.2	198.3	174.4	61.6	64.2	59.0	210.1	225.1	195.7
Lip, oral cavity and pharynx	2.7	3.8	1.7	0.8	1.2	0.5	3.1	4.4	1.9
Esophagus	4.7	7.5	2.0	1.2	1.9	0.5	5.4	8.7	2.2
Stomach	3.7	4.4	3.0	3.1	3.4	2.7	3.8	4.6	3.0
Colon, rectum and anus	17.0	18.0	16.1	6.3	7.0	5.6	19.1	20.2	18.1
Liver and intrahepatic bile ducts	6.6	9.0	4.2	4.6	6.2	3.0	6.9	9.5	4.5
Pancreas	11.9	12.3	11.6	4.2	4.1	4.4	13.4	14.0	12.9
Larynx	1.2	1.9	0.5	0.4	0.7	0.1	1.3	2.2	0.5
Trachea, bronchus and lung	51.3	57.8	45.0	9.8	11.9	7.7	59.3	67.0	51.9
Melanoma of skin	3.0	4.0	2.0	0.4	0.5	0.4	3.5	4.7	2.3
Breast	13.4	0.3	26.1	4.6	*	9.2	15.1	0.3	29.2
Cervix uteri	1.3	X	2.5	0.9	X	1.9	1.3	X	2.6
Corpus uteri and uterus, part unspecified	2.7	X	5.4	1.0	X	2.1	3.0	X	5.9
Ovary	4.7	X	9.3	1.7	X	3.4	5.3	X	10.4
Prostate	9.3	18.8	X	3.0	6.0	X	10.4	21.4	X
Kidney and renal pelvis	4.3	5.6	3.0	1.9	2.3	1.4	4.7	6.2	3.3
Bladder	4.8	6.9	2.7	1.0	1.4	0.7	5.5	8.0	3.1
Meninges, brain and other parts of central nervous system	4.6	5.3	3.9	1.8	2.0	1.5	5.1	5.9	4.4
Lymphoid, hematopoietic and related tissue	18.0	20.3	15.8	7.2	7.7	6.7	20.1	22.8	17.5
Hodgkin's disease	0.4	0.5	0.3	0.3	0.3	0.2	0.4	0.5	0.4
Non-Hodgkin's lymphoma	6.6	7.3	5.9	2.6	2.8	2.5	7.3	8.2	6.5
Leukemia	7.3	8.5	6.2	2.9	3.1	2.7	8.2	9.6	6.8
Multiple myeloma and immunoproliferative neoplasms	3.7	4.0	3.4	1.4	1.5	1.4	4.1	4.5	3.8
Other and unspecified malignant neoplasms of lymphoid, hematopoietic and related tissue	0.0	0.0	0.0	*	*	*	0.0	0.0	0.0
All other and unspecified malignant neoplasms	21.0	22.5	19.5	7.6	8.0	7.2	23.6	25.4	21.8
In situ neoplasms, benign neoplasms and neoplasms of uncertain or unknown behavior	4.8	5.1	4.6	1.6	1.6	1.5	5.5	5.8	5.2
Anemias	1.6	1.3	1.8	0.5	0.5	0.5	1.8	1.5	2.1
Diabetes mellitus	22.4	23.4	21.4	13.0	13.2	12.8	24.1	25.4	23.0
Nutritional deficiencies	1.0	0.8	1.2	0.3	0.3	0.4	1.1	0.8	1.3
Malnutrition	0.9	0.7	1.1	0.3	0.3	0.4	1.0	0.8	1.2
Other nutritional deficiencies	0.1	0.0	0.1	*	*	*	0.1	0.0	0.1
Meningitis	0.2	0.2	0.2	0.1	0.1	0.2	0.2	0.2	0.2
Parkinson's disease	7.1	8.5	5.8	1.9	2.2	1.7	8.1	9.8	6.6
Alzheimer's disease	27.0	16.7	37.0	6.8	4.6	9.1	31.0	19.2	42.3
Major cardiovascular diseases	252.7	252.7	252.7	79.5	82.8	76.2	285.8	286.3	285.3
Diseases of heart	193.6	202.5	184.9	59.4	64.1	54.6	219.2	229.9	209.0
Acute rheumatic fever and chronic rheumatic heart diseases	1.0	0.7	1.3	0.3	0.2	0.4	1.1	0.7	1.4
Hypertensive heart disease	10.9	10.7	11.1	4.1	4.6	3.7	12.2	11.9	12.4
Hypertensive heart and renal disease	0.9	0.8	1.0	0.4	0.4	0.4	1.0	0.9	1.1
Ischemic heart diseases	122.9	136.8	109.6	40.6	45.1	36.0	138.6	154.8	123.1
Acute myocardial infarction	39.5	44.4	34.8	13.0	14.5	11.4	44.6	50.4	39.1
Other acute ischemic heart diseases	1.4	1.4	1.3	0.3	0.2	0.3	1.6	1.7	1.5
Other forms of chronic ischemic heart disease	82.0	90.9	73.5	27.4	30.3	24.3	92.4	102.8	82.5
Atherosclerotic cardiovascular disease, so described	18.6	22.2	15.1	6.8	8.8	4.7	20.8	24.7	17.0
All other forms of chronic ischemic heart disease	63.4	68.7	58.4	20.6	21.5	19.6	71.6	78.1	65.5
Other heart diseases	57.9	53.6	62.0	14.0	13.8	14.1	66.3	61.5	71.0
Acute and subacute endocarditis	0.4	0.4	0.3	0.2	0.2	0.1	0.4	0.5	0.3
Diseases of pericardium and acute myocarditis	0.3	0.3	0.2	0.1	0.1	0.1	0.3	0.3	0.3
Heart failure	18.7	16.1	21.3	4.0	3.7	4.4	21.6	18.6	24.4
All other forms of heart disease	38.6	36.8	40.2	9.7	9.9	9.5	44.1	42.2	45.9
Essential hypertension and hypertensive renal disease	8.6	7.1	10.1	3.4	3.0	3.8	9.6	8.0	11.2
Cerebrovascular diseases	41.9	34.5	49.1	14.4	13.2	15.7	47.2	38.8	55.3
Atherosclerosis	2.3	1.9	2.7	0.5	0.5	0.6	2.7	2.2	3.1
Other diseases of circulatory system	6.2	6.6	5.8	1.8	2.1	1.5	7.1	7.5	6.6
Aortic aneurysm and dissection	3.4	4.0	2.8	0.9	1.2	0.6	3.9	4.6	3.2
Other diseases of arteries, arterioles and capillaries	2.8	2.6	3.1	0.9	0.9	0.9	3.2	2.9	3.5
Other disorders of circulatory system	1.4	1.4	1.4	0.5	0.5	0.5	1.5	1.5	1.6
Influenza and pneumonia	16.2	15.6	16.9	6.0	6.1	5.9	18.2	17.4	18.9
Influenza	0.2	0.2	0.2	0.2	0.2	0.2	0.2	0.2	0.2
Pneumonia	16.1	15.4	16.7	5.8	5.9	5.7	18.0	17.3	18.7
Other acute lower respiratory infections	0.1	0.1	0.1	*	*	*	0.1	0.1	0.1
Acute bronchitis and bronchiolitis	0.1	0.0	0.1	*	*	*	0.1	0.1	0.1
Other and unspecified acute lower respiratory infections	0.0	0.0	*	*	*	*	0.0	*	*
Chronic lower respiratory diseases	44.7	43.1	46.3	8.3	8.5	8.0	51.7	50.0	53.4
Bronchitis, chronic and unspecified	0.2	0.2	0.2	0.1	0.1	0.1	0.2	0.2	0.2
Emphysema	3.2	3.4	3.1	0.5	0.6	0.4	3.8	4.0	3.6
Asthma	1.1	0.8	1.4	0.6	0.5	0.7	1.2	0.9	1.5
Other chronic lower respiratory diseases	40.2	38.6	41.7	7.1	7.3	6.9	46.5	44.9	48.1

Table 2-16A. Death Rates from Selected Causes, by Hispanic Origin and Sex, 2010—*Continued*

(Rates per 100,000 population in specified group.)

Cause of death (based on ICD-10, 2004)	All origins[1]			Hispanic[2]			Non-Hispanic		
	Both sexes	Male	Female	Both sexes	Male	Female	Both sexes	Male	Female
Pneumoconioses and chemical effects	0.3	0.5	0.0	0.0	0.1	*	0.3	0.6	0.0
Pneumonitis due to solids and liquids	5.5	6.1	5.0	1.4	1.5	1.2	6.3	7.0	5.7
Other diseases of respiratory system	10.1	10.4	9.8	4.0	4.0	4.1	11.3	11.7	10.9
Peptic ulcer	1.0	1.0	1.0	0.3	0.3	0.3	1.1	1.1	1.1
Diseases of appendix	0.1	0.2	0.1	0.1	0.1	*	0.1	0.2	0.1
Hernia	0.6	0.5	0.6	0.2	0.2	0.3	0.7	0.6	0.7
Chronic liver disease and cirrhosis	10.3	13.7	7.1	8.6	12.0	5.2	10.6	14.0	7.4
Alcoholic liver disease	5.2	7.5	2.9	4.7	7.6	1.8	5.2	7.5	3.1
Other chronic liver disease and cirrhosis	5.2	6.2	4.2	3.9	4.4	3.3	5.4	6.5	4.3
Cholelithiasis and other disorders of gallbladder	1.1	1.0	1.1	0.5	0.5	0.5	1.2	1.1	1.3
Nephritis, nephrotic syndrome and nephrosis	16.3	16.4	16.3	6.4	6.5	6.4	18.2	18.3	18.2
Acute and rapidly progressive nephritic and nephrotic syndrome	0.1	0.1	0.1	*	*	*	0.1	0.1	0.1
Chronic glomerulonephritis, nephritis and nephropathy not specified as acute or chronic, and renal sclerosis unspecified	1.9	1.8	2.0	0.6	0.6	0.7	2.1	2.1	2.2
Renal failure	14.4	14.5	14.3	5.8	5.9	5.7	16.0	16.2	15.8
Other disorders of kidney	*	*	*	*	*	*	*	*	*
Infections of kidney	0.2	0.1	0.3	0.1	*	0.1	0.2	0.1	0.3
Hyperplasia of prostate	0.2	0.3	X	0.1	0.1	X	0.2	0.4	X
Inflammatory diseases of female pelvic organs	0.0	X	0.1	*	X	*	0.0	X	0.1
Pregnancy, childbirth and the puerperium	0.3	X	0.5	0.3	X	0.6	0.3	X	0.5
Pregnancy with abortive outcome	0.0	X	0.0	*	X	*	0.0	X	0.0
Other complications of pregnancy, childbirth and the puerperium	0.3	X	0.5	0.3	X	0.6	0.2	X	0.5
Certain conditions originating in the perinatal period	3.9	4.5	3.4	5.0	5.7	4.3	3.7	4.2	3.2
Congenital malformations, deformations and chromosomal abnormalities	3.1	3.3	3.0	3.5	3.5	3.6	3.0	3.2	2.9
Symptoms, signs and abnormal clinical and laboratory findings, not elsewhere classified	12.4	10.6	14.2	4.1	4.2	4.0	14.0	11.8	16.1
All other diseases (Residual)	87.4	72.2	102.1	27.7	25.6	29.8	98.9	81.4	115.6
Accidents (unintentional injuries)	39.1	50.0	28.6	20.8	29.6	11.6	42.6	53.9	31.7
Transport accidents	12.3	17.6	7.1	9.5	13.7	5.1	12.8	18.4	7.5
Motor vehicle accidents	11.4	16.3	6.8	8.9	12.8	4.9	11.9	16.9	7.1
Other land transport accidents	0.3	0.5	0.1	0.3	0.6	0.1	0.3	0.5	0.2
Water, air and space, and other and unspecified transport accidents and their sequelae	0.5	0.8	0.2	0.2	0.3	*	0.6	0.9	0.2
Nontransport accidents	26.8	32.4	21.5	11.3	15.9	6.5	29.8	35.6	24.3
Falls	8.4	8.6	8.3	2.5	3.1	1.9	9.6	9.7	9.4
Accidental discharge of firearms	0.2	0.3	0.1	0.1	0.1	*	0.2	0.4	0.1
Accidental drowning and submersion	1.2	1.9	0.5	1.0	1.7	0.3	1.3	2.0	0.6
Accidental exposure to smoke, fire and flames	0.9	1.1	0.7	0.3	0.4	0.2	1.0	1.2	0.8
Accidental poisoning and exposure to noxious substances	10.7	13.9	7.6	5.2	7.5	2.7	11.7	15.1	8.5
Other and unspecified nontransport accidents and their sequelae	5.4	6.5	4.3	2.2	3.0	1.3	6.0	7.2	4.9
Intentional Self-Harm (Suicide)	12.4	19.9	5.2	5.3	8.5	2.0	13.8	22.2	5.7
By discharge of firearms	6.3	11.2	1.5	1.9	3.4	0.4	7.1	12.7	1.8
By other and unspecified means and their sequelae	6.1	8.8	3.6	3.4	5.1	1.6	6.7	9.5	4.0
Assault (Homicide)	5.3	8.4	2.2	5.7	9.5	1.8	5.1	8.1	2.3
By discharge of firearms	3.6	6.2	1.1	3.8	6.7	0.9	3.5	6.0	1.1
By other and unspecified means and their sequelae	1.7	2.3	1.1	1.9	2.8	1.0	1.6	2.1	1.1
Legal intervention	0.1	0.3	*	0.1	0.3	*	0.1	0.3	*
Events of undetermined intent	1.6	1.9	1.3	0.7	0.9	0.4	1.8	2.1	1.4
Discharge of firearms, undetermined intent	0.1	0.1	0.0	0.0	0.1	*	0.1	0.1	0.0
Other and unspecified events of undetermined intent and their sequelae	1.5	1.8	1.2	0.6	0.9	0.4	1.7	2.0	1.4
Operations of war and their sequelae	*	*	*	*	*	*	*	*	*
Complications of medical and surgical care	0.8	0.8	0.8	0.3	0.3	0.3	0.9	0.9	0.9
Enterocolitis due to Clostridium difficile[3]	2.4	1.9	2.8	0.8	0.6	0.9	2.7	2.2	3.2
Drug-induced deaths[4,5]	13.1	16.1	10.2	5.5	7.6	3.4	14.5	17.7	11.4
Alcohol-induced deaths[4,6]	8.3	12.5	4.2	6.6	10.8	2.3	8.6	12.8	4.6
Injury by firearms[4,7]	10.3	18.0	2.7	6.0	10.5	1.3	11.0	19.4	3.0

X = Not applicable. - = Quantity zero. * = Figure does not meet standards of reliability or precision. [1]Figures for origin not stated are included in "All origins" but not distributed among specified origins. [2]Includes races other than White and Black. [3]Included in certain other intestinal infections (A04, A07–A09). Beginning with data year 2006, Enterocolitis due to Clostridium difficile (A04.7) is shown separately at the bottom of the table and is included in the list of rankable causes. [4]Included in selected categories above. [5]Includes ICD–10 codes D52.1, D59.0, D59.2, D61.1, D64.2, E06.4, E16.0, E23.1, E24.2, E27.3, E66.1, F11.1–F11.5, F11.7–F11.9, F12.1–F12.5, F12.7–F12.9, F13.1–F13.5, F13.7–F13.9, F14.1–F14.5, F14.7–F14.9, F15.1–F15.5, F15.7–F15.9, F16.1–F16.5, F16.7–F16.9, F17.3–F17.5, F17.7–F17.9, F18.1–F18.5, F18.7–F18.9, F19.1–F19.5, F19.7–F19.9, G21.1, G24.0, G25.1, G25.4, G25.6, G44.4, G62.0, G72.0, I95.2, J70.2–J70.4, K85.3, L10.5, L27.0–L27.1, M10.2, M32.0, M80.4, M81.4, M83.5, M87.1, R50.2, R78.1–R78.5, X40–X44, X60–X64, X85, and Y10–Y14. Trend data for drug-induced deaths, previously shown in this report, can be found at http://www.cdc.gov/nchs/deaths.htm. [6]Includes ICD–10 codes E24.4, F10, G31.2, G62.1, G72.1, I42.6, K29.2, K70, K85.2, K86.0, R78.0, X45, X65, and Y15. Trend data for alcohol-induced deaths, previously shown in this report, can be found at http://www.cdc.gov/nchs/deaths.htm. [7]Includes ICD–10 codes *U01.4, W32–W34, X72–X74, X93–X95, Y22–Y24, and Y35.0. Trend data for Injury by firearms, previously shown in this report, can be found at http://www.cdc.gov/nchs/deaths.htm.

Table 2-16B. Death Rates from Selected Causes, by Race for Non-Hispanic Population and Sex, 2010

(Rates per 100,000 population in specified group.)

Cause of death (based on ICD-10, 2004)	Non-Hispanic White[1]			Non-Hispanic Black[1]		
	Both sexes	Male	Female	Both sexes	Male	Female
All Causes	984.3	987.5	981.2	718.7	764.5	676.9
Salmonella infections	*	*	*	*	*	*
Shigellosis and amebiasis	*	*	*	*	*	*
Certain other intestinal infections	4.3	3.4	5.2	2.0	1.9	2.2
Tuberculosis	0.1	0.1	0.1	0.3	0.5	0.2
Respiratory tuberculosis	0.1	0.1	0.1	0.2	0.4	*
Other tuberculosis	0.0	0.0	0.0	0.1	*	*
Whooping cough	*	*	*	*	*	*
Scarlet fever and erysipelas	*	*	*	*	*	*
Meningococcal infection	0.0	0.0	0.0	*	*	*
Septicemia	13.0	12.2	13.7	15.1	14.2	15.9
Syphilis	*	*	*	*	*	*
Acute poliomyelitis	*	*	*	*	*	*
Arthropod-borne viral encephalitis	*	*	*	*	*	*
Measles	*	*	*	*	*	*
Viral hepatitis	2.5	3.4	1.6	2.8	3.7	1.9
Human immunodeficiency virus (HIV) disease	1.2	2.1	0.4	11.7	15.9	7.7
Malaria	*	*	*	*	*	*
Other and unspecified infectious and parasitic diseases and their sequelae	2.2	2.2	2.1	2.0	2.1	1.8
Malignant Neoplasms	230.1	245.8	215.0	165.5	178.6	153.5
Lip, oral cavity and pharynx	3.4	4.7	2.1	2.5	3.8	1.3
Esophagus	6.1	9.8	2.5	3.6	5.5	1.9
Stomach	3.5	4.2	2.8	5.0	6.2	3.9
Colon, rectum and anus	20.3	21.3	19.4	17.6	19.1	16.3
Liver and intrahepatic bile ducts	6.8	9.2	4.5	7.1	10.4	4.0
Pancreas	14.6	15.3	14.0	10.9	11.1	10.7
Larynx	1.4	2.3	0.6	1.5	2.5	0.6
Trachea, bronchus and lung	66.3	73.8	59.0	41.9	51.6	33.1
Melanoma of skin	4.4	5.9	2.9	0.3	0.3	0.4
Breast	15.9	0.3	31.0	15.4	0.4	29.0
Cervix uteri	1.3	X	2.5	2.0	X	3.8
Corpus uteri and uterus, part unspecified	3.1	X	6.1	3.6	X	6.9
Ovary	6.0	X	11.8	3.2	X	6.1
Prostate	10.8	22.0	X	12.2	25.5	X
Kidney and renal pelvis	5.4	7.0	3.8	3.0	3.7	2.3
Bladder	6.4	9.4	3.5	2.7	3.2	2.2
Meninges, brain and other parts of central nervous system	6.0	6.9	5.1	2.2	2.4	2.1
Lymphoid, hematopoietic and related tissue	22.5	25.5	19.5	13.7	14.8	12.6
Hodgkin's disease	0.5	0.6	0.4	0.3	0.3	0.3
Non-Hodgkin's lymphoma	8.4	9.3	7.5	3.8	4.3	3.3
Leukemia	9.3	10.9	7.8	4.5	5.0	4.1
Multiple myeloma and immunoproliferative neoplasms	4.2	4.7	3.8	5.0	5.2	4.9
Other and unspecified malignant neoplasms of lymphoid, hematopoietic and related tissue	0.0	0.0	*	*	*	*
All other and unspecified malignant neoplasms	26.1	28.1	24.1	17.1	18.0	16.3
In situ neoplasms, benign neoplasms and neoplasms of uncertain or unknown behavior	6.2	6.7	5.8	3.1	2.9	3.2
Anemias	1.8	1.4	2.1	2.5	2.3	2.7
Diabetes mellitus	23.9	25.5	22.2	30.4	29.6	31.1
Nutritional deficiencies	1.2	0.9	1.4	0.9	0.7	1.1
Malnutrition	1.1	0.9	1.3	0.9	0.7	1.1
Other nutritional deficiencies	0.1	0.1	0.1	*	*	*
Meningitis	0.2	0.2	0.2	0.3	0.3	0.4
Parkinson's disease	9.9	11.8	8.1	2.0	2.4	1.7
Alzheimer's disease	36.7	22.6	50.3	13.1	7.8	17.9
Major cardiovascular diseases	313.1	310.9	315.2	232.8	239.2	227.0
Diseases of heart	241.8	251.8	232.2	173.0	183.9	163.0
Acute rheumatic fever and chronic rheumatic heart diseases	1.2	0.8	1.6	0.6	0.4	0.7
Hypertensive heart disease	11.5	10.7	12.2	19.3	21.3	17.5
Hypertensive heart and renal disease	0.9	0.8	1.0	1.9	2.0	1.8
Ischemic heart diseases	154.6	172.4	137.5	99.0	107.8	91.0
Acute myocardial infarction	49.8	56.3	43.4	31.9	33.8	30.2
Other acute ischemic heart diseases	1.7	1.8	1.6	1.4	1.6	1.2
Other forms of chronic ischemic heart disease	103.2	114.3	92.4	65.7	72.4	59.6
Atherosclerotic cardiovascular disease, so described	21.9	25.8	18.1	20.8	25.7	16.4
All other forms of chronic ischemic heart disease	81.3	88.5	74.3	44.8	46.7	43.1
Other heart diseases	73.6	67.1	79.9	52.2	52.4	52.0
Acute and subacute endocarditis	0.4	0.5	0.3	0.5	0.5	0.4
Diseases of pericardium and acute myocarditis	0.3	0.3	0.3	0.3	0.3	0.3
Heart failure	24.6	20.9	28.2	13.9	12.9	14.9
All other forms of heart disease	48.3	45.4	51.1	37.5	38.6	36.5
Essential hypertension and hypertensive renal disease	9.4	7.6	11.2	12.8	11.7	13.9
Cerebrovascular diseases	50.9	40.7	60.8	40.1	36.6	43.4
Atherosclerosis	3.1	2.5	3.7	1.5	1.3	1.6
Other diseases of circulatory system	7.8	8.3	7.4	5.4	5.6	5.1
Aortic aneurysm and dissection	4.3	5.1	3.6	2.4	2.9	2.0
Other diseases of arteries, arterioles and capillaries	3.5	3.1	3.8	2.9	2.7	3.1
Other disorders of circulatory system	1.6	1.5	1.6	1.9	2.0	1.8
Influenza and pneumonia	20.1	19.0	21.2	12.3	12.4	12.2
Influenza	0.2	0.2	0.2	0.2	0.2	0.2
Pneumonia	19.9	18.8	21.1	12.1	12.3	12.0
Other acute lower respiratory infections	0.1	0.1	0.1	0.1	*	*
Acute bronchitis and bronchiolitis	0.1	0.1	0.1	0.1	*	*
Other and unspecified acute lower respiratory infections	0.0	*	*	*	*	*
Chronic lower respiratory diseases	61.4	58.3	64.4	21.8	23.8	20.0
Bronchitis, chronic and unspecified	0.3	0.2	0.3	0.1	0.1	0.1
Emphysema	4.5	4.7	4.4	1.5	1.9	1.1
Asthma	1.0	0.7	1.4	2.2	2.1	2.2
Other chronic lower respiratory diseases	55.6	52.8	58.3	18.0	19.7	16.6

Table 2-16B. Death Rates from Selected Causes, by Race for Non-Hispanic Population and Sex, 2010—*Continued*

(Rates per 100,000 population in specified group.)

Cause of death (based on ICD-10, 2004)	Non-Hispanic White[1]			Non-Hispanic Black[1]		
	Both sexes	Male	Female	Both sexes	Male	Female
Pneumoconioses and chemical effects	0.4	0.8	0.0	0.1	0.2	*
Pneumonitis due to solids and liquids	7.3	8.0	6.6	3.5	3.8	3.2
Other diseases of respiratory system	12.7	13.2	12.2	7.4	7.2	7.5
Peptic ulcer	1.2	1.2	1.3	0.7	0.9	0.6
Diseases of appendix	0.2	0.2	0.1	0.1	0.1	*
Hernia	0.8	0.7	0.8	0.4	0.4	0.4
Chronic liver disease and cirrhosis	11.8	15.5	8.2	6.6	9.0	4.4
Alcoholic liver disease	5.8	8.3	3.4	3.1	4.3	1.9
Other chronic liver disease and cirrhosis	6.0	7.2	4.9	3.5	4.7	2.5
Cholelithiasis and other disorders of gallbladder	1.3	1.3	1.4	0.8	0.6	0.9
Nephritis, nephrotic syndrome and nephrosis	18.5	18.8	18.1	22.2	21.2	23.2
Acute and rapidly progressive nephritic and nephrotic syndrome	0.1	0.1	0.1	0.1	*	*
Chronic glomerulonephritis, nephritis and nephropathy not specified as acute or chronic, and renal sclerosis unspecified	2.2	2.1	2.3	2.4	2.3	2.5
Renal failure	16.2	16.6	15.8	19.8	18.8	20.6
Other disorders of kidney	*	*	*	*	*	*
Infections of kidney	0.2	0.1	0.3	0.2	0.1	0.2
Hyperplasia of prostate	0.2	0.4	X	0.1	0.2	X
Inflammatory diseases of female pelvic organs	0.1	X	0.1	0.1	X	0.1
Pregnancy, childbirth and the puerperium	0.2	X	0.4	0.7	X	1.3
Pregnancy with abortive outcome	*	X	*	*	X	*
Other complications of pregnancy, childbirth and the puerperium	0.2	X	0.3	0.6	X	1.2
Certain conditions originating in the perinatal period	2.5	2.9	2.2	9.8	11.2	8.4
Congenital malformations, deformations and chromosomal abnormalities	2.9	3.0	2.8	4.1	4.5	3.7
Symptoms, signs and abnormal clinical and laboratory findings, not elsewhere classified	15.3	12.4	18.0	12.3	12.2	12.3
All other diseases (Residual)	110.6	89.8	130.8	71.6	62.5	79.9
Accidents (unintentional injuries)	47.2	58.7	36.0	30.1	42.1	19.1
Transport accidents	13.4	19.2	7.9	11.8	17.9	6.4
Motor vehicle accidents	12.4	17.6	7.5	11.2	16.7	6.1
Other land transport accidents	0.3	0.5	0.2	0.3	0.6	0.1
Water, air and space, and other and unspecified transport accidents and their sequelae	0.7	1.0	0.3	0.3	0.6	0.1
Nontransport accidents	33.8	39.5	28.2	18.2	24.3	12.7
Falls	11.4	11.4	11.5	2.9	3.5	2.4
Accidental discharge of firearms	0.2	0.4	0.1	0.3	0.5	*
Accidental drowning and submersion	1.2	1.9	0.6	1.4	2.4	0.4
Accidental exposure to smoke, fire and flames	1.0	1.1	0.8	1.4	1.8	1.2
Accidental poisoning and exposure to noxious substances	13.3	17.0	9.7	7.4	9.9	5.2
Other and unspecified nontransport accidents and their sequelae	6.6	7.8	5.5	4.7	6.1	3.5
Intentional Self-Harm (Suicide)	16.0	25.7	6.7	5.3	9.1	1.8
By discharge of firearms	8.5	15.0	2.1	2.7	5.0	0.5
By other and unspecified means and their sequelae	7.5	10.6	4.5	2.6	4.1	1.3
Assault (Homicide)	2.5	3.3	1.7	19.5	35.0	5.3
By discharge of firearms	1.4	1.9	0.9	15.3	29.0	2.9
By other and unspecified means and their sequelae	1.1	1.4	0.9	4.1	6.0	2.5
Legal intervention	0.1	0.2	*	0.2	0.5	*
Events of undetermined intent	1.9	2.2	1.6	1.5	2.0	1.0
Discharge of firearms, undetermined intent	0.1	0.2	0.0	0.1	0.1	*
Other and unspecified events of undetermined intent and their sequelae	1.8	2.1	1.5	1.4	1.9	1.0
Operations of war and their sequelae	*	*	*	*	*	*
Complications of medical and surgical care	0.9	0.9	1.0	1.0	0.9	1.1
Enterocolitis due to Clostridium difficile[2]	3.1	2.5	3.8	1.2	1.0	1.4
Drug-induced deaths[3,4]	16.6	20.0	13.2	8.9	11.5	6.5
Alcohol-induced deaths[3,5]	9.4	14.0	5.0	5.8	8.8	3.1
Injury by firearms[3,6]	10.2	17.6	3.1	18.6	35.1	3.5

X = Not applicable.   - = Quantity zero.   * = Figure does not meet standards of reliability or precision.   [1]Race categories are consistent with the 1977 Office of Management and Budget (OMB) standards. Multiple-race data were reported by 37 states and the District of Columbia in 2010. The multiple-race data for these reporting areas were bridged to the single-race categories of the 1977 OMB standards for comparability with other reporting areas.   [2]Included in certain other intestinal infections (A04, A07–A09). Beginning with data year 2006, Enterocolitis due to Clostridium difficile (A04.7) is shown separately at the bottom of the table and is included in the list of rankable causes. [3]Included in selected categories above. [4]Includes ICD–10 codes D52.1, D59.0, D59.2, D61.1, D64.2, E06.4, E16.0, E23.1, E24.2, E27.3, E66.1, F11.1–F11.5, F11.7–F11.9, F12.1–F12.5, F12.7–F12.9, F13.1–F13.5, F13.7–F13.9, F14.1–F14.5, F14.7–F14.9, F15.1–F15.5, F15.7–F15.9, F16.1–F16.5, F16.7–F16.9, F17.3–F17.5, F17.7–F17.9, F18.1–F18.5, F18.7–F18.9, F19.1–F19.5, F19.7–F19.9, G21.1, G24.0, G25.1, G25.4, G25.6, G44.4, G62.0, G72.0, I95.2, J70.2–J70.4, K85.3, L10.5, L27.0–L27.1, M10.2, M32.0, M80.4, M81.4, M83.5, M87.1, R50.2, R78.1–R78.5, X40–X44, X60–X64, X85, and Y10–Y14. Trend data for drug-induced deaths, previously shown in this report, can be found at http://www.cdc.gov/nchs/deaths.htm. [5]Includes ICD–10 codes E24.4, F10, G31.2, G62.1, G72.1, I42.6, K29.2, K70, K85.2, K86.0, R78.0, X45, X65, and Y15. Trend data for alcohol-induced deaths, previously shown in this report, can be found at http://www.cdc.gov/nchs/deaths.htm. [6]Includes ICD–10 codes *U01.4, W32–W34, X72–X74, X93–X95, Y22–Y24, and Y35.0. Trend data for injury by firearms, previously shown in this report, can be found at http://www.cdc.gov/nchs/deaths.htm.

Figure 2-4. Age-Adjusted Death Rates for Selected Causes, 2010

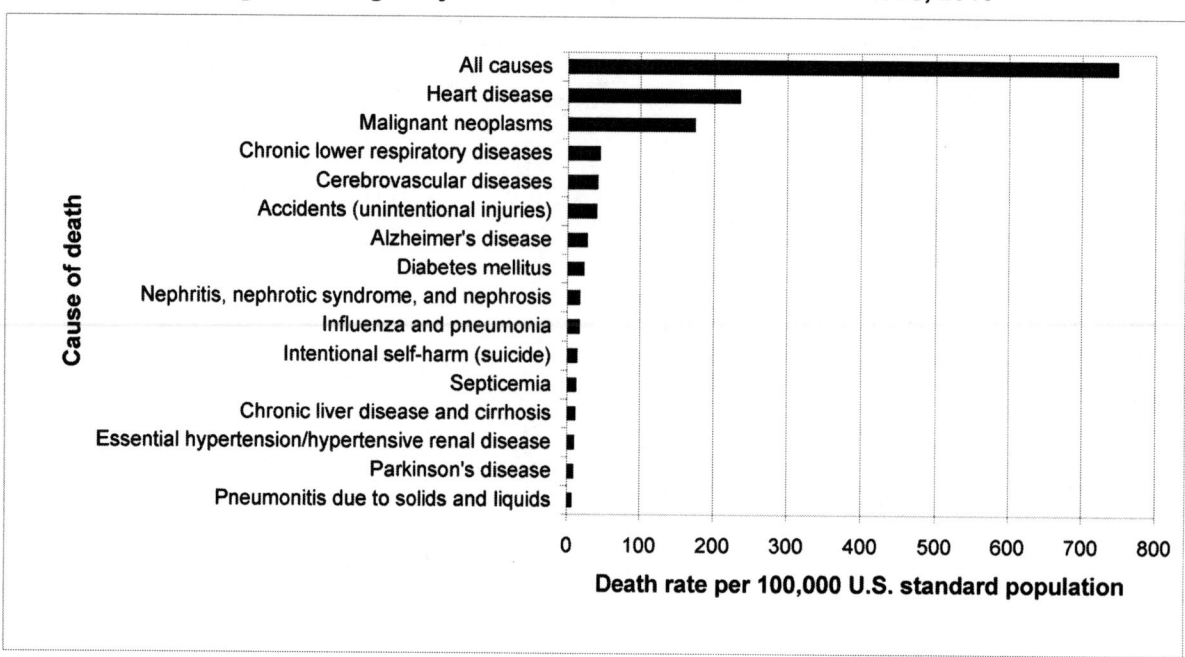

Figure 2-5. Age-Adjusted Death Rates for Injury Deaths, by Mechanism, 2010

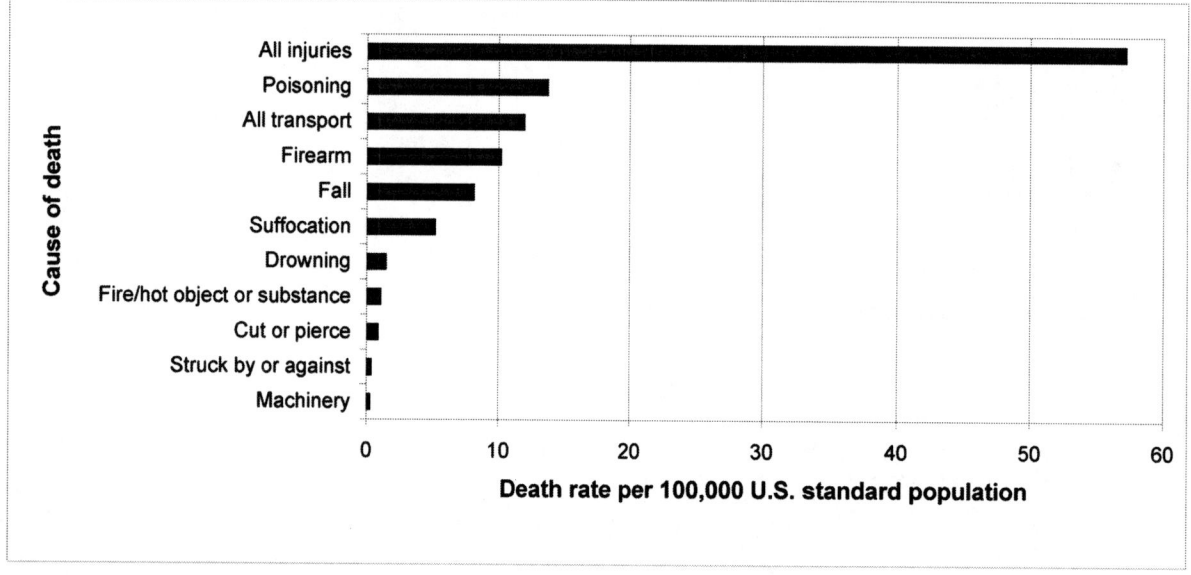

Table 2-17A. Age-Adjusted Death Rates from Selected Causes, by Race and Sex, 2010

(Age-adjusted rates per 100,000 U.S. standard population.)

Cause of death (based on ICD-10, 2004)	All races			White[1]			Black[1]		
	Both sexes	Male	Female	Both sexes	Male	Female	Both sexes	Male	Female
All Causes	747.0	887.1	634.9	741.8	878.5	630.8	898.2	1,104.0	752.5
Salmonella infections	0.0	*	*	*	*	*	*	*	*
Shigellosis and amebiasis									
Certain other intestinal infections	3.1	3.1	3.2	3.2	3.1	3.3	2.6	2.9	2.5
Tuberculosis	0.2	0.2	0.1	0.1	0.2	0.1	0.3	0.6	0.2
Respiratory tuberculosis	0.1	0.2	0.1	0.1	0.1	0.0	0.3	0.5	0.1
Other tuberculosis	0.0	0.0	0.0	0.0	0.0	0.0	0.1	*	*
Whooping cough	0.0	*	*	0.0	*	*	*	*	*
Scarlet fever and erysipelas									
Meningococcal infection	0.0	0.0	0.0	0.0	0.0	0.0	*	*	*
Septicemia	10.6	11.7	9.7	9.8	10.9	9.0	19.4	22.0	17.9
Syphilis	0.0	0.0	*	*	*	*	*	*	*
Acute poliomyelitis	*	*	*	*	*	*	*	*	*
Arthropod-borne viral encephalitis	*	*	*	*	*	*	*	*	*
Measles									
Viral hepatitis	2.1	2.9	1.4	2.1	2.9	1.3	2.8	3.9	1.9
Human immunodeficiency virus (HIV) disease	2.6	3.8	1.4	1.4	2.3	0.5	11.6	16.5	7.5
Malaria	*	*	*	*	*	*	*	*	*
Other and unspecified infectious and parasitic diseases and their sequelae	1.8	2.1	1.5	1.7	2.0	1.5	2.3	2.8	1.9
Malignant Neoplasms	172.8	209.9	146.7	172.4	208.2	146.9	203.8	264.8	167.1
Lip, oral cavity and pharynx	2.5	3.8	1.4	2.5	3.7	1.4	2.8	4.8	1.4
Esophagus	4.3	7.6	1.6	4.4	7.8	1.6	4.2	7.4	2.0
Stomach	3.4	4.6	2.5	3.0	4.0	2.2	6.3	9.3	4.4
Colon, rectum and anus	15.8	19.0	13.3	15.3	18.4	12.9	21.8	27.8	17.9
Liver and intrahepatic bile ducts	6.0	8.8	3.6	5.5	8.1	3.3	7.8	12.4	4.3
Pancreas	11.0	12.8	9.6	10.9	12.7	9.5	13.7	15.8	12.1
Larynx	1.1	2.0	0.4	1.1	1.9	0.4	1.8	3.4	0.7
Trachea, bronchus and lung	47.6	60.3	38.1	48.3	60.1	39.3	51.4	73.7	36.5
Melanoma of skin	2.8	4.1	1.7	3.2	4.7	2.0	0.4	0.5	0.4
Breast	12.4	0.3	22.1	12.0	0.3	21.5	17.8	0.6	30.3
Cervix uteri	1.2	X	2.3	1.1	X	2.1	2.2	X	3.9
Corpus uteri and uterus, part unspecified	2.5	X	4.5	2.3	X	4.2	4.5	X	7.6
Ovary	4.4	X	7.9	4.5	X	8.2	3.9	X	6.7
Prostate	8.7	21.9	X	8.1	20.2	X	17.2	48.0	X
Kidney and renal pelvis	3.9	5.7	2.5	4.1	5.9	2.6	3.6	5.2	2.6
Bladder	4.5	7.8	2.2	4.7	8.2	2.2	3.7	5.6	2.5
Meninges, brain and other parts of central nervous system	4.3	5.2	3.4	4.6	5.6	3.7	2.5	3.1	2.2
Lymphoid, hematopoietic and related tissue	17.0	22.0	13.2	17.2	22.4	13.3	17.1	21.6	14.1
Hodgkin's disease	0.4	0.5	0.3	0.4	0.5	0.3	0.3	0.4	0.3
Non-Hodgkin's lymphoma	6.2	7.9	4.9	6.4	8.1	5.1	4.6	5.9	3.7
Leukemia	6.9	9.2	5.2	7.2	9.6	5.4	5.7	7.3	4.6
Multiple myeloma and immunoproliferative neoplasms	3.4	4.3	2.8	3.2	4.1	2.6	6.5	8.0	5.6
Other and unspecified malignant neoplasms of lymphoid, hematopoietic and related tissue	0.0	0.0	0.0	0.0	0.0	*	*	*	*
All other and unspecified malignant neoplasms	19.5	23.9	16.3	19.7	24.1	16.3	20.8	25.5	17.7
In situ neoplasms, benign neoplasms and neoplasms of uncertain or unknown behavior	4.6	5.8	3.7	4.7	6.0	3.8	4.0	4.5	3.6
Anemias	1.5	1.5	1.4	1.3	1.3	1.2	3.0	3.0	2.9
Diabetes mellitus	20.8	24.9	17.6	19.0	23.1	15.6	38.7	43.6	35.1
Nutritional deficiencies	0.9	0.9	0.9	0.9	0.8	0.9	1.3	1.2	1.3
Malnutrition	0.8	0.8	0.8	0.8	0.8	0.8	1.2	1.2	1.3
Other nutritional deficiencies	0.0	0.0	0.0	0.0	0.0	0.0	*	*	*
Meningitis	0.2	0.2	0.2	0.2	0.2	0.1	0.4	0.4	0.4
Parkinson's disease	6.8	10.4	4.6	7.3	11.0	4.9	3.0	4.9	2.1
Alzheimer's disease	25.1	21.0	27.3	26.0	21.7	28.4	20.6	17.9	21.7
Major cardiovascular diseases	234.2	282.0	196.1	229.6	277.1	191.1	304.1	366.6	258.5
Diseases of heart	179.1	225.1	143.3	176.9	222.9	140.4	224.9	280.6	185.3
Acute rheumatic fever and chronic rheumatic heart diseases	0.9	0.7	1.0	0.9	0.8	1.0	0.7	0.5	0.8
Hypertensive heart disease	10.0	11.2	8.7	8.6	9.5	7.5	23.6	29.0	19.3
Hypertensive heart and renal disease	0.8	0.9	0.7	0.7	0.7	0.6	2.4	2.8	2.0
Ischemic heart diseases	113.6	151.3	84.9	113.5	151.9	83.8	131.2	169.0	104.9
Acute myocardial infarction	36.5	48.0	27.5	36.6	48.5	27.1	41.8	51.8	34.7
Other acute ischemic heart diseases	1.3	1.5	1.0	1.2	1.5	1.0	1.7	2.2	1.4
Other forms of chronic ischemic heart disease	75.9	101.8	56.4	75.7	101.9	55.7	87.6	115.0	68.8
Atherosclerotic cardiovascular disease, so described	17.0	23.1	11.8	16.3	22.2	11.3	26.0	36.6	18.4
All other forms of chronic ischemic heart disease	58.9	78.7	44.5	59.4	79.8	44.4	61.6	78.4	50.4
Other heart diseases	53.7	60.9	48.0	53.1	60.1	47.5	67.1	79.2	58.4
Acute and subacute endocarditis	0.3	0.4	0.3	0.3	0.4	0.2	0.5	0.6	0.4
Diseases of pericardium and acute myocarditis	0.2	0.3	0.2	0.2	0.2	0.2	0.3	0.4	0.3
Heart failure	17.3	19.2	15.9	17.4	19.2	16.0	19.3	22.3	17.3
All other forms of heart disease	35.9	41.0	31.6	35.2	40.1	31.0	46.9	55.9	40.4
Essential hypertension and hypertensive renal disease	8.0	8.0	7.8	7.0	7.0	6.9	17.0	18.3	15.8
Cerebrovascular diseases	39.1	39.3	38.3	37.7	37.6	37.2	53.0	56.6	49.6
Atherosclerosis	2.2	2.3	2.0	2.2	2.3	2.1	2.1	2.4	1.9
Other diseases of circulatory system	5.8	7.3	4.7	5.8	7.3	4.6	7.1	8.7	5.9
Aortic aneurysm and dissection	3.2	4.4	2.3	3.2	4.5	2.3	3.0	4.0	2.3
Other diseases of arteries, arterioles and capillaries	2.6	2.9	2.4	2.6	2.8	2.3	4.0	4.7	3.6
Other disorders of circulatory system	1.3	1.4	1.2	1.2	1.3	1.1	2.2	2.6	2.0
Influenza and pneumonia	15.1	18.2	13.1	14.9	17.8	13.0	16.8	21.3	14.1
Influenza	0.1	0.2	0.2	0.1	0.2	0.2	0.2	0.2	0.2
Pneumonia	14.9	18.0	12.9	14.7	17.6	12.8	16.7	21.1	14.0
Other acute lower respiratory infections	0.1	0.1	0.1	0.0	0.1	0.1	0.1	*	*
Acute bronchitis and bronchiolitis	0.0	0.0	0.0	0.0	0.0	0.1	0.1	*	*
Other and unspecified acute lower respiratory infections	0.0	0.0	*	0.0	0.0	*	*	*	*
Chronic lower respiratory diseases	42.2	48.7	38.0	44.6	50.6	40.8	29.0	39.8	22.8
Bronchitis, chronic and unspecified	0.2	0.2	0.2	0.2	0.2	0.2	0.1	0.2	0.1
Emphysema	3.1	3.8	2.6	3.3	4.0	2.8	2.0	3.1	1.3
Asthma	1.0	0.9	1.2	0.9	0.7	1.0	2.3	2.2	2.3
Other chronic lower respiratory diseases	37.9	43.8	34.1	40.3	45.8	36.8	24.5	34.3	19.1

Table 2-17A. Age-Adjusted Death Rates from Selected Causes, by Race and Sex, 2010—*Continued*

(Age-adjusted rates per 100,000 U.S. standard population.)

Cause of death (based on ICD-10, 2004)	All races Both sexes	All races Male	All races Female	White[1] Both sexes	White[1] Male	White[1] Female	Black[1] Both sexes	Black[1] Male	Black[1] Female
Pneumoconioses and chemical effects	0.3	0.6	0.0	0.3	0.7	0.0	0.1	0.4	*
Pneumonitis due to solids and liquids	5.1	7.3	3.8	5.2	7.4	3.9	4.9	6.9	3.7
Other diseases of respiratory system	9.5	11.7	8.0	9.7	11.9	8.1	9.2	11.0	8.2
Peptic ulcer	0.9	1.0	0.8	0.9	1.0	0.8	0.9	1.3	0.7
Diseases of appendix	0.1	0.2	0.1	0.1	0.2	0.1	0.1	0.2	*
Hernia	0.5	0.6	0.5	0.6	0.6	0.5	0.6	0.6	0.5
Chronic liver disease and cirrhosis	9.4	12.9	6.2	9.9	13.6	6.5	6.7	9.8	4.3
Alcoholic liver disease	4.7	7.0	2.6	5.0	7.4	2.8	3.1	4.5	1.9
Other chronic liver disease and cirrhosis	4.7	5.9	3.6	4.9	6.2	3.8	3.7	5.2	2.5
Cholelithiasis and other disorders of gallbladder	1.0	1.2	0.9	1.0	1.2	0.9	1.1	1.2	1.0
Nephritis, nephrotic syndrome and nephrosis	15.3	18.7	13.0	14.0	17.5	11.6	29.3	34.0	26.4
Acute and rapidly progressive nephritic and nephrotic syndrome	0.0	0.1	0.0	0.0	0.0	0.0	0.1	*	*
Chronic glomerulonephritis, nephritis and nephropathy not specified as acute or chronic, and renal sclerosis unspecified	1.8	2.2	1.5	1.6	2.0	1.4	3.3	4.0	2.9
Renal failure	13.4	16.5	11.5	12.2	15.4	10.2	25.9	29.8	23.5
Other disorders of kidney	*	*	*	*	*	*	*	*	*
Infections of kidney	0.2	0.1	0.2	0.2	0.1	0.2	0.2	0.2	0.2
Hyperplasia of prostate	0.1	0.4	X	0.1	0.4	X	0.1	0.4	X
Inflammatory diseases of female pelvic organs	0.0	X	0.1	0.0	X	0.1	0.1	X	0.1
Pregnancy, childbirth and the puerperium	0.3	X	0.6	0.2	X	0.5	0.6	X	1.2
Pregnancy with abortive outcome	0.0	X	0.0	*	X	*	*	X	*
Other complications of pregnancy, childbirth and the puerperium	0.3	X	0.5	0.2	X	0.4	0.6	X	1.2
Certain conditions originating in the perinatal period	4.2	4.7	3.8	3.5	3.8	3.1	8.3	9.0	7.6
Congenital malformations, deformations and chromosomal abnormalities	3.2	3.3	3.1	3.2	3.3	3.1	3.6	3.9	3.4
Symptoms, signs and abnormal clinical and laboratory findings, not elsewhere classified	11.7	11.9	11.1	11.5	11.6	11.0	14.9	16.5	13.4
All other diseases (Residual)	81.1	80.9	79.6	81.3	80.8	79.8	94.3	98.9	90.2
Accidents (unintentional injuries)	38.0	51.5	25.6	40.3	54.0	27.3	31.3	46.0	19.3
Transport accidents	12.1	17.6	6.9	12.5	18.1	7.2	11.6	17.9	6.1
Motor vehicle accidents	11.3	16.2	6.5	11.7	16.7	6.8	10.9	16.7	5.9
Other land transport accidents	0.3	0.5	0.1	0.3	0.5	0.2	0.3	0.6	0.2
Water, air and space, and other and unspecified transport accidents and their sequelae	0.5	0.8	0.2	0.5	0.9	0.2	0.3	0.6	0.1
Nontransport accidents	25.9	33.9	18.7	27.7	35.9	20.1	19.7	28.1	13.2
Falls	7.9	9.9	6.4	8.4	10.4	6.8	3.8	5.5	2.7
Accidental discharge of firearms	0.2	0.3	0.1	0.2	0.3	0.1	0.2	0.5	*
Accidental drowning and submersion	1.2	1.9	0.5	1.2	1.9	0.6	1.3	2.3	0.4
Accidental exposure to smoke, fire and flames	0.9	1.1	0.7	0.8	1.0	0.6	1.6	2.1	1.2
Accidental poisoning and exposure to noxious substances	10.6	13.8	7.5	11.9	15.3	8.5	7.3	10.0	5.0
Other and unspecified nontransport accidents and their sequelae	5.2	7.0	3.6	5.2	7.1	3.6	5.5	7.7	3.7
Intentional Self-Harm (Suicide)	12.1	19.8	5.0	13.6	22.0	5.6	5.2	9.1	1.8
By discharge of firearms	6.1	11.2	1.5	6.9	12.5	1.8	2.7	5.0	0.5
By other and unspecified means and their sequelae	6.0	8.7	3.5	6.7	9.5	3.9	2.6	4.0	1.3
Assault (Homicide)	5.3	8.4	2.3	3.3	4.7	1.8	17.7	31.5	5.0
By discharge of firearms	3.6	6.1	1.1	1.9	2.9	0.9	13.8	25.7	2.6
By other and unspecified means and their sequelae	1.7	2.2	1.1	1.3	1.7	0.9	3.9	5.7	2.3
Legal intervention	0.1	0.3	*	0.1	0.2	*	0.2	0.5	*
Events of undetermined intent	1.6	1.9	1.2	1.7	2.0	1.3	1.4	2.0	1.0
Discharge of firearms, undetermined intent	0.1	0.1	0.0	0.1	0.1	0.0	0.1	0.1	*
Other and unspecified events of undetermined intent and their sequelae	1.5	1.8	1.2	1.6	1.9	1.3	1.4	1.9	0.9
Operations of war and their sequelae	*	*	*	*	*	*	*	*	*
Complications of medical and surgical care	0.8	0.8	0.7	0.7	0.8	0.7	1.2	1.2	1.2
Enterocolitis due to Clostridium difficile[2]	2.2	2.3	2.2	2.3	2.3	2.3	1.7	1.9	1.6
Drug-induced deaths[3,4]	12.9	15.9	10.0	14.6	17.7	11.4	8.7	11.6	6.2
Alcohol-induced deaths[3,5]	7.6	11.7	3.9	8.0	12.2	4.0	5.9	9.6	3.0
Injury by firearms[3,6]	10.1	17.9	2.7	9.2	16.1	2.7	16.9	31.8	3.3

X = Not applicable.   0.0 = Quantity more than zero but less than 0.05.   * = Figure does not meet standards of reliability or precision.   [1]Race categories are consistent with the 1977 Office of Management and Budget (OMB) standards. Multiple-race data were reported by 37 states and the District of Columbia in 2010. The multiple-race data for these reporting areas were bridged to the single-race categories of the 1977 OMB standards for comparability with other reporting areas.   [2]Included in certain other intestinal infections (A04, A07–A09). Beginning with data year 2006, Enterocolitis due to Clostridium difficile (A04.7) is shown separately at the bottom of the table and is included in the list of rankable causes.   [3]Included in selected categories above.   [4]Includes ICD–10 codes D52.1, D59.0, D59.2, D61.1, D64.2, E06.4, E16.0, E23.1, E24.2, E27.3, E66.1, F11.1–F11.5, F11.7–F11.9, F12.1–F12.5, F12.7–F12.9, F13.1–F13.5, F13.7–F13.9, F14.1–F14.5, F14.7–F14.9, F15.1–F15.5, F15.7–F15.9, F16.1–F16.5, F16.7–F16.9, F17.3–F17.5, F17.7–F17.9, F18.1–F18.5, F18.7–F18.9, F19.1–F19.5, F19.7–F19.9, G21.1, G24.0, G25.1, G25.4, G25.6, G44.4, G62.0, G72.0, I95.2, J70.2–J70.4, K85.3, L10.5, L27.0–L27.1, M10.2, M32.0, M80.4, M81.4, M83.5, M87.1, R50.2, R78.1–R78.5, X40–X44, X60–X64, X85, and Y10–Y14. Trend data for drug-induced deaths, previously shown in this report, can be found at http://www.cdc.gov/nchs/deaths.htm.   [5]Includes ICD–10 codes E24.4, F10, G31.2, G62.1, G72.1, I42.6, K29.2, K70, K85.2, K86.0, R78.0, X45, X65, and Y15. Trend data for alcohol-induced deaths, previously shown in this report, can be found at http://www.cdc.gov/nchs/deaths.htm.   [6]Includes ICD–10 codes *U01.4, W32–W34, X72–X74, X93–X95, Y22–Y24, and Y35.0. Trend data for Injury by firearms, previously shown in this report, can be found at http://www.cdc.gov/nchs/deaths.htm.

Table 2-17B. Age-Adjusted Death Rates from Selected Causes, by Race and Sex, 2010

(Age-adjusted rates per 100,000 U.S. standard population.)

Cause of death (based on ICD-10, 2004)	American Indian or Alaska Native[1,2]			Asian or Pacific Islander[1,3]		
	Both sexes	Male	Female	Both sexes	Male	Female
All Causes	628.3	730.2	541.7	424.3	512.1	359.0
Salmonella infections	*	*	*	*	*	*
Shigellosis and amebiasis	*	*	*	*	*	*
Certain other intestinal infections	3.0	4.1	2.5	1.3	1.4	1.2
Tuberculosis	*	*	*	0.8	1.1	0.5
Respiratory tuberculosis	*	*	*	0.6	1.0	0.4
Other tuberculosis	*	*	*	*	*	*
Whooping cough	*	*	*	*	*	*
Scarlet fever and erysipelas	*	*	*	*	*	*
Meningococcal infection	*	*	*	*	*	*
Septicemia	10.5	9.8	10.7	5.0	6.2	4.2
Syphilis	*	*	*	*	*	*
Acute poliomyelitis	*	*	*	*	*	*
Arthropod-borne viral encephalitis	*	*	*	*	*	*
Measles	*	*	*	*	*	*
Viral hepatitis	2.8	3.6	1.9	2.1	2.5	1.8
Human immunodeficiency virus (HIV) disease	1.6	2.6	*	0.4	0.7	*
Malaria	*	*	*	*	*	*
Other and unspecified infectious and parasitic diseases and their sequelae	1.9	2.1	1.6	1.3	1.6	1.1
Malignant Neoplasms	122.4	151.0	102.0	108.9	131.0	93.5
Lip, oral cavity and pharynx	1.5	2.1	*	2.0	2.9	1.3
Esophagus	2.5	4.2	*	1.7	3.0	0.7
Stomach	3.5	5.1	2.3	6.1	8.3	4.6
Colon, rectum and anus	11.7	14.2	9.8	11.4	13.3	9.9
Liver and intrahepatic bile ducts	7.8	12.1	4.2	10.0	14.8	6.1
Pancreas	7.1	8.1	6.1	7.8	8.1	7.5
Larynx	1.1	2.1	*	0.4	0.8	*
Trachea, bronchus and lung	33.1	41.6	26.3	24.8	33.8	18.3
Melanoma of skin	0.8	*	*	0.4	0.4	0.4
Breast	6.4	*	11.5	6.7	*	11.9
Cervix uteri	1.2	X	2.2	1.0	X	1.7
Corpus uteri and uterus, part unspecified	1.5	X	2.7	1.7	X	3.0
Ovary	2.9	X	5.2	2.6	X	4.8
Prostate	6.1	15.3	X	3.8	9.6	X
Kidney and renal pelvis	4.7	6.9	3.0	1.9	3.0	1.2
Bladder	2.2	3.6	*	1.8	2.9	1.1
Meninges, brain and other parts of central nervous system	2.3	2.6	2.1	2.2	2.6	1.9
Lymphoid, hematopoietic and related tissue	9.9	13.2	7.8	10.3	13.5	8.0
Hodgkin's disease	*	*	*	0.2	*	*
Non-Hodgkin's lymphoma	3.1	3.6	2.6	4.1	5.1	3.4
Leukemia	4.4	6.4	3.3	4.2	5.5	3.3
Multiple myeloma and immunoproliferative neoplasms	2.2	2.8	1.8	1.8	2.6	1.3
Other and unspecified malignant neoplasms of lymphoid, hematopoietic and related tissue	*	*	*	*	*	*
All other and unspecified malignant neoplasms	16.1	18.5	14.4	12.2	13.8	11.0
In situ neoplasms, benign neoplasms and neoplasms of uncertain or unknown behavior	2.7	3.4	2.0	3.0	3.6	2.6
Anemias	*	*	*	0.7	0.8	0.6
Diabetes mellitus	36.4	39.2	34.1	15.5	18.0	13.6
Nutritional deficiencies	1.6	*	1.8	0.5	0.5	0.4
Malnutrition	1.5	*	*	0.4	0.5	0.4
Other nutritional deficiencies	*	*	*	*	*	*
Meningitis	*	*	*	0.1	*	*
Parkinson's disease	3.8	6.1	2.2	3.6	4.9	2.7
Alzheimer's disease	17.2	14.4	18.6	10.9	9.0	12.2
Major cardiovascular diseases	169.1	200.3	142.8	145.9	175.6	123.4
Diseases of heart	128.6	158.7	103.5	100.9	127.2	81.2
Acute rheumatic fever and chronic rheumatic heart diseases	*	*	*	0.8	0.5	1.0
Hypertensive heart disease	6.6	8.3	5.2	5.8	6.6	5.2
Hypertensive heart and renal disease	*	*	*	0.7	0.7	0.7
Ischemic heart diseases	84.9	109.6	64.9	68.7	91.0	52.2
Acute myocardial infarction	26.8	35.3	20.0	22.1	28.9	16.9
Other acute ischemic heart diseases	1.6	1.9	*	0.5	0.7	0.3
Other forms of chronic ischemic heart disease	56.5	72.5	43.6	46.2	61.4	34.9
Atherosclerotic cardiovascular disease, so described	15.7	21.2	11.2	10.0	13.4	7.3
All other forms of chronic ischemic heart disease	40.8	51.3	32.4	36.1	48.1	27.5
Other heart diseases	35.4	38.9	32.0	24.9	28.4	22.1
Acute and subacute endocarditis	*	*	*	0.1	*	*
Diseases of pericardium and acute myocarditis	*	*	*	0.1	*	*
Heart failure	12.7	11.8	13.1	6.7	7.1	6.4
All other forms of heart disease	21.9	26.2	18.3	17.8	20.9	15.4
Essential hypertension and hypertensive renal disease	6.9	6.6	7.1	7.5	7.6	7.5
Cerebrovascular diseases	28.1	29.8	26.5	33.2	35.2	31.4
Atherosclerosis	*	*	*	1.0	1.3	0.8
Other diseases of circulatory system	4.4	4.5	4.3	3.3	4.3	2.5
Aortic aneurysm and dissection	2.5	3.0	2.1	2.3	3.1	1.7
Other diseases of arteries, arterioles and capillaries	1.9	*	2.2	1.0	1.2	0.8
Other disorders of circulatory system	0.8	*	*	0.6	0.9	0.5
Influenza and pneumonia	15.9	19.2	13.7	14.4	19.1	11.3
Influenza	*	*	*	*	*	*
Pneumonia	15.8	19.1	13.6	14.3	18.9	11.2
Other acute lower respiratory infections	*	*	*	*	*	*
Acute bronchitis and bronchiolitis	*	*	*	*	*	*
Other and unspecified acute lower respiratory infections	*	*	*	*	*	*
Chronic lower respiratory diseases	33.8	38.8	30.3	13.9	21.0	9.1
Bronchitis, chronic and unspecified	*	*	*	*	*	*
Emphysema	1.9	2.1	1.7	0.9	1.8	0.3
Asthma	0.8	*	*	1.0	1.3	0.9
Other chronic lower respiratory diseases	31.0	35.8	27.7	11.8	17.8	7.8

Table 2-17B. Age-Adjusted Death Rates from Selected Causes, by Race and Sex, 2010—*Continued*

(Age-adjusted rates per 100,000 U.S. standard population.)

Cause of death (based on ICD-10, 2004)	American Indian or Alaska Native[1,2]			Asian or Pacific Islander[1,3]		
	Both sexes	Male	Female	Both sexes	Male	Female
Pneumoconioses and chemical effects	*	*	*	*	*	*
Pneumonitis due to solids and liquids	4.0	4.2	3.7	3.0	4.4	2.1
Other diseases of respiratory system	11.4	12.9	10.4	5.6	6.8	4.7
Peptic ulcer	1.0	*	*	0.8	1.1	0.6
Diseases of appendix	*	*	*	*	*	*
Hernia	*	*	*	*	*	*
Chronic liver disease and cirrhosis	22.8	25.5	20.3	3.2	4.4	2.2
Alcoholic liver disease	16.2	20.1	12.7	1.0	1.9	0.3
Other chronic liver disease and cirrhosis	6.6	5.5	7.6	2.2	2.5	1.9
Cholelithiasis and other disorders of gallbladder	0.8	*	*	0.9	1.1	0.7
Nephritis, nephrotic syndrome and nephrosis	16.4	16.7	16.2	9.6	11.0	8.6
Acute and rapidly progressive nephritic and nephrotic syndrome						
Chronic glomerulonephritis, nephritis and nephropathy not specified as acute or chronic, and renal sclerosis unspecified	2.3	2.7	2.1	1.2	1.2	1.3
Renal failure	14.0	14.0	14.0	8.3	9.8	7.2
Other disorders of kidney	*	*	*	*	*	*
Infections of kidney	*	*	*	*	*	*
Hyperplasia of prostate	*	*	X	*	*	X
Inflammatory diseases of female pelvic organs	*	X	*	*	X	*
Pregnancy, childbirth and the puerperium	*	X	*	0.2	X	0.4
Pregnancy with abortive outcome	*	X	*	*	X	*
Other complications of pregnancy, childbirth and the puerperium	*	X	*	0.2	X	0.4
Certain conditions originating in the perinatal period	2.1	2.7	1.5	2.9	3.3	2.4
Congenital malformations, deformations and chromosomal abnormalities	2.5	2.6	2.3	2.0	1.9	2.0
Symptoms, signs and abnormal clinical and laboratory findings, not elsewhere classified	8.1	8.6	7.4	4.3	4.8	3.9
All other diseases (Residual)	65.8	63.1	66.1	38.2	40.7	36.1
Accidents (unintentional injuries)	46.9	64.5	30.7	15.0	20.3	10.7
Transport accidents	16.9	23.0	11.0	5.5	7.2	4.0
Motor vehicle accidents	15.7	21.1	10.6	5.1	6.5	3.9
Other land transport accidents	0.5	*	*	0.2	0.3	*
Water, air and space, and other and unspecified transport accidents and their sequelae	0.6	*	*	0.2	0.4	*
Nontransport accidents	30.1	41.5	19.6	9.5	13.0	6.7
Falls	7.4	9.5	5.7	4.9	6.7	3.6
Accidental discharge of firearms	*	*	*	*	*	*
Accidental drowning and submersion	1.6	2.8	*	1.1	1.6	0.5
Accidental exposure to smoke, fire and flames	1.3	1.5	*	0.2	*	*
Accidental poisoning and exposure to noxious substances	13.0	16.8	9.3	1.4	2.1	0.8
Other and unspecified nontransport accidents and their sequelae	6.5	10.3	3.2	1.9	2.5	1.5
Intentional Self-Harm (Suicide)	10.8	15.5	6.1	6.2	9.5	3.4
By discharge of firearms	4.3	6.7	1.8	1.3	2.5	0.2
By other and unspecified means and their sequelae	6.6	8.8	4.3	4.9	7.1	3.2
Assault (Homicide)	5.7	8.8	2.5	1.8	2.6	1.2
By discharge of firearms	2.5	4.1	*	0.9	1.5	0.3
By other and unspecified means and their sequelae	3.2	4.7	1.8	0.9	1.0	0.8
Legal intervention	*	*	*	*	*	*
Events of undetermined intent	2.0	2.3	1.9	0.5	0.7	0.3
Discharge of firearms, undetermined intent	*	*	*	*	*	*
Other and unspecified events of undetermined intent and their sequelae	1.9	2.1	1.8	0.5	0.7	0.3
Operations of war and their sequelae	*	*	*	*	*	*
Complications of medical and surgical care	0.8	*	*	0.3	*	0.4
Enterocolitis due to Clostridium difficile[4]	2.0	2.8	*	0.9	1.0	0.9
Drug-induced deaths[5,6]	11.4	12.3	10.4	2.0	2.7	1.5
Alcohol-induced deaths[5,7]	25.4	34.9	16.7	1.6	2.8	0.5
Injury by firearms[5,8]	7.3	11.7	2.6	2.3	4.2	0.6

X = Not applicable.   0.0 = Quantity more than zero but less than 0.05.   * = Figure does not meet standards of reliability or precision.   [1]Race categories are consistent with the 1977 Office of Management and Budget (OMB) standards. Multiple-race data were reported by 37 states and the District of Columbia in 2010. The multiple-race data for these reporting areas were bridged to the single-race categories of the 1977 OMB standards for comparability with other reporting areas.   [2]Includes Aleuts and Eskimos.   [3]Includes Chinese, Filipinos, Hawaiians, Japanese, and other Asian and Pacific Islander persons.   [4]Included in certain other intestinal infections (A04, A07–A09). Beginning with data year 2006, Enterocolitis due to Clostridium difficile (A04.7) is shown separately at the bottom of the table and is included in the list of rankable causes.   [5]Included in selected categories above.   [6]Includes ICD–10 codes D52.1, D59.0, D59.2, D61.1, D64.2, E06.4, E16.0, E23.1, E24.2, E27.3, E66.1, F11.1–F11.5, F11.7–F11.9, F12.1–F12.5, F12.7–F12.9, F13.1–F13.5, F13.7–F13.9, F14.1–F14.5, F14.7–F14.9, F15.1–F15.5, F15.7–F15.9, F16.1–F16.5, F16.7–F16.9, F17.3–F17.5, F17.7–F17.9, F18.1–F18.5, F18.7–F18.9, F19.1–F19.5, F19.7–F19.9, G21.1, G24.0, G25.1, G25.4, G25.6, G44.4, G62.0, G72.0, I95.2, J70.2–J70.4, K85.3, L10.5, L27.0–L27.1, M10.2, M32.0, M80.4, M81.4, M83.5, M87.1, R50.2, R78.1–R78.5, X40–X44, X60–X64, X85, and Y10–Y14. Trend data for drug-induced deaths, previously shown in this report, can be found at http://www.cdc.gov/nchs/deaths.htm.   [7]Includes ICD–10 codes E24.4, F10, G31.2, G62.1, G72.1, I42.6, K29.2, K70, K85.2, K86.0, R78.0, X45, X65, and Y15. Trend data for alcohol-induced deaths, previously shown in this report, can be found at http://www.cdc.gov/nchs/deaths.htm.   [8]Includes ICD–10 codes *U01.4, W32–W34, X72–X74, X93–X95, Y22–Y24, and Y35.0. Trend data for Injury by firearms, previously shown in this report, can be found at http://www.cdc.gov/nchs/deaths.htm.

Table 2-18A. Age-Adjusted Death Rates from Selected Causes, by Hispanic Origin and Sex, 2010

(Age-adjusted rates per 100,000 U.S. standard population.)

Cause of death (based on ICD-10, 2004)	All origins[1]			Hispanic (of any race)			Non-Hispanic[2]		
	Both sexes	Male	Female	Both sexes	Male	Female	Both sexes	Male	Female
All Causes	747.0	887.1	634.9	558.6	677.7	463.4	762.6	904.6	649.2
Salmonella infections	0.0	*	*	*	*	*	0.0	*	*
Shigellosis and amebiasis	*	*	*	*	*	*	*	*	*
Certain other intestinal infections	3.1	3.1	3.2	2.5	2.6	2.5	3.2	3.1	3.2
Tuberculosis	0.2	0.2	0.1	0.3	0.5	0.2	0.2	0.2	0.1
Respiratory tuberculosis	0.1	0.2	0.1	0.3	0.4	0.1	0.1	0.2	0.1
Other tuberculosis	0.0	0.0	0.0	0.1	*	*	0.0	0.0	0.0
Whooping cough	0.0	*	*	*	*	*	*	*	*
Scarlet fever and erysipelas	*	*	*	*	*	*	*	*	*
Meningococcal infection	0.0	0.0	0.0	0.0	*	*	0.0	0.0	0.0
Septicemia	10.6	11.7	9.7	8.3	9.3	7.4	10.7	11.8	10.0
Syphilis	0.0	0.0	*	*	*	*	0.0	*	*
Acute poliomyelitis	*	*	*	*	*	*	*	*	*
Arthropod-borne viral encephalitis	*	*	*	*	*	*	*	*	*
Measles	*	*	*	*	*	*	*	*	*
Viral hepatitis	2.1	2.9	1.4	3.3	4.6	2.1	2.0	2.8	1.3
Human immunodeficiency virus (HIV) disease	2.6	3.8	1.4	2.8	4.6	1.1	2.6	3.8	1.5
Malaria	*	*	*	*	*	*	*	*	*
Other and unspecified infectious and parasitic diseases and their sequelae	1.8	2.1	1.5	1.5	1.6	1.3	1.8	2.1	1.6
Malignant Neoplasms	172.8	209.9	146.7	119.7	149.4	99.4	177.1	214.6	150.7
Lip, oral cavity and pharynx	2.5	3.8	1.4	1.5	2.4	0.8	2.6	3.9	1.5
Esophagus	4.3	7.6	1.6	2.3	4.1	0.8	4.5	7.9	1.7
Stomach	3.4	4.6	2.5	5.8	7.6	4.4	3.2	4.4	2.3
Colon, rectum and anus	15.8	19.0	13.3	12.3	15.9	9.7	16.1	19.2	13.6
Liver and intrahepatic bile ducts	6.0	8.8	3.6	8.8	12.9	5.4	5.7	8.5	3.4
Pancreas	11.0	12.8	9.6	8.6	9.4	8.0	11.2	13.0	9.8
Larynx	1.1	2.0	0.4	0.8	1.8	0.2	1.1	2.0	0.4
Trachea, bronchus and lung	47.6	60.3	38.1	20.4	29.6	13.8	49.9	62.8	40.2
Melanoma of skin	2.8	4.1	1.7	0.8	1.0	0.6	2.9	4.4	1.8
Breast	12.4	0.3	22.1	8.0	*	14.4	12.7	0.3	22.8
Cervix uteri	1.2	X	2.3	1.4	X	2.6	1.2	X	2.2
Corpus uteri and uterus, part unspecified	2.5	X	4.5	1.9	X	3.4	2.5	X	4.5
Ovary	4.4	X	7.9	3.1	X	5.6	4.4	X	8.0
Prostate	8.7	21.9	X	7.3	18.4	X	8.8	22.1	X
Kidney and renal pelvis	3.9	5.7	2.5	3.6	5.0	2.5	4.0	5.8	2.6
Bladder	4.5	7.8	2.2	2.3	3.8	1.3	4.6	8.1	2.3
Meninges, brain and other parts of central nervous system	4.3	5.2	3.4	2.8	3.5	2.3	4.4	5.4	3.6
Lymphoid, hematopoietic and related tissue	17.0	22.0	13.2	13.5	16.5	11.2	17.2	22.3	13.3
Hodgkin's disease	0.4	0.5	0.3	0.4	0.5	0.3	0.4	0.5	0.3
Non-Hodgkin's lymphoma	6.2	7.9	4.9	5.2	6.2	4.5	6.2	8.0	4.9
Leukemia	6.9	9.2	5.2	4.9	6.0	4.0	7.0	9.4	5.3
Multiple myeloma and immunoproliferative neoplasms	3.4	4.3	2.8	3.0	3.7	2.4	3.5	4.4	2.8
Other and unspecified malignant neoplasms of lymphoid, hematopoietic and related tissue	0.0	0.0	0.0	*	*	*	0.0	0.0	0.0
All other and unspecified malignant neoplasms	19.5	23.9	16.3	14.5	17.3	12.3	20.0	24.4	16.6
In situ neoplasms, benign neoplasms and neoplasms of uncertain or unknown behavior	4.6	5.8	3.7	3.2	4.0	2.7	4.7	5.9	3.8
Anemias	1.5	1.5	1.4	1.0	1.1	0.8	1.5	1.6	1.5
Diabetes mellitus	20.8	24.9	17.6	27.1	31.2	23.7	20.4	24.4	17.2
Nutritional deficiencies	0.9	0.9	0.9	0.8	0.9	0.8	0.9	0.9	0.9
Malnutrition	0.8	0.8	0.8	0.8	0.9	0.7	0.8	0.8	0.8
Other nutritional deficiencies	0.0	0.0	0.0	*	*	*	0.0	0.0	0.0
Meningitis	0.2	0.2	0.2	0.2	0.2	0.2	0.2	0.2	0.2
Parkinson's disease	6.8	10.4	4.6	5.1	7.2	3.7	7.0	10.6	4.7
Alzheimer's disease	25.1	21.0	27.3	18.5	16.6	19.5	25.5	21.3	27.8
Major cardiovascular diseases	234.2	282.0	196.1	177.9	213.8	149.6	238.3	287.1	199.3
Diseases of heart	179.1	225.1	143.3	132.8	165.1	107.8	182.6	229.6	145.8
Acute rheumatic fever and chronic rheumatic heart diseases	0.9	0.7	1.0	0.6	0.4	0.8	0.9	0.7	1.1
Hypertensive heart disease	10.0	11.2	8.7	8.5	10.1	7.1	10.1	11.3	8.8
Hypertensive heart and renal disease	0.8	0.9	0.7	0.9	1.0	0.8	0.8	0.9	0.7
Ischemic heart diseases	113.6	161.2	93.0	90.0	111.5	72.0	125.0	164.9	94.4
Acute myocardial infarction	36.5	151.3	84.9	92.3	119.0	72.0	115.2	153.7	85.8
Other acute ischemic heart diseases	1.3	48.0	27.5	28.8	37.2	22.3	37.2	48.9	27.9
Other forms of chronic ischemic heart disease	75.9	1.5	1.0	0.6	0.5	0.6	1.3	1.6	1.0
Atherosclerotic cardiovascular disease, so described	17.0	101.8	56.4	62.9	81.2	49.1	76.7	103.2	56.8
All other forms of chronic ischemic heart disease		23.1	11.8	13.8	19.6	9.1	17.2	23.3	12.0
Other heart diseases	58.9	78.7	44.5	49.1	61.6	39.9	59.5	79.9	44.8
Acute and subacute endocarditis	53.7	60.9	48.0	30.5	34.6	27.1	55.5	62.9	49.5
Diseases of pericardium and acute myocarditis	0.3	0.4	0.3	0.3	0.3	0.2	0.4	0.4	0.3
Heart failure	0.2	0.3	0.2	0.1	0.2	0.1	0.2	0.3	0.2
All other forms of heart disease	17.3	19.2	15.9	10.0	11.4	9.0	17.7	19.7	16.3
Essential hypertension and hypertensive renal disease	35.9	41.0	31.6	20.1	22.7	17.8	37.1	42.5	32.7
Cerebrovascular diseases	8.0	8.0	7.8	7.8	8.1	7.5	8.0	8.0	7.8
Atherosclerosis	39.1	39.3	38.3	32.1	33.9	30.2	39.6	39.6	38.9
Other diseases of circulatory system	2.2	2.3	2.0	1.3	1.6	1.2	2.2	2.4	2.1
Aortic aneurysm and dissection	5.8	7.3	4.7	3.8	5.1	2.9	6.0	7.5	4.8
Other diseases of arteries, arterioles and capillaries	3.2	4.4	2.3	1.8	2.6	1.1	3.3	4.5	2.3
Other disorders of circulatory system	2.6	2.9	2.4	2.1	2.5	1.7	2.7	2.9	2.5
Influenza and pneumonia	1.3	1.4	1.2	0.9	1.0	0.8	1.3	1.4	1.2
Influenza	15.1	18.2	13.1	13.7	17.0	11.4	15.2	18.3	13.2
Pneumonia	0.1	0.2	0.2	0.2	0.3	0.2	0.1	0.1	0.1
Other acute lower respiratory infections	14.9	18.0	12.9	13.4	16.7	11.2	15.1	18.1	13.0
Acute bronchitis and bronchiolitis	0.1	0.1	0.1	*	*	*	0.1	0.1	0.1
Other and unspecified acute lower respiratory infections	0.0	0.0	0.0	*	*	*	0.0	0.0	0.0
Chronic lower respiratory diseases	0.0	0.0		*	*	*	0.0		
Bronchitis, chronic and unspecified	42.2	48.7	38.0	19.6	25.2	15.9	43.9	50.4	39.7
Emphysema	0.2	0.2	0.2	0.2	0.2	0.1	0.2	0.2	0.2
Asthma	3.1	3.8	2.6	1.1	1.7	0.8	3.2	3.9	2.7
Other chronic lower respiratory diseases	1.0	0.9	1.2	0.9	0.7	1.1	1.1	0.9	1.2

Table 2-18A. Age-Adjusted Death Rates from Selected Causes, by Hispanic Origin and Sex, 2010—*Continued*

(Age-adjusted rates per 100,000 U.S. standard population.)

Cause of death (based on ICD-10, 2004)	All origins[1]			Hispanic (of any race)[2]			Non-Hispanic[3]		
	Both sexes	Male	Female	Both sexes	Male	Female	Both sexes	Male	Female
Pneumoconioses and chemical effects	37.9	43.8	34.1	17.3	22.5	13.9	39.4	45.3	35.6
Pneumonitis due to solids and liquids	5.1	7.3	3.8	3.3	4.7	2.4	5.3	7.4	3.9
Other diseases of respiratory system	9.5	11.7	8.0	8.5	9.8	7.5	9.6	11.8	8.1
Peptic ulcer	0.9	1.0	0.8	0.6	0.7	0.5	0.9	1.1	0.8
Diseases of appendix	0.1	0.2	0.1	0.1	0.1	*	0.1	0.2	0.1
Hernia	0.5	0.6	0.5	0.5	0.4	0.6	0.6	0.6	0.5
Chronic liver disease and cirrhosis	9.4	12.9	6.2	13.7	19.8	8.2	9.0	12.2	6.1
Alcoholic liver disease	4.7	7.0	2.6	6.8	11.7	2.4	4.5	6.5	2.7
Other chronic liver disease and cirrhosis	4.7	5.9	3.6	6.9	8.1	5.7	4.5	5.7	3.4
Cholelithiasis and other disorders of gallbladder	1.0	1.2	0.9	1.1	1.4	0.9	1.0	1.2	0.9
Nephritis, nephrotic syndrome and nephrosis	15.3	18.7	13.0	14.1	17.3	11.9	15.3	18.8	13.1
Acute and rapidly progressive nephritic and nephrotic syndrome	0.0	0.1	0.0	*	*	*	0.0	0.1	0.0
Chronic glomerulonephritis, nephritis and nephropathy not specified as acute or chronic, and renal sclerosis unspecified	1.8	2.2	1.5	1.5	1.8	1.3	1.8	2.2	1.5
Renal failure	13.4	16.5	11.5	12.5	15.5	10.6	13.5	16.5	11.5
Other disorders of kidney	*	*	*	*	*	*	*	*	*
Infections of kidney	0.2	0.1	0.2	0.2	*	0.2	0.2	0.1	0.2
Hyperplasia of prostate	0.1	0.4	X	0.1	0.4	X	0.1	0.4	X
Inflammatory diseases of female pelvic organs	0.0	X	0.1	*	X	*	0.0	X	0.1
Pregnancy, childbirth and the puerperium	0.3	X	0.6	0.3	X	0.6	0.3	X	0.6
Pregnancy with abortive outcome	0.0	X	0.0	*	X	*	0.0	X	0.0
Other complications of pregnancy, childbirth and the puerperium	0.3	X	0.5	0.3	X	0.5	0.3	X	0.5
Certain conditions originating in the perinatal period	4.2	4.7	3.8	3.4	3.9	3.0	4.4	4.8	4.0
Congenital malformations, deformations and chromosomal abnormalities	3.2	3.3	3.1	2.7	2.8	2.7	3.3	3.4	3.2
Symptoms, signs and abnormal clinical and laboratory findings, not elsewhere classified	11.7	11.9	11.1	7.0	7.2	6.6	12.1	12.3	11.5
All other diseases (Residual)	81.1	80.9	79.6	58.1	60.3	55.3	82.8	82.5	81.3
Accidents (unintentional injuries)	38.0	51.5	25.6	25.8	37.2	14.9	39.7	53.6	27.1
Transport accidents	12.1	17.6	6.9	10.2	15.0	5.5	12.4	18.0	7.1
Motor vehicle accidents	11.3	16.2	6.5	9.6	14.0	5.3	11.5	16.6	6.8
Other land transport accidents	0.3	0.5	0.1	0.4	0.6	0.1	0.3	0.5	0.2
Water, air and space, and other and unspecified transport accidents and their sequelae	0.5	0.8	0.2	0.2	0.4	*	0.5	0.9	0.2
Nontransport accidents	25.9	33.9	18.7	15.6	22.2	9.4	27.4	35.7	19.9
Falls	7.9	9.9	6.4	5.2	7.0	3.8	8.0	10.0	6.5
Accidental discharge of firearms	0.2	0.3	0.1	0.1	0.1	*	0.2	0.4	0.1
Accidental drowning and submersion	1.2	1.9	0.5	1.0	1.7	0.3	1.3	1.9	0.6
Accidental exposure to smoke, fire and flames	0.9	1.1	0.7	0.5	0.7	0.3	0.9	1.2	0.7
Accidental poisoning and exposure to noxious substances	10.6	13.8	7.5	5.6	8.1	3.1	11.6	14.9	8.3
Other and unspecified nontransport accidents and their sequelae	5.2	7.0	3.6	3.1	4.6	1.8	5.3	7.2	3.7
Intentional Self-Harm (Suicide)	12.1	19.8	5.0	5.9	9.9	2.1	13.1	21.4	5.4
By discharge of firearms	6.1	11.2	1.5	2.2	4.2	0.4	6.6	12.2	1.6
By other and unspecified means and their sequelae	6.0	8.7	3.5	3.6	5.6	1.7	6.4	9.2	3.8
Assault (Homicide)	5.3	8.4	2.3	5.3	8.7	1.8	5.3	8.2	2.3
By discharge of firearms	3.6	6.1	1.1	3.4	5.8	0.9	3.7	6.1	1.2
By other and unspecified means and their sequelae	1.7	2.2	1.1	1.9	2.9	0.9	1.6	2.1	1.2
Legal intervention	0.1	0.3	*	0.2	0.3	*	0.1	0.3	*
Events of undetermined intent	1.6	1.9	1.2	0.7	1.0	0.5	1.7	2.1	1.4
Discharge of firearms, undetermined intent	0.1	0.1	0.0	0.0	0.1	*	0.1	0.1	0.0
Other and unspecified events of undetermined intent and their sequelae	1.5	1.8	1.2	0.7	0.9	0.4	1.6	1.9	1.3
Operations of war and their sequelae	*	*	*	*	*	*	*	*	*
Complications of medical and surgical care	0.8	0.8	0.7	0.5	0.6	0.4	0.8	0.8	0.8
Enterocolitis due to Clostridium difficile[4]	2.2	2.3	2.2	1.8	1.8	1.8	2.2	2.3	2.2
Drug-induced deaths[5,6]	12.9	15.9	10.0	6.1	8.4	3.8	14.2	17.3	11.1
Alcohol-induced deaths[5,7]	7.6	11.7	3.9	9.1	16.0	3.0	7.4	11.2	4.0
Injury by firearms[5,8]	10.1	17.9	2.7	5.9	10.5	1.3	10.7	19.1	2.9

X = Not applicable.   - = Quantity zero.   * = Figure does not meet standards of reliability or precision.   [1]Figures for origin not stated are included in "All origins" but not distributed among specified origins.   [2]Includes races other than White and Black.   [3]Race categories are consistent with the 1977 Office of Management and Budget (OMB) standards. Multiple-race data were reported by 37 states and the District of Columbia in 2010. The multiple-race data for these reporting areas were bridged to the single-race categories of the 1977 OMB standards for comparability with other reporting areas.   [4]Included in certain other intestinal infections (A04, A07–A09). Beginning with data year 2006, Enterocolitis due to Clostridium difficile (A04.7) is shown separately at the bottom of the table and is included in the list of rankable causes.   [5]Included in selected categories above.   [6]Includes ICD-10 codes D52.1, D59.0, D59.2, D61.1, D64.2, E06.4, E16.0, E23.1, E24.2, E27.3, E66.1, F11.1–F11.5, F11.7–F11.9, F12.1–F12.5, F12.7–F12.9, F13.1–F13.5, F13.7–F13.9, F14.1–F14.5, F14.7–F14.9, F15.1–F15.5, F15.7–F15.9, F16.1–F16.5, F16.7–F16.9, F17.3–F17.5, F17.7–F17.9, F18.1–F18.5, F18.7–F18.9, F19.1–F19.5, F19.7–F19.9, G21.1, G24.0, G25.1, G25.4, G25.6, G44.4, G62.0, G72.0, I95.2, J70.2–J70.4, K85.3, L10.5, L27.0–L27.1, M10.2, M32.0, M80.4, M81.4, M83.5, M87.1, R50.2, R78.1–R78.5, X40–X44, X60–X64, X85, and Y10–Y14. Trend data for drug-induced deaths, previously shown in this report, can be found at http://www.cdc.gov/nchs/deaths.htm.   [7]Includes ICD-10 codes E24.4, F10, G31.2, G62.1, G72.1, I42.6, K29.2, K70, K85.2, K86.0, R78.0, X45, X65, and Y15. Trend data for alcohol-induced deaths, previously shown in this report, can be found at http://www.cdc.gov/nchs/deaths.htm.   [8]Includes ICD-10 codes *U01.4, W32–W34, X72–X74, X93–X95, Y22–Y24, and Y35.0. Trend data for Injury by firearms, previously shown in this report, can be found at http://www.cdc.gov/nchs/deaths.htm.

Table 2-18B. Age-Adjusted Death Rates from Selected Causes, by Race for Non-Hispanic Population and Sex, 2010

(Age-adjusted rates per 100,000 U.S. standard population.)

Cause of death (based on ICD-10, 2004)	Non-Hispanic White[1] Both sexes	Male	Female	Non-Hispanic Black[1] Both sexes	Male	Female
All Causes	755.0	892.5	643.3	920.4	1,131.7	770.8
Salmonella infections	*	*	*	*	*	*
Shigellosis and amebiasis	*	*	*	*	*	*
Certain other intestinal infections	3.2	3.2	3.3	2.7	3.0	2.5
Tuberculosis	0.1	0.1	0.1	0.3	0.6	0.2
Respiratory tuberculosis	0.1	0.1	0.0	0.3	0.5	*
Other tuberculosis	0.0	0.0	0.0	0.1	*	*
Whooping cough	*	*	*	*	*	*
Scarlet fever and erysipelas	*	*	*	*	*	*
Meningococcal infection	0.0	0.0	0.0	*	*	*
Septicemia	9.9	11.0	9.1	20.0	22.6	18.3
Syphilis	*	*	*	*	*	*
Acute poliomyelitis	*	*	*	*	*	*
Arthropod-borne viral encephalitis	*	*	*	*	*	*
Measles	*	*	*	*	*	*
Viral hepatitis	1.9	2.6	1.2	2.8	4.0	1.9
Human immunodeficiency virus (HIV) disease	1.1	1.8	0.4	12.0	17.0	7.9
Malaria	*	*	*	*	*	*
Other and unspecified infectious and parasitic diseases and their sequelae	1.7	2.0	1.5	2.3	2.9	2.0
Malignant Neoplasms	176.5	212.6	150.6	208.8	271.1	171.4
Lip, oral cavity and pharynx	2.6	3.8	1.4	2.9	4.9	1.4
Esophagus	4.6	8.2	1.7	4.3	7.7	2.0
Stomach	2.7	3.6	1.9	6.5	9.5	4.5
Colon, rectum and anus	15.5	18.5	13.1	22.4	28.6	18.4
Liver and intrahepatic bile ducts	5.2	7.5	3.2	8.0	12.7	4.4
Pancreas	11.1	12.9	9.6	14.0	16.2	12.4
Larynx	1.1	1.9	0.4	1.8	3.5	0.7
Trachea, bronchus and lung	50.8	62.7	41.7	52.6	75.6	37.3
Skin	3.4	5.1	2.1	0.4	0.5	0.4
Breast	12.3	0.3	22.1	18.4	0.6	31.3
Cervix uteri	1.0	X	2.0	2.3	X	4.0
Corpus uteri and uterus, part unspecified	2.3	X	4.2	4.6	X	7.7
Ovary	4.6	X	8.3	4.0	X	6.8
Prostate	8.1	20.3	X	17.5	49.0	X
Kidney and renal pelvis	4.1	6.0	2.6	3.8	5.4	2.6
Bladder	4.9	8.5	2.3	3.8	5.7	2.6
Meninges, brain and other parts of central nervous system	4.8	5.9	3.9	2.6	3.1	2.2
Lymphoid, hematopoietic and related tissue	17.4	22.6	13.4	17.5	22.1	14.4
Hodgkin's disease	0.4	0.5	0.3	0.3	0.4	0.3
Non-Hodgkin's lymphoma	6.4	8.2	5.1	4.7	6.0	3.7
Leukemia	7.3	9.8	5.4	5.8	7.5	4.7
Multiple myeloma and immunoproliferative neoplasms	3.2	4.1	2.6	6.6	8.2	5.7
Other and unspecified malignant neoplasms of lymphoid, hematopoietic and related tissue	0.0	0.0	*	*	*	*
All other and unspecified malignant neoplasms	20.1	24.6	16.6	21.3	26.0	18.2
In situ neoplasms, benign neoplasms and neoplasms of uncertain or unknown behavior	4.8	6.1	3.9	4.1	4.6	3.7
Anemias	1.3	1.3	1.3	3.1	3.1	3.0
Diabetes mellitus	18.2	22.3	14.9	39.6	44.6	35.9
Nutritional deficiencies	0.8	0.8	0.9	1.3	1.3	1.3
Malnutrition	0.8	0.8	0.8	1.3	1.2	1.3
Other nutritional deficiencies	0.0	0.0	0.0	*	*	*
Meningitis	0.2	0.2	0.2	0.4	0.4	0.4
Parkinson's disease	7.5	11.2	5.0	3.1	5.0	2.1
Alzheimer's disease	26.4	22.0	28.9	20.9	18.2	22.0
Major cardiovascular diseases	232.8	281.1	193.5	310.5	374.5	263.9
Diseases of heart	179.9	226.9	142.5	229.5	286.3	189.1
Acute rheumatic fever and chronic rheumatic heart diseases	0.9	0.8	1.1	0.7	0.5	0.8
Hypertensive heart disease	8.6	9.4	7.5	24.0	29.6	19.6
Hypertensive heart and renal disease	0.6	0.7	0.6	2.4	2.9	2.1
Ischemic heart diseases	124.8	165.5	93.1	146.2	187.2	117.4
Acute myocardial infarction	115.0	154.2	84.4	133.4	171.9	106.7
Other acute ischemic heart diseases	37.3	49.4	27.5	42.7	52.9	35.4
Other forms of chronic ischemic heart disease	1.3	1.5	1.0	1.8	2.3	1.4
Atherosclerotic cardiovascular disease, so described	76.4	103.2	56.0	89.0	116.7	69.8
All other forms of chronic ischemic heart disease	16.4	22.3	11.4	26.4	37.1	18.7
Other heart diseases	60.0	81.0	44.6	62.5	79.6	51.1
Acute and subacute endocarditis	54.7	61.9	48.9	68.9	81.4	60.0
Diseases of pericardium and acute myocarditis	0.3	0.4	0.3	0.5	0.7	0.4
Heart failure	0.2	0.2	0.2	0.3	0.4	0.3
All other forms of heart disease	17.8	19.7	16.4	19.8	22.8	17.7
Essential hypertension and hypertensive renal disease	36.3	41.4	32.0	48.2	57.5	41.5
Cerebrovascular diseases	6.9	6.9	6.7	17.4	18.8	16.1
Atherosclerosis	37.8	37.5	37.4	54.3	58.1	50.7
Other diseases of circulatory system	2.2	2.4	2.1	2.2	2.5	2.0
Aortic aneurysm and dissection	5.9	7.5	4.7	7.2	8.9	6.0
Other diseases of arteries, arterioles and capillaries	3.3	4.6	2.4	3.1	4.1	2.3
Other disorders of circulatory system	2.6	2.8	2.4	4.1	4.9	3.7
Influenza and pneumonia	1.2	1.3	1.1	2.3	2.6	2.0
Influenza	14.9	17.7	13.1	17.1	21.7	14.3
Pneumonia	0.1	0.1	0.1	0.2	0.2	0.2
Other acute lower respiratory infections	14.8	17.6	12.9	16.9	21.5	14.2
Acute bronchitis and bronchiolitis	0.1	0.1	0.1	0.1	*	*
Other and unspecified acute lower respiratory infections	0.1	0.0	0.0	0.1	*	*
Chronic lower respiratory diseases	0.0	*	*	*	*	*
Bronchitis, chronic and unspecified	46.6	52.5	42.9	29.6	40.7	23.3
Emphysema	0.2	0.2	0.2	0.1	0.2	0.1
Asthma	3.4	4.1	3.0	2.0	3.1	1.3
Other chronic lower respiratory diseases	0.9	0.6	1.0	2.4	2.3	2.4

Table 2-18B. Age-Adjusted Death Rates from Selected Causes, by Race for Non-Hispanic Population and Sex, 2010—*Continued*

(Age-adjusted rates per 100,000 U.S. standard population.)

Cause of death (based on ICD-10, 2004)	Non-Hispanic White[1]			Non-Hispanic Black[1]		
	Both sexes	Male	Female	Both sexes	Male	Female
Pneumoconioses and chemical effects	42.1	47.5	38.7	25.1	35.1	19.5
Pneumonitis due to solids and liquids	5.4	7.6	4.0	5.0	7.1	3.8
Other diseases of respiratory system	9.7	11.9	8.1	9.5	11.3	8.5
Peptic ulcer	0.9	1.1	0.8	0.9	1.3	0.7
Diseases of appendix	0.1	0.2	0.1	0.1	0.2	*
Hernia	0.6	0.6	0.5	0.6	0.6	0.5
Chronic liver disease and cirrhosis	9.4	12.7	6.4	6.9	10.0	4.5
Alcoholic liver disease	4.7	6.8	2.8	3.1	4.6	1.9
Other chronic liver disease and cirrhosis	4.7	5.9	3.6	3.8	5.4	2.6
Cholelithiasis and other disorders of gallbladder	1.0	1.2	0.9	1.1	1.2	1.0
Nephritis, nephrotic syndrome and nephrosis	13.8	17.4	11.5	30.1	34.9	27.0
Acute and rapidly progressive nephritic and nephrotic syndrome	0.0	0.1	0.0	0.1	*	*
Chronic glomerulonephritis, nephritis and nephropathy not specified as acute or chronic, and renal sclerosis unspecified	1.6	2.0	1.4	3.4	4.1	2.9
Renal failure	12.1	15.3	10.1	26.6	30.6	24.0
Other disorders of kidney	*	*	*	*	*	*
Infections of kidney	0.2	0.1	0.2	0.2	0.2	0.2
Hyperplasia of prostate	0.1	0.4	X	0.1	0.4	X
Inflammatory diseases of female pelvic organs	0.0	X	0.1	0.1	X	0.1
Pregnancy, childbirth and the puerperium	0.2	X	0.4	0.7	X	1.3
Pregnancy with abortive outcome	*	X	*	*	X	*
Other complications of pregnancy, childbirth and the puerperium	0.2	X	0.4	0.6	X	1.2
Certain conditions originating in the perinatal period	3.3	3.6	3.0	8.8	9.5	8.0
Congenital malformations, deformations and chromosomal abnormalities	3.2	3.3	3.1	3.8	4.2	3.6
Symptoms, signs and abnormal clinical and laboratory findings, not elsewhere classified	11.9	12.0	11.4	15.3	17.0	13.8
All other diseases (Residual)	82.9	82.2	81.5	96.5	101.3	92.3
Accidents (unintentional injuries)	42.4	56.6	29.2	32.4	47.5	20.0
Transport accidents	12.9	18.5	7.5	12.1	18.6	6.4
Motor vehicle accidents	11.9	17.1	7.0	11.4	17.4	6.1
Other land transport accidents	0.3	0.5	0.2	0.4	0.6	0.2
Water, air and space, and other and unspecified transport accidents and their sequelae	0.6	0.9	0.3	0.3	0.6	0.1
Nontransport accidents	29.6	38.1	21.7	20.3	28.9	13.6
Falls	8.6	10.6	7.0	3.9	5.7	2.8
Accidental discharge of firearms	0.2	0.4	0.1	0.3	0.5	*
Accidental drowning and submersion	1.2	1.8	0.6	1.3	2.3	0.5
Accidental exposure to smoke, fire and flames	0.9	1.1	0.7	1.6	2.2	1.2
Accidental poisoning and exposure to noxious substances	13.3	16.9	9.6	7.5	10.3	5.2
Other and unspecified nontransport accidents and their sequelae	5.4	7.3	3.8	5.6	8.0	3.8
Intentional Self-Harm (Suicide)	15.0	24.2	6.2	5.4	9.4	1.9
By discharge of firearms	7.7	14.0	2.0	2.7	5.3	0.6
By other and unspecified means and their sequelae	7.2	10.3	4.3	2.7	4.2	1.3
Assault (Homicide)	2.5	3.3	1.8	18.6	33.1	5.2
By discharge of firearms	1.4	2.0	0.9	14.6	27.2	2.8
By other and unspecified means and their sequelae	1.1	1.4	0.9	4.1	6.0	2.4
Legal intervention	0.1	0.2	*	0.3	0.5	*
Events of undetermined intent	1.8	2.2	1.5	1.5	2.1	1.0
Discharge of firearms, undetermined intent	0.1	0.2	0.0	0.1	0.1	*
Other and unspecified events of undetermined intent and their sequelae	1.8	2.0	1.5	1.4	2.0	1.0
Operations of war and their sequelae	*	*	*	*	*	*
Complications of medical and surgical care	0.8	0.8	0.7	1.2	1.3	1.2
Enterocolitis due to Clostridium difficile[2]	2.3	2.3	2.3	1.7	1.9	1.6
Drug-induced deaths[3,4]	16.4	19.8	12.9	9.0	11.9	6.5
Alcohol-induced deaths[3,5]	7.8	11.6	4.2	6.1	9.8	3.1
Injury by firearms[3,6]	9.5	16.6	3.0	17.8	33.4	3.4

X = Not applicable.   - = Quantity zero.   * = Figure does not meet standards of reliability or precision.   [1]Race categories are consistent with the 1977 Office of Management and Budget (OMB) standards. Multiple-race data were reported by 37 states and the District of Columbia in 2010. The multiple-race data for these reporting areas were bridged to the single-race categories of the 1977 OMB standards for comparability with other reporting areas.   [2]Included in certain other intestinal infections (A04, A07–A09). Beginning with data year 2006, Enterocolitis due to Clostridium difficile (A04.7) is shown separately at the bottom of the table and is included in the list of rankable causes.   [3]Included in selected categories above.   [4]Includes ICD–10 codes D52.1, D59.0, D59.2, D61.1, D64.2, E06.4, E16.0, E23.1, E24.2, E27.3, E66.1, F11.1–F11.5, F11.7–F11.9, F12.1–F12.5, F12.7–F12.9, F13.1–F13.5, F13.7–F13.9, F14.1–F14.5, F14.7–F14.9, F15.1–F15.5, F15.7–F15.9, F16.1–F16.5, F16.7–F16.9, F17.3–F17.5, F17.7–F17.9, F18.1–F18.5, F18.7–F18.9, F19.1–F19.5, F19.7–F19.9, G21.1, G24.0, G25.1, G25.4, G25.6, G44.4, G62.0, G72.0, I95.2, J70.2–J70.4, K85.3, L10.5, L27.0–L27.1, M10.2, M32.0, M80.4, M81.4, M83.5, M87.1, R50.2, R78.1–R78.5, X40–X44, X60–X64, X85, and Y10–Y14. Trend data for drug-induced deaths, previously shown in this report, can be found at http://www.cdc.gov/nchs/deaths.htm.   [5]Includes ICD–10 codes E24.4, F10, G31.2, G62.1, G72.1, I42.6, K29.2, K70, K85.2, K86.0, R78.0, X45, X65, and Y15. Trend data for alcohol-induced deaths, previously shown in this report, can be found at http://www.cdc.gov/nchs/deaths.htm.   [6]Includes ICD–10 codes *U01.4, W32–W34, X72–X74, X93–X95, Y22–Y24, and Y35.0. Trend data for Injury by firearms, previously shown in this report, can be found at http://www.cdc.gov/nchs/deaths.htm.

Table 2-19. Age-Adjusted Death Rates, by Race, Hispanic Origin, Average Annual 1979–1981, 1989–1991, and 2008–2010

(Age-adjusted death rate per 100,000 population.)

State	All persons			White	Black	American Indian or Alaska Native[1]	Asian or Pacific Islander	Hispanic or Latino[2]	White, not Hispanic or Latino
	1979–1981	1989–1991	2008–2010	2008–2010	2008–2010	2008–2010	2008–2010	2008–2010	2008–2010
United States	1,022.8	942.2	757.0	750.5	919.2	629.3	427.8	565.7	763.1
Alabama	1,091.2	1,037.9	946.5	920.0	1,061.2	337.8	456.7	347.4	926.0
Alaska	1,087.4	944.6	765.8	716.6	740.3	1,156.9	452.8	492.4	720.0
Arizona	951.5	873.5	700.3	694.1	791.8	878.1	409.1	635.1	699.8
Arkansas	1,017.0	996.3	905.4	885.9	1,083.1	368.7	579.5	352.3	897.3
California	975.5	911.0	659.9	685.1	875.3	371.4	432.7	551.0	713.3
Colorado	941.1	856.1	695.8	700.1	805.1	456.0	400.2	699.0	693.4
Connecticut	961.5	857.5	661.3	659.8	731.3	277.8	342.7	540.5	659.1
Delaware	1,069.7	1,001.9	777.1	768.2	862.2	U	325.0	437.9	769.3
District of Columbia	1,243.1	1,255.3	840.8	524.9	1,065.4	U	366.0	411.5	522.1
Florida	960.8	870.9	706.4	696.2	827.7	326.9	368.8	555.3	726.1
Georgia	1,094.3	1,037.4	850.6	826.3	955.2	149.0	405.5	298.2	843.0
Hawaii	801.2	752.2	608.0	649.0	620.4	U	593.6	797.3	656.2
Idaho	936.7	856.6	731.1	731.5	597.9	851.3	526.9	503.9	738.2
Illinois	1,063.7	973.8	755.1	734.9	968.1	187.5	385.0	475.9	747.4
Indiana	1,048.3	962.0	828.3	820.5	973.0	156.3	385.7	460.0	820.9
Iowa	919.9	848.2	732.4	730.5	949.0	736.9	417.7	465.5	733.3
Kansas	940.1	867.2	771.4	761.6	978.8	1,222.9	465.4	543.3	766.6
Kentucky	1,088.9	1,024.5	918.0	917.2	999.5	275.3	432.7	343.9	921.6
Louisiana	1,132.6	1,074.6	919.0	870.9	1,063.2	400.0	467.2	368.0	884.1
Maine	1,002.9	918.7	753.8	755.3	535.3	1,197.9	310.0	452.8	754.2
Maryland	1,063.3	985.2	749.3	719.5	884.3	231.4	374.4	324.8	730.9
Massachusetts	982.6	884.8	687.5	698.4	650.3	288.9	356.1	455.7	699.0
Michigan	1,050.2	966.0	793.7	768.4	998.9	841.2	350.7	684.8	768.1
Minnesota	892.9	825.2	662.5	656.5	706.0	1,082.5	527.9	423.6	657.7
Mississippi	1,108.7	1,071.4	965.0	915.1	1,083.9	725.1	472.2	289.3	920.5
Missouri	1,033.7	952.4	831.8	821.3	971.9	428.3	319.3	368.5	827.2
Montana	1,013.6	890.2	766.9	746.4	U	1,203.0	U	525.7	737.2
Nebraska	930.6	867.9	726.6	719.4	974.3	811.4	379.5	450.8	723.6
Nevada	1,077.4	1,017.4	805.9	832.2	849.9	603.3	438.3	496.2	876.7
New Hampshire	982.3	891.7	699.0	704.5	608.3	U	U	333.1	706.3
New Jersey	1,047.5	956.0	699.5	695.1	863.4	214.4	355.8	496.9	708.1
New Mexico	967.1	891.9	762.2	759.1	779.2	807.1	371.0	733.6	750.1
New York	1,051.8	973.7	677.9	689.3	712.0	207.2	366.2	546.1	685.7
North Carolina	1,050.4	986.0	812.3	788.4	934.1	785.1	351.3	314.3	796.7
North Dakota	922.4	818.4	710.0	687.1	U	1,406.3	U	650.6	685.3
Ohio	1,070.6	967.4	824.8	810.5	981.1	277.5	420.9	488.7	812.4
Oklahoma	1,025.6	961.4	925.1	912.0	1,068.1	990.5	572.1	518.7	924.6
Oregon	953.9	893.0	734.8	741.1	815.0	715.5	453.5	479.2	747.9
Pennsylvania	1,076.4	963.4	780.0	766.5	974.5	197.1	377.1	502.1	767.9
Rhode Island	990.8	889.6	725.1	731.4	627.9	581.6	440.7	416.2	736.1
South Carolina	1,104.6	1,030.0	856.2	816.4	996.7	459.5	439.9	419.9	818.3
South Dakota	941.9	846.4	717.8	682.8	378.0	1,312.9	U	406.6	683.5
Tennessee	1,045.5	1,011.8	896.4	878.1	1,053.5	289.6	456.2	309.5	884.5
Texas	1,014.9	947.6	782.4	778.9	954.8	174.4	376.9	656.3	813.3
Utah	924.9	823.2	697.8	700.0	752.8	750.2	535.3	574.9	704.9
Vermont	990.2	908.6	708.2	711.6	U	U	U	U	709.0
Virginia	1,054.0	963.1	756.2	736.7	922.0	366.4	407.6	412.8	742.6
Washington	947.7	869.4	711.4	719.6	807.1	940.0	469.6	501.1	726.1
West Virginia	1,100.3	1,031.5	948.4	949.1	1,041.2	U	412.7	285.4	952.2
Wisconsin	956.4	879.1	717.4	704.0	982.2	1,068.9	460.7	445.3	707.0
Wyoming	1,016.1	897.4	775.9	770.4	U	1,165.3	U	635.4	773.0

NOTE: The race groups, White, Black, American Indian or Alaska Native, and Asian or Pacific Islander, include persons of Hispanic and non-Hispanic origin. Prior to 2001, age-adjusted rates were calculated using standard million proportions based on rounded population numbers. Starting with 2001 data, unrounded population numbers are used to calculate age-adjusted rates.   U = Prior to 2008–2010, data for states with populations under 10,000 in the middle year of a 3-year period, or fewer than 50 deaths for the 3-year period, are considered unreliable and are not shown.

[1] All data for the American Indian or Alaska Native (AIAN) category should be used with caution. Agreement between self-reported race and death certificate proxy reporting was found to be poor for the AIAN population. For more information, see Arias E, Schauman WS, Eschbach K, et al. The validity of race and Hispanic origin reporting on death certificates in the United States. National Center for Health Statistics. Vital Health Stat 2(148). 2008.   [2] Persons of Hispanic origin may be of any race. Data for Hispanic origin and race among states should be interpreted with caution because of inconsistencies between reporting Hispanic origin and race on death certificates and on censuses and surveys.

Table 2-20. Age-Adjusted Death Rates for Selected Causes of Death, by Sex, Race, and Hispanic Origin, Selected Years, 1950–2010

(Age-adjusted rate per 100,000 population.)

Sex, race, Hispanic origin, and cause of death[1]	1950[2,3]	1960[2,3]	1970[3]	1980[3]	1985[3]	1990[3]	1995[3]	2000[4]	2005[4]	2006[4]	2007[4]	2008[4]	2009[4]	2010[4]
							Age-adjusted death rate per 100,000 population[5]							
All Persons														
All causes	1,446.0	1,339.2	1,222.6	1,039.1	988.1	938.7	909.8	869.0	815.0	791.8	775.3	774.9	749.6	747.0
Diseases of heart	588.8	559.0	492.7	412.1	375.0	321.8	293.4	257.6	216.8	205.5	196.1	192.1	182.8	179.1
Ischemic heart disease	NA	NA	NA	345.2	296.2	249.6	219.7	186.8	148.2	138.3	129.2	126.1	117.7	113.6
Cerebrovascular diseases	180.7	177.9	147.7	96.2	76.4	65.3	63.1	60.9	48.0	44.8	43.5	42.1	39.6	39.1
Malignant neoplasms	193.9	193.9	198.6	207.9	211.3	216.0	209.9	199.6	185.1	181.8	179.3	176.4	173.5	172.8
Trachea, bronchus, and lung	15.0	24.1	37.1	49.9	54.6	59.3	58.4	56.1	52.7	51.5	50.6	49.5	48.4	47.6
Colon, rectum, and anus	NA	30.3	28.9	27.4	26.3	24.5	22.5	20.8	17.7	17.4	17.0	16.6	16.0	15.8
Chronic lower respiratory diseases	NA	NA	NA	28.3	34.5	37.2	40.1	44.2	43.9	41.0	41.4	44.7	42.7	42.2
Influenza and pneumonia	48.1	53.7	41.7	31.4	34.5	36.8	33.4	23.7	21.0	18.4	16.8	17.6	16.5	15.1
Chronic liver disease and cirrhosis	11.3	13.3	17.8	15.1	12.3	11.1	9.9	9.5	8.9	8.8	9.1	9.2	9.1	9.4
Diabetes mellitus	23.1	22.5	24.3	18.1	17.4	20.7	23.2	25.0	24.9	23.6	22.8	22.0	21.0	20.8
Alzheimer's disease	NA	NA	NA	V	V	V	V	18.1	24.0	23.7	23.8	25.8	24.2	25.1
Human immunodeficiency virus (HIV) disease	X	X	X	X	NA	10.2	16.2	5.2	4.2	4.0	3.7	3.3	3.0	2.6
Unintentional injuries	78.0	62.3	60.1	46.4	38.5	36.3	34.4	34.9	39.5	40.2	40.4	39.2	37.5	38.0
Motor vehicle-related injuries	24.6	23.1	27.6	22.3	18.6	18.5	16.3	15.4	15.2	15.0	14.4	12.9	11.6	11.3
Poisoning	2.5	1.7	2.8	1.9	2.2	2.3	3.4	4.5	8.0	9.2	9.9	10.2	10.3	10.6
Suicide[6]	13.2	12.5	13.1	12.2	12.5	12.5	11.8	10.4	10.9	11.0	11.3	11.6	11.8	12.1
Homicide[6]	5.1	5.0	8.8	10.4	7.9	9.4	8.3	5.9	6.1	6.2	6.1	5.9	5.5	5.3
Male														
All causes	1,674.2	1,609.0	1,542.1	1,348.1	1,278.1	1,202.8	1,143.9	1,053.8	971.9	943.5	922.9	918.8	890.9	887.1
Diseases of heart	699.0	687.6	634.0	538.9	488.0	412.4	371.0	320.0	268.2	254.9	243.7	238.5	229.4	225.1
Ischemic heart disease	NA	NA	NA	459.7	393.7	328.2	286.5	241.4	192.3	180.7	169.2	165.1	156.2	151.3
Cerebrovascular diseases	186.4	186.1	157.4	102.2	79.9	68.5	65.9	62.4	48.4	45.2	43.7	42.2	39.9	39.3
Malignant neoplasms	208.1	225.1	247.6	271.2	274.4	280.4	267.5	248.9	227.2	221.7	218.8	214.9	210.9	209.9
Trachea, bronchus, and lung	24.6	43.6	67.5	85.2	88.6	91.1	84.2	76.7	69.1	67.0	64.9	63.5	61.4	60.3
Colon, rectum, and anus	NA	31.8	32.3	32.8	31.8	30.4	27.4	25.1	21.2	20.7	20.3	19.7	19.1	19.0
Prostate	28.6	28.7	28.8	32.8	33.4	38.4	37.0	30.4	25.3	24.2	24.2	23.0	22.1	21.9
Chronic lower respiratory diseases	NA	NA	NA	49.9	56.2	55.4	54.8	55.8	52.2	48.4	48.8	52.3	49.5	48.7
Influenza and pneumonia	55.0	65.8	54.0	42.1	46.8	47.8	42.8	28.9	24.9	22.1	20.2	20.7	19.6	18.2
Chronic liver disease and cirrhosis	15.0	18.5	24.8	21.3	17.4	15.9	14.2	13.4	12.4	12.1	12.7	12.7	12.5	12.9
Diabetes mellitus	18.8	19.9	23.0	18.1	17.7	21.7	25.0	27.8	28.8	27.7	26.6	25.9	25.0	24.9
Alzheimer's disease	NA	NA	NA	V	V	V	V	15.2	19.5	19.4	19.5	21.3	20.2	21.0
Human immunodeficiency virus (HIV) disease	X	X	X	X	NA	18.5	27.3	7.9	6.3	5.9	5.4	4.8	4.4	3.8
Unintentional injuries	101.8	85.5	87.4	69.0	57.1	52.9	49.6	49.3	55.0	56.0	55.9	54.3	51.4	51.5
Motor vehicle-related injuries	38.5	35.4	41.5	33.6	27.2	26.5	22.8	21.7	21.9	21.5	21.0	18.9	16.8	16.2
Poisoning	3.3	2.3	3.9	2.7	3.2	3.5	5.3	6.6	10.8	12.6	13.1	13.6	13.5	13.8
Suicide[6]	21.2	20.0	19.8	19.9	21.1	21.5	20.3	17.7	18.1	18.1	18.5	19.0	19.2	19.8
Homicide[6]	7.9	7.5	14.3	16.6	12.2	14.8	12.8	9.0	9.7	9.8	9.7	9.3	8.6	8.4
Female														
All causes	1,236.0	1,105.3	971.4	817.9	784.5	750.9	739.4	731.4	692.3	672.2	658.1	659.9	636.8	634.9
Diseases of heart	486.6	447.0	381.6	320.8	294.5	257.0	236.6	210.9	177.5	167.2	159.0	155.9	146.6	143.3
Ischemic heart disease	NA	NA	NA	263.1	227.0	193.9	171.3	146.5	115.0	106.3	98.8	96.3	88.4	84.9
Cerebrovascular diseases	175.8	170.7	140.0	91.7	73.3	62.6	60.5	59.1	47.0	43.9	42.7	41.4	38.8	38.3
Malignant neoplasms	182.3	168.7	163.2	166.7	171.2	175.7	173.6	167.6	156.7	154.7	152.3	149.6	147.4	146.7
Trachea, bronchus, and lung	5.8	7.5	13.1	24.4	30.6	37.1	40.4	41.3	40.6	40.1	40.1	39.1	38.6	38.1
Colon, rectum, and anus	NA	29.1	26.5	23.8	22.7	20.6	19.1	17.7	15.0	14.9	14.6	14.2	13.5	13.3
Breast	31.9	31.7	32.1	31.9	33.0	33.3	30.5	26.8	24.2	23.6	23.0	22.6	22.3	22.1
Chronic lower respiratory diseases	NA	NA	NA	14.9	21.7	26.6	31.8	37.4	38.7	36.4	36.6	39.8	38.3	38.0
Influenza and pneumonia	41.9	43.8	32.7	25.1	27.6	30.5	28.1	20.7	18.6	16.1	14.7	15.6	14.5	13.1
Chronic liver disease and cirrhosis	7.8	8.7	11.9	9.9	7.9	7.1	6.2	6.2	5.8	5.8	5.9	6.0	6.1	6.2
Diabetes mellitus	27.0	24.7	25.1	18.0	17.0	19.9	21.8	23.0	21.9	20.4	19.8	19.1	17.9	17.6
Alzheimer's disease	NA	NA	NA	V	V	V	V	19.3	26.2	25.9	26.2	28.2	26.3	27.3
Human immunodeficiency virus (HIV) disease	X	X	X	X	NA	2.2	5.3	2.5	2.3	2.2	2.1	1.9	1.7	1.4
Unintentional injuries	54.0	40.0	35.1	26.1	22.2	21.5	21.0	22.0	25.3	25.8	26.1	25.4	24.8	25.6
Motor vehicle-related injuries	11.5	11.7	14.9	11.8	10.7	11.0	10.3	9.5	8.9	8.8	8.2	7.2	6.7	6.5
Poisoning	1.7	1.1	1.8	1.3	1.2	1.2	1.6	2.5	5.1	5.9	6.6	6.8	7.1	7.5
Suicide[6]	5.6	5.6	7.4	5.7	5.2	4.8	4.3	4.0	4.4	4.5	4.6	4.8	4.9	5.0
Homicide[6]	2.4	2.6	3.7	4.4	3.8	4.0	3.7	2.8	2.5	2.6	2.5	2.4	2.4	2.3
White [7]														
All causes	1,410.8	1,311.3	1,193.3	1,012.7	963.6	909.8	882.3	849.8	801.1	779.3	764.3	767.2	742.8	741.8
Diseases of heart	586.0	559.0	492.2	409.4	371.4	317.0	288.6	253.4	213.2	202.0	192.8	189.3	180.1	176.9
Ischemic heart disease	NA	NA	NA	347.6	298.0	249.7	219.1	185.6	147.3	137.4	128.5	125.8	117.4	113.5
Cerebrovascular diseases	175.5	172.7	143.5	93.2	73.7	62.8	60.7	58.8	46.0	42.9	41.6	40.4	38.1	37.7
Malignant neoplasms	194.6	193.1	196.7	204.2	207.3	211.6	206.2	197.2	183.9	181.0	178.5	175.9	173.3	172.4
Trachea, bronchus, and lung	15.2	24.0	36.7	49.2	53.9	58.6	58.1	56.2	53.2	52.1	51.2	50.2	49.1	48.3
Colon, rectum, and anus	NA	30.9	29.2	27.4	26.1	24.1	22.0	20.3	17.1	16.9	16.6	16.1	15.6	15.3
Chronic lower respiratory diseases	NA	NA	NA	29.3	35.6	38.3	41.5	46.0	46.0	43.1	43.5	47.1	45.1	44.6
Influenza and pneumonia	44.8	50.4	39.8	30.9	34.3	36.4	33.0	23.5	20.9	18.2	16.6	17.4	16.3	14.9
Chronic liver disease and cirrhosis	11.5	13.2	16.6	13.9	11.4	10.5	9.7	9.6	9.2	9.1	9.5	9.6	9.6	9.9
Diabetes mellitus	22.9	21.7	22.9	16.7	15.9	18.8	20.9	22.8	22.8	21.4	20.7	20.2	19.2	19.0
Alzheimer's disease	NA	NA	NA	V	V	V	V	18.8	24.7	24.5	24.6	26.7	25.0	26.0
Human immunodeficiency virus (HIV) disease	X	X	X	X	NA	8.3	11.4	2.8	2.2	2.1	1.9	1.7	1.5	1.4
Unintentional injuries	77.0	60.4	57.8	45.3	37.7	35.5	33.9	35.1	40.7	41.7	42.1	41.4	39.5	40.3
Motor vehicle-related injuries	24.4	22.9	27.1	22.6	18.8	18.5	16.3	15.6	15.7	15.5	14.9	13.4	12.0	11.7
Poisoning	2.4	1.6	2.4	1.8	2.0	2.1	3.1	4.5	8.5	9.8	10.7	11.3	11.4	11.9
Suicide[6]	13.9	13.1	13.8	13.0	13.4	13.4	12.6	11.3	12.1	12.2	12.6	13.0	13.2	13.6
Homicide[6]	2.6	2.7	4.7	6.7	5.3	5.5	5.0	3.6	3.7	3.7	3.7	3.7	3.4	3.3

Table 2-20. Age-Adjusted Death Rates for Selected Causes of Death, by Race, Selected Years, 1950–2010—*Continued*

(Age-adjusted rate per 100,000 population.)

Sex, race, Hispanic origin, and cause of death[1]	1950[2,3]	1960[2,3]	1970[3]	1980[3]	1985[3]	1990[3]	1995[3]	2000[4]	2005[4]	2006[4]	2007[4]	2008[4]	2009[4]	2010[4]
						Age-adjusted death rate per 100,000 population[5]								
Black or African American [5]														
All causes	1,722.1	1,577.5	1,518.1	1,314.8	1,261.2	1,250.3	1,213.9	1,121.4	1,035.1	997.9	972.0	947.7	912.8	898.2
Diseases of heart	588.7	548.3	512.0	455.3	430.6	391.5	363.8	324.8	278.0	263.5	252.5	243.4	231.8	224.9
Ischemic heart disease	NA	NA	NA	334.5	293.4	267.0	244.9	218.3	175.7	165.4	154.0	146.8	137.4	131.2
Cerebrovascular diseases	233.6	235.2	197.1	129.1	105.2	91.6	86.9	81.9	67.0	63.1	61.7	58.8	54.0	53.0
Malignant neoplasms	176.4	199.1	225.3	256.4	266.5	279.5	267.7	248.5	223.5	217.6	215.1	208.5	204.5	203.8
Trachea, bronchus, and lung	11.1	23.7	41.3	59.7	65.8	72.4	69.0	64.0	58.1	56.3	55.1	52.9	51.3	51.4
Colon, rectum, and anus	NA	22.8	26.1	28.3	30.0	30.6	29.3	28.2	25.1	24.4	23.6	22.9	22.0	21.8
Chronic lower respiratory diseases	NA	NA	NA	19.2	24.6	28.1	30.1	31.6	31.1	28.5	28.5	30.8	28.9	29.0
Influenza and pneumonia	76.7	81.1	57.2	34.4	35.8	39.4	36.4	25.6	22.6	20.4	19.2	19.5	18.0	16.8
Chronic liver disease and cirrhosis	9.0	13.6	28.1	25.0	19.3	16.5	12.0	9.4	7.6	6.8	7.2	6.8	6.8	6.7
Diabetes mellitus	23.5	30.9	38.8	32.7	33.0	40.5	46.7	49.5	47.5	45.5	43.1	40.8	39.1	38.7
Alzheimer's disease	NA	NA	NA	V	V	V	V	13.0	20.8	19.7	20.5	21.2	20.6	20.6
Human immunodeficiency virus (HIV) disease	X	X	X	X	NA	26.7	54.2	23.3	19.2	18.3	17.0	14.9	13.7	11.6
Unintentional injuries	79.9	74.0	78.3	57.6	47.1	43.8	41.0	37.7	38.8	38.2	36.5	33.1	31.6	31.3
Motor vehicle-related injuries	26.0	24.2	31.1	20.2	17.8	18.8	16.7	15.7	14.4	14.5	14.0	12.1	11.5	10.9
Poisoning	2.8	2.9	5.8	3.1	3.6	4.1	6.2	6.0	8.1	9.3	8.4	7.7	7.4	7.3
Suicide[6]	4.5	5.0	6.2	6.5	6.6	7.1	6.8	5.5	5.2	5.0	4.9	5.2	5.1	5.2
Homicide[6]	28.3	26.0	44.0	39.0	28.1	36.3	29.7	20.5	21.1	21.5	20.9	19.3	18.1	17.7
American Indian or Alaska Native [5]														
All causes	NA	NA	NA	867.0	731.7	716.3	771.2	709.3	701.1	676.6	661.3	644.0	616.0	628.3
Diseases of heart	NA	NA	NA	240.6	219.0	200.6	204.6	178.2	156.6	153.2	140.5	132.6	130.7	128.6
Ischemic heart disease	NA	NA	NA	173.6	158.3	139.1	141.4	129.1	106.1	107.2	95.9	88.0	86.5	84.9
Cerebrovascular diseases	NA	NA	NA	57.8	46.2	40.7	48.6	45.0	38.8	33.4	34.2	27.7	29.2	28.1
Malignant neoplasms	NA	NA	NA	113.7	113.5	121.8	138.2	127.8	128.8	125.4	124.1	125.0	114.9	122.4
Trachea, bronchus, and lung	NA	NA	NA	20.7	25.8	30.9	37.4	32.3	35.3	32.3	34.1	34.8	29.5	33.1
Colon, rectum, and anus	NA	NA	NA	9.5	10.5	12.0	14.9	13.4	12.6	11.7	12.1	14.6	13.0	11.7
Chronic lower respiratory diseases	NA	NA	NA	14.2	17.6	25.4	27.6	32.8	31.6	29.8	33.9	31.9	30.7	33.8
Influenza and pneumonia	NA	NA	NA	44.4	33.6	36.1	36.1	22.3	23.6	16.3	15.9	19.6	17.9	15.9
Chronic liver disease and cirrhosis	NA	NA	NA	45.3	27.9	24.1	27.4	24.3	21.6	20.9	23.1	23.6	21.3	22.8
Diabetes mellitus	NA	NA	NA	29.6	29.0	34.1	45.9	41.5	44.1	42.2	40.0	36.3	34.9	36.4
Alzheimer's disease	NA	NA	NA	V	V	V	V	9.1	15.0	13.6	14.3	15.1	13.1	17.2
Human immunodeficiency virus (HIV) disease	X	X	X	X	NA	1.8	6.5	2.2	2.5	2.1	2.3	1.8	1.7	1.6
Unintentional injuries	NA	NA	NA	99.0	67.4	62.6	55.3	51.3	51.3	52.6	50.8	49.0	48.7	46.9
Motor vehicle-related injuries	NA	NA	NA	54.5	34.8	32.5	29.1	27.3	22.6	24.1	20.8	18.4	17.2	15.7
Poisoning	NA	NA	NA	2.3	3.1	3.2	4.6	4.7	8.6	9.4	10.3	12.4	13.8	13.0
Suicide[6]	NA	NA	NA	11.9	10.9	11.7	10.6	9.8	10.7	10.4	10.1	10.1	10.0	10.8
Homicide[6]	NA	NA	NA	15.5	11.7	10.4	9.9	6.8	6.8	6.6	5.6	6.2	5.9	5.7
Asian or Pacific Islander [5]														
All causes	NA	NA	NA	589.9	586.5	582.0	554.8	506.4	459.6	450.7	436.2	435.1	424.6	424.3
Diseases of heart	NA	NA	NA	202.1	196.7	181.7	171.3	146.0	119.7	115.8	108.3	107.7	103.8	100.9
Ischemic heart disease	NA	NA	NA	168.2	153.3	139.6	128.0	109.6	85.6	82.2	75.9	75.9	70.7	68.7
Cerebrovascular diseases	NA	NA	NA	66.1	58.7	56.9	55.2	52.9	40.8	39.3	36.6	35.2	33.0	33.2
Malignant neoplasms	NA	NA	NA	126.1	132.3	134.2	131.8	121.9	113.2	109.6	109.5	108.8	106.8	108.9
Trachea, bronchus, and lung	NA	NA	NA	28.4	27.2	30.2	29.9	28.1	26.3	25.9	26.0	25.6	25.2	24.8
Colon, rectum, and anus	NA	NA	NA	16.4	16.6	14.4	14.0	12.7	11.5	11.3	11.2	11.6	10.5	11.4
Chronic lower respiratory diseases	NA	NA	NA	12.9	17.6	19.4	19.3	18.6	15.9	15.4	14.3	15.2	14.3	13.9
Influenza and pneumonia	NA	NA	NA	24.0	26.1	31.4	29.1	19.7	16.8	16.1	14.9	15.7	15.0	14.4
Chronic liver disease and cirrhosis	NA	NA	NA	6.1	5.9	5.2	3.9	3.5	3.6	3.5	3.3	3.4	3.3	3.2
Diabetes mellitus	NA	NA	NA	12.6	12.1	14.6	16.8	16.4	17.3	16.6	17.0	16.8	16.2	15.5
Alzheimer's disease	NA	NA	NA	V	V	V	V	5.5	8.5	9.4	9.1	10.1	10.9	10.9
Human immunodeficiency virus (HIV) disease	X	X	X	X	NA	2.2	3.2	0.6	0.6	0.6	0.5	0.6	0.4	0.4
Unintentional injuries	NA	NA	NA	27.0	24.8	23.9	20.2	17.9	18.1	17.1	16.9	15.3	14.9	15.0
Motor vehicle-related injuries	NA	NA	NA	13.9	12.9	14.0	11.4	8.6	7.5	7.3	6.9	6.0	4.9	5.1
Poisoning	NA	NA	NA	0.5	0.6	0.7	0.8	1.3	1.4	1.4	1.4	1.3	1.5	1.4
Suicide[6]	NA	NA	NA	7.8	7.1	6.7	6.7	5.5	5.1	5.4	5.9	5.5	5.9	6.2
Homicide[6]	NA	NA	NA	5.9	4.1	5.0	4.7	3.0	2.8	2.7	2.2	2.1	2.0	1.8

Table 2-20. Age-Adjusted Death Rates for Selected Causes of Death, by Hispanic Origin, Selected Years, 1950–2010—*Continued*

(Age-adjusted rate per 100,000 population.)

Sex, race, Hispanic origin, and cause of death[1]	1950[2,3]	1960[2,3]	1970[3]	1980[3]	1985[3]	1990[3]	1995[3]	2000[4]	2005[4]	2006[4]	2007[4]	2008[4]	2009[4]	2010[4]
					Age-adjusted death rate per 100,000 population[5]									
Hispanic or Latino [7,8]														
All causes	NA	NA	NA	NA	698.8	692.0	700.2	665.7	627.6	604.0	586.1	579.8	559.7	558.6
Diseases of heart	NA	NA	NA	NA	239.8	217.1	211.0	196.0	170.4	157.8	149.5	141.4	135.8	132.8
Ischemic heart disease	NA	NA	NA	NA	187.9	173.3	166.4	153.2	127.9	116.4	107.5	100.8	94.7	92.3
Cerebrovascular diseases	NA	NA	NA	NA	51.9	45.2	46.3	46.4	38.6	37.2	35.8	34.4	32.2	32.1
Malignant neoplasms	NA	NA	NA	NA	125.9	136.8	138.5	134.9	127.9	123.7	121.8	121.0	119.7	119.7
Trachea, bronchus, and lung	NA	NA	NA	NA	22.9	26.5	25.9	24.8	23.3	21.6	21.9	21.6	20.4	20.4
Colon, rectum, and anus	NA	NA	NA	NA	13.0	14.7	14.1	14.1	13.1	13.4	12.8	12.7	12.7	12.3
Chronic lower respiratory diseases	NA	NA	NA	NA	17.4	19.3	22.6	21.1	20.9	19.0	19.3	20.5	19.8	19.6
Influenza and pneumonia	NA	NA	NA	NA	30.2	29.7	26.2	20.6	18.5	16.7	14.7	15.9	15.6	13.7
Chronic liver disease and cirrhosis	NA	NA	NA	NA	20.3	18.3	17.4	16.5	14.1	13.6	14.0	14.0	14.0	13.7
Diabetes mellitus	NA	NA	NA	NA	23.0	28.2	35.7	36.9	35.4	31.7	30.6	29.8	27.0	27.1
Alzheimer's disease	NA	NA	NA	NA	V	V	V	V	15.6	16.1	15.6	18.0	16.9	18.5
Human immunodeficiency virus (HIV) disease	X	X	X	X	NA	16.3	24.9	6.7	4.8	4.5	4.1	3.6	3.2	2.8
Unintentional injuries	NA	NA	NA	NA	34.3	34.6	32.2	30.1	31.8	32.0	30.5	28.4	26.3	25.8
Motor vehicle-related injuries	NA	NA	NA	NA	17.1	19.5	16.4	14.7	14.6	14.6	13.1	11.2	10.1	9.6
Poisoning	NA	NA	NA	NA	3.2	3.2	4.9	4.1	5.2	5.7	5.8	5.9	5.8	5.6
Suicide[6]	NA	NA	NA	NA	6.3	7.8	7.2	5.9	5.6	5.3	6.0	5.5	5.8	5.9
Homicide[6]	NA	NA	NA	NA	14.6	16.2	12.5	7.5	7.4	7.2	6.8	6.4	6.0	5.3
White, not Hispanic or Latino [8]														
All causes	NA	NA	NA	NA	942.1	914.5	882.3	855.5	810.1	789.1	775.3	779.4	755.1	755.0
Diseases of heart	NA	NA	NA	NA	366.7	319.7	289.9	255.5	215.5	204.5	195.5	192.4	182.9	179.9
Ischemic heart disease	NA	NA	NA	NA	296.0	251.9	219.9	186.6	148.3	138.6	129.9	127.4	118.9	115.0
Cerebrovascular diseases	NA	NA	NA	NA	72.2	63.5	60.8	59.0	46.2	42.9	41.7	40.5	38.3	37.8
Malignant neoplasms	NA	NA	NA	NA	202.1	215.4	208.9	200.6	187.8	185.1	182.6	179.9	177.4	176.5
Trachea, bronchus, and lung	NA	NA	NA	NA	53.2	60.3	59.6	58.2	55.5	54.5	53.7	52.6	51.6	50.8
Colon, rectum, and anus	NA	NA	NA	NA	25.7	24.6	22.3	20.5	17.4	17.1	16.9	16.4	15.8	15.5
Chronic lower respiratory diseases	NA	NA	NA	NA	36.3	39.2	42.1	47.2	47.7	44.8	45.3	49.1	47.1	46.6
Influenza and pneumonia	NA	NA	NA	NA	35.2	36.5	33.0	23.5	21.0	18.3	16.7	17.4	16.2	14.9
Chronic liver disease and cirrhosis	NA	NA	NA	NA	10.9	9.9	9.0	9.0	8.7	8.6	8.9	9.1	9.1	9.4
Diabetes mellitus	NA	NA	NA	NA	14.8	18.3	20.1	21.8	21.8	20.6	19.9	19.3	18.5	18.2
Alzheimer's disease	NA	NA	NA	NA	V	V	V	19.1	25.1	24.9	25.1	27.2	25.4	26.4
Human immunodeficiency virus (HIV) disease	X	X	X	X	NA	7.4	9.8	2.2	1.8	1.7	1.5	1.4	1.2	1.1
Unintentional injuries	NA	NA	NA	NA	35.2	35.0	33.4	35.3	41.5	42.7	43.6	43.2	41.3	42.4
Motor vehicle-related injuries	NA	NA	NA	NA	17.4	18.2	16.1	15.6	15.7	15.4	15.1	13.7	12.2	11.9
Poisoning	NA	NA	NA	NA	2.2	2.0	2.9	4.6	9.1	10.6	11.8	12.4	12.6	13.3
Suicide[6]	NA	NA	NA	NA	13.8	13.8	13.1	12.0	13.0	13.3	13.7	14.3	14.5	15.0
Homicide[6]	NA	NA	NA	NA	4.4	4.0	3.6	2.8	2.7	2.7	2.8	2.9	2.6	2.5

NA = Not available.   V = Data for Alzheimer's disease are only presented for data years 1999 and beyond due to large differences in death rates caused by changes in the coding of the causes of death between ICD-9 and ICD-10.   X = Not applicable.   [1]Underlying cause of death code numbers are based on the applicable revision of the International Classification of Diseases (ICD) for data years shown.   [2]Includes deaths of persons who were not residents of the 50 states and the District of Columbia.   [3]Underlying cause of death was coded according to the 6th Revision of the ICD in 1950, 7th Revision in 1960, 8th Revision in 1970, and 9th Revision in 1980-1998.   [4]Starting with 1999 data, cause of death is coded according to ICD-10.   [5]Age-adjusted rates are calculated using the year 2000 standard population. Prior to 2001, age-adjusted rates were calculated using standard million proportions based on rounded population numbers. Starting with 2001 data, unrounded population numbers are used to calculate age-adjusted rates.   [6]Figures for 2001 include September 11-related deaths, for which death certificates were filed as of October 24, 2002.   [7]The race groups, White, Black, Asian or Pacific Islander, and American Indian or Alaska Native, include persons of Hispanic and non-Hispanic origin. Persons of Hispanic origin may be of any race. Death rates for the American Indian or Alaska Native, Asian or Pacific Islander, and Hispanic populations are known to be underestimated.   [8]Prior to 1997, data from states that did not report Hispanic origin on the death certificate were excluded.

Table 2-21. Number of Deaths, Death Rates, and Age-Adjusted Death Rates for Injury Deaths, by Mechanism and Intent of Death, 2010

(Number; rates per 100,000 population; age-adjusted rates per 100,000 U.S. standard population.)

Mechanism and intent of death (based on the ICD, Tenth Revision)	Number	Rate	Age-adjusted rate[1]
All Injury (*U01'-*U03, V01'-Y36, Y85'-Y87, Y89)	180,811	58.6	57.1
Unintentional (V01'-X59, Y85'-Y86)	120,859	39.1	38.0
Suicide (*U03,X60'-X84, Y87.0)	38,364	12.4	12.1
Homicide (*U01'-*U02, X85'-Y09, Y87.1)	16,259	5.3	5.3
Undetermined (Y10'-Y34, Y87.2, Y89.9)	4,908	1.6	1.6
Legal intervention/war (Y35'-Y36, Y89[.0,.1])	421	0.1	0.2
Cut/Pierce (W25'-W29, W45, X78, X99, Y28, Y35.4)	2,598	0.8	0.8
Unintentional (W25'-W29, W45)	105	0.0	0.0
Suicide (X78)	673	0.2	0.2
Homicide (X99)	1,799	0.6	0.6
Undetermined (Y28)	21	0.0	0.0
Legal intervention/war (Y35.4)	-	*	*
Drowning (W65'-W74, X71, X92, Y21)	4,521	1.5	1.4
Unintentional (W65'-W74)	3,782	1.2	1.2
Suicide (X71)	409	0.1	0.1
Homicide (X92)	52	0.0	0.0
Undetermined (Y21)	278	0.1	0.1
Fall (W00'-W19, X80, Y01, Y30)	26,852	8.7	8.1
Unintentional (W00'-W19)	26,009	8.4	7.9
Suicide (X80)	781	0.3	0.3
Homicide (Y01)	12	*	*
Undetermined (Y30)	50	0.0	0.0
Fire/Hot Object or Substance (*U01.3, X00'-X19, X76'-X77, X97'-X98, Y26'-Y27, Y36.3)[2]	3,194	1.0	1.0
Unintentional (X00'-X19)	2,845	0.9	0.9
Suicide (X76'-X77)	131	0.0	0.0
Homicide (*U01.3, X97'-X98)	92	0.0	0.0
Undetermined (Y26'-Y27)	126	0.0	0.0
Legal intervention/war (Y36.3)	-	*	*
Fire/flame (X00'-X09, X76, X97, Y26)	3,127	1.0	1.0
Unintentional (X00'-X09)	2,782	0.9	0.9
Suicide (X76)	131	0.0	0.0
Homicide (X97)	89	0.0	0.0
Undetermined (Y26)	125	0.0	0.0
Hot object/substance (X10'-X19, X77, X98,Y27)	67	0.0	0.0
Unintentional (X10'-X19)	63	0.0	0.0
Suicide (X77)	-	*	*
Homicide (X98)	3	*	*
Undetermined (Y27)	1	*	*
Firearm (*U01.4, W32'-W34, X72'-X74, X93'-X95, Y22'-Y24, Y35.0)	31,672	10.3	10.1
Unintentional (W32'-W34)	606	0.2	0.2
Suicide (X72'-X74)	19,392	6.3	6.1
Homicide (*U01.4, X93'-X95)	11,078	3.6	3.6
Undetermined (Y22'-Y24)	252	0.1	0.1
Legal intervention/war (Y35.0)	344	0.1	0.1
Machinery (W24,W30'-W31)[3]	590	0.2	0.2
All Transport (*U01.1, V01'-V99, X82, Y03, Y32, Y36.1)	37,402	12.1	11.9
Unintentional (V01'-V99)	37,236	12.1	11.8
Suicide (X82)	114	0.0	0.0
Homicide (*U01.1,Y03)	39	0.0	0.0
Undetermined (Y32)	13	*	*
Legal intervention/war (Y36.1)	-	*	*
Motor vehicle traffic (V02'-V04[.1,.9], V09.2, V12'-V14[.3'-.9], V19[.4'-.6], V20'-V28[.3'-.9], V29'-V79[.4'-.9], V80[.3'-.5],V81.1, V82.1,V83'-V86[.0'-.3], V87[.0'-.8],V89.2)2	33,687	10.9	10.7
Occupant (V30'-V79[.4'-.9], V83'-V86[.0'-.3])2	10,246	3.3	3.3
Motorcyclist (V20'-V28[.3'-.9], V29[.4'-.9])2	4,177	1.4	1.3
Pedal cyclist (V12'-V14[.3'-.9], V19[.4'-.6])2	551	0.2	0.2
Pedestrian (V02'-V04[.1,.9], V09.2)2	4,383	1.4	1.4
Other (V80[.3'-.5], V81.1, V82.1)2	10	*	*
Unspecified (V87[.0'-.8], V89.2)2	14,320	4.6	4.6
Pedal cyclist, other (V10'-V11, V12'-V14[.0'-.2], V15'-V18, V19[.0'-.3,.8,.9])2	242	0.1	0.1
Pedestrian, other (V01, V02'-V04[.0], V05, V06, V09[.0,.1,.3,.9])2	1,074	0.3	0.3
Other land transport (V20'-V28[.0'-.2], V29'-V79[.0'-.3],V80[.0'-.2,.6'-.9], V81'-V82[.0,.2'-.9], V83'-V86[.4'-.9],V87.9,V88[.0'-.9], V89[.0,.1,.3,.9],X82, Y03, Y32)	1,524	0.5	0.5
Unintentional (V20'-V28[.0'-.2], V29'-V79[.0'-.3], V80(.0'-.2,.6'-.9), V81'-V82[.0,.2'-.9], V83'-V86[.4'-.9], V87.9, V88[.0'-.9], V89[.0,.1,.3,.9])	1,358	0.4	0.4
Suicide (X82)	114	0.0	0.0
Homicide (Y03)	39	0.0	0.0
Undetermined (Y32)	13	*	*
Other transport (*U01.1, V90'-V99, Y36.1)	875	0.3	0.3
Unintentional (V90'-V99)	875	0.3	0.3
Homicide (*U01.1)	-	*	*
Legal intervention/war (Y36.1)	-	*	*
Natural/Environmental (W42'-W43, W53'-W64, W92'-W99, X20'-X39, X51'-X57)[2]	1,576	0.5	0.5
Overexertion (X50)[2]	10	*	*
Poisoning (*U01[.6'-.7], X40'-X49, X60'-X69, X85'-X90, Y10'-Y19, Y35.2)	42,917	13.9	13.7
Unintentional (X40'-X49)	33,041	10.7	10.6
Suicide (X60'-X69)	6,599	2.1	2.1
Homicide (*U01[.6'-.7], X85'-X90)	79	0.0	0.0
Undetermined (Y10'-Y19)	3,197	1.0	1.0
Legal intervention/war (Y35.2)	1	*	*

Table 2-21. Number of Deaths, Death Rates, and Age-Adjusted Death Rates for Injury Deaths, by Mechanism and Intent of Death, 2010—*Continued*

(Number; rates per 100,000 population; age-adjusted rates per 100,000 U.S. standard population.)

Mechanism and intent of death (based on the ICD, Tenth Revision)	Number	Rate	Age-adjusted rate[1]
Struck by or Against (W20'-W22, W50'-W52, X79, Y00, Y04, Y29, Y35.3)	912	0.3	0.3
Unintentional (W20'-W22, W50'-W52)	788	0.3	0.2
Suicide (X79)	-	*	*
Homicide (Y00,Y04)	123	0.0	0.0
Undetermined (Y29)	1	*	*
Legal intervention/war (Y35.3)	-	*	*
Suffocation (W75'-W84, X70, X91,Y20)	16,362	5.3	5.2
Unintentional (W75'-W84)	6,165	2.0	1.9
Suicide (X70)	9,493	3.1	3.1
Homicide (X91)	544	0.2	0.2
Undetermined (Y20)	160	0.1	0.0
Other Specified, Classifiable (*U01[.0,.2,.5], *U03.0, W23, W35'-W41, W44,W49, W85'-W91, X75, X81, X96, Y02, Y05'- Y07, Y25, Y31, Y35[.1,.5], Y36[.0,.2,.4'-.8], Y85)	2,002	0.6	0.7
Unintentional (W23, W35'-W41, W44, W49, W85'-W91, Y85)	1,395	0.5	0.5
Suicide (*U03.0, X75, X81)	337	0.1	0.1
Homicide (*U01[.0,.2,.5], X96, Y02, Y05'-Y07)	211	0.1	0.1
Undetermined (Y25, Y31)	15	*	*
Legal intervention/war (Y35[.1,.5], Y36[.0,.2,.4'-.8])	44	0.0	0.0
Other Specified, Not Elsewhere Classified (*U01.8, *U02, X58, X83, Y08, Y33, Y35.6, Y86'-Y87, Y89[.0'-.1])	1,973	0.6	0.6
Unintentional (X58, Y86)	1,023	0.3	0.3
Suicide (X83, Y87.0)	245	0.1	0.1
Homicide (*U01.8, *U02, Y08, Y87.1)	495	0.2	0.2
Undetermined (Y33, Y87.2)	184	0.1	0.1
Legal intervention/war (Y35.6, Y89[.0,.1])	26	0.0	0.0
Unspecified (*U01.9, *U03.9, X59, X84, Y09, Y34, Y35.7, Y36.9, Y89.9)	8,230	2.7	2.5
Unintentional (X59)	5,688	1.8	1.7
Suicide (*U03.9, X84)	190	0.1	0.1
Homicide (*U01.9, Y09)	1,735	0.6	0.6
Undetermined (Y34, Y89.9)	611	0.2	0.2
Legal intervention/war (Y35.7, Y36.9)	6	*	*

- = Quantity zero.   * = Figure does not meet standard of reliability or precision.   0.0 = Quantity more than zero but less than 0.05.   [1]For method of computation, see chapter notes.   [2]Codes *U01.3 and Y36.3 cannot be divided separately into the subcategories shown below; therefore, subcategories may not add to the total.   [3]Intent of death is unintentional.

Table 2-22A. Leading Causes of Death and Numbers of Death, by Sex, 1980 and 2010

(Number.)

Sex and rank order	1980		Sex and rank order	2010	
	Cause of death	Deaths		Cause of death	Deaths
All Persons			**All Persons**		
Rank	All causes	1,989,841	Rank	All causes	2,468,435
1	Diseases of heart	761,085	1	Diseases of heart	597,689
2	Malignant neoplasms	416,509	2	Malignant neoplasms	574,743
3	Cerebrovascular diseases	170,225	3	Chronic lower respiratory diseases	138,080
4	Unintentional injuries	105,718	4	Cerebrovascular diseases	129,476
5	Chronic obstructive pulmonary diseases	56,050	5	Unintentional injuries	120,859
6	Pneumonia and influenza	54,619	6	Alzheimer's disease	83,494
7	Diabetes mellitus	34,851	7	Diabetes mellitus	69,071
8	Chronic liver disease and cirrhosis	30,583	8	Nephritis, nephrotic syndrome and nephrosis	50,476
9	Atherosclerosis	29,449	9	Influenza and pneumonia	50,097
10	Suicide	26,869	10	Suicide	38,364
Male			**Male**		
Rank	All causes	1,075,078	Rank	All causes	1,232,432
1	Diseases of heart	405,661	1	Diseases of heart	307,384
2	Malignant neoplasms	225,948	2	Malignant neoplasms	301,037
3	Unintentional injuries	74,180	3	Unintentional injuries	75,921
4	Cerebrovascular diseases	69,973	4	Chronic lower respiratory diseases	65,423
5	Chronic obstructive pulmonary diseases	38,625	5	Cerebrovascular diseases	52,367
6	Pneumonia and influenza	27,574	6	Diabetes mellitus	35,490
7	Suicide	20,505	7	Suicide	30,277
8	Chronic liver disease and cirrhosis	19,768	8	Alzheimer's disease	25,364
9	Homicide	18,779	9	Nephritis, nephrotic syndrome and nephrosis	24,865
10	Diabetes mellitus	14,325	10	Influenza and pneumonia	23,615
Female			**Female**		
Rank	All causes	914,763	Rank	All causes	1,236,003
1	Diseases of heart	355,424	1	Diseases of heart	290,305
2	Malignant neoplasms	190,561	2	Malignant neoplasms	273,706
3	Cerebrovascular diseases	100,252	3	Cerebrovascular diseases	77,109
4	Unintentional injuries	31,538	4	Chronic lower respiratory diseases	72,657
5	Pneumonia and influenza	27,045	5	Alzheimer's disease	58,130
6	Diabetes mellitus	20,526	6	Unintentional injuries	44,938
7	Atherosclerosis	17,848	7	Diabetes mellitus	33,581
8	Chronic obstructive pulmonary diseases	17,425	8	Influenza and pneumonia	26,482
9	Chronic liver disease and cirrhosis	10,815	9	Nephritis, nephrotic syndrome and nephrosis	25,611
10	Certain conditions originating in the perinatal period	9,815	10	Septicemia	18,743

NA = Not available.

Table 2-22B. Leading Causes of Death and Numbers of Death, by Race, 1980 and 2010

(Number.)

Sex, race, Hispanic origin, and rank order	1980 Cause of death	Deaths	Sex, race, Hispanic origin, and rank order	2010 Cause of death	Deaths
White			**White**		
Rank	All causes	1,738,607	Rank	All causes	2,114,749
1	Diseases of heart	683,347	1	Diseases of heart	514,323
2	Malignant neoplasms	368,162	2	Malignant neoplasms	491,686
3	Cerebrovascular diseases	148,734	3	Chronic lower respiratory diseases	127,176
4	Unintentional injuries	90,122	4	Cerebrovascular diseases	109,119
5	Chronic obstructive pulmonary diseases	52,375	5	Unintentional injuries	104,945
6	Pneumonia and influenza	48,369	6	Alzheimer's disease	76,928
7	Diabetes mellitus	28,868	7	Diabetes mellitus	54,250
8	Atherosclerosis	27,069	8	Influenza and pneumonia	43,296
9	Chronic liver disease and cirrhosis	25,240	9	Nephritis, nephrotic syndrome and nephrosis	40,205
10	Suicide	24,829	10	Suicide	34,690
Black			**Black**		
Rank	All causes	233,135	Rank	All causes	286,959
1	Diseases of heart	72,956	1	Diseases of heart	69,083
2	Malignant neoplasms	45,037	2	Malignant neoplasms	65,930
3	Cerebrovascular diseases	20,135	3	Cerebrovascular diseases	15,965
4	Unintentional injuries	13,480	4	Diabetes mellitus	12,126
5	Homicide	10,172	5	Unintentional injuries	12,069
6	Certain conditions originating in the perinatal period	6,961	6	Nephritis, nephrotic syndrome and nephrosis	8,841
7	Pneumonia and influenza	5,648	7	Chronic lower respiratory diseases	8,715
8	Diabetes mellitus	5,544	8	Homicide	7,818
9	Chronic liver disease and cirrhosis	4,790	9	Septicemia	6,001
10	Nephritis, nephrotic syndrome, and nephrosis	3,416	10	Alzheimer's disease	5,220
American Indian or Alaska Native			**American Indian or Alaska Native**		
Rank	All causes	6,923	Rank	All causes	15,565
1	Diseases of heart	1,494	1	Malignant neoplasms	2,962
2	Unintentional injuries	1,290	2	Diseases of heart	2,793
3	Malignant neoplasms	770	3	Unintentional injuries	1,701
4	Chronic liver disease and cirrhosis	410	4	Diabetes mellitus	857
5	Cerebrovascular diseases	322	5	Chronic liver disease and cirrhosis	787
6	Pneumonia and influenza	257	6	Chronic lower respiratory diseases	702
7	Homicide	217	7	Cerebrovascular diseases	559
8	Diabetes mellitus	210	8	Suicide	469
9	Certain conditions originating in the perinatal period	199	9	Nephritis, nephrotic syndrome and nephrosis	339
10	Suicide	181	10	Influenza and pneumonia	326
Asian or Pacific Islander			**Asian or Pacific Islander**		
Rank	All causes	11,071	Rank	All causes	51,162
1	Diseases of heart	3,265	1	Malignant neoplasms	14,165
2	Malignant neoplasms	2,522	2	Diseases of heart	11,490
3	Cerebrovascular diseases	1,028	3	Cerebrovascular diseases	3,833
4	Unintentional injuries	810	4	Unintentional injuries	2,144
5	Pneumonia and influenza	342	5	Diabetes mellitus	1,838
6	Suicide	249	6	Influenza and pneumonia	1,539
7	Certain conditions originating in the perinatal period	246	7	Chronic lower respiratory diseases	1,487
8	Diabetes mellitus	227	8	Nephritis, nephrotic syndrome and nephrosis	1,091
9	Homicide	211	9	Alzheimer's disease	1,082
10	Chronic obstructive pulmonary diseases	207	10	Suicide	1,061
Hispanic or Latino [1]			**Hispanic or Latino [1]**		
Rank	NA	NA	Rank	All causes	144,490
1	NA	NA	1	Malignant neoplasms	31,119
2	NA	NA	2	Diseases of heart	30,006
3	NA	NA	3	Unintentional injuries	10,476
4	NA	NA	4	Cerebrovascular diseases	7,274
5	NA	NA	5	Diabetes mellitus	6,556
6	NA	NA	6	Chronic liver disease and cirrhosis	4,348
7	NA	NA	7	Chronic lower respiratory diseases	4,172
8	NA	NA	8	Alzheimer's disease	3,427
9	NA	NA	9	Nephritis, nephrotic syndrome and nephrosis	3,252
10	NA	NA	10	Influenza and pneumonia	3,025

NA = Not available.   [1]Persons of Hispanic origin may be of any race.

Table 2-22C. Leading Causes of Death and Numbers of Death, by Race for Males, 1980 and 2010

(Number.)

Sex, race, Hispanic origin, and rank order	1980 Cause of death	Deaths	Sex, race, Hispanic origin, and rank order	2010 Cause of death	Deaths
White Male			**White Male**		
Rank	All causes	933,878	Rank	All causes	1,051,514
1	Diseases of heart	364,679	1	Diseases of heart	264,425
2	Malignant neoplasms	198,188	2	Malignant neoplasms	258,272
3	Unintentional injuries	62,963	3	Unintentional injuries	65,360
4	Cerebrovascular diseases	60,095	4	Chronic lower respiratory diseases	59,632
5	Chronic obstructive pulmonary diseases	35,977	5	Cerebrovascular diseases	43,424
6	Pneumonia and influenza	23,810	6	Diabetes mellitus	28,486
7	Suicide	18,901	7	Suicide	27,422
8	Chronic liver disease and cirrhosis	16,407	8	Alzheimer's disease	23,442
9	Diabetes mellitus	12,125	9	Influenza and pneumonia	20,238
10	Atherosclerosis	10,543	10	Nephritis, nephrotic syndrome and nephrosis	20,172
Black or African American Male			**Black or African American male**		
Rank	All causes	130,138	Rank	All causes	145,802
1	Diseases of heart	37,877	1	Diseases of heart	35,089
2	Malignant neoplasms	25,861	2	Malignant neoplasms	33,967
3	Unintentional injuries	9,701	3	Unintentional injuries	8,074
4	Cerebrovascular diseases	9,194	4	Cerebrovascular diseases	6,938
5	Homicide	8,274	5	Homicide	6,704
6	Certain conditions originating in the perinatal period	3,869	6	Diabetes mellitus	5,640
7	Pneumonia and influenza	3,386	7	Chronic lower respiratory diseases	4,532
8	Chronic liver disease and cirrhosis	3,020	8	Nephritis, nephrotic syndrome and nephrosis	4,016
9	Chronic obstructive pulmonary diseases	2,429	9	Human immunodeficiency virus (HIV) disease	3,047
10	Diabetes mellitus	2,010	10	Septicemia	2,691
American Indian or Alaska Native Male			**American Indian or Alaska Native Male**		
Rank	All causes	4,193	Rank	All causes	8,516
1	Unintentional injuries	946	1	Diseases of heart	1,608
2	Diseases of heart	917	2	Malignant neoplasms	1,588
3	Malignant neoplasms	408	3	Unintentional injuries	1,150
4	Chronic liver disease and cirrhosis	239	4	Diabetes mellitus	432
5	Cerebrovascular diseases	163	5	Chronic liver disease and cirrhosis	429
6	Homicide	162	6	Chronic lower respiratory diseases	349
7	Pneumonia and influenza	148	7	Suicide	344
8	Suicide	147	8	Cerebrovascular diseases	258
9	Certain conditions originating in the perinatal period	107	9	Homicide	204
10	Diabetes mellitus	86	10	Influenza and pneumonia	172
Asian or Pacific Islander Male			**Asian or Pacific Islander Male**		
Rank	All causes	6,809	Rank	All causes	26,600
1	Diseases of heart	2,174	1	Malignant neoplasms	7,210
2	Malignant neoplasms	1,485	2	Diseases of heart	6,262
3	Unintentional injuries	556	3	Cerebrovascular diseases	1,747
4	Cerebrovascular diseases	521	4	Unintentional injuries	1,337
5	Pneumonia and influenza	227	5	Diabetes mellitus	932
6	Suicide	159	6	Chronic lower respiratory diseases	910
7	Chronic obstructive pulmonary diseases	158	7	Influenza and pneumonia	825
8	Homicide	151	8	Suicide	756
9	Certain conditions originating in the perinatal period	128	9	Nephritis, nephrotic syndrome and nephrosis	524
10	Diabetes mellitus	103	10	Alzheimer's disease	345
Hispanic or Latino Male [1]			**Hispanic or Latino Male [1]**		
Rank	NA	NA	Rank	All causes	79,622
1	NA	NA	1	Malignant neoplasms	16,450
2	NA	NA	2	Diseases of heart	16,421
3	NA	NA	3	Unintentional injuries	7,594
4	NA	NA	4	Cerebrovascular diseases	3,382
5	NA	NA	5	Diabetes mellitus	3,372
6	NA	NA	6	Chronic liver disease and cirrhosis	3,067
7	NA	NA	7	Homicide	2,435
8	NA	NA	8	Chronic lower respiratory diseases	2,174
9	NA	NA	9	Suicide	2,168
10	NA	NA	10	Nephritis, nephrotic syndrome and nephrosis	1,670

NA = Not available.   [1] Persons of Hispanic origin may be of any race.

Table 2-22D. Leading Causes of Death and Numbers of Death, by Race for Females, 1980 and 2010

(Number.)

Sex, race, Hispanic origin, and rank order	1980		Sex, race, Hispanic origin, and rank order	2010	
	Cause of death	Deaths		Cause of death	Deaths
White Female			**White Female**		
Rank	All causes	804,729	Rank	All causes	1,063,235
1	Diseases of heart	318,668	1	Diseases of heart	249,898
2	Malignant neoplasms	169,974	2	Malignant neoplasms	233,414
3	Cerebrovascular diseases	88,639	3	Chronic lower respiratory diseases	67,544
4	Unintentional injuries	27,159	4	Cerebrovascular diseases	65,695
5	Pneumonia and influenza	24,559	5	Alzheimer's disease	53,486
6	Diabetes mellitus	16,743	6	Unintentional injuries	39,585
7	Atherosclerosis	16,526	7	Diabetes mellitus	25,764
8	Chronic obstructive pulmonary diseases	16,398	8	Influenza and pneumonia	23,058
9	Chronic liver disease and cirrhosis	8,833	9	Nephritis, nephrotic syndrome and nephrosis	20,033
10	Certain conditions originating in the perinatal period	6,512	10	Septicemia	15,009
Black or African American Female			**Black or African American Female**		
Rank	All causes	102,997	Rank	All causes	141,157
1	Diseases of heart	35,079	1	Diseases of heart	33,994
2	Malignant neoplasms	19,176	2	Malignant neoplasms	31,963
3	Cerebrovascular diseases	10,941	3	Cerebrovascular diseases	9,027
4	Unintentional injuries	3,779	4	Diabetes mellitus	6,486
5	Diabetes mellitus	3,534	5	Nephritis, nephrotic syndrome and nephrosis	4,825
6	Certain conditions originating in the perinatal period	3,092	6	Chronic lower respiratory diseases	4,183
7	Pneumonia and influenza	2,262	7	Unintentional injuries	3,995
8	Homicide	1,898	8	Alzheimer's disease	3,732
9	Chronic liver disease and cirrhosis	1,770	9	Septicemia	3,310
10	Nephritis, nephrotic syndrome, and nephrosis	1,722	10	Essential hypertension and hypertensive renal disease	2,898
American Indian or Alaska Native Female			**American Indian or Alaska Native Female**		
Rank	All causes	2,730	Rank	All causes	7,049
1	Diseases of heart	577	1	Malignant neoplasms	1,374
2	Malignant neoplasms	362	2	Diseases of heart	1,185
3	Unintentional injuries	344	3	Unintentional injuries	551
4	Chronic liver disease and cirrhosis	171	4	Diabetes mellitus	425
5	Cerebrovascular diseases	159	5	Chronic liver disease and cirrhosis	358
6	Diabetes mellitus	124	6	Chronic lower respiratory diseases	353
7	Pneumonia and influenza	109	7	Cerebrovascular diseases	301
8	Certain conditions originating in the perinatal period	92	8	Nephritis, nephrotic syndrome and nephrosis	186
9	Nephritis, nephrotic syndrome, and nephrosis	56	9	Alzheimer's disease	175
10	Homicide	55	10	Influenza and pneumonia	154
Asian or Pacific Islander Female			**Asian or Pacific Islander Female**		
Rank	All causes	4,262	Rank	All causes	24,562
1	Diseases of heart	1,091	1	Malignant neoplasms	6,955
2	Malignant neoplasms	1,037	2	Diseases of heart	5,228
3	Cerebrovascular diseases	507	3	Cerebrovascular diseases	2,086
4	Unintentional injuries	254	4	Diabetes mellitus	906
5	Diabetes mellitus	124	5	Unintentional injuries	807
6	Certain conditions originating in the perinatal period	118	6	Alzheimer's disease	737
7	Pneumonia and influenza	115	7	Influenza and pneumonia	714
8	Congenital anomalies	104	8	Chronic lower respiratory diseases	577
9	Suicide	90	9	Nephritis, nephrotic syndrome and nephrosis	567
10	Homicide	60	10	Essential hypertension and hypertensive renal disease	477
Hispanic or Latina Female [1]			**Hispanic or Latina Female** [1]		
Rank	NA	NA	Rank	All causes	64,868
1	NA	NA	1	Malignant neoplasms	14,669
2	NA	NA	2	Diseases of heart	13,585
3	NA	NA	3	Cerebrovascular diseases	3,892
4	NA	NA	4	Diabetes mellitus	3,184
5	NA	NA	5	Unintentional injuries	2,882
6	NA	NA	6	Alzheimer's disease	2,256
7	NA	NA	7	Chronic lower respiratory diseases	1,998
8	NA	NA	8	Nephritis, nephrotic syndrome and nephrosis	1,582
9	NA	NA	9	Influenza and pneumonia	1,460
10	NA	NA	10	Chronic liver disease and cirrhosis	1,281

NA = Not available.   [1]Persons of Hispanic origin may be of any race.

Table 2-23A. Leading Causes of Death and Numbers of Deaths for Infants to Persons Aged 24 Years, 1980 and 2010

(Number.)

Under 1 Year

Rank	1980 Cause of death	Deaths	2010 Cause of death	Deaths
	All causes	45,526	All causes	24,586
1	Congenital anomalies	9,220	Congenital malformations, deformations and chromosomal abnormalities	5,107
2	Sudden infant death syndrome	5,510	Disorders related to short gestation and low birth weight, not elsewhere classified	4,148
3	Respiratory distress syndrome	4,989	Sudden infant death syndrome	2,063
4	Disorders relating to short gestation and unspecified low birthweight	3,648	Newborn affected by maternal complications of pregnancy	1,561
5	Newborn affected by maternal complications of pregnancy	1,572	Unintentional injuries	1,110
6	Intrauterine hypoxia and birth asphyxia	1,497	Newborn affected by complications of placenta, cord and membranes	1,030
7	Unintentional injuries	1,166	Bacterial sepsis of newborn	583
8	Birth trauma	1,058	Respiratory distress of newborn	514
9	Pneumonia and influenza	1,012	Diseases of circulatory system	507
10	Newborn affected by complications of placenta, cord, and membranes	985	Necrotizing enterocolitis of newborn	472

1 to 4 Years

Rank	1980 Cause of death	Deaths	2010 Cause of death	Deaths
	All causes	8,187	All causes	4,316
1	Unintentional injuries	3,313	Unintentional injuries	1,394
2	Congenital anomalies	1,026	Congenital malformations, deformations and chromosomal abnormalities	507
3	Malignant neoplasms	573	Homicide	385
4	Diseases of heart	338	Malignant neoplasms	346
5	Homicide	319	Diseases of heart	159
6	Pneumonia and influenza	267	Influenza and pneumonia	91
7	Meningitis	223	Septicemia	62
8	Meningococcal infection	110	In situ neoplasms, benign neoplasms and neoplasms of uncertain or unknown behavior	59
9	Certain conditions originating in the perinatal period	84	Certain conditions originating in the perinatal period	52
10	Septicemia	71	Chronic lower respiratory diseases	51

5 to 14 Years

Rank	1980 Cause of death	Deaths	2010 Cause of death	Deaths
	All causes	10,689	All causes	5,279
1	Unintentional injuries	5,224	Unintentional injuries	1,643
2	Malignant neoplasms	1,497	Malignant neoplasms	916
3	Congenital anomalies	561	Congenital malformations, deformations and chromosomal abnormalities	298
4	Homicide	415	Suicide	274
5	Diseases of heart	330	Homicide	261
6	Pneumonia and influenza	194	Diseases of heart	185
7	Suicide	142	Chronic lower respiratory diseases	133
8	Benign neoplasms	104	Cerebrovascular diseases	90
9	Cerebrovascular diseases	95	In situ neoplasms, benign neoplasms and neoplasms of uncertain or unknown behavior	82
10	Chronic obstructive pulmonary diseases	85	Influenza and pneumonia	71

15 to 24 Years

Rank	1980 Cause of death	Deaths	2010 Cause of death	Deaths
	All causes	49,027	All causes	29,551
1	Unintentional injuries	26,206	Unintentional injuries	12,341
2	Homicide	6,537	Homicide	4,678
3	Suicide	5,239	Suicide	4,600
4	Malignant neoplasms	2,683	Malignant neoplasms	1,604
5	Diseases of heart	1,223	Diseases of heart	1,028
6	Congenital anomalies	600	Congenital malformations, deformations and chromosomal abnormalities	412
7	Cerebrovascular diseases	418	Cerebrovascular diseases	190
8	Pneumonia and influenza	348	Influenza and pneumonia	181
9	Chronic obstructive pulmonary diseases	141	Diabetes mellitus	165
10	Anemias	133	Pregnancy, childbirth, and the puerperium	163

Table 2-23B. Leading Causes of Death and Numbers of Deaths for Persons 25 Years of Age and Over, 1980 and 2010

(Number.)

Age and rank order	1980 Cause of death	Deaths	Age and rank order	2010 Cause of death	Deaths
25 to 44 Years			**25 to 44 Years**		
Rank	All causes	108,658	Rank	All causes	112,292
1	Unintentional injuries	26,722	1	Unintentional injuries	29,365
2	Malignant neoplasms	17,551	2	Malignant neoplasms	15,428
3	Diseases of heart	14,513	3	Diseases of heart	13,816
4	Homicide	10,983	4	Suicide	12,306
5	Suicide	9,855	5	Homicide	6,731
6	Chronic liver disease and cirrhosis	4,782	6	Chronic liver disease and cirrhosis	2,910
7	Cerebrovascular diseases	3,154	7	Human immunodeficiency virus (HIV) disease	2,639
8	Diabetes mellitus	1,472	8	Cerebrovascular diseases	2,421
9	Pneumonia and influenza	1,467	9	Diabetes mellitus	2,395
10	Congenital anomalies	817	10	Influenza and pneumonia	1,158
45 to 64 Years			**45 to 64 Years**		
Rank	All causes	425,338	Rank	All causes	494,009
1	Diseases of heart	148,322	1	Malignant neoplasms	159,712
2	Malignant neoplasms	135,675	2	Diseases of heart	104,806
3	Cerebrovascular diseases	19,909	3	Unintentional injuries	33,690
4	Unintentional injuries	18,140	4	Chronic lower respiratory diseases	18,694
5	Chronic liver disease and cirrhosis	16,089	5	Chronic liver disease and cirrhosis	18,415
6	Chronic obstructive pulmonary diseases	11,514	6	Diabetes mellitus	17,287
7	Diabetes mellitus	7,977	7	Cerebrovascular diseases	16,603
8	Suicide	7,079	8	Suicide	15,183
9	Pneumonia and influenza	5,804	9	Nephritis, nephrotic syndrome and nephrosis	7,304
10	Homicide	4,019	10	Septicemia	6,937
65 Years and Over			**65 Years and Over**		
Rank	All causes	1,341,848	Rank	All causes	1,798,276
1	Diseases of heart	595,406	1	Diseases of heart	477,338
2	Malignant neoplasms	258,389	2	Malignant neoplasms	396,670
3	Cerebrovascular diseases	146,417	3	Chronic lower respiratory diseases	118,031
4	Pneumonia and influenza	45,512	4	Cerebrovascular diseases	109,990
5	Chronic obstructive pulmonary diseases	43,587	5	Alzheimer's disease	82,616
6	Atherosclerosis	28,081	6	Diabetes mellitus	49,191
7	Diabetes mellitus	25,216	7	Influenza and pneumonia	42,846
8	Unintentional injuries	24,844	8	Nephritis, nephrotic syndrome and nephrosis	41,994
9	Nephritis, nephrotic syndrome, and nephrosis	12,968	9	Unintentional injuries	41,300
10	Chronic liver disease and cirrhosis	9,519	10	Septicemia	26,310

Table 2-24. Deaths from Selected Occupational Diseases Among Persons 15 Years of Age and Over, Selected Years, 1980–2010

(Number of deaths.)

Cause of death	1980[1]	1985[1]	1990[1]	1995[1]	2000[2]	2005[2]	2006[2]	2007[2]	2008[2]	2009[2]	2010[2]
Multiple Cause of Death											
Angiosarcoma of liver[3]	NA	NA	NA	NA	16	26	23	22	17	27	29
Malignant mesothelioma[4]	699	715	874	897	2,531	2,704	2,588	2,606	2,709	2,753	2,744
Pneumoconiosis[5]	4,151	3,783	3,644	3,151	2,859	2,425	2,308	2,189	2,155	1,993	2,028
Coal workers' pneumoconiosis	2,576	2,615	1,990	1,413	949	652	654	524	470	480	486
Asbestosis	339	534	948	1,169	1,486	1,416	1,340	1,393	1,341	1,255	1,308
Silicosis	448	334	308	242	151	160	126	122	146	121	101
Other (including unspecified)	814	321	413	343	290	222	206	163	215	158	146
Underlying Cause of Death											
Angiosarcoma of liver[3]	NA	NA	NA	NA	15	23	21	20	16	25	28
Malignant mesothelioma[4]	531	573	725	780	2,384	2,553	2,452	2,432	2,538	2,606	2,573
Pneumoconiosis	1,581	1,355	1,335	1,117	1,142	983	907	898	891	830	820
Coal workers' pneumoconiosis	982	958	734	533	389	270	266	209	183	206	213
Asbestosis	101	139	302	355	558	532	485	538	520	485	486
Silicosis	207	143	150	114	71	74	67	72	85	66	52
Other (including unspecified)	291	115	149	115	124	107	89	79	103	73	69

NA = Not available. [1]For the period 1980–1998, underlying cause of death was coded according to the 9th Revision of the International Classification of Diseases (ICD). [2]Starting with 1999 data, ICD-10 was introduced for coding cause of death. Discontinuities exist between 1998 and 1999 due to ICD-10 coding and classification changes. [3]Prior to 1999, there was no discrete code for this condition. [4]Prior to 1999, the combined ICD-9 categories of malignant neoplasm of peritoneum and malignant neoplasm of pleura served as a crude surrogate for malignant mesothelioma category under ICD-10. [5]For multiple cause of death, counts for pneumoconiosis subgroups may sum to slightly more than total pneumoconiosis due to the reporting of more than one type of pneumoconiosis on some death certificates.

Figure 2-6. Number of Fatal Occupational Injuries, by Selected Industry, 2012

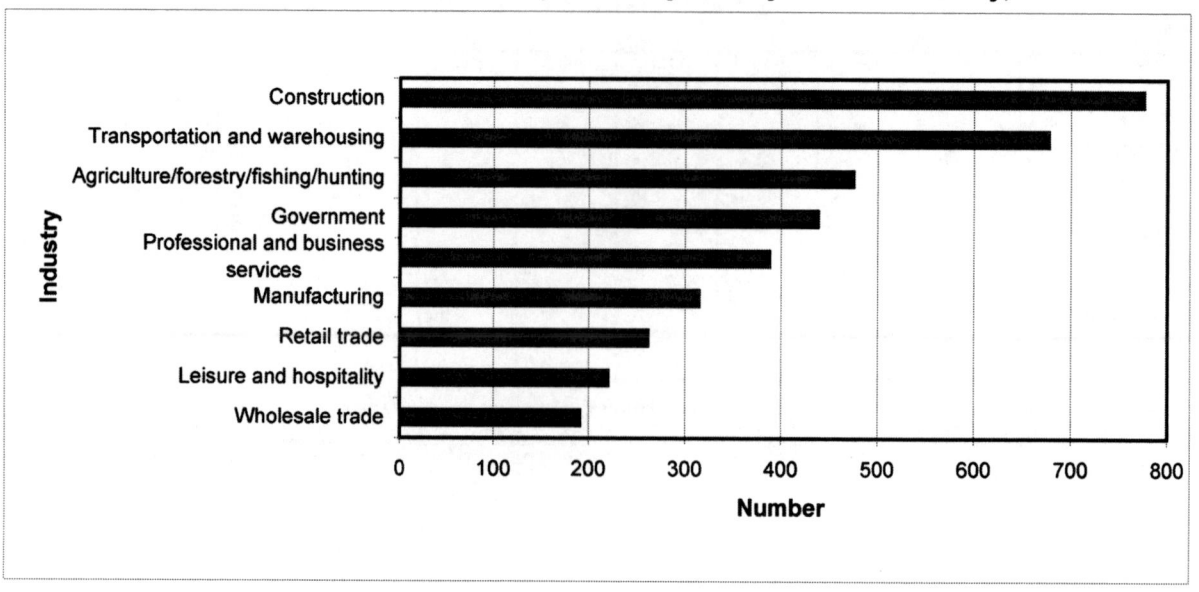

Figure 2-7. Number of Fatal Occupational Injuries, by Selected Occupation, 2012

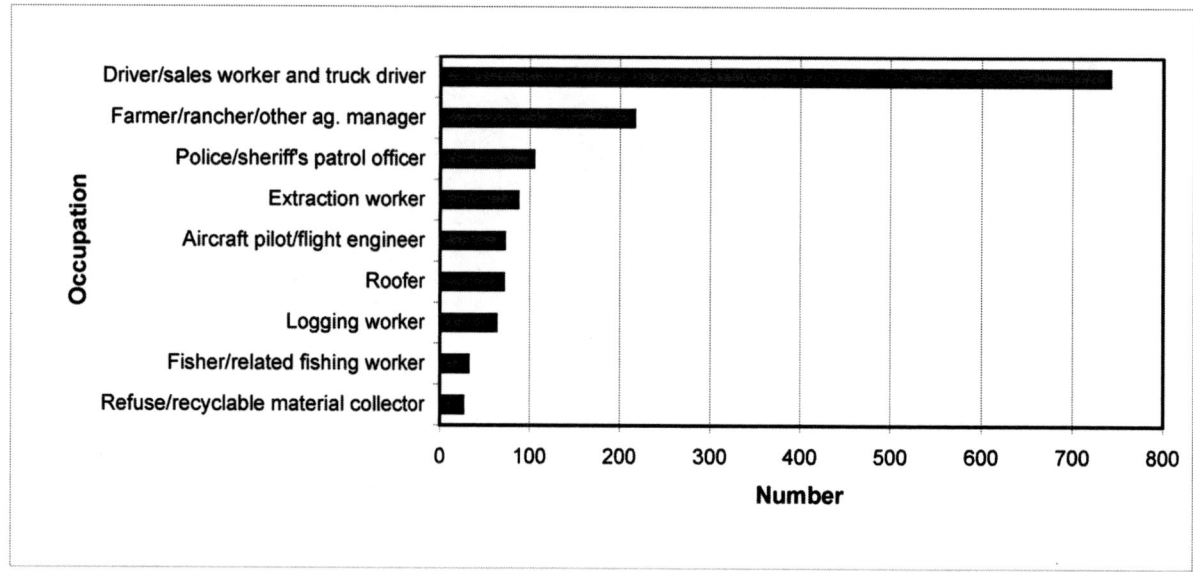

Table 2-25. Death Rates for Motor Vehicle–Related Injuries, by Sex and Age, Selected Years, 1950–2010

(Rate per 100,000 population.)

Sex, race, Hispanic origin, and age	1950[1,2]	1960[1,2]	1970[2]	1980[2]	1985[2]	1990[2]	1995[2]	2000[3]	2005[3]	2006[3]	2007[3]	2008[3]	2009[3]	2010[3]
	Deaths per 100,000 resident population													
All Persons														
All ages, age-adjusted[4]	24.6	23.1	27.6	22.3	18.6	18.5	16.3	15.4	15.2	15.0	14.4	12.9	11.6	11.3
All ages, crude	23.1	21.3	26.9	23.5	19.3	18.8	16.3	15.4	15.3	15.2	14.6	13.1	11.8	11.4
Under 1 year	8.4	8.1	9.8	7.0	4.9	4.9	4.7	4.4	3.6	3.5	3.0	2.5	2.4	2.0
1 to 14 years	9.8	8.6	10.5	8.2	7.0	6.0	5.3	4.3	3.7	3.4	3.2	2.6	2.5	2.3
1 to 4 years	11.5	10.0	11.5	9.2	7.2	6.3	5.2	4.2	3.9	3.7	3.4	2.9	2.9	2.8
5 to 14 years	8.8	7.9	10.2	7.9	6.9	5.9	5.3	4.3	3.6	3.3	3.2	2.5	2.4	2.2
15 to 24 years	34.4	38.0	47.2	44.8	35.7	34.1	28.9	26.9	25.7	25.7	24.5	20.6	17.6	16.6
15 to 19 years	29.6	33.9	43.6	43.0	33.5	33.1	28.1	26.0	23.1	22.6	21.4	17.4	15.2	13.6
20 to 24 years	38.8	42.9	51.3	46.6	37.6	35.0	29.7	28.0	28.3	28.9	27.7	24.0	20.2	19.7
25 to 34 years	24.6	24.3	30.9	29.1	23.0	23.6	19.2	17.3	18.4	18.7	17.8	16.3	14.5	14.0
35 to 44 years	20.3	19.3	24.9	20.9	17.2	16.9	15.3	15.3	15.5	15.4	14.9	13.4	12.2	11.6
45 to 64 years	25.2	23.0	26.5	18.0	15.4	15.7	14.1	14.3	14.8	14.8	14.1	13.3	12.2	11.9
45 to 54 years	22.2	21.4	25.5	18.6	15.2	15.6	13.8	14.2	15.1	15.3	14.9	13.7	12.7	12.0
55 to 64 years	29.0	25.1	27.9	17.4	15.6	15.9	14.5	14.4	14.5	14.1	13.2	12.8	11.5	11.9
65 years and over	43.1	34.7	36.2	22.5	21.7	23.1	22.6	21.4	20.1	19.0	18.7	16.9	15.8	16.0
65 to 74 years	39.1	31.4	32.8	19.2	17.9	18.6	17.5	16.5	16.5	15.2	14.9	13.8	12.7	12.3
75 to 84 years	52.7	41.8	43.5	28.1	27.4	29.1	28.4	25.7	22.9	22.2	21.7	19.2	18.6	18.8
85 years and over	45.1	37.9	34.2	27.6	26.5	31.2	31.0	30.4	27.3	25.5	25.3	23.2	20.9	23.8
Male														
All ages, age-adjusted[4]	38.5	35.4	41.5	33.6	27.2	26.5	22.8	21.7	21.9	21.5	21.0	18.9	16.8	16.2
All ages, crude	35.4	31.8	39.7	35.3	28.0	26.7	22.4	21.3	21.8	21.6	21.0	18.9	16.9	16.3
Under 1 year	9.1	8.6	9.3	7.3	5.0	5.0	4.9	4.6	3.6	3.4	2.7	2.9	2.6	2.2
1 to 14 years	12.3	10.7	13.0	10.0	8.5	7.0	6.1	4.9	4.1	3.7	3.7	3.1	2.9	2.7
1 to 4 years	13.0	11.5	12.9	10.2	8.3	6.9	5.6	4.7	4.3	3.9	3.8	3.2	3.4	3.0
5 to 14 years	11.9	10.4	13.1	9.9	8.6	7.0	6.3	5.0	4.1	3.7	3.7	3.0	2.7	2.5
15 to 24 years	56.7	61.2	73.2	68.4	52.7	49.5	40.5	37.4	36.3	36.3	34.6	29.3	24.5	23.1
15 to 19 years	46.3	51.7	64.1	62.6	46.5	45.5	36.1	33.9	29.9	29.5	27.7	22.6	19.2	17.8
20 to 24 years	66.7	73.2	84.4	74.3	58.2	53.3	45.0	41.2	42.8	43.4	41.9	36.3	30.0	28.5
25 to 34 years	40.8	40.1	49.4	46.3	35.9	35.7	28.1	25.5	27.9	28.5	27.2	25.2	21.7	21.0
35 to 44 years	32.5	29.9	37.7	31.7	25.2	24.7	21.7	22.0	22.5	22.1	22.1	19.9	18.2	16.9
45 to 64 years	37.7	33.3	38.9	26.5	22.0	21.9	19.5	20.2	21.6	21.6	20.9	19.7	18.2	17.9
45 to 54 years	33.6	31.6	37.2	27.6	21.9	22.0	19.3	20.4	22.2	22.6	22.2	20.2	19.0	17.9
55 to 64 years	43.1	35.6	40.9	25.4	22.1	21.7	19.6	19.8	20.7	20.3	19.2	19.0	17.2	17.8
65 years and over	66.6	52.1	54.4	33.9	30.4	32.1	30.7	29.5	28.4	26.4	26.9	24.1	22.0	22.2
65 to 74 years	59.1	45.8	47.3	27.3	23.0	24.2	22.2	21.7	22.8	20.7	21.1	19.4	17.5	17.1
75 to 84 years	85.0	66.0	68.2	44.3	41.3	41.2	39.9	35.6	32.1	30.4	31.4	27.3	25.8	25.9
85 years and over	78.1	62.7	63.1	56.1	55.3	64.5	61.5	57.5	49.0	45.6	44.4	40.2	35.3	40.2
Female														
All ages, age-adjusted[4]	11.5	11.7	14.9	11.8	10.7	11.0	10.3	9.5	8.9	8.8	8.2	7.2	6.7	6.5
All ages, crude	10.9	11.0	14.7	12.3	11.0	11.3	10.4	9.7	9.1	9.0	8.4	7.4	6.9	6.8
Under 1 year	7.6	7.5	10.4	6.7	4.7	4.9	4.5	4.2	3.7	3.5	3.3	2.0	2.1	1.8
1 to 14 years	7.2	6.3	7.9	6.3	5.4	4.9	4.4	3.7	3.1	3.1	2.8	2.2	2.2	2.0
1 to 4 years	10.0	8.4	10.0	8.1	6.0	5.6	4.8	3.8	3.4	3.5	3.1	2.5	2.5	2.5
5 to 14 years	5.7	5.4	7.2	5.7	5.1	4.7	4.2	3.6	3.0	2.9	2.6	2.0	2.0	1.8
15 to 24 years	12.6	15.1	21.6	20.8	18.2	17.9	16.8	15.9	14.5	14.5	13.8	11.5	10.5	9.9
15 to 19 years	12.9	16.0	22.7	22.8	20.1	20.0	19.7	17.5	15.9	15.4	14.8	11.8	10.9	9.2
20 to 24 years	12.2	14.0	20.4	18.9	16.7	16.0	13.8	14.2	13.2	13.6	12.8	11.2	10.0	10.5
25 to 34 years	9.3	9.2	13.0	12.2	10.1	11.5	10.2	8.8	8.9	8.8	8.5	7.4	7.2	6.9
35 to 44 years	8.5	9.1	12.9	10.4	9.4	9.2	9.0	8.8	8.6	8.8	7.8	7.0	6.2	6.2
45 to 64 years	12.6	13.1	15.3	10.3	9.5	10.1	9.0	8.7	8.4	8.3	7.7	7.2	6.5	6.3
45 to 54 years	10.9	11.6	14.5	10.2	9.0	9.6	8.4	8.2	8.2	8.2	7.8	7.4	6.6	6.3
55 to 64 years	14.9	15.2	16.2	10.5	9.9	10.8	9.9	9.5	8.8	8.5	7.5	6.9	6.3	6.3
65 years and over	21.9	20.3	23.1	15.0	15.8	17.2	17.0	15.8	14.1	13.6	12.6	11.5	11.1	11.3
65 to 74 years	20.6	19.0	21.6	13.0	14.0	14.1	13.7	12.3	11.1	10.5	9.6	8.9	8.5	8.2
75 to 84 years	25.2	23.0	27.2	18.5	19.2	21.9	21.2	19.2	16.5	16.5	15.0	13.5	13.5	13.7
85 years and over	22.1	22.0	18.0	15.2	15.0	18.3	19.3	19.3	17.6	16.4	16.5	15.3	14.0	15.9

[1]Includes deaths of persons who were not residents of the 50 states and the District of Columbia. [2]Underlying cause of death was coded according to the 6th Revision of the International Classification of Diseases (ICD) in 1950, 7th Revision in 1960, 8th Revision in 1970, and 9th Revision in 1980–1998. [3]Starting with 1999 data, cause of death is coded according to ICD-10. [4]Age-adjusted rates are calculated using the year 2000 standard population. Prior to 2001, age-adjusted rates were calculated using standard million proportions based on rounded population numbers. Starting with 2001 data, unrounded population numbers are used to calculate age-adjusted rates.

Table 2-26. Occupational Fatal Injuries and Rates, by Industry, Sex, Age, Race, and Hispanic Origin, Selected Years, 1995–2010

(Rate per 100,000 employed workers; number.)

Characteristic	Deaths per 100,000 employed workers[1]					Deaths per full-time equivalent workers[2]		
	1995	2000	2005	2006	2007	2008	2009	2010
Rate								
Total workforce	4.9	4.3	4.0	4.0	3.8	3.7	3.5	3.6
Sex								
Male	8.3	7.4	6.9	6.9	6.6	6.1	5.7	5.8
Female	0.9	0.7	0.6	0.7	0.6	0.6	0.6	0.6
Age [3]								
16 to 17 years	1.6	1.6	1.4	0.9	0.9	2.5	*	3.0
18 to 19 years	3.3	2.7	2.9	2.8	2.6	2.4	2.5	2.8
20 to 24 years	3.8	3.2	2.8	2.7	3.0	2.8	2.4	2.2
25 to 34 years	4.3	3.8	3.3	3.3	3.1	2.8	2.4	2.7
35 to 44 years	4.6	4.0	3.6	3.7	3.4	3.3	3.0	2.9
45 to 54 years	5.2	4.4	4.2	4.2	4.1	3.8	3.6	3.6
55 to 64 years	7.2	6.1	5.1	5.0	4.6	4.7	4.3	4.7
65 years and over	14.0	12.0	11.3	11.2	10.2	12.7	12.1	11.9
Race and Hispanic Origin [4]								
Hispanic or Latino (of any race)	5.5	5.6	4.9	5.0	4.6	4.2	4.0	3.9
Not Hispanic or Latino	NA	NA	NA	NA	NA	NA	NA	NA
White	NA	4.2	3.9	4.0	3.8	3.8	3.5	3.7
Black or African American	NA	3.8	3.9	3.7	3.9	3.7	3.1	3.0
Industry [5]								
Private sector	NA	NA	4.3	4.3	4.1	4.0	3.7	3.8
Agriculture, forestry, fishing, and hunting	NA	NA	32.5	30.0	27.9	30.4	27.2	27.9
Mining	NA	NA	25.6	28.1	25.1	18.1	12.4	19.8
Utilities	NA	NA	3.6	6.3	4.0	3.9	1.7	2.8
Construction	NA	NA	11.1	10.9	10.5	9.7	9.9	9.8
Manufacturing	NA	NA	2.4	2.8	2.5	2.5	2.3	2.3
Wholesale trade	NA	NA	4.6	4.9	4.7	4.4	5.0	4.9
Retail trade	NA	NA	2.4	2.2	2.1	2.0	2.2	2.2
Transportation and warehousing	NA	NA	17.7	16.8	16.9	14.9	13.3	13.7
Information	NA	NA	2.0	2.0	2.3	1.5	1.1	1.5
Finance and insurance	NA	NA	0.6	0.6	0.6	0.3	0.5	0.4
Real estate and rental and leasing	NA	NA	1.9	2.6	2.4	3.1	3.0	3.6
Professional, scientific, and technical services	NA	NA	1.0	0.9	0.9	0.8	1.0	0.9
Management of companies and enterprises	NA	NA	*	*	0.9	*	*	*
Administrative and support and waste management and remediation services	NA	NA	7.2	6.6	6.3	6.1	6.7	5.3
Educational services	NA	NA	1.3	1.3	0.9	0.9	0.7	0.8
Health care and social assistance	NA	NA	0.7	0.8	0.7	0.7	0.8	0.9
Arts, entertainment, and recreation	NA	NA	3.2	3.5	3.9	4.0	3.6	3.6
Accommodation and food services	NA	NA	1.5	2.0	1.7	1.8	1.9	2.0
Other services (except public administration)	NA	NA	3.0	2.6	2.5	2.6	2.8	3.0
Government[6]	NA	NA	2.4	2.4	2.5	2.4	1.9	2.2
Number of Deaths [7]								
Total workforce	6,275	5,920	5,734	5,840	5,657	5,214	4,551	4,690
Sex								
Male	5,736	5,471	5,328	5,396	5,228	4,827	4,216	4,322
Female	539	449	406	444	429	387	335	368
Age [3]								
Under 16 years	26	29	23	11	18	11	13	16
16 to 17 years	42	44	31	21	20	23	14	18
18 to 19 years	130	127	111	106	97	66	57	56
20 to 24 years	486	446	403	390	424	353	275	245
25 to 34 years	1,409	1,163	1,017	1,041	991	850	704	785
35 to 44 years	1,571	1,473	1,243	1,288	1,168	1,113	908	868
45 to 54 years	1,256	1,313	1,389	1,417	1,425	1,292	1,173	1,169
55 to 64 years	827	831	933	963	934	920	853	948
65 years and over	515	488	578	599	574	580	551	582
Unspecified	13	6	6	4	6	6	3	3
Race and Hispanic Origin [4]								
White	5,120	NA	NA	NA	NA	NA	NA	NA
Black or African American	697	NA	NA	NA	NA	NA	NA	NA
Hispanic or Latino (of any race)	619	815	923	990	937	804	713	707
Not Hispanic or Latino	5,656	5,105	4,809	4,850	4,734	4,410	3,838	3,983
White	4,599	4,244	3,977	4,019	3,867	3,663	3,204	3,363
Black or African American	684	575	584	565	609	533	421	412
American Indian or Alaska Native	27	33	50	46	29	32	33	32
Asian[8]	188	171	154	148	166	145	141	143
Native Hawaiian or Other Pacific Islander	NA	14	9	11	6	7	7	6
Multiple races	NA	NA	NA	11	10	6	7	8
Other races or not reported	158	68	35	50	33	24	25	19
Industry [5]								
Private sector	NA	NA	5,214	5,320	5,112	4,670	4,090	4,206
Agriculture, forestry, fishing, and hunting	NA	NA	715	655	585	672	575	621
Mining	NA	NA	159	192	183	176	99	172
Utilities	NA	NA	30	53	34	37	16	26
Construction	NA	NA	1,192	1,239	1,204	975	834	774
Manufacturing	NA	NA	393	456	400	411	319	329
Wholesale trade	NA	NA	209	222	207	180	190	191
Retail trade	NA	NA	400	359	348	301	307	311
Transportation and warehousing	NA	NA	885	860	890	796	633	661
Information	NA	NA	65	66	79	47	33	43
Finance and insurance	NA	NA	42	44	46	24	33	24
Real estate and rental and leasing	NA	NA	57	82	73	82	75	89
Professional, scientific, and technical services	NA	NA	83	78	77	69	85	76
Management of companies and enterprises	NA	NA	*	*	4	*	*	*

Table 2-26. Occupational Fatal Injuries and Rates, by Industry, Sex, Age, Race, and Hispanic Origin, Selected Years, 1995–2010 —Continued

(Rate per 100,000 employed workers; number.)

Characteristic	Deaths per 100,000 employed workers[1]					Deaths per full-time equivalent workers[2]		
	1995	2000	2005	2006	2007	2008	2009	2010
Administrative and support and waste management and remediation services	NA	NA	398	381	395	332	336	288
Educational services	NA	NA	46	49	34	28	27	30
Health care and social assistance	NA	NA	104	129	115	113	123	141
Arts, entertainment, and recreation	NA	NA	77	80	96	92	80	84
Accommodation and food services	NA	NA	136	185	164	146	151	154
Other services (except public administration)	NA	NA	210	183	175	178	173	192
Government[6]	NA	NA	520	520	545	544	461	484

NA = Not available.   * = Estimates are unreliable or data do not meet publication/reliability criteria.   [1]Numerator excludes deaths to workers under age 16. Employment data in denominators are average annual estimates of employed civilians age 16 years and over from the CPS, regardless of the number of hours worked. These data are supplemented by data for the resident military, which was supplied by the U.S. Census Bureau (1995–1998) and the Department of Defense (1999–2008). Starting with 2004 data, rates are taken directly from the U.S. Department of Labor, Bureau of Labor Statistics, Census of Fatal Occupational Injuries, revised annual data. Starting with 2008 data, employment data in denominators are based on hours.   [2]Numerator excludes deaths to workers under 16 years of age, volunteers, and members of the resident military. Starting with 2008 data, fatal injury rates are based on hours, rather than employment, and consequently are not directly comparable with earlier data. Hours-based rates standardize the amount of exposure and are considered more accurate than employment-based rates. Employment- and hours-based rates will be similar for groups of workers who usually work full-time. Differences in these rates are more likely for groups which have a high percentage of part-time workers, such as younger workers. Hours worked are converted to full-time equivalent workers; 200,000,000 hours worked equals 100,000 full-time equivalent workers, working 40 hours per week, 50 weeks per year. Hours worked data are provided by the Current Population Survey (CPS).   [3]Employment data for under 16 years and unspecified were not available for the calculation of rates.   [4]Employment data for American Indian or Alaska Native workers and, prior to 2003, Asian or Pacific Islander workers, were not available for the calculation of rates. Employment data for non-Hispanic White and non-Hispanic Black workers were not available before the year 2000. In 1999 and earlier years, the race groups White and Black included persons of Hispanic and non-Hispanic origin.   [5]Starting with 2003 data, establishments were classified by industry according to the North American Industry Classification System (NAICS). Prior to 2003, the Standard Industrial Classification (SIC) system was used. Because of substantial differences between these systems, industry data classified by these two systems are not comparable. Industry data for 1995 to 2002 classified by SIC are available in *Health, United States, 2004*.   [6]Includes fatal work injuries to workers employed by governmental organizations, regardless of industry.   [7]Includes fatal work injuries to all workers, regardless of age.   [8]In 1999 and earlier years, category also included Native Hawaiian or Other Pacific Islander.

Table 2-27. Number of Fatal Work Injuries, by Most Frequent Type, 1992–Preliminary 2012

(Number.)

Year	Total	Roadway incidents	Homicides	Falls, slips, trips	Struck by object
1992	6,217	1,158	1,044	600	557
1993	6,331	1,242	1,074	618	565
1994	6,632	1,343	1,080	665	591
1995	6,275	1,346	1,036	651	547
1996	6,202	1,346	927	691	582
1997	6,238	1,393	860	716	579
1998	6,055	1,442	714	706	520
1999	6,054	1,496	651	721	585
2000	5,920	1,365	677	734	571
2001	5,915	1,409	643	810	553
2002	5,534	1,373	609	719	505
2003	5,575	1,353	632	696	531
2004	5,764	1,398	559	822	602
2005	5,734	1,437	567	770	607
2006	5,840	1,356	540	827	589
2007	5,657	1,414	628	847	504
2008	5,214	1,215	526	700	520
2009	4,551	985	542	645	420
2010	4,690	1,044	518	646	404
2011	4,693	1,103	468	681	NA
2012[1]	4,383	1,044	463	668	NA

NA = Not available.   [1]Preliminary.

Table 2-28. Number of Fatal Occupational Injuries, by Selected Industry Sector and Occupation, and Percentage of Fatal Incidents, Preliminary 2012

(Number, percent.)

Characteristic	Count	Percent
Total	4,383	100.0
Industry		
Private industry	3,945	90.0
Construction	775	17.7
Transportation and warehousing	677	15.4
Agriculture, forestry, fishing and hunting	475	10.8
Government	438	10.0
Professional and business services	388	8.9
Manufacturing	314	7.2
Retail trade	262	6.0
Leisure and hospitality	220	5.0
Other services (exc. public administration)	183	4.2
Public administration	146	3.3
Wholesale trade	191	4.4
Mining	177	4.0
Educational and health services	139	3.2
Financial activities	81	1.8
Information	38	0.9
Utilities	22	0.5
Occupation		
Fishers and related fishing workers	32	0.7
Logging workers	62	1.4
Aircraft pilots and flight engineers	71	1.6
Farmers, ranchers, and other agricultural managers	216	4.9
Extraction workers	86	2.0
Roofers	70	1.6
Refuse and recyclable material collectors	26	0.6
Driver/sales workers and truck drivers	741	16.9
Industrial machinery installation, repair, and maintenance workers	32	0.7
Police and sheriff's patrol officers	104	2.4

Table 2-29. Number of Fatal Work Injuries, by State, 2011 and Preliminary 2012

(Number.)

State	2011	2012[1]	Net change
Total	4,693	4,383	310
Alabama	75	81	6
Alaska	39	30	9
Arizona	69	37	32
Arkansas	93	63	30
California	390	339	51
Colorado	92	80	12
Connecticut	37	36	1
Delaware	10	14	4
District of Columbia	9	11	2
Florida	226	209	17
Georgia	111	76	35
Hawaii	26	19	7
Idaho	37	18	19
Illinois	177	145	32
Indiana	125	113	12
Iowa	93	84	9
Kansas	78	75	3
Kentucky	93	84	9
Louisiana	111	106	5
Maine	26	19	7
Maryland	71	70	1
Massachusetts	68	33	35
Michigan	141	127	14
Minnesota	60	70	10
Mississippi	63	60	3
Missouri	132	83	49
Montana	49	34	15
Nebraska	39	48	9
Nevada	38	42	4
New Hampshire	9	13	4
New Jersey	99	90	9
New Mexico	52	35	17
New York (incl. New York City)	206	196	10
New York City	72	75	3
North Carolina	148	138	10
North Dakota	44	64	20
Ohio	155	154	1
Oklahoma	86	94	8
Oregon	58	43	15
Pennsylvania	186	163	23
Rhode Island	7	8	1
South Carolina	81	62	19
South Dakota	31	31	0
Tennessee	120	100	20
Texas	433	531	98
Utah	39	39	0
Vermont	8	10	2
Virginia	127	146	19
Washington	60	64	4
West Virginia	43	47	4
Wisconsin	89	114	25
Wyoming	32	35	3

[1]Preliminary data.

Table 2-30A. Years of Potential Life Lost Before Age 75 for Selected Causes of Death, by Sex, Selected Years, 1980–2010

(Years lost before 75 per 100,000 population.)

Sex, race, Hispanic origin, and cause of death[1]	Crude 2010[3]	Age-adjusted[2]									
		1980[2]	1990[2]	1995[2]	2000[3]	2005[3]	2006[3]	2007[3]	2008[3]	2009[3]	2010[3]
ALL PERSONS											
All Causes	6,980.5	10,448.4	9,085.5	8,626.2	7,578.1	7,315.7	7,228.7	7,087.0	6,957.7	6,833.1	6,642.9
Diseases of heart	1,071.0	2,238.7	1,617.7	1,475.4	1,253.0	1,107.5	1,074.8	1,037.8	1,022.9	992.6	972.4
Ischemic heart disease	649.2	1,729.3	1,153.6	1,013.2	841.8	698.9	672.5	638.2	624.4	591.5	577.3
Cerebrovascular diseases	184.3	357.5	259.6	246.5	223.3	192.9	189.7	183.7	177.9	172.8	169.3
Malignant neoplasms	1,563.1	2,108.8	2,003.8	1,841.6	1,674.1	1,519.8	1,484.6	1,452.7	1,427.8	1,413.9	1,395.8
Trachea, bronchus, and lung	384.6	548.5	561.4	497.3	443.1	390.5	376.1	363.5	350.5	341.7	331.3
Colorectal	139.1	190.0	164.7	152.0	141.9	124.3	125.6	126.0	126.8	124.3	125.0
Prostate[4]	59.0	84.9	96.8	83.5	63.6	54.4	54.1	52.7	52.2	50.1	52.2
Breast[5]	291.0	463.2	451.6	398.6	332.6	295.4	285.9	274.0	269.2	269.6	262.4
Chronic lower respiratory diseases	196.4	169.1	187.4	190.4	188.1	180.1	169.7	170.5	179.8	177.2	172.4
Influenza and pneumonia	75.5	160.2	141.5	126.9	87.1	83.6	76.5	71.6	80.7	108.7	71.4
Chronic liver disease and cirrhosis	177.1	300.3	196.9	173.7	164.1	152.5	149.8	157.3	158.7	160.1	163.9
Diabetes mellitus	174.8	134.4	155.9	174.7	178.4	179.4	176.0	169.3	164.4	161.2	158.2
Alzheimer's disease	13.3	V	V	V	10.9	11.7	11.7	11.9	12.3	11.4	11.7
Human immunodeficiency virus (HIV) disease	75.9	X	383.8	595.3	174.6	134.5	126.9	115.8	100.2	89.2	76.6
Unintentional injuries	1,010.2	1,543.5	1,162.1	1,057.2	1,026.5	1,137.2	1,173.3	1,162.1	1,095.8	1,028.2	1,025.2
Motor vehicle-related injuries	395.6	912.9	716.4	616.3	574.3	565.9	563.0	538.4	473.2	421.7	400.6
Poisoning	370.9	68.0	81.2	123.1	163.6	289.1	335.1	356.1	364.0	365.7	379.7
Suicide[6]	381.7	392.0	393.1	384.7	334.5	348.9	350.6	358.6	367.4	372.5	385.2
Homicide[6]	233.6	425.5	417.4	378.6	266.5	278.2	283.4	279.0	267.6	248.0	239.0
MALE											
All Causes	8,667.9	13,777.2	11,973.5	11,289.2	9,572.2	9,244.2	9,130.1	8,945.0	8,764.7	8,560.7	8,329.5
Diseases of heart	1,478.6	3,352.1	2,356.0	2,117.4	1,766.0	1,559.0	1,514.5	1,463.3	1,433.5	1,399.2	1,370.8
Ischemic heart disease	946.8	2,715.1	1,766.3	1,531.5	1,255.4	1,040.6	1,005.2	956.9	927.8	886.5	864.8
Cerebrovascular diseases	203.8	396.7	286.6	276.9	244.6	213.3	211.5	205.4	197.7	195.7	190.7
Malignant neoplasms	1,652.9	2,360.8	2,214.6	2,008.5	1,810.8	1,632.9	1,587.4	1,554.7	1,540.7	1,515.6	1,500.8
Trachea, bronchus, and lung	440.7	821.1	764.8	645.6	554.9	472.8	450.6	429.5	418.8	403.4	390.5
Colorectal	161.1	214.9	194.3	179.4	167.3	145.7	144.7	147.6	148.8	145.6	148.0
Prostate	59.0	84.9	96.8	83.5	63.6	54.4	54.1	52.7	52.2	50.1	52.2
Chronic lower respiratory diseases	201.5	235.1	224.8	213.1	206.0	194.3	180.8	185.6	192.2	186.9	182.8
Influenza and pneumonia	86.3	202.5	180.0	155.7	102.8	98.0	89.0	83.6	91.7	119.5	82.6
Chronic liver disease and cirrhosis	242.2	415.0	283.9	254.8	236.9	216.4	211.1	222.4	223.2	222.8	226.9
Diabetes mellitus	210.9	140.4	170.4	194.6	203.8	216.1	212.8	206.3	200.7	201.2	194.8
Alzheimer's disease	11.5	V	V	V	10.6	10.8	11.4	11.0	11.5	11.0	10.7
Human immunodeficiency virus (HIV) disease	108.6	X	686.2	991.2	258.9	194.0	180.3	162.6	141.0	126.7	109.5
Unintentional injuries	1,420.3	2,342.7	1,715.1	1,531.6	1,475.6	1,622.6	1,675.9	1,652.0	1,562.6	1,449.8	1,432.1
Motor vehicle-related injuries	567.8	1,359.7	1,018.4	851.1	796.4	802.0	797.8	771.0	683.8	600.5	569.2
Poisoning	493.5	96.4	123.6	193.1	242.1	400.4	468.1	486.4	499.6	493.0	503.8
Suicide[6]	603.6	605.6	634.8	628.4	539.1	553.4	555.0	566.6	578.6	585.6	607.0
Homicide[6]	377.7	675.0	658.0	589.6	410.5	443.6	452.0	443.2	426.6	390.3	380.3
FEMALE											
All Causes	5,306.6	7,350.3	6,333.1	6,057.5	5,644.6	5,429.0	5,365.9	5,267.2	5,188.6	5,143.7	4,994.0
Diseases of heart	666.6	1,246.0	948.5	883.9	774.6	680.2	658.1	634.2	633.2	605.5	593.6
Ischemic heart disease	353.9	852.1	600.3	537.8	457.6	377.2	358.7	337.3	338.0	312.7	305.2
Cerebrovascular diseases	164.9	324.0	235.9	218.7	203.9	173.9	169.2	163.5	159.4	151.1	149.1
Malignant neoplasms	1,473.9	1,896.8	1,826.6	1,698.9	1,555.3	1,419.0	1,393.1	1,361.9	1,325.8	1,322.6	1,301.0
Trachea, bronchus, and lung	328.9	310.4	382.2	365.2	342.1	315.2	307.8	303.1	287.7	285.0	276.9
Colorectal	117.2	168.7	138.7	127.5	118.7	104.5	107.9	105.9	106.2	104.5	103.4
Breast	291.0	463.2	451.6	398.6	332.6	295.4	285.9	274.0	269.2	269.6	262.4
Chronic lower respiratory diseases	191.4	114.0	155.9	171.0	172.3	167.2	159.5	156.7	168.5	168.3	162.8
Influenza and pneumonia	64.8	122.0	106.2	100.2	72.3	69.9	64.7	60.1	70.3	98.4	60.7
Chronic liver disease and cirrhosis	112.6	194.5	115.1	96.6	94.5	91.4	91.1	95.0	96.9	99.9	103.5
Diabetes mellitus	139.0	128.5	142.3	155.9	154.4	144.5	141.1	134.1	129.9	123.2	123.5
Alzheimer's disease	15.1	V	V	V	11.1	12.5	11.9	12.7	13.0	11.8	12.6
Human immunodeficiency virus (HIV) disease	43.4	X	87.8	205.7	92.0	76.4	74.7	70.1	63.1	52.7	44.4
Unintentional injuries	603.3	755.3	607.4	580.1	573.2	647.9	666.3	668.5	625.8	604.6	616.4
Motor vehicle-related injuries	224.7	470.4	411.6	378.4	348.5	326.4	324.9	302.8	260.1	241.3	230.5
Poisoning	249.3	40.2	39.1	53.6	85.0	177.3	201.4	225.0	227.6	237.8	255.1
Suicide[6]	161.6	184.2	153.3	140.8	129.1	144.1	145.8	150.4	156.2	159.6	163.7
Homicide[6]	90.6	181.3	174.3	163.2	118.9	108.8	110.5	111.0	105.1	102.8	94.9

NA = Not available.   V = Data for Alzheimer's disease are only presented for data years 1999 and beyond due to large differences in death rates caused by changes in the coding of the causes of death between ICD-9 and ICD-10.   X = Not applicable.   * = Figure does not meet standards of reliability or precision.   [1]Underlying cause of death code was coded according to the 9th Revision of the International Classification of Diseases (ICD) in 1980-1998.   [2]Age-adjusted rates are calculated using the year 2000 standard population. Prior to 2001, age-adjusted rates were calculated using standard million proportions based on rounded population numbers. Starting with 2001 data, unrounded population numbers are used to calculate age-adjusted rates.   [3]Starting with 1999 data, cause of death is coded according to ICD-10.   [4]Rate for male population only.   [5]Rate for female population only.   [6]Figures for 2001 include September 11th-related deaths for which death certificates were filed as of October 24, 2002.

Table 2-30B. Years of Potential Life Lost Before Age 75 for Selected Causes of Death, by Race, Selected Years, 1980–2010

(Years lost before 75 per 100,000 population.)

Sex, race, Hispanic origin, and cause of death[1]	Crude 2010[3]	Age-adjusted[2] 1980[2]	1990[2]	1995[2]	2000[3]	2005[3]	2006[3]	2007[3]	2008[3]	2009[3]	2010[3]
WHITE[4]											
All Causes	6,794.6	9,554.1	8,159.5	7,744.9	6,949.5	6,823.2	6,763.4	6,664.3	6,590.9	6,486.5	6,342.8
Diseases of heart	1,032.4	2,100.8	1,490.3	1,353.0	1,149.4	1,012.4	987.0	952.8	941.9	912.2	900.9
Ischemic heart disease	661.0	1,682.7	1,113.4	975.2	805.3	671.4	647.8	616.4	606.6	573.7	563.7
Cerebrovascular diseases	161.2	300.7	213.1	205.2	187.1	160.5	158.3	154.1	149.5	147.2	142.7
Malignant neoplasms	1,601.4	2,035.9	1,929.3	1,780.5	1,627.8	1,485.8	1,456.8	1,427.3	1,404.5	1,396.1	1,375.8
Trachea, bronchus, and lung	405.3	529.9	544.2	487.1	436.3	388.1	373.4	363.1	351.9	343.7	332.8
Colorectal	136.8	186.8	157.8	145.0	134.1	117.3	118.9	119.6	120.0	118.6	118.4
Prostate[5]	54.4	74.8	86.6	73.0	54.3	46.6	46.8	45.6	45.6	42.6	45.3
Breast[6]	282.1	460.2	441.7	381.5	315.6	275.2	269.3	256.9	253.5	255.7	245.0
Chronic lower respiratory diseases	212.7	165.4	182.3	185.7	185.3	181.5	171.2	173.1	182.9	180.4	176.1
Influenza and pneumonia	72.5	130.8	116.9	108.3	77.7	76.7	70.8	65.6	74.6	103.4	66.7
Chronic liver disease and cirrhosis	192.8	257.3	175.8	164.6	162.7	157.2	156.0	164.3	166.8	169.0	173.5
Diabetes mellitus	159.9	115.7	133.7	149.4	155.6	156.3	153.0	147.7	145.6	142.7	139.0
Alzheimer's disease	15.1	V	V	V	11.4	12.3	12.4	12.6	13.0	12.1	12.4
Human immunodeficiency virus (HIV) disease	39.9	X	309.0	422.6	94.7	70.5	65.4	58.8	51.8	44.5	39.9
Unintentional injuries	1,071.4	1,520.4	1,139.7	1,040.9	1,031.8	1,183.1	1,225.2	1,223.0	1,167.6	1,092.1	1,098.6
Motor vehicle-related injuries	407.8	939.9	726.7	623.6	586.1	591.1	587.2	563.4	497.3	438.5	419.0
Poisoning	421.4	64.9	74.4	115.4	167.2	314.4	366.0	397.4	412.4	415.7	435.4
Suicide[7]	425.2	414.5	417.7	411.6	362.0	385.1	388.3	398.5	409.4	417.1	430.8
Homicide[7]	132.5	271.7	234.9	220.2	156.6	161.7	162.4	164.7	160.9	147.6	138.7
BLACK OR AFRICAN AMERICAN[4]											
All Causes	9,689.4	17,873.4	16,593.0	15,809.7	12,897.1	11,788.4	11,515.2	11,098.2	10,611.2	10,319.6	9,832.5
Diseases of heart	1,600.9	3,619.9	2,891.8	2,681.8	2,275.2	2,011.1	1,929.1	1,859.8	1,813.4	1,766.6	1,691.1
Ischemic heart disease	771.2	2,305.1	1,676.1	1,510.2	1,300.1	1,058.3	1,009.8	945.0	905.2	859.5	818.8
Cerebrovascular diseases	337.8	883.2	656.4	583.6	507.0	434.1	422.8	406.0	386.6	362.3	358.1
Malignant neoplasms	1,708.8	2,946.1	2,894.8	2,597.1	2,294.7	2,030.4	1,957.5	1,913.4	1,864.2	1,823.3	1,796.7
Trachea, bronchus, and lung	386.7	776.0	811.3	683.0	593.0	500.4	483.4	456.3	426.7	417.6	405.6
Colorectal	179.0	232.3	241.8	226.9	222.4	195.7	194.4	193.9	192.8	185.3	188.6
Prostate[5]	107.0	200.3	223.5	210.0	171.0	139.6	134.2	132.1	125.6	129.6	127.3
Breast[6]	408.0	524.2	592.9	577.4	500.0	480.1	444.0	437.7	421.6	415.1	420.8
Chronic lower respiratory diseases	178.6	203.7	240.6	244.0	232.7	207.4	193.6	188.0	197.9	195.9	187.7
Influenza and pneumonia	106.3	384.9	330.8	269.8	161.2	143.7	125.8	121.6	129.4	152.2	109.8
Chronic liver disease and cirrhosis	116.3	644.0	371.8	250.3	185.6	136.0	124.3	126.9	122.1	119.7	120.2
Diabetes mellitus	297.4	305.3	361.5	400.8	383.4	373.1	367.6	349.6	323.2	317.0	316.4
Alzheimer's disease	8.0	V	V	V	8.3	10.9	10.2	9.6	10.8	10.4	10.0
Human immunodeficiency virus (HIV) disease	308.2	X	1,014.7	1,945.4	763.3	590.3	561.1	514.8	435.4	397.3	329.5
Unintentional injuries	907.0	1,751.5	1,392.7	1,272.1	1,152.8	1,129.7	1,163.6	1,106.2	979.2	934.0	896.7
Motor vehicle-related injuries	403.1	750.2	699.5	621.8	580.8	530.4	538.7	516.7	443.6	420.0	393.4
Poisoning	210.0	99.4	144.3	209.6	196.6	252.2	293.3	259.8	230.0	221.3	218.9
Suicide[7]	197.4	238.0	261.4	254.2	208.7	193.6	186.5	185.9	195.3	189.1	196.4
Homicide[7]	865.2	1,580.8	1,612.9	1,352.8	941.6	967.5	996.2	961.8	897.2	834.8	821.2
AMERICAN INDIAN OR ALASKAN NATIVE[4]											
All Causes	6,352.4	13,390.9	9,506.2	9,332.5	7,758.2	7,705.7	7,449.2	7,233.7	7,121.7	7,000.8	6,771.3
Diseases of heart	694.8	1,819.9	1,391.0	1,296.3	1,030.1	945.6	927.9	887.0	853.9	839.3	820.6
Ischemic heart disease	398.4	1,208.2	901.8	877.3	709.3	591.1	572.7	536.8	510.2	502.3	487.6
Cerebrovascular diseases	110.7	269.3	223.3	255.3	198.1	195.8	161.9	153.5	137.3	130.6	129.7
Malignant neoplasms	777.4	1,101.3	1,141.1	1,099.5	995.7	1,021.4	913.5	909.3	940.2	925.5	929.5
Trachea, bronchus, and lung	165.9	181.1	268.1	267.7	227.8	255.5	213.3	212.8	207.3	196.8	211.0
Colorectal	79.7	78.8	82.4	103.5	93.8	102.9	82.5	92.2	107.2	102.5	95.8
Prostate[5]	25.8	66.7	42.0	51.1	44.5	36.3	37.6	31.9	41.5	36.2	36.8
Breast[6]	126.9	205.5	213.4	195.9	174.1	139.2	158.2	149.0	142.7	135.4	145.0
Chronic lower respiratory diseases	126.0	89.3	129.0	145.3	151.8	146.8	134.3	157.6	156.1	138.4	154.5
Influenza and pneumonia	90.8	307.9	206.3	199.7	124.0	102.5	89.4	94.1	141.5	174.5	99.3
Chronic liver disease and cirrhosis	442.7	1,190.3	535.1	604.8	519.4	459.3	433.2	509.7	504.0	477.1	510.8
Diabetes mellitus	221.3	305.5	292.3	360.6	305.6	327.7	301.7	268.3	264.5	260.4	267.6
Alzheimer's disease	5.3	V	V	V	*	*	*	9.9	5.8	6.7	8.8
Human immunodeficiency virus (HIV) disease	41.7	X	70.1	246.9	68.4	81.4	67.4	69.3	57.3	49.5	46.1
Unintentional injuries	1,394.0	3,541.0	2,183.9	1,980.9	1,700.1	1,670.0	1,637.4	1,581.6	1,482.0	1,481.4	1,377.7
Motor vehicle-related injuries	597.8	2,102.4	1,301.5	1,210.3	1,032.2	894.0	891.4	790.8	698.6	667.4	570.6
Poisoning	430.3	92.9	119.5	161.5	180.1	302.0	317.6	359.3	433.5	479.0	449.6
Suicide[7]	464.6	515.0	495.9	445.2	403.1	446.5	427.4	403.5	411.9	415.3	437.9
Homicide[7]	273.1	628.9	434.2	432.7	278.5	298.4	284.7	237.4	264.2	253.3	256.4
ASIAN OR PACIFIC ISLANDER[4]											
All Causes	3,029.3	5,378.4	4,705.2	4,333.2	3,811.1	3,433.5	3,361.3	3,262.2	3,154.7	3,114.2	3,061.2
Diseases of heart	393.5	952.8	702.2	664.9	567.9	505.8	465.0	443.0	431.6	433.2	400.1
Ischemic heart disease	244.9	697.7	486.6	440.6	381.1	322.5	302.2	289.2	275.4	270.5	250.6
Cerebrovascular diseases	145.0	266.9	233.5	220.0	199.4	160.5	161.9	149.6	152.5	141.7	148.3
Malignant neoplasms	866.0	1,218.6	1,166.4	1,122.1	1,033.8	931.0	899.0	871.2	854.5	834.4	874.7
Trachea, bronchus, and lung	144.9	238.2	204.7	197.0	185.8	167.1	169.3	158.9	156.2	144.6	148.2
Colorectal	87.2	115.9	105.1	99.5	91.6	77.7	80.3	80.2	83.7	78.3	87.6
Prostate[5]	15.4	17.0	32.4	25.3	18.8	20.3	18.1	16.3	16.1	16.3	17.0
Breast[6]	162.1	222.2	216.5	237.8	200.8	175.0	169.7	151.0	155.2	149.7	156.9
Chronic lower respiratory diseases	31.6	56.4	72.8	65.8	56.5	35.4	36.6	34.8	33.8	34.3	33.2
Influenza and pneumonia	37.1	79.3	74.0	64.3	48.6	39.3	36.0	35.5	39.9	61.5	38.4
Chronic liver disease and cirrhosis	41.9	85.6	72.4	48.4	44.8	43.2	44.0	40.5	40.6	45.2	41.7
Diabetes mellitus	67.7	83.1	74.0	83.5	77.0	77.1	79.7	77.5	74.9	72.8	69.5
Alzheimer's disease	2.8	V	V	V	3.5	3.1	2.0	2.8	3.4	2.3	3.2
Human immunodeficiency virus (HIV) disease	10.8	X	77.0	110.4	19.9	16.6	15.4	14.6	18.0	11.6	10.7
Unintentional injuries	312.2	742.7	636.6	525.7	425.7	393.5	389.4	385.3	332.3	308.0	303.0
Motor vehicle-related injuries	154.7	472.6	445.5	351.9	263.4	228.9	229.0	210.7	184.2	154.0	147.9
Suicide[7]	210.0	217.1	200.6	24.5	25.9	40.6	45.1	49.8	43.7	50.5	46.5
Homicide[7]	71.4	201.1	205.8	211.1	168.6	158.0	175.8	190.3	170.4	182.0	199.7

Table 2-30B. Years of Potential Life Lost Before Age 75 for Selected Causes of Death, by Race, Selected Years, 1980–2010—*Continued*

(Years lost before 75 per 100,000 population.)

Sex, race, Hispanic origin, and cause of death[1]	Crude 2010[3]	Age-adjusted[2]									
		1980[2]	1990[2]	1995[2]	2000[3]	2005[3]	2006[3]	2007[3]	2008[3]	2009[3]	2010[3]
HISPANIC OR LATINO[4,8]											
All Causes	4,375.2	NA	7,963.3	7,426.7	6,037.6	5,701.1	5,556.2	5,377.7	5,153.6	5,055.4	4,795.1
Diseases of heart	444.8	NA	1,082.0	962.0	821.3	726.9	687.8	664.6	629.0	630.2	598.1
Ischemic heart disease	255.5	NA	756.6	665.8	564.6	483.5	447.0	417.0	396.6	381.9	366.6
Cerebrovascular diseases	114.8	NA	238.0	232.0	207.8	184.8	184.6	175.4	162.5	155.8	150.4
Malignant neoplasms	725.5	NA	1,232.2	1,172.0	1,098.2	1,016.7	988.5	986.6	971.7	955.1	951.2
Trachea, bronchus, and lung	78.0	NA	193.7	173.9	152.1	138.2	125.1	125.7	122.9	117.4	115.0
Colorectal	68.7	NA	100.2	97.9	101.4	86.5	91.7	92.6	92.8	92.3	94.0
Prostate[5]	21.1	NA	47.7	60.8	42.9	42.1	44.3	43.9	41.5	37.3	38.2
Breast[6]	140.3	NA	299.3	257.7	230.7	194.9	200.6	190.7	184.0	186.0	180.0
Chronic lower respiratory diseases	43.7	NA	78.8	82.1	68.5	62.2	56.9	56.2	59.1	58.6	59.6
Influenza and pneumonia	47.7	NA	130.1	108.5	76.0	69.1	64.8	54.7	65.8	114.1	57.5
Chronic liver disease and cirrhosis	153.9	NA	329.1	281.4	252.1	210.7	202.2	210.2	208.4	207.5	201.6
Diabetes mellitus	112.4	NA	177.8	228.8	215.6	202.4	181.4	178.1	171.8	161.6	158.5
Alzheimer's disease	4.7	NA	V	V	6.9	7.8	8.9	7.7	8.5	7.2	8.4
Human immunodeficiency virus (HIV) disease	64.2	X	600.1	865.0	209.4	140.2	130.2	115.9	98.5	86.5	74.9
Unintentional injuries	734.6	NA	1,190.6	1,017.9	920.1	966.1	980.6	907.4	812.0	755.5	708.7
Motor vehicle-related injuries	366.3	NA	740.8	593.0	540.2	558.0	553.9	493.3	414.2	379.5	340.3
Poisoning	184.7	NA	121.9	173.9	145.9	179.5	196.4	200.4	200.5	194.7	191.2
Suicide[7]	198.3	NA	256.2	245.1	188.5	190.9	183.2	196.5	179.9	191.9	193.6
Homicide[7]	265.9	NA	720.8	575.4	335.1	336.2	328.1	311.5	289.7	267.9	238.0

NA = Not available. V = Data for Alzheimer's disease are only presented for data years 1999 and beyond due to large differences in death rates caused by changes in the coding of the causes of death between ICD-9 and ICD-10. X = Not applicable. * = Figure does not meet standards of reliability or precision. [1]Underlying cause of death code was coded according to the 9th Revision of the International Classification of Diseases (ICD) in 1980-1998. [2]Age-adjusted rates are calculated using the year 2000 standard population. Prior to 2001, age-adjusted rates were calculated using standard million proportions based on rounded population numbers. Starting with 2001 data, unrounded population numbers are used to calculate age-adjusted rates. [3]Starting with 1999 data, cause of death is coded according to ICD-10. [4]The race groups, White, Black, Asian or Pacific Islander, and American Indian or Alaska Native, include persons of Hispanic and non-Hispanic origin. Persons of Hispanic origin may be of any race. Death rates for the American Indian or Alaska Native, Asian or Pacific Islander, and Hispanic populations are known to be Indian or Alaska Native, Asian or Pacific Islander, and Hispanic populations are known to be underestimated. [5]Rate for male population only. [6]Rate for female population only. [7]Figures for 2001 include September 11th-related deaths for which death certificates were filed as of October 24, 2002. [8]Prior to 1997, excludes data from states lacking an Hispanic origin item on the death certificate.

Table 2-31. Number of Deaths, Death Rates, and Age-Adjusted Death Rates for Major Causes of Death, by State and Territory, 2010

(Number, rates per 100,000 population, age-adjusted rates per 100,000 U.S. standard population.)

State and territory	All causes			Human immunodeficiency virus (HIV) disease (B20–B24)			Malignant neoplasms (C00–C97)			Diabetes mellitus (E10–E14)		
	Number	Rate	Age-adjusted rate[1]	Number	Rate	Age-adjusted rate[1]	Number	Rate	Age-adjusted rate[1]	Number	Rate	Age-adjusted rate[1]
United States [2]	2,468,435	799.5	747.0	8,369	2.7	2.6	574,743	186.2	172.8	69,071	22.4	20.8
Alabama	48,038	1,005.0	939.7	153	3.2	3.2	10,196	213.3	191.7	1,302	27.2	25.0
Alaska	3,728	524.9	771.5	6	*	*	884	124.5	176.9	86	12.1	19.6
Arizona	46,762	731.6	693.1	102	1.6	1.6	10,678	167.1	154.2	1,389	21.7	20.3
Arkansas	28,916	991.7	892.7	64	2.2	2.2	6,475	222.1	194.7	850	29.2	25.8
California	234,012	628.2	646.7	742	2.0	1.9	56,453	151.5	156.9	7,061	19.0	19.7
Colorado	31,465	625.6	682.7	67	1.3	1.2	7,035	139.9	149.5	721	14.3	15.2
Connecticut	28,692	802.8	652.9	83	2.3	2.0	6,954	194.6	163.4	662	18.5	15.4
Delaware	7,706	858.2	769.9	46	5.1	4.9	1,909	212.6	185.7	196	21.8	19.2
District of Columbia	4,672	776.4	792.4	121	20.1	20.4	1,041	173.0	178.3	145	24.1	24.9
Florida	173,791	924.4	701.1	1,068	5.7	5.4	41,467	220.6	165.6	5,024	26.7	20.1
Georgia	71,263	735.6	845.4	495	5.1	5.0	15,435	159.3	174.8	1,996	20.6	23.1
Hawaii	9,617	707.0	589.6	13	*	*	2,266	166.6	140.9	272	20.0	16.6
Idaho	11,429	729.1	731.6	9	*	*	2,530	161.4	159.9	353	22.5	22.5
Illinois	99,931	778.8	736.9	300	2.3	2.3	24,070	187.6	178.6	2,507	19.5	18.5
Indiana	56,743	875.2	820.6	91	1.4	1.5	13,164	203.0	188.6	1,587	24.5	22.7
Iowa	27,745	910.8	721.7	15	*	*	6,358	208.7	171.9	733	24.1	19.3
Kansas	24,502	858.8	762.2	27	0.9	0.9	5,377	188.5	171.3	655	23.0	20.5
Kentucky	41,983	967.5	915.0	53	1.2	1.2	9,930	228.8	208.3	1,212	27.9	26.0
Louisiana	40,667	897.1	903.8	225	5.0	5.0	9,203	203.0	197.6	1,205	26.6	26.4
Maine	12,750	959.8	749.6	9	*	*	3,248	244.5	187.9	376	28.3	21.8
Maryland	43,325	750.4	728.6	316	5.5	5.0	10,269	177.9	171.2	1,191	20.6	19.9
Massachusetts	52,583	803.1	675.0	120	1.8	1.6	12,993	198.4	171.3	1,028	15.7	13.3
Michigan	88,021	890.6	786.2	150	1.5	1.5	20,620	208.6	182.9	2,697	27.3	24.0
Minnesota	38,972	734.8	661.5	48	0.9	0.9	9,612	181.2	167.2	1,037	19.6	17.7
Mississippi	28,965	976.1	962.0	118	4.0	4.2	6,271	211.3	201.4	926	31.2	30.3
Missouri	55,281	923.1	819.5	105	1.8	1.8	12,626	210.8	185.6	1,425	23.8	21.2
Montana	8,827	892.1	754.7	7	*	*	1,923	194.4	161.0	227	22.9	19.1
Nebraska	15,171	830.7	717.8	12	*	*	3,438	188.2	167.4	452	24.7	21.7
Nevada	19,623	726.6	795.4	60	2.2	2.2	4,529	167.7	174.2	350	13.0	13.8
New Hampshire	10,201	774.9	690.4	9	*	*	2,525	191.8	167.9	236	17.9	16.1
New Jersey	69,495	790.4	691.1	378	4.3	3.9	16,815	191.3	169.5	2,098	23.9	21.0
New Mexico	15,931	773.7	749.0	33	1.6	1.6	3,358	163.1	152.4	643	31.2	29.8
New York	146,432	755.7	665.5	990	5.1	4.7	35,431	182.8	163.1	3,642	18.8	16.7
North Carolina	78,773	826.1	804.9	328	3.4	3.3	18,061	189.4	179.0	2,042	21.4	20.5
North Dakota	5,944	883.7	704.3	2	*	*	1,269	188.7	157.1	192	28.5	22.2
Ohio	108,711	942.3	815.7	138	1.2	1.1	25,083	217.4	187.7	3,470	30.1	25.8
Oklahoma	36,529	973.8	915.5	50	1.3	1.4	7,831	208.8	191.3	1,089	29.0	26.9
Oregon	31,890	832.4	723.1	47	1.2	1.2	7,638	199.4	173.9	1,052	27.5	23.7
Pennsylvania	124,596	980.9	765.9	266	2.1	1.9	29,055	228.7	181.6	3,242	25.5	20.0
Rhode Island	9,579	910.1	721.7	20	1.9	1.8	2,266	215.3	178.3	211	20.0	16.0
South Carolina	41,614	899.7	854.8	184	4.0	3.9	9,356	202.3	183.6	1,128	24.4	22.6
South Dakota	7,100	872.0	715.1	10	*	*	1,655	203.3	171.0	240	29.5	24.5
Tennessee	59,578	938.8	890.8	207	3.3	3.2	13,593	214.2	195.7	1,687	26.6	24.7
Texas	166,527	662.3	772.3	773	3.1	3.2	36,717	146.0	165.9	4,744	18.9	21.6
Utah	14,776	534.6	703.2	13	*	*	2,810	101.7	133.7	471	17.0	22.7
Vermont	5,380	859.8	718.7	7	*	*	1,392	222.5	183.2	151	24.1	20.7
Virginia	59,032	737.8	741.6	142	1.8	1.7	14,080	176.0	172.4	1,530	19.1	18.8
Washington	48,146	716.0	692.3	76	1.1	1.0	11,874	176.6	170.5	1,499	22.3	21.6
West Virginia	21,275	1,148.1	933.6	14	*	*	4,685	252.8	198.0	776	41.9	32.9
Wisconsin	47,308	831.9	719.0	51	0.9	0.8	11,279	198.3	174.5	1,158	20.4	17.7
Wyoming	4,438	787.4	778.8	6	*	*	1,016	180.3	172.6	105	18.6	18.5
Puerto Rico	29,153	783.3	712.8	334	9.0	9.0	5,174	139.0	123.3	2,951	79.3	70.2
Virgin Islands	715	672.8	663.2	7	*	*	131	123.3	109.3	45	42.3	42.3
Guam	857	537.5	810.6	2	*	*	141	88.4	133.6	41	25.7	37.1
American Samoa	224	403.8	932.9	1	*	*	29	52.3	152.5	23	41.5	104.2
Northern Marianas	174	325.1	863.3	-	*	*	26	48.6	123.0	10	*	*

Table 2-31. Number of Deaths, Death Rates, and Age-Adjusted Death Rates for Major Causes of Death, by State and Territory, 2010—Continued

(Number, rates per 100,000 population, age-adjusted rates per 100,000 U.S. standard population.)

State and territory	Parkinson's disease (G20–G21)			Alzheimer's disease (G30)			Disease of the heart (I00–I09, I11, I13, I20–I51)			Essential hypertension and hypertensive renal disease (I10, I12, I15)		
	Number	Rate	Age-adjusted rate[1]	Number	Rate	Age-adjusted rate[1]	Number	Rate	Age-adjusted rate[1]	Number	Rate	Age-adjusted rate[1]
United States [2]	22,032	7.1	6.8	83,494	27.0	25.1	597,689	193.6	179.1	26,634	8.6	8.0
Alabama	342	7.2	6.9	1,523	31.9	31.2	12,083	252.8	236.0	549	11.5	10.6
Alaska	32	4.5	9.2	85	12.0	25.9	707	99.5	151.5	25	3.5	6.4
Arizona	489	7.7	7.4	2,327	36.4	35.3	9,954	155.7	146.7	508	7.9	7.6
Arkansas	206	7.1	6.4	955	32.8	29.6	7,274	249.5	222.5	221	7.6	6.8
California	2,238	6.0	6.5	10,856	29.1	30.1	58,641	157.4	161.9	3,733	10.0	10.4
Colorado	305	6.1	7.2	1,334	26.5	31.1	6,038	120.1	132.8	261	5.2	5.9
Connecticut	237	6.6	5.3	820	22.9	17.1	7,127	199.4	155.7	321	9.0	7.0
Delaware	57	6.3	5.8	215	23.9	21.9	1,776	197.8	175.7	62	6.9	6.2
District of Columbia	26	4.3	4.6	114	18.9	18.7	1,306	217.0	222.4	57	9.5	9.6
Florida	1,755	9.3	6.7	4,831	25.7	18.1	41,737	222.0	162.3	1,821	9.7	7.1
Georgia	472	4.9	6.3	2,080	21.5	28.3	15,987	165.0	192.6	1,076	11.1	12.9
Hawaii	84	6.2	5.0	189	13.9	10.5	2,239	164.6	134.7	98	7.2	5.9
Idaho	123	7.8	8.3	410	26.2	26.8	2,495	159.2	159.3	121	7.7	7.6
Illinois	909	7.1	6.9	2,927	22.8	20.9	24,959	194.5	181.7	871	6.8	6.3
Indiana	485	7.5	7.2	1,940	29.9	27.8	13,388	206.5	191.8	454	7.0	6.5
Iowa	320	10.5	8.1	1,411	46.3	32.9	6,880	225.8	173.3	318	10.4	7.8
Kansas	256	9.0	7.9	825	28.9	24.2	5,433	190.4	164.9	157	5.5	4.6
Kentucky	296	6.8	6.8	1,464	33.7	33.5	9,662	222.7	210.1	295	6.8	6.5
Louisiana	265	5.8	6.2	1,295	28.6	30.7	10,282	226.8	229.4	390	8.6	8.9
Maine	137	10.3	8.2	502	37.8	28.5	2,628	197.8	151.1	87	6.5	5.0
Maryland	389	6.7	6.9	986	17.1	16.8	10,915	189.1	182.2	433	7.5	7.3
Massachusetts	459	7.0	5.9	1,773	27.1	21.2	12,043	183.9	150.0	433	6.6	5.3
Michigan	816	8.3	7.4	2,736	27.7	24.0	23,326	236.0	204.2	815	8.2	7.1
Minnesota	512	9.7	8.9	1,451	27.4	23.4	7,185	135.5	119.4	439	8.3	7.3
Mississippi	174	5.9	6.1	927	31.2	32.6	7,542	254.2	251.1	531	17.9	17.6
Missouri	477	8.0	7.2	1,986	33.2	28.8	13,840	231.1	201.8	437	7.3	6.3
Montana	94	9.5	8.1	302	30.5	25.2	1,849	186.9	154.2	76	7.7	6.3
Nebraska	183	10.0	8.7	565	30.9	24.9	3,355	183.7	154.2	176	9.6	8.0
Nevada	149	5.5	6.6	296	11.0	14.2	4,811	178.1	197.3	128	4.7	5.7
New Hampshire	116	8.8	8.0	396	30.1	26.9	2,290	174.0	152.7	80	6.1	5.4
New Jersey	645	7.3	6.5	1,878	21.4	17.7	18,730	213.0	182.0	750	8.5	7.2
New Mexico	171	8.3	8.3	343	16.7	16.8	3,224	156.6	151.2	122	5.9	5.7
New York	972	5.0	4.5	2,616	13.5	11.3	44,981	232.1	199.9	2,048	10.6	9.1
North Carolina	636	6.7	6.8	2,817	29.5	30.3	17,154	179.9	174.9	844	8.9	8.7
North Dakota	61	9.1	7.0	361	53.7	37.2	1,395	207.4	158.0	64	9.5	7.0
Ohio	920	8.0	6.9	4,109	35.6	29.7	26,164	226.8	192.4	1,220	10.6	8.9
Oklahoma	249	6.6	6.4	1,015	27.1	26.1	9,426	251.3	235.2	343	9.1	8.6
Oregon	356	9.3	8.3	1,300	33.9	28.5	6,198	161.8	137.9	444	11.6	9.8
Pennsylvania	1,184	9.3	7.1	3,591	28.3	20.0	31,556	248.4	187.0	977	7.7	5.7
Rhode Island	96	9.1	7.1	338	32.1	22.6	2,322	220.6	167.1	70	6.7	4.9
South Carolina	381	8.2	8.3	1,570	33.9	34.7	9,295	201.0	189.9	417	9.0	8.5
South Dakota	86	10.6	8.3	398	48.9	35.9	1,616	198.5	155.2	96	11.8	9.1
Tennessee	435	6.9	6.9	2,440	38.4	38.5	14,582	229.8	217.4	594	9.4	9.0
Texas	1,492	5.9	7.6	5,209	20.7	26.8	38,253	152.1	181.1	1,722	6.8	8.3
Utah	170	6.2	8.9	375	13.6	19.3	2,889	104.5	143.2	125	4.5	6.1
Vermont	70	11.2	9.6	238	38.0	30.8	1,172	187.3	153.6	49	7.8	6.5
Virginia	520	6.5	7.0	1,848	23.1	24.4	13,404	167.5	168.5	588	7.3	7.5
Washington	514	7.6	7.9	3,025	45.0	43.6	10,602	157.7	151.5	506	7.5	7.1
West Virginia	142	7.7	6.2	594	32.1	26.0	4,897	264.3	211.2	264	14.2	11.3
Wisconsin	492	8.7	7.4	1,762	31.0	25.3	11,115	195.4	165.1	399	7.0	5.9
Wyoming	37	6.6	6.8	146	25.9	27.2	962	170.7	169.8	19	*	*
Puerto Rico	137	3.7	3.4	1,860	50.0	46.0	5,176	139.1	124.9	496	13.3	12.0
Virgin Islands	4	*	*	18	*	*	174	163.7	149.7	20	18.8	21.5
Guam	2	*	*	3	*	*	245	153.7	254.9	20	12.5	16.6
American Samoa	-	*	*	-	*	*	42	75.7	168.9	7	*	*
Northern Marianas	1	*	*	-	*	*	37	69.1	167.0	3	*	*

Table 2-31. Number of Deaths, Death Rates, and Age-Adjusted Death Rates for Major Causes of Death, by State and Territory, 2010—*Continued*

(Number, rates per 100,000 population, age-adjusted rates per 100,000 U.S. standard population.)

State and territory	Cerebrovascular disease (I60–I69)			Influenza and pneumonia (J09–J18)			Chronic lower respiratory disease (J40–J47)			Chronic liver disease and cirrhosis (K70,K73–K74)		
	Number	Rate	Age-adjusted rate[1]	Number	Rate	Age-adjusted rate[1]	Number	Rate	Age-adjusted rate[1]	Number	Rate	Age-adjusted rate[1]
United States [2]	129,476	41.9	39.1	50,097	16.2	15.1	138,080	44.7	42.2	31,903	10.3	9.4
Alabama	2,619	54.8	51.6	942	19.7	18.7	2,866	60.0	55.4	504	10.5	9.4
Alaska	167	23.5	40.9	64	9.0	15.8	176	24.8	41.5	70	9.9	9.8
Arizona	2,138	33.4	31.9	768	12.0	11.4	2,926	45.8	43.1	870	13.6	12.7
Arkansas	1,741	59.7	53.8	647	22.2	19.9	1,773	60.8	53.5	327	11.2	9.9
California	13,662	36.7	38.1	5,882	15.8	16.4	12,987	34.9	37.0	4,287	11.5	11.3
Colorado	1,607	32.0	36.1	550	10.9	12.3	2,199	43.7	49.7	599	11.9	11.2
Connecticut	1,349	37.7	29.4	568	15.9	12.1	1,289	36.1	29.4	303	8.5	7.3
Delaware	407	45.3	40.7	138	15.4	13.8	441	49.1	44.0	93	10.4	8.8
District of Columbia	196	32.6	32.7	80	13.3	13.5	147	24.4	25.7	54	9.0	8.9
Florida	8,432	44.8	32.8	2,259	12.0	8.9	10,337	55.0	40.1	2,480	13.2	10.6
Georgia	3,762	38.8	46.3	1,456	15.0	18.3	3,816	39.4	46.7	743	7.7	7.5
Hawaii	605	44.5	35.8	289	21.2	17.0	296	21.8	18.0	102	7.5	6.5
Idaho	642	41.0	42.0	208	13.3	13.5	727	46.4	47.0	150	9.6	9.3
Illinois	5,349	41.7	39.2	2,212	17.2	16.1	5,231	40.8	39.3	1,123	8.8	8.2
Indiana	3,082	47.5	44.5	1,175	18.1	16.8	3,794	58.5	55.3	634	9.8	9.0
Iowa	1,537	50.5	38.0	560	18.4	13.7	1,698	55.7	44.7	277	9.1	7.9
Kansas	1,370	48.0	41.2	550	19.3	16.4	1,580	55.4	50.0	244	8.6	7.8
Kentucky	1,992	45.9	44.1	943	21.7	21.0	2,779	64.0	60.0	463	10.7	9.4
Louisiana	1,977	43.6	44.9	878	19.4	20.2	1,939	42.8	43.6	390	8.6	7.9
Maine	602	45.3	34.5	234	17.6	13.4	809	60.9	47.4	154	11.6	8.8
Maryland	2,279	39.5	38.8	925	16.0	15.7	2,039	35.3	35.0	453	7.8	7.0
Massachusetts	2,516	38.4	31.3	1,291	19.7	16.0	2,383	36.4	31.0	584	8.9	7.7
Michigan	4,474	45.3	39.5	1,529	15.5	13.6	5,079	51.4	45.6	1,130	11.4	10.0
Minnesota	2,167	40.9	36.1	595	11.2	9.7	2,016	38.0	35.1	414	7.8	7.0
Mississippi	1,520	51.2	51.2	567	19.1	19.2	1,661	56.0	55.2	291	9.8	9.0
Missouri	3,001	50.1	44.0	1,188	19.8	17.4	3,557	59.4	52.6	530	8.8	7.8
Montana	494	49.9	41.8	168	17.0	13.6	602	60.8	51.3	124	12.5	10.7
Nebraska	876	48.0	40.5	266	14.6	11.9	1,008	55.2	48.8	160	8.8	8.1
Nevada	796	29.5	33.3	471	17.4	19.8	1,186	43.9	49.5	316	11.7	11.1
New Hampshire	500	38.0	33.5	191	14.5	12.6	609	46.3	41.7	103	7.8	6.4
New Jersey	3,402	38.7	33.3	1,128	12.8	11.0	3,106	35.3	31.4	732	8.3	7.3
New Mexico	806	39.1	38.4	294	14.3	14.2	1,022	49.6	47.7	377	18.3	17.0
New York	6,213	32.1	27.9	4,642	24.0	20.6	6,847	35.3	31.4	1,434	7.4	6.6
North Carolina	4,298	45.1	44.7	1,700	17.8	17.7	4,495	47.1	46.1	932	9.8	8.9
North Dakota	382	56.8	42.9	128	19.0	13.9	356	52.9	43.1	70	10.4	10.1
Ohio	5,755	49.9	42.6	1,975	17.1	14.6	6,717	58.2	50.5	1,244	10.8	9.4
Oklahoma	1,980	52.8	50.0	778	20.7	19.7	2,720	72.5	67.4	501	13.4	12.5
Oregon	1,793	46.8	40.1	417	10.9	9.2	1,971	51.4	45.3	509	13.3	11.3
Pennsylvania	6,701	52.8	39.3	2,324	18.3	13.6	6,202	48.8	37.9	1,200	9.4	7.8
Rhode Island	431	40.9	31.4	197	18.7	13.8	507	48.2	38.5	123	11.7	9.7
South Carolina	2,293	49.6	47.9	747	16.2	15.9	2,264	48.9	46.3	571	12.3	10.8
South Dakota	416	51.1	39.9	169	20.8	15.8	451	55.4	46.0	85	10.4	10.1
Tennessee	3,205	50.5	48.7	1,352	21.3	20.5	3,551	56.0	52.7	735	11.6	10.2
Texas	9,180	36.5	44.4	3,022	12.0	14.6	8,921	35.5	43.0	2,873	11.4	11.7
Utah	739	26.7	37.1	348	12.6	17.1	671	24.3	33.1	167	6.0	7.3
Vermont	265	42.3	35.3	60	9.6	7.9	335	53.5	45.3	55	8.8	7.2
Virginia	3,293	41.2	42.1	1,195	14.9	15.5	2,969	37.1	38.1	693	8.7	7.9
Washington	2,548	37.9	37.0	578	8.6	8.3	2,737	40.7	40.4	783	11.6	10.5
West Virginia	1,104	59.6	47.8	436	23.5	19.0	1,482	80.0	62.7	244	13.2	10.7
Wisconsin	2,609	45.9	38.7	904	15.9	13.3	2,474	43.5	38.0	528	9.3	8.2
Wyoming	204	36.2	37.2	109	19.3	19.5	332	58.9	59.5	75	13.3	12.5
Puerto Rico	1,500	40.3	36.4	818	22.0	19.9	1,089	29.3	26.5	201	5.4	4.6
Virgin Islands	34	32.0	33.4	2	.	.	5	.	.	12	.	.
Guam	66	41.4	71.6	11	.	.	24	15.1	24.5	19	.	.
American Samoa	21	37.9	94.5	7	.	.	10	.	.	-	.	.
Northern Marianas	17	.	.	5	.	.	6	.	.	1	.	.

Table 2-31. Number of Deaths, Death Rates, and Age-Adjusted Death Rates for Major Causes of Death, by State and Territory, 2010—Continued

(Number, rates per 100,000 population, age-adjusted rates per 100,000 U.S. standard population.)

State and territory	Nephritis, nephrotic syndrome, and nephrosis (N00–N07, N–17–N19, N–25–N27)			Accidents (V01–X59, Y85–Y86)			Motor vehicle accidents[3]			Intentional self–harm (suicide) (*U03, X60–X84, Y87.0)		
	Number	Rate	Age-adjusted rate[1]	Number	Rate	Age-adjusted rate[1]	Number	Rate	Age-adjusted rate[1]	Number	Rate	Age-adjusted rate[1]
United States [2]	50,476	16.3	15.3	120,859	39.1	38.0	35,332	11.4	11.3	38,364	12.4	12.1
Alabama	1,184	24.8	23.1	2,394	50.1	49.6	931	19.5	19.4	679	14.2	14.0
Alaska	56	7.9	13.5	366	51.5	58.7	71	10.0	10.4	164	23.1	22.8
Arizona	537	8.4	7.9	3,018	47.2	46.7	792	12.4	12.3	1,093	17.1	17.0
Arkansas	737	25.3	22.8	1,461	50.1	49.4	608	20.9	20.7	447	15.3	15.5
California	3,112	8.4	8.7	10,435	28.0	27.8	2,922	7.8	7.7	3,913	10.5	10.3
Colorado	426	8.5	9.6	2,106	41.9	43.5	483	9.6	9.5	865	17.2	16.8
Connecticut	599	16.8	13.4	1,337	37.4	33.6	331	9.3	9.1	353	9.9	9.4
Delaware	158	17.6	15.4	357	39.8	39.2	111	12.4	12.5	106	11.8	11.3
District of Columbia	84	14.0	14.4	212	35.2	35.1	38	6.3	6.0	41	6.8	6.9
Florida	3,297	17.5	12.9	8,875	47.2	43.1	2,536	13.5	13.0	2,789	14.8	13.7
Georgia	1,753	18.1	21.3	3,745	38.7	40.7	1,324	13.7	13.9	1,133	11.7	11.7
Hawaii	208	15.3	12.8	432	31.8	29.6	124	9.1	9.1	207	15.2	15.0
Idaho	186	11.9	12.1	654	41.7	42.1	214	13.7	13.8	290	18.5	18.8
Illinois	2,612	20.4	19.3	3,997	31.2	30.4	1,033	8.1	7.9	1,178	9.2	9.0
Indiana	1,516	23.4	22.0	2,534	39.1	38.5	768	11.8	11.8	864	13.3	13.1
Iowa	323	10.6	8.1	1,273	41.8	37.2	400	13.1	12.7	372	12.2	12.1
Kansas	577	20.2	17.7	1,317	46.2	44.0	482	16.9	16.6	401	14.1	13.9
Kentucky	1,079	24.9	23.8	2,632	60.7	60.5	821	18.9	18.8	631	14.5	14.2
Louisiana	1,218	26.9	27.3	1,999	44.1	44.4	718	15.8	15.8	557	12.3	12.3
Maine	272	20.5	15.8	540	40.7	36.5	171	12.9	12.2	186	14.0	13.2
Maryland	803	13.9	13.6	1,446	25.0	24.7	513	8.9	8.8	502	8.7	8.3
Massachusetts	1,381	21.1	17.5	2,060	31.5	28.5	387	5.9	5.5	598	9.1	8.8
Michigan	1,720	17.4	15.3	3,770	38.1	36.2	1,051	10.6	10.3	1,263	12.8	12.5
Minnesota	897	16.9	15.0	2,103	39.6	36.7	515	9.7	9.5	606	11.4	11.2
Mississippi	738	24.9	24.7	1,685	56.8	56.8	682	23.0	22.9	388	13.1	13.0
Missouri	1,305	21.8	19.2	2,975	49.7	47.9	871	14.5	14.4	856	14.3	14.0
Montana	133	13.4	11.3	548	55.4	53.2	192	19.4	19.6	227	22.9	21.8
Nebraska	290	15.9	13.4	700	38.3	35.8	211	11.6	11.3	193	10.6	10.4
Nevada	471	17.4	19.5	1,088	40.3	41.3	286	10.6	10.7	547	20.3	19.8
New Hampshire	206	15.6	14.2	517	39.3	37.2	135	10.3	10.1	196	14.9	14.1
New Jersey	1,580	18.0	15.6	2,486	28.3	26.7	579	6.6	6.5	719	8.2	7.7
New Mexico	276	13.4	13.1	1,233	59.9	60.7	331	16.1	16.4	413	20.1	20.1
New York	2,439	12.6	11.0	5,004	25.8	24.2	1,323	6.8	6.6	1,547	8.0	7.7
North Carolina	1,892	19.8	19.5	4,144	43.5	43.2	1,383	14.5	14.5	1,174	12.3	12.0
North Dakota	104	15.5	11.5	285	42.4	38.8	97	14.4	14.5	106	15.8	15.6
Ohio	2,066	17.9	15.4	5,124	44.4	42.4	1,251	10.8	10.6	1,439	12.5	12.2
Oklahoma	595	15.9	15.0	2,288	61.0	60.3	716	19.1	19.0	618	16.5	16.5
Oregon	400	10.4	8.9	1,566	40.9	37.8	324	8.5	8.1	685	17.9	17.1
Pennsylvania	2,982	23.5	17.8	5,751	45.3	41.1	1,441	11.3	11.0	1,576	12.4	11.9
Rhode Island	199	18.9	14.5	475	45.1	40.0	91	8.6	8.2	129	12.3	12.3
South Carolina	963	20.8	19.9	2,274	49.2	48.9	812	17.6	17.5	637	13.8	13.5
South Dakota	74	9.1	7.3	393	48.3	44.5	144	17.7	17.3	140	17.2	17.5
Tennessee	983	15.5	14.8	3,539	55.8	54.9	1,099	17.3	17.1	943	14.9	14.6
Texas	3,878	15.4	18.4	9,212	36.6	39.0	3,331	13.2	13.4	2,891	11.5	11.7
Utah	263	9.5	13.1	970	35.1	40.6	272	9.8	10.6	473	17.1	18.3
Vermont	50	8.0	6.7	298	47.6	42.7	76	12.1	11.8	106	16.9	15.7
Virginia	1,595	19.9	20.2	2,527	31.6	31.6	724	9.0	9.0	963	12.0	11.7
Washington	552	8.2	8.0	2,609	38.8	37.6	549	8.2	7.9	957	14.2	13.9
West Virginia	475	25.6	20.3	1,234	66.6	63.7	310	16.7	16.2	279	15.1	14.1
Wisconsin	1,163	20.5	17.5	2,525	44.4	40.8	620	10.9	10.6	793	13.9	13.4
Wyoming	69	12.2	12.5	346	61.4	59.8	138	24.5	23.1	131	23.2	22.4
Puerto Rico	987	26.5	23.7	1,018	27.4	25.9	352	9.5	9.1	286	7.7	7.6
Virgin Islands	14	*	*	25	23.5	22.5	7	*	*	8	*	*
Guam	20	12.5	19.0	45	28.2	36.7	17	*	*	31	19.4	19.2
American Samoa	4	*	*	14	*	*	2	*	*	-	*	*
Northern Marianas	7	*	*	10	*	*	4	*	*	3	*	*

Table 2-31. Number of Deaths, Death Rates, and Age-Adjusted Death Rates for Major Causes of Death, by State and Territory, 2010—*Continued*

(Number, rates per 100,000 population, age-adjusted rates per 100,000 U.S. standard population.)

State and territory	Assault (homicide) (*U01–*U02,X85–Y09, Y87.1)			Alcohol–induced causes[4]			Drug–induced causes[5]			Injury by firearms[6]		
	Number	Rate	Age-adjusted rate[1]	Number	Rate	Age-adjusted rate[1]	Number	Rate	Age-adjusted rate[1]	Number	Rate	Age-adjusted rate[1]
United States[2]	16,259	5.3	5.3	25,692	8.3	7.6	40,393	13.1	12.9	31,672	10.3	10.1
Alabama	391	8.2	8.3	267	5.6	5.0	585	12.2	12.6	782	16.4	16.2
Alaska	44	6.2	6.1	122	17.2	16.3	84	11.8	11.9	144	20.3	20.4
Arizona	418	6.5	6.7	987	15.4	14.7	1,141	17.9	18.2	931	14.6	14.6
Arkansas	188	6.4	6.6	179	6.1	5.7	374	12.8	13.3	419	14.4	14.4
California	1,954	5.2	5.1	4,292	11.5	11.2	4,258	11.4	11.1	2,935	7.9	7.7
Colorado	172	3.4	3.4	733	14.6	13.5	676	13.4	13.1	555	11.0	10.8
Connecticut	144	4.0	4.2	192	5.4	4.8	372	10.4	10.3	209	5.8	5.9
Delaware	61	6.8	7.0	74	8.2	7.3	147	16.4	16.8	88	9.8	9.9
District of Columbia	119	19.8	17.2	87	14.5	14.1	90	15.0	15.0	99	16.5	14.2
Florida	1,114	5.9	6.2	1,751	9.3	7.8	3,181	16.9	17.0	2,268	12.1	11.5
Georgia	640	6.6	6.6	630	6.5	6.2	1,124	11.6	11.4	1,223	12.6	12.6
Hawaii	24	1.8	1.7	87	6.4	5.5	154	11.3	11.1	45	3.3	3.2
Idaho	23	1.5	1.5	162	10.3	9.9	184	11.7	12.2	198	12.6	12.8
Illinois	783	6.1	6.1	690	5.4	5.0	1,344	10.5	10.4	1,064	8.3	8.2
Indiana	315	4.9	4.9	435	6.7	6.3	964	14.9	14.9	709	10.9	10.8
Iowa	55	1.8	1.9	233	7.6	6.7	258	8.5	8.8	213	7.0	6.8
Kansas	105	3.7	3.8	201	7.0	6.5	288	10.1	10.2	300	10.5	10.5
Kentucky	199	4.6	4.7	302	7.0	6.2	1,036	23.9	24.2	555	12.8	12.4
Louisiana	541	11.9	12.0	235	5.2	4.8	616	13.6	13.7	864	19.1	19.2
Maine	26	2.0	2.0	132	9.9	7.6	140	10.5	10.7	113	8.5	7.9
Maryland	438	7.6	7.7	291	5.0	4.5	674	11.7	11.4	538	9.3	9.3
Massachusetts	204	3.1	3.2	485	7.4	6.5	836	12.8	12.5	270	4.1	4.1
Michigan	610	6.2	6.4	928	9.4	8.3	1,723	17.4	17.3	1,076	10.9	11.0
Minnesota	112	2.1	2.1	429	8.1	7.3	427	8.1	7.9	365	6.9	6.8
Mississippi	284	9.6	9.8	167	5.6	5.3	353	11.9	12.0	475	16.0	16.1
Missouri	438	7.3	7.5	399	6.7	6.0	1,024	17.1	17.4	846	14.1	14.0
Montana	30	3.0	3.0	147	14.9	13.0	123	12.4	13.3	164	16.6	15.4
Nebraska	60	3.3	3.4	145	7.9	7.4	130	7.1	7.3	152	8.3	8.2
Nevada	164	6.1	6.1	336	12.4	11.4	581	21.5	20.8	395	14.6	14.5
New Hampshire	19	*	*	127	9.6	7.9	164	12.5	12.1	118	9.0	8.2
New Jersey	388	4.4	4.6	548	6.2	5.6	903	10.3	10.1	456	5.2	5.2
New Mexico	152	7.4	7.6	425	20.6	19.7	487	23.7	24.3	301	14.6	14.9
New York	898	4.6	4.6	1,217	6.3	5.7	1,760	9.1	8.8	1,011	5.2	5.1
North Carolina	539	5.7	5.7	669	7.0	6.3	1,125	11.8	11.7	1,123	11.8	11.6
North Dakota	14	*	*	78	11.6	11.4	26	3.9	3.9	65	9.7	9.5
Ohio	569	4.9	5.1	840	7.3	6.5	1,911	16.6	16.7	1,148	10.0	9.9
Oklahoma	214	5.7	5.7	440	11.7	11.1	728	19.4	19.7	538	14.3	14.4
Oregon	115	3.0	2.9	572	14.9	12.9	576	15.0	14.6	458	12.0	11.4
Pennsylvania	689	5.4	5.6	728	5.7	5.0	1,980	15.6	15.8	1,307	10.3	10.1
Rhode Island	27	2.6	2.6	102	9.7	8.2	176	16.7	16.3	49	4.7	4.6
South Carolina	322	7.0	7.1	394	8.5	7.5	697	15.1	15.0	648	14.0	14.0
South Dakota	17	*	*	89	10.9	10.7	48	5.9	6.6	75	9.2	9.2
Tennessee	410	6.5	6.5	542	8.5	7.5	1,132	17.8	17.7	932	14.7	14.4
Texas	1,363	5.4	5.4	1,579	6.3	6.3	2,492	9.9	10.0	2,714	10.8	11.0
Utah	52	1.9	1.9	182	6.6	7.7	457	16.5	17.9	314	11.4	12.2
Vermont	8	*	*	59	9.4	7.9	68	10.9	10.3	70	11.2	10.3
Virginia	373	4.7	4.7	414	5.2	4.7	571	7.1	7.0	875	10.9	10.8
Washington	180	2.7	2.7	850	12.6	11.4	962	14.3	13.8	609	9.1	8.9
West Virginia	86	4.6	5.0	139	7.5	6.3	520	28.1	29.3	273	14.7	14.1
Wisconsin	159	2.8	2.8	500	8.8	7.8	635	11.2	11.0	501	8.8	8.6
Wyoming	9	*	*	80	14.2	13.5	88	15.6	15.5	92	16.3	15.6
Puerto Rico	959	25.8	26.1	200	5.4	4.7	148	4.0	4.1	923	24.8	25.2
Virgin Islands	56	52.7	63.3	15	*	*	2	*	*	53	49.9	59.7
Guam	4	*	*	1	*	*	2	*	*	3	*	*
American Samoa	5	*	*	-	*	*	-	*	*	1	*	*
Northern Marianas	1	*	*	3	*	*	-	*	*	-	*	*

- = Quantity zero.   * = Figure does not meet standards of reliability or precision.   [1]Death rates are affected by the population composition of the area. Age-adjusted death rates should be used for comparisons between areas.   [2]Excludes data for Puerto Rico, Virgin Islands, Guam, American Samoa and Northern Marianas.   [3]ICD-10 codes for Motor vehicle accidents are V02–V04, V09.0, V09.2, V12–V14, V19.0–V19.2, V19.4–V19.6, V20–V79, V80.3–V80.5, V81.0–V81.1, V82.0–V82.1, V83–V86, V87.0–V87.8, V88.0–V88.8, V89.0, and V89.2.   [4]Causes of death attributable to alcohol-induced mortality include ICD-10 codes E24.4, F10, G31.2, G62.1, G72.1, I42.6, K29.2, K70, K85.2, K86.0, R78.0, X45, X65, and Y15.   [5]Causes of death attributable to drug-induced mortality include ICD-10 codes D52.1, D59.0, D59.2, D61.1, D64.2, E06.4, E16.0, E23.1, E24.2, E27.3, E66.1, F11.1–F11.5, F11.7–F11.9, F12.1–F12.5, F12.7–F12.9, F13.1–F13.5, F13.7–F13.9, F14.1–F14.5, F14.7–F14.9, F15.1–F15.5, F15.7–F15.9, F16.1–F16.5, F16.7–F16.9, F17.3–F17.5, F17.7–F17.9, F18.1–F18.5, F18.7–F18.9, F19.1–F19.5, F19.7–F19.9, G21.1, G24.0, G25.1, G25.4, G25.6, G44.4, G62.0, G72.0, I95.2, J70.2–J70.4, K85.3,L10.5, L27.0–L27.1, M10.2, M32.0, M80.4, M81.4, M83.5, M87.1, R50.2, R78.1–R78.5, X40–X44, X60–X64, X85, and Y10–Y14.   [6]ICD–10 codes for Injury by firearms are *U01.4, W32–W34, X72–X74, X93–X95, Y22–Y24, and Y35.0.

Table 2-32A. Death Rates for All Causes, by Sex and Age, Selected Years, 1950–2010

(Deaths per 100,000 resident population.)

Sex, race, Hispanic origin, and age	1950[1]	1960[1]	1970	1980	1985	1990	1995	2000	2005	2006	2007	2008	2009	2010
All Persons														
All ages, age-adjusted[2]	1,446.0	1,339.2	1,222.6	1,039.1	988.1	938.7	909.8	869.0	815.0	791.8	775.3	774.9	749.6	747.0
All ages, crude	963.8	954.7	945.3	878.3	876.9	863.8	868.3	854.0	828.4	813.1	804.6	812.9	794.5	799.5
Under 1 year	3,299.2	2,696.4	2,142.4	1,288.3	1,088.1	971.9	780.3	736.7	710.2	705.8	702.5	678.9	659.7	623.4
1 to 4 years	139.4	109.1	84.5	63.9	51.8	46.8	40.4	32.4	29.9	29.1	29.4	29.3	27.4	26.5
5 to 14 years	60.1	46.6	41.3	30.6	26.5	24.0	22.2	18.0	16.3	15.2	15.2	13.9	13.8	12.9
15 to 24 years	128.1	106.3	127.7	115.4	94.9	99.2	93.4	79.9	80.7	81.4	78.8	74.2	69.8	67.7
25 to 34 years	178.7	146.4	157.4	135.5	124.4	139.2	137.3	101.4	106.8	109.0	107.2	105.1	104.4	102.9
35 to 44 years	358.7	299.4	314.5	227.9	207.7	223.2	239.4	198.9	194.9	192.0	186.0	181.0	180.0	170.5
45 to 54 years	853.9	756.0	730.0	584.0	519.3	473.4	454.3	425.6	431.9	427.5	420.3	419.6	418.1	407.1
55 to 64 years	1,901.0	1,735.1	1,658.8	1,346.3	1,294.2	1,196.9	1,104.7	992.2	898.5	881.3	866.7	867.1	856.7	851.9
65 to 74 years	4,104.3	3,822.1	3,582.7	2,994.9	2,862.8	2,648.6	2,549.0	2,399.1	2,109.7	2,031.4	1,976.0	1,958.4	1,888.7	1,875.1
75 to 84 years	9,331.1	8,745.2	8,004.4	6,692.6	6,398.7	6,007.2	5,811.3	5,666.5	5,251.8	5,096.1	4,987.1	4,998.1	4,820.2	4,790.2
85 years and over	20,196.9	19,857.5	16,344.9	15,980.3	15,712.4	15,327.4	15,248.6	15,524.4	14,982.4	14,426.7	14,160.9	14,332.4	13,660.1	13,934.3
Male														
All ages, age-adjusted[2]	1,674.2	1,609.0	1,542.1	1,348.1	1,278.1	1,202.8	1,143.9	1,053.8	971.9	943.5	922.9	918.8	890.9	887.1
All ages, crude	1,106.1	1,104.5	1,090.3	976.9	948.6	918.4	900.8	853.0	831.7	819.6	813.1	820.3	807.2	812.0
Under 1 year	3,728.0	3,059.3	2,410.0	1,428.5	1,219.9	1,082.8	856.3	806.5	782.2	773.5	768.2	742.7	725.0	680.2
1 to 4 years	151.7	119.5	93.2	72.6	58.5	52.4	44.5	35.9	34.0	31.3	32.3	32.7	30.1	29.6
5 to 14 years	70.9	55.7	50.5	36.7	31.8	28.5	26.4	20.9	18.5	17.5	17.3	15.8	15.6	14.6
15 to 24 years	167.9	152.1	188.5	172.3	138.9	147.4	137.4	114.9	117.1	118.5	114.3	108.0	100.0	97.6
25 to 34 years	216.5	187.9	215.3	196.1	179.6	204.3	198.0	138.6	148.6	152.7	149.5	146.8	142.7	141.5
35 to 44 years	428.8	372.8	402.6	299.2	278.9	310.4	331.0	255.2	246.3	242.4	235.3	227.1	225.5	212.5
45 to 54 years	1,067.1	992.2	958.5	767.3	671.6	610.3	589.9	542.8	548.2	541.4	529.8	526.2	520.3	505.9
55 to 64 years	2,395.3	2,309.5	2,282.7	1,815.1	1,711.4	1,553.4	1,400.7	1,230.7	1,119.8	1,097.5	1,086.5	1,089.8	1,078.4	1,075.5
65 to 74 years	4,931.4	4,914.4	4,873.8	4,105.2	3,856.3	3,491.5	3,263.8	2,979.6	2,566.0	2,464.5	2,398.6	2,372.3	2,290.5	2,275.1
75 to 84 years	10,426.0	10,178.4	10,010.2	8,816.7	8,501.6	7,888.6	7,399.6	6,972.6	6,300.3	6,103.8	5,948.6	5,939.4	5,725.8	5,693.7
85 years and over	21,636.0	21,186.3	17,821.5	18,801.1	18,614.1	18,056.6	17,861.0	17,501.4	16,538.9	15,910.1	15,620.2	15,709.6	15,142.9	15,414.3
Female														
All ages, age-adjusted[2]	1,236.0	1,105.3	971.4	817.9	784.5	750.9	739.4	731.4	692.3	672.2	658.1	659.9	636.8	634.9
All ages, crude	823.5	809.2	807.8	785.3	809.1	812.0	837.2	855.0	825.1	806.9	796.4	805.8	782.1	787.4
Under 1 year	2,854.6	2,321.3	1,863.7	1,141.7	950.6	855.7	700.5	663.4	634.9	635.0	633.6	612.5	591.5	564.0
1 to 4 years	126.7	98.4	75.4	54.7	44.8	41.0	36.0	28.7	25.6	26.9	26.5	25.8	24.6	23.3
5 to 14 years	48.9	37.3	31.8	24.2	21.0	19.3	17.9	15.0	13.9	12.7	12.9	11.9	12.0	11.1
15 to 24 years	89.1	61.3	68.1	57.5	49.6	49.0	47.3	43.1	42.2	42.3	41.3	38.6	38.1	36.4
25 to 34 years	142.7	106.6	101.6	75.9	69.4	74.2	76.1	63.5	64.7	65.0	64.6	63.1	65.6	64.0
35 to 44 years	290.3	229.4	231.1	159.3	138.7	137.9	149.3	143.2	144.0	142.2	137.2	135.3	134.9	128.9
45 to 54 years	641.5	526.7	517.2	412.9	375.2	342.7	324.1	312.5	319.5	317.4	314.4	316.4	319.1	311.4
55 to 64 years	1,404.8	1,196.4	1,098.9	934.3	925.6	878.8	835.2	772.2	692.4	680.0	661.8	659.6	650.1	643.5
65 to 74 years	3,333.2	2,871.8	2,579.7	2,144.7	2,096.9	1,991.2	1,975.8	1,921.2	1,721.3	1,661.0	1,612.8	1,601.0	1,540.5	1,527.5
75 to 84 years	8,399.6	7,633.1	6,677.6	5,440.1	5,162.1	4,883.1	4,818.6	4,814.7	4,532.3	4,397.2	4,313.2	4,331.8	4,172.2	4,137.7
85 years and over	19,194.7	19,008.4	15,518.0	14,746.9	14,553.9	14,274.3	14,242.3	14,719.2	14,290.8	13,753.8	13,486.3	13,684.3	12,951.6	13,219.2

[1]Includes deaths of persons who were not residents of the 50 states and the District of Columbia (DC).   [2]Age-adjusted rates are calculated using the year 2000 standard population. Prior to 2001, age-adjusted rates were calculated using standard million proportions based on rounded population numbers. Starting with 2001 data, unrounded population numbers are used to calculate age-adjusted rates.

Table 2-32B. Death Rates for All Causes, by Race, Age, and Hispanic Origin for Males, Selected Years, 1950–2010

(Deaths per 100,000 resident population.)

Sex, race, Hispanic origin, and age	1950[1]	1960[1]	1970	1980	1985	1990	1995	2000	2005	2006	2007	2008	2009	2010
White Male [2]														
All ages, age-adjusted[3]	1,642.5	1,586.0	1,513.7	1,317.6	1,249.8	1,165.9	1,107.5	1,029.4	952.9	925.8	907.1	907.1	880.5	878.5
All ages, crude	1,089.5	1,098.5	1,086.7	983.3	963.6	930.9	921.0	887.8	873.5	862.3	857.8	870.6	858.2	866.1
Under 1 year	3,400.5	2,694.1	2,113.2	1,230.3	1,056.5	896.1	720.7	667.6	664.5	653.2	653.2	635.8	611.2	584.3
1 to 4 years	135.5	104.9	83.6	66.1	52.8	45.9	39.0	32.6	31.7	28.4	29.4	30.5	28.3	27.4
5 to 14 years	67.2	52.7	48.0	35.0	30.1	26.4	24.3	19.8	17.1	16.5	16.2	14.6	14.5	13.8
15 to 24 years	152.4	143.7	170.8	167.0	134.2	131.3	120.1	105.8	110.6	112.2	108.1	102.4	94.9	91.8
25 to 34 years	185.3	163.2	176.6	171.3	158.8	176.1	171.9	124.1	136.2	141.7	140.4	139.3	135.9	135.6
35 to 44 years	380.9	332.6	343.5	257.4	243.1	268.2	286.8	233.6	232.4	228.8	222.7	218.3	216.8	206.6
45 to 54 years	984.5	932.2	882.9	698.9	611.7	548.7	528.3	496.9	512.1	508.6	501.9	504.8	502.3	491.9
55 to 64 years	2,304.4	2,225.2	2,202.6	1,728.5	1,625.8	1,467.2	1,319.3	1,163.3	1,061.3	1,043.2	1,034.7	1,044.0	1,032.2	1,033.0
65 to 74 years	4,864.9	4,848.4	4,810.1	4,035.7	3,770.7	3,397.7	3,173.3	2,905.7	2,511.6	2,409.6	2,345.4	2,324.8	2,245.3	2,232.4
75 to 84 years	10,526.3	10,299.6	10,098.8	8,829.8	8,486.1	7,844.9	7,347.3	6,933.1	6,277.9	6,089.7	5,939.7	5,938.3	5,737.1	5,703.6
85 years and over	22,116.3	21,750.0	18,551.7	19,097.3	18,980.1	18,268.3	18,050.7	17,716.4	16,693.3	16,059.2	15,776.0	15,922.9	15,362.2	15,640.3
Black or African American Male [2]														
All ages, age-adjusted[3]	1,909.1	1,811.1	1,873.9	1,697.8	1,634.5	1,644.5	1,585.7	1,403.5	1,281.3	1,239.5	1,204.8	1,168.0	1,123.1	1,104.0
All ages, crude	1,257.7	1,181.7	1,186.6	1,034.1	989.3	1,008.0	960.2	834.1	796.1	781.4	768.1	750.6	735.3	725.4
Under 1 year	---	5,306.8	4,298.9	2,586.7	2,219.9	2,112.4	1,664.7	1,567.6	1,478.6	1,449.5	1,406.0	1,343.0	1,357.2	1,206.5
1 to 4 years[4]	1,412.6	208.5	150.5	110.5	90.1	85.8	73.1	54.5	48.7	49.3	47.6	48.2	41.9	42.9
5 to 14 years	95.1	75.1	67.1	47.4	42.3	41.2	38.5	28.2	26.4	24.2	23.9	22.6	22.2	19.6
15 to 24 years	289.7	212.0	320.6	209.1	173.6	252.2	246.6	181.4	170.8	169.5	165.5	156.2	142.5	142.8
25 to 34 years	503.5	402.5	559.5	407.3	351.9	430.8	407.4	261.0	264.8	265.0	251.0	235.7	226.1	216.7
35 to 44 years	878.1	762.0	956.6	689.8	630.2	699.6	716.8	453.0	394.1	389.1	374.3	342.0	336.8	307.5
45 to 54 years	1,905.0	1,624.8	1,777.5	1,479.9	1,292.9	1,261.0	1,238.9	1,017.7	923.1	891.5	842.5	790.7	760.4	716.3
55 to 64 years	3,773.2	3,316.4	3,256.9	2,873.0	2,779.8	2,618.4	2,382.0	2,080.1	1,877.9	1,805.8	1,774.9	1,723.4	1,707.1	1,662.1
65 to 74 years	5,310.3	5,798.7	5,803.2	5,131.1	5,172.4	4,946.1	4,707.8	4,253.5	3,606.8	3,511.6	3,428.7	3,347.9	3,250.1	3,205.6
75 to 84 years[5]	10,101.9	8,605.1	9,454.9	9,231.6	9,262.3	9,129.5	8,862.0	8,486.0	7,674.6	7,381.4	7,142.9	7,084.2	6,727.9	6,721.5
85 years and over	NA	14,844.8	12,222.3	16,098.8	15,774.2	16,954.9	17,016.0	16,791.0	16,769.2	16,110.0	15,879.4	15,380.0	14,562.9	14,715.3
American Indian or Alaska Native Male [2]														
All ages, age-adjusted[3]	NA	NA	NA	1,111.5	926.1	916.2	932.0	841.5	824.5	780.8	780.3	757.2	709.0	730.2
All ages, crude	NA	NA	NA	597.1	492.5	476.4	459.4	415.6	428.4	413.7	411.1	408.7	389.9	397.5
Under 1 year	NA	NA	NA	1,598.1	1,080.0	1,056.6	696.0	700.2	600.5	706.2	646.4	600.1	548.7	542.5
1 to 4 years	NA	NA	NA	82.7	105.3	77.4	73.3	44.9	49.8	39.5	42.0	34.6	31.2	34.3
5 to 14 years	NA	NA	NA	43.7	39.2	33.4	27.0	20.2	19.7	14.1	17.9	14.7	15.5	18.1
15 to 24 years	NA	NA	NA	311.1	214.4	219.8	182.1	136.2	126.7	133.1	119.2	122.0	121.0	116.4
25 to 34 years	NA	NA	NA	360.6	275.0	256.1	263.6	179.1	191.6	176.3	175.6	171.3	154.9	156.2
35 to 44 years	NA	NA	NA	556.8	363.5	365.4	377.4	295.2	304.7	298.7	285.4	262.9	275.6	258.2
45 to 54 years	NA	NA	NA	871.3	687.9	619.9	601.0	520.0	541.6	534.2	507.1	535.2	486.7	496.1
55 to 64 years	NA	NA	NA	1,547.5	1,319.1	1,211.3	1,276.0	1,090.4	1,076.6	974.9	973.7	961.8	941.0	951.2
65 to 74 years	NA	NA	NA	2,968.4	2,692.3	2,461.7	2,660.8	2,478.3	2,243.8	2,127.5	2,105.8	2,128.4	1,969.9	1,971.0
75 to 84 years	NA	NA	NA	5,607.0	5,572.7	5,389.2	5,787.7	5,351.2	4,877.8	4,722.6	4,737.9	4,729.6	4,342.4	4,451.8
85 years and over	NA	NA	NA	12,635.2	8,900.0	11,243.9	10,604.7	10,725.8	11,841.9	10,735.7	11,274.5	9,880.9	9,174.7	10,268.1
Asian or Pacific Islander Male [2]														
All ages, age-adjusted[3]	NA	NA	NA	786.5	755.4	716.4	693.4	624.2	560.6	544.9	525.9	518.5	509.2	512.1
All ages, crude	NA	NA	NA	375.3	344.6	334.3	341.4	332.9	326.6	323.4	318.7	320.0	321.2	327.0
Under 1 year	NA	NA	NA	816.5	750.0	605.3	468.3	529.4	439.3	457.8	462.5	443.8	412.0	434.4
1 to 4 years	NA	NA	NA	50.9	43.4	45.0	28.0	23.3	19.7	17.4	24.3	16.8	19.3	19.3
5 to 14 years	NA	NA	NA	23.4	22.5	20.7	19.6	12.9	13.5	10.7	11.4	11.5	11.0	8.4
15 to 24 years	NA	NA	NA	80.8	76.0	76.0	73.0	55.2	51.2	54.7	52.2	41.5	41.3	43.0
25 to 34 years	NA	NA	NA	83.5	77.3	79.6	75.4	55.0	54.9	53.5	47.9	50.9	50.3	52.6
35 to 44 years	NA	NA	NA	128.3	114.4	130.8	124.9	104.9	96.5	92.3	92.0	89.1	93.7	83.5
45 to 54 years	NA	NA	NA	342.3	284.8	287.1	273.0	249.7	242.4	232.9	227.6	219.3	226.5	213.7
55 to 64 years	NA	NA	NA	881.1	869.4	789.1	714.2	642.4	540.4	546.1	514.8	516.3	509.9	519.0
65 to 74 years	NA	NA	NA	2,236.1	2,102.0	2,041.4	1,894.8	1,661.0	1,388.9	1,315.0	1,278.2	1,273.1	1,218.8	1,226.0
75 to 84 years	NA	NA	NA	5,389.5	5,551.2	5,008.6	4,729.9	4,328.2	3,875.2	3,730.6	3,650.5	3,595.7	3,456.9	3,438.7
85 years and over	NA	NA	NA	13,753.6	12,750.0	12,446.3	13,252.0	12,125.3	11,343.4	11,154.9	10,580.0	10,492.8	10,477.3	10,824.5
Hispanic or Latino Male [2,6]														
All ages, age-adjusted[3]	NA	NA	NA	NA	889.2	886.4	897.6	818.1	771.2	732.3	711.4	695.3	675.5	677.7
All ages, crude	NA	NA	NA	NA	374.6	411.6	391.6	331.3	335.6	326.1	321.6	316.0	311.8	310.8
Under 1 year	NA	NA	NA	NA	1,044.6	921.8	684.6	637.1	637.6	613.6	616.5	605.0	569.5	556.8
1 to 4 years	NA	NA	NA	NA	53.8	53.8	39.3	31.5	33.0	28.9	28.4	29.0	25.9	25.0
5 to 14 years	NA	NA	NA	NA	23.0	26.0	24.6	17.9	15.1	16.0	15.3	12.3	14.1	11.4
15 to 24 years	NA	NA	NA	NA	147.5	159.3	147.3	107.7	112.3	111.8	104.2	91.9	87.6	79.4
25 to 34 years	NA	NA	NA	NA	202.1	234.0	196.7	120.2	123.0	121.7	117.4	112.3	107.1	100.9
35 to 44 years	NA	NA	NA	NA	290.1	341.8	333.6	211.0	188.8	184.6	173.7	165.5	158.5	146.2
45 to 54 years	NA	NA	NA	NA	495.7	533.9	528.5	439.0	421.7	409.6	404.3	377.2	376.9	351.9
55 to 64 years	NA	NA	NA	NA	1,129.4	1,123.7	1,076.9	965.7	880.2	849.4	836.0	837.0	818.9	815.1
65 to 74 years	NA	NA	NA	NA	2,484.9	2,368.2	2,429.3	2,287.9	2,052.2	1,936.1	1,884.2	1,854.9	1,789.2	1,775.0
75 to 84 years	NA	NA	NA	NA	5,696.1	5,369.1	5,557.4	5,395.3	5,096.5	4,739.5	4,612.2	4,563.6	4,396.7	4,461.9
85 years and over	NA	NA	NA	NA	12,156.2	12,272.1	13,295.9	13,086.2	12,746.1	12,135.6	11,719.4	11,453.4	11,225.7	11,779.8

Table 2-32B. Death Rates for All Causes, by Race, Age, and Hispanic Origin for Males, Selected Years, 1950–2010—*Continued*

(Deaths per 100,000 resident population.)

Sex, race, Hispanic origin, and age	1950[1]	1960[1]	1970	1980	1985	1990	1995	2000	2005	2006	2007	2008	2009	2010
White, not Hispanic or Latino Male [6]														
All ages, age-adjusted[2]	NA	NA	NA	NA	1,215.6	1,170.9	1,105.6	1,035.4	961.5	935.7	918.4	920.2	893.7	892.5
All ages, crude	NA	NA	NA	NA	956.3	985.9	984.8	978.5	978.1	969.4	968.3	987.5	975.7	987.5
Under 1 year	NA	NA	NA	NA	1,002.0	865.4	703.8	658.7	656.4	647.8	647.5	627.9	604.4	575.9
1 to 4 years	NA	NA	NA	NA	48.8	43.8	37.8	32.4	30.6	27.4	29.1	30.3	28.3	27.5
5 to 14 years	NA	NA	NA	NA	28.9	25.7	23.5	20.0	17.5	16.2	16.1	15.1	14.2	14.3
15 to 24 years	NA	NA	NA	NA	125.0	123.4	111.5	103.5	107.6	109.6	106.8	103.2	94.4	93.4
25 to 34 years	NA	NA	NA	NA	151.2	165.3	163.5	123.0	137.7	145.0	145.0	145.1	142.1	143.6
35 to 44 years	NA	NA	NA	NA	231.8	257.1	276.5	233.9	238.4	235.3	230.7	227.9	227.9	219.1
45 to 54 years	NA	NA	NA	NA	587.7	544.5	520.7	497.7	518.8	516.8	510.5	518.2	515.4	508.1
55 to 64 years	NA	NA	NA	NA	1,550.7	1,479.7	1,322.7	1,170.9	1,070.8	1,054.0	1,046.7	1,056.2	1,045.1	1,046.2
65 to 74 years	NA	NA	NA	NA	3,648.1	3,434.5	3,188.5	2,930.5	2,536.0	2,435.4	2,372.1	2,350.7	2,269.9	2,256.9
75 to 84 years	NA	NA	NA	NA	8,361.0	7,920.4	7,367.4	6,977.8	6,329.5	6,154.5	6,008.4	6,009.9	5,810.0	5,770.3
85 years and over	NA	NA	NA	NA	18,635.3	18,505.4	18,132.6	17,853.2	16,840.7	16,206.8	15,946.0	16,114.4	15,552.9	15,816.6

NA = Not available.   [1]Includes deaths of persons who were not residents of the 50 states and the District of Columbia (DC).   [2]The race groups, White, Black, Asian or Pacific Islander, and American Indian and Alaska Native, include persons of Hispanic and non-Hispanic origin. Persons of Hispanic origin may be of any race. Death rates for the American Indian and Alaska Native, Asian or Pacific Islander, and Hispanic populations are known to be underestimated.   [3]Age-adjusted rates are calculated using the year 2000 standard population. Prior to 2001, age-adjusted rates were calculated using standard million proportions based on rounded population numbers. Starting with 2001 data, unrounded population numbers are used to calculate age-adjusted rates.   [4]In 1950, rate is for the age group under 5 years.   [5]In 1950, rate is for the age group 75 years and over.   [6]Prior to 1997, excludes data from states lacking an Hispanic-origin item on the death certificate.

Table 2-32C. Death Rates for All Causes, by Race, Age, and Hispanic Origin for Females, Selected Years, 1950–2010

(Deaths per 100,000 resident population.)

Sex, race, Hispanic origin, and age	1950[1]	1960[1]	1970	1980	1985	1990	1995	2000	2005	2006	2007	2008	2009	2010
White Female [2]														
All ages, age-adjusted[3]	1,198.0	1,074.4	944.0	796.1	764.3	728.8	718.7	715.3	680.9	662.3	649.4	653.7	631.3	630.8
All ages, crude	803.3	800.9	812.6	806.1	840.1	846.9	883.2	912.3	888.1	870.3	860.6	874.6	849.3	857.3
Under 1 year	2,566.8	2,007.7	1,614.6	962.5	799.3	690.0	574.4	550.5	535.5	533.3	537.1	525.0	502.3	488.0
1 to 4 years	112.2	85.2	66.1	49.3	40.0	36.1	31.3	25.5	23.5	24.3	24.1	23.8	22.6	21.6
5 to 14 years	45.1	34.7	29.9	22.9	19.5	17.9	16.5	14.1	12.9	12.0	12.5	11.4	11.1	10.6
15 to 24 years	71.5	54.9	61.6	55.5	48.1	45.9	43.7	41.1	41.5	41.8	41.1	37.6	37.1	36.2
25 to 34 years	112.8	85.0	84.1	65.4	59.4	61.5	62.9	55.1	59.0	60.2	60.7	59.2	62.9	61.4
35 to 44 years	235.8	191.1	193.3	138.2	121.9	117.4	125.5	125.7	131.3	130.1	127.2	126.8	128.2	122.8
45 to 54 years	546.4	458.8	462.9	372.7	341.7	309.3	291.9	281.4	291.8	292.6	291.4	296.1	301.6	295.1
55 to 64 years	1,293.8	1,078.9	1,014.9	876.2	869.1	822.7	783.4	730.9	659.7	649.9	632.5	633.2	624.8	617.8
65 to 74 years	3,242.8	2,779.3	2,470.7	2,066.6	2,027.1	1,923.5	1,913.2	1,868.3	1,687.6	1,631.5	1,584.0	1,577.5	1,517.9	1,504.9
75 to 84 years	8,481.5	7,696.6	6,698.7	5,401.7	5,111.6	4,839.1	4,775.2	4,785.3	4,526.1	4,397.1	4,319.4	4,352.9	4,190.9	4,165.4
85 years and over	19,679.5	19,477.7	15,980.2	14,979.6	14,745.4	14,400.6	14,405.8	14,890.7	14,438.0	13,905.7	13,636.6	13,868.7	13,132.7	13,419.3
Black or African American Female [2]														
All ages, age-adjusted[3]	1,545.5	1,369.7	1,228.7	1,033.3	994.4	975.1	955.9	927.6	862.7	828.4	808.1	792.0	763.3	752.5
All ages, crude	1,002.0	905.0	829.2	733.3	734.2	747.9	743.2	733.0	699.2	678.3	668.2	661.8	645.6	642.7
Under 1 year	NA	4,162.2	3,368.8	2,123.7	1,821.4	1,735.5	1,399.9	1,279.8	1,203.3	1,215.9	1,160.8	1,105.1	1,070.0	994.4
1 to 4 years[4]	1,139.3	173.3	129.4	84.4	71.1	67.6	59.5	45.3	38.2	41.2	41.0	36.3	37.7	33.2
5 to 14 years	72.8	53.8	43.8	30.5	28.6	27.5	25.4	20.0	19.0	17.0	16.6	15.8	16.6	14.5
15 to 24 years	213.1	107.5	111.9	70.5	59.6	68.7	68.9	58.3	50.3	50.2	47.5	48.8	46.6	43.3
25 to 34 years	393.3	273.2	231.0	150.0	137.6	159.5	162.8	121.8	110.2	107.0	102.1	97.2	97.5	92.9
35 to 44 years	758.1	568.5	533.0	323.9	276.5	298.6	324.9	271.9	248.4	243.0	226.4	218.2	207.7	199.3
45 to 54 years	1,576.4	1,177.0	1,043.9	768.2	667.6	639.4	612.1	588.3	562.0	540.9	528.3	515.1	500.5	481.0
55 to 64 years	3,089.4	2,510.9	1,986.2	1,561.0	1,532.5	1,452.6	1,354.3	1,227.2	1,083.0	1,052.9	1,021.0	1,000.1	983.7	972.2
65 to 74 years	4,000.2	4,064.2	3,860.9	2,967.8	2,865.7	2,837.5	2,689.6	2,300.8	2,196.1	2,159.9	2,101.7	2,041.2	2,021.2	
75 to 84 years[5]	8,347.0	6,730.0	6,691.5	6,212.1	6,078.0	5,688.3	5,671.9	5,696.5	5,278.5	5,042.4	4,918.6	4,843.3	4,694.0	4,580.9
85 years and over	---	13,052.6	10,706.6	12,367.2	12,703.0	13,309.5	13,073.3	13,941.3	14,183.6	13,535.1	13,323.3	13,177.9	12,378.5	12,589.9
American Indian or Alaska Native Female [3]														
All ages, age-adjusted[3]	NA	NA	NA	662.4	577.2	561.8	643.9	604.5	601.8	589.0	565.2	548.7	536.4	541.7
All ages, crude	NA	NA	NA	380.1	342.5	330.4	360.1	346.1	354.8	347.6	339.0	332.9	332.4	332.4
Under 1 year	NA	NA	NA	1,352.6	910.5	688.7	780.6	492.2	500.1	453.5	528.3	437.3	444.2	366.4
1 to 4 years	NA	NA	NA	87.5	54.8	37.8	54.4	39.8	31.3	34.0	30.3	35.8	23.5	24.4
5 to 14 years	NA	NA	NA	33.5	23.0	25.5	20.0	17.7	14.5	13.6	9.9	13.1	16.2	10.5
15 to 24 years	NA	NA	NA	90.3	72.8	69.0	60.4	58.9	61.5	56.3	53.1	49.4	56.3	43.6
25 to 34 years	NA	NA	NA	178.5	121.5	102.3	106.3	84.8	80.8	80.7	77.8	83.6	81.9	85.6
35 to 44 years	NA	NA	NA	286.0	185.6	156.4	171.9	171.9	171.2	176.1	164.3	177.6	171.8	146.6
45 to 54 years	NA	NA	NA	491.4	415.5	380.9	349.1	284.9	338.9	311.6	309.8	300.0	346.5	326.2
55 to 64 years	NA	NA	NA	837.1	851.9	805.9	876.2	772.1	675.6	656.8	659.0	626.3	603.9	623.8
65 to 74 years	NA	NA	NA	1,765.5	1,630.3	1,679.4	1,935.6	1,899.8	1,770.0	1,639.8	1,589.6	1,528.3	1,472.4	1,481.7
75 to 84 years	NA	NA	NA	3,612.9	3,200.0	3,073.2	4,067.6	3,850.0	3,812.8	3,967.9	3,656.9	3,472.8	3,332.7	3,391.9
85 years and over	NA	NA	NA	8,567.4	7,740.0	8,201.1	9,201.8	9,118.2	9,752.1	9,413.5	9,155.0	9,024.2	8,619.3	9,277.9
Asian or Pacific Islander Female [2]														
All ages, age-adjusted[3]	NA	NA	NA	425.9	456.7	469.3	446.7	416.8	385.2	381.2	369.2	372.4	361.1	359.0
All ages, crude	NA	NA	NA	222.5	224.9	234.3	250.4	262.3	271.4	273.4	269.5	277.0	273.5	277.3
Under 1 year	NA	NA	NA	755.8	622.0	518.2	396.6	434.3	373.8	348.6	380.0	360.7	373.7	341.8
1 to 4 years	NA	NA	NA	35.4	36.8	32.0	24.9	20.0	16.2	19.8	16.8	19.3	12.7	16.3
5 to 14 years	NA	NA	NA	21.5	19.1	13.0	15.4	11.7	11.4	9.8	9.0	7.9	10.0	7.9
15 to 24 years	NA	NA	NA	32.3	30.7	28.8	31.1	22.4	23.1	22.2	20.5	19.1	21.1	17.0
25 to 34 years	NA	NA	NA	45.4	36.5	37.5	35.6	27.6	27.1	26.9	25.4	30.4	26.0	27.1
35 to 44 years	NA	NA	NA	89.7	77.8	69.9	66.2	65.6	57.9	56.8	54.3	48.0	50.8	49.0
45 to 54 years	NA	NA	NA	214.1	184.9	182.7	184.1	155.5	140.1	142.1	131.7	129.9	122.0	127.9
55 to 64 years	NA	NA	NA	440.8	468.0	483.4	457.7	390.9	342.8	321.9	315.0	310.2	294.8	298.8
65 to 74 years	NA	NA	NA	1,027.7	1,130.8	1,089.2	1,037.8	996.4	896.0	887.7	813.6	835.8	776.8	788.7
75 to 84 years	NA	NA	NA	2,833.6	2,873.9	3,127.9	3,089.9	2,882.4	2,613.2	2,623.3	2,566.2	2,531.2	2,472.3	2,445.5
85 years and over	NA	NA	NA	7,923.3	9,808.3	10,254.0	9,406.1	9,052.2	8,769.0	8,664.5	8,546.0	8,859.2	8,685.4	8,590.1
Hispanic or Latina Female [2,6]														
All ages, age-adjusted[3]	NA	NA	NA	NA	546.1	537.1	546.1	546.0	513.8	500.2	484.4	484.7	466.1	463.4
All ages, crude	NA	NA	NA	NA	251.9	285.4	281.9	274.6	272.7	269.0	264.0	265.8	261.4	260.9
Under 1 year	NA	NA	NA	NA	791.4	746.6	572.0	553.6	526.3	512.0	522.8	499.2	480.1	462.9
1 to 4 years	NA	NA	NA	NA	42.3	42.1	33.1	27.5	24.3	24.0	24.1	22.8	23.4	20.2
5 to 14 years	NA	NA	NA	NA	16.0	17.3	15.0	13.4	11.8	11.6	11.9	11.0	11.8	8.9
15 to 24 years	NA	NA	NA	NA	36.2	40.6	37.5	31.7	34.5	33.0	30.8	28.4	29.1	26.3
25 to 34 years	NA	NA	NA	NA	56.3	62.9	58.6	43.4	40.5	42.6	42.0	40.2	42.5	38.9
35 to 44 years	NA	NA	NA	NA	100.0	109.3	118.9	100.5	89.1	85.7	80.7	79.3	81.0	75.2
45 to 54 years	NA	NA	NA	NA	251.3	253.3	238.8	223.8	213.7	212.5	199.9	195.4	200.0	193.9
55 to 64 years	NA	NA	NA	NA	619.7	607.5	602.3	548.4	489.0	481.0	468.8	467.0	456.8	450.1
65 to 74 years	NA	NA	NA	NA	1,449.5	1,453.8	1,457.2	1,423.2	1,285.1	1,216.0	1,149.2	1,137.4	1,106.7	1,085.5
75 to 84 years	NA	NA	NA	NA	3,551.8	3,351.3	3,506.4	3,624.5	3,464.7	3,329.0	3,299.5	3,244.7	3,160.1	3,067.4
85 years and over	NA	NA	NA	NA	10,228.6	10,098.7	10,540.5	11,202.8	10,769.7	10,682.9	10,276.7	10,636.2	9,794.3	10,237.3

Table 2-32C. Death Rates for All Causes, by Race, Age, and Hispanic Origin for Females, Selected Years, 1950–2010—*Continued*

(Deaths per 100,000 resident population.)

Sex, race, Hispanic origin, and age	1950[1]	1960[1]	1970	1980	1985	1990	1995	2000	2005	2006	2007	2008	2009	2010
White, not Hispanic or Latina Female [6]														
All ages, age-adjusted[2]	NA	NA	NA	NA	754.3	734.6	721.1	721.5	690.7	672.4	660.6	665.4	643.1	643.3
All ages, crude	NA	NA	NA	NA	861.7	903.6	951.7	1,007.3	999.7	982.8	976.1	995.6	969.1	981.2
Under 1 year	NA	NA	NA	NA	763.0	655.3	553.9	530.9	522.3	526.7	525.3	516.0	494.2	480.4
1 to 4 years	NA	NA	NA	NA	36.5	34.0	30.3	24.4	22.7	23.8	23.5	23.5	21.6	21.8
5 to 14 years	NA	NA	NA	NA	19.0	17.6	16.4	13.9	13.0	11.8	12.4	11.1	10.5	10.9
15 to 24 years	NA	NA	NA	NA	47.9	46.0	44.0	42.6	42.6	43.3	43.2	39.6	38.6	38.4
25 to 34 years	NA	NA	NA	NA	59.0	60.6	62.2	56.8	63.3	64.0	65.0	63.8	67.5	66.8
35 to 44 years	NA	NA	NA	NA	122.8	116.8	124.1	128.1	138.1	137.7	135.8	136.1	137.7	133.1
45 to 54 years	NA	NA	NA	NA	335.7	312.1	293.0	285.0	299.4	300.8	301.6	308.0	313.5	307.7
55 to 64 years	NA	NA	NA	NA	853.3	834.5	789.8	742.1	672.7	662.8	645.5	646.2	638.5	631.5
65 to 74 years	NA	NA	NA	NA	1,998.1	1,940.2	1,925.9	1,891.0	1,715.2	1,660.9	1,616.4	1,609.8	1,548.1	1,535.9
75 to 84 years	NA	NA	NA	NA	5,059.1	4,887.3	4,794.9	4,819.3	4,577.1	4,451.4	4,375.2	4,416.1	4,252.4	4,232.6
85 years and over	NA	NA	NA	NA	14,560.4	14,533.1	14,450.9	14,971.7	14,560.9	14,014.9	13,761.8	13,984.1	13,264.8	13,543.5

NA = Not available. [1]Includes deaths of persons who were not residents of the 50 states and the District of Columbia (DC). [2]The race groups, White, Black, Asian or Pacific Islander, and American Indian and Alaska Native, include persons of Hispanic and non-Hispanic origin. Persons of Hispanic origin may be of any race. Death rates for the American Indian and Alaska Native, Asian or Pacific Islander, and Hispanic populations are known to be underestimated. [3]Age-adjusted rates are calculated using the year 2000 standard population. Prior to 2001, age-adjusted rates were calculated using standard million proportions based on rounded population numbers. Starting with 2001 data, unrounded population numbers are used to calculate age-adjusted rates. [4]In 1950, rate is for the age group under 5 years. [5]In 1950, rate is for the age group 75 years and over. [6]Prior to 1997, excludes data from states lacking an Hispanic-origin item on the death certificate.

Table 2-33. Death Rates for Diseases of the Heart, by Sex, Race, Hispanic Origin, and Age, Selected Years, 1950–2010

(Deaths per 100,000 resident population.)

Sex, race, Hispanic origin, and age	1950[1,2]	1960[1,2]	1970[2]	1980[2]	1985[2]	1990[2]	1995[2]	2000[3]	2005[3]	2006[3]	2007[3]	2008[3]	2009[3]	2010[3]
All Persons														
All ages, age-adjusted[4]	588.8	559.0	492.7	412.1	375.0	321.8	293.4	257.6	216.8	205.5	196.1	192.1	182.8	179.1
All ages, crude	356.8	369.0	362.0	336.0	324.1	289.5	277.0	252.6	220.7	211.7	204.5	202.8	195.4	193.6
Under 1 year	4.1	6.6	13.1	22.8	25.0	20.1	17.4	13.0	8.9	8.6	10.2	9.6	9.6	8.3
1 to 4 years	1.6	1.3	1.7	2.6	2.2	1.9	1.6	1.2	0.9	1.0	1.1	1.2	0.9	1.0
5 to 14 years	3.9	1.3	0.8	0.9	1.0	0.9	0.8	0.7	0.6	0.6	0.6	0.6	0.5	0.5
15 to 24 years	8.2	4.0	3.0	2.9	2.8	2.5	2.8	2.6	2.6	2.5	2.5	2.5	2.4	2.4
25 to 34 years	20.9	15.6	11.4	8.3	8.3	7.6	8.2	7.4	8.3	8.4	8.1	8.1	7.8	7.8
35 to 44 years	88.3	74.6	66.7	44.6	38.1	31.4	31.8	29.2	29.2	28.5	27.7	26.9	26.7	25.8
45 to 54 years	309.2	271.8	238.4	180.2	153.8	120.5	109.6	94.2	89.7	88.0	85.2	85.2	82.3	81.6
55 to 64 years	804.3	737.9	652.3	494.1	443.0	367.3	320.1	261.2	212.8	205.1	197.8	195.3	190.0	186.6
65 to 74 years	1,857.2	1,740.5	1,558.2	1,218.6	1,089.8	894.3	795.4	665.6	512.3	483.0	454.8	441.4	422.8	409.2
75 to 84 years	4,311.0	4,089.4	3,683.8	2,993.1	2,693.1	2,295.7	2,050.5	1,780.3	1,458.5	1,378.0	1,308.6	1,271.7	1,210.8	1,172.0
85 years and over	9,152.5	9,317.8	7,891.3	7,777.1	7,384.1	6,739.9	6,391.5	5,926.1	5,188.3	4,877.6	4,668.1	4,598.4	4,316.9	4,285.2
Male														
All ages, age-adjusted[4]	699.0	687.6	634.0	538.9	488.0	412.4	371.0	320.0	268.2	254.9	243.7	238.5	229.4	225.1
All ages, crude	424.7	439.5	422.5	368.6	344.1	297.6	278.5	249.8	222.3	215.3	209.2	208.2	203.7	202.5
Under 1 year	4.7	7.8	15.1	25.5	27.8	21.9	17.7	13.3	9.6	9.1	11.2	10.3	10.5	9.8
1 to 4 years	1.7	1.4	1.9	2.8	2.2	1.9	1.7	1.4	1.0	1.1	1.0	1.2	0.9	1.1
5 to 14 years	3.5	1.4	0.9	1.0	0.9	0.9	0.8	0.8	0.6	0.7	0.6	0.6	0.5	0.5
15 to 24 years	8.3	4.2	3.7	3.7	3.5	3.1	3.5	3.2	3.5	3.2	3.2	3.3	3.1	3.2
25 to 34 years	24.4	20.1	15.2	11.4	11.6	10.3	11.0	9.6	11.2	11.6	10.9	10.8	10.6	10.7
35 to 44 years	120.4	112.7	103.2	68.7	58.6	48.1	46.9	41.4	41.3	40.1	39.2	37.4	37.5	36.0
45 to 54 years	441.2	420.4	376.4	282.6	237.8	183.0	166.1	140.2	131.6	128.9	124.6	122.9	119.8	117.8
55 to 64 years	1,100.5	1,066.9	987.2	746.8	659.1	537.3	460.1	371.7	303.9	293.4	285.1	280.8	274.1	269.5
65 to 74 years	2,310.2	2,291.3	2,170.3	1,728.0	1,535.8	1,250.0	1,095.3	898.3	680.1	646.9	610.0	594.0	571.1	553.0
75 to 84 years	4,825.8	4,742.4	4,534.8	3,834.3	3,496.9	2,968.2	2,622.9	2,248.1	1,815.1	1,722.7	1,631.9	1,584.3	1,514.8	1,475.7
85 years and over	9,661.4	9,788.9	8,426.2	8,752.7	8,251.8	7,418.4	6,993.5	6,430.0	5,713.2	5,359.2	5,154.3	5,083.6	4,862.8	4,833.6
Female														
All ages, age-adjusted[4]	486.6	447.0	381.6	320.8	294.5	257.0	236.6	210.9	177.5	167.2	159.0	155.9	146.6	143.3
All ages, crude	289.7	300.6	304.5	305.1	305.2	281.8	275.5	255.3	219.0	208.2	199.9	197.7	187.3	184.9
Under 1 year	3.4	5.4	10.9	20.0	22.0	18.3	17.0	12.5	8.2	8.0	9.2	8.8	8.8	6.8
1 to 4 years	1.6	1.1	1.6	2.5	2.2	1.9	1.5	1.0	0.9	0.9	1.2	1.1	1.0	0.9
5 to 14 years	4.3	1.2	0.8	0.9	1.0	0.8	0.7	0.5	0.6	0.6	0.5	0.5	0.5	0.4
15 to 24 years	8.2	3.7	2.3	2.1	2.1	1.8	2.1	2.1	1.7	1.8	1.8	1.6	1.6	1.5
25 to 34 years	17.6	11.3	7.7	5.3	5.0	5.0	5.4	5.2	5.3	5.1	5.3	5.4	5.0	4.9
35 to 44 years	57.0	38.2	32.2	21.4	18.3	15.1	17.0	17.2	17.2	17.1	16.2	16.4	16.0	15.6
45 to 54 years	177.8	127.5	109.9	84.5	74.4	61.0	55.4	49.8	49.1	48.4	47.1	48.8	46.0	46.5
55 to 64 years	507.0	429.4	351.6	272.1	252.1	215.7	192.6	159.3	128.0	122.8	116.4	115.6	111.6	109.3
65 to 74 years	1,434.9	1,261.3	1,082.7	828.6	746.1	616.8	554.9	474.0	369.5	342.8	321.4	309.7	294.2	284.2
75 to 84 years	3,873.0	3,582.7	3,120.8	2,497.0	2,220.4	1,893.8	1,692.7	1,475.1	1,213.8	1,139.0	1,082.0	1,050.4	993.3	952.7
85 years and over	8,798.1	9,016.8	7,591.8	7,350.5	7,037.6	6,478.1	6,159.6	5,720.9	4,955.1	4,659.1	4,443.3	4,370.0	4,056.0	4,020.3
White Male[5]														
All ages, age-adjusted[4]	701.4	694.5	640.2	539.6	487.3	409.2	367.0	316.7	264.8	251.1	240.3	235.8	226.6	222.9
All ages, crude	434.2	454.6	438.3	384.0	360.3	312.7	294.4	265.8	237.3	229.5	223.6	223.3	218.4	217.8
45 to 54 years	424.1	413.2	365.7	269.8	225.5	170.6	153.9	130.7	122.0	120.0	117.0	117.1	113.1	111.2
55 to 64 years	1,082.6	1,056.0	979.3	730.6	640.1	516.7	439.2	351.8	286.4	276.9	269.3	266.9	258.9	257.0
65 to 74 years	2,309.4	2,297.9	2,177.2	1,729.7	1,522.7	1,230.5	1,071.8	877.8	661.1	624.6	590.1	573.9	551.1	536.3
75 to 84 years	4,908.0	4,839.9	4,617.6	3,883.2	3,527.0	2,983.4	2,625.6	2,247.0	1,812.9	1,717.2	1,629.3	1,580.9	1,516.2	1,475.1
85 years and over	9,952.3	10,135.8	8,818.0	8,958.0	8,481.7	7,558.7	7,125.1	6,560.8	5,824.6	5,450.2	5,252.0	5,192.6	4,972.4	4,943.1
Black or African American Male[5]														
All ages, age-adjusted[4]	641.5	615.2	607.3	561.4	533.9	485.4	451.3	392.5	338.8	328.3	312.4	301.2	289.0	280.6
All ages, crude	348.4	330.6	330.3	301.0	288.6	256.8	239.1	211.1	194.0	190.5	184.7	180.5	178.1	174.6
45 to 54 years	624.1	514.0	512.8	433.4	385.2	328.9	308.6	247.2	231.1	222.2	207.9	192.4	194.1	190.9
55 to 64 years	1,434.0	1,236.8	1,135.4	987.2	935.3	824.0	740.5	631.2	527.6	502.5	489.8	465.5	463.2	437.8
65 to 74 years	2,140.1	2,281.4	2,237.8	1,847.2	1,839.2	1,632.9	1,514.1	1,268.8	1,002.5	999.7	941.0	925.0	893.3	847.8
75 to 84 years[6]	4,107.9	3,533.6	3,783.4	3,578.8	3,436.6	3,107.1	2,908.7	2,597.6	2,206.2	2,126.5	1,992.0	1,958.6	1,821.7	1,807.1
85 years and over	NA	6,037.9	5,367.6	6,819.5	6,393.5	6,479.6	6,088.5	5,633.5	5,137.1	4,968.8	4,751.8	4,519.0	4,260.8	4,202.7
American Indian or Alaska Native Male[6]														
All ages, age-adjusted[4]	NA	NA	NA	320.5	280.5	264.1	256.4	222.2	191.7	186.1	175.5	163.5	162.2	158.7
All ages, crude	NA	NA	NA	130.6	117.9	108.0	101.0	90.1	82.8	83.1	79.3	76.5	76.5	75.0
45 to 54 years	NA	NA	NA	238.1	209.1	173.8	136.2	108.5	103.2	107.8	99.5	106.1	86.4	98.0
55 to 64 years	NA	NA	NA	496.3	438.3	411.0	375.7	285.0	263.4	242.6	221.4	219.4	230.2	217.2
65 to 74 years	NA	NA	NA	1,009.4	984.6	839.1	938.2	748.2	551.9	568.4	515.2	520.5	518.1	425.1
75 to 84 years	NA	NA	NA	2,062.2	2,118.2	1,788.8	1,858.5	1,655.7	1,253.6	1,323.6	1,276.2	1,058.5	1,097.2	1,042.6
85 years and over	NA	NA	NA	4,413.7	2,766.7	3,860.3	3,306.5	3,318.3	3,529.4	2,942.8	2,805.9	2,684.7	2,560.7	2,833.1
Asian or Pacific Islander Male[5]														
All ages, age-adjusted[4]	NA	NA	NA	286.9	258.9	220.7	214.5	185.5	149.4	145.4	134.4	133.0	130.2	127.2
All ages, crude	NA	NA	NA	119.8	103.5	88.7	93.2	90.6	81.7	80.6	76.6	77.3	78.4	77.0
45 to 54 years	NA	NA	NA	112.0	81.1	70.4	69.8	61.1	58.1	55.8	51.1	50.8	54.1	49.2
55 to 64 years	NA	NA	NA	306.7	291.2	226.1	205.4	182.6	143.9	144.1	129.4	131.3	129.2	119.3
65 to 74 years	NA	NA	NA	852.4	753.5	623.5	581.0	482.5	370.9	340.7	314.8	308.0	307.6	294.4
75 to 84 years	NA	NA	NA	2,010.9	2,025.6	1,642.2	1,533.8	1,354.7	1,014.6	996.4	935.0	924.3	874.4	855.5
85 years and over	NA	NA	NA	5,923.0	4,937.5	4,617.8	4,888.9	4,154.2	3,518.6	3,497.0	3,162.6	3,170.9	3,080.5	3,132.9

Table 2-33. Death Rates for Diseases of the Heart, by Sex, Race, Hispanic Origin, and Age, Selected Years, 1950–2010—*Continued*

(Deaths per 100,000 resident population.)

Sex, race, Hispanic origin, and age	1950[1,2]	1960[1,2]	1970[2]	1980[2]	1985[2]	1990[2]	1995[2]	2000[3]	2005[3]	2006[3]	2007[3]	2008[3]	2009[3]	2010[3]
Hispanic or Latino Male [5,7]														
All ages, age-adjusted[4]	NA	NA	NA	NA	296.6	270.0	260.8	238.2	210.5	193.7	183.1	171.2	169.4	165.1
All ages, crude	NA	NA	NA	NA	92.1	91.0	83.1	74.7	72.3	68.2	66.5	63.7	65.0	64.1
45 to 54 years	NA	NA	NA	NA	128.1	116.4	102.0	84.3	78.7	76.7	74.3	68.4	71.0	66.1
55 to 64 years	NA	NA	NA	NA	398.8	363.0	311.2	264.8	220.4	203.7	203.0	196.6	195.5	185.9
65 to 74 years	NA	NA	NA	NA	971.1	829.9	784.6	684.8	567.9	512.3	482.5	459.1	452.0	424.5
75 to 84 years	NA	NA	NA	NA	2,150.0	1,971.3	1,854.0	1,733.2	1,541.7	1,380.2	1,303.4	1,219.9	1,211.9	1,160.9
85 years and over	NA	NA	NA	NA	4,912.5	4,711.9	5,104.0	4,897.5	4,442.3	4,190.2	3,875.4	3,569.9	3,486.6	3,577.9
White, Not Hispanic or Latino Male [7]														
All ages, age-adjusted[4]	NA	NA	NA	NA	480.4	413.6	369.1	319.9	267.9	254.6	244.0	240.0	230.4	226.9
All ages, crude	NA	NA	NA	NA	362.8	336.5	320.6	297.5	269.9	262.3	256.4	257.3	251.8	251.8
45 to 54 years	NA	NA	NA	NA	219.9	172.8	155.9	134.3	126.6	124.9	122.0	123.0	118.4	117.2
55 to 64 years	NA	NA	NA	NA	610.6	521.3	443.2	356.3	290.6	281.8	273.8	271.5	263.1	261.9
65 to 74 years	NA	NA	NA	NA	1,471.3	1,243.4	1,077.0	885.1	664.8	630.1	595.7	579.8	555.4	542.2
75 to 84 years	NA	NA	NA	NA	3,512.8	3,007.7	2,635.3	2,261.9	1,823.1	1,732.6	1,645.5	1,599.4	1,531.7	1,491.4
85 years and over	NA	NA	NA	NA	8,538.4	7,663.4	7,156.4	6,606.6	5,876.4	5,495.9	5,310.7	5,263.8	5,042.8	5,006.6
White Female [5]														
All ages, age-adjusted[4]	479.2	441.7	376.7	315.9	289.1	250.9	230.8	205.6	173.2	163.4	155.4	152.5	143.4	140.4
All ages, crude	290.5	306.5	313.8	319.2	321.8	298.4	294.7	274.5	236.9	225.9	216.9	215.0	203.7	201.5
45 to 54 years	142.4	103.4	91.4	71.2	62.5	50.2	45.5	40.9	40.9	40.9	40.2	41.3	39.5	40.7
55 to 64 years	460.7	383.0	317.7	248.1	227.1	192.4	172.0	141.3	113.8	110.6	104.4	103.4	99.7	98.2
65 to 74 years	1,401.6	1,229.8	1,044.0	796.7	713.3	583.6	523.2	445.2	349.2	323.0	301.1	292.6	276.8	268.4
75 to 84 years	3,926.2	3,629.7	3,143.5	2,493.6	2,207.5	1,874.3	1,670.3	1,452.4	1,195.1	1,124.4	1,069.4	1,038.5	982.3	941.6
85 years and over	9,086.9	9,280.8	7,839.9	7,501.6	7,170.0	6,563.4	6,251.3	5,801.4	5,017.5	4,721.8	4,496.0	4,437.7	4,119.8	4,086.7
Black or African American Female [5]														
All ages, age-adjusted[4]	538.9	488.9	435.6	378.6	357.7	327.5	304.0	277.6	234.5	218.1	209.8	202.5	191.0	185.3
All ages, crude	289.9	268.5	261.0	249.7	250.3	237.0	226.3	212.6	184.0	172.9	168.1	164.8	157.6	154.8
45 to 54 years	526.8	360.7	290.9	202.4	176.2	155.3	141.5	125.0	114.1	109.6	105.3	109.7	99.5	96.6
55 to 64 years	1,210.7	952.3	710.5	530.1	510.7	442.0	386.0	332.8	266.9	245.8	236.4	234.1	228.5	218.6
65 to 74 years	1,659.4	1,680.5	1,553.2	1,210.3	1,149.9	1,017.5	938.2	815.2	604.2	567.1	550.8	514.0	498.5	475.9
75 to 84 years[6]	3,499.3	2,926.9	2,964.1	2,707.2	2,533.4	2,250.9	2,100.7	1,913.1	1,599.6	1,465.7	1,388.4	1,342.1	1,272.0	1,227.2
85 years and over	NA	5,650.0	5,003.8	5,796.5	5,686.5	5,766.1	5,448.5	5,298.7	4,841.3	4,493.7	4,399.9	4,153.1	3,833.3	3,783.8
American Indian or Alaska Native Female [5]														
All ages, age-adjusted[4]	NA	NA	NA	175.4	170.0	153.1	164.8	143.6	129.3	126.1	112.2	106.8	104.6	103.5
All ages, crude	NA	NA	NA	80.3	84.3	77.5	80.2	71.9	66.8	65.3	59.0	56.9	56.9	55.9
45 to 54 years	NA	NA	NA	65.2	59.2	62.0	62.4	40.2	48.2	38.0	32.8	35.1	42.0	37.7
55 to 64 years	NA	NA	NA	193.5	230.8	197.0	200.7	149.4	118.0	119.8	103.3	99.9	102.1	89.0
65 to 74 years	NA	NA	NA	577.2	472.7	492.8	514.2	391.8	346.6	318.9	284.5	260.0	262.7	248.1
75 to 84 years	NA	NA	NA	1,364.3	1,258.8	1,050.3	1,184.3	1,044.1	896.3	993.4	829.1	764.1	734.4	684.7
85 years and over	NA	NA	NA	2,893.3	3,180.0	2,868.7	3,118.1	3,146.3	2,962.1	2,672.2	2,487.8	2,469.0	2,352.1	2,614.1
Asian or Pacific Islander Female [5]														
All ages, age-adjusted[4]	NA	NA	NA	132.3	149.4	149.2	137.6	115.7	97.5	93.7	88.5	88.5	83.6	81.2
All ages, crude	NA	NA	NA	57.0	60.3	62.0	66.3	65.0	63.6	62.1	60.0	61.7	59.4	59.0
45 to 54 years	NA	NA	NA	28.6	23.8	17.5	20.8	15.9	15.5	15.6	11.7	12.7	11.4	10.6
55 to 64 years	NA	NA	NA	92.9	103.0	99.0	89.5	68.8	55.2	46.8	44.8	48.5	38.6	40.6
65 to 74 years	NA	NA	NA	313.3	341.0	323.9	288.3	229.6	192.3	185.3	164.6	158.0	150.2	141.6
75 to 84 years	NA	NA	NA	1,053.2	1,056.5	1,130.9	1,001.8	866.2	705.4	664.5	635.0	637.8	594.4	574.3
85 years and over	NA	NA	NA	3,211.0	4,208.3	4,161.2	3,942.4	3,367.2	2,881.1	2,856.6	2,733.3	2,730.3	2,644.6	2,581.8
Hispanic or Latina Female [5,7]														
All ages, age-adjusted[4]	NA	NA	NA	NA	195.9	177.2	173.8	163.7	139.9	130.1	123.2	117.6	109.6	107.8
All ages, crude	NA	NA	NA	NA	75.0	79.4	76.5	71.5	64.9	61.4	59.0	57.3	54.9	54.6
45 to 54 years	NA	NA	NA	NA	46.6	43.5	32.0	28.2	25.9	26.9	22.9	23.7	23.8	24.5
55 to 64 years	NA	NA	NA	NA	184.7	153.2	141.0	111.2	91.7	85.9	80.0	77.9	74.0	72.3
65 to 74 years	NA	NA	NA	NA	534.1	460.4	419.0	366.3	304.3	271.5	246.9	242.4	224.5	212.2
75 to 84 years	NA	NA	NA	NA	1,457.3	1,259.7	1,231.3	1,169.4	1,002.0	924.0	884.3	799.9	793.7	756.0
85 years and over	NA	NA	NA	NA	4,528.6	4,440.3	4,653.1	4,605.8	3,968.1	3,735.5	3,568.0	3,486.5	3,080.0	3,140.3
White, not Hispanic or Latina Female [7]														
All ages, age-adjusted[4]	NA	NA	NA	NA	287.2	252.6	231.5	206.8	174.8	165.2	157.3	154.6	145.4	142.5
All ages, crude	NA	NA	NA	NA	334.2	320.0	319.7	304.9	268.3	256.8	247.7	246.5	234.3	232.2
45 to 54 years	NA	NA	NA	NA	61.3	50.2	46.1	41.9	42.5	42.4	42.2	43.5	41.5	42.9
55 to 64 years	NA	NA	NA	NA	219.6	193.6	172.0	142.9	115.3	112.3	106.2	105.3	101.7	100.3
65 to 74 years	NA	NA	NA	NA	700.5	584.7	525.2	448.5	351.7	325.9	304.6	295.6	279.9	271.9
75 to 84 years	NA	NA	NA	NA	2,201.7	1,890.2	1,674.9	1,458.9	1,202.9	1,133.4	1,078.5	1,052.0	992.3	951.5
85 years and over	NA	NA	NA	NA	7,164.2	6,615.2	6,265.8	5,822.7	5,049.4	4,753.9	4,528.6	4,470.5	4,161.5	4,122.8

NA = Not available. [1]Includes deaths of persons who were not residents of the 50 states and the District of Columbia. [2]Underlying cause of death was coded according to the 6th Revision of the International Classification of Diseases (ICD) in 1950, 7th Revision in 1960, 8th Revision in 1970, and 9th Revision in 1980–1998. [3]Starting with 1999 data, cause of death is coded according to ICD-10. [4]Age-adjusted rates are calculated using the year 2000 standard population. Prior to 2001, age-adjusted rates were calculated using standard million proportions based on rounded population numbers. Starting with 2001 data, unrounded population numbers are used to calculate age-adjusted rates. [5]The race groups, White, Black, Asian or Pacific Islander, and American Indian or Alaska Native, include persons of Hispanic and non-Hispanic origin. Persons of Hispanic origin may be of any race. Death rates for the American Indian or Alaska Native, Asian or Pacific Islander, and Hispanic populations are known to be underestimated. [6]In 1950, rate is for the age group 75 years and over. [7]Prior to 1997, excludes data from states lacking an Hispanic-origin item on the death certificate.

Table 2-34. Death Rates for Cerebrovascular Diseases, by Sex, Race, Hispanic Origin, and Age, Selected Years, 1950–2010

(Deaths per 100,000 resident population.)

Sex, race, Hispanic origin, and age	1950[1,2]	1960[1,2]	1970[2]	1980[2]	1985[2]	1990[2]	1995[2]	2000[3]	2005[3]	2006[3]	2007[3]	2008[3]	2009[3]	2010[3]
All Persons														
All ages, age-adjusted[4]	180.7	177.9	147.7	96.2	76.4	65.3	63.1	60.9	48.0	44.8	43.5	42.1	39.6	39.1
All ages, crude	104.0	108.0	101.9	75.0	64.2	57.8	59.2	59.6	48.6	46.0	45.1	44.1	42.0	41.9
Under 1 year	5.1	4.1	5.0	4.4	3.6	3.8	5.9	3.3	3.1	3.5	3.2	3.4	3.7	3.3
1 to 4 years	0.9	0.8	1.0	0.5	0.3	0.3	0.4	0.3	0.4	0.3	0.3	0.4	0.3	0.3
5 to 14 years	0.5	0.7	0.7	0.3	0.2	0.2	0.2	0.2	0.2	0.2	0.2	0.2	0.2	0.2
15 to 24 years	1.6	1.8	1.6	1.0	0.8	0.6	0.5	0.5	0.5	0.5	0.5	0.4	0.4	0.4
25 to 34 years	4.2	4.7	4.5	2.6	2.2	2.2	1.7	1.5	1.4	1.3	1.3	1.3	1.3	1.3
35 to 44 years	18.7	14.7	15.6	8.5	7.2	6.4	6.5	5.8	5.2	5.1	5.0	4.8	4.6	4.6
45 to 54 years	70.4	49.2	41.6	25.2	21.2	18.7	17.4	16.0	15.0	14.6	14.5	13.7	13.7	13.1
55 to 64 years	194.2	147.3	115.8	65.1	54.7	47.9	45.6	41.0	32.7	32.9	31.7	30.6	29.7	29.3
65 to 74 years	554.7	469.2	384.1	219.0	172.4	144.2	136.2	128.6	99.8	94.9	91.4	87.3	82.8	81.7
75 to 84 years	1,499.6	1,491.3	1,254.2	786.9	600.1	498.0	477.1	461.3	358.4	333.9	320.8	313.3	294.9	288.3
85 years and over	2,990.1	3,680.5	3,014.3	2,283.7	1,858.5	1,628.9	1,607.2	1,589.2	1,239.7	1,131.7	1,110.7	1,071.0	992.2	993.8
Male														
All ages, age-adjusted[4]	186.4	186.1	157.4	102.2	79.9	68.5	65.9	62.4	48.4	45.2	43.7	42.2	39.9	39.3
All ages, crude	102.5	104.5	94.5	63.4	52.4	46.7	47.2	46.9	39.0	37.2	36.5	35.8	34.5	34.5
Under 1 year	6.4	5.0	5.8	5.0	4.6	4.4	6.4	3.8	3.6	4.0	3.6	3.3	4.4	3.2
1 to 4 years	1.1	0.9	1.2	0.4	0.4	0.3	0.4	*	0.5	0.3	0.2	0.4	0.3	0.3
5 to 14 years	0.5	0.7	0.8	0.3	0.2	0.2	0.2	0.2	0.3	0.3	0.2	0.2	0.2	0.3
15 to 24 years	1.8	1.9	1.8	1.1	0.7	0.7	0.5	0.5	0.4	0.5	0.5	0.5	0.5	0.5
25 to 34 years	4.2	4.5	4.4	2.6	2.2	2.1	1.8	1.5	1.5	1.5	1.3	1.5	1.5	1.3
35 to 44 years	17.5	14.6	15.7	8.7	7.4	6.8	7.0	5.8	5.3	5.4	5.4	5.2	5.1	5.0
45 to 54 years	67.9	52.2	44.4	27.2	23.1	20.5	19.5	17.5	16.5	16.4	16.2	15.3	15.3	14.9
55 to 64 years	205.2	163.8	138.7	74.6	63.4	54.3	52.7	47.2	38.2	38.3	37.5	35.5	35.0	34.7
65 to 74 years	589.6	530.7	449.5	258.6	201.0	166.6	154.7	145.0	111.6	105.8	102.7	97.6	94.2	92.0
75 to 84 years	1,543.6	1,555.9	1,361.6	866.3	659.4	551.1	517.7	490.8	370.0	341.4	328.2	320.4	300.9	295.2
85 years and over	3,048.6	3,643.1	2,895.2	2,193.6	1,723.8	1,528.5	1,522.1	1,484.3	1,136.7	1,036.8	998.9	965.2	891.6	892.0
Female														
All ages, age-adjusted[4]	175.8	170.7	140.0	91.7	73.3	62.6	60.5	59.1	47.0	43.9	42.7	41.4	38.8	38.3
All ages, crude	105.6	111.4	109.0	85.9	75.3	68.4	70.7	71.8	57.9	54.4	53.4	52.1	49.2	49.1
Under 1 year	3.7	3.2	4.0	3.8	2.7	3.1	5.3	2.7	2.7	3.0	2.7	3.6	3.0	3.4
1 to 4 years	0.7	0.7	0.7	0.5	0.3	0.3	0.3	0.4	0.3	0.4	0.4	0.4	0.3	0.3
5 to 14 years	0.4	0.6	0.6	0.3	0.3	0.2	0.1	0.2	0.2	0.2	0.2	0.2	0.1	0.2
15 to 24 years	1.5	1.6	1.4	0.8	0.8	0.6	0.4	0.5	0.5	0.5	0.4	0.4	0.4	0.4
25 to 34 years	4.3	4.9	4.7	2.6	2.1	2.2	1.6	1.5	1.3	1.2	1.3	1.2	1.2	1.2
35 to 44 years	19.9	14.8	15.6	8.4	6.9	6.1	6.0	5.7	5.1	4.9	4.6	4.5	4.2	4.2
45 to 54 years	72.9	46.3	39.0	23.3	19.4	17.0	15.3	14.5	13.6	13.0	12.9	12.2	12.2	11.4
55 to 64 years	183.1	131.8	95.3	56.8	47.1	42.2	39.1	35.3	27.7	28.0	26.3	26.1	24.8	24.3
65 to 74 years	522.1	415.7	333.3	188.7	150.4	126.7	121.4	115.1	89.7	85.6	81.7	78.4	72.9	72.8
75 to 84 years	1,462.2	1,441.1	1,183.1	740.1	565.1	466.2	451.8	442.1	350.4	328.6	315.5	308.2	290.6	283.4
85 years and over	2,949.4	3,704.4	3,081.0	2,323.1	1,912.3	1,667.6	1,640.0	1,632.0	1,285.5	1,174.8	1,162.4	1,120.8	1,040.2	1,043.0
White Male [5]														
All ages, age-adjusted[4]	182.1	181.6	153.7	98.7	77.1	65.5	62.9	59.8	46.0	42.8	41.3	40.2	38.0	37.6
All ages, crude	100.5	102.7	93.5	63.1	52.5	46.9	48.0	48.4	40.1	38.1	37.5	37.0	35.7	35.8
45 to 54 years	53.7	40.9	35.6	21.7	18.0	15.4	14.7	13.6	12.9	12.9	13.1	12.0	12.7	12.2
55 to 64 years	182.2	139.0	119.9	64.0	54.5	45.7	44.2	39.7	31.5	31.3	31.2	29.9	29.3	29.0
65 to 74 years	569.7	501.0	420.0	239.8	185.9	152.9	142.1	133.8	101.3	95.3	92.3	88.2	86.2	83.3
75 to 84 years	1,556.3	1,564.8	1,361.6	852.7	648.1	539.2	503.8	480.0	361.0	333.4	317.3	313.3	292.9	288.3
85 years and over	3,127.1	3,734.8	3,018.1	2,230.8	1,758.7	1,545.4	1,536.0	1,490.7	1,138.5	1,037.0	999.3	968.9	896.0	903.2
Black or African American Male [5]														
All ages, age-adjusted[4]	228.8	238.5	206.4	142.0	112.5	102.2	97.0	89.6	72.7	68.8	68.7	63.5	58.8	56.6
All ages, crude	122.0	122.9	108.8	73.0	59.2	53.0	49.8	46.1	40.1	39.0	39.1	36.8	35.0	34.5
45 to 54 years	211.9	166.1	136.1	82.1	71.1	68.4	62.3	49.5	43.6	42.1	39.4	39.4	34.5	33.6
55 to 64 years	522.8	439.9	343.4	189.7	160.5	141.7	130.8	115.4	99.6	101.1	94.7	85.1	84.5	83.2
65 to 74 years	783.6	899.2	780.1	472.3	379.4	326.9	297.0	268.5	215.9	209.3	212.4	195.0	182.8	182.6
75 to 84 years[6]	1,504.9	1,475.2	1,445.7	1,066.3	813.2	721.5	705.9	659.2	504.2	470.4	490.1	443.5	412.7	398.0
85 years and over	NA	2,700.0	1,963.1	1,873.2	1,427.4	1,421.5	1,410.1	1,458.8	1,194.3	1,076.0	1,061.7	1,002.8	887.4	804.5
American Indian or Alaska Native Male [5]														
All ages, age-adjusted[4]	NA	NA	NA	66.4	48.4	44.3	51.7	46.1	35.0	28.4	35.6	27.5	32.0	29.8
All ages, crude	NA	NA	NA	23.1	18.4	16.0	18.4	16.8	14.0	12.5	13.9	11.7	12.7	12.0
45 to 54 years	NA	NA	NA	*	*	*	25.5	13.3	12.6	14.7	12.3	13.0	14.4	11.7
55 to 64 years	NA	NA	NA	72.0	0.0	39.8	42.6	48.6	34.5	33.2	34.8	28.1	25.2	22.1
65 to 74 years	NA	NA	NA	170.5	196.2	120.3	156.4	144.7	112.5	82.1	82.2	94.5	68.4	68.0
75 to 84 years	NA	NA	NA	523.9	372.7	325.9	351.2	373.3	255.8	196.1	300.5	193.8	288.5	267.5
85 years and over	NA	NA	NA	1,384.7	733.3	949.8	1,072.4	834.9	655.7	490.5	709.9	492.5	629.2	580.4
Asian or Pacific Islander Male [5]														
All ages, age-adjusted[4]	NA	NA	NA	71.4	65.2	59.1	64.0	58.0	43.9	42.5	37.9	36.2	35.4	35.2
All ages, crude	NA	NA	NA	28.7	24.0	23.3	27.5	27.2	23.3	23.1	21.2	20.9	20.8	21.5
45 to 54 years	NA	NA	NA	17.0	13.9	15.6	16.5	15.0	14.4	13.5	14.6	13.1	12.9	14.7
55 to 64 years	NA	NA	NA	59.9	48.8	51.8	59.6	49.3	33.1	36.0	31.0	31.3	31.1	31.7
65 to 74 years	NA	NA	NA	197.9	155.6	167.9	155.6	135.6	103.9	107.7	88.9	88.2	76.2	84.9
75 to 84 years	NA	NA	NA	619.5	583.7	483.9	521.9	438.7	347.8	305.1	282.8	265.1	278.0	260.0
85 years and over	NA	NA	NA	1,399.0	1,387.5	1,196.6	1,382.1	1,415.6	1,007.2	1,014.1	888.2	835.2	800.0	778.7

Table 2-34. Death Rates for Cerebrovascular Diseases, by Sex, Race, Hispanic Origin, and Age, Selected Years, 1950–2010—*Continued*

(Deaths per 100,000 resident population.)

Sex, race, Hispanic origin, and age	1950[1,2]	1960[1,2]	1970[2]	1980[2]	1985[2]	1990[2]	1995[2]	2000[3]	2005[3]	2006[3]	2007[3]	2008[3]	2009[3]	2010[3]
Hispanic or Latino Male [5,7]														
All ages, age-adjusted[4]	NA	NA	NA	NA	57.5	46.5	51.2	50.5	41.6	39.4	38.1	37.3	34.0	33.9
All ages, crude	NA	NA	NA	NA	17.2	15.6	16.2	15.8	14.5	14.4	14.1	13.9	13.1	13.2
45 to 54 years	NA	NA	NA	NA	23.6	20.0	20.3	18.1	18.0	17.3	16.7	15.4	14.7	14.3
55 to 64 years	NA	NA	NA	NA	64.0	49.2	46.9	48.8	40.5	41.4	43.2	35.3	33.7	31.9
65 to 74 years	NA	NA	NA	NA	163.3	126.4	138.1	136.1	107.4	101.4	95.6	90.6	92.6	84.4
75 to 84 years	NA	NA	NA	NA	394.7	356.6	373.3	392.9	308.5	308.9	278.6	292.2	253.0	266.5
85 years and over	NA	NA	NA	NA	1,181.2	866.3	1,079.5	1,029.9	870.3	748.4	778.3	758.4	678.8	679.1
White, Not Hispanic or Latino Male [7]														
All ages, age-adjusted[4]	NA	NA	NA	NA	74.8	66.3	62.8	59.9	46.0	42.7	41.1	40.0	37.9	37.5
All ages, crude	NA	NA	NA	NA	52.1	50.6	51.9	53.9	45.1	42.9	42.3	41.9	40.6	40.7
45 to 54 years	NA	NA	NA	NA	15.9	14.9	13.9	13.0	12.1	12.2	12.4	11.3	12.1	11.6
55 to 64 years	NA	NA	NA	NA	50.4	45.1	43.3	38.7	30.5	30.0	29.7	29.1	28.6	28.4
65 to 74 years	NA	NA	NA	NA	178.2	154.5	141.4	133.1	100.5	94.3	91.5	87.4	85.1	82.6
75 to 84 years	NA	NA	NA	NA	635.2	547.3	506.2	482.3	363.0	333.7	318.6	313.6	294.7	288.6
85 years and over	NA	NA	NA	NA	1,729.1	1,578.7	1,544.8	1,505.9	1,148.7	1,048.5	1,008.2	976.7	906.2	913.2
White Female [5]														
All ages, age-adjusted[4]	169.7	165.0	135.5	89.0	70.7	60.3	58.6	57.3	45.3	42.3	41.2	39.9	37.6	37.2
All ages, crude	103.3	110.1	109.8	88.6	78.2	71.6	75.1	76.9	62.0	58.3	57.3	56.0	53.1	53.0
45 to 54 years	55.0	33.8	30.5	18.6	15.5	13.5	12.6	11.2	10.5	10.4	10.0	9.5	9.6	9.1
55 to 64 years	156.9	103.0	78.1	48.6	39.9	35.8	33.3	30.2	23.7	23.9	22.3	21.9	21.1	20.6
65 to 74 years	498.1	383.3	303.2	172.5	137.6	116.1	111.7	107.3	82.6	78.6	75.0	72.8	67.5	66.8
75 to 84 years	1,471.3	1,444.7	1,176.8	728.8	551.7	456.5	443.4	434.2	343.4	321.6	310.6	302.0	286.4	280.2
85 years and over	3,017.9	3,795.7	3,167.6	2,362.7	1,938.0	1,685.9	1,656.7	1,646.7	1,292.6	1,182.1	1,168.7	1,129.7	1,052.0	1,052.8
Black or African American Female [5]														
All ages, age-adjusted[4]	238.4	232.5	189.3	119.6	99.2	84.0	79.4	76.2	62.4	58.4	56.4	54.8	50.0	49.6
All ages, crude	128.3	127.7	112.2	77.8	68.5	60.7	59.1	58.3	48.8	46.2	45.1	44.2	41.0	41.1
45 to 54 years	248.9	166.2	119.4	61.8	50.8	44.1	36.0	38.1	34.6	30.9	32.4	30.1	28.8	26.7
55 to 64 years	567.7	452.0	272.4	138.4	113.5	96.9	85.6	76.4	58.7	59.8	57.0	57.5	53.5	51.3
65 to 74 years	754.4	830.5	673.5	361.7	285.1	236.7	222.3	190.9	151.0	146.0	140.5	127.4	122.5	126.2
75 to 84 years[6]	1,496.7	1,413.1	1,338.3	917.5	752.4	595.0	565.1	549.2	451.5	416.8	389.1	399.3	360.1	347.2
85 years and over	NA	2,578.9	2,210.5	1,891.6	1,653.4	1,495.2	1,518.4	1,556.5	1,282.5	1,176.9	1,166.7	1,106.4	989.6	1,001.5
American Indian or Alaska Native Female [5]														
All ages, age-adjusted[4]	NA	NA	NA	51.2	44.3	38.4	46.3	43.7	41.1	35.4	32.8	27.2	27.0	26.5
All ages, crude	NA	NA	NA	22.0	21.5	19.3	22.0	21.5	21.3	17.2	16.7	14.2	14.4	14.2
45 to 54 years	NA	NA	NA	*	*	*	*	14.4	16.3	*	8.9	9.3	11.6	10.6
55 to 64 years	NA	NA	NA	*	40.4	40.7	41.5	37.9	34.6	15.5	22.5	24.4	24.6	22.4
65 to 74 years	NA	NA	NA	128.3	118.2	100.5	114.8	79.5	114.5	78.0	82.2	54.5	69.3	59.4
75 to 84 years	NA	NA	NA	404.2	317.6	282.0	364.4	391.1	304.7	283.4	211.4	221.3	169.7	173.6
85 years and over	NA	NA	NA	1,095.5	980.0	776.2	983.9	931.5	865.8	919.7	879.0	615.3	692.2	700.0
Asian or Pacific Islander Female [5]														
All ages, age-adjusted[4]	NA	NA	NA	60.8	54.8	54.9	48.3	49.1	38.3	37.0	35.5	34.2	31.2	31.4
All ages, crude	NA	NA	NA	26.4	23.3	24.3	24.2	28.7	25.6	25.5	24.8	24.7	22.9	23.5
45 to 54 years	NA	NA	NA	20.3	15.1	19.7	15.6	13.3	9.7	10.2	9.6	10.2	9.4	7.9
55 to 64 years	NA	NA	NA	43.7	49.0	42.1	37.6	33.3	26.4	27.8	24.1	24.6	20.6	22.1
65 to 74 years	NA	NA	NA	136.1	129.9	124.0	101.0	102.8	80.1	79.9	70.9	74.9	61.4	65.6
75 to 84 years	NA	NA	NA	446.6	387.0	396.6	381.8	386.0	278.1	295.2	269.8	247.2	237.1	218.4
85 years and over	NA	NA	NA	1,545.2	1,383.3	1,395.0	1,197.0	1,246.6	1,044.6	890.5	935.0	898.2	814.3	872.8
Hispanic or Latina Female [5,7]														
All ages, age-adjusted[4]	NA	NA	NA	NA	47.5	43.7	42.7	43.0	36.0	35.0	33.5	32.0	30.4	30.2
All ages, crude	NA	NA	NA	NA	18.2	20.1	19.4	19.4	17.3	17.1	16.6	16.0	15.6	15.7
45 to 54 years	NA	NA	NA	NA	15.8	15.2	15.1	12.4	11.9	11.6	10.8	10.0	9.1	9.2
55 to 64 years	NA	NA	NA	NA	35.3	38.5	36.5	31.9	26.9	27.5	25.0	20.7	22.9	22.1
65 to 74 years	NA	NA	NA	NA	108.6	102.6	102.3	95.2	75.4	76.5	70.8	65.9	58.4	60.6
75 to 84 years	NA	NA	NA	NA	340.0	308.5	307.3	311.3	270.3	248.5	252.1	248.9	234.0	221.6
85 years and over	NA	NA	NA	NA	1,185.7	1,055.3	1,021.0	1,108.9	905.5	901.5	845.7	804.0	774.8	799.3
White, not Hispanic or Latina Female [7]														
All ages, age-adjusted[4]	NA	NA	NA	NA	69.7	61.0	58.7	57.6	45.6	42.5	41.5	40.2	37.8	37.4
All ages, crude	NA	NA	NA	NA	80.8	77.2	81.5	85.5	70.1	66.0	65.3	64.0	60.8	60.8
45 to 54 years	NA	NA	NA	NA	14.3	13.2	12.3	10.9	10.2	10.1	9.8	9.3	9.6	9.0
55 to 64 years	NA	NA	NA	NA	37.8	35.7	32.6	29.9	23.2	23.4	21.9	21.8	20.7	20.3
65 to 74 years	NA	NA	NA	NA	133.2	116.9	111.4	107.6	82.9	78.3	75.0	73.1	68.0	66.9
75 to 84 years	NA	NA	NA	NA	550.8	461.9	445.9	438.3	347.0	325.2	313.7	304.6	289.1	283.4
85 years and over	NA	NA	NA	NA	1,920.7	1,714.7	1,666.8	1,661.6	1,306.0	1,192.2	1,181.4	1,142.1	1,062.9	1,063.0

NA = Not available.   * = Rates based on fewer than 20 deaths are considered unreliable and are not shown.   [1]Includes deaths of persons who were not residents of the 50 states and the District of Columbia.   [2]Underlying cause of death was coded according to the 6th Revision of the International Classification of Diseases (ICD) in 1950, 7th Revision in 1960, 8th Revision in 1970, and 9th Revision in 1980–1998.   [3]Starting with 1999 data, cause of death is coded according to ICD-10.   [4]Age-adjusted rates are calculated using the year 2000 standard population. Prior to 2001, age-adjusted rates were calculated using standard million proportions based on rounded population numbers. Starting with 2001 data, unrounded population numbers are used to calculate age-adjusted rates.   [5]The race groups, White, Black, Asian or Pacific Islander, and American Indian or Alaska Native, include persons of Hispanic and non-Hispanic origin. Persons of Hispanic origin may be of any race. Death rates for the American Indian or Alaska Native, Asian or Pacific Islander, and Hispanic populations are known to be underestimated.   [6]In 1950, rate is for the age group 75 years and over.   [7]Prior to 1997, excludes data from states lacking an Hispanic-origin item on the death certificate.

Figure 2-8. Age-Adjusted Death Rates for Heart Disease, by Race and Sex, Selected Years, 1950–2010

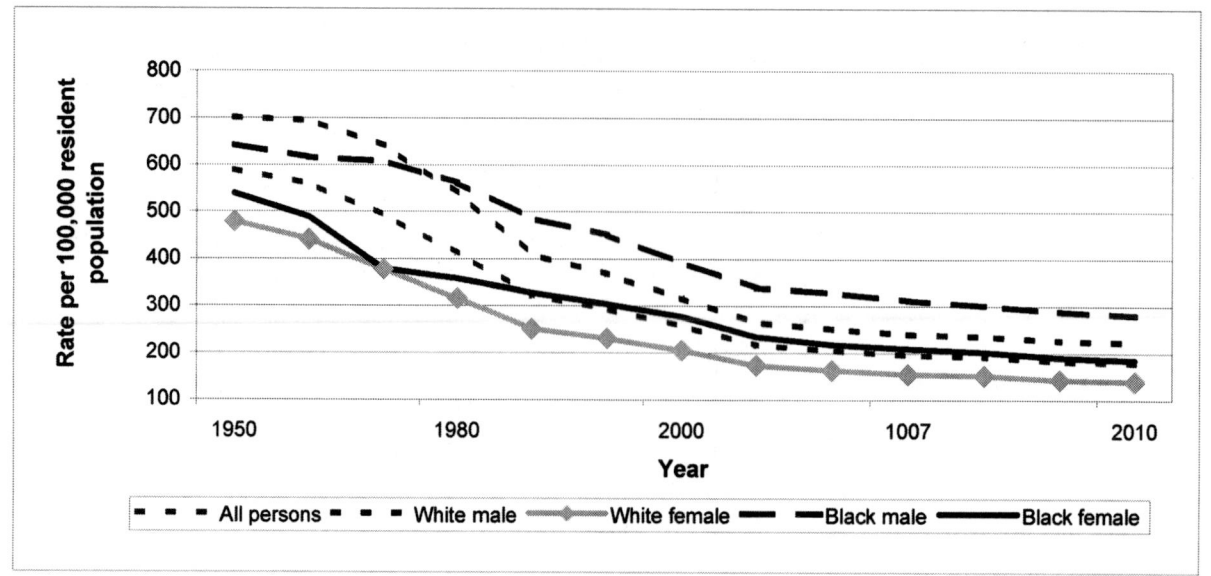

Figure 2-9. Age-Adjusted Death Rates for Malignant Neoplasms, by Race and Sex, Selected Years, 1950–2010

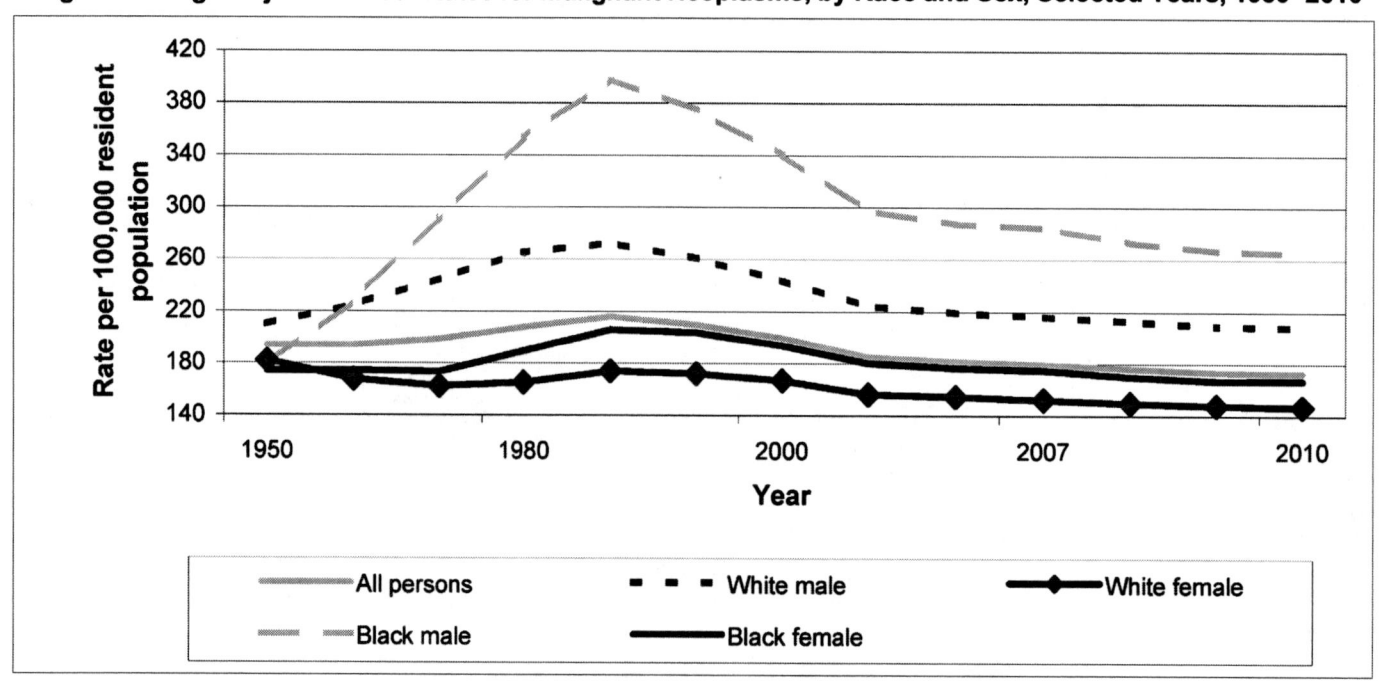

Table 2-35A. Death Rates for Malignant Neoplasms, by Sex and Age, Selected Years, 1950–2010

(Deaths per 100,000 resident population.)

Sex, race, Hispanic origin, and age	1950[1,2]	1960[1,2]	1970[2]	1980[2]	1985[2]	1990[2]	1995[2]	2000[3]	2005[3]	2006[3]	2007[3]	2008[3]	2009[3]	2010[3]
All Persons														
All ages, age-adjusted[4]	193.9	193.9	198.6	207.9	211.3	216.0	209.9	199.6	185.1	181.8	179.3	176.4	173.5	172.8
All ages, crude	139.8	149.2	162.8	183.9	194.0	203.2	202.2	196.5	189.3	187.6	186.9	186.0	185.0	186.2
Under 1 year	8.7	7.2	4.7	3.2	3.1	2.3	1.8	2.4	1.9	1.9	1.7	1.7	1.8	1.6
1 to 4 years	11.7	10.9	7.5	4.5	3.8	3.5	3.1	2.7	2.4	2.4	2.3	2.4	2.2	2.1
5 to 14 years	6.7	6.8	6.0	4.3	3.5	3.1	2.7	2.5	2.5	2.2	2.4	2.2	2.2	2.2
15 to 24 years	8.6	8.3	8.3	6.3	5.4	4.9	4.5	4.4	4.0	3.8	3.8	3.8	3.8	3.7
25 to 34 years	20.0	19.5	16.5	13.7	13.2	12.6	11.6	9.8	9.2	9.3	8.7	8.8	9.0	8.8
35 to 44 years	62.7	59.7	59.5	48.6	45.9	43.3	40.1	36.6	33.5	32.2	31.0	30.1	30.2	28.8
45 to 54 years	175.1	177.0	182.5	180.0	170.1	158.9	140.4	127.5	118.6	116.3	114.2	113.4	112.8	111.6
55 to 64 years	390.7	396.8	423.0	436.1	454.6	449.6	412.3	366.7	323.9	317.7	311.4	304.7	301.7	300.1
65 to 74 years	698.8	713.9	754.2	817.9	845.5	872.3	863.3	816.3	733.2	716.3	702.9	688.4	668.2	666.1
75 to 84 years	1,153.3	1,127.4	1,169.2	1,232.3	1,271.8	1,348.5	1,355.4	1,335.6	1,272.8	1,259.2	1,250.1	1,230.9	1,213.0	1,202.2
85 years and over	1,451.0	1,450.0	1,320.7	1,594.6	1,615.4	1,752.9	1,797.7	1,819.4	1,778.2	1,748.3	1,739.4	1,724.6	1,699.3	1,729.5
Male														
All ages, age-adjusted[4]	208.1	225.1	247.6	271.2	274.4	280.4	267.5	248.9	227.2	221.7	218.8	214.9	210.9	209.9
All ages, crude	142.9	162.5	182.1	205.3	213.4	221.3	216.3	207.2	200.0	197.8	197.8	197.5	196.8	198.3
Under 1 year	9.7	7.7	4.4	3.7	3.0	2.4	1.9	2.6	2.2	1.9	1.8	2.3	2.2	1.5
1 to 4 years	12.5	12.4	8.3	5.2	4.3	3.7	3.6	3.0	2.7	2.5	2.3	2.6	2.2	2.4
5 to 14 years	7.4	7.6	6.7	4.9	3.9	3.5	3.0	2.7	2.7	2.4	2.4	2.2	2.3	2.3
15 to 24 years	9.7	10.2	10.4	7.8	6.4	5.7	5.4	5.1	4.8	4.6	4.5	4.6	4.5	4.5
25 to 34 years	17.7	18.8	16.3	13.4	13.2	12.6	11.3	9.2	9.2	9.0	8.5	8.8	8.8	8.6
35 to 44 years	45.6	48.9	53.0	44.0	42.4	38.5	36.3	32.7	29.3	27.8	26.8	26.2	26.1	25.2
45 to 54 years	156.2	170.8	183.5	188.7	175.2	162.5	141.5	130.9	121.7	119.1	117.4	117.7	115.3	113.8
55 to 64 years	413.1	459.9	511.8	520.8	536.9	532.9	475.1	415.8	365.8	359.4	353.9	349.3	345.9	344.9
65 to 74 years	791.5	890.5	1,006.8	1,093.2	1,105.2	1,122.2	1,083.0	1,001.9	883.1	852.5	834.1	817.0	790.4	789.2
75 to 84 years	1,332.6	1,389.4	1,588.3	1,790.5	1,839.7	1,914.4	1,847.9	1,760.6	1,636.8	1,611.8	1,593.3	1,563.1	1,538.3	1,514.2
85 years and over	1,668.3	1,741.2	1,720.8	2,369.5	2,451.8	2,739.9	2,818.7	2,710.7	2,576.2	2,500.3	2,508.4	2,444.4	2,412.2	2,452.6
Female														
All ages, age-adjusted[4]	182.3	168.7	163.2	166.7	171.2	175.7	173.6	167.6	156.7	154.7	152.3	149.6	147.4	146.7
All ages, crude	136.8	136.4	144.4	163.6	175.7	186.0	188.8	186.2	178.9	177.8	176.3	174.8	173.7	174.4
Under 1 year	7.6	6.8	5.0	2.7	3.2	2.2	1.8	2.3	1.5	1.9	1.6	1.1	1.5	1.6
1 to 4 years	10.8	9.3	6.7	3.7	3.4	3.2	2.6	2.5	2.1	2.2	2.2	2.2	2.1	1.9
5 to 14 years	6.0	6.0	5.2	3.6	3.1	2.8	2.3	2.2	2.2	2.0	2.3	2.2	2.0	2.2
15 to 24 years	7.6	6.5	6.2	4.8	4.3	4.1	3.5	3.6	3.3	3.1	3.2	3.0	3.0	2.8
25 to 34 years	22.2	20.1	16.7	14.0	13.2	12.6	11.9	10.4	9.2	9.6	8.9	8.7	9.1	9.0
35 to 44 years	79.3	70.0	65.6	53.1	49.2	48.1	43.8	40.4	37.6	36.5	35.3	34.0	34.2	32.3
45 to 54 years	194.0	183.0	181.5	171.8	165.3	155.5	139.3	124.2	115.7	113.5	111.0	109.2	110.4	109.4
55 to 64 years	368.2	337.7	343.2	361.7	381.8	375.2	355.1	321.3	284.8	278.9	271.8	263.3	260.6	258.5
65 to 74 years	612.3	560.2	557.9	607.1	645.3	677.4	687.1	663.6	605.6	599.8	590.3	577.3	562.2	559.1
75 to 84 years	1,000.7	924.1	891.9	903.1	937.8	1,010.3	1,047.5	1,058.5	1,023.0	1,014.6	1,009.6	995.9	980.1	977.0
85 years and over	1,299.7	1,263.9	1,096.7	1,255.7	1,281.4	1,372.1	1,404.4	1,456.4	1,423.6	1,407.2	1,383.9	1,385.9	1,358.6	1,380.1

NA = Not available. * = Rates based on fewer than 20 deaths are considered unreliable and are not shown. [1]Includes deaths of persons who were not residents of the 50 states and the District of Columbia. [2]Underlying cause of death was coded according to the 6th Revision of the International Classification of Diseases (ICD) in 1950, 7th Revision in 1960, 8th Revision in 1970, and 9th Revision in 1980–1998. [3]Starting with 1999 data, cause of death is coded according to ICD-10. [4]Age-adjusted rates are calculated using the year 2000 standard population. Prior to 2001, age-adjusted rates were calculated using standard million proportions based on rounded population numbers. Starting with 2001 data, unrounded population numbers are used to calculate age-adjusted rates.

Table 2-35B. Death Rates for Malignant Neoplasms, by Race, Hispanic Origin, and Age for Males, Selected Years, 1950–2010

(Deaths per 100,000 resident population.)

Sex, race, Hispanic origin, and age	1950[1,2]	1960[1,2]	1970[2]	1980[2]	1985[2]	1990[2]	1995[2]	2000[3]	2005[3]	2006[3]	2007[3]	2008[3]	2009[3]	2010[3]
White Male [4]														
All ages, age-adjusted[5]	210.0	224.7	244.8	265.1	267.1	272.2	260.6	243.9	224.3	219.3	216.3	212.9	209.2	208.2
All ages, crude	147.2	166.1	185.1	208.7	218.1	227.7	225.3	218.1	212.8	211.1	211.2	211.5	211.0	212.7
25 to 34 years	17.7	18.8	16.2	13.6	13.1	12.3	11.0	9.2	8.8	9.0	8.5	8.8	8.9	8.8
35 to 44 years	44.5	46.3	50.1	41.1	39.8	35.8	34.1	30.9	28.9	27.2	26.4	25.6	25.9	25.2
45 to 54 years	150.8	164.1	172.0	175.4	162.0	149.9	132.7	123.5	116.3	114.3	112.8	113.9	112.5	111.6
55 to 64 years	409.4	450.9	498.1	497.4	512.0	508.2	456.0	401.9	354.2	350.4	344.1	340.4	335.8	334.9
65 to 74 years	798.7	887.3	997.0	1,070.7	1,076.5	1,090.7	1,056.1	984.3	875.6	845.8	827.3	811.1	784.2	782.8
75 to 84 years	1,367.6	1,413.7	1,592.7	1,779.7	1,817.1	1,883.2	1,817.4	1,736.0	1,629.2	1,606.9	1,588.2	1,560.4	1,538.3	1,511.6
85 years and over	1,732.7	1,791.4	1,772.2	2,375.6	2,449.1	2,715.1	2,789.4	2,693.7	2,558.2	2,487.9	2,488.1	2,437.8	2,412.5	2,453.5
Black or African American Male [4]														
All ages, age-adjusted[5]	178.9	227.6	291.9	353.4	373.9	397.9	374.3	340.3	297.2	287.2	284.2	273.1	266.7	264.8
All ages, crude	106.6	136.7	171.6	205.5	214.9	221.9	204.8	188.5	174.7	171.2	171.3	168.4	168.2	169.0
25 to 34 years	18.0	18.4	18.8	14.1	14.9	15.7	14.8	10.1	12.4	10.4	9.9	9.9	10.4	9.2
35 to 44 years	55.7	72.9	81.3	73.8	69.9	64.3	57.2	48.4	36.1	36.2	33.6	33.7	31.3	30.1
45 to 54 years	211.7	244.7	311.2	333.0	315.9	302.6	243.9	214.2	181.1	176.1	171.1	165.4	157.4	150.9
55 to 64 years	490.8	579.7	689.2	812.5	851.3	859.2	738.1	626.4	546.0	518.2	516.3	501.3	502.0	496.7
65 to 74 years[6]	636.5	938.5	1,168.9	1,417.2	1,532.8	1,613.9	1,541.4	1,363.8	1,139.4	1,106.8	1,083.8	1,047.3	1,038.6	1,027.8
75 to 84 years	853.5	1,053.3	1,624.8	2,029.6	2,229.6	2,478.3	2,449.8	2,351.8	2,019.5	1,976.0	1,929.9	1,875.6	1,835.3	1,826.8
85 years and over	NA	1,155.2	1,387.0	2,393.9	2,629.0	3,238.3	3,395.5	3,264.8	3,258.8	3,102.5	3,230.0	2,956.8	2,791.3	2,854.6
American Indian or Alaska Native Male [4]														
All ages, age-adjusted[5]	NA	NA	NA	140.5	142.1	145.8	169.0	155.8	158.5	146.0	150.7	151.8	132.8	151.0
All ages, crude	NA	NA	NA	58.1	62.8	61.4	67.8	67.0	73.0	66.0	70.1	72.7	66.4	74.1
25 to 34 years	NA	NA	NA	*	*	*	*	*	*	*	*	*	6.5	7.4
35 to 44 years	NA	NA	NA	*	28.8	22.8	14.3	21.4	24.3	13.3	13.7	17.7	12.3	13.4
45 to 54 years	NA	NA	NA	86.9	89.4	86.9	79.2	70.3	75.2	67.3	69.3	82.5	73.2	70.0
55 to 64 years	NA	NA	NA	213.4	276.6	246.2	279.8	255.6	257.7	211.0	248.4	225.4	229.6	249.5
65 to 74 years	NA	NA	NA	613.0	584.6	530.6	684.7	648.0	619.3	578.3	558.7	620.8	541.3	597.7
75 to 84 years	NA	NA	NA	936.4	963.6	1,038.4	1,346.3	1,152.5	1,138.4	1,143.9	1,112.3	1,144.2	936.9	1,104.4
85 years and over	NA	NA	NA	1,471.2	1,133.3	1,654.4	1,549.0	1,584.2	1,832.2	1,653.0	1,876.3	1,588.6	1,390.1	1,741.3
Asian or Pacific Islander Male [4]														
All ages, age-adjusted[5]	NA	NA	NA	165.2	173.4	172.5	164.3	150.8	137.4	131.6	134.8	132.8	131.0	131.0
All ages, crude	NA	NA	NA	81.9	82.6	82.7	83.7	85.2	84.8	82.6	85.5	86.3	86.7	88.6
25 to 34 years	NA	NA	NA	6.3	10.0	9.2	8.2	7.4	7.1	6.9	6.2	6.8	5.7	6.5
35 to 44 years	NA	NA	NA	29.4	25.7	27.7	26.1	26.1	20.6	20.4	19.5	18.9	21.2	18.2
45 to 54 years	NA	NA	NA	108.2	98.0	92.6	82.4	78.5	75.9	70.3	72.9	69.5	67.5	67.4
55 to 64 years	NA	NA	NA	298.5	315.0	274.6	244.8	229.2	197.5	195.6	187.0	189.4	193.4	195.2
65 to 74 years	NA	NA	NA	581.2	631.3	687.2	614.3	559.4	487.0	455.0	461.2	464.1	425.8	446.2
75 to 84 years	NA	NA	NA	1,147.6	1,251.2	1,229.9	1,167.2	1,086.1	1,022.0	974.7	1,046.7	1,004.1	988.2	980.4
85 years and over	NA	NA	NA	1,798.7	1,800.0	1,837.0	2,081.3	1,823.2	1,716.2	1,685.3	1,693.4	1,689.0	1,762.0	1,707.2
Hispanic or Latino Male [4,7]														
All ages, age-adjusted[4]	NA	NA	NA	NA	161.3	174.7	180.9	171.7	162.4	153.5	151.7	151.4	148.6	149.4
All ages, crude	NA	NA	NA	NA	56.1	65.5	65.4	61.3	63.2	60.9	61.6	62.8	62.9	64.2
25 to 34 years	NA	NA	NA	NA	9.7	8.0	8.4	6.9	6.9	6.5	6.7	8.0	7.7	7.2
35 to 44 years	NA	NA	NA	NA	22.9	22.5	24.7	20.1	18.5	16.8	18.2	18.2	18.0	16.5
45 to 54 years	NA	NA	NA	NA	83.5	96.6	85.0	79.4	76.7	72.4	75.2	71.7	70.7	69.7
55 to 64 years	NA	NA	NA	NA	259.0	294.0	281.6	253.1	238.1	226.4	223.1	228.8	222.9	225.4
65 to 74 years	NA	NA	NA	NA	598.2	655.5	697.9	651.2	610.3	582.5	566.8	565.5	545.9	552.0
75 to 84 years	NA	NA	NA	NA	1,210.5	1,233.4	1,359.8	1,306.4	1,219.2	1,158.8	1,133.4	1,137.6	1,128.7	1,118.7
85 years and over	NA	NA	NA	NA	1,743.8	2,019.4	2,018.6	2,049.7	2,013.0	1,852.2	1,855.9	1,820.3	1,794.7	1,861.2
White, Not Hispanic or Latino Male [7]														
All ages, age-adjusted[4]	NA	NA	NA	NA	259.0	276.7	263.5	247.7	228.4	223.7	220.8	217.2	213.6	212.6
All ages, crude	NA	NA	NA	NA	217.4	246.2	246.0	244.4	242.5	241.7	242.6	243.3	243.5	245.8
25 to 34 years	NA	NA	NA	NA	13.5	12.8	11.2	9.7	9.3	9.5	8.9	8.9	9.1	9.1
35 to 44 years	NA	NA	NA	NA	39.1	36.8	34.8	32.3	30.8	29.2	28.0	27.1	27.6	27.0
45 to 54 years	NA	NA	NA	NA	159.9	153.9	135.6	127.2	120.7	119.1	117.2	119.3	117.9	117.2
55 to 64 years	NA	NA	NA	NA	496.4	520.6	464.9	412.0	363.1	360.0	354.0	349.4	345.4	344.2
65 to 74 years	NA	NA	NA	NA	1,044.2	1,109.0	1,069.9	1,002.1	893.3	863.5	845.7	827.6	800.4	798.5
75 to 84 years	NA	NA	NA	NA	1,765.5	1,906.6	1,825.4	1,750.2	1,650.0	1,630.1	1,614.0	1,583.8	1,561.8	1,534.4
85 years and over	NA	NA	NA	NA	2,327.3	2,744.4	2,810.8	2,714.1	2,578.7	2,511.9	2,514.5	2,464.5	2,440.5	2,480.8

NA = Not available.   * = Rates based on fewer than 20 deaths are considered unreliable and are not shown.   [1]Includes deaths of persons who were not residents of the 50 states and the District of Columbia.   [2]Underlying cause of death was coded according to the 6th Revision of the International Classification of Diseases (ICD) in 1950, 7th Revision in 1960, 8th Revision in 1970, and 9th Revision in 1980-1998.   [3]Starting with 1999 data, cause of death is coded according to ICD-10.   [4]The race groups, White, Black, Asian or Pacific Islander, and American Indian or Alaska Native, include persons of Hispanic and non-Hispanic origin. Persons of Hispanic origin may be of any race. Death rates for the American Indian or Alaska Native, Asian or Pacific Islander, and Hispanic populations are known to be underestimated.   [5]Age-adjusted rates are calculated using the year 2000 standard population. Prior to 2001, age-adjusted rates were calculated using standard million proportions based on rounded population numbers. Starting with 2001 data, unrounded population numbers are used to calculate age-adjusted rates.   [6]In 1950, rate is for the age group 75 years and over.   [7]Prior to 1997, excludes data from states lacking an Hispanic-origin item on the death certificate.

Table 2-35C. Death Rates for Malignant Neoplasms, by Race, Hispanic Origin, and Age for Females, Selected Years, 1950–2010

(Deaths per 100,000 resident population.)

Sex, race, Hispanic origin, and age	1950[1,2]	1960[1,2]	1970[2]	1980[2]	1985[2]	1990[2]	1995[2]	2000[3]	2005[3]	2006[3]	2007[3]	2008[3]	2009[3]	2010[3]
White Female[4]														
All ages, age-adjusted[5]	182.0	167.7	162.5	165.2	169.9	174.0	172.1	166.9	156.4	154.7	152.3	149.8	147.9	146.9
All ages, crude	139.9	139.8	149.4	170.3	184.4	196.1	200.6	199.4	192.3	191.5	190.0	188.7	187.8	188.2
25 to 34 years	20.9	18.8	16.3	13.5	12.7	11.9	11.2	10.1	8.8	9.3	8.8	8.6	9.1	8.8
35 to 44 years	74.5	66.6	62.4	50.9	47.3	46.2	41.9	38.2	36.2	35.2	34.2	32.8	33.6	31.3
45 to 54 years	185.8	175.7	177.3	166.4	161.6	150.9	135.0	120.1	110.9	109.9	107.4	106.0	108.4	106.5
55 to 64 years	362.5	329.0	338.6	355.5	376.3	368.5	350.3	319.7	282.2	277.1	269.5	261.7	258.9	255.3
65 to 74 years	616.5	562.1	554.7	605.2	644.9	675.1	685.6	665.6	611.5	606.1	595.9	581.9	567.1	563.7
75 to 84 years	1,026.6	939.3	903.5	905.4	938.2	1,011.8	1,047.9	1,063.4	1,032.0	1,023.5	1,018.1	1,008.3	991.2	988.6
85 years and over	1,348.3	1,304.9	1,126.6	1,266.8	1,285.4	1,372.3	1,405.4	1,459.1	1,426.4	1,413.0	1,392.7	1,393.2	1,370.0	1,389.8
Black or African American Female[4]														
All ages, age-adjusted[5]	174.1	174.3	173.4	189.5	195.5	205.9	203.8	193.8	180.3	176.6	174.9	170.1	167.0	167.1
All ages, crude	111.8	113.8	117.3	136.5	145.2	156.1	155.8	151.8	148.1	146.5	146.5	144.2	143.5	145.5
25 to 34 years	34.3	31.0	20.9	18.3	17.2	18.7	16.5	13.5	12.7	12.6	12.0	10.4	11.4	10.8
35 to 44 years	119.8	102.4	94.6	73.5	69.0	67.4	61.7	58.9	52.1	50.3	47.9	47.7	44.6	44.5
45 to 54 years	277.0	254.8	228.6	230.2	212.4	209.9	190.6	173.9	164.5	156.6	153.5	149.0	145.7	146.4
55 to 64 years	484.6	442.7	404.8	450.4	474.9	482.4	444.9	391.0	358.6	349.1	343.6	330.7	327.2	331.1
65 to 74 years	477.3	541.6	615.8	662.4	704.2	773.2	803.5	753.1	667.7	659.8	665.7	652.1	638.2	631.0
75 to 84 years[6]	605.3	696.3	763.3	923.9	986.3	1,059.9	1,120.8	1,124.0	1,074.9	1,068.2	1,075.1	1,021.3	1,026.7	1,008.2
85 years and over	NA	728.9	791.5	1,159.9	1,284.2	1,431.3	1,446.2	1,527.7	1,514.6	1,469.8	1,405.0	1,427.8	1,345.7	1,418.6
American Indian or Alaska Native Female[5]														
All ages, age-adjusted[4]	NA	NA	NA	94.0	93.0	106.9	117.7	108.3	108.9	111.9	105.8	105.6	102.2	102.0
All ages, crude	NA	NA	NA	50.4	52.5	62.1	64.5	61.3	65.7	66.7	63.6	64.2	64.4	64.8
25 to 34 years	NA	NA	NA	*	*	*	10.2	*	*	*	*	*	6.6	6.3
35 to 44 years	NA	NA	NA	36.9	23.4	31.0	29.7	23.7	20.7	21.8	17.0	22.5	20.4	14.2
45 to 54 years	NA	NA	NA	96.9	90.1	104.5	76.9	59.7	79.1	66.3	67.6	64.3	70.5	68.7
55 to 64 years	NA	NA	NA	198.4	192.3	213.3	213.2	200.9	194.6	185.3	180.8	169.8	183.1	185.9
65 to 74 years	NA	NA	NA	350.8	378.8	438.9	437.0	458.3	473.0	464.9	438.2	443.9	414.4	432.2
75 to 84 years	NA	NA	NA	446.4	505.9	554.3	819.9	714.0	742.4	801.6	757.7	732.5	696.4	682.3
85 years and over	NA	NA	NA	786.5	700.0	843.7	1,039.4	983.2	802.0	971.7	937.1	986.0	863.4	885.7
Asian or Pacific Islander Female[4]														
All ages, age-adjusted[5]	NA	NA	NA	93.0	99.6	103.0	107.4	100.7	96.2	94.2	91.7	91.8	89.6	93.5
All ages, crude	NA	NA	NA	54.1	57.5	60.5	69.5	72.1	75.0	74.5	73.4	74.4	73.7	78.5
25 to 34 years	NA	NA	NA	9.5	9.9	7.3	9.9	8.1	7.3	6.9	5.4	7.8	5.8	7.1
35 to 44 years	NA	NA	NA	38.7	33.1	29.8	27.6	28.9	25.0	24.7	23.7	20.5	21.3	21.7
45 to 54 years	NA	NA	NA	99.8	91.3	93.9	94.4	78.2	73.9	72.0	67.7	67.1	60.2	69.5
55 to 64 years	NA	NA	NA	174.7	195.5	196.2	203.5	176.5	166.2	155.0	155.2	145.6	144.9	152.6
65 to 74 years	NA	NA	NA	301.9	330.8	346.2	343.3	357.4	324.7	327.1	301.7	316.1	300.8	314.4
75 to 84 years	NA	NA	NA	522.1	589.1	641.4	681.0	650.1	626.8	625.7	624.4	633.4	618.7	654.5
85 years and over	NA	NA	NA	800.0	908.3	971.7	1,092.7	988.5	1,060.1	1,006.7	1,019.8	1,027.2	1,053.5	994.4
Hispanic or Latina Female[4,7]														
All ages, age-adjusted[5]	NA	NA	NA	NA	101.5	111.9	110.8	110.8	104.9	103.8	101.7	100.1	99.8	99.4
All ages, crude	NA	NA	NA	NA	49.8	60.7	58.7	58.5	58.3	58.5	58.1	57.8	58.4	59.0
25 to 34 years	NA	NA	NA	NA	9.7	9.7	8.5	7.8	7.0	8.4	8.6	7.7	7.4	8.4
35 to 44 years	NA	NA	NA	NA	30.9	34.8	30.7	30.7	26.6	27.5	25.9	25.0	24.4	23.5
45 to 54 years	NA	NA	NA	NA	90.1	100.5	89.7	84.7	78.9	77.1	74.0	69.8	70.8	74.0
55 to 64 years	NA	NA	NA	NA	199.2	205.4	203.0	192.5	170.8	172.5	172.7	175.2	170.0	165.9
65 to 74 years	NA	NA	NA	NA	356.4	404.8	398.0	410.0	380.6	368.2	360.4	346.3	351.7	355.2
75 to 84 years	NA	NA	NA	NA	600.0	663.0	706.2	716.5	708.7	687.8	687.2	684.5	665.4	657.6
85 years and over	NA	NA	NA	NA	907.1	1,022.7	1,028.6	1,056.5	1,045.6	1,073.8	1,005.8	1,020.6	1,061.0	1,043.4
White, not Hispanic or Latina Female[7]														
All ages, age-adjusted[5]	NA	NA	NA	NA	167.1	177.5	174.7	170.0	160.1	158.4	156.1	153.6	151.8	150.6
All ages, crude	NA	NA	NA	NA	187.1	210.6	217.3	220.6	216.6	216.5	215.6	214.7	214.2	215.0
25 to 34 years	NA	NA	NA	NA	12.2	11.9	11.5	10.5	9.1	9.4	8.6	8.7	9.3	8.8
35 to 44 years	NA	NA	NA	NA	47.2	47.0	42.7	38.9	37.8	36.3	35.6	34.1	35.4	32.8
45 to 54 years	NA	NA	NA	NA	158.8	154.9	137.8	123.0	114.2	113.4	111.3	110.3	113.1	110.5
55 to 64 years	NA	NA	NA	NA	372.7	379.5	359.3	328.9	291.7	286.3	278.1	269.2	266.9	263.4
65 to 74 years	NA	NA	NA	NA	638.4	688.5	697.9	681.0	629.1	625.1	615.2	600.9	584.6	580.4
75 to 84 years	NA	NA	NA	NA	917.8	1,027.2	1,056.1	1,075.3	1,048.9	1,042.3	1,037.7	1,028.1	1,012.4	1,010.4
85 years and over	NA	NA	NA	NA	1,241.5	1,385.7	1,411.6	1,468.7	1,440.0	1,424.6	1,407.8	1,407.4	1,382.3	1,403.8

NA = Not available.   * = Rates based on fewer than 20 deaths are considered unreliable and are not shown.   [1]Includes deaths of persons who were not residents of the 50 states and the District of Columbia.   [2]Underlying cause of death was coded according to the 6th Revision of the International Classification of Diseases (ICD) in 1950, 7th Revision in 1960, 8th Revision in 1970, and 9th Revision in 1980-1998.   [3]Starting with 1999 data, cause of death is coded according to ICD-10.   [4]The race groups, White, Black, Asian or Pacific Islander, and American Indian or Alaska Native, include persons of Hispanic and non-Hispanic origin. Persons of Hispanic origin may be of any race. Death rates for the American Indian or Alaska Native, Asian or Pacific Islander, and Hispanic populations are known to be underestimated.   [5]Age-adjusted rates are calculated using the year 2000 standard population. Prior to 2001, age-adjusted rates were calculated using standard million proportions based on rounded population numbers. Starting with 2001 data, unrounded population numbers are used to calculate age-adjusted rates.   [6]In 1950, rate is for the age group 75 years and over.   [7]Prior to 1997, excludes data from states lacking an Hispanic-origin item on the death certificate.

Table 2-36. Death Rates for Malignant Neoplasm of Breast Among Females, by Race, Hispanic Origin, and Age, Selected Years, 1950–2010

(Deaths per 100,000 resident population.)

Sex, race, Hispanic origin, and age	1950[1,2]	1960[1,2]	1970[2]	1980[2]	1985[2]	1990[2]	1995[2]	2000[3]	2005[3]	2006[3]	2007[3]	2008[3]	2009[3]	2010[3]
All Females														
All ages, age-adjusted[4]	31.9	31.7	32.1	31.9	33.0	33.3	30.5	26.8	24.2	23.6	23.0	22.6	22.3	22.1
All ages, crude	24.7	26.1	28.4	30.6	32.8	34.0	32.2	29.2	27.4	26.9	26.5	26.3	26.1	26.1
Under 25 years	*	*	*	*	*	*	*	*	*	*	*	*	*	*
25 to 34 years	3.8	3.8	3.9	3.3	3.0	2.9	2.6	2.3	1.8	1.9	1.7	1.6	1.7	1.6
35 to 44 years	20.8	20.2	20.4	17.9	17.5	17.8	14.9	12.4	11.4	10.8	10.1	10.1	10.5	9.8
45 to 54 years	46.9	51.4	52.6	48.1	47.1	45.4	41.0	33.0	28.7	27.6	26.7	26.2	26.2	25.7
55 to 64 years	69.9	70.8	77.6	80.5	84.2	78.6	69.4	59.3	54.0	53.1	50.7	49.2	47.9	47.7
65 to 74 years	95.0	90.0	93.8	101.1	107.8	111.7	102.8	88.3	78.5	76.1	76.3	75.6	73.4	73.9
75 to 84 years	139.8	129.9	127.4	126.4	136.2	146.3	140.1	128.9	119.6	119.4	116.6	113.8	112.6	109.1
85 years and over	195.5	191.9	157.1	169.3	178.5	196.8	200.2	205.7	191.2	183.1	184.7	182.7	178.0	185.8
White [5]														
All ages, age-adjusted[4]	32.4	32.0	32.5	32.1	33.1	33.2	30.1	26.3	23.6	23.1	22.5	22.1	21.9	21.5
All ages, crude	25.7	27.2	29.9	32.3	34.7	35.9	33.8	30.7	28.5	28.2	27.7	27.4	27.4	27.3
35 to 44 years	20.8	19.7	20.2	17.3	16.8	17.1	14.0	11.3	10.3	9.9	9.2	9.1	9.8	8.8
45 to 54 years	47.1	51.2	53.0	48.1	46.8	44.3	38.9	31.2	26.3	25.7	24.8	24.5	24.8	23.9
55 to 64 years	70.9	71.8	79.3	81.3	84.7	78.5	68.3	57.9	52.1	51.6	49.0	47.8	46.4	45.9
65 to 74 years	96.3	91.6	95.9	103.7	109.9	113.3	103.3	89.3	78.7	76.4	76.5	74.9	73.2	73.3
75 to 84 years	143.6	132.8	129.6	128.4	138.8	148.2	141.4	130.2	120.9	120.4	117.4	114.4	113.1	110.2
85 years and over	204.2	199.7	161.9	171.7	180.9	198.0	202.6	205.5	191.6	182.7	185.5	182.9	179.2	186.8
Black or African American [5]														
All ages, age-adjusted[4]	25.3	27.9	28.9	31.7	34.6	38.1	38.0	34.5	32.8	31.6	31.3	30.9	30.2	30.3
All ages, crude	16.4	18.7	19.7	22.9	25.9	29.0	29.6	27.9	28.2	27.3	27.4	27.3	26.9	27.5
35 to 44 years	21.0	24.8	24.4	24.1	26.1	25.8	22.9	20.9	20.1	18.8	18.0	17.7	17.6	18.3
45 to 54 years	46.5	54.4	52.0	52.7	55.5	60.5	61.9	51.5	49.5	44.0	43.6	42.2	40.6	40.9
55 to 64 years	NA	NA	NA	NA	NA	NA	NA	NA	NA	NA	NA	NA	NA	NA
65 to 74 years	67.0	72.3	77.3	84.3	100.7	112.2	89.1	80.9	79.6	74.6	73.8	69.2	68.5	70.5
75 to 84 years[6]	81.0	87.5	101.8	114.1	117.6	140.5	117.9	98.6	94.5	89.5	93.8	97.8	92.4	97.4
85 years and over	NA	92.1	112.1	149.9	159.4	201.5	147.2	139.8	126.9	138.6	135.6	133.4	136.4	123.2
American Indian or Alaska Native [5]														
All ages, age-adjusted[4]	NA	NA	NA	10.8	12.1	13.7	15.0	13.6	15.5	13.0	13.0	12.5	12.2	11.5
All ages, crude	NA	NA	NA	6.1	6.9	8.6	9.0	8.7	9.3	8.7	8.8	8.6	8.4	8.0
35 to 44 years	NA	NA	NA	*	*	*	*	*	*	*	*	*	*	*
45 to 54 years	NA	NA	NA	*	*	23.9	21.6	14.4	11.9	14.4	16.2	12.1	12.0	13.2
55 to 64 years	NA	NA	NA	*	*	*	37.4	40.0	20.3	29.6	33.1	33.1	29.9	25.2
65 to 74 years	NA	NA	NA	*	*	*	46.3	42.5	65.4	42.5	37.8	50.7	51.3	34.3
75 to 84 years	NA	NA	NA	*	*	*	*	71.8	124.2	57.3	54.9	55.3	53.2	61.1
85 years and over	NA	NA	NA	*	*	*	*	*	*	*	*	*	*	*
Asian or Pacific Islander [5]														
All ages, age-adjusted[4]	NA	NA	NA	11.9	13.2	13.7	13.9	12.3	12.2	12.1	11.0	11.5	11.1	11.9
All ages, crude	NA	NA	NA	8.2	8.6	9.3	10.8	10.2	10.6	10.6	9.7	10.3	10.1	10.8
35 to 44 years	NA	NA	NA	10.4	7.2	8.4	8.0	8.1	6.7	5.2	5.7	6.2	5.4	5.4
45 to 54 years	NA	NA	NA	23.4	21.9	26.4	29.1	22.3	18.2	19.2	14.9	15.2	15.5	17.0
55 to 64 years	NA	NA	NA	35.7	39.5	33.8	37.9	31.3	34.0	32.0	27.6	29.2	28.8	28.4
65 to 74 years	NA	NA	NA	*	32.5	38.5	36.6	34.7	31.7	38.7	34.9	39.5	34.6	37.9
75 to 84 years	NA	NA	NA	*	50.0	48.0	42.3	37.5	53.9	44.1	50.7	52.3	46.4	53.2
85 years and over	NA	NA	NA	*	*	*	*	68.2	69.7	78.9	61.0	56.5	72.9	77.5
Hispanic or Latina [5,7]														
All ages, age-adjusted[4]	NA	NA	NA	NA	16.3	19.5	18.7	16.9	15.3	15.2	14.8	14.6	14.8	14.4
All ages, crude	NA	NA	NA	NA	8.8	11.5	10.6	9.7	9.2	9.4	9.2	9.1	9.4	9.2
35 to 44 years	NA	NA	NA	NA	10.4	11.7	9.5	8.7	7.9	7.8	7.2	7.2	7.0	6.2
45 to 54 years	NA	NA	NA	NA	26.4	32.8	27.7	23.9	19.7	19.4	19.0	17.0	19.0	18.6
55 to 64 years	NA	NA	NA	NA	43.5	45.8	45.0	39.1	34.4	36.0	33.4	34.6	32.6	32.7
65 to 74 years	NA	NA	NA	NA	40.9	64.8	58.0	54.9	46.7	47.0	47.7	45.9	46.3	49.0
75 to 84 years	NA	NA	NA	NA	64.5	67.2	80.9	74.9	75.4	71.1	68.6	69.7	72.4	61.8
85 years and over	NA	NA	NA	NA	85.7	102.8	115.6	105.8	113.0	109.1	109.0	111.5	111.4	117.8
White, not Hispanic or Latina [7]														
All ages, age-adjusted[4]	NA	NA	NA	NA	33.0	33.9	30.6	26.8	24.2	23.6	23.1	22.6	22.5	22.1
All ages, crude	NA	NA	NA	NA	35.6	38.5	36.6	33.8	32.0	31.7	31.3	31.1	31.0	31.0
35 to 44 years	NA	NA	NA	NA	16.9	17.5	14.4	11.6	10.7	10.1	9.4	9.4	10.3	9.3
45 to 54 years	NA	NA	NA	NA	46.8	45.2	39.5	31.7	26.9	26.4	25.4	25.3	25.4	24.5
55 to 64 years	NA	NA	NA	NA	85.1	80.6	69.5	59.2	53.5	53.0	50.4	48.9	47.6	47.1
65 to 74 years	NA	NA	NA	NA	108.6	115.7	105.4	91.4	81.2	78.8	78.9	77.2	75.3	75.1
75 to 84 years	NA	NA	NA	NA	139.4	151.4	143.2	132.2	123.3	123.3	120.4	117.2	115.9	113.6
85 years and over	NA	NA	NA	NA	175.6	201.5	204.4	208.3	194.7	185.5	188.8	185.8	182.3	189.9

NA = Not available.   * = Rates based on fewer than 20 deaths are considered unreliable and are not shown.   [1]Includes deaths of persons who were not residents of the 50 states and the District of Columbia.   [2]Underlying cause of death was coded according to the 6th Revision of the International Classification of Diseases (ICD) in 1950, 7th Revision in 1960, 8th Revision in 1970, and 9th Revision in 1980-1998.   [3]Starting with 1999 data, cause of death is coded according to ICD-10.   [4]Age-adjusted rates are calculated using the year 2000 standard population. Prior to 2001, age-adjusted rates were calculated using standard million proportions based on rounded population numbers. Starting with 2001 data, unrounded population numbers are used to calculate age-adjusted rates.   [5]The race groups, White, Black, Asian or Pacific Islander, and American Indian or Alaska Native, include persons of Hispanic and non-Hispanic origin. Persons of Hispanic origin may be of any race. Death rates for the American Indian or Alaska Native, Asian or Pacific Islander, and Hispanic populations are known to be underestimated.   [6]In 1950, rate is for the age group 75 years and over.   [7]Prior to 1997, excludes data from states lacking an Hispanic-origin item on the death certificate.

Table 2-37. Death Rates for Malignant Neoplasms of the Trachea, Bronchus, and Lung, by Sex, Race, Hispanic Origin, and Age, Selected Years, 1950–2010

(Deaths per 100,000 resident population.)

Sex, race, Hispanic origin, and age	1950[1,2]	1960[1,2]	1970[2]	1980[2]	1985[2]	1990[2]	1995[2]	2000[3]	2005[3]	2006[3]	2007[3]	2008[3]	2009[3]	2010[3]
All Persons														
All ages, age-adjusted[4]	15.0	24.1	37.1	49.9	54.6	59.3	58.4	56.1	52.7	51.5	50.6	49.5	48.4	47.6
All ages, crude	12.2	20.3	32.1	45.8	51.5	56.8	56.8	55.3	53.9	53.2	52.7	52.2	51.6	51.3
Under 25 years	0.1	0.0	0.1	0.0	0.0	0.0	0.0	0.0	0.0	0.0	0.0	0.0	0.0	0.0
25 to 34 years	0.8	1.0	0.9	0.6	0.6	0.7	0.6	0.5	0.3	0.4	0.3	0.4	0.4	0.4
35 to 44 years	4.5	6.8	11.0	9.2	7.8	6.8	6.0	6.1	5.3	4.7	4.3	3.8	3.7	3.3
45 to 54 years	20.4	29.6	43.4	54.1	50.9	46.8	37.5	31.6	29.7	29.1	28.4	28.2	27.8	26.9
55 to 64 years	48.7	75.3	109.1	138.2	153.8	160.6	141.6	122.4	102.4	98.1	94.2	90.2	87.5	85.4
65 to 74 years	59.7	108.1	164.5	233.3	261.2	288.4	295.4	284.2	256.3	249.3	244.5	235.5	228.6	223.9
75 to 84 years	55.8	91.5	163.2	240.5	282.0	333.3	358.9	370.8	375.0	372.1	369.5	366.7	359.8	357.2
85 years and over	42.3	65.6	101.7	176.0	195.2	242.5	279.9	302.1	328.2	327.1	328.0	332.9	328.0	332.4
Male														
All ages, age-adjusted[4]	24.6	43.6	67.5	85.2	88.6	91.1	84.2	76.7	69.1	67.0	64.9	63.5	61.4	60.3
All ages, crude	19.9	35.4	53.4	68.6	72.5	75.1	70.5	65.5	62.1	60.9	59.7	59.3	58.2	57.8
Under 25 years	0.0	0.0	0.1	0.1	*	0.0	0.1	*	*	*	0.0	0.1	0.0	*
25 to 34 years	1.1	1.4	1.3	0.8	0.7	0.9	0.7	0.5	0.4	0.4	0.4	0.4	0.4	0.4
35 to 44 years	7.1	10.5	16.1	11.9	10.0	8.5	7.0	6.9	5.5	4.8	4.3	4.0	3.7	3.2
45 to 54 years	35.0	50.6	67.5	76.0	67.5	59.7	46.3	38.5	35.1	33.8	32.1	32.3	31.0	30.0
55 to 64 years	83.8	139.3	189.7	213.6	223.5	222.9	185.3	154.0	126.3	120.2	114.7	111.1	107.9	104.9
65 to 74 years	98.7	204.3	320.8	403.9	416.2	430.4	414.3	377.9	324.8	312.9	302.8	291.2	279.4	274.9
75 to 84 years	82.6	167.1	330.8	488.8	537.6	572.9	553.8	532.2	511.1	503.8	490.9	482.0	470.5	461.9
85 years and over	62.5	107.7	194.0	368.1	433.2	513.2	540.3	521.2	519.9	508.9	505.2	511.0	489.1	492.3
Female														
All ages, age-adjusted[4]	5.8	7.5	13.1	24.4	30.6	37.1	40.4	41.3	40.6	40.1	40.1	39.1	38.6	38.1
All ages, crude	4.5	6.4	11.9	24.3	31.7	39.4	43.6	45.4	46.0	45.7	46.0	45.3	45.1	45.0
Under 25 years	0.1	0.0	0.0	*	*	*	*	*	*	*	*	*	*	0.0
25 to 34 years	NA	NA	NA	NA	NA	NA	NA	NA	NA	NA	NA	NA	NA	NA
35 to 44 years	1.9	3.2	6.1	6.5	5.6	5.2	5.0	5.3	5.1	4.6	4.4	3.6	3.6	3.3
45 to 54 years	5.8	9.2	21.0	33.7	35.2	34.5	29.1	25.0	24.5	24.6	24.8	24.3	24.7	23.8
55 to 64 years	13.6	15.4	36.8	72.0	92.1	105.0	101.9	93.3	80.0	77.4	75.2	70.7	68.4	67.2
65 to 74 years	23.3	24.4	43.1	102.7	141.8	177.6	200.0	206.9	197.9	195.0	194.3	187.4	184.5	179.5
75 to 84 years	32.9	32.8	52.4	94.1	131.7	190.1	237.2	265.6	281.6	280.8	284.4	285.1	280.6	281.7
85 years and over	28.2	38.8	50.0	91.9	100.2	138.1	179.6	212.8	243.1	244.6	246.0	249.1	251.0	255.2
White Male[5]														
All ages, age-adjusted[4]	25.1	43.6	67.1	83.8	86.8	89.0	82.6	75.7	68.8	66.7	64.6	63.4	61.3	60.1
All ages, crude	20.8	36.4	54.6	70.2	74.5	77.8	74.0	69.4	66.6	65.4	64.1	63.9	62.8	62.3
45 to 54 years	35.1	49.2	63.3	70.9	62.7	55.2	43.2	35.7	33.5	31.9	30.4	31.0	30.3	28.8
55 to 64 years	85.4	139.2	186.8	205.6	214.2	213.7	178.9	150.8	122.6	117.4	112.2	108.9	105.2	101.8
65 to 74 years	101.5	207.5	325.0	401.0	409.5	422.1	408.0	374.9	326.5	313.8	303.8	293.3	280.7	275.7
75 to 84 years	85.5	170.4	336.7	493.5	540.3	572.2	550.8	529.9	514.5	506.9	493.6	484.0	474.3	465.5
85 years and over	67.4	109.4	199.6	374.1	440.0	516.3	539.3	522.4	517.6	511.1	500.5	509.4	489.5	495.0
Black or African American Male[5]														
All ages, age-adjusted[4]	17.8	42.6	75.4	107.6	117.2	125.4	115.1	101.1	86.1	83.0	81.5	77.8	75.0	73.7
All ages, crude	12.1	28.1	47.7	66.6	71.2	73.7	65.6	58.3	52.8	51.7	51.0	49.2	48.7	48.7
45 to 54 years	34.4	68.4	115.4	133.8	122.5	114.9	85.2	70.7	55.4	55.0	52.0	48.7	45.1	45.2
55 to 64 years	68.3	146.8	234.3	321.1	351.5	358.6	288.5	223.5	191.3	175.9	168.6	159.0	158.1	155.4
65 to 74 years	53.8	168.3	300.5	472.3	539.6	585.4	559.5	488.8	393.5	385.4	376.3	345.5	348.8	341.3
75 to 84 years	36.2	107.3	271.6	472.9	556.4	645.4	667.1	642.5	565.7	563.0	544.2	544.3	516.0	509.1
85 years and over	NA	82.8	137.0	311.3	382.3	499.5	583.0	562.8	601.6	539.6	618.3	591.2	526.6	521.8
American Indian or Alaska Native Male[5]														
All ages, age-adjusted[4]	NA	NA	NA	31.7	41.2	47.5	53.6	42.9	42.6	39.6	43.7	44.3	35.4	41.6
All ages, crude	NA	NA	NA	14.2	18.4	20.0	21.8	18.1	20.1	18.4	20.0	20.8	17.7	20.8
45 to 54 years	NA	NA	NA	*	*	26.6	23.8	14.5	18.2	16.5	12.8	16.7	14.4	19.7
55 to 64 years	NA	NA	NA	72.0	85.1	97.8	98.9	86.0	79.5	61.0	77.4	66.2	65.4	67.6
65 to 74 years	NA	NA	NA	202.8	223.1	194.3	261.5	184.8	190.3	200.4	200.2	221.0	183.2	213.2
75 to 84 years	NA	NA	NA	*	263.6	356.2	409.7	367.9	341.1	330.9	339.5	361.5	249.4	325.8
85 years and over	NA	NA	NA	*	*	*	*	*	*	*	422.6	333.6	*	276.4
Asian or Pacific Islander Male[5]														
All ages, age-adjusted[4]	NA	NA	NA	43.3	42.7	44.2	41.0	40.9	37.1	36.6	35.9	36.1	34.8	33.8
All ages, crude	NA	NA	NA	22.1	20.4	20.7	20.7	22.7	22.4	22.7	22.0	22.9	22.3	22.5
45 to 54 years	NA	NA	NA	33.3	21.7	18.8	18.6	17.2	15.6	18.1	17.0	16.3	13.1	13.8
55 to 64 years	NA	NA	NA	94.4	98.1	74.4	64.4	61.4	56.7	55.7	43.4	49.5	49.6	51.1
65 to 74 years	NA	NA	NA	174.3	180.8	215.8	184.0	183.2	142.6	139.7	132.5	136.5	117.7	127.0
75 to 84 years	NA	NA	NA	301.3	295.3	307.5	296.6	323.2	295.0	295.5	311.1	303.2	304.9	286.4
85 years and over	NA	NA	NA	*	350.0	421.3	439.0	378.0	439.5	401.3	423.9	416.6	429.9	382.0
Hispanic or Latino Male[5,7]														
All ages, age-adjusted[4]	NA	NA	NA	NA	39.2	44.1	42.2	39.0	35.2	32.3	31.6	32.2	29.8	29.6
All ages, crude	NA	NA	NA	NA	12.9	16.2	14.8	13.3	13.1	12.1	12.0	12.4	11.8	11.9
45 to 54 years	NA	NA	NA	NA	16.7	21.5	17.5	14.8	12.1	10.6	10.4	9.8	10.3	9.0
55 to 64 years	NA	NA	NA	NA	68.6	80.7	69.9	58.6	52.5	45.1	42.3	43.5	38.5	40.1
65 to 74 years	NA	NA	NA	NA	169.9	195.5	192.0	167.3	153.1	142.0	142.4	137.2	128.6	126.2
75 to 84 years	NA	NA	NA	NA	292.1	313.4	324.4	327.5	295.5	268.2	260.0	278.1	263.3	256.3
85 years and over	NA	NA	NA	NA	393.8	420.7	382.8	368.8	338.1	339.4	335.3	337.7	290.7	307.9

Table 2-37. Death Rates for Malignant Neoplasms of the Trachea, Bronchus, and Lung, by Sex, Race, Hispanic Origin, and Age, Selected Years, 1950–2010—*Continued*

(Deaths per 100,000 resident population.)

Sex, race, Hispanic origin, and age	1950[1,2]	1960[1,2]	1970[2]	1980[2]	1985[2]	1990[2]	1995[2]	2000[3]	2005[3]	2006[3]	2007[3]	2008[3]	2009[3]	2010[3]
White, Not Hispanic or Latino Male[7]														
All ages, age-adjusted[4]	NA	NA	NA	NA	84.2	91.1	84.1	77.9	71.3	69.3	67.2	65.9	63.9	62.7
All ages, crude	NA	NA	NA	NA	74.5	84.7	81.5	78.9	77.4	76.4	75.2	75.1	74.2	73.8
45 to 54 years	NA	NA	NA	NA	62.6	57.8	44.9	37.7	36.2	34.6	33.1	34.0	33.2	31.8
55 to 64 years	NA	NA	NA	NA	209.8	221.0	184.8	157.7	128.6	123.7	118.6	114.9	111.6	107.8
65 to 74 years	NA	NA	NA	NA	398.4	431.4	416.0	387.3	339.1	326.6	316.1	305.0	292.3	287.3
75 to 84 years	NA	NA	NA	NA	518.2	580.4	554.8	537.7	526.6	520.7	508.2	496.7	487.7	479.3
85 years and over	NA	NA	NA	NA	413.8	520.9	542.7	527.3	525.1	517.8	508.0	517.1	499.5	504.4
White Female[5]														
All ages, age-adjusted[4]	5.9	6.8	13.1	24.5	31.0	37.6	41.1	42.3	41.7	41.2	41.3	40.4	40.0	39.3
All ages, crude	4.7	5.9	12.3	25.6	33.9	42.4	47.5	49.9	50.7	50.6	51.0	50.5	50.4	50.0
45 to 54 years	5.7	9.0	20.9	33.0	35.4	34.6	29.3	24.8	24.1	24.1	24.8	24.7	25.2	24.3
55 to 64 years	13.7	15.1	37.2	71.9	92.4	105.7	104.0	96.1	82.2	79.9	77.6	73.1	70.1	68.9
65 to 74 years	23.7	24.8	42.9	104.6	145.5	181.3	203.8	213.2	205.6	203.3	202.5	195.6	193.6	187.4
75 to 84 years	34.0	32.7	52.6	95.2	134.8	194.6	243.3	272.7	288.9	288.9	293.1	294.1	289.8	290.5
85 years and over	29.3	39.1	50.6	92.4	99.3	138.3	181.0	215.9	245.9	248.8	250.5	253.1	257.3	258.3
Black or African American Female[5]														
All ages, age-adjusted[4]	4.5	6.8	13.7	24.8	29.7	36.8	38.8	39.8	39.9	38.8	37.9	36.8	35.8	36.5
All ages, crude	2.8	4.3	9.4	18.3	22.5	28.1	29.5	30.8	32.5	32.0	31.5	30.8	30.5	31.4
45 to 54 years	7.5	11.3	23.9	43.4	39.1	41.3	34.5	32.9	33.2	34.2	31.9	28.3	29.0	27.7
55 to 64 years	12.9	17.9	33.5	79.9	103.5	117.9	106.9	95.3	86.3	80.8	76.6	74.1	76.3	74.0
65 to 74 years	14.0	18.1	46.1	88.0	117.2	164.3	196.2	194.1	181.3	175.6	176.3	168.3	161.4	163.1
75 to 84 years	*	31.3	49.1	79.4	101.2	148.1	183.2	224.3	254.2	252.0	250.1	249.0	243.2	249.2
85 years and over	NA	34.2	44.8	85.8	114.3	134.9	158.9	185.9	228.4	213.0	212.0	226.3	197.6	249.3
American Indian or Alaska Native Female[5]														
All ages, age-adjusted[4]	NA	NA	NA	11.7	14.2	19.3	25.9	24.8	30.0	26.9	27.4	27.4	25.1	26.3
All ages, crude	NA	NA	NA	6.0	8.2	11.2	13.8	14.0	17.8	16.1	16.3	15.9	15.5	16.0
45 to 54 years	NA	NA	NA	*	*	22.9	*	12.1	17.2	11.0	9.7	10.9	12.7	13.2
55 to 64 years	NA	NA	NA	*	38.5	53.7	45.7	54.9	57.1	49.7	41.2	50.5	40.3
65 to 74 years	NA	NA	NA	*	93.9	78.5	134.6	151.5	165.1	143.1	157.7	126.8	119.4	141.8
75 to 84 years	NA	NA	NA	*	*	111.8	209.5	136.3	204.1	183.2	192.2	218.7	197.5	185.9
85 years and over	NA	NA	NA	*	*	*	*	*	*	236.6	*	200.0
Asian or Pacific Islander Female[5]														
All ages, age-adjusted[4]	NA	NA	NA	15.4	14.4	18.9	21.4	18.4	18.5	18.1	18.9	18.1	18.3	18.3
All ages, crude	NA	NA	NA	8.4	7.9	10.5	13.0	12.6	13.9	13.9	14.8	14.2	14.5	14.9
45 to 54 years	NA	NA	NA	13.5	12.5	11.3	11.6	9.9	10.6	10.0	10.3	9.5	8.7	8.8
55 to 64 years	NA	NA	NA	24.6	26.0	38.3	37.6	30.4	27.3	26.6	31.8	25.8	25.1	28.0
65 to 74 years	NA	NA	NA	62.4	60.7	71.6	84.2	77.0	73.9	74.2	73.0	73.8	68.0	67.0
75 to 84 years	NA	NA	NA	117.7	97.8	137.9	153.5	135.0	144.6	135.0	145.2	148.6	153.9	160.3
85 years and over	NA	NA	NA	*	*	172.9	235.5	175.3	184.4	190.7	193.6	168.3	203.9	171.1
Hispanic or Latina Female[5,7]														
All ages, age-adjusted[4]	NA	NA	NA	NA	10.9	14.1	14.3	14.7	14.8	14.0	14.9	14.2	13.6	13.8
All ages, crude	NA	NA	NA	NA	4.9	7.2	7.1	7.2	7.7	7.4	7.9	7.7	7.5	7.7
45 to 54 years	NA	NA	NA	NA	6.8	8.7	7.1	7.1	7.0	6.2	6.5	7.1	5.9	7.1
55 to 64 years	NA	NA	NA	NA	17.4	25.1	25.5	22.2	20.2	18.8	21.8	20.8	20.5	19.3
65 to 74 years	NA	NA	NA	NA	49.1	66.8	59.2	66.0	62.8	64.9	65.9	62.0	58.5	51.7
75 to 84 years	NA	NA	NA	NA	73.6	94.3	111.0	112.3	118.3	111.1	115.3	111.2	104.0	117.3
85 years and over	NA	NA	NA	NA	110.7	118.2	128.3	137.5	153.2	128.7	152.0	137.7	144.9	143.4
White, not Hispanic or Latina Female[7]														
All ages, age-adjusted[4]	NA	NA	NA	NA	31.7	39.0	42.5	44.1	43.8	43.5	43.5	42.7	42.3	41.7
All ages, crude	NA	NA	NA	NA	35.6	46.2	52.3	56.4	58.7	58.9	59.5	59.2	59.3	59.0
45 to 54 years	NA	NA	NA	NA	36.6	36.6	31.0	26.4	26.1	26.4	27.2	27.1	28.0	26.9
55 to 64 years	NA	NA	NA	NA	93.4	111.3	109.4	102.2	87.9	85.7	83.0	78.3	75.1	74.0
65 to 74 years	NA	NA	NA	NA	149.4	186.4	210.4	222.9	217.5	215.2	214.3	207.3	205.6	199.5
75 to 84 years	NA	NA	NA	NA	138.1	199.1	247.2	279.2	298.6	299.8	304.5	306.5	303.1	303.0
85 years and over	NA	NA	NA	NA	100.9	139.0	181.6	218.0	249.1	253.4	254.5	258.2	262.3	263.8

NA = Not available.   * = Rates based on fewer than 20 deaths are considered unreliable and are not shown.   0.0 = Quantity more than zero but less than 0.05.   [1]Includes deaths of persons who were not residents of the 50 states and the District of Columbia.   [2]Underlying cause of death was coded according to the 6th Revision of the International Classification of Diseases (ICD) in 1950, 7th Revision in 1960, 8th Revision in 1970, and 9th Revision in 1980–1998.   [3]Starting with 1999 data, cause of death is coded according to ICD-10.   [4]Age-adjusted rates are calculated using the year 2000 standard population. Prior to 2001, age-adjusted rates were calculated using standard million proportions based on rounded population numbers. Starting with 2001 data, unrounded population numbers are used to calculate age-adjusted rates.   [5]The race groups, White, Black, Asian or Pacific Islander, and American Indian or Alaska Native, include persons of Hispanic and non-Hispanic origin. Persons of Hispanic origin may be of any race. Death rates for the American Indian or Alaska Native, Asian or Pacific Islander, and Hispanic populations are known to be underestimated.   [6]In 1950, rate is for the age group 75 years and over.   [7]Prior to 1997, excludes data from states lacking an Hispanic-origin item on the death certificate.

Table 2-38. Death Rates for Human Immunodeficiency Virus (HIV) Disease, by Sex, Race, Hispanic Origin, and Age, Selected Years, 1987–2010

(Deaths per 100,000 resident population.)

Sex, race, Hispanic origin, and age[1]	1987[2]	1990[2]	1995[2]	2000[3]	2005[3]	2009[3]	2010[3]
All Persons							
All ages, age-adjusted[4]	5.6	10.2	16.2	5.2	4.2	3.0	2.6
All ages, crude	5.6	10.1	16.2	5.1	4.2	3.1	2.7
Under 1 year	2.3	2.7	1.5	*	*	*	*
1 to 4 years	0.7	0.8	1.3	*	*	*	*
5 to 14 years	0.1	0.2	0.5	0.1	*	*	*
15 to 24 years	1.3	1.5	1.7	0.5	0.4	0.3	0.3
25 to 34 years	11.7	19.7	28.3	6.1	3.4	2.2	1.8
35 to 44 years	14.0	27.4	44.2	13.1	10.0	5.8	4.6
45 to 54 years	8.0	15.2	26.0	11.0	10.6	7.6	6.9
55 to 64 years	3.5	6.2	10.9	5.1	5.3	5.2	5.0
65 to 74 years	1.3	2.0	3.6	2.2	2.3	2.6	2.2
75 to 84 years	0.8	0.7	0.7	0.7	0.8	0.9	0.9
85 years and over	*	*	*	*	*	0.4	0.4
Male							
All ages, age-adjusted[4]	10.4	18.5	27.3	7.9	6.3	4.4	3.8
All ages, crude	10.2	18.5	27.6	7.9	6.3	4.5	4.0
Under 1 year	2.2	2.4	1.7	*	*	*	*
1 to 4 years	0.7	0.8	1.2	*	*	*	*
5 to 14 years	0.2	0.3	0.5	0.1	*	*	*
15 to 24 years	2.2	2.2	2.0	0.5	0.4	0.4	0.4
25 to 34 years	20.7	34.5	45.5	8.0	4.1	2.7	2.3
35 to 44 years	26.3	50.2	75.5	19.8	14.5	8.2	6.3
45 to 54 years	15.5	29.1	46.2	17.8	16.4	11.2	10.6
55 to 64 years	6.8	12.0	19.7	8.7	8.7	8.5	7.9
65 to 74 years	2.4	3.7	6.4	3.8	4.0	4.4	3.8
75 to 84 years	1.2	1.1	1.3	1.3	1.4	1.6	1.7
85 years and over	*	*	*	*	*	*	*
Female							
All ages, age-adjusted[4]	1.1	2.2	5.3	2.5	2.3	1.7	1.4
All ages, crude	1.1	2.2	5.3	2.5	2.2	1.7	1.4
Under 1 year	2.5	3.0	1.2	*	*	*	*
1 to 4 years	0.7	0.8	1.5	*	*	*	*
5 to 14 years	*	0.2	0.5	0.1	*	*	*
15 to 24 years	0.3	0.7	1.4	0.4	0.3	0.3	0.2
25 to 34 years	2.8	4.9	10.9	4.2	2.6	1.6	1.3
35 to 44 years	2.1	5.2	13.3	6.5	5.6	3.5	2.9
45 to 54 years	0.8	1.9	6.6	4.4	5.1	4.0	3.4
55 to 64 years	0.5	1.1	2.8	1.8	2.0	2.2	2.3
65 to 74 years	0.5	0.8	1.4	0.8	0.9	1.1	0.9
75 to 84 years	0.5	0.4	0.3	0.3	0.4	0.4	0.4
85 years and over	*	*	*	*	*	*	*
All Ages, Age-Adjusted[4]							
White male	8.7	15.7	20.4	4.6	3.7	2.5	2.3
Black or African American male	26.2	46.3	89.0	35.1	27.7	19.5	16.5
American Indian or Alaska Native male	*	3.3	10.5	3.5	3.7	2.4	2.6
Asian or Pacific Islander male	2.5	4.3	6.0	1.2	1.0	0.7	0.7
Hispanic or Latino male[5]	18.8	28.8	40.8	10.6	7.7	5.0	4.6
White, not Hispanic or Latino male[5]	10.7	14.1	17.9	3.8	3.0	2.0	1.8
White female	0.6	1.1	2.5	1.0	0.8	0.6	0.5
Black or African American female	4.6	10.1	24.4	13.2	11.9	8.8	7.5
American Indian or Alaska Native female	*	*	2.5	1.0	1.3	*	*
Asian or Pacific Islander female	*	*	0.6	0.2	*	*	*
Hispanic or Latina female[5]	2.1	3.8	8.8	2.9	1.9	1.4	1.1
White, not Hispanic or Latina female[5]	0.5	0.7	1.7	0.7	0.6	0.4	0.4
Age 25 to 44 Years							
All persons	12.7	23.2	36.3	9.8	6.9	4.0	3.2
White male	19.2	35.0	46.1	8.8	5.9	3.1	2.5
Black or African American male	60.2	102.0	179.4	55.4	36.9	22.3	17.1
American Indian or Alaska Native male	*	7.7	28.5	5.5	5.6	*	*
Asian or Pacific Islander male	4.1	8.1	12.1	1.9	1.4	0.8	*
Hispanic or Latino male[5]	36.8	59.3	73.9	14.3	8.8	4.8	4.1
White, not Hispanic or Latino male[5]	23.3	31.6	41.2	7.4	5.0	2.5	1.9
White female	1.2	2.3	5.9	2.1	1.5	0.8	0.7
Black or African American female	11.6	23.6	53.6	26.7	20.6	13.1	10.3
American Indian or Alaska Native female	*	*	1.2	*	*	*	*
Asian or Pacific Islander female	*	*	*	*	*	*	*
Hispanic or Latina female[5]	4.9	8.9	17.2	4.6	2.6	1.3	1.2
White, not Hispanic or Latina female[5]	1.0	1.5	4.2	1.6	1.2	0.6	0.6
Age 45 to 64 Years							
All persons	5.8	11.1	19.9	8.7	8.4	6.5	6.1
White male	9.9	18.6	26.0	8.1	7.3	5.7	5.6
Black or African American male	27.3	53.0	133.2	71.6	64.1	45.3	39.8
American Indian or Alaska Native male	*	*	*	*	8.3	6.7	7.0
Asian or Pacific Islander male	*	6.5	9.1	2.1	2.0	1.6	1.9
Hispanic or Latino male[5]	25.8	37.9	67.1	23.3	18.1	12.6	11.5
White, not Hispanic or Latino male[5]	12.6	16.9	22.4	6.5	6.0	4.7	4.7
White female	0.5	0.9	2.4	1.3	1.4	1.2	1.0
Black or African American female	2.6	7.5	27.0	19.6	21.7	17.7	16.3
American Indian or Alaska Native female	*	*	*	*	*	*	*
Asian or Pacific Islander female	*	*	*	*	*	*	*
Hispanic or Latina female[5]	*	3.1	12.6	5.8	4.0	3.4	2.5
White, not Hispanic or Latina female[5]	0.5	0.7	1.5	0.9	1.1	0.8	0.8

* = Rates based on fewer than 20 deaths are considered unreliable and are not shown.   [1]The race groups, White, Black, Asian or Pacific Islander, and American Indian or Alaska Native, include persons of Hispanic and non-Hispanic origin. Persons of Hispanic origin may be of any race. Death rates for the American Indian or Alaska Native, Asian or Pacific Islander, and Hispanic populations are known to be underestimated.   [2]Categories for the coding and classification of human immunodeficiency virus (HIV) disease were introduced in the United States in 1987.   [3]Starting with 1999 data, cause of death is coded according to ICD-10.   [4]Age-adjusted rates are calculated using the year 2000 standard population. Prior to 2001, age-adjusted rates were calculated using standard million proportions based on rounded population numbers. Starting with 2001 data, unrounded population numbers are used to calculate age-adjusted rates.   [5]Prior to 1997, excludes data from states lacking an Hispanic-origin item on the death certificate.

Table 2-39. Death Rates for Motor Vehicle–Related Injuries, by Sex, Race, Hispanic Origin, and Age, Selected Years, 1950–2010

(Deaths per 100,000 resident population.)

Sex, race, Hispanic origin, and age	1950[1,2]	1960[1,2]	1970[2]	1980[2]	1985	1990[2]	1995	2000[3]	2005[3]	2006[3]	2007[3]	2008[3]	2009[3]	2010[3]
All Persons														
All ages, age-adjusted[4]	24.6	23.1	27.6	22.3	18.6	18.5	16.3	15.4	15.2	15.0	14.4	12.9	11.6	11.3
All ages, crude	23.1	21.3	26.9	23.5	19.3	18.8	16.3	15.4	15.3	15.2	14.6	13.1	11.8	11.4
Under 1 year	8.4	8.1	9.8	7.0	4.9	4.9	4.7	4.4	3.6	3.5	3.0	2.5	2.4	2.0
1 to 14 years	9.8	8.6	10.5	8.2	7.0	6.0	5.3	4.3	3.7	3.4	3.2	2.6	2.5	2.3
1 to 4 years	11.5	10.0	11.5	9.2	7.2	6.3	5.2	4.2	3.9	3.7	3.4	2.9	2.9	2.8
5 to 14 years	8.8	7.9	10.2	7.9	6.9	5.9	5.3	4.3	3.6	3.3	3.2	2.5	2.4	2.2
15 to 24 years	34.4	38.0	47.2	44.8	35.7	34.1	28.9	26.9	25.7	25.7	24.5	20.6	17.6	16.6
15 to 19 years	29.6	33.9	43.6	43.0	33.5	33.1	28.1	26.0	23.1	22.6	21.4	17.4	15.2	13.6
20 to 24 years	38.8	42.9	51.3	46.6	37.6	35.0	29.7	28.0	28.3	28.9	27.7	24.0	20.2	19.7
25 to 34 years	24.6	24.3	30.9	29.1	23.0	23.6	19.2	17.3	18.4	18.7	17.8	16.3	14.5	14.0
35 to 44 years	20.3	19.3	24.9	20.9	17.2	16.9	15.3	15.3	15.5	15.4	14.9	13.4	12.2	11.6
45 to 64 years	25.2	23.0	26.5	18.0	15.4	15.7	14.1	14.3	14.8	14.8	14.1	13.3	12.2	11.9
45 to 54 years	22.2	21.4	25.5	18.6	15.2	15.6	13.8	14.2	15.1	15.3	14.9	13.7	12.7	12.0
55 to 64 years	29.0	25.1	27.9	17.4	15.6	15.9	14.5	14.4	14.5	14.1	13.2	12.8	11.5	11.9
65 years and over	43.1	34.7	36.2	22.5	21.7	23.1	22.6	21.4	20.1	19.0	18.7	16.9	15.8	16.0
65 to 74 years	39.1	31.4	32.8	19.2	17.9	18.6	17.5	16.5	16.5	15.2	14.9	13.8	12.7	12.3
75 to 84 years	52.7	41.8	43.5	28.1	27.4	29.1	28.4	25.7	22.9	22.2	21.7	19.2	18.6	18.8
85 years and over	45.1	37.9	34.2	27.6	26.5	31.2	31.0	30.4	27.3	25.5	25.3	23.2	20.9	23.8
Male														
All ages, age-adjusted[4]	38.5	35.4	41.5	33.6	27.2	26.5	22.8	21.7	21.9	21.5	21.0	18.9	16.8	16.2
All ages, crude	35.4	31.8	39.7	35.3	28.0	26.7	22.4	21.3	21.8	21.6	21.0	18.9	16.9	16.3
Under 1 year	9.1	8.6	9.3	7.3	5.0	5.0	4.9	4.6	3.6	3.4	2.7	2.9	2.6	2.2
1 to 14 years	12.3	10.7	13.0	10.0	8.5	7.0	6.1	4.9	4.1	3.7	3.7	3.1	2.9	2.7
1 to 4 years	13.0	11.5	12.9	10.2	8.3	6.9	5.6	4.7	4.3	3.9	3.8	3.2	3.4	3.0
5 to 14 years	11.9	10.4	13.1	9.9	8.6	7.0	6.3	5.0	4.1	3.7	3.7	3.0	2.7	2.5
15 to 24 years	56.7	61.2	73.2	68.4	52.7	49.5	40.5	37.4	36.3	36.3	34.6	29.3	24.5	23.1
15 to 19 years	46.3	51.7	64.1	62.6	46.5	45.5	36.1	33.9	29.9	29.5	27.7	22.6	19.2	17.8
20 to 24 years	66.7	73.2	84.4	74.3	58.2	53.3	45.0	41.2	42.8	43.4	41.9	36.3	30.0	28.5
25 to 34 years	40.8	40.1	49.4	46.3	35.9	35.7	28.1	25.5	27.9	28.5	27.2	25.2	21.7	21.0
35 to 44 years	32.5	29.9	37.7	31.7	25.2	24.7	21.7	22.0	22.5	22.1	22.1	19.9	18.2	16.9
45 to 64 years	37.7	33.3	38.9	26.5	22.0	21.9	19.5	20.2	21.6	21.6	20.9	19.7	18.2	17.9
45 to 54 years	33.6	31.6	37.2	27.6	21.9	22.0	19.3	20.4	22.2	22.6	22.2	20.2	19.0	17.9
55 to 64 years	43.1	35.6	40.9	25.4	22.1	21.7	19.6	19.8	20.7	20.3	19.2	19.0	17.2	17.8
65 years and over	66.6	52.1	54.4	33.9	30.4	32.1	30.7	29.5	28.4	26.4	26.9	24.1	22.0	22.2
65 to 74 years	59.1	45.8	47.3	27.3	23.0	24.2	22.2	21.7	22.8	20.7	21.1	19.4	17.5	17.1
75 to 84 years	85.0	66.0	68.2	44.3	41.3	41.2	39.9	35.6	32.1	30.4	31.4	27.3	25.8	25.9
85 years and over	78.1	62.7	63.1	56.1	55.3	64.5	61.5	57.5	49.0	45.6	44.4	40.2	35.3	40.2
Female														
All ages, age-adjusted[4]	11.5	11.7	14.9	11.8	10.7	11.0	10.3	9.5	8.9	8.8	8.2	7.2	6.7	6.5
All ages, crude	10.9	11.0	14.7	12.3	11.0	11.3	10.4	9.7	9.1	9.0	8.4	7.4	6.9	6.8
Under 1 year	7.6	7.5	10.4	6.7	4.7	4.9	4.5	4.2	3.7	3.5	3.3	2.0	2.1	1.8
1 to 14 years	7.2	6.3	7.9	6.3	5.4	4.9	4.4	3.7	3.1	3.1	2.8	2.2	2.2	2.0
1 to 4 years	10.0	8.4	10.0	8.1	6.0	5.6	4.8	3.8	3.4	3.5	3.1	2.5	2.5	2.5
5 to 14 years	5.7	5.4	7.2	5.7	5.1	4.7	4.2	3.6	3.0	2.9	2.6	2.0	2.0	1.8
15 to 24 years	12.6	15.1	21.6	20.8	18.2	17.9	16.8	15.9	14.5	14.5	13.8	11.5	10.5	9.9
15 to 19 years	12.9	16.0	22.7	22.8	20.1	20.0	19.7	17.5	15.9	15.4	14.8	11.8	10.9	9.2
20 to 24 years	12.2	14.0	20.4	18.9	16.7	16.0	13.8	14.2	13.2	13.6	12.8	11.2	10.0	10.5
25 to 34 years	9.3	9.2	13.0	12.2	10.1	11.5	10.2	8.8	8.9	8.8	8.5	7.4	7.2	6.9
35 to 44 years	8.5	9.1	12.9	10.4	9.4	9.2	9.0	8.8	8.6	8.8	7.8	7.0	6.2	6.2
45 to 64 years	12.6	13.1	15.3	10.3	9.5	10.1	9.0	8.7	8.4	8.3	7.7	7.2	6.5	6.3
45 to 54 years	10.9	11.6	14.5	10.2	9.0	9.6	8.4	8.2	8.2	8.2	7.8	7.4	6.6	6.3
55 to 64 years	14.9	15.2	16.2	10.5	9.9	10.8	9.9	9.5	8.8	8.5	7.5	6.9	6.3	6.3
65 years and over	21.9	20.3	23.1	15.0	15.8	17.2	17.0	15.8	14.1	13.6	12.6	11.5	11.1	11.3
65 to 74 years	20.6	19.0	21.6	13.0	14.0	14.1	13.7	12.3	11.1	10.5	9.6	8.9	8.5	8.2
75 to 84 years	25.2	23.0	27.2	18.5	19.2	21.9	21.2	19.2	16.5	16.5	15.0	13.5	13.5	13.7
85 years and over	22.1	22.0	18.0	15.2	15.0	18.3	19.3	19.3	17.6	16.4	16.5	15.3	14.0	15.9
White Male [5]														
All ages, age-adjusted[4]	37.9	34.8	40.4	33.8	27.2	26.3	22.6	21.8	22.4	22.1	21.6	19.6	17.3	16.7
All ages, crude	35.1	31.5	39.1	35.9	28.3	26.7	22.4	21.6	22.5	22.2	21.7	19.7	17.5	17.0
Under 1 year	9.1	8.8	9.1	7.0	4.6	4.8	4.3	4.2	3.4	3.3	2.9	2.9	2.5	2.0
1 to 14 years	12.4	10.6	12.5	9.8	8.3	6.6	5.9	4.8	4.1	3.6	3.8	3.1	2.8	2.7
15 to 24 years	58.3	62.7	75.2	73.8	56.5	52.5	42.4	39.6	39.2	39.3	37.4	31.7	26.6	24.6
25 to 34 years	39.1	38.6	47.0	46.6	35.8	35.4	27.9	25.1	28.4	28.8	27.8	26.2	21.8	21.4
35 to 44 years	30.9	28.4	35.2	30.7	24.3	23.7	21.1	21.8	22.8	22.6	22.2	20.3	18.5	17.4
45 to 64 years	36.2	31.7	36.5	25.2	20.8	20.6	18.7	19.7	21.7	21.6	21.1	20.1	18.7	18.3
65 years and over	67.1	52.1	54.2	32.7	29.9	31.4	30.1	29.4	28.7	26.6	27.0	24.5	22.3	22.7
Black or African American Male [5]														
All ages, age-adjusted[4]	34.8	39.6	51.0	34.2	29.0	29.9	26.1	24.4	22.5	22.6	22.3	18.9	17.8	16.7
All ages, crude	37.2	33.1	44.3	31.1	27.1	28.1	24.1	22.5	21.1	21.4	21.0	18.0	16.7	15.9
Under 1 year	NA	*	10.6	7.8	*	*	8.7	6.7	*	*	*	*	*	*
1 to 14 years[6]	10.4	11.2	16.3	11.4	9.7	8.9	7.5	5.5	4.4	4.8	4.0	3.1	3.5	3.0
15 to 24 years	42.5	46.4	58.1	34.9	32.0	36.1	33.9	30.2	27.8	26.9	26.9	22.4	18.5	19.4
25 to 34 years	54.4	51.0	70.4	44.9	37.7	39.5	32.2	32.6	32.1	34.4	32.0	27.0	26.9	24.9
35 to 44 years	46.7	43.6	59.5	41.2	34.7	33.5	28.7	27.2	25.8	25.1	27.2	23.0	21.9	19.4
45 to 64 years	54.6	47.8	61.7	39.5	32.9	33.3	26.2	27.1	24.1	25.2	24.0	21.5	19.3	19.1
65 years and over	52.6	48.2	53.4	42.4	35.2	36.3	36.9	32.1	29.1	26.1	27.4	22.9	22.8	20.0

Table 2-39. Death Rates for Motor Vehicle–Related Injuries, by Sex, Race, Hispanic Origin, and Age, Selected Years, 1950–2010 —Continued

(Deaths per 100,000 resident population.)

Sex, race, Hispanic origin, and age	1950[1,2]	1960[1,2]	1970[2]	1980[2]	1985	1990[2]	1995	2000[3]	2005[3]	2006[3]	2007[3]	2008[3]	2009[3]	2010[3]
American Indian or Alaska Native Male [5]														
All ages, age-adjusted[4]	NA	NA	NA	78.9	50.9	48.3	40.7	35.8	31.5	33.5	28.6	24.1	22.7	21.1
All ages, crude	NA	NA	NA	74.6	51.7	47.6	40.1	33.6	31.3	32.2	27.3	23.5	22.0	19.8
1 to 14 years	NA	NA	NA	15.1	16.2	11.6	7.6	7.8	9.6	4.6	4.4	4.6	4.8	*
15 to 24 years	NA	NA	NA	126.1	77.3	75.2	69.0	56.8	44.1	47.9	40.0	37.5	35.2	31.9
25 to 34 years	NA	NA	NA	107.0	84.0	78.2	67.8	49.8	49.0	45.2	42.7	30.5	29.3	23.8
35 to 44 years	NA	NA	NA	82.8	55.8	57.0	45.2	36.3	36.9	34.3	32.0	29.3	28.5	24.5
45 to 64 years	NA	NA	NA	77.4	52.2	45.9	38.8	32.0	31.9	41.4	27.9	25.8	22.8	23.2
65 years and over	NA	NA	NA	97.0	*	43.0	*	48.5	27.8	37.4	38.5	24.5	22.2	26.6
Asian or Pacific Islander Male [5]														
All ages, age-adjusted[4]	NA	NA	NA	19.0	17.3	17.9	14.5	10.6	9.5	9.3	9.1	7.9	6.2	6.5
All ages, crude	NA	NA	NA	17.1	16.0	15.8	12.6	9.8	8.7	8.6	8.3	7.5	5.8	6.2
1 to 14 years	NA	NA	NA	8.2	5.2	6.3	4.5	2.5	1.7	2.6	1.8	1.6	1.5	*
15 to 24 years	NA	NA	NA	27.2	28.1	25.7	18.5	17.0	14.5	14.9	15.7	11.6	8.8	9.6
25 to 34 years	NA	NA	NA	18.8	18.4	17.0	12.4	10.4	8.9	8.4	7.0	8.5	7.3	7.8
35 to 44 years	NA	NA	NA	13.1	12.0	12.2	9.9	6.9	6.6	6.0	6.1	6.4	4.5	4.1
45 to 64 years	NA	NA	NA	13.7	13.4	15.1	14.3	10.1	9.0	8.6	7.7	7.4	5.6	6.0
65 years and over	NA	NA	NA	37.3	37.3	33.6	32.1	21.1	20.8	19.7	20.9	16.1	11.9	14.6
Hispanic or Latino Male [5,7]														
All ages, age-adjusted[4]	NA	NA	NA	NA	25.4	29.5	24.4	21.3	21.4	21.4	19.4	16.7	14.7	14.0
All ages, crude	NA	NA	NA	NA	25.6	29.2	22.4	20.1	20.8	20.9	18.6	16.1	14.2	12.8
1 to 14 years	NA	NA	NA	NA	7.7	7.2	5.7	4.4	4.6	4.6	4.1	2.9	3.0	2.5
15 to 24 years	NA	NA	NA	NA	44.9	48.2	37.1	34.7	37.6	38.1	32.8	26.9	24.1	20.2
25 to 34 years	NA	NA	NA	NA	31.2	41.0	28.8	24.9	28.0	27.6	25.9	24.7	20.1	18.0
35 to 44 years	NA	NA	NA	NA	26.3	28.0	23.2	21.6	20.9	21.6	18.6	16.4	15.5	13.9
45 to 64 years	NA	NA	NA	NA	25.9	28.9	23.0	21.7	20.2	21.6	18.8	16.9	14.4	14.3
65 years and over	NA	NA	NA	NA	22.9	35.3	37.0	28.9	27.6	24.8	25.6	19.7	16.9	20.7
White, Not Hispanic or Latino Male [7]														
All ages, age-adjusted[4]	NA	NA	NA	NA	24.9	25.7	22.1	21.7	22.2	21.8	21.6	19.8	17.4	17.1
All ages, crude	NA	NA	NA	NA	25.9	26.0	21.9	21.5	22.5	22.1	22.0	20.2	17.9	17.6
1 to 14 years	NA	NA	NA	NA	7.8	6.4	5.8	4.9	3.9	3.2	3.5	3.1	2.6	2.7
15 to 24 years	NA	NA	NA	NA	53.3	52.3	42.7	40.3	38.8	38.8	37.9	32.5	26.6	25.4
25 to 34 years	NA	NA	NA	NA	33.2	34.0	27.1	24.7	27.8	28.5	27.6	26.1	21.8	21.9
35 to 44 years	NA	NA	NA	NA	21.6	23.1	20.3	21.6	22.9	22.4	22.7	20.9	18.9	18.0
45 to 64 years	NA	NA	NA	NA	18.0	19.8	18.1	19.3	21.7	21.4	21.1	20.2	19.0	18.6
65 years and over	NA	NA	NA	NA	27.6	31.1	29.4	29.3	28.6	26.6	27.0	24.7	22.6	22.7
White Female [5]														
All ages, age-adjusted[4]	11.4	11.7	14.9	12.2	10.9	11.2	10.4	9.8	9.3	9.2	8.6	7.5	6.9	6.8
All ages, crude	10.9	11.2	14.8	12.8	11.4	11.6	10.7	10.0	9.6	9.4	8.8	7.8	7.2	7.1
Under 1 year	7.8	7.5	10.2	7.1	3.9	4.7	4.5	3.5	3.0	3.1	2.9	1.8	1.5	1.9
1 to 14 years	7.2	6.2	7.5	6.2	5.4	4.8	4.3	3.7	3.2	3.1	2.7	2.1	2.1	2.1
15 to 24 years	12.6	15.6	22.7	23.0	20.0	19.5	18.1	17.1	15.7	15.9	15.1	12.6	11.3	10.8
25 to 34 years	9.0	9.0	12.7	12.2	10.1	11.6	10.2	8.9	9.4	9.1	9.0	7.6	7.4	7.1
35 to 44 years	8.1	8.9	12.3	10.6	9.4	9.2	8.9	8.9	9.0	9.2	8.1	7.4	6.5	6.5
45 to 64 years	12.7	13.1	15.1	10.4	9.5	9.9	8.9	8.7	8.6	8.3	7.8	7.3	6.6	6.4
65 years and over	22.2	20.8	23.7	15.3	16.2	17.4	17.5	16.2	14.5	14.0	13.0	11.8	11.4	11.5
Black or African American Female [5]														
All ages, age-adjusted[4]	9.3	10.4	14.1	8.5	8.5	9.6	9.0	8.4	7.6	7.7	7.0	6.4	6.2	5.9
All ages, crude	10.2	9.7	13.4	8.3	8.3	9.4	8.8	8.2	7.5	7.6	6.9	6.3	6.1	5.8
Under 1 year	NA	8.1	11.9	*	8.1	7.0	*	*	6.9	*	*	*	*	*
1 to 14 years[6]	7.2	6.9	10.2	6.3	5.1	5.3	4.9	3.9	3.4	3.4	3.3	2.5	2.6	2.0
15 to 24 years	11.6	9.9	13.4	8.0	9.1	9.9	10.5	11.7	10.5	9.8	9.5	8.4	8.1	7.8
25 to 34 years	10.8	9.8	13.3	10.6	9.3	11.1	10.3	9.4	7.6	8.7	7.5	7.1	7.6	6.8
35 to 44 years	11.1	11.0	16.1	8.3	9.1	9.4	9.7	8.2	7.7	8.0	7.0	6.7	6.0	5.8
45 to 64 years	11.8	12.7	16.7	9.2	9.0	10.7	9.3	9.0	8.2	8.8	7.4	7.0	6.5	6.3
65 years and over	14.3	13.2	15.7	9.5	11.2	13.5	11.4	10.4	9.9	9.5	8.7	8.4	7.9	8.6
American Indian or Alaska Native Female [5]														
All ages, age-adjusted[4]	NA	NA	NA	32.0	19.8	17.5	18.2	19.5	14.0	15.1	13.5	12.8	11.8	10.6
All ages, crude	NA	NA	NA	32.0	20.6	17.3	18.8	18.6	13.8	14.9	13.5	12.4	11.7	10.0
1 to 14 years	NA	NA	NA	15.0	9.2	8.1	8.1	6.5	*	*	*	*	*	*
15 to 24 years	NA	NA	NA	42.3	29.5	31.4	30.4	30.3	22.0	24.5	21.4	17.4	19.8	13.4
25 to 34 years	NA	NA	NA	52.5	30.2	18.8	33.7	22.3	22.1	19.1	19.4	19.2	13.8	17.7
35 to 44 years	NA	NA	NA	38.1	27.0	18.2	17.2	22.0	15.7	17.7	18.8	15.3	16.9	13.1
45 to 64 years	NA	NA	NA	32.6	19.5	17.6	15.7	17.8	10.6	13.5	10.8	10.3	11.7	8.4
65 years and over	NA	NA	NA	*	*	*	*	24.0	*	17.1	*	17.8	*	14.8

Table 2-39. Death Rates for Motor Vehicle–Related Injuries, by Sex, Race, Hispanic Origin, and Age, Selected Years, 1950–2010 —Continued

(Deaths per 100,000 resident population.)

Sex, race, Hispanic origin, and age	1950[1,2]	1960[1,2]	1970[2]	1980[2]	1985	1990[2]	1995	2000[3]	2005[3]	2006[3]	2007[3]	2008[3]	2009[3]	2010[3]
Asian or Pacific Islander Female [5]														
All ages, age-adjusted[4]	NA	NA	NA	9.3	8.8	10.4	8.6	6.7	5.7	5.4	5.0	4.2	3.8	3.9
All ages, crude	NA	NA	NA	8.2	7.9	9.0	7.7	5.9	5.3	5.1	4.6	3.9	3.5	3.6
1 to 14 years	NA	NA	NA	7.4	5.0	3.6	3.2	2.3	1.5	1.7	*	1.4	1.5	*
15 to 24 years	NA	NA	NA	7.4	7.4	11.4	11.5	6.0	7.0	6.3	6.7	4.5	4.3	3.3
25 to 34 years	NA	NA	NA	7.3	8.4	7.3	4.8	4.5	3.4	3.2	2.9	3.1	2.9	3.1
35 to 44 years	NA	NA	NA	8.6	7.0	7.5	5.9	4.9	4.3	4.1	2.7	2.2	2.1	2.0
45 to 64 years	NA	NA	NA	8.5	8.6	11.8	10.4	6.4	6.4	6.0	5.4	4.4	3.0	4.3
65 years and over	NA	NA	NA	18.6	20.5	24.3	18.9	18.5	13.9	13.6	13.4	12.1	11.4	12.2
Hispanic or Latina Female[5,7]														
All ages, age-adjusted[4]	NA	NA	NA	NA	8.8	9.6	8.8	7.9	7.8	7.6	6.8	5.5	5.5	5.3
All ages, crude	NA	NA	NA	NA	7.9	8.9	8.0	7.2	7.3	7.0	6.3	5.0	5.1	4.9
1 to 14 years	NA	NA	NA	NA	4.8	4.8	4.3	3.9	3.3	3.1	2.7	2.1	2.3	2.0
15 to 24 years	NA	NA	NA	NA	10.1	11.6	11.8	10.6	12.7	10.9	10.1	7.8	7.8	7.7
25 to 34 years	NA	NA	NA	NA	7.5	9.4	7.2	6.5	7.1	6.8	6.6	5.4	5.5	5.0
35 to 44 years	NA	NA	NA	NA	8.8	8.0	7.9	7.3	7.3	7.1	6.7	4.8	4.6	4.5
45 to 64 years	NA	NA	NA	NA	9.4	11.4	9.3	8.3	7.4	8.0	6.7	5.1	5.5	5.6
65 years and over	NA	NA	NA	NA	14.8	14.9	14.6	13.4	11.4	12.0	10.5	10.7	9.5	9.4
White, not Hispanic or Latina Female[7]														
All ages, age-adjusted[4]	NA	NA	NA	NA	10.4	11.3	10.5	10.0	9.5	9.4	8.8	7.9	7.1	7.0
All ages, crude	NA	NA	NA	NA	10.9	11.7	10.9	10.3	9.9	9.8	9.2	8.3	7.5	7.5
1 to 14 years	NA	NA	NA	NA	4.9	4.7	4.2	3.5	3.0	3.0	2.6	2.1	1.9	2.0
15 to 24 years	NA	NA	NA	NA	20.2	20.4	19.0	18.4	16.3	16.9	16.2	13.7	12.0	11.4
25 to 34 years	NA	NA	NA	NA	9.8	11.7	10.5	9.3	9.9	9.6	9.5	8.1	7.7	7.6
35 to 44 years	NA	NA	NA	NA	8.6	9.3	8.9	9.0	9.2	9.4	8.3	7.9	6.8	6.9
45 to 64 years	NA	NA	NA	NA	8.6	9.7	8.6	8.7	8.6	8.3	7.9	7.6	6.7	6.4
65 years and over	NA	NA	NA	NA	15.3	17.5	17.5	16.3	14.7	14.1	13.1	11.8	11.5	11.6

NA = Not available.   * = Rates based on fewer than 20 deaths are considered unreliable and are not shown.   [1]Includes deaths of persons who were not residents of the 50 states and the District of Columbia.   [2]Underlying cause of death was coded according to the 6th Revision of the International Classification of Diseases (ICD) in 1950, 7th Revision in 1960, 8th Revision in 1970, and 9th Revision in 1980–1998.   [3]Starting with 1999 data, cause of death is coded according to ICD-10.   [4]Age-adjusted rates are calculated using the year 2000 standard population. Prior to 2001, age-adjusted rates were calculated using standard million proportions based on rounded population numbers. Starting with 2001 data, unrounded population numbers are used to calculate age-adjusted rates.   [5]The race groups, White, Black, Asian or Pacific Islander, and American Indian or Alaska Native, include persons of Hispanic and non-Hispanic origin. Persons of Hispanic origin may be of any race. Death rates for the American Indian or Alaska Native, Asian or Pacific Islander, and Hispanic populations are known to be underestimated.   [6]In 1950, rate is for the age group under 15 years.   [7]Prior to 1997, excludes data from states lacking an Hispanic-origin item on the death certificate.

Table 2-40. Unintentional Motor Vehicle Deaths by States, Annual Averages, 2000–2007

(Deaths per 100,000 population.)

State	Deaths per 100,000 population	State	Deaths per 100,000 population
United States	14.7	Alaska	14.9
Mississippi	30.6	Indiana	14.9
Wyoming	25.7	Colorado	14.7
Montana	24.9	Wisconsin	14.2
Arkansas	24.7	Iowa	14.1
Alabama	24.6	Maine	13.8
South Carolina	23.8	Utah	13.2
New Mexico	22.5	Oregon	13.2
South Dakota	21.9	Virginia	12.9
Louisiana	21.9	Michigan	12.6
Tennessee	21.8	Pennsylvania	12.5
Kentucky	20.9	Vermont	12.3
West Virginia	20.9	Maryland	12.1
Oklahoma	20.6	Ohio	12.0
North Carolina	19.3	Minnesota	12.0
Missouri	19.2	California	11.7
Idaho	19.0	Illinois	11.5
Arizona	19.0	Washington	11.2
Florida	18.4	New Hampshire	10.4
Georgia	17.8	Hawaii	10.3
Kansas	17.7	Connecticut	9.1
Texas	17.2	New Jersey	8.7
Nevada	16.7	District of Columbia	8.3
North Dakota	16.5	Rhode Island	8.1
Nebraska	15.6	New York	7.8
Delaware	15.2	Massachusetts	7.4

NOTE: States listed are where deaths occurred, not state of residence.

Table 2-41. Death Rates for Drug Poisoning and Drug Poisoning Involving Opioid Analgesics, by Sex, Race, Hispanic Origin, and Age, Selected Years, 1999–2010

(Deaths per 100,000 resident population.)

Sex, race, Hispanic origin, and age	1999	2000	2005	2006	2007	2008	2009	2010
Drug Poisoning Deaths per 100,000 Resident Population [1]								
All Persons								
All ages, age-adjusted[2]	6.1	6.2	10.1	11.5	11.9	11.9	11.9	12.3
All ages, crude	6.0	6.2	10.1	11.5	12.0	12.0	12.1	12.4
Under 15 years	0.1	0.1	0.2	0.2	0.2	0.2	0.2	0.2
15 to 24 years	3.2	3.7	6.9	8.1	8.2	8.0	7.7	8.2
25 to 34 years	8.1	7.9	13.6	16.1	16.8	16.8	17.2	18.4
35 to 44 years	14.0	14.3	19.6	21.7	21.4	21.1	20.5	20.8
45 to 54 years	11.1	11.6	21.1	24.1	25.1	25.2	25.4	25.1
55 to 64 years	4.2	4.2	9.0	10.5	12.2	12.9	13.7	15.0
65 to 74 years	2.4	2.0	3.2	3.5	4.0	4.6	4.7	4.7
75 to 84 years	2.8	2.4	3.1	3.3	3.2	3.3	3.8	3.4
85 years and over	3.8	4.4	4.1	4.4	4.5	4.1	4.4	4.7
Male								
All ages, age-adjusted[2]	8.2	8.3	12.8	14.8	14.9	14.9	14.8	15.0
All ages, crude	8.2	8.4	12.9	14.9	15.1	15.0	15.0	15.2
Under 15 years	0.1	0.2	0.2	0.2	0.3	0.2	0.2	0.3
15 to 24 years	4.5	5.3	10.0	12.0	12.0	11.9	11.3	11.6
25 to 34 years	11.5	11.3	18.7	22.7	23.4	23.6	24.0	25.0
35 to 44 years	19.2	19.5	24.4	27.5	26.7	25.6	25.2	24.9
45 to 54 years	15.2	15.7	25.8	29.7	29.2	29.6	29.1	28.5
55 to 64 years	4.9	4.4	10.6	12.3	14.0	14.8	16.0	17.3
65 to 74 years	2.7	2.1	3.3	3.5	4.4	4.8	4.8	4.5
75 to 84 years	2.5	2.5	3.4	3.2	3.2	3.2	3.5	3.6
85 years and over	4.4	5.9	5.2	4.7	4.9	4.4	5.2	5.1
Female								
All ages, age-adjusted[2]	3.9	4.1	7.3	8.2	8.8	8.9	9.1	9.6
All ages, crude	3.9	4.1	7.4	8.3	9.0	9.0	9.2	9.8
Under 15 years	0.1	0.1	0.2	0.2	0.2	0.2	0.2	0.2
15 to 24 years	1.8	1.9	3.5	3.9	4.2	4.0	4.1	4.6
25 to 34 years	4.6	4.6	8.5	9.5	10.1	9.9	10.4	11.9
35 to 44 years	8.7	9.2	14.8	15.9	16.1	16.5	16.0	16.8
45 to 54 years	7.2	7.7	16.5	18.6	21.0	21.0	21.8	21.8
55 to 64 years	3.5	3.9	7.5	8.8	10.5	11.1	11.6	12.9
65 to 74 years	2.1	2.0	3.1	3.6	3.7	4.4	4.6	4.8
75 to 84 years	3.0	2.3	2.9	3.3	3.2	3.3	3.9	3.3
85 years and over	3.5	3.9	3.7	4.2	4.3	4.0	3.9	4.5
All Ages, Age-Adjusted [2,3]								
White male	8.1	8.4	13.6	15.7	16.3	16.5	16.4	16.8
Black or African American male	11.5	10.8	12.8	15.2	13.0	11.3	10.8	10.1
American Indian or Alaska Native male	5.7	6.1	10.8	13.0	10.5	13.5	14.2	11.8
Asian or Pacific Islander male	1.5	1.4	2.2	2.3	2.2	2.1	2.8	2.5
Hispanic or Latino male	8.6	7.1	8.4	9.1	8.7	8.4	8.2	7.6
White, not Hispanic or Latino male	8.0	8.6	14.7	17.2	18.0	18.3	18.3	19.0
White female	4.0	4.3	8.0	9.0	9.8	10.1	10.3	10.9
Black or African American female	3.9	4.1	6.0	6.3	6.3	5.4	5.6	5.7
American Indian or Alaska Native female	4.6	3.7	8.6	7.9	9.9	8.8	9.6	9.7
Asian or Pacific Islander female	1.0	0.8	1.3	1.4	1.6	1.3	1.3	1.5
Hispanic or Latina female	2.2	2.0	3.0	3.4	3.1	3.2	3.5	3.6
White, not Hispanic or Latina female	4.3	4.5	8.8	10.0	11.0	11.4	11.6	12.5
Drug Poisoning Deaths Involving Opioid Analgesics per 100,000 Resident Population [4]								
All Persons								
All ages, age-adjusted[2]	1.4	1.5	3.7	4.6	4.8	4.8	5.0	5.4
All ages, crude	1.4	1.6	3.7	4.6	4.8	4.9	5.1	5.4
Under 15 years	*	0.0	0.1	0.1	0.1	0.1	0.1	0.1
15 to 24 years	0.7	0.8	2.7	3.8	3.9	3.7	3.6	3.9
25 to 34 years	1.9	1.9	5.3	6.9	7.3	7.2	7.6	8.5
35 to 44 years	3.5	3.7	6.9	8.3	8.3	8.4	8.6	9.1
45 to 54 years	2.9	3.2	7.9	9.6	9.8	10.4	10.6	10.9
55 to 64 years	1.0	1.1	3.1	3.9	4.7	4.9	5.8	6.2
65 to 74 years	0.4	0.4	1.0	1.1	1.2	1.4	1.7	1.5
75 to 84 years	0.3	0.2	0.6	0.6	0.6	0.6	0.8	0.7
85 years and over	*	*	0.9	0.7	0.9	0.6	0.7	1.1
Male								
All ages, age-adjusted[2]	2.0	2.0	4.6	5.8	5.9	6.0	6.2	6.5
All ages, crude	2.0	2.1	4.6	5.9	5.9	6.1	6.2	6.6
Under 15 years	*	*	0.1	0.1	0.1	0.1	0.1	0.2
15 to 24 years	1.0	1.2	4.2	5.8	5.8	5.6	5.3	5.6
25 to 34 years	2.7	2.7	7.2	9.7	10.2	10.2	10.6	11.7
35 to 44 years	5.0	4.9	8.3	10.4	10.0	10.0	10.4	10.9
45 to 54 years	3.9	4.3	9.4	11.3	10.8	11.8	11.6	12.0
55 to 64 years	1.1	1.0	3.5	4.2	5.1	5.3	6.3	7.0
65 to 74 years	0.5	0.3	0.7	1.0	1.1	1.5	1.6	1.2
75 to 84 years	*	*	0.6	0.6	0.5	0.5	0.6	0.7
85 years and over	*	*	*	*	*	1.3	1.2	1.3
Female								
All ages, age-adjusted[2]	0.9	1.1	2.8	3.3	3.6	3.7	3.9	4.2
All ages, crude	0.9	1.1	2.8	3.3	3.7	3.7	4.0	4.2
Under 15 years	*	*	*	0.1	0.1	0.1	0.1	0.1
15 to 24 years	0.3	0.4	1.2	1.6	1.8	1.6	1.7	2.1
25 to 34 years	1.1	1.2	3.4	4.0	4.4	4.2	4.7	5.3
35 to 44 years	2.1	2.5	5.6	6.2	6.6	6.8	6.9	7.3
45 to 54 years	1.9	2.2	6.5	8.0	8.9	9.0	9.7	9.8
55 to 64 years	0.8	1.1	2.8	3.6	4.2	4.6	5.2	5.5
65 to 74 years	0.3	0.4	1.2	1.1	1.2	1.4	1.7	1.7
75 to 84 years	0.4	*	0.6	0.6	0.7	0.7	0.9	0.7
85 years and over	*	*	0.8	0.8	0.7	0.8	*	1.1

Table 2-41. Death Rates for Drug Poisoning and Drug Poisoning Involving Opioid Analgesics, by Sex, Race, Hispanic Origin, and Age, Selected Years, 1999–2010—*Continued*

(Deaths per 100,000 resident population.)

Sex, race, Hispanic origin, and age	1999	2000	2005	2006	2007	2008	2009	2010
All Ages, Age-Adjusted [2,3]								
White male	2.2	2.3	5.3	6.6	6.8	7.0	7.2	7.7
Black or African American male	1.2	1.2	2.1	3.5	2.3	2.2	2.4	2.2
American Indian or Alaska Native male	*	1.9	4.4	5.4	4.0	5.9	7.5	5.3
Asian or Pacific Islander male	*	*	0.5	0.6	0.4	0.5	0.7	0.8
Hispanic or Latino male	2.9	1.7	2.2	2.7	2.8	2.9	2.6	2.4
White, not Hispanic or Latino male	2.1	2.3	5.9	7.5	7.8	8.0	8.2	9.0
White female	1.0	1.2	3.2	3.8	4.2	4.3	4.5	4.8
Black or African American female	0.6	0.6	1.4	1.8	1.7	1.6	1.8	2.0
American Indian or Alaska Native female	*	*	3.8	3.2	4.5	4.6	4.7	4.9
Asian or Pacific Islander female	*	*	0.4	0.4	0.3	0.5	0.4	0.5
Hispanic or Latina female	0.5	0.5	1.0	1.3	1.2	1.2	1.3	1.3
White, not Hispanic or Latina female	1.1	1.3	3.5	4.2	4.8	4.8	5.2	5.6

0.0 = Rate more than zero but less than 0.05.   * = Rates based on fewer than 20 deaths are considered unreliable and are not shown.   [1]Drug poisoning was coded using underlying cause of death according to the 10th Revision of the International Classification of Diseases (ICD-10).   [2]Age-adjusted rates are calculated using the year 2000 standard population with unrounded population numbers.   [3]The race groups, White, Black, Asian or Pacific Islander, and American Indian or Alaska Native, include persons of Hispanic and non-Hispanic origin. Persons of Hispanic origin may be of any race. Death rates for the American Indian or Alaska Native, Asian or Pacific Islander, and Hispanic populations are known to be underestimated.   [4]Opioid analgesics include pharmaceutical opioids such as hydrocodone, codeine, and methadone, and synthetic narcotics such as fentanyl and propoxyphene. Drug poisoning deaths involving opioid analgesics include those with an underlying cause of drug poisoning and with opioid analgesics mentioned in the ICD-10 multiple causes of death.

Figure 2-10. Age-Adjusted Death Rates for Homicide, by Race and Sex, Selected Years, 1950–2010

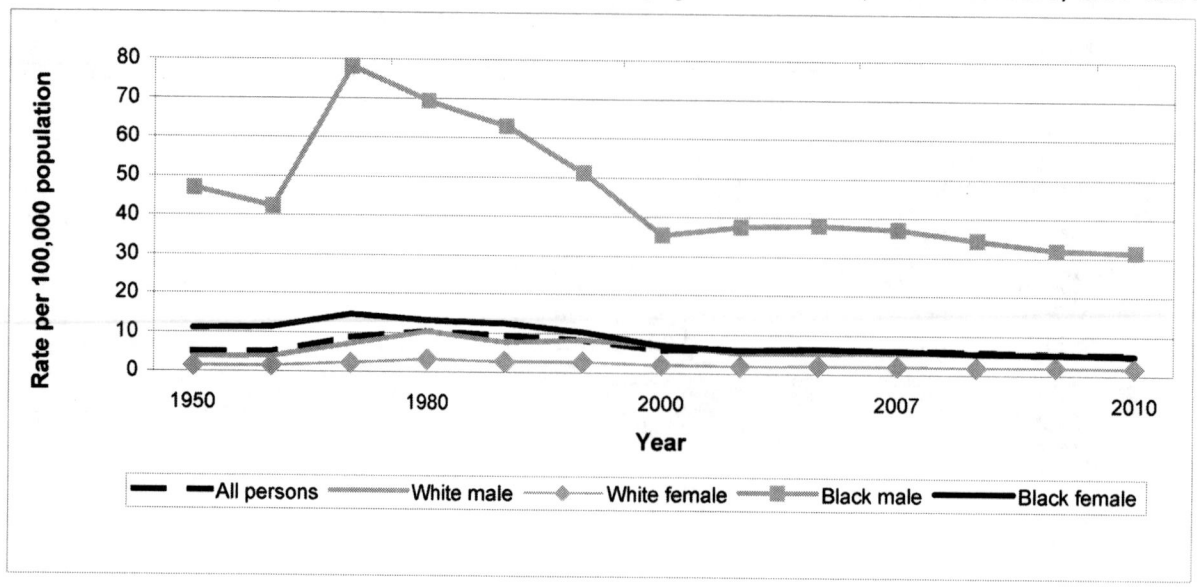

Figure 2-11. Age-Adjusted Death Rates for Suicide, by Race and Sex, Selected Years, 1950–2010

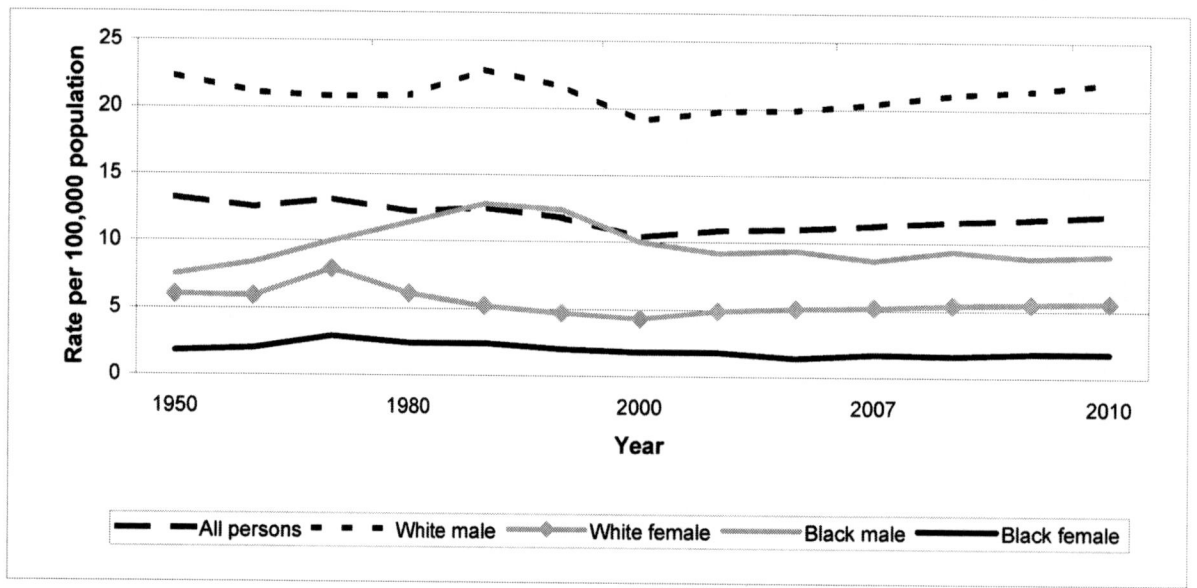

Table 2-42. Death Rates for Homicide, by Sex, Race, Hispanic Origin, and Age, Selected Years, 1950–2010

(Deaths per 100,000 resident population.)

Sex, race, Hispanic origin, and age	1950[1,2]	1960[1,2]	1970[2]	1980[2]	1985	1990[2]	1995	2000[3]	2005[3]	2006[3]	2007[3]	2008[3]	2009[3]	2010[3]
All Persons														
All ages, age-adjusted[4]	5.1	5.0	8.8	10.4	7.9	9.4	8.3	5.9	6.1	6.2	6.1	5.9	5.5	5.3
All ages, crude	5.0	4.6	8.1	10.6	8.2	9.9	8.5	6.0	6.1	6.2	6.1	5.9	5.5	5.3
Under 1 year	4.4	4.8	4.3	5.9	5.4	8.4	8.2	9.2	7.6	8.3	8.5	8.2	7.9	7.9
1 to 14 years	0.6	0.6	1.1	1.5	1.6	1.8	1.9	1.3	1.3	1.3	1.3	1.3	1.2	1.1
1 to 4 years	0.6	0.7	1.9	2.5	2.5	2.5	2.9	2.3	2.4	2.3	2.5	2.6	2.3	2.4
5 to 14 years	0.5	0.5	0.9	1.2	1.2	1.5	1.5	0.9	0.8	1.0	0.9	0.8	0.7	0.6
15 to 24 years	5.8	5.6	11.3	15.4	11.7	19.7	19.6	12.6	12.9	13.3	12.9	12.2	11.2	10.7
15 to 19 years	3.9	3.9	7.7	10.5	8.4	16.9	17.8	9.5	9.7	10.5	10.1	9.4	8.6	8.3
20 to 24 years	8.5	7.7	15.6	20.2	14.6	22.2	21.5	16.0	16.2	16.3	15.8	15.0	13.8	13.2
25 to 44 years	8.9	8.5	14.9	17.5	13.1	14.7	11.9	8.7	9.5	9.4	9.5	9.1	8.5	8.2
25 to 34 years	9.3	9.2	16.2	19.3	14.6	17.4	14.4	10.4	12.1	12.0	12.0	11.5	10.4	10.4
35 to 44 years	8.4	7.8	13.5	14.9	11.1	11.6	9.4	7.1	7.1	7.0	7.1	6.9	6.7	6.0
45 to 64 years	5.0	5.3	8.7	9.0	6.9	6.3	5.4	4.0	4.0	4.3	4.0	4.0	3.8	3.8
45 to 54 years	5.9	6.1	10.0	11.0	8.1	7.5	6.0	4.7	4.8	5.1	4.9	4.8	4.6	4.4
55 to 64 years	3.9	4.1	7.1	7.0	5.7	5.0	4.4	3.0	2.8	3.2	3.0	2.9	2.9	2.9
65 years and over	3.0	2.7	4.6	5.5	4.3	4.0	3.1	2.4	2.3	2.1	2.0	2.1	2.2	2.0
65 to 74 years	3.2	2.8	4.9	5.7	4.3	3.8	3.2	2.4	2.3	2.1	2.1	2.3	2.2	2.1
75 to 84 years	2.5	2.3	4.0	5.2	4.3	4.3	3.0	2.4	2.2	2.1	2.0	1.8	2.0	1.9
85 years and over	2.3	2.4	4.2	5.3	4.1	4.6	3.2	2.4	2.3	2.1	1.6	2.3	2.3	2.0
Male														
All ages, age-adjusted[4]	7.9	7.5	14.3	16.6	12.2	14.8	12.8	9.0	9.7	9.8	9.7	9.3	8.6	8.4
All ages, crude	7.7	6.8	13.1	17.1	12.8	15.9	13.4	9.3	9.9	10.0	9.8	9.5	8.7	8.4
Under 1 year	4.5	4.7	4.5	6.3	5.6	8.8	9.0	10.4	8.4	9.6	9.7	9.3	9.0	8.8
1 to 14 years	0.6	0.6	1.2	1.6	1.8	2.0	2.2	1.5	1.4	1.6	1.5	1.5	1.3	1.4
1 to 4 years	0.5	0.7	1.9	2.7	2.5	2.7	3.1	2.5	2.6	2.6	2.6	2.8	2.3	2.8
5 to 14 years	0.6	0.5	1.0	1.2	1.4	1.7	1.9	1.1	1.0	1.2	1.0	0.9	0.9	0.8
15 to 24 years	8.6	8.4	18.2	24.0	18.2	32.5	32.8	20.9	21.9	22.7	21.8	20.6	18.8	18.2
15 to 19 years	5.5	5.7	12.1	15.9	12.8	27.8	29.1	15.5	16.4	17.8	17.0	15.9	14.5	14.0
20 to 24 years	13.5	11.8	25.6	32.2	23.0	36.9	36.5	26.7	27.5	27.8	26.8	25.5	23.4	22.6
25 to 44 years	13.8	12.8	24.4	28.9	20.6	23.5	18.2	13.3	15.3	15.1	15.3	14.9	13.6	13.3
25 to 34 years	14.4	13.9	26.8	31.9	22.8	27.7	22.5	16.7	20.3	20.1	20.2	19.3	17.0	17.3
35 to 44 years	13.2	11.7	21.7	24.5	17.6	18.6	14.0	10.3	10.7	10.5	10.7	10.7	10.3	9.2
45 to 64 years	8.1	8.1	14.8	15.2	11.0	10.2	8.3	6.0	6.2	6.5	6.1	6.1	5.7	5.6
45 to 54 years	9.5	9.4	16.8	18.4	12.7	11.9	9.2	6.9	7.6	7.7	7.3	7.3	6.8	6.7
55 to 64 years	6.3	6.4	12.1	11.8	9.1	8.0	7.0	4.6	4.3	4.8	4.5	4.4	4.2	4.3
65 years and over	4.8	4.3	7.7	8.8	6.2	5.8	4.2	3.3	3.0	2.8	2.8	2.8	3.0	2.6
65 to 74 years	5.2	4.6	8.5	9.2	6.5	5.8	4.5	3.4	3.2	2.9	3.1	3.1	3.2	2.9
75 to 84 years	3.9	3.7	5.9	8.1	5.7	5.7	3.7	3.2	2.6	2.6	2.8	2.4	2.6	2.1
85 years and over	2.5	3.6	7.4	7.5	5.0	6.7	4.1	3.3	3.0	2.5	1.6	2.5	3.1	2.2
Female														
All ages, age-adjusted[4]	2.4	2.6	3.7	4.4	3.8	4.0	3.7	2.8	2.5	2.6	2.5	2.4	2.4	2.3
All ages, crude	2.4	2.4	3.4	4.5	3.9	4.2	3.8	2.8	2.5	2.5	2.5	2.4	2.4	2.2
Under 1 year	4.2	4.9	4.1	5.6	5.2	8.0	7.4	7.9	6.8	6.9	7.2	7.1	6.8	6.9
1 to 14 years	0.6	0.5	1.0	1.4	1.4	1.6	1.5	1.1	1.1	1.1	1.2	1.1	1.1	0.9
1 to 4 years	0.7	0.7	1.9	2.2	2.4	2.3	2.6	2.1	2.1	2.0	2.4	2.4	2.4	1.9
5 to 14 years	0.5	0.4	0.7	1.1	1.0	1.2	1.0	0.7	0.7	0.7	0.7	0.6	0.5	0.5
15 to 24 years	3.0	2.8	4.6	6.6	5.1	6.2	5.9	3.9	3.4	3.5	3.4	3.3	3.1	2.9
15 to 19 years	2.4	1.9	3.2	4.9	3.9	5.4	5.8	3.1	2.5	2.8	2.7	2.6	2.5	2.3
20 to 24 years	3.7	3.8	6.2	8.2	6.1	7.0	6.0	4.7	4.3	4.2	4.2	4.0	3.7	3.4
25 to 44 years	4.2	4.3	5.8	6.4	5.7	6.0	5.6	4.0	3.7	3.6	3.6	3.3	3.4	3.1
25 to 34 years	4.5	4.6	6.0	6.9	6.4	7.1	6.3	4.1	3.8	3.8	3.7	3.6	3.7	3.3
35 to 44 years	3.8	4.0	5.7	5.7	4.9	4.8	4.9	4.0	3.6	3.5	3.5	3.1	3.1	2.9
45 to 64 years	1.9	2.5	3.1	3.4	3.2	2.8	2.6	2.1	1.9	2.2	2.1	2.0	2.1	2.0
45 to 54 years	2.3	2.9	3.7	4.1	3.7	3.2	2.9	2.5	2.2	2.6	2.5	2.4	2.4	2.3
55 to 64 years	1.4	2.0	2.5	2.8	2.7	2.3	2.1	1.6	1.4	1.7	1.5	1.5	1.6	1.7
65 years and over	1.4	1.3	2.3	3.3	3.0	2.8	2.4	1.8	1.7	1.6	1.4	1.6	1.6	1.6
65 to 74 years	1.3	1.3	2.2	3.0	2.6	2.2	2.1	1.6	1.5	1.3	1.2	1.6	1.5	1.4
75 to 84 years	1.4	1.3	2.7	3.5	3.4	3.4	2.6	2.0	1.9	1.8	1.5	1.3	1.5	1.8
85 years and over	2.1	1.6	2.5	4.3	3.8	3.8	2.9	2.0	2.0	1.9	1.6	2.3	2.0	2.0
White Male [5]														
All ages, age-adjusted[4]	3.8	3.9	7.2	10.4	7.7	8.3	7.3	5.2	5.4	5.5	5.5	5.5	4.9	4.7
All ages, crude	3.6	3.6	6.6	10.7	8.1	8.8	7.5	5.2	5.5	5.5	5.5	5.5	4.9	4.7
Under 1 year	4.3	3.8	2.9	4.3	3.8	6.4	7.1	8.2	6.9	7.6	8.1	7.7	7.1	8.5
1 to 14 years	0.4	0.5	0.7	1.2	1.3	1.3	1.5	1.2	1.0	1.1	1.0	1.1	1.0	1.0
15 to 24 years	3.2	5.0	7.6	15.1	10.7	15.2	15.9	9.9	10.6	10.7	10.5	10.2	9.1	8.2
25 to 44 years	5.4	5.5	11.6	17.2	12.7	13.0	10.4	7.4	8.2	8.0	8.4	8.3	7.3	6.9
25 to 34 years	4.9	5.7	12.5	18.5	13.7	14.7	12.1	8.4	10.2	9.8	10.4	9.9	8.3	8.3
35 to 44 years	6.1	5.2	10.8	15.2	11.3	11.1	8.7	6.5	6.5	6.5	6.5	6.9	6.3	5.5
45 to 64 years	4.8	4.6	8.3	9.8	7.4	6.9	5.5	4.1	4.3	4.4	4.2	4.4	4.1	4.1
65 years and over	3.8	3.1	5.4	6.7	4.4	4.1	2.9	2.5	2.2	2.1	2.2	2.3	2.5	2.1
Black or African American Male [5]														
All ages, age-adjusted[4]	47.0	42.3	78.2	69.4	48.4	63.1	51.1	35.4	37.6	38.0	37.1	34.4	32.0	31.5
All ages, crude	44.7	35.0	66.0	65.7	48.3	68.5	54.5	37.2	39.6	40.4	39.3	36.5	33.8	33.4
Under 1 year	NA	10.3	14.3	18.6	16.7	21.4	20.3	23.3	16.4	21.4	19.8	17.5	18.7	12.3
1 to 14 years[6]	1.8	1.5	4.4	4.1	4.2	5.8	5.8	3.1	3.9	4.0	3.9	3.7	3.2	3.4
15 to 24 years	53.8	43.2	98.3	82.6	64.8	137.1	129.4	85.3	83.5	87.3	83.9	76.7	70.7	71.0
25 to 44 years	92.8	80.5	140.2	130.0	86.1	105.4	75.8	55.8	64.6	64.2	63.3	60.1	56.4	55.9
25 to 34 years	104.3	86.4	154.5	142.9	94.0	123.7	95.1	73.9	89.8	89.9	86.2	82.2	74.1	76.1
35 to 44 years	80.0	74.4	124.0	109.3	74.0	81.2	54.9	38.5	40.5	39.5	40.7	38.0	38.0	34.5

Table 2-42. Death Rates for Homicide, by Sex, Race, Hispanic Origin, and Age, Selected Years, 1950–2010—*Continued*

(Deaths per 100,000 resident population.)

Sex, race, Hispanic origin, and age	1950[1,2]	1960[1,2]	1970[2]	1980[2]	1985	1990[2]	1995	2000[3]	2005[3]	2006[3]	2007[3]	2008[3]	2009[3]	2010[3]
45 to 64 years	46.0	44.6	82.3	70.6	46.0	41.4	33.4	21.9	21.6	22.5	21.5	19.9	18.0	17.6
65 years and over	16.5	17.3	33.3	30.9	26.1	25.7	20.3	12.8	11.8	9.9	10.6	8.4	8.8	8.0
American Indian or Alaska Native Male [5]														
All ages, age-adjusted[4]	NA	NA	NA	23.3	19.1	16.7	14.4	10.7	10.1	10.5	7.9	9.2	8.9	8.8
All ages, crude	NA	NA	NA	23.1	18.4	16.6	15.7	10.7	10.9	11.2	8.5	9.6	9.3	9.5
15 to 24 years	NA	NA	NA	35.4	27.1	25.1	28.0	17.0	19.3	19.2	12.2	13.2	15.8	17.6
25 to 44 years	NA	NA	NA	39.2	28.2	25.7	24.6	17.0	14.7	16.1	15.0	16.1	15.0	14.8
45 to 64 years	NA	NA	NA	22.1	21.2	14.8	12.0	*	10.0	8.4	5.8	7.8	7.5	6.5
Asian or Pacific Islander Male [5]														
All ages, age-adjusted[4]	NA	NA	NA	9.1	5.5	7.3	7.2	4.3	4.3	4.2	3.1	2.9	2.8	2.6
All ages, crude	NA	NA	NA	8.3	5.7	7.9	7.5	4.4	4.5	4.4	3.3	3.1	3.0	2.7
15 to 24 years	NA	NA	NA	9.3	8.0	14.9	17.2	7.8	9.7	10.2	6.3	5.9	4.4	4.0
25 to 44 years	NA	NA	NA	11.3	8.6	9.6	7.4	4.6	4.9	4.1	3.9	3.5	3.2	3.3
45 to 64 years	NA	NA	NA	10.4	5.2	7.0	7.7	6.1	4.1	4.7	3.3	2.8	3.7	3.1
Hispanic or Latino Male [4,6]														
All ages, age-adjusted[4]	NA	NA	NA	NA	24.9	27.4	20.4	11.8	12.1	11.7	11.1	10.3	9.7	8.7
All ages, crude	NA	NA	NA	NA	27.2	31.0	23.5	13.4	13.7	13.2	12.4	11.4	10.5	9.5
Under 1 year	NA	NA	NA	NA	*	8.7	5.9	6.6	6.0	9.7	8.1	7.4	5.7	7.0
1 to 14 years	NA	NA	NA	NA	1.5	3.1	3.2	1.7	1.5	1.6	1.2	1.2	1.2	1.1
15 to 24 years	NA	NA	NA	NA	42.1	55.4	54.7	28.5	29.0	28.7	27.1	24.5	22.9	19.7
25 to 44 years	NA	NA	NA	NA	46.7	46.4	28.8	17.2	19.0	17.6	16.9	15.8	14.2	13.2
25 to 34 years	NA	NA	NA	NA	50.6	50.9	33.0	19.9	23.7	21.3	21.3	18.8	16.5	16.8
35 to 44 years	NA	NA	NA	NA	39.8	39.3	22.8	13.5	13.2	13.1	11.7	12.3	11.5	8.9
45 to 64 years	NA	NA	NA	NA	19.6	20.5	14.7	9.1	8.3	8.4	7.7	7.5	6.9	6.9
65 years and over	NA	NA	NA	NA	8.9	9.4	5.8	4.4	4.6	3.3	3.9	3.1	4.9	3.2
White, not Hispanic or Latino Male [6]														
All ages, age-adjusted[4]	NA	NA	NA	NA	6.1	5.6	4.8	3.6	3.6	3.6	3.8	3.9	3.4	3.3
All ages, crude	NA	NA	NA	NA	6.2	5.8	4.9	3.6	3.6	3.7	3.7	3.9	3.4	3.3
Under 1 year	NA	NA	NA	NA	4.6	5.4	6.8	8.3	7.3	6.8	7.6	7.4	7.3	8.7
1 to 14 years	NA	NA	NA	NA	1.2	0.9	1.1	1.0	0.8	0.9	0.9	1.0	0.8	0.9
15 to 24 years	NA	NA	NA	NA	7.6	7.5	7.2	4.7	4.8	4.8	5.0	5.2	4.1	4.1
25 to 44 years	NA	NA	NA	NA	9.2	8.7	7.2	5.2	5.2	5.2	5.7	5.9	4.9	4.7
25 to 34 years	NA	NA	NA	NA	9.3	9.3	7.7	5.2	5.6	5.6	6.4	6.6	5.2	5.0
35 to 44 years	NA	NA	NA	NA	9.1	8.0	6.7	5.2	4.9	4.9	5.1	5.3	4.7	4.4
45 to 64 years	NA	NA	NA	NA	6.3	5.7	4.6	3.6	3.8	3.9	3.7	3.9	3.7	3.6
65 years and over	NA	NA	NA	NA	4.4	3.7	2.6	2.3	2.1	2.1	2.0	2.2	2.3	2.0
White Female [4]														
All ages, age-adjusted[4]	1.4	1.5	2.3	3.2	2.9	2.7	2.7	2.1	1.9	2.0	2.0	1.9	1.9	1.8
All ages, crude	1.4	1.4	2.1	3.2	2.9	2.8	2.7	2.1	1.9	1.9	1.9	1.9	1.9	1.8
Under 1 year	3.9	3.5	2.9	4.3	4.3	5.1	5.1	5.0	5.7	6.6	6.4	5.6	5.1	5.8
1 to 14 years	0.4	0.4	0.7	1.1	1.1	1.0	1.1	0.8	0.8	0.8	0.9	0.8	0.9	0.7
15 to 24 years	1.3	1.5	2.7	4.7	3.6	4.0	4.0	2.7	2.3	2.4	2.5	2.2	2.1	2.0
25 to 44 years	2.0	2.1	3.3	4.2	4.1	3.8	3.7	2.9	2.8	2.5	2.8	2.7	2.7	2.4
45 to 64 years	1.5	1.7	2.1	2.6	2.6	2.3	2.2	1.8	1.5	1.8	1.7	1.8	1.8	1.7
65 years and over	1.2	1.2	1.9	2.9	2.6	2.2	2.0	1.6	1.6	1.5	1.3	1.5	1.5	1.6
Black or African American Female [4]														
All ages, age-adjusted[4]	11.1	11.4	14.7	13.2	10.6	12.5	10.4	7.1	6.0	6.4	6.0	5.4	5.2	5.0
All ages, crude	11.5	10.4	13.2	13.5	11.0	13.4	10.9	7.2	6.1	6.5	6.1	5.5	5.3	5.1
Under 1 year	NA	13.8	10.7	12.8	10.7	22.8	20.1	22.2	12.9	11.3	11.7	15.4	15.4	13.9
1 to 14 years[6]	1.8	1.2	3.1	3.3	3.3	4.7	3.4	2.7	2.3	2.5	2.7	2.5	2.2	2.0
15 to 24 years	16.5	11.9	17.7	18.4	14.2	18.9	16.4	10.7	8.7	9.3	8.6	9.3	8.0	7.5
25 to 44 years	22.5	22.7	25.3	22.6	17.8	21.0	17.1	11.0	9.3	10.1	9.1	7.6	7.8	7.4
45 to 64 years	6.8	10.3	13.4	10.8	7.9	6.5	5.9	4.5	4.8	5.1	4.8	3.7	4.0	4.2
65 years and over	3.6	3.0	7.4	8.0	7.8	9.4	6.8	3.5	3.0	2.5	2.6	2.3	2.2	1.8
American Indian or Alaska Native Female [4]														
All ages, age-adjusted[4]	NA	NA	NA	8.1	4.8	4.6	5.3	3.0	3.5	2.6	3.1	3.1	2.9	2.5
All ages, crude	NA	NA	NA	7.7	4.5	4.8	5.1	2.9	3.6	2.6	3.0	3.2	3.0	2.5
15 to 24 years	NA	NA	NA	*	*	*	*	*	*	*	*	*	*	*
25 to 44 years	NA	NA	NA	13.7	*	6.9	8.3	5.9	5.4	5.2	4.4	3.9	*	4.7
45 to 64 years	NA	NA	NA	*	*	*	*	*	*	*	*	*	*	*
Asian or Pacific Islander Female [5]														
All ages, age-adjusted[4]	NA	NA	NA	3.1	2.6	2.8	2.4	1.7	1.5	1.3	1.3	1.2	1.3	1.2
All ages, crude	NA	NA	NA	3.1	2.8	2.8	2.6	1.7	1.5	1.4	1.3	1.2	1.3	1.2
15 to 24 years	NA	NA	NA	*	*	*	*	*	2.5	*	*	*	*	*
25 to 44 years	NA	NA	NA	4.6	2.9	3.8	3.6	2.2	1.6	1.6	1.8	1.3	1.5	1.3
45 to 64 years	NA	NA	NA	*	*	*	2.2	2.0	1.2	1.9	1.5	1.1	1.6	1.4

Table 2-42. Death Rates for Homicide, by Sex, Race, Hispanic Origin, and Age, Selected Years, 1950–2010—Continued

(Deaths per 100,000 resident population.)

Sex, race, Hispanic origin, and age	1950[1,2]	1960[1,2]	1970[2]	1980[2]	1985	1990[2]	1995	2000[3]	2005[3]	2006[3]	2007[3]	2008[3]	2009[3]	2010[3]
Hispanic or Latina Female[5,7]														
All ages, age-adjusted[4]	NA	NA	NA	NA	4.1	4.3	4.0	2.8	2.3	2.3	2.2	2.3	2.2	1.8
All ages, crude	NA	NA	NA	NA	4.3	4.7	4.2	2.8	2.4	2.4	2.4	2.4	2.2	1.8
Under 1 year	NA	NA	NA	NA	*	*	*	7.4	6.2	6.2	7.1	5.4	6.1	6.6
1 to 14 years	NA	NA	NA	NA	1.5	1.9	1.8	1.0	1.0	1.0	1.2	1.1	1.1	0.5
15 to 24 years	NA	NA	NA	NA	5.7	8.1	6.4	3.7	3.4	3.6	3.2	3.3	3.0	2.6
25 to 44 years	NA	NA	NA	NA	6.8	6.1	5.6	3.7	3.3	3.1	3.2	3.1	2.9	2.5
45 to 64 years	NA	NA	NA	NA	3.2	3.3	3.4	2.9	1.9	1.8	1.7	2.0	2.0	1.6
65 years and over	NA	NA	NA	NA	*	*	2.4	2.4	*	*	*	1.6	1.3	1.3
White, not Hispanic or Latina Female														
All ages, age-adjusted[4]	NA	NA	NA	NA	2.9	2.5	2.3	1.9	1.8	1.8	1.9	1.8	1.8	1.8
All ages, crude	NA	NA	NA	NA	2.9	2.5	2.3	1.9	1.8	1.8	1.8	1.8	1.8	1.7
Under 1 year	NA	NA	NA	NA	4.1	4.4	4.4	4.1	5.3	6.5	5.9	5.7	4.2	5.3
1 to 14 years	NA	NA	NA	NA	1.0	0.8	0.9	0.8	0.7	0.8	0.8	0.7	0.8	0.7
15 to 24 years	NA	NA	NA	NA	3.5	3.3	3.4	2.3	2.0	2.1	2.2	1.8	1.7	1.8
25 to 44 years	NA	NA	NA	NA	3.9	3.5	3.3	2.7	2.7	2.3	2.6	2.5	2.5	2.4
45 to 64 years	NA	NA	NA	NA	3.6	2.2	1.9	1.6	1.4	1.8	1.7	1.7	1.7	1.7
65 years and over	NA	NA	NA	NA	2.6	2.2	1.9	1.6	1.6	1.5	1.3	1.5	1.5	1.6

NA = Not available.   * = Rates based on fewer than 20 deaths are considered unreliable and are not shown.   [1]Includes deaths of persons who were not residents of the 50 states and the District of Columbia.   [2]Underlying cause of death was coded according to the 6th Revision of the International Classification of Diseases (ICD) in 1950, 7th Revision in 1960, 8th Revision in 1970, and 9th Revision in 1980-1998.   [3]Starting with 1999 data, cause of death is coded according to ICD-10.   [4]Age-adjusted rates are calculated using the year 2000 standard population. Prior to 2001, age-adjusted rates were calculated using standard million proportions based on rounded population numbers. Starting with 2001 data, unrounded population numbers are used to calculate age-adjusted rates.   [5]The race groups, White, Black, Asian or Pacific Islander, and American Indian or Alaska Native, include persons of Hispanic and non-Hispanic origin. Persons of Hispanic origin may be of any race. Death rates for the American Indian or Alaska Native, Asian or Pacific Islander, and Hispanic populations are known to be underestimated.   [6]In 1950, rate is for the age group under 15 years.   [7]Prior to 1997, excludes data from states lacking an Hispanic-origin item on the death certificate.

Table 2-43. Death Rates for Suicide, by Sex, Race, Hispanic Origin, and Age, Selected Years, 1950–2010

(Deaths per 100,000 resident population.)

Sex, race, Hispanic origin, and age	1950[1,2]	1960[1,2]	1970[2]	1980[2]	1985	1990[2]	1995	2000[3]	2005[3]	2006[3]	2007[3]	2008[3]	2009[3]	2010[3]
All Persons														
All ages, age-adjusted[4]	13.2	12.5	13.1	12.2	12.5	12.5	11.8	10.4	10.9	11.0	11.3	11.6	11.8	12.1
All ages, crude	11.4	10.6	11.6	11.9	12.4	12.4	11.7	10.4	11.0	11.2	11.5	11.8	12.0	12.4
Under 1 year	X	X	X	X	X	X	X	X	X	X	X	X	X	X
1 to 4 years	X	X	X	X	X	X	X	X	X	X	X	X	X	X
5 to 14 years	0.2	0.3	0.3	0.4	0.8	0.8	0.9	0.7	0.7	0.5	0.5	0.5	0.6	0.7
15 to 24 years	4.5	5.2	8.8	12.3	12.8	13.2	13.0	10.2	9.9	9.8	9.6	9.9	10.0	10.5
15 to 19 years	2.7	3.6	5.9	8.5	9.9	11.1	10.3	8.0	7.5	7.1	6.7	7.2	7.5	7.5
20 to 24 years	6.2	7.1	12.2	16.1	15.4	15.1	15.8	12.5	12.4	12.5	12.6	12.7	12.6	13.6
25 to 44 years	11.6	12.2	15.4	15.6	15.0	15.2	15.1	13.4	13.9	14.0	14.5	14.6	14.6	15.0
25 to 34 years	9.1	10.0	14.1	16.0	15.3	15.2	15.0	12.0	12.7	12.7	13.3	13.2	13.1	14.0
35 to 44 years	14.3	14.2	16.9	15.4	14.6	15.3	15.1	14.5	15.1	15.2	15.7	15.9	16.1	16.0
45 to 64 years	23.5	22.0	20.6	15.9	16.3	15.3	13.9	13.5	15.3	16.0	16.7	17.5	17.9	18.6
45 to 54 years	20.9	20.7	20.0	15.9	15.7	14.8	14.4	14.4	16.5	17.2	17.7	18.6	19.2	19.6
55 to 64 years	26.8	23.7	21.4	15.9	16.8	16.0	13.2	12.1	13.7	14.4	15.3	16.0	16.4	17.5
65 years and over	30.0	24.5	20.8	17.6	20.4	20.5	17.9	15.2	14.7	14.3	14.3	14.8	14.8	14.9
65 to 74 years	29.6	23.0	20.8	16.9	18.7	17.9	15.7	12.5	12.4	12.4	12.4	13.6	13.7	13.7
75 to 84 years	31.1	27.9	21.2	19.1	23.9	24.9	20.6	17.6	16.8	15.8	16.2	16.1	15.8	15.7
85 years and over	28.8	26.0	19.0	19.2	19.4	22.2	21.3	19.6	18.3	17.3	17.0	16.4	16.4	17.6
Male														
All ages, age-adjusted[4]	21.2	20.0	19.8	19.9	21.1	21.5	20.3	17.7	18.1	18.1	18.5	19.0	19.2	19.8
All ages, crude	17.8	16.5	16.8	18.6	20.0	20.4	19.5	17.1	17.8	17.9	18.4	19.0	19.3	19.9
Under 1 year	X	X	X	X	X	X	X	X	X	X	X	X	X	X
1 to 4 years	X	X	X	X	X	X	X	X	X	X	X	X	X	X
5 to 14 years	0.3	0.4	0.5	0.6	1.2	1.1	1.3	1.2	1.0	0.7	0.6	0.7	0.8	0.9
15 to 24 years	6.5	8.2	13.5	20.2	21.0	22.0	22.0	17.1	16.1	16.0	15.7	16.0	16.1	16.9
15 to 19 years	3.5	5.6	8.8	13.8	15.8	18.1	17.1	13.0	11.8	11.3	10.8	11.3	11.6	11.7
20 to 24 years	9.3	11.5	19.3	26.8	25.7	25.7	27.0	21.4	20.4	21.0	20.9	21.0	20.8	22.2
25 to 44 years	17.2	17.9	20.9	24.0	23.7	24.4	24.4	21.3	22.1	22.1	22.9	22.8	23.0	23.6
25 to 34 years	13.4	14.7	19.8	25.0	24.7	24.8	24.8	19.6	20.6	20.5	21.5	21.2	21.0	22.5
35 to 44 years	21.3	21.0	22.1	22.5	22.3	23.9	24.0	22.8	23.4	23.5	24.2	24.4	24.9	24.6
45 to 64 years	37.1	34.4	30.0	23.7	25.3	24.3	22.2	21.3	23.9	24.6	25.7	27.4	27.9	29.2
45 to 54 years	32.0	31.6	27.9	22.9	23.6	23.2	22.5	22.4	25.2	26.2	27.0	28.6	29.3	30.4
55 to 64 years	43.6	38.1	32.7	24.5	27.1	25.7	21.8	19.4	22.0	22.5	23.9	25.8	26.1	27.7
65 years and over	52.8	44.0	38.4	35.0	40.9	41.6	36.2	31.1	29.5	28.4	28.4	29.2	29.1	29.0
65 to 74 years	50.5	39.6	36.0	30.4	33.9	32.2	28.5	22.7	22.3	22.2	22.0	24.3	24.3	23.9
75 to 84 years	58.3	52.5	42.8	42.3	53.1	56.1	44.9	38.6	35.5	32.9	33.8	33.5	32.9	32.3
85 years and over	58.3	57.4	42.4	50.6	56.2	65.9	62.7	57.5	49.9	48.0	46.6	43.0	44.0	47.3
Female														
All ages, age-adjusted[4]	5.6	5.6	7.4	5.7	5.2	4.8	4.3	4.0	4.4	4.5	4.6	4.8	4.9	5.0
All ages, crude	5.1	4.9	6.6	5.5	5.2	4.8	4.3	4.0	4.5	4.6	4.8	4.9	5.0	5.2
Under 1 year	X	X	X	X	X	X	X	X	X	X	X	X	X	X
1 to 4 years	X	X	X	X	X	X	X	X	X	X	X	X	X	X
5 to 14 years	0.1	0.1	0.2	0.2	0.4	0.4	0.4	0.3	0.3	0.3	0.3	0.3	0.5	0.4
15 to 24 years	2.6	2.2	4.2	4.3	4.3	3.9	3.6	3.0	3.5	3.2	3.1	3.5	3.6	3.9
15 to 19 years	1.8	1.6	2.9	3.0	3.7	3.7	3.1	2.7	3.0	2.8	2.4	3.0	3.2	3.1
20 to 24 years	3.3	2.9	5.7	5.5	4.9	4.1	4.2	3.2	4.0	3.6	3.9	4.0	4.1	4.7
25 to 44 years	6.2	6.6	10.2	7.7	6.5	6.2	5.8	5.4	5.8	5.9	6.2	6.3	6.2	6.4
25 to 34 years	4.9	5.5	8.6	7.1	5.9	5.6	5.1	4.3	4.7	4.7	5.0	5.1	5.1	5.3
35 to 44 years	7.5	7.7	11.9	8.5	7.1	6.8	6.4	6.4	6.8	7.0	7.3	7.4	7.4	7.5
45 to 64 years	9.9	10.2	12.0	8.9	8.0	7.1	6.1	6.2	7.2	7.7	8.1	8.1	8.5	8.6
45 to 54 years	9.9	10.2	12.6	9.4	8.3	6.9	6.6	6.7	8.0	8.4	8.7	9.0	9.3	9.0
55 to 64 years	9.9	10.2	11.4	8.4	7.8	7.3	5.3	5.4	6.0	6.8	7.2	6.9	7.4	8.0
65 years and over	9.4	8.4	8.1	6.1	6.6	6.4	5.4	4.0	4.0	3.9	3.9	4.1	4.0	4.2
65 to 74 years	10.1	8.4	9.0	6.5	6.9	6.7	5.4	4.0	4.0	4.0	4.2	4.4	4.6	4.8
75 to 84 years	8.1	8.9	7.0	5.5	6.7	6.3	5.4	4.0	4.0	4.0	3.8	3.8	3.6	3.7
85 years and over	8.2	6.0	5.9	5.5	4.7	5.4	5.4	4.2	4.3	3.3	3.4	3.8	3.2	3.3
White Male [5]														
All ages, age-adjusted[4]	22.3	21.1	20.8	20.9	22.4	22.8	21.6	19.1	19.8	19.9	20.4	21.1	21.4	22.0
All ages, crude	19.0	17.6	18.0	19.9	21.6	22.0	21.1	18.8	19.9	20.0	20.7	21.5	21.9	22.6
15 to 24 years	6.6	8.6	13.9	21.4	22.3	23.2	23.1	17.9	17.3	17.2	16.9	17.2	17.6	18.3
25 to 44 years	17.9	18.5	21.5	24.6	24.8	25.4	25.8	22.9	24.2	24.2	25.3	25.4	25.7	26.2
45 to 64 years	39.3	36.5	31.9	25.0	27.0	26.0	23.9	23.2	26.6	27.5	28.8	30.8	31.4	33.0
65 years and over	55.8	46.7	41.1	37.2	43.7	44.2	38.5	33.3	32.0	30.8	30.9	31.6	31.5	31.7
65 to 74 years	53.2	42.0	38.7	32.5	35.8	34.2	30.1	24.3	24.5	24.3	24.1	26.3	26.6	26.3
75 to 84 years	61.9	55.7	45.5	45.5	57.0	60.2	47.7	41.1	38.0	35.4	36.2	36.1	35.3	34.9
85 years and over	61.9	61.3	45.8	52.8	60.9	70.3	67.9	61.6	53.1	50.8	50.1	45.8	46.9	50.8

Table 2-43. Death Rates for Suicide, by Sex, Race, Hispanic Origin, and Age, Selected Years, 1950–2010—*Continued*

(Deaths per 100,000 resident population.)

Sex, race, Hispanic origin, and age	1950[1,2]	1960[1,2]	1970[2]	1980[2]	1985	1990[2]	1995	2000[3]	2005[3]	2006[3]	2007[3]	2008[3]	2009[3]	2010[3]
Black or African American Male[5]														
All ages, age-adjusted[4]	7.5	8.4	10.0	11.4	11.8	12.8	12.4	10.0	9.2	9.4	8.7	9.4	8.9	9.1
All ages, crude	6.3	6.4	8.0	10.3	11.0	12.0	11.7	9.4	8.7	8.8	8.3	9.0	8.5	8.7
15 to 24 years	4.9	4.1	10.5	12.3	13.3	15.1	17.8	14.2	11.4	10.5	10.1	12.0	10.4	11.1
25 to 44 years	9.8	12.6	16.1	19.2	17.8	19.6	18.3	14.3	14.0	14.5	13.9	13.9	13.2	14.5
45 to 64 years	12.7	13.0	12.4	11.8	12.9	13.1	11.5	9.9	9.1	9.5	9.0	9.8	9.6	9.5
65 years and over	9.0	9.9	8.7	11.4	15.8	14.9	14.6	11.5	10.2	10.3	8.5	10.8	9.6	8.3
65 to 74 years	10.0	11.3	8.7	11.1	16.7	14.7	13.8	11.1	8.1	8.4	7.9	10.4	8.0	7.6
75 to 84 years[6]	*	*	*	10.5	15.6	14.4	16.7	12.1	12.9	11.6	11.2	11.8	11.9	9.9
85 years and over	NA	*	*	*	*	*	*	*	*	*	*	*	*	*
American Indian or Alaska Native Male[5]														
All ages, age-adjusted[4]	NA	NA	NA	19.3	17.9	20.1	17.4	16.0	17.3	16.5	15.9	15.4	14.6	15.5
All ages, crude	NA	NA	NA	20.9	20.3	20.9	18.0	15.9	17.6	16.8	16.2	15.4	15.1	16.1
15 to 24 years	NA	NA	NA	45.3	42.0	49.1	30.8	26.2	28.6	30.6	26.8	29.0	28.9	30.6
25 to 44 years	NA	NA	NA	31.2	30.2	27.8	29.1	24.5	27.0	23.3	24.9	22.7	20.4	20.9
45 to 64 years	NA	NA	NA	*	*	*	13.6	15.4	15.6	16.5	14.4	11.1	15.4	17.8
65 years and over	NA	NA	NA	*	*	*	*	*	*	*	*	*	*	*
Asian or Pacific Islander Male[5]														
All ages, age-adjusted[4]	NA	NA	NA	10.7	9.3	9.6	9.6	8.6	7.3	7.8	8.8	7.9	8.7	9.5
All ages, crude	NA	NA	NA	8.8	8.4	8.7	9.0	7.9	7.1	7.8	8.4	7.5	8.4	9.3
15 to 24 years	NA	NA	NA	10.8	14.2	13.5	14.4	9.1	6.5	10.6	11.4	7.1	8.0	10.9
25 to 44 years	NA	NA	NA	11.0	9.3	10.6	10.8	9.9	9.6	9.3	9.7	8.5	9.7	10.6
45 to 64 years	NA	NA	NA	13.0	10.4	9.7	8.7	9.7	8.9	9.7	10.6	10.9	12.1	12.8
65 years and over	NA	NA	NA	18.6	16.7	16.8	18.9	15.4	11.2	10.8	13.1	14.8	15.3	14.9
Hispanic or Latino Male[5,7]														
All ages, age-adjusted[4]	NA	NA	NA	NA	11.0	13.7	12.7	10.3	9.6	9.0	10.3	9.5	9.9	9.9
All ages, crude	NA	NA	NA	NA	9.8	11.4	10.9	8.4	8.4	8.0	8.8	8.0	8.5	8.5
15 to 24 years	NA	NA	NA	NA	13.8	14.7	16.0	10.9	11.3	10.7	10.4	9.5	10.7	10.7
25 to 44 years	NA	NA	NA	NA	14.8	16.2	14.5	11.2	11.8	11.5	12.5	11.2	11.4	11.2
45 to 64 years	NA	NA	NA	NA	12.3	16.1	14.2	12.0	10.8	10.4	13.1	11.6	12.6	12.9
65 years and over	NA	NA	NA	NA	14.7	23.4	21.0	19.5	14.7	12.7	16.6	16.7	16.0	15.7
White, not Hispanic or Latino Male[7]														
All ages, age-adjusted[4]	NA	NA	NA	NA	22.9	23.5	22.3	20.2	21.4	21.6	22.1	23.1	23.4	24.2
All ages, crude	NA	NA	NA	NA	22.3	23.1	22.2	20.4	22.1	22.4	23.1	24.3	24.7	25.7
15 to 24 years	NA	NA	NA	NA	22.6	24.4	24.0	19.5	18.8	18.8	18.6	19.2	19.4	20.4
25 to 44 years	NA	NA	NA	NA	25.1	26.4	27.1	25.1	27.1	27.4	28.6	29.1	29.5	30.3
45 to 64 years	NA	NA	NA	NA	27.3	26.8	24.5	24.0	28.2	29.3	30.5	33.0	33.6	35.4
65 years and over	NA	NA	NA	NA	46.4	45.4	39.0	33.9	33.0	31.9	31.8	32.5	32.5	32.7
White Female[5]														
All ages, age-adjusted[4]	6.0	5.9	7.9	6.1	5.7	5.2	4.7	4.3	4.9	5.1	5.2	5.4	5.5	5.6
All ages, crude	5.5	5.3	7.1	5.9	5.6	5.3	4.8	4.4	5.0	5.3	5.4	5.6	5.7	5.9
15 to 24 years	2.7	2.3	4.2	4.6	4.7	4.2	3.8	3.1	3.7	3.4	3.4	3.6	3.8	4.2
25 to 44 years	6.6	7.0	11.0	8.1	7.0	6.6	6.3	6.0	6.6	6.9	7.0	7.2	7.1	7.3
45 to 64 years	10.6	10.9	13.0	9.6	8.7	7.7	6.7	6.9	8.1	8.8	9.3	9.4	9.6	9.9
65 years and over	9.9	8.8	8.5	6.4	6.9	6.8	5.7	4.3	4.2	4.1	4.2	4.4	4.4	4.5
Black or African American Female[5]														
All ages, age-adjusted[4]	1.8	2.0	2.9	2.4	2.3	2.4	2.0	1.8	1.8	1.4	1.7	1.6	1.8	1.8
All ages, crude	1.5	1.6	2.6	2.2	2.1	2.3	2.0	1.7	1.8	1.4	1.7	1.6	1.8	1.8
15 to 24 years	1.8	*	3.8	2.3	2.0	2.3	2.2	2.2	1.7	1.7	1.6	2.4	2.1	2.0
25 to 44 years	2.3	3.0	4.8	4.3	3.2	3.8	3.3	2.6	2.8	2.0	2.7	2.5	2.7	2.8
45 to 64 years	2.7	3.1	2.9	2.5	2.8	2.9	2.0	2.1	2.4	1.9	2.2	1.6	2.5	2.1
65 years and over	*	*	2.6	*	2.7	1.9	2.1	1.3	1.5	*	*	1.2	1.0	*

Table 2-43. Death Rates for Suicide, by Sex, Race, Hispanic Origin, and Age, Selected Years, 1950–2010—*Continued*

(Deaths per 100,000 resident population.)

Sex, race, Hispanic origin, and age	1950[1,2]	1960[1,2]	1970[2]	1980[2]	1985	1990[2]	1995	2000[3]	2005[3]	2006[3]	2007[3]	2008[3]	2009[3]	2010[3]
American Indian or Alaska Native Female[5]														
All ages, age-adjusted[4]	NA	NA	NA	4.7	4.1	3.6	3.9	3.8	4.2	4.5	4.3	4.9	5.4	6.1
All ages, crude	NA	NA	NA	4.7	4.4	3.7	3.8	4.0	4.4	4.7	4.3	5.1	5.6	5.9
15 to 24 years	NA	NA	NA	*	*	*	*	*	9.1	7.9	6.7	8.6	11.1	10.4
25 to 44 years	NA	NA	NA	10.7	*	*	6.4	7.2	6.6	6.9	5.8	6.2	7.5	7.4
45 to 64 years	NA	NA	NA	*	*	*	*	*	*	*	*	6.5	5.9	6.2
65 years and over	NA	NA	NA	*	*	*	*	*	*	*	*	*	*	*
Asian or Pacific Islander Female[5]														
All ages, age-adjusted[4]	NA	NA	NA	5.5	5.0	4.1	4.1	2.8	3.2	3.3	3.4	3.5	3.5	3.4
All ages, crude	NA	NA	NA	4.7	4.3	3.4	3.7	2.7	3.1	3.2	3.4	3.5	3.5	3.4
15 to 24 years	NA	NA	NA	*	5.8	3.9	4.8	2.7	3.2	3.5	3.2	3.9	4.4	3.5
25 to 44 years	NA	NA	NA	5.4	4.2	3.8	3.6	3.3	3.3	3.2	4.3	4.5	3.9	4.1
45 to 64 years	NA	NA	NA	7.9	5.4	5.0	4.7	3.2	3.7	4.1	3.9	3.7	4.7	4.7
65 years and over	NA	NA	NA	*	13.6	8.5	8.6	5.2	6.9	7.0	5.3	5.8	4.8	4.3
Hispanic or Latina Female[5,7]														
All ages, age-adjusted[4]	NA	NA	NA	NA	1.9	2.3	2.0	1.7	1.8	1.8	1.8	1.8	2.0	2.1
All ages, crude	NA	NA	NA	NA	1.6	2.2	1.8	1.5	1.6	1.7	1.7	1.7	1.8	2.0
15 to 24 years	NA	NA	NA	NA	2.1	3.1	2.4	2.0	2.5	2.5	2.0	2.2	2.3	3.1
25 to 44 years	NA	NA	NA	NA	2.1	3.1	2.5	2.1	2.2	2.3	2.6	2.2	2.5	2.4
45 to 64 years	NA	NA	NA	NA	3.2	2.5	2.8	2.5	2.1	2.4	2.7	2.7	2.5	2.8
65 years and over	NA	NA	NA	NA	*	*	*	*	2.0	1.7	*	1.6	2.3	2.2
White, not Hispanic or Latina Female[7]														
All ages, age-adjusted[4]	NA	NA	NA	NA	6.1	5.4	4.9	4.7	5.3	5.6	5.8	6.0	6.1	6.2
All ages, crude	NA	NA	NA	NA	6.2	5.6	5.1	4.9	5.6	5.9	6.1	6.3	6.5	6.7
15 to 24 years	NA	NA	NA	NA	4.7	4.3	4.0	3.3	4.0	3.5	3.7	3.9	4.1	4.4
25 to 44 years	NA	NA	NA	NA	7.7	7.0	6.6	6.7	7.5	7.9	8.1	8.4	8.3	8.6
45 to 64 years	NA	NA	NA	NA	9.2	8.0	6.9	7.3	8.7	9.5	10.0	10.1	10.5	10.7
65 years and over	NA	NA	NA	NA	7.5	7.0	5.8	4.4	4.4	4.3	4.4	4.6	4.5	4.7

NA = Not available. X = Not applicable. * = Rates based on fewer than 20 deaths are considered unreliable and are not shown. [1]Includes deaths of persons who were not residents of the 50 states and the District of Columbia. [2]Underlying cause of death was coded according to the 6th Revision of the International Classification of Diseases (ICD) in 1950, 7th Revision in 1960, 8th Revision in 1970, and 9th Revision in 1980–1998. [3]Starting with 1999 data, cause of death is coded according to ICD-10. [4]Age-adjusted rates are calculated using the year 2000 standard population. Prior to 2001, age-adjusted rates were calculated using standard million proportions based on rounded population numbers. Starting with 2001 data, unrounded population numbers are used to calculate age-adjusted rates. [5]The race groups, White, Black, Asian or Pacific Islander, and American Indian or Alaska Native, include persons of Hispanic and non-Hispanic origin. Persons of Hispanic origin may be of any race. Death rates for the American Indian or Alaska Native, Asian or Pacific Islander, and Hispanic populations are known to be underestimated. [6]In 1950, rate is for the age group 75 years and over. [7]Prior to 1997, excludes data from states lacking an Hispanic-origin item on the death certificate.

Table 2-44. Death Rates for Firearm-Related Injuries, by Sex, Race, Hispanic Origin, and Age, Selected Years, 1970–2010

(Deaths per 100,000 resident population.)

Sex, race, Hispanic origin, and age	1970[1]	1980[1]	1985	1990[1]	1995[1]	2000[2]	2005[2]	2006[2]	2007[2]	2008[2]	2009[2]	2010[2]
All Persons												
All ages, age-adjusted[3]	14.3	14.8	13.1	14.6	13.4	10.2	10.3	10.3	10.3	10.3	10.1	10.1
All ages, crude	13.1	14.9	13.3	14.9	13.5	10.2	10.4	10.4	10.4	10.4	10.2	10.3
Under 1 year	*	*	*	*	*	*	*	*	*	*	*	*
1 to 14 years	1.6	1.4	1.4	1.5	1.6	0.7	0.7	0.7	0.7	0.6	0.6	0.6
1 to 4 years	1.0	0.7	0.7	0.6	0.6	0.3	0.4	0.4	0.4	0.5	0.4	0.4
5 to 14 years	1.7	1.6	1.8	1.9	1.9	0.9	0.8	0.9	0.8	0.7	0.7	0.7
15 to 24 years	15.5	20.6	17.2	25.8	26.7	16.8	16.1	16.7	16.0	15.4	14.4	14.2
15 to 19 years	11.4	14.7	13.3	23.3	24.1	12.9	12.2	12.9	12.1	11.7	11.1	10.6
20 to 24 years	20.3	26.4	20.6	28.1	29.2	20.9	20.0	20.7	20.1	19.3	18.0	17.9
25 to 44 years	20.9	22.5	17.9	19.3	16.9	13.1	13.8	13.6	13.8	13.5	13.2	13.3
25 to 34 years	22.2	24.3	19.3	21.8	19.6	14.5	16.1	15.7	15.9	15.4	14.5	15.0
35 to 44 years	19.6	20.0	16.0	16.3	14.3	11.9	11.7	11.6	12.0	11.8	11.9	11.7
45 to 64 years	17.6	15.2	14.3	13.6	11.7	10.0	10.6	10.6	10.6	11.2	11.4	11.6
45 to 54 years	18.1	16.4	14.7	13.9	12.0	10.5	11.2	11.2	11.1	11.5	11.8	12.0
55 to 64 years	17.0	13.9	13.9	13.3	11.3	9.4	9.7	9.7	10.1	10.8	10.8	11.1
65 years and over	13.8	13.5	15.6	16.0	14.1	12.2	11.8	11.3	11.3	11.8	11.9	11.7
65 to 74 years	14.5	13.8	15.1	14.4	12.8	10.6	10.2	9.9	9.8	10.7	10.9	10.7
75 to 84 years	13.4	13.4	17.7	19.4	16.3	13.9	13.6	12.9	13.1	13.2	13.3	12.7
85 years and over	10.2	11.6	12.2	14.7	14.4	14.2	13.0	12.5	12.7	12.5	12.5	13.2
Male												
All ages, age-adjusted[3]	24.8	25.9	23.1	26.1	23.8	18.1	18.5	18.2	18.3	18.3	17.8	17.9
All ages, crude	22.2	25.7	22.8	26.2	23.6	17.8	18.4	18.2	18.3	18.3	17.9	18.0
Under 1 year	*	*	*	*	*	*	*	*	*	*	*	*
1 to 14 years	2.3	2.0	2.1	2.2	2.3	1.1	1.0	1.0	1.0	0.9	0.9	1.0
1 to 4 years	1.2	0.9	0.8	0.7	0.8	0.4	0.5	0.5	0.5	0.6	0.5	0.6
5 to 14 years	2.7	2.5	2.7	2.9	2.9	1.4	1.2	1.2	1.1	1.0	1.0	1.1
15 to 24 years	26.4	34.8	29.1	44.7	46.5	29.4	28.5	29.5	28.2	27.0	25.3	25.0
15 to 19 years	19.2	24.5	22.4	40.1	41.6	22.4	21.5	22.7	21.2	20.4	19.3	18.4
20 to 24 years	35.1	45.2	35.0	49.1	51.5	37.0	35.7	36.6	35.5	34.0	31.6	31.8
25 to 44 years	34.1	38.1	29.7	32.6	28.4	22.0	23.7	23.2	23.8	23.3	22.4	22.9
25 to 34 years	36.5	41.4	32.1	37.0	33.2	24.9	28.2	27.6	28.0	27.1	25.0	26.4
35 to 44 years	31.6	33.2	26.6	27.4	23.6	19.4	19.5	19.2	19.8	19.6	19.9	19.3
45 to 64 years	31.0	25.9	24.5	23.4	20.0	17.1	18.2	17.8	18.2	19.2	19.3	19.9
45 to 54 years	30.7	27.3	24.4	23.2	20.1	17.6	18.9	18.6	18.6	19.4	19.6	20.3
55 to 64 years	31.3	24.5	24.6	23.7	19.8	16.3	17.2	16.8	17.7	19.0	19.1	19.3
65 years and over	29.7	29.7	34.2	35.3	30.7	26.4	25.1	24.0	24.0	24.7	24.8	24.1
65 to 74 years	29.5	27.8	30.0	28.2	25.1	20.3	19.3	18.8	18.7	20.3	20.6	20.0
75 to 84 years	31.0	33.0	42.7	46.9	37.8	32.2	30.5	28.8	29.0	29.0	28.8	27.5
85 years and over	26.2	34.9	38.2	49.3	47.1	44.7	39.3	37.3	37.4	35.5	35.7	37.4
Female												
All ages, age-adjusted[3]	4.8	4.7	4.2	4.2	3.8	2.8	2.7	2.7	2.7	2.7	2.8	2.7
All ages, crude	4.4	4.7	4.2	4.3	3.8	2.8	2.7	2.8	2.7	2.8	2.8	2.7
Under 1 year	*	*	*	*	*	*	*	*	*	*	*	*
1 to 14 years	0.8	0.7	0.7	0.8	0.8	0.3	0.4	0.4	0.4	0.4	0.3	0.3
1 to 4 years	0.9	0.5	0.5	0.5	0.5	*	0.3	*	0.4	0.4	0.4	0.3
5 to 14 years	0.8	0.7	0.8	1.0	0.9	0.4	0.4	0.4	0.4	0.4	0.3	0.3
15 to 24 years	4.8	6.1	5.0	6.0	5.9	3.5	3.0	3.1	3.2	3.2	3.1	2.9
15 to 19 years	3.5	4.6	3.9	5.7	5.6	2.9	2.4	2.5	2.5	2.4	2.4	2.3
20 to 24 years	6.4	7.7	5.9	6.3	6.1	4.2	3.6	3.8	3.9	4.0	3.7	3.5
25 to 44 years	8.3	7.4	6.2	6.1	5.5	4.2	3.9	3.9	3.9	3.8	3.9	3.8
25 to 34 years	8.4	7.5	6.6	6.7	5.8	4.0	3.8	3.7	3.6	3.6	3.9	3.5
35 to 44 years	8.2	7.2	5.8	5.4	5.2	4.4	4.0	4.1	4.2	4.0	3.9	4.1
45 to 64 years	5.4	5.4	5.0	4.5	3.9	3.4	3.3	3.6	3.4	3.6	3.8	3.7
45 to 54 years	6.4	6.2	5.6	4.9	4.2	3.6	3.7	4.0	3.7	3.9	4.3	3.8
55 to 64 years	4.2	4.6	4.5	4.0	3.5	3.0	2.8	3.1	3.0	3.1	3.2	3.4
65 years and over	2.4	2.5	3.2	3.1	2.8	2.2	2.1	1.9	2.0	2.1	2.2	2.2
65 to 74 years	2.8	3.1	3.6	3.6	3.0	2.5	2.5	2.2	2.2	2.4	2.6	2.6
75 to 84 years	1.7	1.7	3.0	2.9	2.8	2.0	2.1	1.8	2.0	2.0	2.2	2.1
85 years and over	*	1.3	1.8	1.3	1.8	1.7	1.4	1.2	1.2	1.6	1.3	1.5
White Male [4]												
All ages, age-adjusted[3]	19.7	22.1	21.0	22.0	20.1	15.9	15.9	15.5	15.8	16.1	15.9	16.1
All ages, crude	17.6	21.8	20.7	21.8	19.9	15.6	16.0	15.6	15.9	16.4	16.2	16.5
1 to 14 years	1.8	1.9	2.1	1.9	1.9	1.0	0.8	0.8	0.7	0.7	0.8	0.8
15 to 24 years	16.9	28.4	24.1	29.5	30.8	19.6	18.3	18.4	17.5	17.7	16.9	16.2
25 to 44 years	24.2	29.5	25.0	25.7	23.2	18.0	18.4	17.9	18.9	18.6	18.1	18.6
25 to 34 years	24.3	31.1	26.3	27.8	25.2	18.1	19.4	18.5	19.8	19.1	17.9	19.1
35 to 44 years	24.1	27.1	23.3	23.3	21.2	17.9	17.5	17.3	18.0	18.2	18.2	18.0
45 to 64 years	27.4	23.3	23.6	22.8	19.5	17.4	19.0	18.4	19.0	20.5	20.5	21.3
65 years and over	29.9	30.1	35.4	36.8	32.2	28.2	27.0	25.8	26.0	26.6	26.9	26.5
Black or African American Male [4]												
All ages, age-adjusted[3]	70.8	60.1	40.9	56.3	49.2	34.2	36.7	37.6	36.2	34.3	32.3	31.8
All ages, crude	60.8	57.7	41.3	61.9	52.9	36.1	38.6	39.8	38.5	36.2	33.7	33.4
1 to 14 years	5.3	3.0	2.7	4.4	4.4	1.8	2.1	2.2	2.2	2.0	1.6	1.9
15 to 24 years	97.3	77.9	61.3	138.0	138.7	89.3	86.2	90.9	87.7	79.7	72.8	73.2
25 to 44 years	126.2	114.1	71.8	90.3	70.2	54.1	64.8	64.8	63.3	60.8	57.2	57.3
25 to 34 years	145.6	128.4	79.8	108.6	92.3	74.8	92.1	92.8	88.5	85.3	76.0	78.2
35 to 44 years	104.2	92.3	59.2	66.1	46.3	34.3	38.6	37.8	38.4	36.2	37.7	35.2
45 to 64 years	71.1	55.6	36.9	34.5	28.3	18.4	17.2	18.5	18.1	16.9	17.1	16.5
65 years and over	30.6	29.7	26.3	23.9	21.8	13.8	13.5	13.2	10.9	13.2	12.1	9.4
American Indian or Alaska Native Male [4]												
All ages, age-adjusted[3]	NA	24.0	23.6	19.4	19.4	13.1	14.4	13.3	11.0	11.7	11.4	11.7
All ages, crude	NA	27.5	24.4	20.5	20.9	13.2	14.9	13.7	11.1	11.7	11.6	12.5
15 to 24 years	NA	55.3	39.8	49.1	40.9	26.9	28.6	27.8	20.8	22.2	22.2	26.0
25 to 44 years	NA	43.9	40.3	25.4	31.2	16.6	21.3	19.0	14.2	17.3	16.3	16.9
45 to 64 years	NA	*	21.2	*	14.2	12.2	12.1	10.1	10.6	7.1	11.1	11.1
65 years and over	NA	*	*	*	*	*	*	*	*	*	*	*

Table 2-44. Death Rates for Firearm-Related Injuries, by Sex, Race, Hispanic Origin, and Age, Selected Years, 1970–2010—*Continued*

(Deaths per 100,000 resident population.)

Sex, race, Hispanic origin, and age	1970[1]	1980[1]	1985	1990[1]	1995[1]	2000[2]	2005[2]	2006[2]	2007[2]	2008[2]	2009[2]	2010[2]
Asian or Pacific Islander Male [4]												
All ages, age-adjusted[3]	NA	7.8	7.3	8.8	9.2	6.0	5.1	5.2	5.0	4.2	4.4	4.2
All ages, crude	NA	8.2	7.3	9.4	10.0	6.2	5.4	5.5	5.1	4.4	4.5	4.4
15 to 24 years	NA	10.8	12.6	21.0	24.3	9.3	10.9	12.9	9.7	7.5	5.4	6.8
25 to 44 years	NA	12.8	9.8	10.9	10.6	8.1	6.4	5.7	5.9	5.2	6.2	6.0
45 to 64 years	NA	10.4	6.7	8.1	8.2	7.4	5.7	5.6	5.6	4.7	5.2	4.4
65 years and over	NA	*	*	*	*	*	*	*	4.5	4.4	4.7	3.9
Hispanic or Latino Male [4]												
All ages, age-adjusted[3]	NA	NA	24.2	27.6	23.8	13.6	13.4	12.8	12.9	11.7	11.4	10.5
All ages, crude	NA	NA	26.0	29.9	26.2	14.2	14.3	13.8	13.4	12.0	11.4	10.5
1 to 14 years	NA	NA	1.4	2.6	2.8	1.0	0.7	1.1	0.8	0.5	0.7	0.6
15 to 24 years	NA	NA	42.0	55.5	61.7	30.8	30.8	31.1	28.4	24.9	23.3	20.9
25 to 44 years	NA	NA	43.2	42.7	31.4	17.3	19.7	18.5	18.2	16.6	15.5	14.4
25 to 34 years	NA	NA	47.3	47.3	36.4	20.3	24.4	22.5	22.5	19.4	18.0	18.0
35 to 44 years	NA	NA	35.9	35.4	24.2	13.2	13.9	13.5	12.9	13.2	12.4	10.2
45 to 64 years	NA	NA	19.2	21.4	17.2	12.0	9.2	8.6	9.7	9.0	9.5	9.1
65 years and over	NA	NA	12.4	19.1	16.5	12.2	10.2	8.0	11.2	10.3	10.8	9.9
White, not Hispanic or Latino Male [5]												
All ages, age-adjusted[3]	NA	NA	20.2	20.6	18.6	15.5	15.5	15.1	15.5	16.2	16.1	16.6
All ages, crude	NA	NA	19.9	20.4	18.5	15.7	16.1	15.8	16.3	17.1	17.0	17.6
1 to 14 years	NA	NA	2.0	1.6	1.6	1.0	0.9	0.7	0.7	0.7	0.7	0.9
15 to 24 years	NA	NA	22.0	24.1	23.5	16.2	14.1	14.1	13.7	14.9	14.2	14.2
25 to 44 years	NA	NA	23.0	23.3	21.4	17.9	17.7	17.4	18.7	18.9	18.4	19.4
25 to 34 years	NA	NA	23.7	24.7	22.5	17.2	17.4	16.7	18.5	18.5	17.4	18.9
35 to 44 years	NA	NA	22.0	21.6	20.4	18.4	17.9	18.0	18.8	19.2	19.4	19.9
45 to 64 years	NA	NA	23.0	22.7	19.5	17.8	20.0	19.5	20.0	21.8	21.8	22.8
65 years and over	NA	NA	37.3	37.4	32.5	29.0	28.1	27.0	27.0	27.7	27.9	27.6
White Female [4]												
All ages, age-adjusted[3]	4.0	4.2	3.9	3.8	3.5	2.7	2.6	2.6	2.6	2.7	2.8	2.7
All ages, crude	3.7	4.1	4.0	3.8	3.5	2.7	2.6	2.7	2.7	2.8	2.9	2.8
15 to 24 years	3.4	5.1	4.4	4.8	4.5	2.8	2.3	2.3	2.6	2.3	2.4	2.3
25 to 44 years	6.9	6.2	5.6	5.3	4.9	3.9	3.8	3.6	3.8	3.8	3.8	3.7
45 to 64 years	5.0	5.1	5.0	4.5	4.0	3.5	3.5	3.9	3.7	4.0	4.2	4.1
65 years and over	2.2	2.5	3.2	3.1	2.8	2.4	2.3	2.1	2.1	2.3	2.5	2.5
Black or African American Female [4]												
All ages, age-adjusted[3]	11.1	8.7	6.4	7.3	6.2	3.9	3.6	3.9	3.8	3.4	3.4	3.3
All ages, crude	10.0	8.8	6.5	7.8	6.5	4.0	3.7	4.1	3.8	3.5	3.5	3.3
15 to 24 years	15.2	12.3	8.3	13.3	13.2	7.6	6.6	7.5	6.9	7.9	6.7	6.4
25 to 44 years	19.4	16.1	11.4	12.4	9.8	6.5	6.0	6.9	6.3	5.3	5.7	5.6
45 to 64 years	10.2	8.2	5.8	4.8	4.1	3.1	2.7	2.6	2.7	2.0	2.4	2.2
65 years and over	4.3	3.1	3.7	3.1	2.6	1.3	1.3	1.0	1.2	1.3	*	*
American Indian or Alaska Native Female [4]												
All ages, age-adjusted[3]	NA	5.8	3.9	3.3	3.8	2.9	2.2	2.1	1.8	2.3	2.5	2.6
All ages, crude	NA	5.8	4.1	3.4	4.1	2.9	2.3	2.1	1.7	2.3	2.4	2.4
15 to 24 years	NA	*	*	*	*	*	*	*	*	*	*	*
25 to 44 years	NA	10.2	*	*	7.0	5.5	*	*	*	3.5	3.6	3.7
45 to 64 years	NA	*	*	*	*	*	*	*	*	*	*	*
65 years and over	NA	*	*	*	*	*	*	*	*	*	*	*
Asian or Pacific Islander Female [4]												
All ages, age-adjusted[3]	NA	2.0	1.5	1.9	2.0	1.1	0.9	0.9	0.7	0.7	0.9	0.6
All ages, crude	NA	2.1	1.7	2.1	2.1	1.2	0.9	1.0	0.7	0.8	0.9	0.6
15 to 24 years	NA	*	*	*	3.9	*	2.0	*	*	*	*	*
25 to 44 years	NA	3.2	2.2	2.7	2.7	1.5	0.9	1.2	0.9	1.1	1.1	1.1
45 to 64 years	NA	*	*	*	*	*	*	1.2	*	*	1.2	*
65 years and over	NA	*	*	*	*	*	*	*	*	*	*	*
Hispanic or Latina Female [4]												
All ages, age-adjusted[3]	NA	NA	2.9	3.3	3.1	1.8	1.5	1.4	1.5	1.5	1.4	1.3
All ages, crude	NA	NA	3.2	3.6	3.3	1.8	1.5	1.5	1.5	1.5	1.4	1.3
15 to 24 years	NA	NA	5.1	6.9	6.1	2.9	2.4	2.5	2.6	2.6	2.6	2.1
25 to 44 years	NA	NA	5.5	5.1	4.7	2.5	2.6	2.2	2.2	1.9	1.9	1.8
45 to 64 years	NA	NA	2.2	2.4	2.4	2.2	1.2	1.3	1.4	1.6	1.4	1.5
65 years and over	NA	NA	*	*	*	*	*	*	*	*	*	*
White, not Hispanic or Latina Female [4]												
All ages, age-adjusted[3]	NA	NA	4.0	3.7	3.4	2.8	2.7	2.7	2.8	2.9	3.0	3.0
All ages, crude	NA	NA	4.1	3.7	3.5	2.9	2.8	2.9	2.9	3.0	3.1	3.1
15 to 24 years	NA	NA	4.5	4.3	4.1	2.7	2.2	2.2	2.5	2.2	2.2	2.3
25 to 44 years	NA	NA	5.6	5.1	4.8	4.2	4.0	3.8	4.1	4.2	4.3	4.2
45 to 64 years	NA	NA	5.1	4.6	4.1	3.6	3.8	4.2	3.9	4.2	4.5	4.4
65 years and over	NA	NA	3.4	3.2	2.8	2.4	2.4	2.2	2.2	2.4	2.6	2.6

Figure 2-12. Infant Mortality Rates, by Race of Mother, 1980–2010

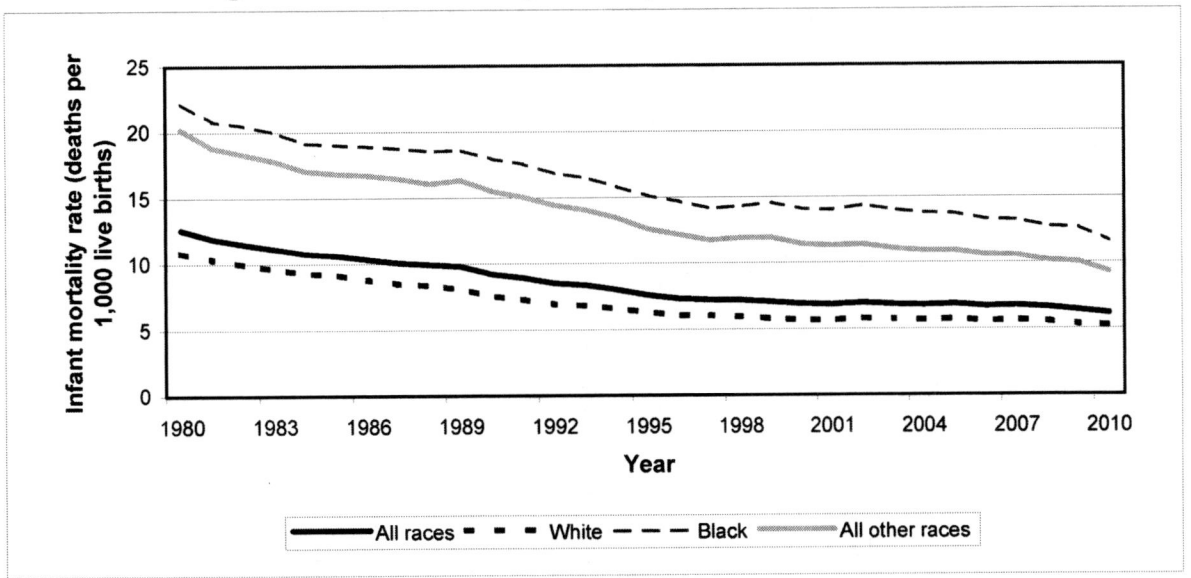

Figure 2-13. States with the Highest and Lowest Infant Death Rates, 2010

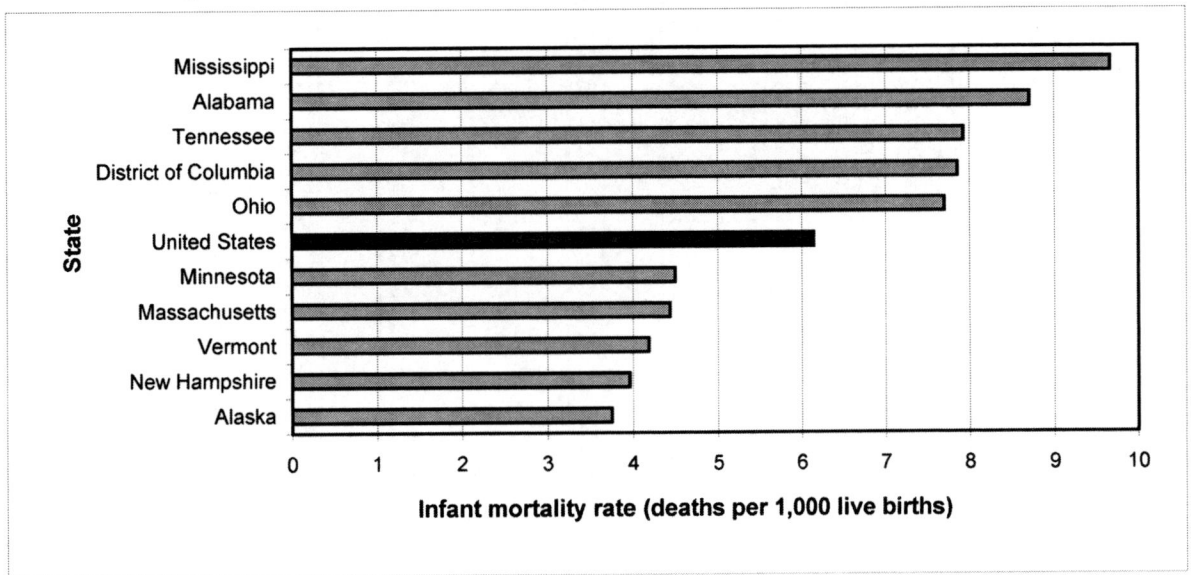

Table 2-45. Infant, Neonatal, and Postneonatal Mortality Rates, by Race and Sex, Selected Years, 1940–2010

(Rates are infant [under 1 year], neonatal [under 28 days], and postneonatal [28 days to 11 months]; deaths per 1,000 live births in specified group.)

Year	All races			White[1]			All other[1]					
							Total[1]			Black[1]		
	Both sexes	Male	Female	Both sexes	Male	Female	Both sexes	Male	Female	Both sexes	Male	Female
INFANT MORTALITY RATE												
Race of Mother [2]												
1980	12.6	13.9	11.2	10.9	12.1	9.5	20.2	21.9	18.4	22.2	24.2	20.2
1981	11.9	13.1	10.7	10.3	11.5	9.1	18.8	20.4	17.2	20.8	22.5	19.0
1982	11.5	12.8	10.2	9.9	11.1	8.7	18.3	20.1	16.5	20.5	22.5	18.4
1983	11.2	12.3	10.0	9.6	10.7	8.5	17.8	19.4	16.1	20.0	22.0	18.0
1984	10.8	11.9	9.6	9.3	10.4	8.2	17.1	18.4	15.7	19.2	20.7	17.6
1985	10.6	11.9	9.3	9.2	10.4	7.9	16.8	18.3	15.3	19.0	20.8	17.2
1986	10.4	11.6	9.1	8.8	9.9	7.7	16.7	18.5	14.9	18.9	20.9	16.8
1987	10.1	11.2	8.9	8.5	9.5	7.5	16.5	18.1	14.8	18.8	20.6	16.8
1988	10.0	11.0	8.9	8.4	9.4	7.3	16.1	17.3	14.8	18.5	20.0	17.0
1989	9.8	10.8	8.8	8.1	9.0	7.1	16.3	17.6	15.0	18.6	20.0	17.2
1990	9.2	10.3	8.1	7.6	8.5	6.6	15.5	17.0	14.0	18.0	19.6	16.3
1991	8.9	10.0	7.8	7.3	8.3	6.3	15.1	16.5	13.6	17.6	19.4	15.7
1992	8.5	9.4	7.6	6.9	7.7	6.1	14.4	15.7	13.1	16.9	18.4	15.3
1993	8.4	9.3	7.4	6.8	7.6	6.1	14.1	15.6	12.5	16.5	18.3	14.7
1994	8.0	8.8	7.2	6.6	7.2	5.9	13.5	14.8	12.1	15.8	17.5	14.1
1995	7.6	8.3	6.8	6.3	7.0	5.6	12.6	13.5	11.7	15.1	16.3	13.9
1996	7.3	8.0	6.6	6.1	6.7	5.4	12.2	13.3	11.0	14.7	16.0	13.3
1997	7.2	8.0	6.5	6.0	6.7	5.4	11.8	12.8	10.7	14.2	15.5	12.8
1998	7.2	7.8	6.5	6.0	6.5	5.4	11.9	13.0	10.8	14.3	15.8	12.8
1999	7.1	7.7	6.4	5.8	6.4	5.2	11.9	12.9	10.9	14.6	15.9	13.2
2000	6.9	7.6	6.2	5.7	6.2	5.1	11.4	12.6	10.3	14.1	15.5	12.6
2001	6.9	7.5	6.1	5.7	6.2	5.1	11.3	12.4	10.2	14.0	15.5	12.5
2002	7.0	7.6	6.3	5.8	6.4	5.1	11.4	12.2	10.6	14.4	15.4	13.3
2003	6.9	7.6	6.1	5.7	6.4	5.1	11.1	12.2	9.9	14.0	15.5	12.4
2004	6.8	7.5	6.1	5.7	6.2	5.1	10.9	12.0	9.8	13.8	15.2	12.3
2005	6.9	7.6	6.2	5.7	6.3	5.1	10.9	12.0	9.8	13.7	15.2	12.3
2006	6.7	7.3	6.0	5.6	6.1	5.0	10.6	11.5	9.6	13.3	14.4	12.2
2007	6.8	7.4	6.1	5.6	6.2	5.1	10.6	11.5	9.5	13.2	14.5	11.9
2008	6.6	7.2	6.0	5.6	6.1	5.0	10.2	11.1	9.2	12.7	13.9	11.5
2009	6.4	7.0	5.8	5.3	5.8	4.8	10.0	11.1	8.9	12.6	14.1	11.2
2010	6.2	6.7	5.6	5.2	5.7	4.7	9.3	10.2	8.4	11.6	12.7	10.5
Race of Child [3]												
1940	47.0	52.5	41.3	43.2	48.3	37.8	73.8	82.2	65.2	72.9	81.1	64.6
1950	29.2	32.8	25.5	26.8	30.2	23.1	44.5	48.9	39.9	43.9	48.3	39.4
1960	26.0	29.3	22.6	22.9	26.0	19.6	43.2	47.9	38.5	44.3	49.1	39.4
1970	20.0	22.4	17.5	17.8	20.0	15.4	30.9	34.2	27.5	32.7	36.2	29.0
1975	16.1	17.9	14.2	14.2	15.9	12.3	24.2	26.2	22.2	26.2	28.3	24.0
1976	15.2	16.8	13.6	13.3	14.8	11.7	23.5	25.5	21.4	25.5	27.8	23.2
1977	14.1	15.8	12.4	12.3	13.9	10.7	21.7	23.7	19.6	23.6	25.9	21.3
1978	13.8	15.3	12.2	12.0	13.4	10.6	21.1	23.2	18.9	23.1	25.4	20.8
1979	13.1	14.5	11.6	11.4	12.8	9.9	19.8	21.5	18.1	21.8	23.7	19.9
1980	12.6	13.9	11.2	11.0	12.3	9.7	19.1	20.7	17.5	21.4	23.3	19.4
NEONATAL MORTALITY RATE												
Race of Mother [2]												
1980	8.5	9.3	7.6	7.4	8.2	6.5	13.2	14.3	12.1	14.6	15.9	13.3
1981	8.0	8.8	7.2	7.0	7.7	6.2	12.5	13.5	11.5	14.0	15.2	12.8
1982	7.7	8.5	6.9	6.7	7.4	5.9	12.0	13.2	10.9	13.6	14.9	12.3
1983	7.3	8.0	6.5	6.3	7.0	5.6	11.4	12.5	10.3	12.9	14.2	11.6
1984	7.0	7.7	6.3	6.1	6.7	5.4	10.9	11.7	10.1	12.3	13.2	11.4
1985	7.0	7.8	6.1	6.0	6.8	5.2	11.0	12.0	10.0	12.6	13.8	11.4
1986	6.7	7.4	6.0	5.7	6.3	5.1	10.8	11.8	9.7	12.3	13.6	11.0
1987	6.5	7.1	5.8	5.4	6.0	4.8	10.7	11.7	9.6	12.3	13.5	11.1
1988	6.3	7.0	5.7	5.3	5.8	4.7	10.3	11.2	9.4	12.1	13.1	10.9
1989	6.2	6.8	5.6	5.2	5.7	4.6	10.3	11.1	9.5	11.9	12.8	11.0
1990	5.9	6.5	5.2	4.8	5.4	4.2	9.9	10.8	8.9	11.6	12.7	10.4
1991	5.6	6.2	5.0	4.5	5.0	4.0	9.5	10.5	8.5	11.3	12.6	9.9
1992	5.4	5.8	4.9	4.4	4.7	4.0	9.2	10.0	8.3	10.8	11.8	9.8
1993	5.3	5.8	4.8	4.3	4.6	3.9	9.0	9.9	8.1	10.7	11.8	9.6
1994	5.1	5.6	4.6	4.2	4.6	3.8	8.6	9.5	7.7	10.2	11.3	9.1
1995	4.9	5.4	4.4	4.1	4.5	3.6	8.1	8.7	7.5	9.9	10.6	9.1
1996	4.8	5.2	4.3	4.0	4.3	3.6	7.9	8.6	7.1	9.6	10.5	8.7
1997	4.8	5.2	4.3	4.0	4.4	3.6	7.7	8.4	7.1	9.4	10.1	8.7
1998	4.8	5.2	4.4	4.0	4.3	3.6	7.9	8.6	7.2	9.6	10.5	8.6
1999	4.7	5.1	4.3	3.9	4.2	3.6	7.9	8.6	7.3	9.8	10.7	8.8
2000	4.6	5.1	4.2	3.8	4.2	3.5	7.6	8.4	6.8	9.4	10.4	8.4
2001	4.5	5.0	4.1	3.8	4.2	3.4	7.4	8.1	6.7	9.2	10.2	8.3
2002	4.7	5.1	4.3	3.9	4.3	3.5	7.6	8.0	7.1	9.5	10.1	8.9
2003	4.6	5.1	4.1	3.9	4.3	3.5	7.4	8.1	6.6	9.4	10.4	8.4
2004	4.5	4.9	4.1	3.8	4.1	3.4	7.2	7.8	6.5	9.1	10.0	8.3
2005	4.5	4.9	4.1	3.8	4.1	3.5	7.2	7.9	6.5	9.1	10.0	8.1
2006	4.5	4.8	4.1	3.7	4.1	3.4	7.0	7.6	6.4	8.8	9.5	8.1
2007	4.4	4.8	4.0	3.7	4.0	3.4	6.9	7.5	6.2	8.7	9.5	7.8
2008	4.3	4.7	3.9	3.6	3.9	3.3	6.5	7.1	5.9	8.2	9.0	7.5
2009	4.2	4.5	3.8	3.5	3.8	3.2	6.5	7.1	5.8	8.2	9.0	7.3
2010	4.1	4.4	3.7	3.5	3.7	3.2	6.0	6.5	5.5	7.5	8.1	6.9

Table 2-45. Infant, Neonatal, and Postneonatal Mortality Rates, by Race and Sex, Selected Years, 1940–2010—*Continued*

(Rates are infant [under 1 year], neonatal [under 28 days], and postneonatal [28 days to 11 months]; deaths per 1,000 live births in specified group.)

Year	All races			White[1]			All other[1]					
							Total[1]			Black[1]		
	Both sexes	Male	Female	Both sexes	Male	Female	Both sexes	Male	Female	Both sexes	Male	Female
Race of Child[3]												
1940	28.8	32.6	24.7	27.2	30.9	23.3	39.7	44.9	34.5	39.9	44.8	34.9
1950	20.5	23.3	17.5	19.4	22.2	16.4	27.5	30.8	24.2	27.8	31.1	24.4
1960	18.7	21.2	16.1	17.2	19.7	14.7	26.9	30.0	23.6	27.8	31.1	24.5
1970	15.1	17.0	13.1	13.8	15.6	11.9	21.4	23.9	18.9	22.8	25.4	20.1
1975	11.6	12.9	10.2	10.4	11.7	9.0	16.8	18.2	15.3	18.3	19.8	16.8
1976	10.9	12.0	9.8	9.7	10.7	8.5	16.3	17.7	14.9	17.9	19.5	16.3
1977	9.9	11.0	8.7	8.8	9.8	7.6	14.7	16.0	13.3	16.1	17.6	14.5
1978	9.5	10.5	8.4	8.4	9.3	7.4	14.0	15.5	12.4	15.5	17.2	13.7
1979	8.9	9.8	7.9	7.9	8.8	6.9	12.9	13.9	11.8	14.3	15.5	13.1
1980	8.5	9.3	7.6	7.5	8.3	6.6	12.5	13.5	11.5	14.1	15.3	12.8
POSTNEONATAL MORTALITY RATE												
Race of Mother[2]												
1980	4.1	4.6	3.6	3.5	3.9	3.0	7.0	7.6	6.3	7.6	8.3	6.9
1981	3.9	4.3	3.5	3.4	3.8	2.9	6.3	6.8	5.8	6.8	7.4	6.3
1982	3.8	4.3	3.3	3.3	3.7	2.8	6.3	6.9	5.6	6.9	7.6	6.1
1983	3.9	4.3	3.4	3.3	3.7	2.9	6.4	7.0	5.8	7.1	7.8	6.3
1984	3.8	4.2	3.3	3.2	3.7	2.8	6.2	6.7	5.6	6.8	7.5	6.2
1985	3.7	4.2	3.2	3.2	3.6	2.7	5.8	6.3	5.3	6.4	7.0	5.8
1986	3.6	4.1	3.1	3.1	3.5	2.6	5.9	6.6	5.2	6.6	7.3	5.8
1987	3.6	4.1	3.2	3.1	3.5	2.6	5.8	6.3	5.2	6.5	7.1	5.8
1988	3.6	4.0	3.2	3.1	3.5	2.7	5.8	6.1	5.4	6.5	6.9	6.1
1989	3.6	4.0	3.1	2.9	3.4	2.5	6.0	6.5	5.5	6.7	7.2	6.2
1990	3.4	3.8	3.0	2.8	3.1	2.4	5.7	6.2	5.1	6.4	6.9	5.9
1991	3.4	3.8	2.9	2.8	3.3	2.3	5.6	6.0	5.1	6.3	6.8	5.8
1992	3.1	3.6	2.7	2.6	3.0	2.2	5.3	5.7	4.8	6.0	6.5	5.5
1993	3.1	3.5	2.6	2.5	2.9	2.1	5.1	5.7	4.4	5.8	6.6	5.1
1994	2.9	3.2	2.6	2.4	2.7	2.1	4.9	5.3	4.4	5.6	6.2	5.0
1995	2.7	3.0	2.4	2.2	2.5	1.9	4.5	4.8	4.1	5.3	5.7	4.8
1996	2.6	2.8	2.2	2.1	2.4	1.8	4.3	4.7	3.9	5.1	5.6	4.6
1997	2.5	2.8	2.1	2.0	2.3	1.8	4.0	4.5	3.6	4.8	5.3	4.2
1998	2.4	2.6	2.2	2.0	2.2	1.8	4.0	4.4	3.6	4.8	5.2	4.3
1999	2.3	2.6	2.0	1.9	2.2	1.6	4.0	4.3	3.6	4.8	5.2	4.4
2000	2.3	2.5	2.0	1.9	2.1	1.7	3.8	4.2	3.5	4.7	5.1	4.3
2001	2.3	2.6	2.1	1.9	2.1	1.7	4.0	4.4	3.5	4.8	5.3	4.3
2002	2.3	2.6	2.0	1.9	2.2	1.6	3.9	4.2	3.5	4.9	5.3	4.4
2003	2.2	2.5	1.9	1.8	2.1	1.6	3.7	4.1	3.3	4.6	5.1	4.1
2004	2.3	2.5	2.0	1.9	2.1	1.7	3.7	4.2	3.2	4.7	5.2	4.1
2005	2.3	2.6	2.0	1.9	2.2	1.7	3.7	4.1	3.4	4.7	5.2	4.1
2006	2.2	2.5	2.0	1.8	2.1	1.6	3.6	4.0	3.2	4.5	4.9	4.0
2007	2.3	2.6	2.1	1.9	2.2	1.7	3.7	4.0	3.3	4.6	5.0	4.2
2008	2.3	2.5	2.1	1.9	2.1	1.7	3.6	4.0	3.3	4.5	4.9	4.1
2009	2.1	2.3	1.9	1.7	1.9	1.6	3.3	3.7	2.9	4.1	4.6	3.6
2010	2.2	2.5	1.9	1.8	2.0	1.6	3.6	4.0	3.1	4.5	5.1	3.9
Race of Child[3]												
1940	18.3	19.9	16.6	16.0	17.5	14.5	34.1	37.4	30.7	33.1	36.3	29.7
1950	8.7	9.4	8.0	7.4	8.0	6.7	16.9	18.1	15.7	16.1	17.2	15.0
1960	7.3	8.1	6.5	5.7	6.4	4.9	16.4	17.8	14.8	16.5	18.0	15.0
1970	4.9	5.4	4.4	4.0	4.4	3.5	9.5	10.3	8.6	9.9	10.8	8.9
1975	4.5	5.0	4.0	3.8	4.2	3.3	7.5	8.0	6.9	7.9	8.5	7.2
1976	4.3	4.8	3.8	3.7	4.1	3.2	7.2	7.8	6.5	7.6	8.4	6.9
1977	4.2	4.8	3.7	3.6	4.1	3.1	7.0	7.7	6.3	7.6	8.3	6.8
1978	4.3	4.7	3.9	3.6	4.0	3.2	7.1	7.6	6.5	7.6	8.2	7.1
1979	4.2	4.7	3.7	3.5	4.0	3.0	6.9	7.6	6.3	7.5	8.2	6.7
1980	4.1	4.6	3.6	3.5	4.0	3.0	6.6	7.2	6.0	7.3	8.0	6.6

[1]Multiple-race data were reported by 34 states and the District of Columbia in 2008, by 27 states and the District of Columbia in 2007, by 25 states and the District of Columbia in 2006, by 21 states and the District of Columbia in 2005, by 15 states in 2004, and by 7 states in 2003. Multiple-race data were reported for births by 38 states and the District of Columbia in 2010, by 32 states and the District of Columbia in 2009, by 30 areas in 2008, by 27 areas in 2007, by 23 areas in 2006, by 19 areas in 2005, by 15 areas in 2004, and by 6 areas in 2003. The multiple-race data for these reporting areas were bridged to the single-race categories of the 1977 OMB standards for comparability with other reporting areas.   [2]Infant deaths are based on race of child as stated on the death certificate; live births are based on race of mother as stated on the birth certificate.   [3]Infant deaths are based on race of child as stated on the death certificate; live births are based on race of parents as stated on the birth certificate.

Table 2-46. Number of Infant Deaths and Infant Mortality Rates, by Selected Cause and Race, 2010

(Infant deaths [under 1 year] per 100,000 live births in specified group. Infant deaths based on race of decedent; live births based on race of mother.)

Cause of death (based on ICD–10, 2004)	Number			Rate		
	All races[1]	White[2]	Black[2]	All races[1]	White[2]	Black[2]
All Causes	24,586	15,954	7,401	614.7	519.8	1,162.9
Certain infectious and parasitic diseases (A00-B99)	696	401	266	17.4	13.1	41.8
Certain intestinal infectious diseases (A00-A08)	7	4	2	*	*	*
Diarrhea and gastroenteritis of infectious origin (A09)	316	170	133	7.9	5.5	20.9
Tuberculosis (A16-A19)	-	-	-	*	*	*
Tetanus (A33,A35)	-	-	-	*	*	*
Diphtheria (A36)	-	-	-	*	*	*
Whooping cough (A37)	25	23	2	0.6	0.7	*
Meningococcal infection (A39)	11	9	2	*	*	*
Septicemia (A40-A41)	215	114	90	5.4	3.7	14.1
Congenital syphilis (A50)	2	1	1	*	*	*
Gonococcal infection (A54)	-	-	-	*	*	*
Viral diseases (A80-B34)	92	58	30	2.3	1.9	4.7
Acute poliomyelitis (A80)	-	-	-	*	*	*
Varicella (chicken pox) (B01)	-	-	-	*	*	*
Measles (B05)	-	-	-	*	*	*
Human immunodeficiency virus (HIV) disease (B20-B24)	-	-	-	*	*	*
Mumps (B26)	-	-	-	*	*	*
Other and unspecified viral diseases (A81-B00,B02-B04,B06-B19,B25,B27-B34)	92	58	30	2.3	1.9	4.7
Candidiasis (B37)	6	5	1	*	*	*
Malaria (B50-B54)	-	-	-	*	*	*
Pneumocystosis (B59)	-	-	-	*	*	*
All other and unspecified infectious and parasitic diseases (A51-A53,A55-A79,B35-B36,B38-B49,B55-B58,B60-B99)	22	17	5	0.6	*	*
Neoplasms (C00-D48)	110	84	16	2.8	2.7	*
Malignant neoplasms (C00-C97)	62	47	8	1.6	1.5	*
Hodgkin's disease and non-Hodgkin's lymphomas (C81-C85)	2	2	-	*	*	*
Leukemia (C91-C95)	25	19	4	0.6	*	*
Other and unspecified malignant neoplasms (C00-C80,C88,C90,C96-C97)	35	26	4	0.9	0.8	*
In situ neoplasms, benign neoplasms and neoplasms of uncertain or unknown behavior (D00-D48)	48	37	8	1.2	1.2	*
Diseases of the blood and blood-forming organs and certain disorders involving the immune mechanism (D50-D89)	95	65	26	2.4	2.1	4.1
Anemias (D50-D64)	15	5	9	*	*	*
Hemorrhagic conditions and other diseases of blood and blood-forming organs (D65-D76)	60	43	14	1.5	1.4	*
Certain disorders involving the immune mechanism (D80-D89)	20	17	3	0.5	*	*
Endocrine, nutritional and metabolic diseases (E00-E88)	188	135	43	4.7	4.4	6.8
Short stature, not elsewhere classified (E343)	2	2	-	*	*	*
Nutritional deficiencies (E40-E64)	3	2	-	*	*	*
Cystic fibrosis (E84)	5	5	-	*	*	*
Volume depletion, disorders of fluid, electrolyte and acid-base balance (E86-E87)	48	27	19	1.2	0.9	*
All other endocrine, nutritional and metabolic diseases (E344-E349,E65-E83,E85,E88)	130	99	24	3.3	3.2	3.8
Diseases of the nervous system (G00-G98)	345	244	75	8.6	7.9	11.8
Meningitis (G00,G03)	58	33	19	1.5	1.1	*
Infantile spinal muscular atrophy, type I (Werdnig-Hoffman) (G120)	4	4	-	*	*	*
Infantile cerebral palsy (G80)	3	2	1	*	*	*
Anoxic brain damage, not elsewhere classified (G931)	39	25	11	1.0	0.8	*
Other diseases of nervous system (G04, G06-G11, G12.1-G12.9, G20-G72, G81-G92,G930,G932-G939,G95-G98)	241	180	44	6.0	5.9	6.9
Diseases of the ear and mastoid process (H60-H93)	3	2	-	*	*	*
Diseases of the circulatory system (I00-I99)	507	326	152	12.7	10.6	23.9
Pulmonary heart disease and diseases of pulmonary circulation (I26-I28)	90	52	32	2.3	1.7	5.0
Pericarditis, endocarditis and myocarditis (I30,I33,I40)	14	9	4	*	*	*
Cardiomyopathy (I42)	79	62	12	2.0	2.0	*
Cardiac arrest (I46)	18	11	6	*	*	*
Cerebrovascular diseases (I60-I69)	130	74	48	3.3	2.4	7.5
All other diseases of circulatory system (I00-I25,I31,I34-I38,I44-I45,I47-I51,I70-I99)	176	118	50	4.4	3.8	7.9
Diseases of the respiratory system (J00-J98,U04)	574	306	221	14.4	10.0	34.7
Acute upper respiratory infections (J00-J06)	15	12	2	*	*	*
Influenza and pneumonia (J09-J18)	195	101	73	4.9	3.3	11.5
Influenza (J09-J11)	16	6	6	*	*	*
Pneumonia (J12-J18)	179	95	67	4.5	3.1	10.5
Acute bronchitis and acute bronchiolitis (J20–J21)	27	14	10	0.7	*	*
Bronchitis, chronic and unspecified (J40–J42)	25	13	6	0.6	*	*
Asthma (J45–J46)	6	5	1	*	*	*
Pneumonitis due to solids and liquids (J69)	18	8	9	*	*	*
Other and unspecified diseases of respiratory system (J22, J30–J39, J43–J44, J47–J68, J70–J98, U04)4	288	153	120	7.2	5.0	18.9
Diseases of the digestive system (K00–K92)	204	141	53	5.1	4.6	8.3
Gastritis, duodenitis, and noninfective enteritis and colitis (K29,K50–K55)	29	20	8	0.7	0.7	*
Hernia of abdominal cavity and intestinal obstruction without hernia (K40–K46,K56)	51	39	11	1.3	1.3	*
All other and unspecified diseases of digestive system (K00–K28,K30–K38,K57–K92)	124	82	34	3.1	2.7	5.3
Diseases of the genitourinary system (N00–N95)	126	73	42	3.2	2.4	6.6
Renal failure and other disorders of kidney (N17–N19,N25,N27)	100	56	35	2.5	1.8	5.5
Other and unspecified diseases of genitourinary system (N00–N15,N20–N23,N26,N28–N95)	26	17	7	0.7	*	*
Certain conditions originating in the perinatal period (P00–P96)	12,008	7,423	4,005	300.2	241.8	629.3
Newborn affected by maternal factors and by complications of pregnancy, labor, and delivery (P00–P04)	2,920	1,842	922	73.0	60.0	144.9
Newborn affected by maternal hypertensive disorders (P00)	85	49	34	2.1	1.6	5.3
Newborn affected by other maternal conditions which may be unrelated to present pregnancy (P00.1–P00.9)	87	56	27	2.2	1.8	4.2
Newborn affected by maternal complications of pregnancy (P01)	1,561	991	486	39.0	32.3	76.4
Newborn affected by incompetent cervix (P01. 0)	431	242	154	10.8	7.9	24.2
Newborn affected by premature rupture of membranes (P01.1)	781	520	225	19.5	16.9	35.4
Newborn affected by multiple pregnancy (P01.5)	163	99	60	4.1	3.2	9.4
Newborn affected by other maternal complications of pregnancy (P01.2–P01.4,P01.6–P01.9)	186	130	47	4.7	4.2	7.4
Newborn affected by complications of placenta, cord, and membranes (P02)	1,030	643	327	25.8	20.9	51.4
Newborn affected by complications involving placenta (P02.0–P02.3)	492	334	121	12.3	10.9	19.0
Newborn affected by complications involving cord (P02.4–P02.6)	39	26	10	1.0	0.8	*
Newborn affected by chorioamnionitis (P02.7)	497	281	196	12.4	9.2	30.8
Newborn affected by other and unspecified abnormalities of membranes (P02.8–P02.9)	2	2	-	*	*	*
Newborn affected by other complications of labor and delivery (P03)	110	73	33	2.8	2.4	5.2
Newborn affected by noxious influences transmitted via placenta or breast milk (P04)	47	30	15	1.2	1.0	*
Disorders related to length of gestation and fetal malnutrition (P05–P08)	4,233	2,362	1,669	105.8	77.0	262.2
Slow fetal growth and fetal malnutrition (P05)	85	48	34	2.1	1.6	5.3
Disorders related to short gestation and low birth weight, not elsewhere classified (P07)	4,148	2,314	1,635	103.7	75.4	256.9
Extremely low birth weight or extreme immaturity (P07.0, P07.2)	3,176	1,770	1,248	79.4	57.7	196.1
Other low birth weight or preterm (P07.1, P07.3)	972	544	387	24.3	17.7	60.8
Disorders related to long gestation and high birth weight (P08)	-	-	-	*	*	*
Birth trauma (P10–P15)	19	12	4	*	*	*
Intrauterine hypoxia and birth asphyxia (P20–P21)	314	214	76	7.9	7.0	11.9
Intrauterine hypoxia (P20)	136	92	35	3.4	3.0	5.5
Birth asphyxia (P21)	178	122	41	4.5	4.0	6.4

Table 2-46. Number of Infant Deaths and Infant Mortality Rates, by Selected Cause and Race, 2010—*Continued*

(Infant deaths [under 1 year] per 100,000 live births in specified group. Infant deaths based on race of decedent; live births based on race of mother.)

Cause of death (based on ICD–10, 2004)	Number			Rate		
	All races[1]	White[2]	Black[2]	All races[1]	White[2]	Black[2]
Respiratory distress of newborn (P22)	514	318	176	12.9	10.4	27.7
Other respiratory conditions originating in the perinatal period (P23–P28)	812	556	221	20.3	18.1	34.7
Congenital pneumonia (P23)	71	49	22	1.8	1.6	3.5
Neonatal aspiration syndromes (P24)	51	42	6	1.3	1.4	*
Interstitial emphysema and related conditions originating in the perinatal period (P25)	106	83	22	2.7	2.7	3.5
Pulmonary hemorrhage originating in the perinatal period (P26)	167	98	60	4.2	3.2	9.4
Chronic respiratory disease originating in the perinatal period (P27)	106	58	40	2.7	1.9	6.3
Atelectasis (P28.0–P28.1)	248	180	58	6.2	5.9	9.1
All other respiratory conditions originating in the perinatal period (P28.2–P28.9)	63	46	13	1.6	1.5	*
Infections specific to the perinatal period (P35–P39)	745	480	234	18.6	15.6	36.8
Bacterial sepsis of newborn (P36)	583	382	176	14.6	12.4	27.7
Omphalitis of newborn with or without mild hemorrhage (P38)	1	1	-	*	*	*
All other infections specific to the perinatal period (P35,P37,P39)	161	97	58	4.0	3.2	9.1
Hemorrhagic and hematological disorders of newborn (P50–P61)	556	396	140	13.9	12.9	22.0
Neonatal hemorrhage (P50–P52, P54)	469	337	118	11.7	11.0	18.5
Hemorrhagic disease of newborn (P53)	1	1	-	*	*	*
Hemolytic disease of newborn due to isoimmunization and other perinatal jaundice (P55–P59)	7	5	-	*	*	*
Syndrome of infant of a diabetic mother and neonatal diabetes mellitus (P70.0–P70.2)	79	53	22	2.0	1.7	3.5
Necrotizing enterocolitis of newborn (P77)	3	2	1	*	*	*
Hydrops fetalis not due to hemolytic disease (P83.2)	472	282	174	11.8	9.2	27.3
Other perinatal conditions (P29,P70.3–P70.9,P71–P76,P78–P81,P83.0–P83.1, P83.3–P83.9,P90–P96)	150	122	15	3.8	4.0	*
Congenital malformations, deformations and chromosomal abnormalities (Q00–Q99)	5,107	3,822	1,010	127.7	124.5	158.7
Anencephaly and similar malformations (Q00)	293	246	33	7.3	8.0	5.2
Congenital hydrocephalus (Q03)	105	79	17	2.6	2.6	*
Spina bifida (Q05)	15	11	4	*	*	*
Other congenital malformations of nervous system (Q01–Q02,Q04,Q06–Q07)	318	242	58	8.0	7.9	9.1
Congenital malformations of heart (Q20–Q24)	1,148	861	233	28.7	28.1	36.6
Other congenital malformations of circulatory system (Q25–Q28)	176	120	42	4.4	3.9	6.6
Congenital malformations of respiratory system (Q30–Q34)	399	284	95	10.0	9.3	14.9
Congenital malformations of digestive system (Q35–Q45)	88	58	18	2.2	1.9	*
Congenital malformations of genitourinary system (Q50–Q64)	457	346	88	11.4	11.3	13.8
Congenital malformations and deformations of musculoskeletal system, limbs and integument (Q65–Q85)	577	439	106	14.4	14.3	16.7
Down syndrome (Q90)	85	60	16	2.1	2.0	*
Edward's syndrome (Q91.0–Q91.3)	470	363	83	11.8	11.8	13.0
Patau's syndrome (Q91.4–Q91.7)	244	170	63	6.1	5.5	9.9
Other congenital malformations and deformations (Q10–Q18,Q86–Q89)	542	397	116	13.6	12.9	18.2
Other chromosomal abnormalities, not elsewhere classified (Q92–Q99)	190	146	38	4.8	4.8	6.0
Symptoms, signs, and abnormal clinical and laboratory findings, not elsewhere classified (R00–R99)	3,052	1,930	994	76.3	62.9	156.2
Sudden infant death syndrome (R95)	2,063	1,311	668	51.6	42.7	105.0
Other symptoms, signs, and abnormal clinical and laboratory findings, not elsewhere classified R00–R53,R55–R94,R96–R99)	989	619	326	24.7	20.2	51.2
All other diseases (residual)	20	12	8	0.5	*	*
External causes of mortality (*U01,V01–Y84)	1,551	990	490	38.8	32.3	77.0
Accidents (unintentional injuries) (V01–X59)	1,110	703	354	27.8	22.9	55.6
Transport accidents (V01–V99)	81	60	16	2.0	2.0	*
Motor vehicle accidents (V02–V04,V09.0,V09.2,V12–V14,V19.0–V19.2,V19.4–V19.6,V20–V79,V80.3–V80.5, V81.0–V81.1,V82.0–V82.1,V83–V86, V87.0–V87.8,V88.0–V88.8,V89.0,V89.2)	79	58	16	2.0	1.9	*
Other and unspecified transport accidents (V01,V05–V06,V09.1,V09.3–V09.9,V10–V11,V15–V18,V19.3,V19.8– V19.9,V80.0–V80.2,V80.6–V80.9,V81.2–V81.9,V82.2–V82.9,V87.9,V88.9,V89.1,V89.3,V89.9,V90–V99)	2	2	-	*	*	*
Falls (W00–W19)	10	5	5	*	*	*
Accidental discharge of firearms (W32–W34)	-	-	-	*	*	*
Accidental drowning and submersion (W65–W74)	39	31	8	1.0	1.0	*
Accidental suffocation and strangulation in bed (W75)	629	386	217	15.7	12.6	34.1
Other accidental suffocation and strangulation (W76–W77,W81–W84)	218	134	74	5.5	4.4	11.6
Accidental inhalation and ingestion of food or other objects causing obstruction of respiratory tract (W78–W80)	58	33	17	1.5	1.1	*
Accidents caused by exposure to smoke, fire, and flames (X00–X09)	21	17	4	0.5	*	*
Accidental poisoning and exposure to noxious substances (X40–X49)	6	4	1	*	*	*
Other and unspecified accidents (W20–W31,W35–W64,W85–W99,X10–X39,X50–X59)	48	33	12	1.2	1.1	*
Assault (homicide) (*U01,X85–Y09)	311	213	88	7.8	6.9	13.8
Assault (homicide) by hanging, strangulation, and suffocation (X91)	15	14	1	*	*	*
Assault (homicide) by discharge of firearms (*U01.4,X93–X95)	11	8	3	*	*	*
Neglect, abandonment, and other maltreatment syndromes (Y06–Y07)	82	47	32	2.1	1.5	5.0
Assault (homicide) by other and unspecified means (*U01.0–*U01.3,*U01.5–*U01.9,X85–X90,X92,X96–X99, Y00–Y05,Y08–Y09)	203	144	52	5.1	4.7	8.2
Complications of medical and surgical care (Y40–Y84)	22	15	5	0.6	*	*
Other external causes (Y10–Y36)	108	59	43	2.7	1.9	6.8

- = Quantity zero.   * = Figure does not meet standards of reliability or precision.   [1]Includes races other than White and Black.   [2]Race categories are consistent with the 1977 Office of Management and Budget (OMB) births, by 38 states and the District of Columbia. The multiple-race comparability with other reporting areas were bridged to the single-race categories of the 1977 OMB standards for comparability with other reporting areas.

Table 2-47. Number of Infant and Neonatal Deaths and Mortality Rates, by Race, Sex, State, and Territory, 2010

(Infant [under 1 year] and neonatal [under 28 days] deaths per 1,000 live births in specified group. Infant and neonatal deaths are based on race of decedent; live births are based on race of mother.)

Sex, state, and territory	Infant deaths						Neonatal deaths					
	All races[1]		White[2]		Black[2]		All races[1]		White[2]		Black[2]	
	Number	Rate	Number	Rate	Number	Rate	Number	Rate	Number	Rate	Number	Rate
United States [3]	24,586	6.15	15,954	5.20	7,401	11.63	16,188	4.05	10,612	3.46	4,769	7.49
Male	13,702	6.69	8,871	5.65	4,116	12.71	8,953	4.37	5,856	3.73	2,616	8.08
Female	10,884	5.57	7,083	4.73	3,285	10.51	7,235	3.71	4,756	3.18	2,153	6.89
Alabama	523	8.71	269	6.63	250	13.66	326	5.43	159	3.92	164	8.96
Alaska	43	3.75	23	3.26	5	*	22	1.92	13	*	5	*
Arizona	522	5.97	403	5.47	54	12.14	332	3.80	262	3.56	35	7.87
Arkansas	282	7.32	201	6.66	77	10.34	160	4.15	109	3.61	47	6.31
California	2,420	4.74	1,853	4.58	324	9.84	1,682	3.30	1,320	3.26	200	6.07
Colorado	392	5.91	330	5.55	47	13.13	287	4.33	239	4.02	36	10.06
Connecticut	199	5.28	134	4.50	61	11.59	150	3.98	104	3.49	45	8.55
Delaware	87	7.66	49	6.36	37	11.87	58	5.10	30	3.89	27	8.66
District of Columbia	72	7.86	16	*	56	10.48	50	5.46	11	*	39	7.30
Florida	1,403	6.54	773	5.04	610	11.33	934	4.35	514	3.35	406	7.54
Georgia	860	6.42	397	5.05	448	9.11	523	3.90	247	3.14	264	5.37
Hawaii	117	6.16	23	3.92	11	*	76	4.00	14	*	9	*
Idaho	112	4.83	105	4.75	1	*	63	2.72	61	2.76	1	*
Illinois	1,118	6.77	680	5.39	394	13.58	769	4.65	496	3.93	238	8.20
Indiana	640	7.62	476	6.65	153	14.96	417	4.97	321	4.48	87	8.51
Iowa	189	4.88	163	4.61	22	11.18	103	2.66	89	2.52	12	*
Kansas	253	6.22	204	5.71	40	12.35	174	4.28	139	3.89	28	8.65
Kentucky	379	6.79	316	6.43	61	11.12	185	3.32	160	3.25	24	4.38
Louisiana	474	7.60	176	4.86	287	11.75	265	4.25	96	2.65	163	6.67
Maine	70	5.40	66	5.39	3	*	49	3.78	46	3.76	2	*
Maryland	498	6.75	184	4.35	297	11.55	350	4.74	127	3.00	212	8.25
Massachusetts	323	4.43	231	4.03	68	7.22	241	3.31	172	3.00	50	5.31
Michigan	817	7.13	481	5.51	318	14.08	550	4.80	321	3.68	219	9.69
Minnesota	308	4.49	231	4.20	44	6.35	209	3.05	157	2.86	29	4.18
Mississippi	387	9.67	144	6.61	242	13.80	220	5.50	75	3.44	145	8.27
Missouri	507	6.61	362	5.78	139	11.84	318	4.14	220	3.51	93	7.92
Montana	71	5.89	61	5.86	–	*	42	3.48	37	3.55	–	*
Nebraska	136	5.25	107	4.72	26	13.40	96	3.70	72	3.18	21	10.82
Nevada	201	5.59	137	4.76	52	13.83	126	3.51	83	2.88	36	9.57
New Hampshire	51	3.96	47	3.90	3	*	27	2.10	25	2.07	1	*
New Jersey	514	4.81	275	3.64	202	10.39	369	3.45	196	2.60	142	7.30
New Mexico	157	5.64	126	5.48	5	*	95	3.41	79	3.43	2	*
New York	1,243	5.09	731	4.24	439	9.21	866	3.54	527	3.05	285	5.98
North Carolina	858	7.01	461	5.35	367	12.28	603	4.93	320	3.71	265	8.87
North Dakota	62	6.81	42	5.43	3	*	46	5.05	33	4.26	3	*
Ohio	1,072	7.71	695	6.27	360	14.78	728	5.23	486	4.38	230	9.44
Oklahoma	404	7.59	255	6.28	62	12.38	227	4.26	143	3.52	35	6.99
Oregon	225	4.94	192	4.72	14	*	153	3.36	129	3.17	9	*
Pennsylvania	1,039	7.25	696	6.28	325	12.62	736	5.14	503	4.54	218	8.47
Rhode Island	79	7.07	60	6.67	17	*	59	5.28	44	4.89	13	*
South Carolina	430	7.37	199	5.32	221	11.32	266	4.56	120	3.21	138	7.07
South Dakota	82	6.94	57	6.03	1	*	55	4.66	39	4.12	–	*
Tennessee	630	7.93	393	6.55	232	13.28	367	4.62	222	3.70	141	8.07
Texas	2,368	6.13	1,788	5.58	533	11.23	1,508	3.91	1,162	3.62	320	6.74
Utah	254	4.86	223	4.53	8	*	176	3.37	161	3.27	3	*
Vermont	26	4.18	26	4.35	–	*	14	*	14	*	–	*
Virginia	700	6.80	347	4.81	328	14.27	475	4.61	233	3.23	224	9.75
Washington	389	4.50	283	4.02	40	8.22	266	3.07	194	2.76	27	5.55
West Virginia	149	7.28	138	7.08	11	*	81	3.96	74	3.79	7	*
Wisconsin	400	5.84	280	4.88	102	14.61	263	3.84	185	3.22	69	9.88
Wyoming	51	6.75	45	6.37	1	*	31	4.10	29	4.10	–	*
Puerto Rico	341	8.09	330	8.75	10	*	242	5.74	233	6.18	8	*
Virgin Islands	13	*	3	*	10	*	9	*	2	*	7	*
Guam	48	14.05	1	*	–	*	29	8.49	–	*	–	*
American Samoa	14	*	–	*	–	*	8	*	–	*	–	*
Northern Marianas	4	*	–	*	–	*	2	*	–	*	–	*

- = Quantity zero.   * = Figure does not meet standards of reliability or precision.   [1]Includes races other than White and Black.   [2]Race categories are consistent with the 1977 Office of Management and Budget (OMB) births, by 38 states and the District of Columbia. The multiple-race comparability with other reporting areas were bridged to the single-race categories of the 1977 OMB standards for comparability with other reporting areas.   [3]Excludes data for Puerto Rico, Virgin Islands, Guam, American Samoa, and Northern Marianas.

NOTES AND DEFINITIONS

SOURCES OF DATA

Four different publications were used to obtain the mortality data. A significant number of tables came from Murphy SL, Xu JQ, Kochanek KD. *Deaths: Final Data for 2010.* National Vital Statistics Reports; vol. 61, no. 14 Hyattsville, MD: National Center for Health Statistics. 2013. In these tables, the asterisks (*) preceding the cause-of-death codes indicate that they are not part of the *International Classification of Diseases, Tenth Revision (ICD–10), Second Edition.*

Tables 2-9, 2-19, 2-20, 2-22 through 2-26, 2-30, 2-32 through 2-39, and 2-41 through 2-44 are from National Center for Health Statistics. *Health, United States, 2011: With Special Feature on Socioeconomic Status and Health.* Hyattsville, MD. 2012. Some tables have been updated since the publication of this document and are available at http://www.cdc.gov/nchs/hus/contents2011.htm#023.

Tables 2-27 through 2-29 come from the Census of Fatal Occupational Injuries, which can be found on the Web site of the U.S. Department of Commerce's Bureau of Labor Statistics.

Tables 2-40 and 2-48 through 2-52 were derived from National Center for Health Statistics. *Health, United States, 2010: With Special Feature on Death and Dying.* Hyattsville, MD. 2011.

NOTES ON THE DATA

Final data in Part B are based on information from all resident death certificates filed in the 50 states and the District of Columbia. It is believed that more than 99 percent of all deaths that occur in the United States are registered. Data for 2010 are based on records of deaths that occurred during 2010 and were received as of April 12, 2012.

Data shown for geographic areas are by place of residence. Beginning with 1970, mortality statistics for the United States exclude deaths of nonresidents of the United States. All data exclude fetal deaths. Mortality statistics for Puerto Rico, Virgin Islands, American Samoa, and Northern Marianas exclude deaths of nonresidents for each area. For Guam, however, mortality statistics exclude deaths that occurred to a resident of any place other than Guam or the United States.

Race and Hispanic origin are reported separately on the death certificate. Therefore, data shown by race include persons of Hispanic and non-Hispanic origin, and data for Hispanic origin include persons of any race. Unless otherwise specified, deaths of Hispanic origin are included in the totals for each

race group—White, Black, American Indian or Alaska Native (AIAN), and Asian or Pacific Islander (API)—according to the decedent's race as reported on the death certificate. Data shown for Hispanic persons include all persons of Hispanic origin of any race.

Age-adjusted rates are used to compare relative mortality risks among groups and over time. However, they should be viewed as relative indexes rather than as actual measures of mortality risk. They were computed by the direct method—that is, by applying age-specific death rates to the U.S. standard population age distribution. Beginning with the 1999 data year, NCHS adopted a new population standard for use in age-adjusting death rates. Based on the projected year 2000 population of the United States, the new standard replaced the 1940 standard population that had been used for more than 50 years. The new population standard affects levels of mortality and, to some extent, trends and group comparisons. Of particular note are the effects on race mortality comparisons. Beginning with 2003 data, the traditional standard million population along with corresponding standard weights to six decimal places were replaced by the projected year 2000 population age distribution. The effect of the change is negligible and does not significantly affect comparability with age-adjusted rates calculated using the previous method. All age-adjusted rates shown in this report are based on the 2000 U.S. standard population.

Infant mortality rates are the most commonly used index for measuring the risk of dying during the first year of life. The rates presented in this report are calculated by dividing the number of infant deaths in a calendar year by the number of live births registered for the same period, and are presented as rates per 1,000 or per 100,000 live births. For final birth figures used in the denominator for infant mortality rates, see the CDC's *Births: Final Data for 2010* report. In contrast to infant mortality rates based on live births, infant death rates are based on the estimated population under age 1 year. Infant death rates that appear in tabulations of age-specific death rates in this report are calculated by dividing the number of infant deaths by the April 1, 2010, population estimate of persons under age 1, based on 2010 census populations. These rates are presented per 100,000 population in this age group. Because of differences in the denominators, infant death rates may differ from infant mortality rates.

Race and Hispanic origin are reported separately on the death certificate. Therefore, data shown by race include persons of Hispanic and non-Hispanic origin, and data for Hispanic origin include persons of any race. In this report, unless otherwise specified, deaths of persons of Hispanic origin are included in the totals for each race group (White, Black, American Indian and Alaska Native, and Asian or Pacific

Islander) according to the decedent's race as reported on the death certificate. Mortality data for the Hispanic-origin population are based on deaths of residents of all 50 states and the District of Columbia. Death rates for Hispanic, American Indian and Alaska Native, and Asian or Pacific Islander persons should be interpreted with caution because of inconsistencies in reporting Hispanic origin or race on the death certificate compared with censuses, surveys, and birth certificates. Studies have shown underreporting on death certificates of American Indian and Alaska Native, Asian or Pacific Islander, and Hispanic decedents, as well as undercounts of these groups in censuses.

Cause of death statistics are in accordance with the *International Classification of Diseases, Tenth Revision (ICD-10)*.

CONCEPTS AND DEFINITIONS

Age-adjusted death rate—the death rate used to make comparisons of relative mortality risks across groups and over time. This rate should be viewed as a construct or an index rather than as a direct or actual measure of mortality risk. Statistically, it is a weighted average of the age-specific death rates, where the weights represent the fixed population proportions by age.

Age-specific death rate—deaths per 100,000 population in a specified age group, such as 1–4 years or 5–9 years for a specified period.

Cause of death—for the purpose of national mortality statistics, every death is attributed to one underlying condition, based on information reported on the death certificate and using the international rules for selecting the underlying cause of death from the conditions stated on the death certificate. The underlying cause is defined by the World Health Organization as the disease or injury that initiated the train of events leading directly to death, or the circumstances of the accident or violence that produced the fatal injury. Generally more medical information is reported on death certificates than is directly reflected in the underlying cause of death. The conditions that are not selected as underlying cause of death constitute the nonunderlying causes of death, also known as multiple cause of death.

Cause-of-death ranking—selected causes of death of public health and medical importance comprise tabulation lists and are ranked according to the number of deaths assigned to these causes. The top-ranking causes determine the leading causes of death. Certain causes on the tabulation lists are not ranked if, for example, the category title represents a group title (such as major cardiovascular diseases and symptoms,

signs, and abnormal clinical and laboratory findings, not elsewhere classified); or the category title begins with the words "other" and "all other". In addition, when one of the titles that represents a subtotal (such as malignant neoplasms) is ranked, its component parts are not ranked.

Crude death rate—total deaths per 100,000 population for a specified period. The crude death rate represents the average chance of dying during a specified period for persons in the entire population.

Fetal death rate—the number of fetal deaths with stated or presumed gestation of 20 weeks or more, divided by the sum of live births plus fetal deaths, per 1,000 live births plus fetal deaths.

Infant deaths—deaths of infants under 1 year of age.

International Classification of Diseases (ICD)—used to code and classify cause-of-death data. It is developed collaboratively by the World Health Organization and 10 international centers, one of which is housed at NCHS. The purpose of it is to promote international comparability in the collection, classification, processing, and presentation of health statistics. Since 1900, it has been modified about once every 10 years, except for the 20-year interval between the ninth and tenth editions. The purpose of the revisions is to stay abreast with advances in medical science. New revisions usually introduce major disruptions in time series of mortality statistics.

Hispanic origin—includes persons of Mexican, Puerto Rican, Cuban, Central and South American, and other or unknown Latin American or Spanish origins. Persons of Hispanic origin may be of any race.

Late fetal death rate—the number of fetal deaths with stated or presumed gestation of 28 weeks or more, divided by the sum of live births plus late fetal deaths per 1,000 live births plus late fetal deaths.

Life expectancy—the average number of years of life remaining to a person at a particular age and is based on a given set of age-specific death rates, generally the mortality conditions existing in the period mentioned.

Maternal mortality rate—the number of maternal deaths per 100,000 live births. The maternal mortality rate is the measure of the likelihood that a pregnant woman will die from maternal causes.

Neonatal deaths—deaths of infants aged 0–27 days.

Perinatal mortality rate—the sum of late fetal deaths plus infant deaths within 7 days of birth divided by the sum of live births plus late fetal deaths, per 1,000 live births plus late fetal deaths.

Perinatal mortality ratio—the sum of late fetal deaths plus infant deaths within 7 days of birth divided by the number of live births, per 1,000 live births.

Postneonatal deaths—deaths of infants aged 28 days–1 year old.

Years of potential life lost (YPLL)—a measure of premature mortality. YPLL is presented for persons under 75 years of age because the average life expectancy in the United States is over 75 years. YPLL-75 is calculated using the following eight age groups: under 1 year, 1–14 years, 15–24 years, 25–34 years, 35–44 years, 45–54 years, 55–64 years, and 65–74 years. The number of deaths for each age group is multiplied by years of life lost, calculated as the difference between age 75 years and the midpoint of the age group. For the eight age groups, the midpoints are 0.5, 7.5, 19.5, 29.5, 39.5, 49.5, 59.5, and 69.5. For example, the death of a person 15–24 years of age counts as 55.5 years of life lost. Years of potential life lost is derived by summing years of life lost over all age groups.

PART C

HEALTH

CHAPTER 3: DETERMINANTS AND MEASURES OF HEALTH

Figure 3-1. Age-Adjusted Prevalence of Heart Disease, Cancer, and Stroke Among Persons Age 18 Years and Over, Selected Years, 1997–1998 Through 2010–2011

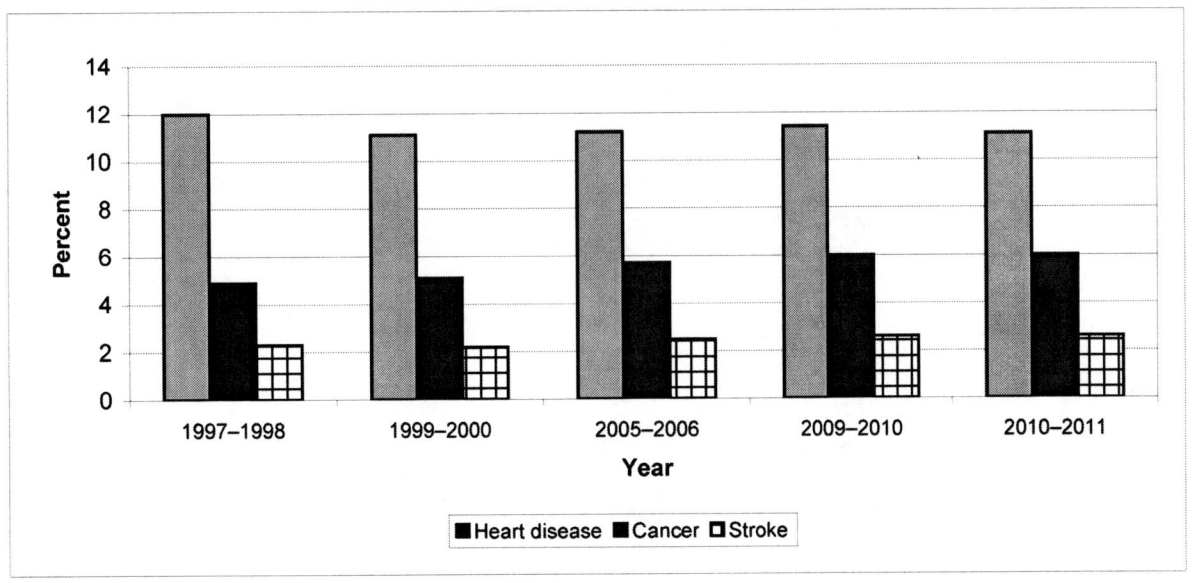

HIGHLIGHTS

- In 2010–2011, according to age-adjusted data, 11.1 percent of people suffered from heart disease, a decline from 12.0 percent in 1997–1998. Although the percent of people with heart disease declined, the percent of people suffering from cancer increased from 4.9 percent to 6.0 percent while and the percent of people suffering from a stroke increased from 2.3 percent to 2.6 percent in the same time period. (Tables 3-6A, 3-6B, and 3-6C)

- In 2010, 41.2 percent of high school seniors reported using alcohol, 21.4 percent of high school students reported using marijuana, 19.2 percent reported using cigarettes, and 1.3 percent reported using cocaine. The percentage of students using each of these drugs declined significantly from 1980 to 2010. (Table 3-32)

- Nearly 23 percent of American Indian or Alaska Natives and Blacks or African Americans had no usual source of health care, compared to 18.9 percent of Whites. (Table 3-34)

- The average length of stay in the hospital declined 7.5 days in 1990 to 4.8 days in 2009–2010. (Table 3-57)

- The mean annual wage for healthcare practitioners and technical occupations in May 2012 was $91,890. Anesthesiologists earned the most at $232,820, while home health aides earned the least at $21,830. (Table 3-63)

- National health care expenditures continued to climb in 2010, increasing to $2.6 billion dollars and representing 17.9 percent of the gross domestic product (GDP). (Table 3-70)

- In 2009–2010, 15.8 percent of people in the United States did not have health insurance. Massachusetts had the highest percentage of insured residents, with only 5.0 percent lacking insurance, while Texas had the highest percentage of uninsured residents at 24.8 percent. (Table 3-84)

Table 3-1. Nonfatal Occupational Injuries and Illnesses with Days Away from Work, Job Transfer, or Restriction, by Industry, Selected Years, 2005–2009

(Cases per 100 full-time workers, number.)

Industry	Injuries and illnesses with days away from work, job transfer, or restriction									
	Cases per 100 full-time workers[1]					Number of cases in thousands[2]				
	2005	2006	2007	2008	2009	2005	2006	2007	2008	2009
Total Private Sector[3]	2.4	2.3	2.1	2.0	1.8	2,184.8	2,114.6	2,036.0	1,900.8	1,667.4
Agriculture, forestry, fishing, and hunting[4]	3.3	3.2	2.8	2.9	2.9	29.5	27.6	26.6	26.0	24.2
Mining	2.2	2.1	2.0	2.0	1.5	13.7	14.0	14.1	16.4	10.7
Utilities	2.4	2.2	2.1	1.9	1.8	12.9	11.8	11.4	10.6	10.0
Construction	3.4	3.2	2.8	2.5	2.3	222.5	223.7	197.5	171.6	136.5
Manufacturing	3.5	3.3	3.0	2.7	2.3	490.8	473.4	427.1	372.9	285.6
Wholesale trade	2.7	2.5	2.4	2.2	2.0	146.8	140.6	139.3	130.9	112.2
Retail trade	2.6	2.6	2.5	2.3	2.2	314.2	308.6	309.1	283.4	254.3
Transportation and warehousing	4.6	4.3	4.3	3.9	3.5	185.6	176.3	179.4	164.3	141.0
Information	1.1	1.0	1.1	1.1	1.0	30.9	28.3	29.1	28.0	25.1
Finance and insurance	0.4	0.3	0.4	0.3	0.2	19.1	17.7	20.7	18.7	12.3
Real estate and rental and leasing	2.1	1.8	1.6	1.8	1.9	37.1	33.0	29.0	32.1	33.3
Professional, scientific, and technical services	0.6	0.5	0.5	0.5	0.5	38.4	34.5	31.8	33.5	34.0
Management of companies and enterprises	1.3	1.1	0.9	0.7	0.8	20.8	17.9	15.1	12.7	14.0
Administrative and support and waste management and remediation services	2.0	1.9	1.8	1.8	1.6	89.5	87.0	89.2	87.0	74.7
Educational services	1.0	0.9	1.0	1.0	0.8	14.8	14.5	15.8	16.0	14.5
Health care and social assistance	2.8	2.7	2.5	2.5	2.4	318.4	310.0	303.7	302.6	304.0
Arts, entertainment, and recreation	2.9	2.5	2.5	2.4	2.3	34.1	28.7	31.9	31.9	29.5
Accommodation and food services	1.7	1.7	1.6	1.5	1.5	120.8	124.6	119.6	116.0	108.5
Other services, except public administration	1.5	1.4	1.5	1.5	1.4	44.8	42.4	45.7	46.2	43.0

[1]Incidence rate calculated as (N/EH) x 200,000, where N = total number of injuries and illnesses, EH = total hours worked by all employees during the calendar year, and 200,000 = base for 100 full-time equivalent employees working 40 hours per week, 50 weeks per year. [2]Because of rounding, components may not add to total number of cases in private sector. [3]Totals include data for industries not shown separately. Excludes self-employed, private households, and employees in federal, state, and local government agencies. [4]Excludes farms with fewer than 11 employees.

Table 3-2A. Selected Notifiable Disease Rates and Number of New Cases, Selected Years, 1950–1995

(Cases per 100,000 population.)

Disease	1950	1960	1970	1980	1990	1995
Rate						
Diphtheria	3.83	0.51	0.21	0.00	0.00	-
Haemophilus influenzae, invasive	NA	NA	NA	NA	NA	0.45
Hepatitis A	NA	NA	27.87	12.84	12.64	12.13
Hepatitis B	NA	NA	4.08	8.39	8.48	4.19
Lyme disease[1]	NA	NA	NA	NA	NA	4.49
Meningococcal disease	NA	NA	1.23	1.25	0.99	1.25
Mumps	NA	NA	55.55	3.86	2.17	0.35
Pertussis (whooping cough)	79.82	8.23	2.08	0.76	1.84	1.97
Poliomyelitis, paralytic[2]	NA	1.40	0.02	0.00	0.00	0.00
Rocky Mountain spotted fever[3]	NA	NA	0.19	0.52	0.26	0.23
Rubella (German measles)	NA	NA	27.75	1.72	0.45	0.05
Rubeola (measles)	211.01	245.42	23.23	5.96	11.17	0.12
Salmonellosis, excluding typhoid fever	NA	3.85	10.84	14.88	19.54	17.66
Shigellosis	15.45	6.94	6.79	8.41	10.89	12.32
Tuberculosis[4]	NA	30.83	18.28	12.25	10.33	8.70
Sexually transmitted diseases[5]						
Syphilis[6]	146.02	68.78	44.80	30.30	54.32	26.05
Primary and secondary	16.73	9.06	10.80	12.00	20.26	6.21
Early latent	39.71	10.11	8.00	8.90	22.19	10.01
Late and late latent[7]	70.22	45.91	24.70	9.20	10.32	9.12
Congenital[8]	368.30	103.70	52.30	7.70	92.95	47.77
Chlamydia[9]	NA	NA	NA	NA	160.19	187.84
Gonorrhea[10]	192.50	145.40	294.20	442.10	276.43	147.46
Chancroid	3.34	0.94	0.70	0.30	1.69	0.23
Number						
Diphtheria	5,796	918	435	3	4	-
Haemophilus influenzae, invasive	NA	NA	NA	NA	NA	1,180
Hepatitis A	NA	NA	56,797	29,087	31,441	31,582
Hepatitis B	NA	NA	8,310	19,015	21,102	10,805
Lyme disease[1]	NA	NA	NA	NA	NA	11,700
Meningococcal disease	NA	NA	2,505	2,840	2,451	3,243
Mumps	NA	NA	104,953	8,576	5,292	906
Pertussis (whooping cough)	120,718	14,809	4,249	1,730	4,570	5,137
Poliomyelitis, paralytic[2]	NA	2,525	31	9	6	7
Rocky Mountain spotted fever[3]	NA	NA	380	1,163	651	590
Rubella (German measles)	NA	NA	56,552	3,904	1,125	128
Rubeola (measles)	319,124	441,703	47,351	13,506	27,786	309
Salmonellosis, excluding typhoid fever	NA	6,929	22,096	33,715	48,603	45,970
Shigellosis	23,367	12,487	13,845	19,041	27,077	32,080
Tuberculosis[4]	NA	55,494	37,137	27,749	25,701	22,860
Sexually transmitted diseases[5]						
Syphilis[6]	217,558	122,538	91,382	68,832	135,590	69,359
Primary and secondary	23,939	16,145	21,982	27,204	50,578	16,543
Early latent	59,256	18,017	16,311	20,297	55,397	26,657
Late and late latent[7]	113,569	81,798	50,348	20,979	25,750	24,296
Congenital[8]	13,377	4,416	1,953	277	3,865	1,863
Chlamydia[9]	NA	NA	NA	NA	323,663	478,577
Gonorrhea[10]	286,746	258,933	600,072	1,004,029	690,042	392,651
Chancroid	4,977	1,680	1,416	788	4,212	607

NOTE: The total resident population was used to calculate all rates except sexually transmitted diseases (STDs), which used the civilian resident population prior to 1991.

NA = Not available.   - = Quantity zero.   0.00 = Rate more than zero but less than 0.005.   [1]National surveillance case definition revised in 2008; probable cases not previously reported.   [2]Cases of vaccine-associated paralytic poliomyelitis caused by polio vaccine virus.   [3]Revision of national surveillance case definition distinguishing between confirmed and probable cases; total case count includes two case reports with unknown case status.   [4]Case reporting for tuberculosis began in 1953. Data prior to 1975 are not comparable with subsequent years because of changes in reporting criteria effective in 1975. Data from 1993 to 2009 were updated through the Division of Tuberculosis Elimination, National Center for HIV/AIDS, Viral Hepatitis, STD, and TB Prevention (NCHHSTP), as of May 14, 2010.   [5]Starting with 1991, data include both civilian and military cases. Adjustments to the number of cases reported from state health departments were made for hardcopy forms and for electronic data submissions through June 9, 2010. For 1950, data for Alaska and Hawaii were not included. Cases and rates shown do not include outlying areas of Guam, Puerto Rico, and the Virgin Islands.   [6]Includes stage of syphilis not stated.   [7]Includes cases of unknown duration.   [8]Rates include all cases of congenitally acquired syphilis per 100,000 live births. Cases of congenitally acquired syphilis were reported through 1994; starting with 1995 data, only congenital syphilis for cases less than 1 year of age were reported.   [9]Prior to 1994, chlamydia was not notifiable. In 1994–1999, cases for New York were exclusively reported by New York City. Starting with 2000 data, includes for New York were exclusively reported by New York City. Starting with 2000 data, includes cases for the entire state.   [10]Data for 1994 do not include cases from Georgia.

Table 3-2B. Selected Notifiable Disease Rates and Number of New Cases, 2005–2009

(Cases per 100,000 population.)

Disease	2005	2006	2007	2008	2009
Rate					
Diphtheria	-	-	-	-	-
Haemophilus influenzae, invasive	0.78	0.82	0.85	0.96	0.99
Hepatitis A	1.53	1.21	1.00	0.86	0.65
Hepatitis B	1.78	1.62	1.51	1.34	1.12
Lyme disease[1]	7.94	6.75	9.21	11.67	12.71
Meningococcal disease	0.42	0.40	0.36	0.39	0.32
Mumps	0.11	2.22	0.27	0.15	0.65
Pertussis (whooping cough)	8.72	5.27	3.49	4.40	5.54
Poliomyelitis, paralytic[2]	-	-	-	-	0.00
Rocky Mountain spotted fever[3]	0.66	0.80	0.77	0.85	0.60
Rubella (German measles)	0.00	0.00	0.00	0.01	0.00
Rubeola (measles)	0.02	0.02	0.01	0.05	0.02
Salmonellosis, excluding typhoid fever	15.43	15.45	16.03	16.92	16.18
Shigellosis	5.51	5.23	6.60	7.50	5.24
Tuberculosis[4]	4.80	4.65	4.44	4.28	3.80
Sexually transmitted diseases[5]					
Syphilis[6]	11.23	12.34	13.57	15.22	14.74
Primary and secondary	2.94	3.26	3.80	4.44	4.60
Early latent	2.76	3.07	3.57	4.08	4.30
Late and late latent[7]	5.41	5.89	6.05	6.56	5.70
Congenital[8]	8.19	8.72	10.20	10.43	10.01
Chlamydia[9]	329.42	344.33	367.47	398.12	409.19
Gonorrhea[10]	114.57	119.70	118.03	110.75	99.05
Chancroid	0.01	0.01	0.01	0.01	0.01
Number					
Diphtheria	-	-	0	0	0
Haemophilus influenzae, invasive	2,304	2,496	2,541	2,886	3,022
Hepatitis A	4,488	3,579	2,979	2,585	1,987
Hepatitis B	5,119	4,713	4,519	4,033	3,405
Lyme disease[1]	23,305	19,931	27,444	35,198	38,468
Meningococcal disease	1,245	1,194	1,077	1,172	980
Mumps	314	6,584	800	454	1,991
Pertussis (whooping cough)	25,616	15,632	10,454	13,278	16,858
Poliomyelitis, paralytic[2]	0	0	0	0	1
Rocky Mountain spotted fever[3]	1,936	2,288	2,221	2,563	1,815
Rubella (German measles)	11	11	12	16	3
Rubeola (measles)	66	55	43	140	71
Salmonellosis, excluding typhoid fever	45,322	45,808	47,995	51,040	49,192
Shigellosis	16,168	15,503	19,758	22,625	15,931
Tuberculosis[4]	14,097	13,779	13,299	12,904	11,545
Sexually transmitted diseases[5]					
Syphilis[6]	33,288	36,958	40,925	46,291	44,828
Primary and secondary	8,724	9,756	11,466	13,500	13,997
Early latent	8,176	9,186	10,768	12,401	13,066
Late and late latent[7]	16,049	17,644	18,256	19,945	17,338
Congenital[8]	339	372	435	445	427
Chlamydia[9]	976,445	1,030,911	1,108,374	1,210,523	1,244,180
Gonorrhea[10]	339,593	358,366	355,991	336,742	301,174
Chancroid	17	19	23	25	28

NOTE: The total resident population was used to calculate all rates except sexually transmitted diseases (STDs), which used the civilian resident population prior to 1991.

NA = Not available.   - = Quantity zero.   0.00 = Rate more than zero but less than 0.005.   [1]National surveillance case definition revised in 2008; probable cases not previously reported.   [2]Cases of vaccine-associated paralytic poliomyelitis caused by polio vaccine virus.   [3]Revision of national surveillance case definition distinguishing between confirmed and probable cases; total case count includes two case reports with unknown case status.   [4]Case reporting for tuberculosis began in 1953. Data prior to 1975 are not comparable with subsequent years because of changes in reporting criteria effective in 1975. Data from 1993 to 2009 were updated through the Division of Tuberculosis Elimination, National Center for HIV/AIDS, Viral Hepatitis, STD, and TB Prevention (NCHHSTP), as of May 14, 2010.   [5]Starting with 1991, data include both civilian and military cases. Adjustments to the number of cases reported from state health departments were made for hardcopy forms and for electronic data submissions through June 9, 2010. For 1950, data for Alaska and Hawaii were not included. Cases and rates shown do not include outlying areas of Guam, Puerto Rico, and the Virgin Islands.   [6]Includes stage of syphilis not stated.   [7]Includes cases of unknown duration.   [8]Rates include all cases of congenitally acquired syphilis per 100,000 live births. Cases of congenitally acquired syphilis were reported through 1994; starting with 1995 data, only congenital syphilis for cases less than 1 year of age were reported.   [9]Prior to 1994, chlamydia was not notifiable. In 1994–1999, cases for New York were exclusively reported by New York City. Starting with 2000 data, includes for New York were exclusively reported by New York City. Starting with 2000 data, includes cases for the entire state.   [10]Data for 1994 do not include cases from Georgia.

Table 3-3. Acquired Immunodeficiency Syndrome (AIDS) Cases, by Year of Diagnosis and Selected Characteristics, 2007–2010

(Number, percent distribution.)

Characteristic	Year of diagnosis				
	All years[1]	2007	2008	2009	2010
Estimated Number of AIDS Diagnoses [2]					
All persons[3]	1,129,127	34,319	33,613	32,942	33,015
Sex and Age					
Male, 13 years and over	893,058	24,979	24,735	24,507	24,749
Female, 13 years and over	226,593	9,304	8,839	8,421	8,242
Children, under 13 years	9,475	36	39	14	23
Region of Residence					
Northeast	343,357	8,824	7,909	7,742	7,824
Midwest	118,260	3,811	3,962	4,019	4,178
South	440,261	15,843	15,721	15,018	14,722
West	227,249	5,840	6,021	6,163	6,292
Male, 13 Years and Over					
Hispanic origin and race	385,023	8,196	7,886	7,683	7,596
Not Hispanic or Latino					
White	327,877	10,450	10,497	10,319	10,754
Black or African American	7,436	360	399	358	408
Asian[4]	723	39	37	46	34
Native Hawaiian or Other Pacific Islander	2,881	86	132	108	126
American Indian or Alaska Native	157,853	5,295	5,268	5,449	5,406
Hispanic or Latino[5]	11,120	552	515	543	426
Multiple race					
Age at Diagnosis					
13 to 14 years	745	28	27	22	20
15 to 24 years	36,920	1,686	1,756	2,000	2,250
25 to 34 years	275,806	5,222	5,304	5,454	5,641
35 to 44 years	349,525	8,803	8,219	7,430	7,110
45 to 54 years	165,995	6,631	6,548	6,723	6,750
55 to 64 years	49,926	2,065	2,278	2,287	2,329
65 years and over	14,140	544	603	591	650
Female, 13 Years and Over					
Hispanic origin and race	43,182	1,474	1,353	1,291	1,275
Not Hispanic or Latina					
White	139,621	5,981	5,783	5,468	5,422
Black or African American	1,274	85	84	87	70
Asian[4]	140	8	4	6	10
Native Hawaiian or Other Pacific Islander	809	41	35	28	44
American Indian or Alaska Native	37,667	1,490	1,371	1,349	1,224
Hispanic or Latina[5]	3,877	224	210	193	197
Multiple race					
Age at Diagnosis					
13 to 14 years	653	51	33	30	31
15 to 24 years	15,611	590	536	547	541
25 to 34 years	72,469	2,060	2,062	1,834	1,746
35 to 44 years	82,599	3,168	2,930	2,676	2,552
45 to 54 years	38,745	2,385	2,295	2,300	2,269
55 to 64 years	12,226	835	802	805	864
65 years and over	4,291	215	181	229	239
Children, Under 13 Years					
Hispanic origin and race	1,599	4	5	1	4
Not Hispanic or Latino					
White	5,731	27	25	8	12
Black or African American	49	0	2	0	1
Asian[4]	7	0	0	0	0
Native Hawaiian or Other Pacific Islander	31	0	0	0	0
American Indian or Alaska Native	1,929	4	3	4	6
Hispanic or Latino[5]	129	0	4	0	0
Multiple race					
Percent Distribution [6]					
All Persons[3]	100.0	100.0	100.0	100.0	100.0
Sex and Age					
Male, 13 years and over	79.1	72.8	73.6	74.4	75.0
Female, 13 years and over	20.1	27.1	26.3	25.6	25.0
Children, under 13 years	0.8	0.1	0.1	0.0	0.1
Region of Residence					
Northeast	30.4	25.7	23.5	23.5	23.7
Midwest	10.5	11.1	11.8	12.2	12.7
South	39.0	46.2	46.8	45.6	44.6
West	20.1	17.0	17.9	18.7	19.1
Male, 13 Years and Over					
Hispanic origin and race	43.1	32.8	31.9	31.4	30.7
Not Hispanic or Latino					
White	36.7	41.8	42.4	42.1	43.5
Black or African American	0.8	1.4	1.6	1.5	1.6
Asian[4]	0.1	0.2	0.2	0.2	0.1
Native Hawaiian or Other Pacific Islander	0.3	0.3	0.5	0.4	0.5
American Indian or Alaska Native	17.7	21.2	21.3	22.2	21.8
Hispanic or Latino[5]	1.2	2.2	2.1	2.2	1.7
Multiple race					
Age at Diagnosis					
13 to 14 years	0.1	0.1	0.1	0.1	0.1
15 to 24 years	4.1	6.8	7.1	8.2	9.1
25 to 34 years	30.9	20.9	21.4	22.3	22.8
35 to 44 years	39.1	35.2	33.2	30.3	28.7
45 to 54 years	18.6	26.5	26.5	27.4	27.3
55 to 64 years	5.6	8.3	9.2	9.3	9.4
65 years and over	1.6	2.2	2.4	2.4	2.6

**Table 3-3. Acquired Immunodeficiency Syndrome (AIDS) Cases, by Year of Diagnosis and Selected Characteristics, 2007–2010
—Continued**

(Number, percent distribution.)

Characteristic	Year of diagnosis				
	All years[1]	2007	2008	2009	2010
Female, 13 Years and Over					
Hispanic origin and race					
Not Hispanic or Latina	19.1	15.8	15.3	15.3	15.5
White					
Black or African American	61.6	64.3	65.4	64.9	65.8
Asian[4]	0.6	0.9	0.9	1.0	0.9
Native Hawaiian or Other Pacific Islander	0.1	0.1	0.0	0.1	0.1
American Indian or Alaska Native	0.4	0.4	0.4	0.3	0.5
Hispanic or Latina[5]	16.6	16.0	15.5	16.0	14.9
Multiple race	1.7	2.4	2.4	2.3	2.4
Age at Diagnosis					
13 to 14 years	0.3	0.5	0.4	0.4	0.4
15 to 24 years	6.9	6.3	6.1	6.5	6.6
25 to 34 years	32.0	22.1	23.3	21.8	21.2
35 to 44 years	36.5	34.1	33.2	31.8	31.0
45 to 54 years	17.1	25.6	26.0	27.3	27.5
55 to 64 years	5.4	9.0	9.1	9.6	10.5
65 years and over	1.9	2.3	2.0	2.7	2.9
Children, Under 13 Years					
Hispanic origin and race					
Not Hispanic or Latino	16.9	11.7	13.3	7.6	15.9
White					
Black or African American	60.5	76.5	62.7	60.3	52.4
Asian[4]	0.5	-	5.4	-	6.2
Native Hawaiian or Other Pacific Islander	0.1	-	-	-	-
American Indian or Alaska Native	0.3	-	-	-	-
Hispanic or Latino[5]	20.4	11.7	8.1	32.1	25.5
Multiple race	1.4	-	10.5	-	-

0.0 = Quantity more than zero but less than 0.05.   - =Quantity zero.   [1]Based on diagnoses reported to CDC from the beginning of the epidemic (1981) through June 30, 2011.   [2]Numbers are point estimates that result from statistical adjustments for reporting delays and missing risk factor information. The estimates do not include adjustments for incomplete reporting.   [3]Total for all years includes 170 persons of unknown race and Hispanic origin. All persons totals were calculated independent of values for subpopulations.   [4]Includes Asian and Pacific Islander legacy cases.   [5]Persons of Hispanic origin may be of any race.   [6]Percents may not sum to 100% due to rounding and because persons of unknown race and Hispanic origin are included in the totals.

Table 3-4. Age-Adjusted Cancer Incidence Rates[1] for Selected Cancer Sites, by Sex, Race, and Hispanic Origin, Selected Geographic Areas, Selected Years, 1990–2009

(Number of new cases per 100,000 population.)

Site, sex, race, and Hispanic origin	1990	1995	2000	2001	2002	2003	2004	2005	2006	2007	2008	2009	2000–2009 APC[2]
All Sites													
All persons	475.6	470.9	474.1	477.6	473.0	461.8	462.7	457.8	457.4	463.7	455.9	450.9	^-0.4
White	483.3	477.5	485.5	489.7	483.4	472.0	472.3	468.7	468.0	472.7	464.4	457.5	^-0.4
Black or African American	513.2	535.1	519.5	511.8	519.6	508.0	512.3	495.8	491.9	500.4	492.4	487.0	^-0.6
American Indian or Alaska Native[3]	347.9	368.1	362.1	393.4	353.2	374.4	399.7	400.1	385.3	366.3	383.2	386.9	0.3
Asian or Pacific Islander	334.2	336.8	336.5	342.9	344.0	333.0	336.8	331.6	327.6	338.7	332.0	324.6	^-0.3
Hispanic or Latino[4]	357.3	359.7	360.7	363.3	368.6	354.8	363.1	360.0	349.5	355.0	349.5	343.6	^-0.3
White, not Hispanic or Latino[4]	495.0	491.3	503.4	508.4	501.1	490.5	490.1	487.2	488.6	493.9	485.5	479.4	^-0.2
Male	583.9	564.1	564.1	565.1	557.0	543.8	543.5	531.5	532.7	543.5	523.1	511.2	^-0.9
White	591.0	563.5	569.1	571.8	562.4	548.4	548.7	538.7	538.6	547.9	526.6	513.3	^-0.9
Black or African American	686.4	736.1	698.9	684.3	685.0	664.1	663.4	627.6	621.0	640.5	629.9	604.5	^-1.2
American Indian or Alaska Native[3]	394.5	421.6	373.0	451.9	378.8	434.4	401.2	421.8	388.7	400.2	416.6	429.2	-0.2
Asian or Pacific Islander	385.2	395.2	393.9	388.7	386.4	383.7	381.3	369.1	369.9	376.4	358.0	344.0	^-0.8
Hispanic or Latino[4]	416.2	439.1	432.4	430.2	434.1	413.0	424.2	412.6	400.2	407.9	392.7	385.1	^-0.7
White, not Hispanic or Latino[4]	606.6	577.5	588.5	591.4	581.0	568.2	567.8	558.5	561.1	572.0	550.4	537.1	^-0.8
Female	411.3	410.3	413.3	417.9	416.2	406.0	407.5	407.6	405.3	407.6	409.7	409.8	-0.1
White	421.4	423.4	430.1	434.6	430.7	420.9	420.4	421.7	419.4	420.3	422.3	420.2	0.0
Black or African American	404.4	400.7	398.7	395.1	409.9	403.9	412.6	407.9	404.3	406.0	399.3	408.3	0.0
American Indian or Alaska Native[3]	316.5	334.0	360.6	356.1	333.1	334.7	404.7	385.5	387.8	346.5	365.4	361.0	^0.8
Asian or Pacific Islander	294.1	293.9	297.1	312.5	317.5	300.1	308.8	308.5	301.3	315.4	318.1	316.2	^0.4
Hispanic or Latina[4]	325.8	311.3	318.5	321.8	328.6	319.6	326.0	327.8	318.7	322.9	324.6	319.3	0.1
White, not Hispanic or Latina[4]	430.3	436.7	446.0	452.1	447.1	437.8	436.4	438.5	437.8	438.0	440.5	439.8	0.1
Lung and Bronchus													
Male	95.0	86.9	77.7	77.2	75.6	75.4	71.6	71.4	69.6	68.7	66.7	64.9	^-2.0
White	94.2	85.0	76.4	76.3	74.9	74.2	70.3	70.6	68.3	68.0	65.3	63.9	^-2.0
Black or African American	133.9	136.7	110.6	112.5	108.9	111.5	102.1	98.3	98.3	94.4	95.6	91.5	^-2.3
American Indian or Alaska Native[3]	74.9	83.0	62.8	81.5	46.2	71.4	59.4	67.0	64.2	60.3	68.0	58.0	-0.9
Asian or Pacific Islander	64.2	60.0	63.2	57.1	57.7	58.4	59.5	57.9	57.5	55.1	55.5	52.0	^-1.0
Hispanic or Latino[4]	59.3	52.3	45.3	42.4	48.1	45.4	39.6	42.4	38.2	42.1	37.7	35.7	^-2.1
White, not Hispanic or Latino[4]	97.5	88.4	80.3	80.8	78.4	78.0	74.7	74.7	72.8	72.0	69.6	68.4	^-1.8
Female	47.2	49.3	48.6	48.8	49.4	49.7	48.9	49.7	49.0	48.9	47.4	47.5	0.0
White	48.5	51.8	50.8	50.8	51.6	52.3	50.4	51.6	50.9	51.4	49.7	49.2	0.0
Black or African American	52.9	49.7	54.6	54.7	55.0	54.4	57.1	57.4	56.6	53.8	52.5	54.2	0.2
American Indian or Alaska Native[3]	Y	46.2	38.7	36.6	39.7	40.6	56.6	45.3	44.0	34.4	44.9	33.1	^1.6
Asian or Pacific Islander	28.3	27.1	27.2	30.0	29.3	29.1	31.0	30.9	30.2	28.6	27.8	30.7	^0.4
Hispanic or Latina[4]	26.4	25.1	24.1	25.2	24.9	25.0	26.2	23.7	23.6	25.0	24.3	25.1	^-0.5
White, not Hispanic or Latina[4]	50.8	54.9	54.4	54.4	55.5	56.5	54.2	56.0	55.3	55.8	54.0	53.4	0.2
Colon and Rectum													
Male	72.3	63.2	62.6	61.6	60.0	58.3	56.6	54.4	53.1	52.7	51.2	48.3	^-1.8
White	73.0	62.5	62.2	61.1	58.9	57.0	55.6	53.9	51.8	51.3	49.9	46.5	^-2.0
Black or African American	72.7	74.5	72.7	71.4	72.6	75.8	73.7	66.4	65.3	66.6	65.7	60.4	^-0.9
American Indian or Alaska Native[3]	62.0	65.3	48.2	62.0	49.7	68.1	53.9	65.6	47.5	52.1	48.6	63.1	-0.5
Asian or Pacific Islander	60.8	58.2	57.3	56.4	58.4	52.8	50.0	47.4	51.4	49.1	46.9	46.3	^-1.4
Hispanic or Latino[4]	47.3	45.7	50.1	49.0	45.1	46.2	47.1	45.6	45.2	44.0	45.5	42.9	^-0.6
White, not Hispanic or Latino[4]	75.1	64.0	63.6	62.5	60.4	58.3	56.6	54.9	52.8	52.2	50.5	47.0	^-2.1
Female	50.2	45.9	46.0	45.3	45.1	43.4	41.9	41.2	41.0	39.9	39.3	37.7	^-1.3
White	49.7	45.5	45.6	44.4	44.1	42.8	40.7	40.0	40.0	38.8	38.4	36.0	^-1.4
Black or African American	61.1	54.7	57.8	56.2	55.9	55.0	53.6	53.3	53.1	51.6	47.9	49.7	^-0.8
American Indian or Alaska Native[3]	45.9	46.7	39.2	49.9	49.6	44.1	66.6	47.6	48.4	43.8	46.8	43.5	0.2
Asian or Pacific Islander	37.7	38.4	37.2	41.0	41.6	36.5	37.5	37.2	35.8	35.6	35.6	34.8	^-0.7
Hispanic or Latina[4]	34.9	32.1	34.2	32.9	31.8	34.4	33.0	33.1	32.5	34.0	31.6	30.8	^-0.3
White, not Hispanic or Latina[4]	50.8	46.7	46.8	45.8	45.5	43.7	41.7	41.0	41.0	39.3	39.5	36.8	^-1.4
Prostate													
Male	166.8	166.3	178.4	179.6	177.6	165.0	164.9	153.3	163.2	166.1	151.2	146.7	^-1.4
White	168.4	161.3	174.5	177.1	174.1	160.9	161.4	148.6	159.0	159.7	145.6	140.0	^-1.6
Black or African American	218.9	275.9	287.8	270.1	278.8	251.7	249.6	237.9	239.0	250.6	234.5	229.0	^-1.3
American Indian or Alaska Native[3]	99.6	92.6	69.8	97.7	92.4	108.8	88.2	92.0	87.8	91.7	79.4	91.3	^-1.5
Asian or Pacific Islander	88.4	103.5	106.0	107.5	102.6	103.6	101.7	95.0	96.2	98.8	86.6	82.0	^-1.1
Hispanic or Latino[4]	118.7	140.2	148.5	145.3	149.0	135.5	145.7	128.9	129.1	127.4	120.7	116.8	^-1.1
White, not Hispanic or Latino[4]	172.1	163.7	178.5	181.5	177.6	164.8	163.9	151.7	163.9	165.7	150.6	145.0	^-1.5
Breast													
Female	129.3	130.8	134.0	135.7	132.7	124.0	124.7	124.1	122.6	125.6	125.9	127.2	-0.3
White	134.3	136.4	140.8	142.7	138.7	128.9	128.8	129.2	126.6	129.2	128.7	130.3	^-0.3
Black or African American	116.7	122.3	120.5	116.6	122.2	121.8	122.0	117.0	121.9	124.5	123.4	126.0	0.2
American Indian or Alaska Native[3]	69.9	94.5	98.8	96.7	79.3	93.2	101.9	106.1	87.9	91.7	90.5	99.6	0.5
Asian or Pacific Islander	87.5	86.6	93.4	100.6	100.3	92.1	97.3	95.5	94.3	101.3	104.9	102.0	^0.9
Hispanic or Latina[4]	91.8	90.1	96.9	91.9	94.0	88.0	91.6	93.4	91.7	91.7	93.7	91.4	0.1
White, not Hispanic or Latina[4]	138.5	141.9	147.2	150.4	145.7	135.5	135.3	135.7	132.8	136.0	135.2	138.0	-0.2
Cervix uteri													
Female	11.9	9.9	8.9	8.8	8.4	8.2	7.8	7.9	7.6	7.4	7.5	7.4	^-2.5
White	11.2	9.2	8.9	8.4	8.3	7.9	7.7	7.7	7.6	7.3	7.4	7.4	^-2.2
Black or African American	16.4	14.7	10.6	10.8	10.0	10.6	9.8	9.1	8.1	8.2	9.0	7.9	^-3.8
American Indian or Alaska Native[3]	Y	Y	Y	Y	Y	Y	Y	Y	Y	Y	Y	Y	Y
Asian or Pacific Islander	12.1	11.0	7.9	9.6	8.2	8.1	7.2	8.0	7.1	7.1	6.4	7.0	^-3.8
Hispanic or Latina[4]	21.4	17.4	17.1	15.1	14.7	14.3	13.3	13.9	11.9	10.9	11.9	10.4	^-3.6
White, not Hispanic or Latina[4]	9.7	7.8	7.1	7.0	6.9	6.4	6.5	6.3	6.6	6.4	6.3	6.5	^-2.2

Table 3-4. Age-Adjusted Cancer Incidence Rates[1] for Selected Cancer Sites, by Sex, Race, and Hispanic Origin, Selected Geographic Areas, Selected Years, 1990–2009—*Continued*

(Number of new cases per 100,000 population.)

Site, sex, race, and Hispanic origin	1990	1995	2000	2001	2002	2003	2004	2005	2006	2007	2008	2009	2000–2009 APC[2]
Corpus and Uterus, Not Otherwise Specified													
Female	24.7	24.9	23.8	24.7	24.0	23.6	24.0	24.1	24.1	24.5	25.3	26.5	0.1
White	26.4	26.4	25.6	26.1	24.8	24.9	25.2	25.4	25.5	25.3	26.1	27.1	-0.1
Black or African American	16.9	17.7	17.2	20.3	22.0	20.2	20.6	21.3	18.9	22.9	23.6	25.4	^2.0
American Indian or Alaska Native[3]	Y	Y	Y	19.6	18.8	19.6	17.3	Y	22.7	22.0	19.8	30.2	Y
Asian or Pacific Islander	13.5	17.7	16.5	17.8	19.0	16.9	19.2	19.2	18.4	19.8	20.8	21.6	^1.8
Hispanic or Latina[4]	18.0	16.5	16.2	17.3	17.7	18.0	19.6	19.6	18.3	19.2	19.4	21.1	^1.0
White, not Hispanic or Latina[4]	27.0	27.5	26.8	27.3	25.7	25.9	25.8	26.1	26.5	26.2	27.2	28.0	-0.1
Ovary													
Female	15.5	14.6	14.2	14.2	13.9	13.5	13.1	13.1	12.8	13.0	12.8	12.4	^-1.0
White	16.4	15.4	15.1	15.4	14.7	14.2	13.8	13.8	13.5	13.6	13.5	13.1	^-1.1
Black or African American	11.3	10.9	10.7	9.4	9.8	11.4	11.0	10.5	8.9	11.3	9.9	9.8	-0.4
American Indian or Alaska Native[3]	Y	Y	19.0	Y	Y	Y	Y	Y	16.0	Y	Y	16.8	Y
Asian or Pacific Islander	11.2	10.4	10.2	9.7	12.1	10.3	10.0	11.0	10.6	10.6	10.2	9.7	-0.1
Hispanic or Latina[4]	12.3	11.7	10.9	13.4	13.9	12.0	11.9	11.8	10.9	11.2	12.0	10.0	-0.5
White, not Hispanic or Latina[4]	16.7	15.9	15.6	15.7	14.6	14.6	14.0	14.0	14.1	14.0	13.7	13.5	^-1.1
Oral Cavity and Pharynx													
Male	18.5	16.5	15.8	15.1	15.7	15.2	15.3	15.0	14.8	15.3	15.7	15.6	^-1.0
White	18.0	16.3	15.6	15.4	15.8	15.2	15.6	15.3	14.9	15.6	16.1	16.0	^-0.7
Black or African American	25.4	22.3	19.3	18.1	17.9	17.3	16.2	15.8	15.8	16.0	14.4	14.6	^-2.8
American Indian or Alaska Native[3]	Y	Y	Y	Y	Y	Y	Y	Y	Y	Y	Y	Y	Y
Asian or Pacific Islander	14.8	11.7	13.2	9.9	12.8	11.7	11.4	11.5	11.4	11.2	12.8	11.5	^-1.0
Hispanic or Latino[4]	10.8	12.3	9.0	9.2	9.4	8.8	10.1	9.3	7.5	8.9	9.9	10.7	^-1.1
White, not Hispanic or Latino[4]	18.8	16.9	16.7	16.3	16.9	16.3	16.6	16.4	16.2	17.0	17.3	17.1	^-0.5
Female	7.3	7.0	6.2	6.6	6.5	5.9	6.1	6.1	6.2	6.0	6.2	6.0	^-1.0
White	7.4	7.1	6.2	6.6	6.5	5.8	6.1	6.0	6.2	6.1	6.3	6.0	^-1.1
Black or African American	6.4	6.6	5.3	6.5	6.3	6.7	5.9	6.8	5.4	5.5	4.9	6.1	^-1.1
American Indian or Alaska Native[3]	Y	Y	Y	Y	Y	Y	Y	Y	Y	Y	Y	Y	Y
Asian or Pacific Islander	6.1	5.2	6.1	5.8	6.0	5.2	5.7	6.0	5.3	5.2	5.8	4.6	^-0.9
Hispanic or Latina[4]	4.1	3.7	3.7	4.1	3.7	3.9	3.6	3.4	4.0	4.1	4.4	4.1	-0.5
White, not Hispanic or Latina[4]	7.8	7.6	6.6	7.0	7.1	6.2	6.5	6.4	6.6	6.5	6.6	6.4	^-1.0
Stomach													
Male	14.6	13.5	12.6	11.8	12.0	11.7	11.9	11.4	11.2	11.4	10.5	11.1	^-1.7
White	12.8	11.9	10.7	10.3	10.4	10.1	10.3	9.6	9.7	9.7	9.2	9.7	^-1.7
Black or African American	21.4	18.6	18.4	17.5	15.8	18.5	16.4	17.4	16.2	17.5	16.7	15.1	^-2.0
American Indian or Alaska Native[3]	Y	Y	Y	Y	Y	Y	Y	Y	Y	Y	Y	Y	Y
Asian or Pacific Islander	26.8	24.5	22.7	19.1	20.4	19.1	20.1	20.0	18.0	18.1	15.6	17.1	^-2.7
Hispanic or Latino[4]	20.2	19.4	16.0	15.7	16.1	15.8	16.6	15.0	14.9	16.7	14.9	15.0	^-1.8
White, not Hispanic or Latino[4]	12.1	11.1	10.0	9.4	9.6	9.2	9.3	8.7	8.8	8.5	8.1	8.7	^-2.0
Female	6.7	6.2	6.1	5.8	6.2	6.0	5.9	5.7	5.9	5.6	5.5	5.7	^-0.9
White	5.7	5.1	5.0	4.7	5.1	4.9	5.0	4.7	5.0	4.5	4.5	4.4	^-1.1
Black or African American	9.9	9.8	8.6	9.0	9.9	9.5	7.5	8.0	9.5	7.7	8.0	8.8	^-1.2
American Indian or Alaska Native[3]	Y	Y	Y	Y	Y	Y	Y	Y	Y	Y	Y	Y	Y
Asian or Pacific Islander	15.4	13.0	12.9	12.2	11.3	11.2	11.2	10.5	9.3	10.6	10.0	10.6	^-2.4
Hispanic or Latina[4]	10.8	11.3	10.8	10.3	10.6	10.2	10.2	10.3	9.8	9.4	8.5	8.1	^-1.1
White, not Hispanic or Latina[4]	5.1	4.4	4.2	3.8	4.2	4.1	4.1	3.7	4.1	3.5	3.6	3.7	^-1.8
Pancreas													
Male	13.0	12.7	12.8	12.8	12.8	12.5	13.4	13.6	13.6	13.9	13.8	13.8	^0.5
White	12.7	12.4	12.6	12.9	13.0	12.3	13.2	13.4	13.8	13.8	13.6	13.8	^0.6
Black or African American	19.3	19.1	18.1	15.6	13.7	17.2	18.1	18.2	17.3	16.6	18.5	18.2	-0.4
American Indian or Alaska Native[3]	Y	Y	Y	Y	Y	Y	Y	Y	Y	Y	Y	Y	Y
Asian or Pacific Islander	11.0	10.3	10.7	9.8	9.8	10.1	11.9	11.7	10.5	11.9	11.7	10.4	0.0
Hispanic or Latino[4]	10.7	12.0	12.2	9.6	10.7	9.7	11.2	11.8	12.2	11.4	11.0	12.7	0.7
White, not Hispanic or Latino[4]	12.8	12.4	12.7	13.3	13.3	12.7	13.4	13.5	14.0	14.2	14.0	13.9	^0.7
Female	10.0	9.9	9.9	9.8	10.4	10.3	10.3	10.8	10.9	10.6	10.8	10.9	^0.5
White	9.7	9.6	9.6	9.5	10.1	10.2	10.1	10.5	10.5	10.4	10.5	10.7	^0.5
Black or African American	12.9	15.5	12.6	13.5	15.8	14.3	14.4	16.2	15.1	14.5	15.1	14.4	-0.1
American Indian or Alaska Native[3]	Y	Y	Y	Y	Y	Y	Y	Y	Y	Y	Y	Y	Y
Asian or Pacific Islander	9.9	8.1	9.2	9.1	8.9	8.2	9.0	8.1	9.7	8.9	9.1	9.6	^0.8
Hispanic or Latina[4]	9.9	8.9	9.2	9.9	10.8	8.8	9.2	11.4	9.6	10.6	9.5	9.2	0.0
White, not Hispanic or Latina[4]	9.7	9.7	9.6	9.5	10.0	10.4	10.3	10.4	10.6	10.3	10.7	11.0	^0.6
Urinary bladder													
Male	37.2	35.4	36.8	36.9	35.7	36.8	36.9	36.8	35.9	37.1	35.2	34.4	-0.2
White	40.7	38.9	40.8	41.1	39.3	40.6	40.9	40.6	39.5	41.0	38.5	37.5	-0.1
Black or African American	19.5	19.3	20.2	19.3	20.5	22.7	22.6	22.7	19.7	21.6	22.5	21.3	0.5
American Indian or Alaska Native[3]	Y	Y	Y	Y	Y	Y	Y	Y	Y	Y	Y	Y	Y
Asian or Pacific Islander	15.4	16.4	16.5	17.0	19.4	17.7	17.0	17.0	18.6	17.9	18.1	17.1	^1.0
Hispanic or Latino[4]	22.1	17.8	20.3	21.5	20.5	19.6	18.9	19.3	19.7	19.7	16.1	17.4	^-0.7
White, not Hispanic or Latino[4]	42.4	41.0	43.2	43.5	41.7	43.3	43.8	43.5	42.3	44.2	41.9	40.7	0.1
Female	9.5	9.3	9.1	9.1	9.1	9.2	9.2	8.9	8.8	8.5	8.7	8.3	^-0.5
White	10.0	10.1	9.9	10.0	10.1	9.9	10.0	9.6	9.4	9.3	9.5	9.0	^-0.4
Black or African American	8.6	7.2	7.7	7.2	8.5	7.7	8.2	7.7	8.6	7.5	6.3	6.7	-0.3
American Indian or Alaska Native[3]	Y	Y	Y	Y	Y	Y	Y	Y	Y	Y	Y	Y	Y
Asian or Pacific Islander	5.3	4.4	4.1	4.6	3.2	4.9	3.9	5.1	3.7	3.8	5.0	3.7	-0.3
Hispanic or Latina[4]	6.0	5.3	5.7	5.3	6.4	4.4	5.7	6.2	5.3	5.2	5.4	4.6	-0.6
White, not Hispanic or Latina[4]	10.3	10.6	10.5	10.6	10.6	10.8	10.6	10.1	10.1	10.0	10.2	9.7	-0.2

Table 3-4. Age-Adjusted Cancer Incidence Rates[1] for Selected Cancer Sites, by Sex, Race, and Hispanic Origin, Selected Geographic Areas, Selected Years, 1990–2009—Continued

(Number of new cases per 100,000 population.)

Site, sex, race, and Hispanic origin	1990	1995	2000	2001	2002	2003	2004	2005	2006	2007	2008	2009	2000–2009 APC[2]
Non-Hodgkin's Lymphoma													
Male	22.6	25.0	23.5	24.0	23.8	24.1	25.0	24.4	23.7	24.7	24.4	24.2	0.2
White	23.6	26.2	24.9	25.1	25.0	25.6	26.2	25.6	25.1	26.3	25.5	25.2	^0.2
Black or African American	17.4	21.4	17.5	18.2	18.0	19.1	22.0	19.3	19.4	17.5	18.0	18.8	0.0
American Indian or Alaska Native[3]	Y	Y	Y	Y	Y	Y	Y	Y	Y	Y	Y	Y	Y
Asian or Pacific Islander	16.7	16.5	15.9	17.6	16.3	16.3	16.3	17.9	15.2	16.7	17.8	16.7	0.1
Hispanic or Latino[4]	17.3	21.0	20.3	18.5	20.2	19.1	21.0	19.1	18.5	20.1	20.2	18.8	0.1
White, not Hispanic or Latino[4]	24.3	26.7	25.4	25.9	25.7	26.4	26.9	26.7	26.2	27.4	26.4	26.4	^0.4
Female	14.5	15.2	16.0	16.2	16.4	17.1	17.3	16.3	16.8	16.6	16.4	16.6	^0.8
White	15.4	16.0	16.9	17.0	17.4	17.9	18.2	17.5	17.9	17.5	17.1	17.5	^0.8
Black or African American	10.3	10.1	11.7	12.5	11.7	13.2	13.4	13.0	12.3	13.0	12.8	11.9	^1.6
American Indian or Alaska Native[3]	Y	Y	Y	Y	Y	Y	Y	Y	Y	Y	Y	Y	Y
Asian or Pacific Islander	9.1	11.8	11.4	12.8	12.2	12.7	12.4	9.7	11.1	11.6	12.3	11.6	0.7
Hispanic or Latina[4]	13.8	13.2	13.6	14.4	13.9	15.3	15.7	15.1	15.3	14.6	14.6	17.0	^1.1
White, not Hispanic or Latina[4]	15.6	16.2	17.3	17.5	18.0	18.3	18.6	17.8	18.3	18.1	17.4	17.6	^0.9
Leukemia													
Male	17.1	17.6	16.9	17.7	16.9	17.1	16.9	16.9	16.0	16.7	16.5	16.1	^-0.2
White	18.0	18.9	18.0	19.0	18.3	18.1	17.8	18.3	17.1	18.1	17.4	16.9	-0.2
Black or African American	16.0	13.3	13.8	13.3	12.6	14.5	16.3	12.4	13.9	13.0	13.6	13.4	-0.1
American Indian or Alaska Native[3]	Y	Y	Y	Y	Y	Y	Y	Y	Y	Y	Y	Y	Y
Asian or Pacific Islander	8.5	10.0	10.3	10.4	9.3	10.3	10.1	9.1	8.7	9.3	9.8	9.1	-0.4
Hispanic or Latino[4]	12.1	14.6	12.9	11.0	12.1	11.9	12.4	12.7	12.6	11.2	11.6	11.3	-0.2
White, not Hispanic or Latino[4]	18.2	19.2	18.5	19.7	18.9	18.7	18.3	18.7	17.3	18.8	17.9	17.7	-0.1
Female	9.9	10.2	10.3	10.4	9.9	9.9	10.2	9.8	10.5	9.7	10.3	9.5	0.0
White	10.3	10.8	10.9	11.2	10.7	10.4	10.8	10.2	11.2	10.4	10.7	9.9	0.0
Black or African American	8.5	8.2	9.7	9.1	7.4	8.9	9.6	9.1	8.2	7.5	7.4	7.3	-0.5
American Indian or Alaska Native[3]	Y	Y	Y	Y	Y	Y	Y	Y	Y	Y	Y	Y	Y
Asian or Pacific Islander	5.7	6.3	6.3	5.2	6.3	6.4	6.4	6.4	6.5	6.1	7.0	6.7	0.2
Hispanic or Latina[4]	8.6	8.2	7.8	7.6	8.5	7.0	9.1	8.3	8.9	7.7	9.3	8.0	0.2
White, not Hispanic or Latina[4]	10.2	11.0	10.9	11.6	10.7	10.9	10.9	10.2	11.5	10.7	10.7	10.0	0.1

NOTE: Estimates are based on 13 SEER areas, November 2011 submission and differ from published estimates based on 9 SEER areas or other submission dates. The site variable distinguishes Kaposi Sarcoma and Mesothelioma as individual cancer sites. As a result, Kaposi Sarcoma and Mesothelioma cases do not contribute to other cancer sites.

^ =Annual percent change (APC) is significantly different from 0 (p<0.05).   0.0 = APC is greater than -0.05 but less than 0.05.   Y = Estimate not shown. Rate based on less than 25 cases for the time interval. Trend based on less than 10 cases.   [1] Age adjusted by 5-year age groups to the year 2000 U.S. standard population. Age-adjusted rates are based on at least 25 cases.   [2] APC has been calculated by fitting a linear regression model to the natural logarithm of the yearly rates from 1990–2009.   [3] Starting with Health, United States, 2007, estimates for American Indian or Alaska Native population are based on the Contract Health Service Delivery Area (CHSDA) counties within SEER areas.   [4] Hispanic data exclude cases from Alaska. The race groups White, Black, Asian or Pacific Islander, and American Indian or Alaska Native, include persons of Hispanic and non-Hispanic origin. Persons of Hispanic origin may be of any race. The North American Association of Central Cancer Registries (NAACCR) Hispanic Identification Algorithm was used on a combination of variables to classify cases as Hispanic for analytic purposes.

Table 3-5. Five-Year Relative Cancer Survival Rates for Selected Cancer Sites, by Sex and Selected Race, Selected Geographic Areas, Selected Years, 1975–1977 Through 2002–2008

(Percent of patients.)

Sex and site	White										Black or African American									
	1975–1977	1978–1980	1981–1983	1984–1986	1987–1989	1990–1992	1993–1995	1996–1998	1999–2001	2002–2008	1975–1977	1978–1980	1981–1983	1984–1986	1987–1989	1990–1992	1993–1995	1996–1998	1999–2001	2002–2008
Both Sexes																				
All sites	50.0	50.1	51.5	53.8	56.8	61.5	62.5	64.5	67.3	68.9	39.2	39.0	39.0	40.2	43.1	47.9	52.8	55.1	57.8	59.9
Oral cavity and pharynx	54.4	55.5	54.2	56.5	56.3	58.1	60.3	60.0	62.3	66.5	36.1	35.0	31.4	35.1	33.9	32.5	38.0	36.3	44.3	45.2
Esophagus	5.5	5.3	7.3	10.4	10.6	13.0	13.5	14.2	18.8	20.5	3.2	4.3	4.3	8.7	6.6	9.2	7.5	10.2	12.9	13.5
Stomach	14.2	15.5	16.2	17.0	18.5	18.8	20.0	20.6	22.5	26.6	16.1	16.5	16.6	19.1	18.8	22.8	19.5	22.4	22.5	28.3
Colon	51.1	52.6	55.7	59.2	60.9	63.0	60.8	63.2	66.9	66.2	45.3	48.9	48.7	49.3	52.5	53.5	51.5	53.5	52.6	55.4
Rectum	48.4	49.9	52.4	57.3	58.8	60.2	60.8	63.9	66.8	68.8	44.6	34.9	39.8	45.8	52.3	51.3	53.9	55.3	59.4	60.7
Pancreas	2.5	2.5	2.6	2.6	3.2	4.4	3.9	4.2	4.9	6.2	2.3	5.6	3.6	4.6	5.5	3.7	3.4	3.4	5.5	4.8
Lung and bronchus	12.3	12.9	13.4	13.1	13.4	14.0	14.6	14.9	15.5	17.3	11.4	11.8	11.4	11.2	11.0	10.5	12.8	12.4	12.6	13.5
Urinary bladder	73.5	74.9	77.7	77.5	80.0	80.6	81.4	80.1	81.4	80.7	50.3	54.6	59.7	59.7	62.5	63.4	60.0	62.1	67.3	62.1
Non-Hodgkin's lymphoma	47.0	48.1	51.1	52.1	51.6	51.7	53.5	59.7	65.1	71.8	48.4	51.1	49.9	47.1	46.4	42.1	42.0	54.0	55.8	62.8
Leukemia	34.8	36.9	38.4	41.8	44.1	46.5	48.4	49.2	50.9	58.8	33.1	28.5	33.9	32.9	35.3	36.0	41.3	37.8	42.0	51.4
Male																				
All sites	42.9	44.5	46.8	48.8	53.0	61.0	62.2	64.2	67.6	69.7	32.9	33.4	34.3	35.6	39.0	47.7	54.4	57.8	60.9	63.6
Oral cavity and pharynx	54.1	54.6	53.1	55.0	54.3	56.6	59.7	59.3	62.3	66.5	29.8	30.0	26.0	29.5	29.8	27.8	33.0	31.3	39.0	41.3
Esophagus	4.8	5.3	6.5	9.2	11.1	12.4	13.7	14.1	18.6	20.6	1.6	3.4	3.7	8.2	5.3	9.4	7.8	8.5	11.1	12.5
Stomach	13.2	13.7	15.4	14.6	15.7	16.1	19.0	18.9	21.3	24.9	16.1	15.6	16.5	17.0	16.6	22.1	17.5	20.3	24.2	22.8
Colon	50.8	51.6	56.4	59.8	61.7	63.2	61.0	63.2	68.0	66.9	43.9	47.5	44.9	48.9	50.9	55.0	51.0	55.3	53.8	53.4
Rectum	47.5	49.5	51.3	56.7	59.1	59.4	59.7	63.2	66.9	69.2	41.8	34.0	37.3	43.5	47.7	53.5	51.6	54.0	60.3	58.1
Pancreas	2.6	2.6	2.2	2.1	3.1	4.2	3.6	4.7	5.3	5.9	2.6	4.1	3.7	3.9	5.1	3.2	3.3	3.1	3.7	4.5
Lung and bronchus	11.1	11.5	11.8	11.4	12.1	12.5	12.7	13.1	13.3	15.2	10.7	9.8	10.2	10.5	10.8	9.3	11.3	10.9	10.8	12.6
Prostate gland	69.0	71.7	73.5	76.8	84.8	94.4	96.1	98.1	99.9	99.9	61.0	62.1	63.2	65.8	71.5	84.7	91.8	95.0	97.4	97.7
Urinary bladder	74.6	75.7	78.9	78.7	82.2	83.0	82.8	81.4	81.9	82.2	56.5	62.7	64.9	62.8	67.6	66.1	67.0	64.8	71.6	66.8
Non-Hodgkin's lymphoma	46.4	46.4	50.7	50.8	48.4	47.7	50.0	57.8	63.0	71.0	42.6	47.1	49.4	44.5	41.7	38.2	36.0	52.5	49.0	58.7
Leukemia	33.8	35.9	38.2	41.5	45.8	46.3	49.3	49.1	51.9	59.0	30.0	27.8	33.4	31.9	33.5	31.0	41.4	38.7	42.6	53.3
Female																				
All sites	56.7	55.7	56.2	58.7	60.8	62.2	63.0	64.8	66.9	68.0	46.4	45.7	44.6	45.5	47.8	48.3	50.7	52.1	54.1	55.8
Colon	51.4	53.5	55.1	58.6	60.2	62.7	60.6	63.1	65.9	65.6	46.1	49.9	51.7	49.5	53.8	52.3	51.8	52.1	51.5	56.9
Rectum	49.5	50.3	53.6	57.9	58.5	61.4	62.2	64.8	66.7	68.3	46.9	35.6	42.4	48.0	57.1	48.7	56.5	56.4	58.3	63.3
Pancreas	2.3	2.5	3.0	3.1	3.3	4.6	4.3	3.6	4.4	6.5	1.9	7.0	3.2	5.1	5.8	4.1	3.5	3.5	7.2	5.0
Lung and bronchus	15.6	16.3	16.7	16.3	15.4	16.2	17.2	17.1	18.1	19.7	13.8	17.9	14.9	12.8	11.2	12.6	15.5	14.9	15.2	14.6
Melanoma of skin	86.3	87.8	87.2	91.0	91.3	91.8	92.6	92.8	94.7	95.3	*	*	*	*	89.5	*	*	78.7	75.3	72.8
Breast	75.9	75.3	77.3	80.3	85.3	86.6	87.8	89.5	91.0	91.7	62.2	63.4	63.8	65.2	71.3	71.7	72.7	76.3	78.8	78.0
Cervix uteri	69.8	68.2	67.9	69.0	72.5	70.9	74.2	73.7	73.4	70.2	64.5	61.0	59.4	57.6	57.4	58.0	63.1	64.9	66.0	61.1
Corpus uteri, not otherwise specified	88.1	83.8	82.2	84.1	84.1	85.8	84.9	85.4	86.2	85.4	60.3	55.0	50.9	56.3	57.0	53.9	58.6	61.5	60.8	62.6
Ovary	35.3	36.9	38.8	37.6	38.2	40.5	40.8	43.3	43.6	42.8	41.9	38.9	37.6	39.4	33.8	36.2	41.9	39.2	35.7	35.6
Non-Hodgkin's lymphoma	47.6	49.9	51.4	53.7	55.4	56.7	57.9	61.8	67.6	72.7	54.9	56.7	50.4	50.4	52.1	47.6	53.5	56.3	63.8	67.4

NOTE: Rates are based on follow-up of patients through 2009. The rate is the ratio of the observed survival rate for the patient group to the expected survival rate for persons in the general population similar to the patient group with respect to age, sex, race, and calendar year of observation. It estimates the chance of surviving the effects of cancer. The site variable distinguishes Kaposi Sarcoma and Mesothelioma as individual cancer sites. As a result, Kaposi Sarcoma and Mesothelioma cases are excluded from each of the sites shown except all sites combined. The race groups White and Black include persons of Hispanic and non-Hispanic origin. Due to death certificate race-ethnicity classification and other methodological issues related to developing life tables, survival rates for race-ethnicity groups other than White and Black are not calculated. * = Figure does not meet standards of reliability or precision.

Table 3-6A. Respondent-Reported Prevalence of Heart Disease Among Adults 18 Years of Age and Over, by Selected Characteristics, Selected Years, 1997–1998 Through 2010–2011

(Percent.)

Characteristic	Heart disease[1]								
	1997–1998	1999–2000	2001–2002	2003–2004	2005–2006	2007–2008	2008–2009	2009–2010	2010–2011
18 years and over, age adjusted[2,3]	12.0	11.1	11.5	11.3	11.2	11.3	11.5	11.4	11.1
18 years and over, crude[3]	11.6	10.9	11.3	11.3	11.4	11.6	11.8	11.8	11.6
Age									
18 to 44 years	4.6	4.3	4.3	4.1	4.0	4.4	4.5	4.4	4.0
18 to 24 years	3.2	3.3	3.3	3.0	3.2	3.1	3.3	3.4	3.0
25 to 44 years	5.0	4.6	4.6	4.5	4.2	4.8	4.9	4.8	4.4
45 to 64 years	13.5	12.6	12.9	12.5	12.9	12.2	12.7	13.1	13.0
45 to 54 years	10.9	10.0	10.0	9.4	9.4	8.8	9.5	10.1	9.6
55 to 64 years	17.4	16.6	17.4	17.0	17.8	16.8	16.8	17.0	17.1
65 years and over	31.8	29.6	31.3	31.8	31.2	31.8	31.7	30.4	30.5
65 to 74 years	27.8	25.8	26.6	27.3	26.5	26.9	26.2	25.1	25.6
75 years and over	37.0	34.3	36.8	36.8	36.6	37.5	38.0	37.0	36.5
Sex [2]									
Male	12.3	11.9	12.4	12.3	12.2	12.5	12.8	12.8	12.4
Female	11.8	10.5	10.8	10.7	10.5	10.5	10.5	10.3	10.2
Sex and Age									
Male									
18 to 44 years	3.7	3.6	3.6	3.6	3.3	3.8	4.4	4.3	3.7
45 to 54 years	11.0	10.0	10.1	8.7	9.8	9.2	10.0	10.4	9.5
55 to 64 years	18.7	19.7	19.9	20.4	20.5	18.3	18.8	19.0	19.1
65 to 74 years	32.0	30.4	31.9	33.1	31.6	32.0	30.5	30.8	31.3
75 years and over	40.8	39.2	43.6	42.6	43.1	46.5	46.6	45.3	44.7
Female									
18 to 44 years	5.5	4.9	4.9	4.7	4.7	4.9	4.7	4.5	4.3
45 to 54 years	10.8	9.9	9.9	10.1	9.1	8.4	9.0	9.8	9.6
55 to 64 years	16.2	13.8	15.2	13.9	15.4	15.4	14.9	15.1	15.3
65 to 74 years	24.5	22.0	22.2	22.5	22.2	22.5	22.6	20.2	20.6
75 years and over	34.6	31.2	32.6	33.1	32.4	31.7	32.3	31.3	30.9
Race [2,4]									
White only	12.2	11.3	11.7	11.6	11.5	11.7	11.9	11.6	11.2
Black or African American only	11.4	10.6	10.6	9.8	10.1	10.2	10.7	11.0	10.7
American Indian or Alaska Native only	18.6	14.7	11.4	12.8	15.9	11.1	10.2	10.3	12.5
Asian only	6.9	6.3	8.8	6.3	6.8	6.0	5.7	6.7	7.2
Native Hawaiian or Other Pacific Islander only	NA	*	*	*	*	*	*	*	*
Two or more races	NA	17.0	16.5	12.5	14.7	16.9	15.2	15.5	16.7
Hispanic Origin and Race [2,4]									
Hispanic or Latino	8.7	8.0	8.0	8.5	8.0	8.5	8.4	8.3	8.4
Mexican	7.5	7.4	7.8	8.9	7.5	8.3	8.4	8.4	8.4
Not Hispanic or Latino	12.2	11.4	11.8	11.6	11.6	11.7	11.9	11.8	11.4
White only	12.5	11.6	12.1	12.0	12.0	12.1	12.4	12.1	11.7
Black or African American only	11.4	10.5	10.5	9.8	10.2	10.2	10.8	11.1	10.8
Education [5,6]									
No high school diploma or GED	15.1	13.8	14.3	14.3	14.2	14.9	14.5	14.5	14.6
High school diploma or GED	12.8	11.9	12.4	12.3	12.6	11.9	12.7	12.7	12.4
Some college or more	12.7	12.0	12.4	12.2	11.9	12.4	12.4	12.2	11.9
Percent of Poverty Level [2,7]									
Below 100 percent	15.3	13.6	14.4	14.3	14.6	14.0	14.1	14.5	13.9
100 percent to 199 percent	13.2	12.0	12.4	12.8	12.5	13.0	13.2	12.8	12.3
200 percent to 399 percent	11.5	11.0	11.3	11.4	11.0	11.7	11.6	11.3	11.3
400 percent or more	11.0	10.2	10.9	10.0	10.1	10.0	10.1	10.0	9.8
Hispanic Origin and Race and Percent of Poverty Level [2,4,7]									
Hispanic or Latino									
Below 100 percent	9.7	9.7	8.7	11.3	11.0	11.0	10.3	10.3	9.4
100 percent to 199 percent	8.7	8.4	9.0	8.0	8.1	9.6	8.8	7.9	8.3
200 percent to 399 percent	8.4	8.2	6.5	8.2	6.9	7.1	7.7	8.4	8.5
400 percent or more	8.4	5.6	6.9	5.4	5.1	8.0	7.1	7.2	7.5
Not Hispanic or Latino									
White only									
Below 100 percent	17.8	15.2	16.5	15.9	16.9	16.0	15.9	16.3	15.8
100 percent to 199 percent	14.1	12.8	13.5	14.8	14.3	14.7	15.6	15.1	13.8
200 percent to 399 percent	12.2	11.6	12.1	12.3	11.9	12.9	12.8	12.1	11.8
400 percent or more	11.3	10.6	11.3	10.3	10.6	10.5	10.6	10.5	10.2
Black or African American only									
Below 100 percent	14.6	13.0	14.1	14.1	13.2	13.2	15.2	15.7	14.7
100 percent to 199 percent	12.9	11.2	12.3	10.5	10.7	11.3	10.9	10.5	11.2
200 percent to 399 percent	9.2	10.2	9.0	8.0	9.1	9.3	9.3	10.2	10.5
400 percent or more	9.5	8.9	8.0	7.7	8.5	7.7	8.9	8.7	7.3
Geographic Region [2]									
Northeast	11.6	10.6	10.9	10.8	11.0	10.9	11.1	10.8	10.1
Midwest	12.1	11.4	12.1	11.8	12.3	12.4	12.4	12.1	11.5
South	12.5	11.5	11.7	11.7	11.5	11.7	12.3	12.3	12.1
West	11.1	10.4	10.9	10.5	9.8	9.9	9.7	9.8	9.9
Location of Residence [2]									
Within MSA[8]	11.7	10.7	11.2	10.9	10.9	10.8	11.2	11.2	10.8
Outside MSA[8]	12.8	12.5	12.7	13.0	13.0	14.1	13.1	12.5	13.0

NA = Not available.   * = Figure does not meet standards of reliability or precision. Data preceded by an asterisk have a relative standard error (RSE) of 20 percent to 30 percent. Data not shown have an RSE of greater than 30 percent.   [1]Heart disease is based on self-reported responses to questions about whether respondents had ever been told by a doctor or other health professional that they had coronary heart disease, angina (angina pectoris), a heart attack (myocardial infarction), or any other kind or heart disease or heart condition.   [2]Estimates are age-adjusted to the year 2000 standard population using five age groups: 18 to 44 years, 45 to 54 years, 55 to 64 years, 65 to 74 years, and 75 years and over. Age-adjusted estimates in this table may differ from other age-adjusted estimates based on the same data and presented elsewhere if different age groups are used in the adjustment procedure.   [3]Includes all other races not shown separately and unknown education level.   [4]The race groups White, Black, American Indian or Alaska Native, Asian, Native Hawaiian or Other Pacific Islander, and two or more races, include persons of Hispanic and non-Hispanic origin. Persons of Hispanic origin may be of any race.   [5]Estimates are for persons 25 years of age and over and are age-adjusted to the year 2000 standard population using five age groups: 25 to 44 years, 45 to 54 years, 55 to 64 years, 65 to 74 years, and 75 years and over.   [6]GED is General Educational Development high school equivalency diploma.   [7]Percent of poverty level is based on family income and family size and composition using U.S. Census Bureau poverty thresholds.   [8]MSA = metropolitan statistical area.

Table 3-6B. Respondent-Reported Prevalence of Cancer Among Adults 18 Years of Age and Over, by Selected Characteristics, Selected Years, 1997–1998 Through 2010–2011

(Percent.)

Characteristic	Cancer[1]								
	1997–1998	1999–2000	2001–2002	2003–2004	2005–2006	2007–2008	2008–2009	2009–2010	2010–2011
18 years and over, age adjusted[2,3]	4.9	5.1	5.3	5.2	5.7	5.6	5.9	6.0	6.0
18 years and over, crude[3]	4.8	4.9	5.2	5.2	5.7	5.8	6.1	6.3	6.3
Age									
18 to 44 years	1.7	1.7	1.7	1.5	1.8	1.7	1.6	1.6	1.7
18 to 24 years	0.8	1.0	0.8	0.7	0.9	0.8	0.8	0.7	0.7
25 to 44 years	2.0	1.9	2.1	1.7	2.2	2.0	1.9	2.0	2.0
45 to 64 years	5.4	5.2	5.7	5.8	6.0	6.3	6.7	7.1	6.9
45 to 54 years	4.0	4.0	4.2	4.2	4.4	4.6	4.9	5.3	4.9
55 to 64 years	7.4	7.2	7.9	8.1	8.2	8.6	9.2	9.3	9.3
65 years and over	14.1	15.2	15.6	15.9	17.1	17.0	17.7	18.1	18.5
65 to 74 years	12.4	13.1	13.9	13.8	14.3	14.6	15.8	16.1	15.9
75 years and over	16.2	17.7	17.6	18.3	20.2	19.8	20.0	20.5	21.7
Sex [2]									
Male	4.1	4.4	4.7	4.7	5.1	4.8	5.0	5.5	5.5
Female	5.8	5.8	6.0	5.9	6.4	6.5	6.8	6.6	6.6
Sex and Age									
Male									
18 to 44 years	0.8	0.8	0.7	0.7	0.8	0.8	0.7	0.8	0.9
45 to 54 years	2.0	2.0	2.2	2.7	2.6	2.6	2.9	3.3	3.1
55 to 64 years	5.8	5.9	6.5	6.7	6.8	7.2	7.0	7.8	7.5
65 to 74 years	12.8	13.9	16.1	14.3	15.5	14.3	16.2	17.6	16.9
75 years and over	18.3	20.3	20.8	22.1	24.3	21.9	22.2	24.8	26.1
Female									
18 to 44 years	2.6	2.5	2.7	2.3	2.9	2.5	2.5	2.4	2.5
45 to 54 years	6.0	5.9	6.1	5.7	6.2	6.4	6.8	7.3	6.6
55 to 64 years	8.8	8.4	9.1	9.5	9.5	10.0	11.2	10.7	10.9
65 to 74 years	12.1	12.5	12.1	13.4	13.3	14.8	15.6	14.9	15.0
75 years and over	14.9	16.1	15.5	15.9	17.6	18.5	18.5	17.6	18.7
Race [2,4]									
White only	5.2	5.4	5.6	5.5	6.0	6.0	6.2	6.3	6.3
Black or African American only	3.5	3.5	3.3	4.0	3.9	4.4	4.3	4.7	5.1
American Indian or Alaska Native only	*6.5	*5.7	*	7.0	*7.4	*4.3	*5.4	7.0	6.5
Asian only	2.4	*2.3	*1.6	3.0	2.9	3.1	3.0	2.9	3.0
Native Hawaiian or Other Pacific Islander only	NA	*	*	*	*	*	*	*	*
Two or more races	NA	*4.7	7.1	*3.4	7.8	5.8	9.1	9.8	7.9
Hispanic Origin and Race [2,4]									
Hispanic or Latino	2.9	3.0	2.9	3.0	3.5	3.7	3.6	3.4	3.4
Mexican	3.0	2.8	2.9	2.6	3.1	3.6	3.3	3.2	3.2
Not Hispanic or Latino	5.1	5.2	5.5	5.5	5.9	5.9	6.1	6.3	6.3
White only	5.4	5.5	5.9	5.8	6.3	6.3	6.5	6.7	6.7
Black or African American only	3.6	3.6	3.3	3.9	3.9	4.3	4.2	4.7	5.1
Education [5,6]									
No high school diploma or GED	5.3	5.5	5.4	5.6	5.7	5.8	6.1	5.9	5.8
High school diploma or GED	5.5	5.8	6.3	5.7	6.4	6.1	6.4	6.7	6.8
Some college or more	6.0	5.9	6.2	6.4	6.9	6.9	7.1	7.4	7.4
Percent of Poverty Level [2,7]									
Below 100 percent	4.9	4.9	5.4	5.6	5.3	6.2	6.2	5.4	5.3
100 percent to 199 percent	4.8	5.3	5.0	5.6	5.7	5.8	6.0	6.1	5.9
200 percent to 399 percent	4.9	5.1	5.6	5.2	5.5	5.4	5.5	5.9	6.2
400 percent or more	5.2	5.1	5.2	5.0	6.1	5.8	6.0	6.3	6.2
Hispanic Origin and Race and Percent of Poverty Level [2,4,7]									
Hispanic or Latino									
Below 100 percent	2.2	2.3	2.9	2.9	3.5	5.0	3.8	2.8	2.9
100 percent to 199 percent	2.8	3.2	2.3	3.7	3.3	3.2	3.2	2.5	2.6
200 percent to 399 percent	2.7	2.7	3.5	2.8	3.6	3.2	3.3	4.3	4.7
400 percent or more	*5.5	*4.5	*3.1	*1.9	*3.4	3.6	4.2	4.2	3.3
Not Hispanic or Latino									
White only									
Below 100 percent	6.3	6.2	7.2	6.9	6.9	8.0	8.1	6.9	6.8
100 percent to 199 percent	5.6	6.2	5.9	6.6	6.7	7.4	7.4	7.3	7.3
200 percent to 399 percent	5.2	5.5	6.1	5.7	6.0	6.0	6.1	6.5	6.8
400 percent or more	5.4	5.3	5.5	5.3	6.5	6.0	6.2	6.6	6.6
Black or African American only									
Below 100 percent	4.4	4.0	3.2	4.6	3.6	4.6	4.9	4.9	4.5
100 percent to 199 percent	3.3	3.2	3.2	4.1	4.3	3.5	3.6	4.9	5.2
200 percent to 399 percent	3.2	3.7	3.6	3.5	4.2	4.4	4.0	4.3	5.3
400 percent or more	4.0	4.3	*3.3	4.5	3.6	5.4	5.0	5.2	5.6
Geographic Region [2]									
Northeast	4.5	5.0	5.0	5.3	5.6	6.1	6.2	5.9	5.6
Midwest	5.1	5.2	5.7	5.3	5.7	5.5	5.8	6.4	6.7
South	5.0	5.0	5.3	5.2	5.6	5.8	5.9	6.1	6.2
West	5.1	5.0	5.1	5.2	5.7	5.3	5.6	5.6	5.5
Location of Residence [2]									
Within MSA[8]	4.9	5.0	5.1	5.1	5.6	5.6	5.7	5.9	5.9
Outside MSA[8]	5.1	5.5	6.0	5.7	6.0	6.2	7.0	6.8	6.7

NA = Not available.   * = Figure does not meet standards of reliability or precision. Data preceded by an asterisk have a relative standard error (RSE) of 20 percent to 30 percent. Data not shown have an RSE of greater than 30 percent.   [1]Cancer is based on self-reported responses to a question about whether respondents had ever been told by a doctor or other health professional that they had cancer or a malignancy of any kind. Excludes squamous cell and basal cell carcinomas.   [2]Estimates are age-adjusted to the year 2000 standard population using five age groups: 18 to 44 years, 45 to 54 years, 55 to 64 years, 65 to 74 years, and 75 years and over. Age-adjusted estimates in this table may differ from other age-adjusted estimates based on the same data and presented elsewhere if different age groups are used in the adjustment procedure.   [3]Includes all other races not shown separately and unknown education level.   [4]The race groups White, Black, American Indian or Alaska Native, Asian, Native Hawaiian or Other Pacific Islander, and two or more races, include persons of Hispanic and non-Hispanic origin. Persons of Hispanic origin may be of any race.   [5]Estimates are for persons 25 years of age and over and are age-adjusted to the year 2000 standard population using five age groups: 25 to 44 years, 45 to 54 years, 55 to 64 years, 65 to 74 years, and 75 years and over.   [6]GED is General Educational Development high school equivalency diploma.   [7]Percent of poverty level is based on family income and family size and composition using U.S. Census Bureau poverty thresholds.   [8]MSA = metropolitan statistical area.

Table 3-6C. Respondent-Reported Prevalence of Stroke Among Adults 18 Years of Age and Over, by Selected Characteristics, Selected Years, 1997–1998 Through 2010–2011

(Percent.)

Characteristic	Stroke[1]								
	1997–1998	1999–2000	2001–2002	2003–2004	2005–2006	2007–2008	2008–2009	2009–2010	2010–2011
18 years and over, age adjusted[2,3]	2.3	2.2	2.4	2.5	2.5	2.6	2.7	2.6	2.6
18 years and over, crude[3]	2.2	2.1	2.4	2.5	2.5	2.7	2.8	2.7	2.7
Age									
18 to 44 years	0.4	0.4	0.4	0.4	0.4	0.5	0.6	0.6	0.6
18 to 24 years	*	*	*	*	*	*	*	*	*
25 to 44 years	0.4	0.5	0.5	0.5	0.5	0.6	0.7	0.7	0.7
45 to 64 years	2.3	2.0	2.4	2.4	2.3	2.9	2.7	2.8	2.9
45 to 54 years	1.4	1.3	1.8	1.5	1.5	2.0	1.8	1.9	2.1
55 to 64 years	3.8	3.1	3.3	3.7	3.5	4.0	3.8	3.8	3.9
65 years and over	8.1	8.1	8.8	9.2	9.2	8.8	9.2	8.6	8.2
65 to 74 years	6.7	6.2	6.6	7.1	6.9	6.3	6.3	6.3	6.3
75 years and over	9.8	10.3	11.2	11.6	11.8	11.8	12.5	11.4	10.6
Sex [2]									
Male	2.6	2.4	2.6	2.7	2.6	2.5	2.7	2.7	2.6
Female	2.1	2.1	2.3	2.4	2.4	2.6	2.7	2.6	2.6
Sex and Age									
Male									
18 to 44 years	0.3	0.3	0.4	0.4	0.4	*0.3	0.5	0.5	0.5
45 to 54 years	1.2	1.3	1.9	1.5	1.5	2.0	1.6	1.6	1.9
55 to 64 years	4.6	3.7	3.5	4.2	3.9	4.2	4.4	4.1	4.0
65 to 74 years	8.1	6.7	7.2	8.3	7.7	7.0	6.7	6.9	6.6
75 years and over	11.2	11.3	12.6	12.5	12.5	11.1	12.8	12.1	10.6
Female									
18 to 44 years	0.4	0.4	0.5	0.5	0.5	0.6	0.8	0.6	0.6
45 to 54 years	1.5	1.4	1.6	1.5	1.4	2.1	2.1	2.3	2.2
55 to 64 years	3.2	2.6	3.2	3.3	3.1	3.8	3.3	3.5	3.9
65 to 74 years	5.5	5.8	6.1	6.1	6.3	5.7	6.0	5.7	6.1
75 years and over	9.0	9.6	10.4	11.0	11.5	12.2	12.3	10.9	10.6
Race [2,4]									
White only	2.2	2.1	2.3	2.4	2.3	2.5	2.6	2.5	2.3
Black or African American only	3.3	3.5	3.3	3.4	4.0	3.6	3.7	3.9	4.1
American Indian or Alaska Native only	*5.0	*5.4	*	*	*	*	*	*	*4.7
Asian only	*1.2	*1.2	*3.1	*2.2	1.9	2.1	1.5	1.6	2.4
Native Hawaiian or Other Pacific Islander only	NA	*	*	*	*	*	*	*	*
Two or more races	NA	*4.0	*4.9	4.0	*4.6	*4.1	*3.5	*3.3	*3.9
Hispanic Origin and Race [2,4]									
Hispanic or Latino	2.1	1.9	2.5	2.6	2.1	2.6	2.3	2.3	2.7
Mexican	2.5	2.0	2.7	2.9	2.5	2.5	2.5	2.4	2.6
Not Hispanic or Latino	2.3	2.2	2.4	2.5	2.5	2.6	2.7	2.6	2.6
White only	2.2	2.1	2.3	2.4	2.3	2.4	2.7	2.5	2.3
Black or African American only	3.3	3.5	3.3	3.4	4.1	3.6	3.7	3.9	4.2
Education [5,6]									
No high school diploma or GED	3.9	3.8	3.8	4.4	4.1	4.4	4.5	4.2	4.4
High school diploma or GED	2.5	2.5	2.9	2.8	2.9	3.2	3.3	3.2	3.4
Some college or more	2.1	1.9	2.3	2.3	2.3	2.3	2.5	2.5	2.3
Percent of Poverty Level [2,7]									
Below 100 percent	4.3	3.7	3.7	4.4	4.1	4.4	4.4	4.4	4.6
100 percent to 199 percent	3.1	3.2	3.3	3.5	3.2	3.9	3.6	3.5	3.7
200 percent to 399 percent	2.1	2.1	2.4	2.3	2.4	2.5	2.7	2.6	2.5
400 percent or more	1.6	1.5	1.9	1.8	1.8	1.6	1.8	1.7	1.5
Hispanic Origin and Race and Percent of Poverty Level [2,4,7]									
Hispanic or Latino									
Below 100 percent	3.0	2.0	2.7	3.9	3.1	3.8	2.6	2.9	3.4
100 percent to 199 percent	2.2	2.2	3.2	2.8	1.8	2.6	2.6	2.3	3.2
200 percent to 399 percent	*1.8	*2.3	2.0	*2.0	*2.0	*2.2	2.4	2.0	2.2
400 percent or more	*	*	*	*	*	*2.7	*	*2.6	*2.1
Not Hispanic or Latino									
White only									
Below 100 percent	4.4	3.8	3.6	4.3	4.1	4.3	4.4	4.4	4.4
100 percent to 199 percent	3.2	3.0	3.2	3.5	3.2	4.1	4.0	3.9	3.6
200 percent to 399 percent	2.1	2.1	2.3	2.3	2.3	2.6	2.8	2.5	2.3
400 percent or more	1.6	1.5	1.8	1.8	1.8	1.5	1.8	1.7	1.4
Black or African American only									
Below 100 percent	5.0	4.5	4.8	5.6	5.3	5.5	6.4	6.2	6.2
100 percent to 199 percent	4.2	5.1	3.9	3.8	4.6	4.7	4.0	3.9	4.6
200 percent to 399 percent	2.5	2.7	2.8	2.4	4.1	2.7	2.8	3.7	3.9
400 percent or more	*	*	*	*2.0	*2.6	*2.6	*2.5	*2.6	*2.1
Geographic Region [2]									
Northeast	1.8	1.8	2.1	2.2	1.9	2.4	2.3	2.1	2.0
Midwest	2.3	2.2	2.4	2.5	2.5	2.5	2.6	2.6	2.6
South	2.6	2.5	2.5	2.8	2.9	3.0	3.2	3.0	2.9
West	2.1	2.0	2.7	2.4	2.1	2.2	2.2	2.3	2.4
Location of Residence [2]									
Within MSA[8]	2.2	2.1	2.4	2.4	2.4	2.5	2.6	2.4	2.4
Outside MSA[8]	2.7	2.5	2.5	2.8	2.9	2.9	3.0	3.3	3.4

NA = Not available.   * = Figure does not meet standards of reliability or precision. Data preceded by an asterisk have a relative standard error (RSE) of 20 percent to 30 percent. Data not shown have an RSE of greater than 30 percent.   [1]Stroke is based on self-reported responses to a question about whether respondents had ever been told by a doctor or other health professional that they had a stroke.   [2]Estimates are age-adjusted to the year 2000 standard population using five age groups: 18 to 44 years, 45 to 54 years, 55 to 64 years, 65 to 74 years, and 75 years and over. Age-adjusted estimates in this table may differ from other age-adjusted estimates based on the same data and presented elsewhere if different age groups are used in the adjustment procedure.   [3]Includes all other races not shown separately and unknown education level.   [4]The race groups White, Black, American Indian or Alaska Native, Asian, Native Hawaiian or Other Pacific Islander, and two or more races, include persons of Hispanic and non-Hispanic origin. Persons of Hispanic origin may be of any race.   [5]Estimates are for persons 25 years of age and over and are age-adjusted to the year 2000 standard population using five age groups: 25 to 44 years, 45 to 54 years, 55 to 64 years, 65 to 74 years, and 75 years and over.   [6]GED is General Educational Development high school equivalency diploma.   [7]Percent of poverty level is based on family income and family size and composition using U.S. Census Bureau poverty thresholds.   [8]MSA = metropolitan statistical area.

Table 3-7A. Diabetes Prevalence and Glycemic Control Among Adults 20 Years of Age and Over, by Sex, Age, Race and Hispanic Origin, Selected Years, 1988–1994 Through 2003–2006

(Percent.)

Age, race, sex, and Hispanic origin[1]	Physician-diagnosed and undiagnosed diabetes[2,3]				Physician-diagnosed diabetes[2]				Undiagnosed diabetes[3]			
	1988–1994	1999–2002	2001–2004	2003–2006	1988–1994	1999–2002	2001–2004	2003–2006	1988–1994	1999–2002	2001–2004	2003–2006
20 Years and Over, Age-Adjusted[4]												
All persons[5]	9.1	9.8	10.7	10.6	5.5	6.6	7.3	7.6	3.6	3.2	3.3	2.9
Sex												
Male	9.6	10.8	12.0	11.5	5.5	7.0	7.5	7.5	4.1	3.8	4.5	4.0
Female	8.7	8.8	9.5	9.8	5.6	6.2	7.2	7.8	3.1	2.6	2.3	2.0
Hispanic Origin												
Not Hispanic or Latino												
White only	8.0	8.3	9.1	9.0	5.1	5.3	6.2	6.3	2.9	3.0	2.9	2.7
Black or African American only	16.0	16.3	15.4	16.4	8.8	11.9	11.3	12.6	7.2	4.4	4.1	3.8
Mexican	14.9	13.2	15.2	16.3	9.8	10.1	11.7	12.1	5.0	*3.1	3.5	4.2
Percent of Poverty Level[6]												
Below 100 percent	14.2	14.5	14.8	15.1	8.8	9.1	10.2	12.8	5.4	5.4	4.6	*
100 percent or more	8.4	8.9	9.8	9.9	5.1	6.0	6.7	6.9	3.3	2.9	3.1	3.0
100 percent to 199 percent	10.9	12.6	12.9	13.3	6.6	9.0	9.2	8.9	4.3	*3.6	3.7	4.4
200 percent or more	7.7	7.7	8.8	8.8	4.6	5.1	5.8	6.2	3.1	2.7	2.9	2.6
200 percent to 399 percent	8.4	10.0	10.5	10.1	4.8	6.8	6.9	7.1	3.6	3.2	3.6	*3.0
400 percent or more	6.8	5.9	7.5	7.4	4.3	3.6	5.2	5.6	2.6	2.3	*2.3	*
20 Years and Over, Crude												
All persons[5]	8.4	9.7	10.4	10.7	5.1	6.5	7.2	7.7	3.3	3.2	3.2	3.0
Sex												
Male	8.6	10.4	11.5	11.4	4.8	6.7	7.2	7.4	3.7	3.7	4.3	4.0
Female	8.3	9.0	9.5	10.1	5.4	6.3	7.1	8.1	3.0	2.7	2.3	2.0
Hispanic Origin												
Not Hispanic or Latino												
White only	7.8	8.7	9.5	9.8	5.0	5.5	6.4	6.9	2.8	3.2	3.1	2.9
Black or African American only	12.9	14.1	13.7	15.2	6.9	10.1	10.1	11.8	6.0	4.0	3.6	3.4
Mexican	9.7	8.5	9.8	11.6	5.6	6.5	7.0	7.9	4.1	1.9	*2.8	*3.6
Percent of Poverty Level[6]												
Below 100 percent	11.3	13.0	11.9	12.8	7.0	8.1	8.2	10.7	4.3	4.9	3.7	*
100 percent or more	7.8	8.8	9.7	10.2	4.7	5.9	6.7	7.1	3.0	2.8	3.0	3.1
100 percent to 199 percent	10.1	12.6	12.8	14.3	6.4	9.1	9.2	9.7	3.8	*3.5	3.6	4.6
200 percent or more	7.0	7.5	8.7	9.0	4.2	4.9	5.8	6.3	2.8	2.6	2.9	2.6
200 percent to 399 percent	7.3	9.6	10.3	10.5	4.3	6.5	6.7	7.3	3.1	*3.1	3.6	*3.2
400 percent or more	6.5	6.0	7.3	7.6	4.1	3.7	5.1	5.5	*2.4	2.2	*2.3	*2.1
Age												
20 to 44 years	2.6	3.4	3.6	3.6	1.6	2.3	2.5	2.6	*1.0	*	*1.1	*1.1
45 to 64 years	13.9	13.0	13.4	13.5	7.9	8.5	9.2	9.9	6.0	4.5	4.2	3.5
65 years and over	19.6	22.4	26.4	25.7	12.9	15.8	18.1	18.3	6.7	6.6	8.3	7.3

* = Figure does not meet standards of reliability or precision. Data preceded by an asterisk have a relative standard error (RSE) of 20 percent to 30 percent. Data not shown have an RSE of greater than 30 percent.   [1]Persons of Mexican origin may be of any race.   [2]Physician-diagnosed diabetes was obtained by self-report and excludes women who reported having diabetes only during pregnancy.   [3]Undiagnosed diabetes is defined as a fasting plasma glucose (FPG) of at least 126 mg/dL or a hemoglobin A1c of at least 6.5 percent and no reported physician diagnosis. Respondents had fasted for at least 8 hours and less than 24 hours.   [4]Estimates are age adjusted to the year 2000 standard population using three age groups: 20 to 44 years, 45 to 64 years, and 65 years and over. Age-adjusted estimates in this table may differ from other age-adjusted estimates based on the same data and presented elsewhere if different age groups are used in the adjustment procedure.   [5]Includes all other races and Hispanic origins not shown separately.   [6]Percent of poverty level is based on family income and family size.

Table 3-7B. Diabetes Prevalence and Glycemic Control Among Adults 20 Years of Age and Over, by Sex, Age, Race and Hispanic Origin, Selected Years, 1988–1994 Through 2003–2006

(Percent.)

Age, race, sex, and Hispanic origin	Poor glycemic control (A1c greater than 9%) among persons with diagnosed diabetes			
	Percent of population with diagnosed diabetes			
	1988–1994	1999–2002	2001–2004	2003–2006
20 Years and Over, Crude [1]				
All persons[2]	23.3	18.4	14.4	13.0
Sex				
Male	20.2	20.2	17.5	14.8
Female	25.8	16.6	11.6	11.4
Hispanic Origin [3]				
Not Hispanic or Latino				
White only	20.6	13.6	11.5	8.6
Black or African American only	34.2	25.4	20.0	21.0
Mexican	29.2	26.5	22.9	24.0
Percent of Poverty Level [4]				
Below 100 percent	30.2	25.6	16.3	17.6
100 percent or more	21.4	15.9	13.8	12.2
100 percent to 199 percent	24.2	*14.9	*10.5	*11.5
200 percent or more	20.0	16.4	15.5	12.5
200 percent to 399 percent	*21.2	*17.3	15.5	*10.6
400 percent or more	*18.3	*	15.5	14.8
Age				
20 to 44 years	29.5	*32.1	*19.7	24.7
45 to 64 years	26.0	19.9	19.5	16.6
65 years and over	18.0	*10.2	*6.3	*4.1

* = Figure does not meet standards of reliability or precision. Data preceded by an asterisk have a relative standard error (RSE) of 20 percent to 30 percent. Data not shown have an RSE of greater than 30 percent.   [1]Age-adjusted estimates are not provided because the 2000 standard population used for age adjustment.   [2]Includes all other races and Hispanic origins not shown separately.   [3]Persons of Hispanic origin may be of any race.   [4]Percent of poverty level is based on family income and family size.

Table 3-8A. Incidence and Prevalence of End-Stage Renal Disease, by Selected Characteristics, Selected Years, 1980–2010

(Number, rate per million population.)

Characteristic	Incidence — Number of new patients					Prevalence — Number of patients alive on December 31				
	1980	1990	2000	2009	2010	1980	1990	2000	2009	2010
Total	17,338	49,766	92,069	114,168	114,281	58,330	182,804	384,246	559,448	580,741
Age										
Under 20 years	737	1,054	1,173	1,304	1,308	2,374	4,494	6,288	7,331	7,388
20 to 44 years	4,702	10,351	12,810	13,940	13,434	20,266	57,214	87,916	97,261	98,277
45 to 64 years	6,950	17,154	32,129	43,769	43,788	23,695	67,162	156,840	251,282	261,940
65 to 74 years	3,644	13,338	23,345	26,519	27,084	9,205	35,616	76,326	114,341	119,875
75 years and over	1,305	7,869	22,612	28,636	28,667	2,790	18,318	56,876	89,233	93,261
Sex										
Male	9,662	26,676	49,161	64,694	65,038	32,211	98,542	209,727	316,015	329,098
Female	7,676	23,090	42,908	49,474	49,243	26,119	84,262	174,519	243,433	251,643
Race [1]										
White	12,293	33,143	61,059	74,944	75,690	41,111	118,694	237,414	342,160	354,460
Black or African American	4,816	14,827	26,660	32,431	31,739	16,442	57,395	126,180	180,330	186,785
American Indian or Alaska Native	124	600	1,202	1,411	1,390	375	2,176	5,402	7,613	7,968
Asian or Pacific Islander	105	1,196	3,148	5,382	5,462	402	4,539	15,250	29,345	31,528
Hispanic Origin [1,2]										
Hispanic	NA	NA	10,731	14,822	15,284	NA	NA	42,443	79,934	85,202
Not Hispanic[3]	NA	NA	81,338	99,346	98,997	NA	NA	341,803	479,514	495,539
Primary Diagnosis										
Diabetes	2,592	17,712	41,118	49,987	50,356	5,586	46,982	136,097	211,003	219,794
Hypertension	3,096	15,196	24,708	32,545	32,537	9,443	47,316	94,929	139,053	145,182
Glomerulonephritis	2,721	6,915	8,445	7,536	7,312	13,371	39,726	67,728	83,047	84,521
Cystic kidney	756	1,551	2,141	2,641	2,605	3,628	9,979	17,879	26,906	27,960
Other urologic	461	1,259	2,664	1,556	1,544	1,587	6,101	11,655	12,845	12,919
Other cause	1,793	4,812	8,920	14,666	14,796	6,624	21,525	39,670	61,733	64,469
Unknown cause	1,508	1,848	3,639	4,231	3,924	5,849	8,182	13,665	20,834	21,361
Missing disease	4,411	473	434	1,006	1,207	12,242	2,993	2,623	4,027	4,535

NA = Not available. [1]The race groups White, Black, American Indian or Alaska Native, and Asian or Pacific Islander, include persons of Hispanic and non-Hispanic origin. Persons of Hispanic origin may be of any race. [2]Centers for Medicare & Medicaid Services began collecting Hispanic ethnicity data in April 1995. [3]Not Hispanic includes unknown ethnicity.

Table 3-8B. End-Stage Renal Disease Patients, by Selected Characteristics, Selected Years, 1980–2010

(Number, rate per million population.)

Characteristic	New patients per million population					Patients alive on December 31 per million population				
	1980	1990	2000	2009	2010	1980	1990	2000	2009	2010
Total	76.3	199.4	326.3	372.2	369.4	255.3	727.4	1,355.1	1,816.0	1,869.5
Age										
Under 20 years	10.2	14.7	14.6	15.7	15.7	32.8	62.2	77.9	88.1	88.8
20 to 44 years	55.6	103.4	123.1	134.6	129.3	237.2	566.7	843.8	937.5	944.5
45 to 64 years	156.2	370.4	514.7	545.3	535.4	531.1	1,441.6	2,471.5	3,101.2	3,173.8
65 to 74 years	232.8	736.7	1,269.9	1,248.9	1,240.0	583.3	1,957.0	4,151.7	5,309.0	5,413.1
75 years and over	129.8	598.7	1,355.2	1,557.1	1,541.6	273.4	1,374.1	3,386.3	4,825.2	4,987.4
Sex										
Male	87.5	219.2	355.1	429.0	427.6	290.1	804.0	1,507.0	2,086.5	2,154.4
Female	65.7	180.5	298.6	317.2	313.2	222.5	654.5	1,208.6	1,554.5	1,593.9
Race [1]										
White	63.0	158.3	264.8	306.7	307.9	209.8	563.9	1,026.1	1,396.0	1,437.9
Black or African American	179.8	483.8	725.8	778.8	752.3	609.3	1,853.3	3,410.9	4,302.2	4,399.0
American Indian or Alaska Native	86.7	291.4	402.9	341.8	325.2	256.4	1,039.7	1,779.5	1,811.8	1,832.6
Asian or Pacific Islander	27.4	158.4	264.7	324.0	319.7	100.1	585.4	1,254.0	1,741.8	1,820.5
Hispanic Origin [1,2]										
Hispanic	NA	NA	300.9	300.5	300.8	NA	NA	1,165.9	1,596.5	1,652.8
Not Hispanic [3]	NA	NA	330.0	385.9	382.9	NA	NA	1,382.9	1,858.6	1,912.6
Primary Diagnosis										
Diabetes	11.4	71.0	145.7	162.9	162.8	24.5	187.0	479.9	684.9	707.6
Hypertension	13.6	60.9	87.6	106.1	105.2	41.3	188.3	334.8	451.4	467.4
Glomerulonephritis	12.0	27.7	29.9	24.6	23.6	58.5	158.1	238.8	269.6	272.1
Cystic kidney	3.3	6.2	7.6	8.6	8.4	15.9	39.7	63.1	87.3	90.0
Other urologic	2.0	5.0	9.4	5.1	5.0	6.9	24.3	41.1	41.7	41.6
Other cause	7.9	19.3	31.6	47.8	47.8	29.0	85.7	139.9	200.4	207.5
Unknown cause	6.6	7.4	12.9	13.8	12.7	25.6	32.6	48.2	67.6	68.8
Missing disease	19.4	1.9	1.5	3.3	3.9	53.6	11.9	9.3	13.1	14.6

NA = Not available.   [1]The race groups White, Black, American Indian or Alaska Native, and Asian or Pacific Islander, include persons of Hispanic and non-Hispanic origin. Persons of Hispanic origin may be of any race.   [2]Centers for Medicare & Medicaid Services began collecting Hispanic ethnicity data in April 1995.   [3]Not Hispanic includes unknown ethnicity.

Figure 3-2. Percent Distribution of Newly Diagnosed AIDS Cases, by Race and Hispanic Origin, 2010

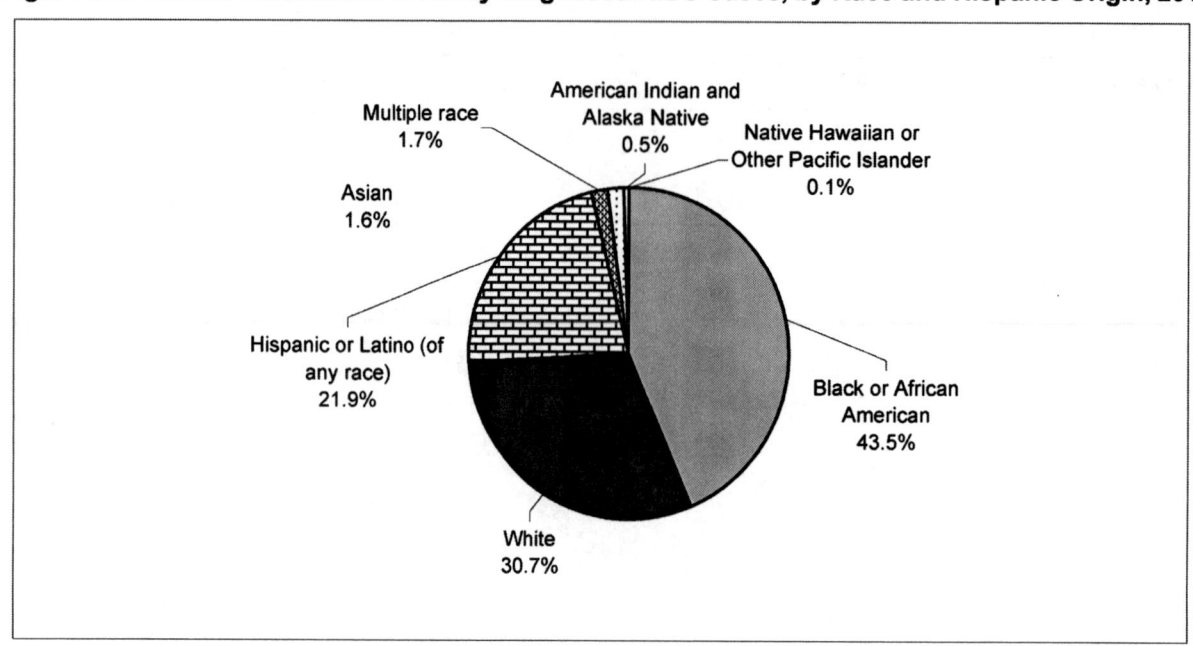

Figure 3-3. Percent of Persons Age 18 Years and Over Suffering from Severe Headache or Migraine, Low Back Pain, and Neck Pain, 1997, 2000, 2010, and 2011

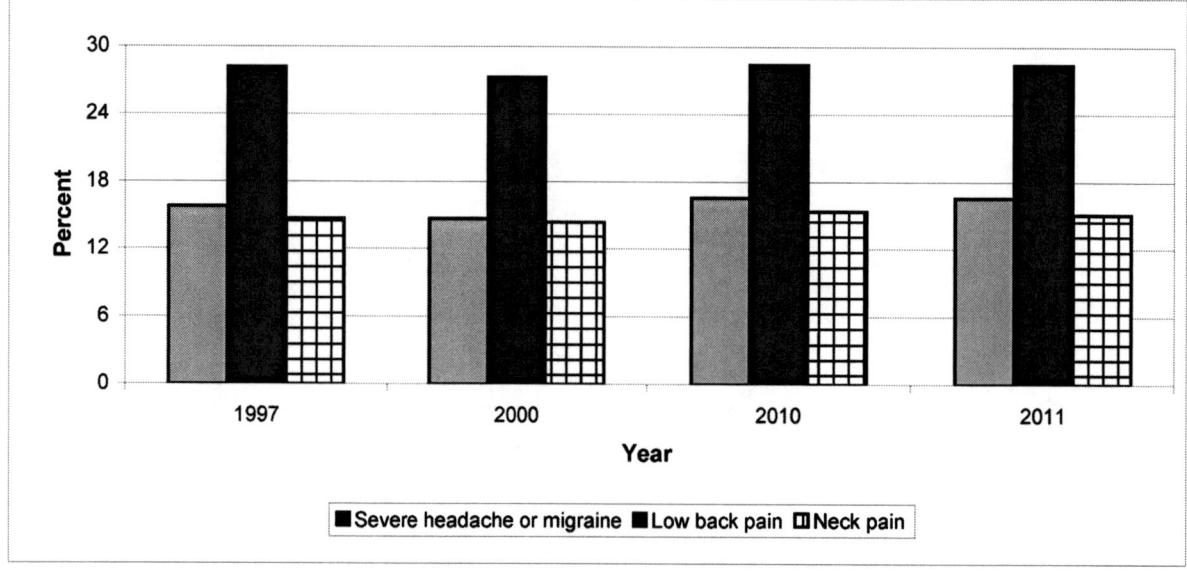

Table 3-9. Severe Headache or Migraine, Low Back Pain, and Neck Pain Among Adults 18 Years of Age and Over, by Selected Characteristics, 1997, 2000, 2010, and 2011

(Percent.)

Characteristic	Severe headache or migraine[1]				Low back pain[1]				Neck pain[1]			
	1997	2000	2010	2011	1997	2000	2010	2011	1997	2000	2010	2011
18 years and over, age-adjusted[2,3]	15.8	14.7	16.6	16.6	28.2	27.3	28.4	28.4	14.7	14.4	15.4	15.1
18 years and over, crude[3]	16.0	14.8	16.4	16.4	28.1	27.2	28.8	28.9	14.6	14.4	15.8	15.5
Age												
18 to 44 years	18.7	17.2	20.4	19.4	26.1	24.6	25.2	24.4	13.3	12.6	13.1	12.4
18 to 24 years	18.7	16.1	19.6	18.4	21.9	20.9	19.4	18.0	9.8	8.7	8.3	7.6
25 to 44 years	18.7	17.6	20.7	19.8	27.3	25.8	27.2	26.8	14.3	13.9	14.8	14.1
45 to 64 years	15.8	14.8	15.6	16.4	31.3	30.4	32.4	33.3	17.0	17.7	20.0	19.4
45 to 54 years	17.8	16.3	16.7	18.4	31.3	29.4	31.3	32.2	17.3	17.8	19.1	19.2
55 to 64 years	12.7	12.3	14.1	14.0	31.2	32.0	33.8	34.5	16.6	17.6	21.0	19.7
65 years and over	7.0	7.0	6.4	8.0	29.5	30.0	31.8	32.7	15.0	14.0	14.8	16.2
65 to 74 years	8.2	7.9	7.4	9.5	30.2	29.6	32.5	33.2	15.0	13.9	15.5	17.7
75 years and over	5.4	6.0	5.1	6.1	28.6	30.6	30.9	32.1	15.0	14.2	14.0	14.4
Sex[2]												
Male	9.9	8.9	11.0	10.8	26.5	25.5	26.3	26.8	12.6	12.1	13.1	12.6
Female	21.4	20.3	22.1	22.3	29.6	28.8	30.3	29.9	16.6	16.5	17.6	17.4
Sex and Age												
Male												
18 to 44 years	11.9	10.4	13.5	12.7	24.8	23.4	23.2	22.7	11.6	10.6	11.0	10.4
45 to 54 years	10.3	9.1	10.4	10.8	29.4	27.4	29.6	31.4	13.9	14.8	16.3	15.3
55 to 64 years	8.8	7.6	9.6	9.7	30.7	29.6	32.8	34.2	14.6	15.1	17.6	16.5
65 to 74 years	5.0	5.1	5.5	6.9	29.0	27.5	28.4	30.7	13.6	12.0	12.8	15.4
75 years and over	*2.4	4.5	4.0	4.6	22.5	26.3	27.4	28.5	12.6	12.4	13.0	12.2
Female												
18 to 44 years	25.4	23.9	27.3	26.1	27.3	25.7	27.1	26.2	14.9	14.6	15.2	14.3
45 to 54 years	24.9	23.2	22.9	25.7	33.1	31.3	33.0	33.0	20.6	20.7	21.8	22.9
55 to 64 years	16.3	16.7	18.2	18.0	31.7	34.2	34.7	34.7	18.4	19.8	24.1	22.8
65 to 74 years	10.7	10.1	9.1	11.8	31.1	31.2	36.1	35.5	16.1	15.5	17.8	19.7
75 years and over	7.4	6.9	5.8	7.1	32.4	33.2	33.2	34.6	16.5	15.2	14.6	15.8
Race[2,4]												
White only	15.9	15.0	16.7	16.9	28.7	28.0	29.1	29.0	15.1	15.0	16.0	15.6
Black or African American only	16.7	13.9	18.2	17.2	26.9	24.3	27.2	27.6	13.3	10.7	13.3	13.0
American Indian or Alaska Native only	18.9	21.1	18.8	21.5	33.3	31.4	33.6	31.0	16.2	19.6	16.9	16.6
Asian only	11.7	12.0	10.1	11.4	21.0	19.0	19.1	19.8	9.2	11.0	9.6	10.6
Native Hawaiian or Other Pacific Islander only	NA	*	*	*	NA	*	*	*	NA	*	*	*
2 or more races	NA	19.9	21.5	19.5	NA	41.8	35.6	37.6	NA	22.1	22.0	20.2
Hispanic Origin and Race[2,4]												
Hispanic or Latino	15.5	13.5	16.2	16.1	26.4	25.0	27.4	27.4	13.9	13.4	15.1	14.7
Mexican	14.6	12.3	15.7	15.7	25.2	21.5	26.5	26.6	12.9	11.6	14.7	13.9
Not Hispanic or Latino	15.9	15.0	16.8	16.9	28.4	27.7	28.7	28.7	14.9	14.7	15.5	15.3
White only	16.1	15.4	17.0	17.3	29.1	28.4	29.7	29.4	15.4	15.4	16.3	16.0
Black or African American only	16.8	13.8	18.4	17.2	26.9	24.2	27.1	27.5	13.3	10.6	13.3	12.9
Education[5,6]												
25 years and over												
No high school diploma or GED	19.2	17.9	18.2	20.2	33.6	32.4	34.5	37.1	16.5	15.9	18.9	19.2
High school diploma or GED	16.0	14.8	17.4	16.7	30.2	29.4	31.9	33.0	15.5	15.4	16.8	16.5
Some college or more	13.8	13.4	15.1	15.3	26.9	26.3	28.0	27.4	14.6	15.0	15.8	15.6
Percent of Poverty Level[2,7]												
Below 100 percent	23.3	19.9	22.7	23.7	35.4	32.4	34.9	37.5	18.6	16.5	20.2	19.9
100 percent to 199 percent	18.9	17.7	19.5	20.7	30.8	30.6	32.5	33.4	16.1	15.3	17.7	18.2
200 percent to 399 percent	15.5	15.4	16.6	16.0	27.9	27.4	28.5	28.4	14.8	14.7	15.2	15.0
400 percent or more	12.4	11.8	13.3	12.7	24.8	24.5	24.7	23.2	12.8	13.4	13.1	12.3
Hispanic Origin and Race and Percent of Poverty Level[2,4,7]												
Hispanic or Latino												
Below 100 percent	18.9	18.1	19.6	21.6	29.5	28.4	29.0	31.6	16.4	15.6	17.4	18.0
100 percent to 199 percent	15.7	12.9	15.1	15.8	26.8	24.8	27.2	29.3	12.9	13.3	15.7	15.9
200 percent to 399 percent	14.0	13.6	16.5	14.4	25.0	23.5	27.5	26.0	13.8	13.6	12.9	13.8
400 percent or more	13.0	9.6	14.0	11.6	21.6	24.1	25.6	20.0	12.1	11.6	15.3	9.5
Not Hispanic or Latino												
White only												
Below 100 percent	26.1	21.3	24.8	25.8	38.9	36.6	40.5	42.1	20.5	18.7	23.7	22.3
100 percent to 199 percent	20.4	20.3	22.0	23.9	33.3	34.6	35.9	36.9	18.0	17.6	19.9	21.4
200 percent to 399 percent	16.3	16.5	16.9	17.1	29.1	28.5	30.5	30.2	15.9	16.0	16.8	16.2
400 percent or more	12.5	12.3	13.8	13.3	25.4	25.2	25.2	23.7	13.1	14.0	13.6	12.9
Black or African American only												
Below 100 percent	22.7	21.1	24.0	23.8	34.5	27.5	32.5	36.0	17.9	13.7	18.6	17.4
100 percent to 199 percent	17.6	16.3	19.6	20.2	27.7	26.2	31.2	30.2	14.0	11.1	14.4	13.8
200 percent to 399 percent	14.0	11.4	17.6	13.6	24.3	23.8	23.7	22.7	10.2	9.8	11.7	11.3
400 percent or more	12.9	8.2	12.2	12.2	21.5	20.3	21.0	23.4	11.9	8.1	8.5	9.6

Table 3-9. Severe Headache or Migraine, Low Back Pain, and Neck Pain Among Adults 18 Years of Age and Over, by Selected Characteristics, 1997, 2000, 2010, and 2011—*Continued*

(Percent.)

Characteristic	Severe headache or migraine[1]				Low back pain[1]				Neck pain[1]			
	1997	2000	2010	2011	1997	2000	2010	2011	1997	2000	2010	2011
Disability Measure [2,8]												
Any basic actions difficulty or complex activity limitation	29.3	28.3	30.1	31.1	48.0	49.0	49.5	51.1	27.2	29.0	28.1	29.1
Any basic actions difficulty	30.0	29.3	30.9	32.1	49.3	50.0	51.1	52.5	27.9	29.9	29.0	30.1
Any complex activity limitation	34.6	32.7	36.0	34.7	55.1	54.3	54.5	57.1	33.1	33.9	34.3	35.7
No disability	11.0	10.4	11.7	11.4	19.4	18.7	19.0	18.6	9.1	9.1	9.7	9.0
Geographic Region [2]												
Northeast	14.5	12.7	15.4	14.0	27.1	26.0	28.0	27.1	14.0	13.5	14.9	13.5
Midwest	15.6	15.1	16.8	16.8	28.7	28.2	28.1	28.1	15.3	14.5	16.0	15.5
South	17.1	14.9	18.2	17.8	27.5	26.5	28.3	29.4	13.9	13.7	14.6	14.8
West	15.3	15.9	15.1	16.7	30.0	28.6	29.3	28.4	16.1	16.5	16.5	16.3
Location of Residence [2]												
Within MSA[9]	15.2	14.4	16.3	16.0	27.0	26.6	27.5	27.6	14.2	14.3	14.9	14.7
Outside MSA[9]	18.1	16.1	18.6	20.0	32.5	29.6	33.8	33.0	16.4	14.9	18.1	17.2

NA = Not available.   * = Figure does not meet standards of reliability or precision. Data preceded by an asterisk have a relative standard error (RSE) of 20 percent to 30 percent. Data not shown have an RSE of greater than 30 percent.   [1]In three separate questions, respondents were asked, "During the past 3 months, did you have a severe headache or migraine? . . . low back pain? . . . neck pain?" Respondents were instructed to report pain that had lasted a whole day or more, and not to report fleeting or minor aches or pains. Persons may be represented in more than one column.   [2]Estimates are age adjusted to the year 2000 standard population using five age groups: 18 to 44 years, 45 to 54 years, 55 to 64 years, 65 to 74 years, and 75 years and over. Age-adjusted estimates in this table may differ from other age-adjusted estimates based on the same data and presented elsewhere if different age groups are used in the adjustment procedure.   [3]Includes all other races not shown separately, unknown education level, and unknown disability status.   [4]The race groups White, Black, American Indian or Alaska Native, Asian, Native Hawaiian or Other Pacific Islander, and two or more races, include persons of Hispanic and non-Hispanic origin. Persons of Hispanic origin may be of any race.   [5]Estimates are for persons 25 years of age and over and are age-adjusted to the year 2000 standard population using five age groups: 25 to 44 years, 45 to 54 years, 55 to 64 years, 65 to 74 years, and 75 years and over.   [6]GED is General Educational Development high school equivalency diploma.   [7]Percent of poverty level is based on family income and family size and composition using U.S. Census Bureau poverty thresholds.   [8]Any basic actions difficulty or complex activity limitation is defined as having one or more of the following limitations or difficulties: movement difficulty, emotional difficulty, sensory (seeing or hearing) difficulty, cognitive difficulty, self-care (activities of daily living or instrumental activities of daily living) limitation, social limitation, or work limitation.   [9]MSA = metropolitan statistical area.

Table 3-10A. Joint Pain Among Adults 18 Years of Age and Over, by Selected Characteristics, Selected Years, 2002–2010

(Percent.)

Characteristic	Any joint pain[1]		
	2002	2005	2010
18 years and over, age-adjusted[2,3]	29.5	30.7	32.1
18 years and over, crude[3]	29.5	31.1	33.3
Age			
18 to 44 years	19.3	19.1	20.6
18 to 24 years	14.2	14.0	15.2
25 to 44 years	21.0	20.9	22.6
45 to 64 years	37.5	39.9	42.9
45 to 54 years	34.3	35.8	39.3
55 to 64 years	42.3	45.7	47.3
65 years and over	47.2	50.9	49.6
65 to 74 years	46.0	49.3	49.5
75 years and over	48.7	52.6	49.8
Sex[2]			
Male	28.0	28.9	30.8
Female	30.7	32.2	33.2
Sex and Age			
Male			
18 to 44 years	20.1	19.3	21.6
45 to 54 years	31.1	33.4	37.3
55 to 64 years	37.3	40.7	42.5
65 to 74 years	41.7	45.1	42.9
75 years and over	43.9	47.0	46.6
Female			
18 to 44 years	18.4	18.9	19.7
45 to 54 years	37.3	38.2	41.3
55 to 64 years	46.8	50.4	51.8
65 to 74 years	49.6	52.9	55.2
75 years and over	51.6	56.2	51.9
Race[2,4]			
White only	29.8	31.3	32.6
Black or African American only	30.8	28.5	32.0
American Indian or Alaska Native only	36.7	34.8	38.1
Asian only	18.1	18.5	20.4
Native Hawaiian or Other Pacific Islander only	*	*	*
2 or more races	42.7	46.2	43.5
Hispanic Origin and Race[2,4]			
Hispanic or Latino	23.4	24.2	25.4
Mexican	24.6	23.8	25.0
Not Hispanic or Latino	30.4	31.7	33.3
White only	30.8	32.8	34.3
Black or African American only	30.8	28.5	32.1
Education[5,6]			
25 years and over			
No high school diploma or GED	33.0	33.3	33.8
High school diploma or GED	32.9	33.1	36.8
Some college or more	31.1	33.2	34.0
Percent of Poverty Level[2,7]			
Below 100 percent	31.7	33.7	35.6
100 percent to 199 percent	31.7	31.9	34.0
200 percent to 399 percent	30.1	31.0	32.2
400 percent or more	27.6	29.3	30.5
Hispanic Origin and Race and Percent of Poverty Level[2,4,7]			
Hispanic or Latino			
Below 100 percent	26.8	24.5	25.3
100 percent to 199 percent	24.5	24.1	25.4
200 percent to 399 percent	21.6	23.6	24.8
400 percent or more	21.9	24.7	27.4
Not Hispanic or Latino			
White only			
Below 100 percent	34.2	39.3	40.1
100 percent to 199 percent	34.9	36.2	38.7
200 percent to 399 percent	32.0	33.6	34.8
400 percent or more	28.2	30.1	31.8
Black or African American only			
Below 100 percent	31.6	33.0	37.6
100 percent to 199 percent	34.0	28.6	33.0
200 percent to 399 percent	29.1	27.2	30.8
400 percent or more	29.8	25.8	26.8

Table 3-10A. Joint Pain Among Adults 18 Years of Age and Over, by Selected Characteristics, Selected Years, 2002–2010—*Continued*

(Percent.)

Characteristic	Any joint pain[1]		
	2002	2005	2010
Disability Measure [2,8]			
Any basic actions difficulty or complex activity limitation	52.5	54.8	54.6
Any basic actions difficulty	54.0	56.7	56.2
Any complex activity limitation	56.4	57.8	56.5
No disability	19.6	20.3	21.5
Geographic Region [2]			
Northeast	27.5	28.6	28.9
Midwest	32.1	34.8	35.7
South	29.3	29.8	32.4
West	28.4	29.2	30.6
Location of Residence [2]			
Within MSA[9]	28.3	29.2	31.1
Outside MSA[9]	33.9	36.3	37.4

* = Figure does not meet standards of reliability or precision. Data preceded by an asterisk have a relative standard error (RSE) of 20 percent to 30 percent. Data not shown have an RSE of greater than 30 percent.   [1]Starting with 2002 data, respondents were asked, "During the past 30 days, have you had any symptoms of pain, aching, or stiffness in or around a joint?" Respondents were instructed not to include the back or neck. To facilitate their responses, respondents were shown a card illustrating the body joints. Respondents reporting more than one type of joint pain were included in each response category. This table shows the most commonly reported joints.   [2]Estimates are age adjusted to the year 2000 standard population using five age groups: 18 to 44 years, 45 to 54 years, 55 to 64 years, 65 to 74 years, and 75 years and over. Age-adjusted estimates in this table may differ from other age-adjusted estimates based on the same data and presented elsewhere if different age groups are used in the adjustment procedure.   [3]Includes all other races not shown separately, unknown education level, and unknown disability status.   [4]The race groups White, Black, American Indian or Alaska Native, Asian, Native Hawaiian or Other Pacific Islander, and two or more races, include persons of Hispanic and non-Hispanic origin. Persons of Hispanic origin may be of any race.   [5]Estimates are for persons 25 years of age and over and are age-adjusted to the year 2000 standard population using five age groups: 25 to 44 years, 45 to 54 years, 55 to 64 years, 65 to 74 years, and 75 years and over.   [6]GED is General Educational Development high school equivalency diploma.   [7]Percent of poverty level is based on family income and family size and composition using U.S. Census Bureau poverty thresholds.   [8]Any basic actions difficulty or complex activity limitation is defined as having one or more of the following limitations or difficulties: movement difficulty, emotional difficulty, sensory (seeing or hearing) difficulty, cognitive difficulty, self-care (activities of daily living or instrumental activities of daily living) limitation, social limitation, or work limitation.   [9]MSA = metropolitan statistical area.

Table 3-10B. Knee and Shoulder Pain Among Adults 18 Years of Age and Over, by Selected Characteristics, Selected Years, 2002–2010

(Percent.)

Characteristic	Knee pain[1]			Shoulder pain[1]		
	2002	2005	2010	2002	2005	2010
18 years and over, age-adjusted[2,3]	16.5	18.2	19.6	8.6	9.2	9.0
18 years and over, crude[3]	16.5	18.5	20.3	8.7	9.3	9.4
Age						
18 to 44 years	10.5	11.6	12.6	4.9	4.9	5.2
18 to 24 years	8.3	8.8	9.8	3.4	2.4	3.5
25 to 44 years	11.2	12.6	13.6	5.4	5.8	5.8
45 to 64 years	20.4	23.2	26.1	12.3	12.9	13.2
45 to 54 years	18.4	20.6	23.5	10.5	11.5	12.0
55 to 64 years	23.4	26.9	29.3	15.1	14.9	14.8
65 years and over	28.6	30.2	30.5	14.1	16.0	13.6
65 to 74 years	27.6	29.7	30.2	14.0	15.7	13.5
75 years and over	29.7	30.8	30.9	14.1	16.2	13.7
Sex [2]						
Male	15.2	16.8	18.7	8.4	9.3	9.3
Female	17.6	19.4	20.3	8.8	9.0	8.6
Sex and Age						
Male						
18 to 44 years	10.7	12.0	12.9	5.5	5.4	6.1
45 to 54 years	16.2	18.9	22.3	9.5	11.4	12.2
55 to 64 years	20.1	23.1	27.4	13.7	14.7	15.3
65 to 74 years	24.1	25.1	25.3	13.3	15.7	11.8
75 years and over	25.7	25.7	28.7	11.4	15.1	13.1
Female						
18 to 44 years	10.2	11.2	12.2	4.2	4.5	4.3
45 to 54 years	20.5	22.3	24.8	11.4	11.5	11.8
55 to 64 years	26.4	30.5	31.0	16.3	15.1	14.3
65 to 74 years	30.5	33.6	34.4	14.7	15.7	15.0
75 years and over	32.1	34.0	32.4	15.7	16.9	14.1
Race [2,4]						
White only	16.3	18.5	19.7	8.8	9.5	9.1
Black or African American only	20.2	18.2	21.0	8.3	7.6	8.9
American Indian or Alaska Native only	24.5	15.0	26.9	*11.3	*8.1	10.1
Asian only	8.5	10.2	12.8	3.9	5.3	6.9
Native Hawaiian or Other Pacific Islander only	*	*	*	*	*	*
2 or more races	28.1	28.6	27.1	15.4	18.9	13.9
Hispanic Origin and Race [2,4]						
Hispanic or Latino	13.6	14.9	15.5	7.6	8.2	7.4
Mexican	14.1	14.9	15.4	8.3	8.5	7.3
Not Hispanic or Latino	17.0	18.9	20.3	8.9	9.4	9.3
White only	16.9	19.4	20.7	9.1	9.8	9.5
Black or African American only	20.1	18.1	21.0	8.3	7.6	8.9
Education [5,6]						
25 years and over						
No high school diploma or GED	19.5	20.7	22.0	10.8	11.7	10.9
High school diploma or GED	18.6	19.7	22.7	10.2	10.5	10.9
Some college or more	16.9	19.2	20.1	8.8	9.7	9.1
Percent of Poverty Level [2,7]						
Below 100 percent	19.9	21.4	22.9	11.2	11.2	11.1
100 percent to 199 percent	19.0	19.8	21.9	10.4	10.5	10.9
200 percent to 399 percent	16.4	18.4	19.3	8.8	9.2	9.0
400 percent or more	14.9	16.6	18.1	7.3	8.1	7.7
Hispanic Origin and Race and Percent of Poverty Level [2,4,7]						
Hispanic or Latino						
Below 100 percent	16.1	15.7	15.9	11.5	10.5	7.6
100 percent to 199 percent	14.4	15.2	16.1	8.2	8.3	8.0
200 percent to 399 percent	11.7	13.1	14.5	5.7	8.2	6.8
400 percent or more	12.3	15.6	16.3	4.9	*6.4	7.4
Not Hispanic or Latino						
White only						
Below 100 percent	21.3	24.7	25.2	12.4	13.4	12.6
100 percent to 199 percent	20.3	22.8	24.8	11.6	12.0	12.2
200 percent to 399 percent	17.0	20.1	20.9	9.6	10.1	10.0
400 percent or more	15.1	17.0	18.8	7.6	8.4	8.0
Black or African American only						
Below 100 percent	20.8	22.5	25.1	9.1	9.0	11.9
100 percent to 199 percent	23.2	18.3	22.6	10.9	8.3	10.0
200 percent to 399 percent	19.1	16.6	19.8	7.4	7.2	7.8
400 percent or more	18.2	15.8	15.7	*8.0	*5.7	6.5

Table 3-10B. Knee and Shoulder Pain Among Adults 18 Years of Age and Over, by Selected Characteristics, Selected Years, 2002–2010—*Continued*

(Percent.)

Characteristic	Knee pain[1]			Shoulder pain[1]		
	2002	2005	2010	2002	2005	2010
Disability Measure [2,8]						
Any basic actions difficulty or complex activity limitation	32.1	35.7	35.9	17.8	18.8	16.8
Any basic actions difficulty	33.4	37.3	37.3	18.3	19.5	17.2
Any complex activity limitation	35.2	38.2	37.5	22.0	23.5	20.6
No disability	9.4	10.4	11.6	4.6	4.8	4.9
Geographic Region [2]						
Northeast	15.8	16.7	17.9	7.9	8.1	8.3
Midwest	18.4	21.6	22.3	8.6	10.1	10.0
South	16.7	17.9	19.8	9.1	8.9	9.0
West	14.6	16.3	17.9	8.6	9.6	8.5
Location of Residence [2]						
Within MSA[9]	16.0	17.2	19.0	8.1	8.4	8.3
Outside MSA[9]	18.7	22.3	23.0	10.8	12.2	12.3

* = Figure does not meet standards of reliability or precision. Data preceded by an asterisk have a relative standard error (RSE) of 20 percent to 30 percent. Data not shown have an RSE of greater than 30 percent.   [1]Starting with 2002 data, respondents were asked, "During the past 30 days, have you had any symptoms of pain, aching, or stiffness in or around a joint?" Respondents were instructed not to include the back or neck. To facilitate their responses, respondents were shown a card illustrating the body joints. Respondents reporting more than one type of joint pain were included in each response category. This table shows the most commonly reported joints.   [2]Estimates are age adjusted to the year 2000 standard population using five age groups: 18 to 44 years, 45 to 54 years, 55 to 64 years, 65 to 74 years, and 75 years and over. Age-adjusted estimates in this table may differ from other age-adjusted estimates based on the same data and presented elsewhere if different age groups are used in the adjustment procedure.   [3]Includes all other races not shown separately, unknown education level, and unknown disability status.   [4]The race groups White, Black, American Indian or Alaska Native, Asian, Native Hawaiian or Other Pacific Islander, and two or more races, include persons of Hispanic and non-Hispanic origin. Persons of Hispanic origin may be of any race.   [5]Estimates are for persons 25 years of age and over and are age-adjusted to the year 2000 standard population using five age groups: 25 to 44 years, 45 to 54 years, 55 to 64 years, 65 to 74 years, and 75 years and over.   [6]GED is General Educational Development high school equivalency diploma.   [7]Percent of poverty level is based on family income and family size and composition using U.S. Census Bureau poverty thresholds.   [8]Any basic actions difficulty or complex activity limitation is defined as having one or more of the following limitations or difficulties: movement difficulty, emotional difficulty, sensory (seeing or hearing) difficulty, cognitive difficulty, self-care (activities of daily living or instrumental activities of daily living) limitation, social limitation, or work limitation.   [9]MSA = metropolitan statistical area.

Table 3-10C. Finger and Hip Pain Among Adults 18 Years of Age and Over, by Selected Characteristics, Selected Years, 2002–2010

(Percent.)

Characteristic	Finger pain[1]			Hip pain[1]		
	2002	2005	2010	2002	2005	2010
18 years and over, age-adjusted[2,3]	7.5	7.4	7.1	6.6	7.1	7.0
18 years and over, crude[3]	7.5	7.6	7.5	6.6	7.2	7.3
Age						
18 to 44 years	3.4	2.8	3.1	3.2	3.2	3.2
18 to 24 years	2.0	*1.0	1.7	1.6	2.1	*1.5
25 to 44 years	3.9	3.5	3.6	3.8	3.6	3.8
45 to 64 years	11.0	11.2	10.5	9.1	9.7	10.0
45 to 54 years	9.1	9.2	8.4	7.8	7.6	9.0
55 to 64 years	13.9	14.0	13.2	11.0	12.6	11.3
65 years and over	13.9	15.2	14.2	12.9	14.6	13.5
65 to 74 years	14.4	14.9	15.3	12.6	13.7	13.3
75 years and over	13.3	15.4	12.8	13.3	15.7	13.7
Sex[2]						
Male	5.8	6.0	5.8	5.1	5.4	5.3
Female	8.9	8.7	8.2	8.0	8.6	8.6
Sex and Age						
Male						
18 to 44 years	3.0	2.6	3.0	2.5	2.4	2.0
45 to 54 years	6.6	7.5	7.3	5.6	5.7	6.8
55 to 64 years	10.5	10.4	9.9	8.0	9.5	8.7
65 to 74 years	11.2	11.4	10.9	10.5	10.8	10.3
75 years and over	10.0	12.1	9.5	10.1	12.7	12.9
Female						
18 to 44 years	3.8	3.0	3.1	3.9	4.0	4.5
45 to 54 years	11.5	10.9	9.4	9.9	9.5	11.1
55 to 64 years	17.0	17.4	16.2	13.7	15.4	13.7
65 to 74 years	17.1	17.9	19.0	14.2	16.2	15.8
75 years and over	15.3	17.5	15.1	15.2	17.5	14.3
Race[2,4]						
White only	7.6	7.8	7.4	6.9	7.4	7.2
Black or African American only	6.5	4.6	5.6	5.6	6.1	6.0
American Indian or Alaska Native only	*12.9	*13.0	*7.2	*10.4	*	*9.9
Asian only	*3.2	4.1	3.3	*2.3	*2.1	*2.4
Native Hawaiian or Other Pacific Islander only	*	*	*	*	*	*
2 or more races	12.8	10.5	12.2	10.0	13.7	11.7
Hispanic Origin and Race[2,4]						
Hispanic or Latino	6.8	6.0	6.0	3.8	4.1	4.3
Mexican	7.8	7.0	6.3	4.0	4.1	3.9
Not Hispanic or Latino	7.6	7.6	7.3	6.9	7.4	7.3
White only	7.8	8.2	7.7	7.3	7.8	7.7
Black or African American only	6.5	4.7	5.6	5.7	6.2	6.1
Education[5,6]						
25 years and over						
No high school diploma or GED	9.5	8.8	8.5	7.3	8.5	7.9
High school diploma or GED	8.3	8.8	9.1	7.3	7.5	9.0
Some college or more	8.2	8.1	7.4	7.5	7.8	7.3
Percent of Poverty Level[2,7]						
Below 100 percent	9.8	8.0	9.1	8.5	8.9	9.7
100 percent to 199 percent	8.9	8.2	8.3	7.5	8.1	8.5
200 percent to 399 percent	7.9	7.9	7.2	6.8	6.9	6.8
400 percent or more	6.2	6.6	6.0	5.8	6.3	5.7
Hispanic Origin and Race and Percent of Poverty Level[2,4,7]						
Hispanic or Latino						
Below 100 percent	8.6	6.4	6.4	5.9	4.4	5.6
100 percent to 199 percent	8.2	5.7	5.2	3.9	3.9	4.5
200 percent to 399 percent	6.2	6.5	6.8	3.2	4.2	3.1
400 percent or more	*5.3	*5.1	5.8	*1.8	*4.3	*5.2
Not Hispanic or Latino						
White only						
Below 100 percent	10.9	9.9	11.1	9.9	11.6	12.0
100 percent to 199 percent	9.9	9.6	9.8	9.1	9.8	10.6
200 percent to 399 percent	8.5	8.9	7.8	7.5	7.8	7.8
400 percent or more	6.5	7.0	6.3	6.2	6.8	6.0
Black or African American only						
Below 100 percent	7.9	5.7	7.8	8.1	7.7	9.0
100 percent to 199 percent	7.4	6.0	6.2	6.4	6.3	5.9
200 percent to 399 percent	6.0	3.9	4.3	4.7	6.0	5.2
400 percent or more	*4.8	*2.8	*4.2	*4.5	*5.5	4.7

Table 3-10C. Finger and Hip Pain Among Adults 18 Years of Age and Over, by Selected Characteristics, Selected Years, 2002–2010—*Continued*

(Percent.)

Characteristic	Finger pain[1]			Hip pain[1]		
	2002	2005	2010	2002	2005	2010
Disability Measure [2,8]						
Any basic actions difficulty or complex activity limitation	14.5	14.2	12.8	13.8	14.6	14.2
Any basic actions difficulty	14.9	14.8	13.3	14.4	15.2	14.6
Any complex activity limitation	17.8	16.9	15.0	17.8	19.7	18.7
No disability	4.0	4.1	4.2	3.1	3.3	3.1
Geographic Region [2]						
Northeast	6.6	6.2	5.5	5.7	6.4	5.5
Midwest	7.5	8.5	7.9	6.9	7.9	8.5
South	7.6	7.3	7.4	7.0	7.1	7.2
West	8.0	7.5	7.1	6.4	6.6	6.3
Location of Residence [2]						
Within MSA[9]	7.2	7.0	7.0	6.2	6.5	6.5
Outside MSA[9]	8.4	9.1	7.9	8.0	9.3	9.4

* = Figure does not meet standards of reliability or precision. Data preceded by an asterisk have a relative standard error (RSE) of 20 percent to 30 percent. Data not shown have an RSE of greater than 30 percent.   [1]Starting with 2002 data, respondents were asked, "During the past 30 days, have you had any symptoms of pain, aching, or stiffness in or around a joint?" Respondents were instructed not to include the back or neck. To facilitate their responses, respondents were shown a card illustrating the body joints. Respondents reporting more than one type of joint pain were included in each response category. This table shows the most commonly reported joints.   [2]Estimates are age adjusted to the year 2000 standard population using five age groups: 18 to 44 years, 45 to 54 years, 55 to 64 years, 65 to 74 years, and 75 years and over. Age-adjusted estimates in this table may differ from other age-adjusted estimates based on the same data and presented elsewhere if different age groups are used in the adjustment procedure.   [3]Includes all other races not shown separately, unknown education level, and unknown disability status.   [4]The race groups White, Black, American Indian or Alaska Native, Asian, Native Hawaiian or Other Pacific Islander, and two or more races, include persons of Hispanic and non-Hispanic origin. Persons of Hispanic origin may be of any race.   [5]Estimates are for persons 25 years of age and over and are age-adjusted to the year 2000 standard population using five age groups: 25 to 44 years, 45 to 54 years, 55 to 64 years, 65 to 74 years, and 75 years and over.   [6]GED is General Educational Development high school equivalency diploma.   [7]Percent of poverty level is based on family income and family size and composition using U.S. Census Bureau poverty thresholds.   [8]Any basic actions difficulty or complex activity limitation is defined as having one or more of the following limitations or difficulties: movement difficulty, emotional difficulty, sensory (seeing or hearing) difficulty, cognitive difficulty, self-care (activities of daily living or instrumental activities of daily living) limitation, social limitation, or work limitation.   [9]MSA = metropolitan statistical area.

Table 3-11. Basic Actions Difficulty and Complex Activity Limitation Among Adults 18 Years of Age and Over, by Selected Characteristics, Selected Years, 1997–2011

(Number, percent.)

Characteristic	18 years and over					18 to 64 years					65 years and over				
	1997	2000	2005	2010[1]	2011	1997	2000	2005	2010[1]	2011	1997	2000	2005	2010[1]	2011
Number in Millions															
At least one basic actions difficulty or complex activity limitation[2,3]	60.9	59.0	66.5	73.7	74.6	41.3	39.3	45.4	50.7	50.9	19.6	19.7	21.1	23.0	23.7
At least one basic actions difficulty[2]	56.7	55.2	62.4	69.2	70.1	38.1	36.4	42.1	47.2	47.3	18.6	18.7	20.3	22.0	22.7
At least one complex activity limitation[3]	29.0	27.2	31.3	35.0	36.4	18.1	16.7	19.9	22.9	23.7	11.0	10.5	11.5	12.1	12.7
Percent with At Least One Basic Actions Difficulty or Complex Activity Limitation[2,3]															
Total, age-adjusted[4,5]	32.5	29.9	31.0	31.9	31.9	X	X	X	X	X	X	X	X	X	X
Total, crude[4]	31.8	29.5	31.2	32.8	32.9	25.8	23.5	25.3	27.1	27.0	62.2	60.8	62.4	61.7	62.0
Percent with At Least One Basic Actions Difficulty[2]															
Total, age-adjusted[4,5]	30.1	27.9	29.1	29.9	29.8	X	X	X	X	X	X	X	X	X	X
Total, crude[4]	29.4	27.5	29.3	30.8	30.8	23.6	21.7	23.5	25.1	25.0	58.8	58.1	60.1	59.3	59.3
Sex															
Male	25.6	23.8	25.2	26.3	26.7	20.7	18.9	20.3	21.4	21.8	54.5	53.4	55.2	53.8	53.5
Female	32.9	31.0	33.1	35.1	34.6	26.4	24.3	26.6	28.8	28.1	61.9	61.5	63.7	63.6	63.9
Race[6]															
White only	29.6	28.1	29.7	31.2	31.0	23.5	21.8	23.5	25.1	24.9	58.5	58.0	60.0	59.2	59.0
Black or African American only	31.4	27.2	30.4	32.3	33.1	26.9	22.7	26.1	28.4	28.9	64.4	60.6	63.2	62.9	64.0
American Indian or Alaska Native only	43.8	36.8	25.6	41.6	40.8	41.9	34.1	25.2	38.5	35.7	66.0	70.2	*	74.0	65.6
Asian only	15.5	15.5	15.7	17.5	19.0	13.0	12.6	11.8	12.8	14.5	46.4	44.7	46.2	50.1	49.4
Native Hawaiian or Other Pacific Islander only	NA	*	*	*	*	NA	*	*	*	*	NA	*	*	*	*
Two or more races	NA	38.0	40.0	36.3	31.6	NA	34.4	34.9	33.9	27.3	NA	70.7	90.4	65.4	76.9
Hispanic Origin and Race[6]															
Hispanic or Latino	23.8	19.6	21.6	24.7	24.4	21.0	16.6	18.7	21.2	20.9	54.6	57.5	56.2	61.5	60.9
Not Hispanic or Latino	30.0	28.5	30.4	31.8	31.8	23.9	22.4	24.3	25.9	25.8	59.0	58.2	60.3	59.1	59.2
White only	30.3	29.1	31.1	32.4	32.4	23.8	22.5	24.5	26.0	25.9	58.7	58.2	60.3	59.0	59.0
Black or African American only	31.5	27.3	30.7	32.6	33.3	27.0	22.9	26.3	28.6	29.2	64.4	60.4	63.5	63.2	63.3
Percent of Poverty Level[7]															
Below 100 percent	41.9	38.4	40.2	40.6	41.0	36.2	31.9	34.9	36.3	36.6	74.1	71.6	73.1	72.7	74.6
100 percent to 199 percent	38.2	37.1	38.4	38.7	40.0	29.2	26.5	29.6	30.5	31.7	66.6	69.4	68.5	69.5	71.3
200 percent to 399 percent	28.4	28.2	29.7	31.1	31.4	22.0	22.1	22.8	24.1	24.6	56.1	53.9	59.0	58.9	58.9
400 percent or more	21.0	19.4	21.4	23.0	21.7	18.2	16.8	18.1	19.3	17.7	45.5	44.7	48.2	47.0	46.1
Location of Residence															
Within MSA[8]	27.7	25.9	27.5	29.2	29.3	22.3	20.3	22.1	23.6	23.8	56.6	56.7	58.3	59.2	58.4
Outside MSA[8]	35.6	33.6	36.3	39.3	38.3	28.6	26.8	29.5	33.8	31.6	65.8	62.6	65.5	59.9	62.8
Percent with At Least One Complex Activity Limitation[3]															
Total, age-adjusted[4,5]	15.6	13.7	14.5	14.9	15.4	X	X	X	X	X	X	X	X	X	X
Total, crude[4]	15.1	13.4	14.6	15.5	16.0	11.2	9.8	11.0	12.1	12.5	35.1	32.0	33.6	32.3	33.2
Sex															
Male	13.7	12.0	12.9	14.0	14.5	10.6	9.4	10.1	11.3	11.8	31.9	28.1	29.4	30.1	29.1
Female	16.5	14.7	16.1	16.8	17.4	11.9	10.3	11.8	12.9	13.1	37.4	34.9	36.7	34.0	36.3
Race[6]															
White only	15.0	13.6	14.4	15.2	15.9	10.9	9.8	10.7	11.7	12.2	34.3	31.5	33.1	31.7	32.4
Black or African American only	19.0	15.0	17.1	19.7	19.0	15.2	11.7	14.0	17.0	16.1	47.1	40.4	40.9	39.9	39.9
American Indian or Alaska Native only	23.7	20.6	14.2	15.4	18.0	22.1	17.8	13.0	14.5	13.6	*42.6	*54.9	*	*	*42.2
Asian only	5.7	4.7	6.6	7.7	8.6	4.9	3.6	4.7	5.0	5.4	*14.8	*15.5	*20.8	26.7	30.2
Native Hawaiian or Other Pacific Islander only	NA	*	*	*	*	NA	*	*	*	*	NA	*	*	*	*
Two or more races	NA	22.5	26.2	19.6	20.6	NA	20.3	21.8	17.0	17.9	NA	*42.2	69.7	53.6	49.8
Hispanic Origin and Race[6]															
Hispanic or Latino	11.9	9.1	9.8	10.4	11.1	9.8	7.3	7.6	7.9	8.6	33.9	32.4	35.0	37.6	37.7
Not Hispanic or Latino	15.5	14.0	15.3	16.3	16.8	11.4	10.2	11.5	12.9	13.2	35.1	32.0	33.5	31.9	32.8
White only	15.4	14.1	15.2	16.1	16.8	11.1	10.1	11.3	12.5	13.0	34.4	31.5	32.9	31.1	32.0
Black or African American only	18.8	15.1	17.3	20.0	19.2	15.0	11.7	14.1	17.3	16.5	46.8	40.3	40.9	40.0	39.1
Percent of Poverty Level[7]															
Below 100 percent	30.0	26.0	27.3	27.5	28.4	25.2	22.0	23.4	24.0	25.1	56.9	46.7	51.5	54.5	53.7
100 percent to 199 percent	23.3	22.0	22.7	23.7	24.0	16.7	15.1	17.2	18.4	18.2	43.9	42.8	41.3	43.7	45.9
200 percent to 399 percent	13.3	12.8	14.0	14.5	15.0	9.3	9.2	9.9	10.8	10.9	30.6	27.5	31.8	29.3	31.3
400 percent or more	7.3	6.4	7.3	7.7	8.1	5.8	5.0	5.5	5.8	6.2	20.2	19.6	21.5	19.8	19.8
Location of Residence															
Within MSA[8]	14.1	12.1	13.2	14.2	14.8	10.6	8.9	9.9	10.9	11.5	32.7	29.8	31.7	31.6	32.5
Outside MSA[8]	19.0	18.2	20.0	22.2	21.8	13.6	13.4	15.4	18.8	18.1	42.8	38.8	39.7	35.2	35.6

NA = Not available.   X = Not applicable.   * = Figure does not meet standards of reliability or precision. Data preceded by an asterisk have a relative standard error (RSE) of 20 percent to 30 percent. Data not shown have an RSE of greater than 30 percent.   [1]Starting with 2007 data, the hearing question, a component of the basic actions difficulty measure, was revised. Consequently, data for basic actions difficulty prior to 2007 are not comparable with 2007 data and beyond.   [2]A basic actions difficulty is defined as having one or more of the following difficulties: movement, emotional, sensory (seeing or hearing), or cognitive.   [3]A complex activity limitation is defined as having one or more of the following limitations: self-care (activities of daily living or instrumental activities of daily living), social, or work.   [4]Includes all other races not shown separately.   [5]Estimates are for persons 25 years of age and over and are age-adjusted to the year 2000 standard population using five age groups: 25 to 44 years, 45 to 54 years, 55 to 64 years, 65 to 74 years, and 75 years and over.   [6]The race groups, White, Black, American Indian or Alaska Native, Asian, Native Hawaiian or Other Pacific Islander, and 2 or more races, include persons of Hispanic and non-Hispanic origin. Persons of Hispanic origin may be of any race.   [7]Percent of poverty level is based on family income and family size and composition using U.S. Census Bureau poverty thresholds.   [8]MSA = metropolitan statistical area.

Table 3-12. Vision and Hearing Limitations Among Adults 18 Years of Age and Over, by Selected Characteristics, Selected Years, 1997–2011

(Percent.)

Characteristic	Any trouble seeing, even with glasses or contacts[1]					A lot of trouble hearing or deaf[2]				
	1997	2000	2005	2010	2011	1997	2000	2005	2010	2011
Percent of Adults										
18 years and over, age-adjusted[3,4]	10.0	9.0	9.2	9.1	8.8	3.2	3.2	3.5	2.1	2.2
18 years and over, crude[4]	9.8	8.9	9.3	9.4	9.2	3.1	3.1	3.5	2.2	2.2
Age										
18 to 44 years	6.2	5.3	5.5	6.2	5.5	1.0	0.9	0.9	0.5	0.6
18 to 24 years	5.4	4.2	5.0	5.8	5.2	*0.5	*0.7	*1.0	*	*
25 to 44 years	6.5	5.7	5.7	6.3	5.6	1.2	1.0	0.9	0.5	0.7
45 to 64 years	12.0	10.7	11.2	11.6	12.0	3.1	3.0	3.4	1.9	1.9
45 to 54 years	12.2	10.9	11.0	10.7	11.7	2.6	2.3	2.3	1.2	1.5
55 to 64 years	11.6	10.5	11.5	12.7	12.4	3.9	4.0	4.8	2.7	2.4
65 years and over	18.1	17.4	17.4	13.9	13.6	9.8	10.5	11.9	7.6	7.7
65 to 74 years	14.2	13.6	13.2	12.2	12.2	6.6	7.4	6.4	4.6	4.6
75 years and over	23.1	21.9	22.0	16.1	15.2	14.1	14.3	18.1	11.1	11.6
Sex[3]										
Male	8.8	7.9	7.9	7.9	7.6	4.2	4.3	4.8	2.8	2.7
Female	11.1	10.1	10.5	10.3	10.1	2.4	2.3	2.5	1.6	1.7
Sex and Age										
Male										
18 to 44 years	5.3	4.4	4.5	5.2	4.2	1.2	1.1	1.2	*0.7	*0.6
45 to 54 years	10.1	8.8	8.8	9.1	10.4	3.6	2.9	3.3	*1.1	*1.8
55 to 64 years	10.5	9.5	10.5	10.7	11.8	5.4	6.2	7.3	3.9	3.2
65 to 74 years	13.2	12.8	11.4	10.5	9.7	9.4	10.8	9.5	6.7	6.0
75 years and over	21.4	20.7	20.4	15.7	14.9	17.7	18.0	23.3	14.5	14.7
Female										
18 to 44 years	7.1	6.2	6.5	7.1	6.9	0.9	0.8	0.7	*0.3	0.5
45 to 54 years	14.2	12.8	13.2	12.3	13.0	1.7	1.8	1.5	*1.3	1.1
55 to 64 years	12.6	11.5	12.4	14.6	13.0	2.6	1.9	2.6	1.6	1.6
65 to 74 years	15.0	14.4	14.8	13.6	14.5	4.4	4.5	3.8	2.9	3.3
75 years and over	24.2	22.7	23.0	16.4	15.4	11.7	12.1	14.7	8.9	9.5
Race[3,5]										
White only	9.7	8.8	9.1	8.8	8.6	3.4	3.4	3.8	2.3	2.3
Black or African American only	12.8	10.6	10.9	12.1	10.8	2.0	1.6	1.4	1.1	1.2
American Indian or Alaska Native only	19.2	16.6	*14.9	15.0	15.0	14.1	*	*	*	*
Asian only	6.2	6.3	5.5	5.3	6.3	*	*2.4	*2.2	*1.0	*1.8
Native Hawaiian or Other Pacific Islander only	NA	*	*	*	*	NA	*	*	*	*
Two or more races	NA	16.2	16.4	13.1	12.4	NA	*5.7	*5.8	*	*
Hispanic Origin and Race[3,5]										
Hispanic or Latino	10.0	9.7	9.6	9.2	9.4	1.5	2.3	2.8	1.4	1.4
Mexican	10.2	8.3	9.9	9.0	10.4	1.8	3.0	3.3	*1.5	1.6
Not Hispanic or Latino	10.0	9.1	9.2	9.2	8.8	3.3	3.3	3.6	2.2	2.3
White only	9.8	8.9	9.1	8.9	8.6	3.5	3.5	3.9	2.4	2.4
Black or African American only	12.8	10.6	10.9	12.2	10.7	2.0	1.6	1.4	1.1	1.2
Education[6,7]										
25 years of age and over										
No high school diploma or GED	15.0	12.2	13.5	14.1	13.9	4.8	4.6	4.6	3.2	3.1
High school diploma or GED	10.6	9.5	10.3	10.5	10.4	3.7	3.9	4.1	2.5	2.8
Some college or more	8.9	8.9	8.6	8.0	7.9	2.9	2.8	3.5	2.0	2.0
Percent of Poverty Level[3,8]										
Below 100 percent	17.0	12.9	15.3	14.8	14.2	4.5	3.7	4.5	2.7	2.7
100 percent to 199 percent	12.9	11.6	11.5	12.2	11.5	3.6	4.2	4.2	2.5	2.5
200 percent to 399 percent	9.1	8.8	8.9	9.0	8.7	3.3	3.3	3.6	2.1	2.4
400 percent or more	7.3	7.1	6.9	6.4	6.0	2.7	2.5	3.0	1.8	1.7
Hispanic Origin and Race and Percent of Poverty Level[3,5,8]										
Hispanic or Latino										
Below 100 percent	12.8	11.0	13.6	10.8	13.9	*1.9	3.3	3.7	*	*1.3
100 percent to 199 percent	11.2	9.4	8.8	10.8	9.6	*1.5	*2.3	*2.7	*2.3	*1.8
200 percent to 399 percent	8.1	9.2	8.2	8.9	8.3	*	*	*	*	*1.3
400 percent or more	*8.1	10.5	8.0	5.3	5.1	*	*	*	*	*
Not Hispanic or Latino										
White only										
Below 100 percent	17.9	13.1	16.2	16.8	14.4	5.8	4.5	5.7	3.7	3.6
100 percent to 199 percent	13.1	12.0	12.7	12.6	12.3	4.3	5.0	5.1	3.0	2.8
200 percent to 399 percent	9.2	9.2	9.0	8.8	9.0	3.7	3.7	4.0	2.3	2.8
400 percent or more	7.3	7.0	6.9	6.7	5.9	2.7	2.6	3.2	2.0	1.8
Black or African American only										
Below 100 percent	17.9	13.6	16.0	15.8	15.5	3.3	*1.6	*1.9	*1.5	*1.6
100 percent to 199 percent	16.0	12.9	11.3	14.9	12.3	*2.0	*2.0	*	*0.7	*1.5
200 percent to 399 percent	9.3	7.7	9.7	12.0	8.5	*	*	*	*	*1.0
400 percent or more	7.7	8.3	6.4	6.6	8.6	*	*	*	*	*
Geographic Region[3]										
Northeast	8.6	7.4	8.1	7.8	7.6	2.2	2.4	2.9	1.4	2.3
Midwest	9.5	9.6	9.7	9.1	8.7	3.5	3.5	3.7	2.3	1.9
South	11.4	9.2	9.8	10.6	9.4	3.5	3.3	3.7	2.6	2.4
West	9.7	9.9	8.6	8.0	9.1	3.4	3.5	3.8	1.9	2.1
Location of Residence[3]										
Within MSA[9]	9.5	8.5	8.6	8.6	8.6	2.9	3.0	3.1	1.9	2.0
Outside MSA[9]	12.0	11.1	11.7	11.6	10.3	4.5	3.9	4.9	3.0	3.0

NA = Not available.   * = Figure does not meet standards of reliability or precision. Data preceded by an asterisk have a relative standard error (RSE) of 20 percent to 30 percent.   [1]Respondents were asked, "Do you have any trouble seeing, even when wearing glasses or contact lenses?" Respondents were also asked, "Are you blind or unable to see at all?" In this analysis, any trouble seeing and blind are combined into one category. In 2011, 0.4 percent of adults 18 years of age and over identified themselves as blind.   [2]Prior to 2007, respondents were asked, "Which statement best describes your hearing without a hearing aid: good, a little trouble, a lot of trouble, or deaf?" In this analysis, a lot of trouble and deaf are combined into one category. Starting with 2007, the question was revised to expand the response categories. Respondents were asked, "Which statement best describes your hearing without a hearing aid: excellent, good, a little trouble, moderate trouble, a lot of trouble, or deaf?" For 2007 and beyond, a lot of trouble and deaf are combined into one category. The decline from 2006 to 2007 in the estimate of those with hearing trouble is likely due to the addition of the "moderate trouble" response category.   [3]Estimates are age adjusted to the year 2000 standard population using five age groups: 18 to 44 years, 45 to 54 years, 55 to 64 years, 65 to 74 years, and 75 years and over. Age-adjusted estimates in this table may differ from other age-adjusted estimates based on the same data and presented elsewhere if different age groups are used in the adjustment procedure.   [4]Includes all other races not shown separately and unknown education level.   [5]The race groups White, Black, American Indian or Alaska Native, Asian, Native Hawaiian or Other Pacific Islander, and two or more races, include persons of Hispanic and non-Hispanic origin. Persons of Hispanic origin may be of any race.   [6]Estimates are for persons 25 years of age and over and are age-adjusted to the year 2000 standard population using five age groups: 25 to 44 years, 45 to 54 years, 55 to 64 years, 65 to 74 years, and 75 years and over.   [7]GED is General Educational Development high school equivalency diploma.   [8]Percent of poverty level is based on family income and family size and composition using U.S. Census Bureau poverty thresholds.   [9]MSA = metropolitan statistical area.

Table 3-13. Respondent-Assessed Health Status, by Selected Characteristics, Selected Years, 1991–2011

(Percent.)

Characteristic	1991[1]	1995[1]	2000	2005	2006	2007	2008	2009	2010	2011
Percent of Persons with Fair or Poor Health										
All ages, age-adjusted[2,3]	10.4	10.6	9.0	9.2	9.2	9.5	9.5	9.4	9.6	9.8
All ages, crude[3]	10.0	10.1	8.9	9.3	9.5	9.8	9.9	9.9	10.1	10.4
Age										
Under 18 years	2.6	2.6	1.7	1.8	1.9	1.7	1.8	1.8	2.0	2.0
Under 6 years	2.7	2.7	1.5	1.6	1.9	1.5	1.2	1.3	1.8	1.5
6 to 17 years	2.6	2.5	1.8	1.9	1.9	1.7	2.1	2.0	2.2	2.2
18 to 44 years	6.1	6.6	5.1	5.5	5.7	5.9	6.3	6.3	6.3	6.5
18 to 24 years	4.8	4.5	3.3	3.3	3.7	3.3	4.0	3.6	3.9	4.2
25 to 44 years	6.4	7.2	5.7	6.3	6.3	6.8	7.2	7.2	7.2	7.3
45 to 54 years	13.4	13.4	11.9	11.6	12.9	13.3	12.9	13.1	13.3	14.1
55 to 64 years	20.7	21.4	17.9	18.3	18.8	17.9	18.8	19.1	19.4	19.1
65 years and over	29.0	28.3	26.9	26.6	24.8	26.8	24.9	24.0	24.4	24.7
65 to 74 years	26.0	25.6	22.5	23.4	21.9	23.4	21.8	19.9	21.2	21.5
75 years and over	33.6	32.2	32.1	30.2	28.1	30.7	28.4	28.9	28.3	28.6
Sex [2]										
Male	10.0	10.1	8.8	8.8	9.0	9.1	9.1	9.1	9.2	9.4
Female	10.8	11.1	9.3	9.5	9.5	9.9	9.8	9.7	10.0	10.1
Race [2,4]										
White only	9.6	9.7	8.2	8.6	8.6	8.8	8.9	8.7	8.8	9.0
Black or African American only	16.8	17.2	14.6	14.3	14.4	14.2	14.6	14.2	14.9	15.0
American Indian or Alaska Native only	18.3	18.7	17.2	13.2	12.1	17.1	14.5	16.3	17.8	14.4
Asian only	7.8	9.3	7.4	6.8	6.9	7.1	6.7	8.4	8.1	8.7
Native Hawaiian or Other Pacific Islander only	NA	NA	*	*	*	*	*	*	*	*
Two or more races	NA	NA	16.2	14.5	13.1	16.8	12.9	15.3	15.6	14.2
Black or African American; White	NA	NA	*14.5	8.3	*15.0	*16.6	20.2	18.0	*16.7	16.7
American Indian and Alaska Native; White	NA	NA	18.7	17.2	13.9	19.2	14.6	15.2	19.0	16.5
Hispanic Origin and Race [2,4]										
Hispanic or Latino	15.6	15.1	12.8	13.3	13.0	13.0	12.8	13.3	13.1	13.2
Mexican	17.0	16.7	12.8	14.3	14.1	13.2	13.4	13.7	13.7	14.0
Not Hispanic or Latino	10.0	10.1	8.7	8.7	8.8	9.1	9.1	8.9	9.2	9.4
White only	9.1	9.1	7.9	8.0	8.0	8.3	8.4	8.0	8.2	8.4
Black or African American only	16.8	17.3	14.6	14.4	14.4	14.1	14.6	14.2	14.9	15.0
Percent of Poverty Level [2,5]										
Below 100 percent	22.8	23.7	19.6	20.4	20.3	21.0	21.8	21.8	20.9	21.5
100 percent to 199 percent	14.7	15.5	14.1	14.4	14.4	15.3	15.4	14.9	15.2	15.0
200 percent to 399 percent	7.9	7.9	8.4	8.3	8.1	9.0	8.7	8.6	8.3	8.7
400 percent or more	4.9	4.7	4.5	4.7	4.5	4.7	4.4	4.3	4.3	4.3
Hispanic Origin and Race and Percent of Poverty Level [2,4,5]										
Hispanic or Latino										
Below 100 percent	23.6	22.7	18.7	20.2	20.6	21.0	21.0	22.1	19.2	21.0
100 percent to 199 percent	18.0	16.9	15.3	15.3	14.4	15.1	14.6	16.2	15.6	14.4
200 percent to 399 percent	10.3	10.1	10.3	10.3	10.5	10.5	10.7	9.7	10.3	10.8
400 percent or more	6.6	4.0	5.5	7.6	5.7	7.2	5.6	5.6	6.4	5.0
Not Hispanic or Latino										
White only										
Below 100 percent	21.9	22.8	18.8	20.1	19.5	20.9	22.1	20.5	20.9	21.2
100 percent to 199 percent	14.0	14.8	13.4	13.8	14.2	15.2	15.7	14.6	14.8	15.0
200 percent to 399 percent	7.5	7.3	7.9	7.9	7.5	8.4	8.3	8.1	7.7	8.1
400 percent or more	4.7	4.6	4.2	4.3	4.2	4.3	4.1	4.0	4.0	4.1
Black or African American only										
Below 100 percent	25.8	27.7	23.8	23.3	23.0	22.6	25.1	25.2	23.9	24.7
100 percent to 199 percent	17.0	19.3	18.2	17.6	16.9	17.7	18.1	16.6	18.3	18.5
200 percent to 399 percent	12.0	11.4	11.7	11.2	11.0	11.3	11.2	11.0	11.2	10.7
400 percent or more	5.9	6.5	7.3	7.1	7.0	7.2	6.9	5.9	6.8	6.9
Disability Measure Among Adults 18 Years and Over [2,6]										
Any basic actions difficulty or complex activity limitation	NA	NA	27.6	28.5	27.2	31.2	28.5	30.3	28.7	30.1
Any basic actions difficulty	NA	NA	27.7	29.1	27.6	31.6	28.7	30.9	28.9	30.6
Any complex activity limitation	NA	NA	45.6	46.3	45.4	50.8	47.9	48.8	46.0	48.3
No disability	NA	NA	3.8	3.6	4.0	4.0	4.2	3.6	3.5	3.6
Geographic Region [2]										
Northeast	8.3	9.1	7.6	7.5	8.2	8.4	8.0	8.4	7.9	8.4
Midwest	9.1	9.7	8.0	8.3	8.8	8.6	8.8	8.6	9.0	8.8
South	13.1	12.3	10.7	11.0	10.4	11.0	11.0	10.9	11.1	11.2
West	9.7	10.1	8.8	8.6	8.5	9.0	9.0	8.8	9.2	9.5
Location of Residence [2]										
Within MSA[7]	9.9	10.1	8.5	8.7	8.7	9.0	9.1	9.1	9.2	9.4
Outside MSA[7]	11.9	12.6	11.1	11.2	11.7	12.0	11.7	11.2	11.9	11.7

NA = Not available.   * = Figure does not meet standards of reliability or precision. Data preceded by an asterisk have a relative standard error (RSE) of 20 percent to 30 percent. Data not shown have an RSE of greater than 30 percent.   [1]Data prior to 1997 are not strictly comparable with data for later years due to the 1997 questionnaire redesign.   [2]Estimates are age-adjusted to the year 2000 standard population using six age groups: under 18 years, 18 to 44 years, 45 to 54 years, 55 to 64 years, 65 to 74 years, and 75 years and over. The disability measure is age-adjusted using the five adult age groups. The disability measure is age-adjusted using the five adult age groups.   [3]Includes all other races not shown separately and unknown disability status.   [4]The race groups White, Black, American Indian or Alaska Native, Asian, Native Hawaiian or Other Pacific Islander, and two or more races, include persons of Hispanic and non-Hispanic origin. Persons of Hispanic origin may be of any race.   [5]Percent of poverty level is based on family income and family size and composition using U.S. Census Bureau poverty thresholds.   [6]Any basic actions difficulty or complex activity limitation is defined as having one or more of the following limitations or difficulties: movement difficulty, emotional difficulty, sensory (seeing or hearing) difficulty, cognitive difficulty, self-care (activities of daily living or instrumental activities of daily living) limitation, social limitation, or work limitation.   [7]MSA = metropolitan statistical area.

Table 3-14. Selected Measures of Disability and Health Status Among Adults 18 to 64 Years of Age, by Urbanization Level and Selected Characteristics, Annual Average, 2002–2004 Through 2009–2011

(Percent.)

Urbanization level[1] and selected characteristic	Any basic actions difficulty or complex activity limitation[2]				Fair or poor respondent-assessed health status[3]			
	2002–2004	2005–2007	2008–2010	2009–2011	2002–2004	2005–2007	2008–2010	2009–2011
PERCENT OF POPULATION, CRUDE								
Geographic Region								
All regions								
Metropolitan counties								
Large central	21.5	21.8	22.8	23.1	8.7	9.0	9.5	9.8
Large fringe	22.4	23.1	24.6	24.9	6.9	7.1	7.9	8.1
Medium and small	27.4	27.3	28.3	28.3	9.6	9.8	10.9	11.0
Nonmetropolitan counties								
Micropolitan	30.4	31.2	33.0	32.6	11.4	12.4	13.3	13.7
Nonmicropolitan	30.9	33.7	36.0	36.1	14.0	14.6	15.7	15.7
Northeast								
Metropolitan counties								
Large central	20.1	21.0	21.5	22.0	9.0	10.1	9.5	9.3
Large fringe	22.3	22.8	23.5	23.5	6.9	6.1	6.8	6.9
Medium and small	25.9	24.6	29.7	28.4	7.6	7.5	9.3	9.3
Nonmetropolitan counties								
Micropolitan	31.0	31.0	37.4	35.5	9.7	9.8	11.4	12.1
Nonmicropolitan	27.4	34.1	33.5	33.0	8.9	10.6	11.5	10.2
Midwest								
Metropolitan counties								
Large central	26.1	25.7	26.6	26.6	8.9	8.8	10.7	10.8
Large fringe	24.4	26.2	26.4	26.1	6.3	8.0	8.3	8.2
Medium and small	28.1	27.1	26.6	27.2	8.1	8.1	9.5	9.8
Nonmetropolitan counties								
Micropolitan	27.0	28.3	29.6	28.7	8.0	9.8	11.2	11.7
Nonmicropolitan	28.6	29.1	30.4	31.7	9.1	10.9	10.1	10.7
South								
Metropolitan counties								
Large fringe	20.9	21.4	23.0	23.7	7.1	7.2	8.3	8.7
Medium and small	27.8	28.0	29.6	29.9	11.9	11.9	12.6	12.9
Nonmetropolitan counties								
Micropolitan	32.3	31.4	32.5	33.7	14.3	14.6	14.7	15.3
Nonmicropolitan	34.7	36.5	42.4	41.9	20.2	18.2	21.8	22.6
West								
Metropolitan counties								
Large central	20.0	19.9	20.4	21.4	8.3	7.9	8.5	9.0
Large fringe	23.1	23.0	27.3	28.1	7.3	7.7	8.3	8.7
Medium and small	26.8	28.3	27.1	26.7	8.7	9.4	10.3	10.0
Nonmetropolitan counties							v	
Micropolitan	30.8	37.1	38.5	35.0	10.9	13.1	14.8	14.1
Nonmicropolitan	*24.2	36.1	33.7	33.0	*7.6	14.1	13.6	12.1
Age								
18 to 44 years								
Metropolitan counties								
Large central	15.4	15.1	16.2	15.9	5.3	5.6	6.0	6.1
Large fringe	16.1	16.2	17.3	17.9	4.3	4.3	5.1	5.2
Medium and small	20.0	19.0	20.2	20.0	6.0	6.0	6.6	6.6
Nonmetropolitan counties								
Micropolitan	22.5	21.6	23.0	21.8	6.6	7.3	7.8	8.1
Nonmicropolitan	21.5	23.4	23.8	24.0	9.3	8.5	9.1	8.8
45 to 64 years								
Metropolitan counties								
Large central	33.2	33.7	33.8	34.9	15.1	15.1	15.2	15.6
Large fringe	32.2	33.0	34.0	33.7	10.9	11.2	11.4	11.9
Medium and small	39.0	39.8	40.1	40.1	15.3	15.3	16.9	17.0
Nonmetropolitan counties								
Micropolitan	42.0	42.8	45.1	45.8	18.4	19.0	19.9	20.4
Nonmicropolitan	42.6	45.2	48.5	49.2	20.0	21.3	22.6	23.3
Sex								
Male								
Metropolitan counties								
Large central	18.2	18.9	19.2	19.7	7.6	8.3	8.5	8.9
Large fringe	19.7	20.3	22.1	21.9	6.3	6.6	7.2	7.6
Medium and small	23.8	24.9	25.1	25.5	8.9	8.9	10.4	10.4
Nonmetropolitan counties								
Micropolitan	28.3	28.2	29.9	29.9	11.2	11.8	12.6	13.0
Nonmicropolitan	28.5	31.0	35.0	33.1	13.5	14.7	14.7	14.3
Female								
Metropolitan counties								
Large central	24.8	24.6	26.4	26.5	9.8	9.7	10.5	10.6
Large fringe	25.0	25.8	27.0	27.8	7.5	7.7	8.5	8.5
Medium and small	30.8	29.7	31.5	31.0	10.3	10.5	11.4	11.5
Nonmetropolitan counties								
Micropolitan	32.3	34.1	35.9	35.1	11.6	13.0	13.9	14.3
Nonmicropolitan	33.2	36.4	36.8	38.9	14.5	14.5	16.6	17.1
Hispanic Origin and Race [4]								
Hispanic or Latino								
Metropolitan counties								
Large central	17.7	17.9	20.5	20.5	10.4	11.3	11.5	11.6
Large fringe	18.3	17.5	21.8	21.5	9.0	8.1	10.2	9.9
Medium and small	21.5	23.6	23.6	24.1	11.6	11.2	11.6	12.2
Nonmetropolitan counties								
Micropolitan	23.1	22.8	22.7	22.0	13.1	10.6	9.9	10.5
Nonmicropolitan	21.8	29.4	30.0	30.8	10.3	13.8	13.8	12.8
White only, not Hispanic or Latino								
Metropolitan counties								
Large central	22.4	23.1	23.2	23.4	6.4	6.5	7.3	7.5
Large fringe	23.5	24.3	25.9	26.3	6.5	6.8	7.2	7.3
Medium and small	27.8	27.8	28.5	28.3	8.7	8.9	9.7	9.8
Nonmetropolitan counties								
Micropolitan	30.6	31.8	33.3	32.7	10.5	11.8	13.0	13.3
Nonmicropolitan	30.9	33.4	35.9	36.0	13.1	13.7	15.3	15.3

Table 3-14. Selected Measures of Disability and Health Status Among Adults 18 to 64 Years of Age, by Urbanization Level and Selected Characteristics, Annual Average, 2002–2004 Through 2009–2011—*Continued*

(Percent.)

Urbanization level[1] and selected characteristic	Any basic actions difficulty or complex activity limitation[2]				Fair or poor respondent-assessed health status[3]			
	2002–2004	2005–2007	2008–2010	2009–2011	2002–2004	2005–2007	2008–2010	2009–2011
Black or African American only, not Hispanic or Latino								
Metropolitan counties								
Large central	26.9	27.5	29.1	30.4	13.6	14.3	14.5	15.0
Large fringe	21.0	23.1	24.5	25.1	8.8	9.1	10.6	11.0
Medium and small	30.5	29.1	33.5	34.2	14.5	15.5	17.2	16.5
Nonmetropolitan counties								
Micropolitan	33.8	31.4	36.1	37.1	18.7	17.4	16.3	18.5
Nonmicropolitan	31.6	37.6	43.7	43.0	23.3	26.4	24.8	28.2
Percent of Poverty Level [5]								
Below 100 percent								
Metropolitan counties								
Large central	31.8	31.4	32.6	32.1	19.7	18.6	19.4	19.4
Large fringe	33.2	38.9	39.4	38.6	17.4	19.1	21.8	20.8
Medium and small	38.8	37.8	41.4	40.2	21.1	20.1	22.6	22.6
Nonmetropolitan counties								
Micropolitan	42.0	46.8	46.5	47.1	23.1	23.8	26.4	26.9
Nonmicropolitan	47.6	51.8	56.5	55.9	27.8	31.3	32.8	31.9
100 percent to 199 percent								
Metropolitan counties								
Large central	24.7	25.2	28.3	28.8	12.7	13.3	14.3	14.5
Large fringe	30.8	31.1	34.5	34.3	13.6	14.1	15.3	15.2
Medium and small	32.9	33.8	34.1	34.6	15.1	15.5	16.8	17.0
Nonmetropolitan counties								
Micropolitan	38.2	39.0	39.6	38.5	17.2	19.3	19.7	18.9
Nonmicropolitan	39.5	40.8	45.4	43.3	19.8	19.6	22.3	22.0
200 percent to 399 percent								
Metropolitan counties								
Large central	20.3	20.4	20.9	21.3	7.9	8.3	8.6	8.7
Large fringe	23.8	23.2	25.7	26.0	7.5	7.3	8.3	8.4
Medium and small	27.3	26.3	27.7	28.0	8.5	8.7	9.8	9.5
Nonmetropolitan counties								
Micropolitan	27.1	28.0	31.2	29.7	8.7	10.1	10.2	11.0
Nonmicropolitan	26.6	29.0	30.5	31.2	10.9	10.8	11.1	11.1
400 percent or more								
Metropolitan counties								
Large central	17.6	17.7	18.0	17.9	4.0	4.4	4.4	4.3
Large fringe	18.4	19.0	19.1	19.2	3.7	3.9	3.7	3.8
Medium and small	21.2	21.1	21.3	20.8	4.5	4.5	4.9	4.7
Nonmetropolitan counties								
Micropolitan	22.8	22.4	22.7	22.6	4.8	5.3	5.0	5.1
Nonmicropolitan	20.0	23.4	22.2	23.2	5.2	5.9	6.0	6.0
PERCENT OF POPULATION, AGE-ADJUSTED [6]								
Geographic Region								
All regions								
Metropolitan counties								
Large central	22.0	22.1	22.8	23.0	8.9	9.1	9.5	9.7
Large fringe	21.9	22.2	23.4	23.6	6.7	6.8	7.4	7.6
Medium and small	27.0	26.7	27.7	27.6	9.4	9.5	10.5	10.6
Nonmetropolitan counties								
Micropolitan	29.8	29.4	31.2	30.8	10.9	11.6	12.3	12.7
Nonmicropolitan	29.1	31.2	32.8	33.2	13.2	13.1	14.0	14.1
Northeast								
Metropolitan counties								
Large central	20.0	20.9	20.9	21.5	8.9	10.1	9.4	9.1
Large fringe	21.3	21.7	21.9	22.0	6.6	5.8	6.3	6.4
Medium and small	24.6	23.1	27.9	26.4	7.1	7.2	8.6	8.6
Nonmetropolitan counties								
Micropolitan	31.0	29.4	34.9	33.3	9.4	9.1	10.4	10.9
Nonmicropolitan	24.8	32.9	28.3	29.0	8.2	9.6	10.7	9.0
Midwest								
Metropolitan counties								
Large central	26.3	26.4	26.9	26.8	9.1	9.0	10.7	10.8
Large fringe	24.0	25.4	25.1	24.7	6.2	7.6	7.8	7.7
Medium and small	28.2	26.9	26.1	26.9	8.1	8.0	9.4	9.5
Nonmetropolitan counties								
Micropolitan	26.5	26.8	28.3	27.3	7.7	9.1	10.5	11.1
Nonmicropolitan	26.9	26.8	27.7	29.5	8.5	9.5	8.8	9.5
South								
Metropolitan counties								
Large central	22.0	22.4	24.5	23.9	9.1	10.3	10.2	10.5
Large fringe	20.7	20.9	21.9	22.6	7.0	6.8	7.8	8.2
Medium and small	27.4	27.4	29.1	29.2	11.6	11.6	12.2	12.3
Nonmetropolitan counties								
Micropolitan	31.4	29.8	31.0	32.0	13.7	13.8	13.6	14.1
Nonmicropolitan	33.1	34.2	39.3	38.9	19.4	16.6	19.7	20.3
West								
Metropolitan counties								
Large central	20.8	19.9	20.3	21.3	8.7	7.9	8.5	8.9
Large fringe	22.6	21.7	26.5	27.2	7.1	7.3	7.9	8.3
Medium and small	26.6	27.8	26.7	26.4	8.6	9.2	10.1	9.8
Nonmetropolitan counties								
Micropolitan	30.1	34.5	35.7	32.4	10.3	12.1	13.6	12.6
Nonmicropolitan	*22.7	32.4	29.8	29.7	*7.3	13.0	12.3	11.1
Sex								
Male								
Metropolitan counties								
Large central	18.7	19.3	19.3	19.9	7.9	8.5	8.6	8.9
Large fringe	19.4	19.7	21.2	20.8	6.1	6.2	6.9	7.2
Medium and small	23.5	24.4	24.6	24.9	8.7	8.7	10.0	10.0
Nonmetropolitan counties								
Micropolitan	27.6	26.6	28.2	28.3	10.7	10.9	11.6	12.0
Nonmicropolitan	27.1	28.5	31.3	30.4	12.8	13.1	13.0	12.7

Table 3-14. Selected Measures of Disability and Health Status Among Adults 18 to 64 Years of Age, by Urbanization Level and Selected Characteristics, Annual Average, 2002–2004 Through 2009–2011—*Continued*

(Percent.)

Urbanization level[1] and selected characteristic	Any basic actions difficulty or complex activity limitation[2]				Fair or poor respondent-assessed health status[3]			
	2002–2004	2005–2007	2008–2010	2009–2011	2002–2004	2005–2007	2008–2010	2009–2011
Female								
Metropolitan counties								
Large central	25.1	24.8	26.2	26.0	9.9	9.8	10.4	10.5
Large fringe	24.2	24.6	25.4	26.3	7.2	7.3	8.0	8.0
Medium and small	30.3	28.9	30.6	30.1	10.1	10.2	11.0	11.1
Nonmetropolitan counties								
Micropolitan	31.7	32.1	34.0	33.3	11.2	12.2	13.0	13.4
Nonmicropolitan	31.1	33.8	34.0	35.9	13.6	13.1	15.1	15.5
Hispanic Origin and Race [4]								
Hispanic or Latino								
Metropolitan counties								
Large central	19.9	19.9	22.0	22.1	12.4	12.8	12.6	12.6
Large fringe	20.9	19.2	22.9	22.7	10.7	9.3	11.3	10.9
Medium and small	24.3	26.1	26.0	26.2	13.7	13.0	13.1	13.5
Nonmetropolitan counties								
Micropolitan	26.0	24.7	26.7	25.7	15.5	12.7	11.5	12.1
Nonmicropolitan	27.5	30.0	32.1	33.0	12.3	14.5	14.9	14.1
White only, not Hispanic or Latino								
Metropolitan counties								
Large central	21.8	22.3	22.5	22.5	6.1	6.2	7.0	7.1
Large fringe	22.3	22.7	24.0	24.4	6.0	6.2	6.6	6.7
Medium and small	26.9	26.6	27.4	27.0	8.3	8.3	9.1	9.1
Nonmetropolitan counties								
Micropolitan	29.6	29.4	31.0	30.4	9.9	10.8	11.8	12.0
Nonmicropolitan	28.7	30.7	32.3	32.7	12.1	12.1	13.4	13.5
Black or African American only, not Hispanic or Latino								
Metropolitan counties								
Large central	27.4	27.8	28.9	30.3	13.8	14.5	14.6	15.0
Large fringe	22.0	23.3	25.0	25.4	9.4	9.2	10.6	11.0
Medium and small	30.9	29.7	33.2	34.0	15.0	16.0	17.2	16.6
Nonmetropolitan counties								
Micropolitan	34.0	31.6	35.5	36.5	18.6	17.3	16.1	18.1
Nonmicropolitan	33.3	32.5	42.3	43.2	24.1	24.6	23.0	26.4
Percent of Poverty Level [5]								
Below 100 percent								
Metropolitan counties								
Large central	36.3	37.2	38.0	37.0	23.5	22.6	22.8	22.4
Large fringe	39.4	43.5	43.1	42.2	20.9	22.0	24.1	23.3
Medium and small	45.3	45.1	47.6	46.6	25.6	25.0	27.6	27.3
Nonmetropolitan counties								
Micropolitan	48.7	51.1	50.6	52.2	27.3	26.3	29.2	29.9
Nonmicropolitan	49.9	51.3	56.7	56.1	29.5	31.5	33.1	31.9
100 percent to 199 percent								
Metropolitan counties								
Large central	27.9	28.2	30.1	30.9	14.6	15.0	15.8	15.7
Large fringe	33.0	31.8	35.8	35.4	14.8	14.7	16.0	15.9
Medium and small	36.0	36.6	36.8	37.1	16.9	17.2	18.4	18.4
Nonmetropolitan counties								
Micropolitan	39.4	39.3	40.3	38.8	18.0	19.9	19.5	18.7
Nonmicropolitan	39.4	39.9	41.6	41.9	19.8	18.6	21.0	21.0
200 percent to 399 percent								
Metropolitan counties								
Large central	21.4	20.9	21.4	21.6	8.4	8.6	8.7	8.8
Large fringe	24.0	23.5	25.3	25.6	7.6	7.3	8.1	8.2
Medium and small	27.6	26.2	27.6	27.6	8.6	8.6	9.6	9.3
Nonmetropolitan counties								
Micropolitan	26.9	26.6	29.5	27.8	8.5	9.5	9.5	9.9
Nonmicropolitan	25.0	26.3	26.8	28.1	10.2	9.5	9.6	9.5
400 percent or more								
Metropolitan counties								
Large central	16.7	16.7	16.7	16.4	3.8	4.0	3.9	3.8
Large fringe	17.0	17.5	16.8	16.9	3.4	3.5	3.2	3.2
Medium and small		18.3	18.7	18.3	3.9	3.7	4.1	4.0
Nonmetropolitan counties								
Micropolitan	19.3	17.8	18.8	18.2	3.9	4.2	4.0	4.3
Nonmicropolitan	19.9	19.1	18.7	18.6	4.3	4.8	4.5	4.6

* = Figure does not meet standards of reliability or precision. Data preceded by an asterisk have a relative standard error (RSE) of 20 percent to 30 percent. Data not shown have an RSE of greater than 30 percent. [1]Urbanization levels were developed by NCHS using information from the Office of Management and Budget, Department of Agriculture, and Census Bureau. [2]Any basic actions difficulty or complex activity limitation is defined as having one or more of the following limitations or difficulties: movement difficulty, emotional difficulty, sensory (seeing or hearing) difficulty, cognitive difficulty, self-care (activities of daily living or instrumental activities of daily living) limitation, social limitation, or work limitation. [3]Based on responses to the question, "Would you say person's health in general is excellent, very good, good, fair, or poor?" [4]Persons of Hispanic origin may be of any race. In this table, data are presented for non-Hispanic White only and non-Hispanic Black only race groups. [5]Percent of poverty level is based on family income and family size and composition using U.S. Census Bureau poverty thresholds. Missing family income data were imputed.

Table 3-15. Serious Psychological Distress[1] in the Past 30 Days Among Adults 18 Years of Age and Over, by Selected Characteristics, Annual Average, Selected Years, 1997–1998 Through 2010–2011

(Percent of persons with serious psychological distress.)

Characteristic	1997–1998	1999–2000	2000–2001	2001–2002	2002–2003	2003–2004	2004–2005	2006–2007	2007–2008	2008–2009	2009–2010	2010–2011
18 years and over, age-adjusted[2,3]	3.2	2.6	3.0	3.1	3.1	3.1	3.0	2.8	2.9	3.2	3.2	3.3
18 years and over, crude[3]	3.2	2.6	3.0	3.1	3.1	3.1	3.0	2.9	2.9	3.2	3.3	3.4
Age												
18 to 44 years	2.9	2.3	2.7	2.9	2.9	2.9	2.8	2.5	2.7	3.1	3.1	2.9
18 to 24 years	2.7	2.2	2.6	2.8	2.8	2.8	2.5	2.0	2.3	2.5	2.4	2.4
25 to 44 years	3.0	2.4	2.8	3.0	2.9	2.9	2.9	2.7	2.8	3.3	3.4	3.1
45 to 64 years	3.7	3.2	3.6	3.9	4.0	3.9	3.7	3.7	3.6	3.7	4.1	4.5
45 to 54 years	3.9	3.5	3.7	4.2	4.2	3.9	3.9	3.7	3.6	3.9	4.1	4.2
55 to 64 years	3.4	2.6	3.4	3.4	3.6	3.9	3.4	3.8	3.6	3.6	4.0	4.7
65 years and over	3.1	2.4	2.7	2.4	2.3	2.4	2.5	2.1	2.4	2.4	2.1	2.4
65 to 74 years	2.5	2.3	2.8	2.4	2.3	2.3	2.2	2.1	2.4	2.2	2.0	2.6
75 years and over	3.8	2.5	2.5	2.4	2.3	2.5	2.9	2.0	2.4	2.6	2.3	2.1
Sex[2]												
Male	2.5	2.0	2.4	2.4	2.3	2.3	2.3	2.1	2.2	2.7	2.8	2.8
Female	3.8	3.1	3.5	3.8	3.9	3.9	3.7	3.4	3.5	3.6	3.7	3.7
Race[2,4]												
White only	3.1	2.5	2.9	3.0	3.0	3.1	2.9	2.7	2.9	3.2	3.2	3.2
Black or African American only	4.0	2.9	3.1	3.5	3.4	3.4	3.6	3.2	3.2	3.7	3.8	3.7
American Indian or Alaska Native only	7.8	*7.2	*7.4	8.1	*7.1	*5.5	*3.5 v	*3.9	*	*3.8	*5.2	5.6
Asian only	2.0	*1.4	*2.0	*1.8	*1.9	*1.8	1.7	2.0	*1.0	*1.1	1.6	1.7
Native Hawaiian or Other Pacific Islander only	NA	*	*	*	*	*	*	*	*	*	*	*
Two or more races	NA	4.8	5.5	5.0	7.3	9.1	7.9	6.5	5.9	*4.9	5.2	5.6
Hispanic Origin and Race[2,4]												
Hispanic or Latino	5.0	3.5	4.0	4.0	3.9	3.9	3.7	3.4	3.6	3.4	3.6	4.0
Mexican	5.2	2.9	3.4	3.8	3.7	3.6	3.6	3.2	3.3	2.9	2.8	3.6
Not Hispanic or Latino	3.0	2.5	2.9	3.1	3.1	3.1	3.0	2.8	2.8	3.1	3.2	3.2
White only	2.9	2.4	2.9	3.0	3.0	3.0	2.9	2.7	2.9	3.2	3.1	3.2
Black or African American only	3.9	2.9	3.1	3.5	3.4	3.3	3.6	3.2	3.1	3.7	3.8	3.7
Percent of Poverty Level[2,5]												
Below 100 percent	9.1	6.8	7.7	8.4	8.6	8.8	8.6	7.2	8.3	9.0	8.4	8.2
100 percent to 199 percent	5.0	4.4	5.0	5.2	5.2	5.2	5.0	5.0	4.7	4.9	4.8	5.0
200 percent to 399 percent	2.5	2.3	2.7	2.8	2.6	2.5	2.5	2.1	2.4	2.7	2.8	2.9
400 percent or more	1.3	1.2	1.2	1.3	1.3	1.2	1.1	1.2	1.1	1.1	1.2	1.2
Hispanic Origin and Race and Percent of Poverty Level[2,4,5]												
Hispanic or Latino												
Below 100 percent	8.6	6.1	6.9	7.5	7.6	7.4	6.6	6.0	7.0	6.7	6.4	7.5
100 percent to 199 percent	5.4	3.8	4.4	4.1	3.8	3.7	3.9	2.9	4.5	4.5	4.1	4.3
200 percent to 399 percent	3.4	2.1	3.0	3.5	3.0	2.5	2.6	2.8	2.2	1.8	2.6	3.1
400 percent or more	*	2.3	*1.6	*	*	*1.8	*1.9	*2.2	*1.6	*1.0	*1.5	*1.4
Not Hispanic or Latino												
White only												
Below 100 percent	9.6	7.8	8.9	9.2	9.6	10.4	10.2	8.8	10.7	11.2	10.1	9.6
100 percent to 199 percent	5.2	4.9	5.5	5.9	6.1	6.1	5.6	6.0	5.4	5.7	5.5	5.6
200 percent to 399 percent	2.5	2.3	2.9	2.9	2.7	2.6	2.6	2.1	2.6	3.1	3.2	3.2
400 percent or more	1.3	1.1	1.2	1.3	1.3	1.2	1.1	1.1	1.0	1.0	1.1	1.1
Black or African American only												
Below 100 percent	8.7	6.0	6.3	7.2	7.1	7.4	7.6	6.2	6.2	8.0	8.3	7.7
100 percent to 199 percent	4.3	3.6	4.3	4.9	4.5	4.1	4.8	4.3	3.6	3.1	3.5	4.4
200 percent to 399 percent	2.2	*1.7	1.9	2.3	2.0	1.9	2.1	2.0	2.4	2.9	2.5	1.9
400 percent or more	*	*1.0	*	*	*1.2	*	*	*	*	*	*1.6	*1.5
Geographic Region[2]												
Northeast	2.7	1.9	2.5	2.8	3.0	2.9	2.5	2.6	2.6	2.9	3.1	3.0
Midwest	2.6	2.5	2.8	2.9	2.7	2.7	2.7	2.9	2.7	3.2	3.3	3.1
South	3.8	2.9	3.2	3.5	3.5	3.5	3.7	3.1	3.3	3.5	3.5	3.6
West	3.3	2.8	3.2	3.0	3.0	3.0	2.8	2.5	2.7	2.8	2.9	3.3
Location of Residence[2]												
Within MSA[6]	3.0	2.3	2.8	3.0	2.9	2.9	2.8	2.6	2.7	3.0	3.1	3.1
Outside MSA[6]	3.9	3.5	3.6	3.8	3.9	3.8	4.0	3.7	3.7	4.0	4.1	4.0

NA = Not available. * = Figure does not meet standards of reliability or precision. Data preceded by an asterisk have a relative standard error (RSE) of 20 percent to 30 percent. Data not shown have an RSE of greater than 30 percent. [1]Serious psychological distress is measured by a six-question scale that asks respondents how often they experienced each of six symptoms of psychological distress in the past 30 days. [2]Estimates are age adjusted to the year 2000 standard population using five age groups: 18 to 44 years, 45 to 54 years, 55 to 64 years, 65 to 74 years, and 75 years and over. [3]Includes all other races not shown separately. [4]The race groups White, Black, American Indian or Alaska Native, Asian, Native Hawaiian or Other Pacific Islander, and two or more races, include persons of Hispanic and non-Hispanic origin. Persons of Hispanic origin may be of any race. [5]Percent of poverty level is based on family income and family size and composition using U.S. Census Bureau poverty thresholds. [6]MSA = metropolitan statistical area.

Table 3-16. Children Under 18 Years of Age Who Suffer from Asthma, by Selected Characteristics, Annual Average, Selected Years, 1997–1999 Through 2009–2011

(Percent of children.)

Characteristic	Current asthma[1]							Asthma attack in the past 12 months[2]						
	1997–1999	2000–2002	2003–2005	2006–2008	2007–2009	2008–2010	2009–2011	1997–1999	2000–2002	2003–2005	2006–2008	2007–2009	2008–2010	2009–2011
Children Under 18 Years [3]	NA	NA	8.7	9.3	9.4	9.5	9.5	5.4	5.7	5.4	5.5	5.4	5.6	5.6
Age														
0 to 4 years	NA	NA	6.1	6.2	6.4	6.2	6.4	4.3	4.7	4.2	4.3	4.3	4.4	4.5
5 to 17 years	NA	NA	9.6	10.5	10.6	10.8	10.7	5.7	6.1	5.8	5.9	5.9	6.1	6.0
5 to 9 years	NA	NA	9.1	10.6	10.2	10.7	10.2	5.6	6.3	6.1	6.8	6.2	6.5	6.2
10 to 17 years	NA	NA	9.9	10.4	10.8	10.9	11.1	5.8	5.9	5.7	5.4	5.7	5.8	5.8
Sex														
Male	NA	NA	9.9	10.7	10.8	11.1	10.7	6.2	6.6	6.3	6.2	6.2	6.5	6.3
Female	NA	NA	7.3	7.8	7.9	7.8	8.3	4.5	4.7	4.4	4.7	4.6	4.6	4.8
Hispanic Origin and Race [4]														
Race [4]														
White only	NA	NA	7.7	8.2	8.0	8.2	8.1	5.0	5.2	4.9	4.9	4.7	4.9	4.8
Black or African American only	NA	NA	13.0	14.6	16.0	16.0	16.4	7.0	8.0	7.6	8.1	8.6	8.7	8.8
American Indian or Alaska Native only	NA	NA	12.2	*10.4	*10.8	*10.3	*6.6	6.4	*8.7	*6.1	*	*	*	*3.5
Asian only	NA	NA	4.8	5.8	6.3	6.7	7.7	4.3	4.7	3.3	3.9	4.1	4.8	5.2
Native Hawaiian or Other Pacific Islander only	NA	NA	*	*	*	*	*	NA	*	*	*	*	*	*
Two or more races	NA	NA	13.5	13.6	13.9	12.8	13.3	NA	7.3	8.8	8.2	9.3	9.0	8.0
Hispanic Origin														
Hispanic or Latino	NA	NA	7.6	8.3	7.9	7.5	8.5	4.8	4.2	4.6	5.0	4.6	4.4	4.7
Not Hispanic or Latino	NA	NA	8.9	9.6	9.8	10.0	9.8	5.5	6.0	5.6	5.6	5.7	5.9	5.8
White only	NA	NA	7.9	8.2	8.2	8.5	8.2	5.1	5.5	5.0	4.9	4.8	5.1	5.0
Black or African American only	NA	NA	13.0	14.6	16.0	16.2	16.4	7.0	7.9	7.5	8.0	8.5	8.8	8.8
Percent of Poverty Level [5]														
Below 100 percent	NA	NA	10.4	11.7	12.2	12.4	12.7	6.1	7.1	6.5	6.8	6.9	7.4	7.5
100 percent to 199 percent	NA	NA	8.6	9.9	9.8	9.9	9.9	5.3	5.4	5.2	5.8	5.7	6.0	5.9
200 percent to 399 percent	NA	NA	8.3	8.8	8.2	8.2	8.3	5.0	5.3	5.2	4.9	4.7	4.6	4.6
400 percent or more	NA	NA	7.9	7.6	8.4	8.2	7.8	5.2	5.5	4.9	4.8	5.0	5.0	4.7
Health Insurance Status at the Time of Interview [6]														
Insured	NA	NA	9.0	9.7	9.7	9.8	9.7	5.6	5.9	5.6	5.7	5.6	5.8	5.7
Private	NA	NA	8.0	8.3	8.4	8.4	8.2	5.0	5.3	5.0	5.0	5.1	5.1	4.9
Medicaid	NA	NA	11.4	12.4	12.1	12.0	12.0	7.7	7.7	7.1	7.0	6.7	7.0	6.9
Uninsured	NA	NA	5.6	6.0	6.3	6.6	6.8	3.9	4.3	3.3	3.7	*3.5	3.6	3.6

NA = Not available.   * = Figure does not meet standards of reliability or precision. Data preceded by an asterisk have a relative standard error (RSE) of 20 percent to 30 percent. Data not shown have an RSE of greater than 30 percent.   [1]Based on parent or knowledgeable adult responding to both questions, "Has a doctor or other health professional ever told you that your child had asthma?" and "Does your child still have asthma?"   [2]Based on parent or knowledgeable adult responding to both questions, "Has a doctor or other health professional ever told you that your child had asthma?" and "During the past 12 months, did your child have an episode of asthma or an asthma attack?"   [3]Includes all other races not shown separately, unknown poverty level, and unknown health insurance status.   [4]The race groups White, Black, American Indian or Alaska Native, Asian, Native Hawaiian or Other Pacific Islander, and two or more races, include persons of Hispanic and non-Hispanic origin. Persons of Hispanic origin may be of any race.   [5]Percent of poverty level is based on family income and family size and composition using U.S. Census Bureau poverty thresholds. Missing family income data were imputed for 1997 and beyond.   [6]Health insurance categories are mutually exclusive. Persons who reported both Medicaid and private coverage are classified as having private coverage. Starting with 1997 data, state-sponsored health plan coverage is included as Medicaid coverage. Starting with 1999 data, coverage by the Children's Health Insurance Program (CHIP) is included as Medicaid coverage. In addition to private and Medicaid, the insured category also includes military, other government, and Medicare coverage. Persons not covered by private insurance, Medicaid, CHIP, state-sponsored or other government-sponsored health plans, Medicare, or military plans are considered to have no health insurance coverage. Persons with only Indian Health Service coverage are considered to have no health insurance coverage.

Table 3-17. Hypertension Among Persons 20 Years of Age and Over, by Selected Characteristics, Selected Years, 1988–1994 Through 2007–2010

(Percent.)

Sex, age, race and Hispanic origin[1], and percent of poverty level	Hypertension[2,3]			Uncontrolled high blood pressure among persons with hypertension[4]		
	1988–1994	2001–2004	2007–2010	1988–1994	2001–2004	2005–2008
20 Years and Over, Age-Adjusted [5]						
Both Sexes [6]	25.5	30.9	30.6	77.2	66.0	59.4
Male	26.4	30.3	31.3	83.2	68.3	63.8
Female	24.4	31.0	29.6	68.5	57.6	48.5
Not Hispanic or Latino						
White only, male	25.6	29.3	31.1	82.6	67.8	60.8
White only, female	23.0	29.0	28.1	67.0	52.7	47.4
Black or African American only, male	37.5	41.5	40.5	84.0	70.8	70.6
Black or African American only, female	38.3	44.3	44.3	71.1	65.4	51.5
Mexican male	26.9	26.1	28.6	87.9	76.4	68.8
Mexican female	25.0	29.7	27.8	77.6	63.8	65.3
Percent of Poverty Level [7]						
Below 100 percent	31.7	35.5	33.8	75.0	66.1	57.7
100 percent to 199 percent	26.6	34.0	33.4	76.0	70.1	65.7
200 percent to 399 percent	24.7	31.4	31.7	76.2	67.8	58.8
400 percent or more	22.6	27.9	28.5	81.5	60.8	56.7
20 Years and Over, Crude						
Both sexes	24.1	30.8	32.2	73.9	63.0	54.1
Male	23.8	29.0	31.7	79.3	62.1	56.3
Female	24.4	32.5	32.8	68.8	63.7	52.1
Not Hispanic or Latino						
White only, male	24.3	29.9	33.7	78.0	59.4	53.6
White only, female	24.6	32.9	33.4	67.8	63.8	51.1
Black or African American only, male	31.1	36.7	37.6	83.3	68.7	64.2
Black or African American only, female	32.5	41.6	44.4	70.0	61.9	51.8
Mexican male	16.4	15.8	19.9	86.5	73.6	64.0
Mexican female	15.9	19.0	21.4	80.6	69.8	62.8
Percent of Poverty Level [7]						
Below 100 percent	25.7	28.3	27.5	74.0	67.3	58.8
100 percent to 199 percent	26.7	34.6	36.2	75.1	64.5	61.9
200 percent to 399 percent	22.4	31.5	34.2	73.4	63.4	52.0
400 percent or more	22.0	28.4	30.6	74.3	59.2	49.5
Male						
20 to 44 years	10.9	12.3	12.5	90.5	71.0	72.5
20 to 34 years	7.1	7.0	6.8	92.6	87.1	81.4
35 to 44 years	17.1	19.2	20.7	89.0	63.2	66.9
45 to 64 years	34.2	39.9	41.2	73.1	61.1	52.8
45 to 54 years	29.2	35.9	35.5	76.2	64.9	55.4
55 to 64 years	40.6	47.5	49.5	70.3	55.5	50.0
65 to 74 years	54.4	61.7	64.1	74.3	49.5	47.7
75 years and over	60.4	67.1	71.7	82.5	68.3	53.5
Female						
20 to 44 years	6.5	7.7	8.3	63.4	51.0	42.6
20 to 34 years	2.9	*2.7	3.8	82.2	*50.2	49.1
35 to 44 years	11.2	14.0	14.2	56.8	51.2	40.9
45 to 64 years	32.8	42.6	39.7	62.1	60.9	49.5
45 to 54 years	23.9	35.2	31.2	58.5	66.1	46.3
55 to 64 years	42.6	54.4	50.4	64.3	55.6	52.4
65 to 74 years	56.2	72.9	69.3	68.7	67.2	51.2
75 years and over	73.6	82.0	81.3	81.9	72.4	62.9

* = Figure does not meet standards of reliability or precision. Data preceded by an asterisk have a relative standard error (RSE) of 20 percent to 30 percent. [1]Persons of Hispanic origin may be of any race. [2]Hypertension is defined as having measured high blood pressure and/or taking antihypertensive medication. High blood pressure is defined as having measured systolic pressure of at least 140 mmHg or diastolic pressure of at least 90 mmHg. Those with high blood pressure also may be taking prescribed medicine for high blood pressure. Those taking antihypertensive medication may not have measured high blood pressure but are still classified as having hypertension. [3]Respondents were asked, "Are you now taking prescribed medicine for your high blood pressure?" [4]Uncontrolled high blood pressure among persons with hypertension is defined as measured systolic pressure of at least 140 mmHg or diastolic pressure of at least 90 mmHg, among those with measured high blood pressure or reporting taking antihypertensive medication. [5]Age-adjusted to the 2000 standard population using five age groups: 20 to 34 years, 35 to 44 years, 45 to 54 years, 55 to 64 years, and 65 years and over. [6]Includes persons of all races and Hispanic origins, not just those shown separately. [7]Percent of poverty level is based on family income and family size. Persons with unknown percent of poverty level are excluded (8 percent in 2007–2010).

Table 3-18. Cholesterol Among Persons 20 Years of Age and Over, by Selected Characteristics, Selected Years, 1988–1994 Through 2007–2010

(Percent, number.)

Sex, age, race and Hispanic origin[1], and percent of poverty level	1988–1994	1999–2002	2003–2006	2007–2010
PERCENT OF POPULATION WITH HIGH CHOLESTEROL (GREATER THAN OR EQUAL TO 240 MG/DL OR TAKING CHOLESTEROL-LOWERING MEDICATIONS) [2]				
20 Years and Over, Age-Adjusted [3]				
Both sexes[4]	22.8	25.0	27.7	27.4
Male	21.1	25.3	27.7	28.0
Female	24.0	24.3	27.4	26.7
Not Hispanic or Latino				
White only, male	21.1	26.0	28.7	28.1
White only, female	24.2	25.1	28.2	27.4
Black or African American only, male	18.6	20.1	22.8	25.4
Black or African American only, female	23.1	22.0	23.3	25.6
Mexican male	19.9	21.6	24.2	28.6
Mexican female	19.8	19.3	24.1	25.5
Percent of Poverty Level [5]				
Below 100 percent	23.0	25.0	27.9	26.5
100 percent to 199 percent	22.1	25.9	27.6	27.6
200 percent to 399 percent	23.1	26.5	27.5	28.9
400 percent or more	21.7	23.1	27.9	26.6
20 Years and Over, Crude				
Both sexes[4]	21.5	25.0	28.0	28.7
Male	19.6	25.1	27.5	28.7
Female	23.2	24.8	28.5	28.7
Not Hispanic or Latino				
White only, male	20.0	26.8	29.7	30.4
White only, female	24.5	27.0	30.8	31.4
Black or African American only, male	16.0	18.5	21.3	24.1
Black or African American only, female	19.7	19.9	21.9	24.7
Mexican male	16.2	17.0	19.3	23.7
Mexican female	14.9	13.8	18.7	21.0
Percent of Poverty Level [5]				
Below 100 percent	19.4	21.6	24.1	22.3
100 percent to 199 percent	21.3	25.4	28.3	28.7
200 percent to 399 percent	21.3	26.2	28.1	30.6
400 percent or more	21.9	24.2	28.7	29.6
Male				
20 to 44 years	13.1	16.1	16.5	14.3
20 to 34 years	8.2	10.4	10.2	8.5
35 to 44 years	21.0	23.1	25.2	22.5
45 to 64 years	30.1	36.0	35.7	39.0
45 to 54 years	29.6	34.1	32.4	34.0
55 to 64 years	30.8	39.1	41.6	46.2
65 to 74 years	27.4	36.3	49.4	48.9
75 years and over	24.4	29.0	37.1	45.2
Female				
20 to 44 years	9.9	11.4	12.9	10.6
20 to 34 years	7.3	9.1	10.8	6.8
35 to 44 years	13.5	14.4	15.8	15.7
45 to 64 years	36.4	31.7	37.3	39.1
45 to 54 years	28.2	27.2	29.6	29.1
55 to 64 years	45.8	39.2	49.2	51.4
65 to 74 years	46.9	51.9	55.3	53.3
75 years and over	41.2	44.0	47.3	52.5

Table 3-18. Cholesterol Among Persons 20 Years of Age and Over, by Selected Characteristics, Selected Years, 1988–1994 Through 2007–2010—*Continued*

(Percent, number.)

Sex, age, race and Hispanic origin[1], and percent of poverty level	1988–1994	1999–2002	2003–2006	2007–2010
PERCENT OF POPULATION WITH HIGH SERUM TOTAL CHOLESTEROL (GREATER THAN OR EQUAL TO 240 MG/DL) [6]				
20 Years and Over, Age-Adjusted [3]				
Both sexes[4]	22.8	25.0	27.7	27.4
Male	21.1	25.3	27.7	28.0
Female	24.0	24.3	27.4	26.7
Not Hispanic or Latino				
White only, male	21.1	26.0	28.7	28.1
White only, female	24.2	25.1	28.2	27.4
Black or African American only, male	18.6	20.1	22.8	25.4
Black or African American only, female	23.1	22.0	23.3	25.6
Mexican male	19.9	21.6	24.2	28.6
Mexican female	19.8	19.3	24.1	25.5
Percent of Poverty Level [5]				
Below 100 percent	23.0	25.0	27.9	26.5
100 percent to 199 percent	22.1	25.9	27.6	27.6
200 percent to 399 percent	23.1	26.5	27.5	28.9
400 percent or more	21.7	23.1	27.9	26.6
20 Years and Over, Crude				
Both sexes[4]	21.5	25.0	28.0	28.7
Male	19.6	25.1	27.5	28.7
Female	23.2	24.8	28.5	28.7
Not Hispanic or Latino				
White only, male	20.0	26.8	29.7	30.4
White only, female	24.5	27.0	30.8	31.4
Black or African American only, male	16.0	18.5	21.3	24.1
Black or African American only, female	19.7	19.9	21.9	24.7
Mexican male	16.2	17.0	19.3	23.7
Mexican female	14.9	13.8	18.7	21.0
Percent of Poverty Level [5]				
Below 100 percent	19.4	21.6	24.1	22.3
100 percent to 199 percent	21.3	25.4	28.3	28.7
200 percent to 399 percent	21.3	26.2	28.1	30.6
400 percent or more	21.9	24.2	28.7	29.6
Male				
20 to 44 years	13.1	16.1	16.5	14.3
20 to 34 years	8.2	10.4	10.2	8.5
35 to 44 years	21.0	23.1	25.2	22.5
45 to 64 years	30.1	36.0	35.7	39.0
45 to 54 years	29.6	34.1	32.4	34.0
55 to 64 years	30.8	39.1	41.6	46.2
65 to 74 years	27.4	36.3	49.4	48.9
75 years and over	24.4	29.0	37.1	45.2
Female				
20 to 44 years	9.9	11.4	12.9	10.6
20 to 34 years	7.3	9.1	10.8	6.8
35 to 44 years	13.5	14.4	15.8	15.7
45 to 64 years	36.4	31.7	37.3	39.1
45 to 54 years	28.2	27.2	29.6	29.1
55 to 64 years	45.8	39.2	49.2	51.4
65 to 74 years	46.9	51.9	55.3	53.3
75 years and over	41.2	44.0	47.3	52.5

Table 3-18. Cholesterol Among Persons 20 Years of Age and Over, by Selected Characteristics, Selected Years, 1988–1994 Through 2007–2010—Continued

(Percent, number.)

Sex, age, race and Hispanic origin[1], and percent of poverty level	1988–1994	1999–2002	2003–2006	2007–2010
MEAN SERUM TOTAL CHOLESTEROL LEVEL, MG/DL [7]				
20 Years and Over, Age-Adjusted [3]				
Both sexes[4]	206	203	200	196
Male	204	202	198	194
Female	207	204	202	198
Not Hispanic or Latino				
White only, male	205	202	198	193
White only, female	208	205	203	199
Black or African American only, male	202	195	193	191
Black or African American only, female	207	202	195	192
Mexican male	206	204	203	200
Mexican female	206	199	200	196
Percent of Poverty Level [5]				
Below 100 percent	205	201	203	196
100 percent to 199 percent	205	204	201	198
200 percent to 399 percent	207	205	199	196
400 percent or more	205	202	201	195
20 Years and Over, Crude				
Both sexes[4]	204	203	200	197
Male	202	202	198	194
Female	206	204	202	199
Not Hispanic or Latino				
White only, male	203	203	198	193
White only, female	208	206	205	201
Black or African American only, male	198	194	192	191
Black or African American only, female	201	199	194	191
Mexican male	199	200	200	200
Mexican female	198	194	196	195
Percent of Poverty Level [5]				
Below 100 percent	200	198	200	194
100 percent to 199 percent	202	202	199	197
200 percent to 399 percent	205	204	199	197
400 percent or more	206	204	203	198
Male				
20 to 44 years	194	196	196	194
20 to 34 years	186	188	186	186
35 to 44 years	206	207	209	205
45 to 64 years	216	213	206	202
45 to 54 years	216	215	208	204
55 to 64 years	216	212	202	199
65 to 74 years	212	202	191	182
75 years and over	205	195	187	176
Female				
20 to 44 years	189	191	192	187
20 to 34 years	184	185	188	181
35 to 44 years	195	198	197	195
45 to 64 years	225	215	213	211
45 to 54 years	217	211	208	208
55 to 64 years	235	221	219	214
65 to 74 years	233	224	214	207
75 years and over	229	217	206	203

[1]Persons of Hispanic origin may be of any race. [2]High cholesterol is defined as measured serum total cholesterol as greater than or equal to 240 mg/dL or reporting taking cholesterol-lowering medications. Respondents were asked, "Are you now following this advice [from a doctor of health professional] to take prescribed medicine [to lower your cholesterol]?" [3]Age adjusted to the 2000 standard population using five age groups: 20 to 34 years, 35 to 44 years, 45 to 54 years, 55 to 64 years, and 65 years and over. [4]Includes persons of all races and Hispanic origins, not just those shown separately. [5]Percent of poverty level is based on family income and family size. Persons with unknown percent of poverty level are excluded (8 percent in 2007–2010). [6]High serum total cholesterol is defined as greater than or equal to 240 mg/dL (6.20 mmol/L), regardless of whether the respondent reported taking cholesterol-lowering medications. [7]Risk levels for cholesterol have been defined by the Third Report of the National Cholesterol Education Program Expert Panel on Detection, Evaluation, and Treatment of High Blood Cholesterol in Adults. National Heart, Lung, and Blood Institute, National Institutes of Health. September 2002.

Table 3-19. Mean Energy and Macronutrient Intake Among Persons 20 Years of Age and Over, by Sex and Age, Selected Years, 1971–1974 Through 2005–2008

(Number, percent.)

Sex and age	1971–1974	1976–1980	1988–1994	1999–2002	2003–2006	2005–2008
Mean Energy Intake in Kilocalories (Kcal)						
Male, age-adjusted[1]	2,450	2,439	2,592	2,570	2,654	2,656
Male, crude	2,461	2,459	2,648	2,593	2,671	2,672
20 to 39 years	2,784	2,753	2,964	2,854	2,978	2,946
40 to 59 years	2,303	2,315	2,567	2,601	2,693	2,702
60 to 74 years	1,918	1,906	2,104	2,124	2,137	2,170
75 years and over	NA	NA	1,814	1,876	1,865	1,941
Female, age-adjusted[1]	1,542	1,522	1,762	1,837	1,836	1,811
Female, crude	1,540	1,525	1,772	1,832	1,828	1,803
20 to 39 years	1,652	1,643	1,956	2,031	2,001	1,973
40 to 59 years	1,510	1,473	1,734	1,823	1,823	1,798
60 to 74 years	1,325	1,322	1,520	1,582	1,633	1,605
75 years and over	NA	NA	1,401	1,435	1,472	1,466
Percent Kcal from Carbohydrates						
Male, age-adjusted[1]	42.4	42.6	48.5	49.1	47.7	47.4
Male, crude	42.4	42.7	48.4	49.0	47.6	47.4
20 to 39 years	42.2	43.1	48.1	50.1	48.5	48.0
40 to 59 years	41.6	41.5	47.8	47.7	46.4	46.5
60 to 74 years	44.8	44.1	49.7	48.9	47.0	47.3
75 years and over	NA	NA	50.9	50.8	50.4	49.0
Female, age-adjusted[1]	45.4	46.0	51.0	51.7	49.7	49.5
Female, crude	45.5	46.1	51.0	51.7	49.7	49.4
20 to 39 years	45.8	46.0	50.6	52.6	50.0	50.0
40 to 59 years	44.4	45.0	50.0	50.4	48.5	48.0
60 to 74 years	46.8	48.6	52.6	51.4	50.2	49.9
75 years and over	NA	NA	54.2	53.5	52.6	52.6
Percent Kcal from Protein						
Male, age-adjusted[1]	16.5	16.1	15.5	15.3	15.5	15.6
Male, crude	16.4	16.0	15.4	15.3	15.5	15.6
20 to 39 years	16.1	15.8	15.0	14.8	15.4	15.5
40 to 59 years	16.9	16.3	15.7	15.5	15.4	15.5
60 to 74 years	16.5	16.3	15.9	16.2	16.0	16.2
75 years and over	NA	NA	16.3	15.7	15.8	15.7
Female, age-adjusted[1]	16.9	16.0	15.4	15.1	15.6	15.8
Female, crude	16.8	16.0	15.4	15.1	15.6	15.9
20 to 39 years	16.4	15.8	14.8	14.6	15.3	15.4
40 to 59 years	17.3	16.3	15.6	15.3	15.7	16.4
60 to 74 years	17.0	16.1	16.4	16.0	15.9	15.9
75 years and over	NA	NA	15.9	15.3	15.6	15.6
Percent Kcal from Total Fat						
Male, age-adjusted[1]	36.9	36.7	33.8	33.0	33.5	33.6
Male, crude	36.9	36.7	33.9	33.0	33.5	33.6
20 to 39 years	37.0	36.2	34.0	32.1	32.5	32.7
40 to 59 years	36.9	37.2	34.2	33.7	34.2	34.1
60 to 74 years	36.4	36.8	32.9	33.8	34.7	34.2
75 years and over	NA	NA	32.9	33.5	33.1	34.1
Female, age-adjusted[1]	36.1	36.0	33.2	33.2	33.9	33.8
Female, crude	36.0	35.9	33.2	33.2	33.9	33.8
20 to 39 years	36.3	36.0	33.6	32.5	33.6	33.6
40 to 59 years	36.3	36.4	34.0	33.9	34.4	34.2
60 to 74 years	34.9	34.7	31.6	33.4	34.2	34.2
75 years and over	NA	NA	31.5	32.8	32.7	32.5
Percent Kcal from Saturated Fat						
Male, age-adjusted[1]	13.5	13.2	11.3	10.8	11.1	11.1
Male, crude	13.5	13.2	11.4	10.8	11.1	11.1
20 to 39 years	13.6	13.1	11.5	10.7	10.9	11.0
40 to 59 years	13.5	13.4	11.3	10.8	11.2	11.2
60 to 74 years	13.3	13.1	10.9	10.7	11.3	11.2
75 years and over	NA	NA	11.2	10.8	11.1	11.5
Female, age-adjusted[1]	13.0	12.5	11.1	10.7	11.2	11.3
Female, crude	12.9	12.5	11.1	10.7	11.2	11.3
20 to 39 years	13.0	12.6	11.4	10.8	11.1	11.2
40 to 59 years	13.1	12.6	11.3	10.9	11.5	11.5
60 to 74 years	12.4	11.8	10.4	10.5	11.1	11.3
75 years and over	NA	NA	10.5	10.2	10.8	10.9

NA = Not available. [1]Age-adjusted to the 2000 standard population using four age groups: 20–39 years, 40–59 years, 60–74 years, and 75 years and over. Age-adjusted estimates in this table may differ from other age-adjusted estimates based on the same data and presented elsewhere if different age groups are used in the adjustment procedure.

Table 3-20. Participation in Leisure-Time Aerobic and Muscle-Strengthening Activities That Meet the 2008 Federal Physical Activity Guidelines for Adults 18 Years of Age and Over, by Selected Characteristics, 2000 and 2011

(Percent.)

Characteristic	2008 Physical Activity Guidelines for Americans[1]							
	Met both aerobic activity and muscle-strengthening guidelines		Met neither aerobic activity nor muscle-strengthening guideline		Met aerobic activity guideline		Met muscle-strengthening guideline	
	2000	2011	2000	2011	2000	2011	2000	2011
18 years and over, age-adjusted[2,3]	15.0	21.0	54.7	47.6	42.2	49.0	18.0	24.4
18 years and over, crude[3]	15.1	20.6	54.6	48.1	42.4	48.4	18.1	24.0
Age								
18 to 44 years	18.9	26.0	49.1	41.4	47.7	55.8	22.1	28.8
18 to 24 years	23.8	30.3	44.5	36.2	52.2	61.2	27.2	32.9
25 to 44 years	17.3	24.5	50.6	43.3	46.3	53.8	20.5	27.3
45 to 64 years	12.8	17.5	57.6	51.5	39.7	44.9	15.5	21.1
45 to 54 years	14.5	18.8	55.4	49.9	42.1	46.4	17.0	22.4
55 to 64 years	10.1	16.1	61.0	53.3	36.1	43.2	13.1	19.5
65 years and over	6.8	11.3	67.0	60.3	30.1	34.9	9.8	16.2
65 to 74 years	8.4	14.3	60.3	54.3	36.8	41.0	11.3	19.2
75 years and over	4.9	7.7	75.0	67.7	22.1	27.4	8.0	12.5
Sex [2]								
Male	17.9	25.0	49.6	43.5	47.4	52.7	20.8	28.7
Female	12.3	17.2	59.4	51.5	37.6	45.6	15.4	20.2
Sex and Age								
Male								
18 to 44 years	23.0	31.9	43.0	36.7	53.6	59.8	26.3	35.4
45 to 54 years	16.0	19.6	52.7	48.4	45.2	47.8	18.0	23.3
55 to 64 years	11.3	17.6	58.7	50.5	38.9	45.8	13.8	21.3
65 to 74 years	9.4	16.8	55.3	50.8	41.8	45.5	12.2	20.5
75 years and over	7.1	11.2	66.7	59.0	30.7	35.5	10.1	16.7
Female								
18 to 44 years	15.0	20.2	55.0	46.1	42.0	51.9	17.9	22.2
45 to 54 years	13.1	17.9	57.9	51.4	39.1	45.1	16.1	21.5
55 to 64 years	9.0	14.7	63.1	56.0	33.5	40.7	12.4	17.9
65 to 74 years	7.7	12.1	64.3	57.2	32.6	37.2	10.5	18.1
75 years and over	3.6	5.3	80.0	73.8	16.8	21.8	6.7	9.6
Race [2,4]								
White only	15.7	21.7	53.1	46.2	44.1	50.4	18.5	25.1
Black or African American only	12.2	17.9	64.6	55.0	31.7	41.5	16.0	21.4
American Indian or Alaska Native only	*10.6	17.0	67.1	51.4	29.7	43.1	13.9	23.4
Asian only	14.1	16.8	55.0	52.6	41.7	44.8	17.2	19.3
Native Hawaiian or Other Pacific Islander only	*	*	*	*	*	*	*	*
Two or more races	19.0	24.1	52.8	45.6	43.9	50.9	22.2	28.3
Hispanic Origin and Race [2,4]								
Hispanic or Latino	9.2	15.4	66.5	56.3	30.8	40.1	11.9	19.0
Mexican	8.1	14.0	67.0	56.7	30.0	39.4	11.3	18.0
Not Hispanic or Latino	15.8	22.0	53.2	46.1	43.7	50.5	18.8	25.3
White only	16.5	23.1	51.4	44.0	45.7	52.6	19.3	26.4
Black or African American only	12.2	18.1	64.6	55.1	31.7	41.3	16.0	21.6
Education [5,6]								
No high school diploma or GED	4.3	7.4	74.0	68.3	23.9	28.7	6.6	10.6
High school diploma or GED	9.5	12.2	61.7	59.0	35.7	37.8	12.1	15.5
Some college or more	18.9	25.4	47.1	40.8	49.4	55.3	22.4	29.1
Percent of Poverty Level [2,7]								
Below 100 percent	9.3	11.7	68.0	61.5	29.3	36.1	12.3	14.2
100 percent to 199 percent	9.0	13.9	65.5	58.7	32.0	37.8	11.5	17.5
200 percent to 399 percent	13.2	19.5	56.8	48.6	39.9	47.8	16.5	23.1
400 percent or more	20.5	29.5	45.0	36.4	52.0	60.1	23.4	32.9
Hispanic Origin and Race and Percent of Poverty Level [2,4,7]								
Hispanic or Latino								
Below 100 percent	4.4	8.4	75.2	66.1	22.1	31.5	7.2	10.8
100 percent to 199 percent	5.0	11.7	72.2	61.8	25.8	34.6	7.1	15.4
200 percent to 399 percent	10.2	17.5	63.1	52.6	33.0	43.1	14.0	21.8
400 percent or more	19.6	27.9	52.8	40.0	45.1	56.1	21.7	32.0
Not Hispanic or Latino								
White only								
Below 100 percent	11.7	14.4	63.5	58.7	34.0	39.1	14.7	16.5
100 percent to 199 percent	10.3	14.9	62.6	56.3	34.8	40.4	12.9	18.3
200 percent to 399 percent	13.9	19.5	54.7	46.9	42.3	49.6	16.9	23.1
400 percent or more	21.0	30.4	43.7	34.6	53.4	61.9	23.8	33.7
Black or African American only								
Below 100 percent	9.5	11.0	72.1	63.4	25.4	33.2	12.1	14.2
100 percent to 199 percent	9.5	13.6	69.2	61.7	28.0	34.2	12.3	17.6
200 percent to 399 percent	11.8	22.8	64.3	51.4	31.4	45.2	16.2	26.2
400 percent or more	17.6	25.1	54.9	44.8	40.3	52.0	22.4	28.4

Table 3-20. Participation in Leisure-Time Aerobic and Muscle-Strengthening Activities That Meet the 2008 Federal Physical Activity Guidelines for Adults 18 Years of Age and Over, by Selected Characteristics, 2000 and 2011—*Continued*

(Percent.)

Characteristic	2008 Physical Activity Guidelines for Americans[1]							
	Met both aerobic activity and muscle-strengthening guidelines		Met neither aerobic activity nor muscle-strengthening guideline		Met aerobic activity guideline		Met muscle-strengthening guideline	
	2000	2011	2000	2011	2000	2011	2000	2011
Disability Measure [2,8]								
Any basic actions difficulty or complex activity limitation	10.3	13.2	62.2	58.7	34.2	37.6	14.0	17.1
Any basic actions difficulty	10.3	12.7	62.1	59.2	34.0	37.0	14.2	16.6
Any complex activity limitation	7.2	9.7	71.2	66.7	24.9	28.8	11.3	14.2
No disability	17.0	24.7	50.6	41.3	46.6	55.5	19.8	27.7
Geographic Region [2]								
Northeast	17.0	19.5	51.8	50.9	45.3	45.8	20.0	22.6
Midwest	16.4	22.0	53.4	47.7	43.5	48.9	19.3	25.4
South	12.1	18.3	59.7	50.8	37.3	46.1	15.1	21.4
West	16.7	25.3	50.1	40.3	46.9	55.9	19.7	29.1
Location of residence [2]								
Within MSA[9]	15.7	22.1	54.1	46.2	42.9	50.3	18.6	25.6
Outside MSA[9]	12.3	14.9	56.9	55.3	39.9	41.9	15.5	17.8

* = Figure does not meet standards of reliability or precision. Data preceded by an asterisk have a relative standard error (RSE) of 20 percent to 30 percent. Data not shown have an RSE of greater than 30 percent.   [1]Starting with Health, United States, 2010, measures of physical activity shown in this table changed to reflect the 2008 federal Physical Activity Guidelines for Americans (available from http://www.health.gov/PAGuidelines/).   [2]Estimates are age adjusted to the year 2000 standard population using five age groups: 18 to 44 years, 45 to 54 years, 55 to 64 years, 65 to 74 years, and 75 years and over.   [3]Includes all other races not shown separately, unknown education level, and unknown disability status.   [4]The race groups White, Black, American Indian or Alaska Native, Asian, Native Hawaiian or Other Pacific Islander, and two or more races, include persons of Hispanic and non-Hispanic origin. Persons of Hispanic origin may be of any race.   [5]Estimates are for persons 25 years of age and over and are age-adjusted to the year 2000 standard population using five age groups: 25–44 years, 45–54 years, 55–64 years, 65–74 years, and 75 years and over.   [7]Percent of poverty level is based on family income and family size and composition using U.S. Census Bureau poverty thresholds.   [8]Any basic actions difficulty or complex activity limitation is defined as having one or more of the following limitations or difficulties: movement difficulty, emotional difficulty, sensory (seeing or hearing) difficulty, cognitive difficulty, self-care (activities of daily living or instrumental activities of daily living) limitation, social limitation, or work limitation.   [9]MSA = metropolitan statistical area.

Figure 3-4. Age-Adjusted Healthy Weight, Overweight, and Obesity Prevalence Among Persons Age 20 to 74 Years, Selected Years, 1960–1962 to 2007–2010

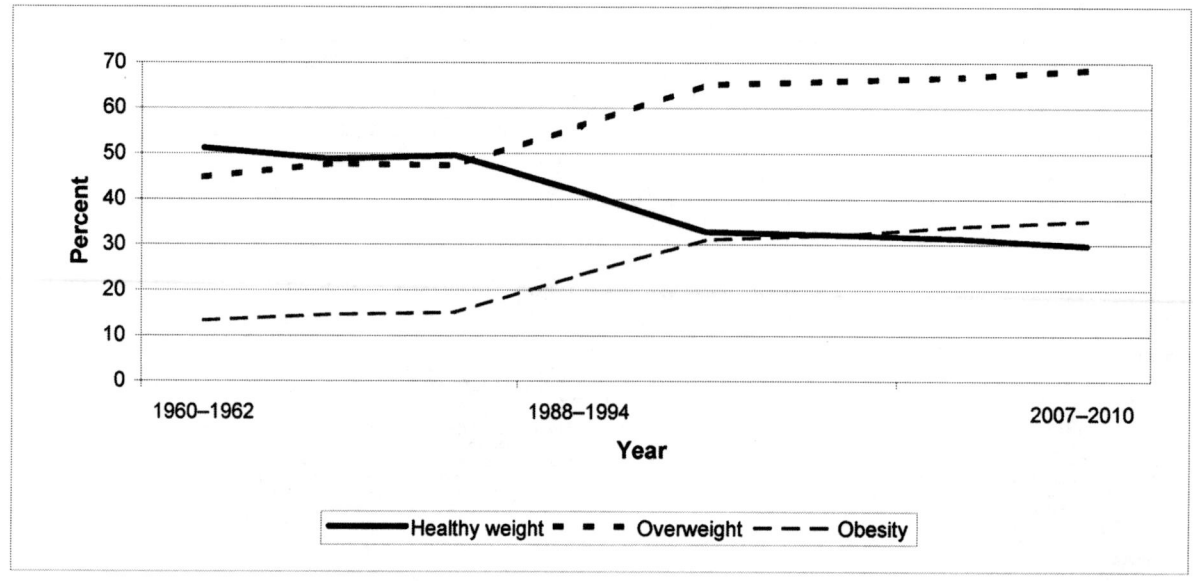

Figure 3-5. Obesity in Children and Adolescents Age 6 to 19 Years, Selected Years, 1971–1974 to 2007–2010

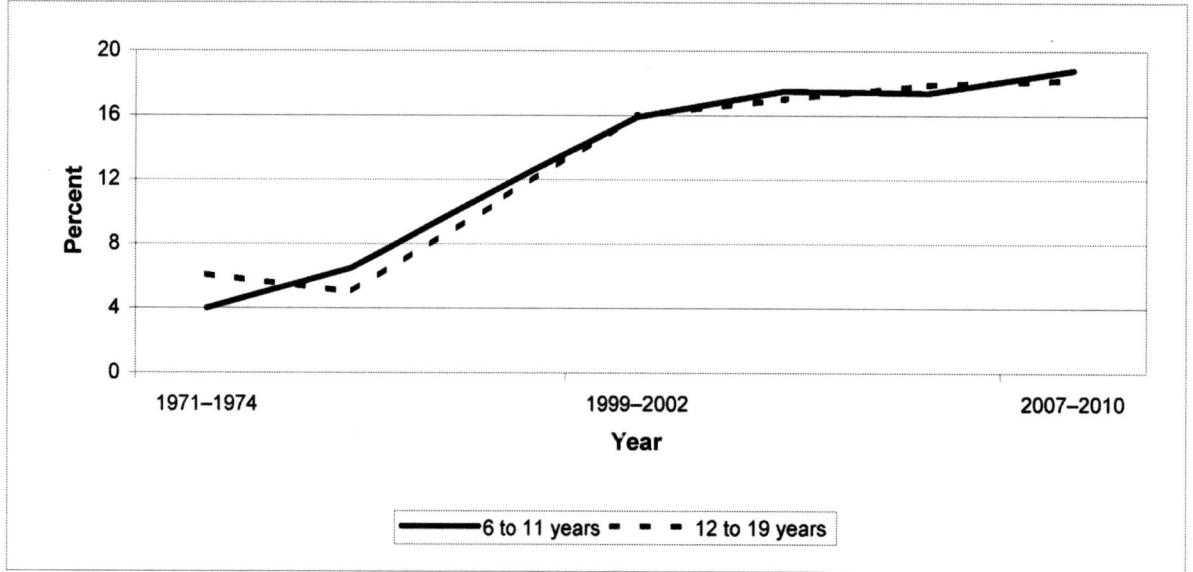

Table 3-21A. Healthy Weight Among Persons 20 Years of Age and Over, by Selected Characteristics, Selected Years, 1960–1962 Through 2007–2010

(Percent.)

Sex, age, race and Hispanic origin[1], and percent of poverty level	Healthy weight (BMI from 18.5 to 24.9)[2]							
	1960–1962	1971–1974	1976–1980[3]	1988–1994	1999–2002	2001–2004	2003–2006	2007–2010
20 to 74 Years, Age-Adjusted [4]								
Both sexes[5]	51.2	48.8	49.6	41.7	32.9	32.2	31.4	29.8
Male	48.3	43.0	45.4	37.9	30.2	28.1	26.1	25.8
Female	54.1	54.3	53.7	45.3	35.6	36.2	36.6	33.6
Not Hispanic or Latino								
White only, male	NA	NA	45.3	37.4	29.5	27.8	26.5	25.6
White only, female	NA	NA	56.7	49.2	39.7	40.2	40.0	36.9
Black or African American only, male	NA	NA	46.6	40.0	35.5	31.3	26.8	28.3
Black or African American only, female	NA	NA	35.0	28.9	21.2	18.9	18.4	17.7
Mexican male	NA	NA	36.6	29.8	25.6	24.2	22.4	18.0
Mexican female	NA	NA	35.9	29.0	27.6	26.3	24.5	20.2
Percent of Poverty Level [6]								
Below 100 percent	NA	45.8	45.1	37.3	32.4	33.7	31.7	27.5
100 percent to 199 percent	NA	45.1	47.6	39.2	29.7	31.8	31.1	27.2
200 percent to 399 percent	NA	48.3	50.1	41.9	29.5	29.3	29.4	29.4
400 percent or more	NA	53.9	53.0	46.0	36.9	35.2	33.8	32.3
20 Years and Over, Age-Adjusted [2]								
Both sexes[5]	NA	NA	NA	41.6	33.0	32.3	31.6	29.8
Male	NA	NA	NA	37.9	30.2	28.3	26.6	25.7
Female	NA	NA	NA	45.0	35.7	36.1	36.5	33.7
Not Hispanic or Latino								
White only, male	NA	NA	NA	37.3	29.6	28.0	26.8	25.5
White only, female	NA	NA	NA	48.7	39.5	39.8	39.6	36.9
Black or African American only, male	NA	NA	NA	40.1	34.7	30.8	27.0	28.5
Black or African American only, female	NA	NA	NA	29.2	21.6	18.9	19.2	17.9
Mexican male	NA	NA	NA	30.2	26.5	25.3	23.8	18.5
Mexican female	NA	NA	NA	29.7	27.5	26.5	25.1	21.3
Percent of Poverty Level [6]								
Below 100 percent	NA	NA	NA	37.5	32.7	34.3	32.1	27.3
100 percent to 199 percent	NA	NA	NA	39.3	30.5	31.9	31.3	27.6
200 percent to 399 percent	NA	NA	NA	41.8	29.6	29.4	29.7	29.7
400 percent or more	NA	NA	NA	45.5	36.5	35.1	33.7	32.1
20 Years and Over, Crude								
Both sexes[5]	NA	NA	NA	42.6	32.9	32.2	31.4	29.6
Male	NA	NA	NA	39.4	30.4	28.4	26.6	25.8
Female	NA	NA	NA	45.7	35.4	35.8	35.9	33.2
Not Hispanic or Latino								
White only, male	NA	NA	NA	38.2	29.2	27.4	26.2	24.8
White only, female	NA	NA	NA	48.8	38.7	38.8	38.2	35.7
Black or African American only, male	NA	NA	NA	41.5	35.9	31.5	27.1	29.4
Black or African American only, female	NA	NA	NA	31.2	21.8	19.3	19.2	17.6
Mexican male	NA	NA	NA	35.2	29.4	28.1	25.2	19.5
Mexican female	NA	NA	NA	32.4	29.5	28.0	25.8	22.3
Percent of Poverty Level [6]								
Below 100 percent	NA	NA	NA	39.8	34.5	36.2	33.2	29.2
100 percent to 199 percent	NA	NA	NA	41.5	31.5	32.6	31.7	28.0
200 percent to 399 percent	NA	NA	NA	42.9	29.7	29.3	29.6	29.5
400 percent or more	NA	NA	NA	44.6	35.3	33.5	32.1	30.5
Male								
20 to 34 years	55.3	54.7	57.1	51.1	40.3	38.3	35.9	37.5
35 to 44 years	45.2	35.2	41.3	33.4	29.0	26.5	24.1	19.8
45 to 54 years	44.8	38.5	38.7	33.6	24.0	21.2	20.8	21.8
55 to 64 years	44.9	38.3	38.7	28.6	23.8	22.2	19.3	19.4
65 to 74 years	46.2	42.1	42.3	30.1	22.8	23.1	21.2	21.6
75 years and over	NA	NA	NA	40.9	32.0	32.1	33.1	25.4
Female								
20 to 34 years	67.6	65.8	65.0	57.9	42.5	44.2	45.1	41.1
35 to 44 years	58.4	56.7	55.6	47.1	37.1	38.3	37.6	34.4
45 to 54 years	47.6	49.3	48.7	37.2	33.1	31.0	31.1	30.7
55 to 64 years	38.1	41.1	43.5	31.5	27.6	29.2	29.5	26.7
65 to 74 years	36.4	40.6	37.8	37.0	26.4	27.0	28.5	23.9
75 years and over	NA	NA	NA	43.0	36.9	34.6	35.4	35.4

NA = Not available.   * = Figure does not meet standards of reliability or precision. Data preceded by an asterisk have a relative standard error (RSE) of 20 percent to 30 percent. Data not shown have an RSE of greater than 30 percent.   [1]Persons of Hispanic origin may be of any race.   [2]Body mass index (BMI) equals weight in kilograms divided by height in meters squared.   [3]Data for Mexican-origin persons are for 1982–1984.   [4]Age adjusted to the year 2000 standard population using five age groups: 20 to 34 years, 35 to 44 years, 45 to 54 years, 55 to 64 years, and 65 years and over (65 to 74 years for estimates for 20 to 74 years).   [5]Includes all other races and origins not shown separately.   [6]Percent of poverty level is based on family income and family size. Persons with unknown percent of poverty level are excluded (8 percent in 2007–2010).

Table 3-21B. Overweight Among Persons 20 Years of Age and Over, by Selected Characteristics, Selected Years, 1960–1962 Through 2007–2010

(Percent.)

Sex, age, race and Hispanic origin[1], and percent of poverty level	Overweight (includes obesity; BMI greater than or equal to 25.0)[2]							
	1960–1962	1971–1974	1976–1980[3]	1988–1994	1999–2002	2001–2004	2003–2006	2007–2010
20 to 74 Years, Age-Adjusted [4]								
Both sexes[5]	44.8	47.7	47.4	56.0	65.2	66.0	66.9	68.5
Male	49.5	54.7	52.9	61.0	68.8	70.7	72.6	73.3
Female	40.2	41.1	42.0	51.2	61.7	61.4	61.2	63.9
Not Hispanic or Latino								
White only, male	NA	NA	53.4	61.6	69.5	71.1	72.1	73.5
White only, female	NA	NA	38.7	47.2	57.0	57.1	57.4	60.2
Black or African American only, male	NA	NA	51.3	58.2	62.0	66.8	72.0	70.2
Black or African American only, female	NA	NA	62.6	68.5	77.6	79.5	80.5	80.3
Mexican male	NA	NA	62.2	69.4	74.1	75.8	77.3	81.8
Mexican female	NA	NA	62.2	69.6	71.4	73.2	74.4	79.2
Percent of Poverty Level [6]								
Below 100 percent	NA	49.3	50.0	59.8	65.2	63.9	66.0	69.5
100 percent to 199 percent	NA	50.9	49.0	58.2	68.0	66.2	66.6	70.9
200 percent to 399 percent	NA	48.4	47.3	56.0	68.7	68.9	69.3	68.8
400 percent or more	NA	43.4	45.0	51.8	61.8	63.5	64.7	66.7
20 Years and Over, Age-Adjusted [2]								
Both sexes[5]	NA	NA	NA	56.0	65.1	66.0	66.7	68.5
Male	NA	NA	NA	60.9	68.8	70.5	72.1	73.3
Female	NA	NA	NA	51.4	61.6	61.6	61.3	63.9
Not Hispanic or Latino								
White only, male	NA	NA	NA	61.6	69.4	71.0	71.8	73.6
White only, female	NA	NA	NA	47.5	57.2	57.6	57.9	60.3
Black or African American only, male	NA	NA	NA	57.8	62.6	67.0	71.6	70.0
Black or African American only, female	NA	NA	NA	68.2	77.2	79.6	79.8	80.0
Mexican male	NA	NA	NA	68.9	73.2	74.6	75.8	81.3
Mexican female	NA	NA	NA	68.9	71.2	73.0	73.9	78.0
Percent of Poverty Level [6]								
Below 100 percent	NA	NA	NA	59.6	64.7	63.4	65.7	69.7
100 percent to 199 percent	NA	NA	NA	58.0	67.3	66.2	66.5	70.5
200 percent to 399 percent	NA	NA	NA	56.0	68.6	68.8	69.0	68.6
400 percent or more	NA	NA	NA	52.4	62.2	63.7	64.7	66.9
20 Years and Over, Crude								
Both sexes[5]	NA	NA	NA	54.9	65.2	66.1	66.9	68.7
Male	NA	NA	NA	59.4	68.6	70.4	72.1	73.2
Female	NA	NA	NA	50.7	62.0	61.9	61.9	64.5
Not Hispanic or Latino								
White only, male	NA	NA	NA	60.6	69.9	71.6	72.5	74.2
White only, female	NA	NA	NA	47.4	58.2	58.7	59.4	61.7
Black or African American only, male	NA	NA	NA	56.7	61.7	66.3	71.6	69.1
Black or African American only, female	NA	NA	NA	66.0	76.9	79.1	79.7	80.2
Mexican male	NA	NA	NA	63.9	70.1	71.8	74.6	80.2
Mexican female	NA	NA	NA	65.9	69.3	71.4	73.0	77.1
Percent of Poverty Level [6]								
Below 100 percent	NA	NA	NA	56.8	62.5	61.4	64.4	67.8
100 percent to 199 percent	NA	NA	NA	55.7	66.2	65.3	66.0	70.1
200 percent to 399 percent	NA	NA	NA	54.9	68.5	69.0	69.0	68.8
400 percent or more	NA	NA	NA	53.3	63.7	65.5	66.5	68.5
Male								
20 to 34 years	42.7	42.8	41.2	47.5	57.4	59.0	61.6	61.1
35 to 44 years	53.5	63.2	57.2	65.5	70.5	72.9	75.2	80.2
45 to 54 years	53.9	59.7	60.2	66.1	75.7	78.5	78.5	76.8
55 to 64 years	52.2	58.5	60.2	70.5	75.4	77.3	79.7	79.8
65 to 74 years	47.8	54.6	54.2	68.5	76.2	76.1	78.0	77.5
75 years and over	NA	NA	NA	56.5	67.4	66.8	65.8	73.2
Female								
20 to 34 years	21.2	25.8	27.9	37.0	52.9	51.6	50.9	55.4
35 to 44 years	37.2	40.5	40.7	49.6	60.6	60.1	60.7	63.9
45 to 54 years	49.3	49.0	48.7	60.3	65.1	67.4	67.3	66.2
55 to 64 years	59.9	54.5	53.7	66.3	72.2	69.9	69.6	72.2
65 to 74 years	60.9	55.9	59.5	60.3	70.9	71.5	70.5	74.2
75 years and over	NA	NA	NA	52.3	59.9	63.7	62.6	63.2

NA = Not available. * = Figure does not meet standards of reliability or precision. Data preceded by an asterisk have a relative standard error (RSE) of 20 percent to 30 percent. Data not shown have an RSE of greater than 30 percent. [1]Persons of Hispanic origin may be of any race. [2]Body mass index (BMI) equals weight in kilograms divided by height in meters squared. [3]Data for Mexican-origin persons are for 1982–1984. [4]Age adjusted to the year 2000 standard population using five age groups: 20 to 34 years, 35 to 44 years, 45 to 54 years, 55 to 64 years, and 65 years and over (65 to 74 years for estimates for 20 to 74 years). [5]Includes all other races and origins not shown separately. [6]Percent of poverty level is based on family income and family size. Persons with unknown percent of poverty level are excluded (8 percent in 2007–2010).

Table 3-21C. Obesity Among Persons 20 Years of Age and Over, by Selected Characteristics, Selected Years, 1960–1962 Through 2007–2010

(Percent.)

Sex, age, race and Hispanic origin[1], and percent of poverty level	Obesity (BMI greater than or equal to 30.0)[2]							
	1960–1962	1971–1974	1976–1980[3]	1988–1994	1999–2002	2001–2004	2003–2006	2007–2010
20 to 74 Years, Age-Adjusted [4]								
Both sexes[5]	13.3	14.6	15.1	23.3	31.1	32.1	34.1	35.3
Male	10.7	12.2	12.8	20.6	28.1	30.2	33.1	34.4
Female	15.7	16.8	17.1	26.0	34.0	34.0	35.2	36.1
Not Hispanic or Latino								
White only, male	NA	NA	12.4	20.7	28.7	31.0	33.0	34.7
White only, female	NA	NA	15.4	23.3	31.3	31.5	32.5	32.9
Black or African American only, male	NA	NA	16.5	21.3	27.9	31.2	36.3	38.7
Black or African American only, female	NA	NA	31.0	39.1	49.4	51.6	54.3	54.4
Mexican male	NA	NA	16.0	24.4	29.0	30.5	30.4	36.5
Mexican female	NA	NA	26.6	36.1	38.9	40.3	42.6	45.8
Percent of Poverty Level [6]								
Below 100 percent	NA	20.7	21.9	29.2	36.0	34.9	35.9	37.9
100 percent to 199 percent	NA	18.4	18.7	26.6	35.4	34.6	36.7	38.2
200 percent to 399 percent	NA	13.7	14.1	23.2	33.0	34.4	36.9	37.6
400 percent or more	NA	10.1	10.0	18.9	25.8	27.4	29.4	31.4
20 Years and Over, Age-Adjusted [2]								
Both sexes[5]	NA	NA	NA	22.9	30.4	31.4	33.4	34.7
Male	NA	NA	NA	20.2	27.5	29.5	32.4	33.9
Female	NA	NA	NA	25.5	33.2	33.2	34.3	35.5
Not Hispanic or Latino								
White only, male	NA	NA	NA	20.3	28.0	30.2	32.4	34.1
White only, female	NA	NA	NA	22.9	30.7	30.7	31.6	32.5
Black or African American only, male	NA	NA	NA	20.9	27.8	30.8	35.7	38.3
Black or African American only, female	NA	NA	NA	38.3	48.6	51.1	53.4	54.0
Mexican male	NA	NA	NA	23.8	27.8	29.1	29.5	36.3
Mexican female	NA	NA	NA	35.2	38.0	39.4	41.8	44.6
Percent of Poverty Level [6]								
Below 100 percent	NA	NA	NA	28.1	34.7	33.7	35.0	37.2
100 percent to 199 percent	NA	NA	NA	26.1	34.1	33.6	35.9	37.3
200 percent to 399 percent	NA	NA	NA	22.7	32.1	33.3	35.7	36.8
400 percent or more	NA	NA	NA	18.7	25.5	27.3	28.9	31.3
20 Years and Over, Crude								
Both sexes[5]	NA	NA	NA	22.3	30.5	31.5	33.5	34.9
Male	NA	NA	NA	19.5	27.5	29.5	32.4	33.9
Female	NA	NA	NA	25.0	33.4	33.3	34.6	35.9
Not Hispanic or Latino								
White only, male	NA	NA	NA	19.9	28.4	30.5	32.6	34.4
White only, female	NA	NA	NA	22.7	31.3	31.2	32.2	33.2
Black or African American only, male	NA	NA	NA	20.7	27.5	30.7	35.8	38.1
Black or African American only, female	NA	NA	NA	36.7	48.7	51.1	53.2	54.2
Mexican male	NA	NA	NA	20.6	26.0	27.8	29.0	35.6
Mexican female	NA	NA	NA	33.3	37.0	38.5	41.2	44.2
Percent of Poverty Level [6]								
Below 100 percent	NA	NA	NA	25.9	33.0	33.0	34.6	36.5
100 percent to 199 percent	NA	NA	NA	24.3	32.8	32.6	35.0	36.8
200 percent to 399 percent	NA	NA	NA	22.1	31.8	33.2	35.5	36.8
400 percent or more	NA	NA	NA	19.3	27.2	28.6	30.7	32.4
Male								
20 to 34 years	9.2	9.7	8.9	14.1	21.7	23.2	26.2	27.1
35 to 44 years	12.1	13.5	13.5	21.5	28.5	33.8	37.0	37.2
45 to 54 years	12.5	13.7	16.7	23.2	30.6	31.8	34.6	36.6
55 to 64 years	9.2	14.1	14.1	27.2	35.5	36.0	39.3	37.3
65 to 74 years	10.4	10.9	13.2	24.1	31.9	32.1	33.0	41.5
75 years and over	NA	NA	NA	13.2	18.0	19.9	24.0	26.6
Female								
20 to 34 years	7.2	9.7	11.0	18.5	28.3	28.6	28.4	30.4
35 to 44 years	14.7	17.7	17.8	25.5	32.1	33.3	36.1	37.1
45 to 54 years	20.3	18.9	19.6	32.4	36.9	38.0	40.0	36.9
55 to 64 years	24.4	24.1	22.9	33.7	42.1	39.0	41.0	43.4
65 to 74 years	23.2	22.0	21.5	26.9	39.3	37.9	36.4	40.3
75 years and over	NA	NA	NA	19.2	23.6	23.2	24.2	28.7

NA = Not available. * = Figure does not meet standards of reliability or precision. Data preceded by an asterisk have a relative standard error (RSE) of 20 percent to 30 percent. Data not shown have an RSE of greater than 30 percent. [1]Persons of Hispanic origin may be of any race. [2]Body mass index (BMI) equals weight in kilograms divided by height in meters squared. [3]Data for Mexican-origin persons are for 1982–1984. [4]Age adjusted to the year 2000 standard population using five age groups: 20 to 34 years, 35 to 44 years, 45 to 54 years, 55 to 64 years, and 65 years and over (65 to 74 years for estimates for 20 to 74 years). [5]Includes all other races and origins not shown separately. [6]Percent of poverty level is based on family income and family size. Persons with unknown percent of poverty level are excluded (8 percent in 2007–2010).

Table 3-22. Obesity Among Children and Adolescents 2 to 19 Years of Age, by Selected Characteristics, Selected Years, 1963–1965 Through 2007–2010

(Percent.)

Sex, age, race and Hispanic origin[1], and percent of poverty level	1963–1965, 1966–1970[2]	1971–1974	1976–1980[3]	1988–1994	1999–2002	2001–2004	2003–2006	2005–2008	2007–2010
2 to 5 Years									
Both sexes[4]									
Not Hispanic or Latino	NA	NA	NA	7.2	10.3	12.4	12.5	10.5	11.1
White only	NA	NA	NA	5.2	8.7	10.2	10.8	9.3	9.0
Black or African American only	NA	NA	NA	7.7	8.8	11.0	14.9	14.0	15.0
Mexican	NA	NA	NA	12.3	13.1	17.7	16.7	14.1	14.6
Boys									
Not Hispanic or Latino	NA	NA	NA	6.1	10.0	13.1	12.8	9.8	11.9
White only	NA	NA	NA	*4.5	*8.2	*11.5	11.1	*7.4	8.8
Black or African American only	NA	NA	NA	7.7	*8.0	9.7	13.3	13.7	15.7
Mexican	NA	NA	NA	12.4	14.1	19.8	18.8	17.1	19.1
Girls									
Not Hispanic or Latino	NA	NA	NA	8.2	10.6	11.7	12.2	11.2	10.2
White only	NA	NA	NA	5.9	*9.0	*9.1	10.4	11.3	*9.2
Black or African American only	NA	NA	NA	7.6	9.6	12.2	16.6	14.3	*14.2
Mexican	NA	NA	NA	12.3	*12.2	*15.7	14.5	10.8	*9.9
Percent of Poverty Level [5]									
Below 100 percent	NA	NA	NA	9.7	10.9	14.4	14.3	12.3	13.2
100 percent to 199 percent	NA	NA	NA	7.2	*13.8	13.3	12.7	10.0	11.8
200 percent to 399 percent	NA	NA	NA	5.6	*7.6	13.6	11.9	11.6	13.9
400 percent or more	NA	NA	NA	*	*	*	*10.0	*	*5.8
6 to 11 Years									
Both sexes[4]	4.2	4.0	6.5	11.3	15.9	17.5	17.0	17.4	18.8
Boys									
Not Hispanic or Latino	4.0	*4.3	6.6	11.6	16.9	18.7	18.0	18.7	20.7
White only	NA	NA	6.1	10.7	14.0	16.9	15.5	16.5	18.6
Black or African American only	NA	NA	6.8	12.3	17.0	17.2	18.6	18.7	23.3
Mexican	NA	NA	13.3	17.5	26.5	25.6	27.5	28.4	24.3
Girls									
Not Hispanic or Latino	4.5	*3.6	6.4	11.0	14.7	16.3	15.8	16.0	16.9
White only	NA	NA	5.2	*9.8	13.1	15.6	14.4	14.5	14.0
Black or African American only	NA	NA	11.2	17.0	22.8	24.8	24.0	21.3	24.5
Mexican	NA	NA	9.8	15.3	17.1	16.6	19.7	21.2	22.4
Percent of Poverty Level [5]									
Below 100 percent	NA	NA	NA	11.4	19.1	20.0	22.0	21.5	22.2
100 percent to 199 percent	NA	NA	NA	11.1	16.4	18.4	19.2	22.2	20.7
200 percent to 399 percent	NA	NA	NA	11.7	15.3	18.2	16.7	16.8	18.9
400 percent or more	NA	NA	NA	*	12.9	11.4	9.2	*9.5	*12.5
12 to 19 Years									
Both sexes[4]	4.6	6.1	5.0	10.5	16.0	17.0	17.6	17.9	18.2
Boys									
Not Hispanic or Latino	4.5	6.1	4.8	11.3	16.7	17.9	18.2	18.7	19.4
White only	NA	NA	3.8	11.6	14.6	17.9	17.3	16.1	17.1
Black or African American only	NA	NA	6.1	10.7	18.8	17.6	18.4	19.1	21.2
Mexican	NA	NA	7.7	14.1	24.7	20.0	22.1	26.2	27.9
Girls									
Not Hispanic or Latino	4.7	6.2	5.3	9.7	15.3	16.0	16.8	17.0	16.9
White only	NA	NA	4.6	8.9	12.6	14.6	14.5	14.0	14.6
Black or African American only	NA	NA	10.7	16.3	23.5	23.8	27.7	29.5	27.1
Mexican	NA	NA	8.8	*13.4	19.6	17.1	19.9	21.3	18.0
Percent of Poverty Level [5]									
Below 100 percent	NA	NA	NA	15.8	19.8	18.2	19.3	23.1	24.3
100 percent to 199 percent	NA	NA	NA	11.2	17.0	17.0	18.4	19.8	20.1
200 percent to 399 percent	NA	NA	NA	9.4	15.7	19.0	19.3	17.2	16.3
400 percent or more	NA	NA	NA	*	13.9	13.2	12.6	14.0	14.0

NA = Not available.   * = Figure does not meet standards of reliability or precision. Data preceded by an asterisk have a relative standard error (RSE) of 20 percent to 30 percent. Data not shown have an RSE of greater than 30 percent.   [1]Persons of Hispanic origin may be of any race.   [2]Data for 1963–1965 are for children 6 to 11 years of age; data for 1966–1970 are for adolescents 12 to 17 years of age, not 12 to 19 years of age.   [3]Data for Mexican-origin persons are for 1982–1984.   [4]Includes all other races and origins not shown separately.   [5]Percent of poverty level is based on family income and family size. Persons with unknown percent of poverty level are excluded (7 percent in 2007–2010).

Table 3-23. Untreated Dental Caries, by Selected Characteristics, Selected Years, 1971–1974 Through 2005–2008

(Percent.)

Sex, race and Hispanic origin[1], and percent of poverty level	Age 2–5 years		Age 6–19 years		Age 20-64 years		Age 65-74 years		Age 75 years and over	
	1971–1974	2005–2008	1971–1974	2005–2008	1971–1974	2005–2008	1971–1974	2005–2008	1971–1974	2005–2008
Total [2]	25.0	X	54.7	16.2	48.0	23.7	29.7	19.6	NA	20.2
Sex										
Male	26.4	X	54.9	17.0	50.5	27.2	32.6	24.8	NA	25.7
Female	23.6	X	54.5	15.3	45.6	20.2	27.4	15.3	NA	16.1
Race and Hispanic Origin										
Not Hispanic or Latino										
White only	23.7	X	51.6	12.9	45.3	19.3	28.3	17.8	NA	17.7
Black or African American only	29.0	X	71.0	22.1	67.3	39.7	41.5	32.4	NA	42.6
Mexican	NA	X	NA	22.2	NA	35.2	NA	33.2	NA	43.4
Percent of Poverty Level [3]										
Below 100 percent	32.0	X	68.0	25.4	63.5	41.9	34.3	42.5	NA	39.3
100 percent to 199 percent	29.9	X	60.3	18.4	56.2	37.7	35.6	22.9	NA	22.1
200 percent or more	17.8	X	46.2	11.9	42.7	16.6	26.2	15.7	NA	14.5
200 percent to 399 percent	NA	X	NA	14.2	NA	24.3	NA	*17.9	NA	14.8
400 percent or more	NA	X	NA	9.3	NA	11.1	NA	12.8	NA	*13.8
Race and Hispanic Origin, and Percent of Poverty Level [3]										
Not Hispanic or Latino										
White only										
Below 100% of poverty level	32.1	X	65.9	25.4	60.2	39.8	33.3	*39.4	NA	*29.6
100% or more of poverty level	22.0	X	49.9	11.0	44.2	17.1	28.3	16.4	NA	15.6
Black or African American only										
Below 100% of poverty level	29.1	X	73.9	27.1	71.9	52.7	39.8	56.2	NA	*
100% or more of poverty level	27.9	X	67.3	19.1	65.3	36.8	41.1	28.1	NA	36.4

NOTE: Root caries are not included. Persons without at least one primary or one permanent tooth or one root tip were classified as edentulous and were excluded from this analysis. The majority of edentulous persons are 65 years of age and over. Estimates of edentulism among persons 65 years of age and over are 46 percent in 1971–1974, 33 percent in 1988–1994, and 23 percent in 2005–2008. For estimates prior to 2005–2008, only dental caries in primary teeth was evaluated for children 2–5 years of age. Caries in both permanent and primary teeth was evaluated for children 6–11 years of age. For children 12–19 years of age and adults, only dental caries in permanent teeth was evaluated. Starting with 2005–2006 data, dental caries data were collected using a simplified examination process that used health technologists to screen for caries instead of using dentists to conduct a comprehensive caries exam. In addition, dental caries data were not collected on children younger than 5 years of age. Because of this change in the examination process and because 2005–2008 dental caries data are based on both primary and permanent teeth, regardless of age, data for 2005–2008 need to be interpreted with caution, especially when comparing with earlier data.

NA = Not available.   X = Not applicable.   * = Figure does not meet standards of reliability or precision. Data preceded by an asterisk have a relative standard error (RSE) of 20 percent to 30 percent. Data not shown have an RSE of greater than 30 percent.   [1]Persons of Hispanic origin may be of any race.   [2]Includes persons of all races and Hispanic origins, not just those shown separately, and those with unknown percent of poverty level.   [3]Percent of poverty level is based on family income and family size. Persons with unknown percent of poverty level are excluded (5 percent in 2005–2008).

Table 3-24. Health-Related Behaviors of Children 6 to 11 Years of Age, by Selected Characteristics, 2003 and 2007

(Percent.)

Characteristic	Did not get daily vigorous physical activity[1]		Greater than 2 hours of screen time per day[2]		Did not get enough sleep nightly[3]	
	2003	2007	2003	2007	2003	2007
Age						
6 to 11 years	68.7	62.3	36.2	39.5	24.5	27.6
6 to 8 years	67.0	59.2	33.8	35.1	22.8	26.1
9 to 11 years	70.3	65.4	38.5	44.0	26.1	29.1
Sex						
Boys	63.7	57.8	37.0	39.4	24.6	27.6
Girls	74.0	67.0	35.4	39.7	24.4	27.6
Sex and Age						
Boys						
6 to 8 years	62.3	55.4	34.9	34.9	22.4	25.2
9 to 11 years	65.0	60.4	39.0	44.1	26.7	30.1
Girls						
6 to 8 years	72.0	63.3	32.8	35.3	23.2	27.0
9 to 11 years	75.8	70.5	37.9	44.0	25.5	28.1
Hispanic Origin and Race [4]						
Hispanic or Latino	70.1	69.3	35.5	41.7	21.7	24.4
Not Hispanic or Latino	68.5	60.4	36.3	38.9	25.2	28.4
White only	68.3	59.7	33.0	34.7	25.8	29.1
Black or African American only	66.2	62.1	48.8	58.2	25.4	27.1
Sex and Hispanic Origin and Race [4]						
Boys						
Hispanic or Latino	66.2	61.7	34.4	39.9	21.1	24.6
Not Hispanic or Latino	63.4	56.8	37.6	39.2	25.4	28.4
White only	62.7	54.9	34.7	35.0	25.8	29.3
Black or African American only	60.3	61.4	49.1	58.3	25.4	27.4
Girls						
Hispanic or Latina	73.9	76.5	36.6	43.4	22.2	24.3
Not Hispanic or Latina	74.0	64.4	35.0	38.6	25.1	28.3
White only	74.4	64.9	31.2	34.4	25.8	29.0
Black or African American only	71.9	62.8	48.6	58.1	25.5	26.8
Percent of Poverty Level [5]						
Below 100 percent	63.3	62.6	38.2	43.9	22.4	25.9
100 percent to 199 percent	66.7	63.1	41.8	44.4	22.8	25.6
200 percent to 399 percent	70.7	60.8	36.8	40.1	25.0	28.9
400 percent or more	71.6	63.1	29.3	32.6	26.8	28.7
Sex and Percent of Poverty Level [5]						
Boys						
Below 100 percent	57.9	59.3	39.0	43.1	21.7	26.7
100 percent to 199 percent	61.2	58.0	42.8	44.6	23.7	26.2
200 percent to 399 percent	65.4	57.6	38.1	40.1	24.6	29.0
400 percent or more	67.6	57.1	29.3	32.6	27.3	27.6
Girls						
Below 100 percent	68.9	66.2	37.5	44.7	23.2	25.1
100 percent to 199 percent	72.4	68.4	40.9	44.2	22.0	24.9
200 percent to 399 percent	76.3	64.4	35.5	40.3	25.4	28.7
400 percent or more	75.8	69.3	29.3	32.8	26.2	29.7

[1]Based on respondent's answer to question, "During the past week, on how many days did CHILD exercise, play a sport, or participate in physical activity for at least 20 minutes that made him/her sweat and breathe hard?" Children whose parent/guardian responded that the child did not exercise, play a sport, or participate in physical activity every day were classified as not getting daily vigorous physical activity. [2]Based on respondent's answer to question, "On an average weekday, about how much time does CHILD use a computer for purposes other than schoolwork?" and "On an average weekday, about how much time does CHILD usually watch TV, watch videos, or play video games?" Children whose parent's/guardian's combined responses to both questions equaled more than 2 hours were classified as watching more than 2 hours of screen time daily. [3]Based on respondent's answer to question, "In the past week, on how many nights did CHILD get enough sleep for a child of his/her age?" Children whose parent/guardian responded that the child did not get enough sleep on at least one night were classified as not getting enough sleep nightly. [4]Persons of Hispanic origin may be of any race. [5]Percent of poverty level is based on total household income and family composition using U.S. Census Bureau poverty thresholds. The poverty categories available in the two survey years used slightly different cut points. In 2003, the available categories were below 100 percent, 100 percent to 199 percent, 200 to 399 percent, and 400 percent or more. In 2007, the categories were at or below 100 percent, above 100 percent to 200 percent, above 200 percent to 400 percent, and above 400 percent. Poverty level was unknown for 1 percent of households in 2003 and 8 percent of households in 2007. Missing household income data were imputed.

Table 3-25. Selected Health Conditions and Risk Factors, Selected Years, 1988–1994 Through 2009–2010

(Percent.)

Health condition	1988–1994	1999–2000	2001–2002	2003–2004	2005–2006	2007–2008	2009–2010
Diabetes [1]							
Total, age-adjusted[2]	9.1	9.0	10.5	10.8	10.4	NA	NA
Total, crude	8.4	8.5	10.1	10.8	10.7	NA	NA
High Cholesterol [3]							
Total, age-adjusted[4]	22.8	25.0	24.4	27.5	27.0	27.2	26.7
Total, crude	21.5	24.0	23.9	27.5	27.6	28.3	27.9
High Serum Total Cholesterol [5]							
Total, age-adjusted[4]	20.8	18.3	16.5	16.9	15.6	14.2	13.2
Total, crude	19.6	17.7	16.4	17.0	15.9	14.6	13.6
Hypertension [6]							
Total, age-adjusted[4]	25.5	30.0	29.7	32.1	30.5	31.2	30.0
Total, crude	24.1	28.9	28.9	32.5	31.7	32.6	31.9
Uncontrolled High Blood Pressure Among Persons with Hypertension [7]							
Total, age-adjusted[4]	77.2	71.9	68.3	63.8	63.0	56.2	55.7
Total, crude	73.9	69.1	65.4	60.8	56.6	51.8	46.7
Overweight (Includes Obesity) [8]							
Total, age-adjusted[4]	56.0	64.5	65.6	66.4	66.9	68.1	68.8
Total, crude	54.9	64.1	65.6	66.5	67.3	68.3	69.2
Obesity [9]							
Total, age-adjusted[4]	22.9	30.5	30.5	32.3	34.4	33.7	35.7
Total, crude	22.3	30.3	30.6	32.3	34.7	33.9	35.9
Untreated Dental Caries [10]							
Total, age-adjusted[4]	27.7	24.3	21.3	30.0	24.4	21.7	NA
Total, crude	28.2	25.0	21.6	30.3	24.5	21.8	NA
Percent of Persons Under 20 Years of Age							
Obesity [11]							
2 to 5 years	7.2	10.3	10.6	14.0	11.0	10.1	12.1
6 to 11 years	11.3	15.1	16.3	18.8	15.1	19.6	18.0
12 to 19 years	10.5	14.8	16.7	17.4	17.8	18.1	18.4
Untreated Dental Caries [10,12]							
6 to 19 years	23.6	22.7	20.6	25.2	NA	16.2	NA

NA = Not available.   [1]Undiagnosed diabetes is defined as a fasting plasma glucose (FPG) of at least 126 mg/dL or a hemoglobin A1c of at least 6.5% and no reported physician diagnosis. Respondents had fasted for at least 8 hours and less than 24 hours.   [2]Age adjusted to the 2000 standard population using three age groups: 20 to 44 years, 45 to 64 years, and 65 years and over.   [3]High cholesterol is defined as measured serum total cholesterol greater than or equal to 240 mg/dL or reporting taking cholesterol-lowering medication. Respondents were asked, "Are you now following this advice [from a doctor of health professional] to take prescribed medicine [to lower your cholesterol]?" Risk levels for cholesterol have been defined by the Third Report of the National Cholesterol Education Program Expert Panel on Detection, Evaluation, and Treatment of High Blood Cholesterol in Adults. National Heart, Lung, and Blood Institute, National Institutes of Health. September 2002.   [4]Age adjusted to the 2000 standard population using five age groups: 20 to 34 years, 35 to 44 years, 45 to 54 years, 55 to 64 years, and 65 years and over.   [5]High serum total cholesterol is defined as greater than or equal to 240 mg/dL (6.20 mmol/L).   [6]Hypertension is defined as having measured high blood pressure and/or taking antihypertensive medication. High blood pressure is defined as having measured systolic pressure of at least 140 mmHg or diastolic pressure of at least 90 mmHg. Those with high blood pressure also may be taking prescribed medicine for high blood pressure. For antihypertensive medication use, respondents were asked, "Are you now taking prescribed medicine for your high blood pressure?"   [7]Uncontrolled high blood pressure among persons with hypertension is defined as measured systolic pressure of at least 140 mmHg or diastolic pressure of at least 90 mmHg, among those with measured high blood pressure or reporting taking antihypertensive medication.   [8]Excludes pregnant women. Overweight is defined as body mass index (BMI) greater than or equal to 25.0.   [9]Excludes pregnant women. Obesity is defined as body mass index (BMI) greater than or equal to 30.0.   [10]Untreated dental caries refers to untreated coronal caries.   [11]Obesity is defined as body mass index (BMI) at or above the sex- and age-specific 5th percentile BMI cutoff points from the 2000 CDC growth charts for the United States.   [12]The estimate in the 2007–2008 column is for 2005–2008. The 4-year estimate is shown for children because it is more reliable than the 2-year estimate.

Table 3-26A. Health Risk Behaviors Among Students in Grades 9 to 12, by Sex, Grade Level, Race, and Hispanic Origin, Selected Years, 1991–2009

(Percent.)

Sex, grade level, race, and Hispanic origin	Seriously considered suicide			In a physical fight[1]			Carried a weapon[2,3]		
	1991	1999	2009	1991	1999	2009	1991	1999	2009
Total	29.0	19.3	13.8	42.5	35.7	31.5	26.1	17.3	17.5
Male									
Total	20.8	13.7	10.5	50.2	44.0	39.3	40.6	28.6	27.1
9th grade	17.6	11.9	10.0	57.8	49.5	45.1	44.4	28.7	27.3
10th grade	19.5	13.7	10.0	50.2	46.0	41.2	41.5	30.7	28.5
11th grade	25.3	13.7	11.4	51.0	38.9	36.2	44.0	26.9	25.6
12th grade	20.7	15.6	10.5	42.3	39.0	32.5	33.1	27.3	26.5
Not Hispanic or Latino									
White	21.7	12.5	10.5	49.1	43.2	36.0	41.2	28.6	29.3
Black or African American	13.3	11.7	7.8	58.4	44.4	48.3	43.4	23.1	21.0
Hispanic or Latino	18.0	13.6	10.7	48.5	50.5	43.8	40.0	29.5	26.5
Female									
Total	37.2	24.9	17.4	34.4	27.3	22.9	10.9	6.0	7.1
9th grade	40.3	24.4	20.3	42.9	32.5	27.8	10.4	6.5	7.6
10th grade	39.7	30.1	17.2	35.4	29.4	24.8	11.2	7.1	7.2
11th grade	38.4	23.0	17.8	34.5	23.4	20.5	12.9	5.2	6.3
12th grade	30.7	21.2	13.6	25.4	21.9	17.0	9.5	4.8	6.4
Not Hispanic or Latina									
White	38.6	23.2	16.1	32.2	22.3	18.2	7.5	3.6	6.5
Black or African American	29.4	18.8	18.1	43.8	38.6	33.9	23.6	11.7	7.8
Hispanic or Latina	34.6	26.1	20.2	34.8	29.7	28.5	12.9	8.4	7.9

NOTE: Only youths attending school participated in the survey. Persons of Hispanic origin may be of any race.

NA = Data not available.   [1]During the last 12 months.   [2]During the last 30 days.   [3]Weapon refers to gun, knife, or club.

Table 3-26B. Health Risk Behaviors Among Students in Grades 9 to 12, by Sex, Grade Level, Race, and Hispanic Origin, Selected Years, 1991–2009

(Percent.)

Sex, grade level, race, and Hispanic origin	Rarely or never wore a seatbelt[1]			Rode with a driver who had been drinking alcohol[2,3]			Drove while drinking alcohol[2,3]		
	1991	1999	2009	1991	1999	2009	1991	1999	2009
Total	25.9	16.4	9.7	39.9	33.1	28.3	16.7	13.1	9.7
Male									
Total	30.0	20.8	11.5	40.0	34.4	27.8	21.5	17.4	11.6
9th grade	30.0	19.8	11.2	40.0	29.9	25.3	8.6	6.1	5.1
10th grade	25.5	17.7	11.7	33.9	34.8	28.3	16.1	15.0	11.0
11th grade	29.5	17.7	11.2	36.6	33.4	29.2	26.4	20.5	13.0
12th grade	34.7	28.1	12.0	45.0	39.7	28.6	34.5	31.2	19.3
Not Hispanic or Latino									
White	28.6	19.6	11.2	40.2	33.0	25.5	23.3	18.7	12.7
Black or African American	37.5	27.9	14.8	37.4	34.0	31.2	14.0	10.6	8.7
Hispanic or Latino	37.1	19.6	9.8	47.2	41.8	33.5	25.1	17.2	11.0
Female									
Total	21.6	11.9	7.7	39.8	31.7	28.8	11.7	8.7	7.6
9th grade	25.0	14.4	9.8	36.0	32.0	30.0	3.3	4.5	4.8
10th grade	20.4	12.3	6.8	38.8	32.0	27.6	7.3	5.3	5.3
11th grade	20.8	9.8	6.0	39.7	28.1	29.6	14.2	12.3	9.6
12th grade	20.2	10.3	8.0	44.8	34.8	27.9	21.7	14.4	11.4
Not Hispanic or Latina									
White	18.7	11.2	7.6	40.9	31.7	26.9	13.6	10.3	8.7
Black or African American	31.9	17.4	8.3	33.8	34.8	28.7	6.2	5.4	4.1
Hispanic or Latina	25.9	9.5	7.8	46.7	37.3	34.9	9.5	8.3	7.9

NOTE: Only youths attending school participated in the survey. Persons of Hispanic origin may be of any race.

NA = Data not available.   [1]When riding in a car driven by someone else.   [2]During the last 30 days.   [3]In car or other vehicle.

Table 3-26C. Health Risk Behaviors Among Students in Grades 9 to 12, by Sex, Grade Level, Race, and Hispanic Origin, Selected Years, 1991–2009

(Percent.)

Sex, grade level, race, and Hispanic origin	Ever had sexual intercourse			Did not use a condom at last sex[1]			Physically forced to have sex		
	1991	1999	2009	1991	1999	2009	1991	1999	2009
Total	54.1	49.9	46.0	53.8	42.0	38.9	NA	8.8	7.4
Male									
Total	57.4	52.2	46.1	45.5	34.5	31.4	NA	5.2	4.5
9th grade	45.6	44.5	33.6	44.1	30.5	30.1	NA	5.6	4.1
10th grade	50.9	51.1	41.9	43.1	30.0	28.1	NA	4.6	4.0
11th grade	64.5	51.4	53.4	43.2	30.7	31.1	NA	5.0	5.4
12th grade	68.3	63.9	59.6	49.3	44.1	35.0	NA	5.6	4.9
Not Hispanic or Latino									
White	52.7	45.4	39.6	44.8	37.0	29.0	NA	3.5	3.2
Black or African American	88.1	75.7	72.1	43.0	24.7	27.5	NA	9.7	7.9
Hispanic or Latino	64.1	62.9	52.8	53.0	33.9	38.2	NA	5.9	5.7
Female									
Total	50.8	47.7	45.7	62.0	49.3	46.1	NA	12.5	10.5
9th grade	32.2	32.5	29.3	49.7	36.9	42.3	NA	10.4	9.4
10th grade	45.3	42.6	39.6	63.6	44.7	36.5	NA	12.4	10.6
11th grade	60.2	53.8	52.5	59.3	50.0	46.0	NA	14.5	11.2
12th grade	65.2	65.8	65.0	67.4	58.9	53.7	NA	12.8	10.8
Not Hispanic or Latina									
White	47.1	44.8	44.7	62.0	52.4	43.9	NA	10.1	10.0
Black or African American	75.9	66.9	58.3	60.6	35.5	48.2	NA	13.5	12.0
Hispanic or Latina	43.3	45.5	45.4	73.1	57.0	52.0	NA	15.1	11.2

NOTE: Only youths attending school participated in the survey. Persons of Hispanic origin may be of any race.

NA = Data not available.   [1]Among students who had sexual intercourse in the last 3 months.

USE OF ADDICTIVE SUBSTANCES

Figure 3-6. Use of Selected Substances in the Past Month Among Persons Age 12 Years and Over, 2002, 2008, and 2009

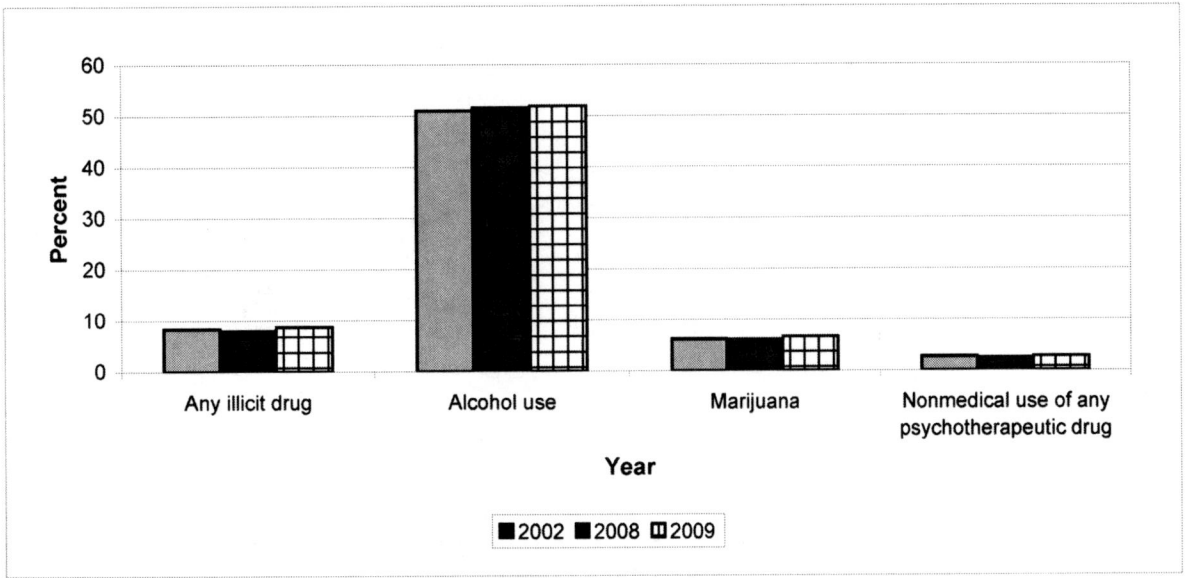

Figure 3-7. Current Cigarette Smoking Among Adults Age 18 Years and Over, by Sex and Selected Race, Selected Years, 1990–1992 to 2009–2011

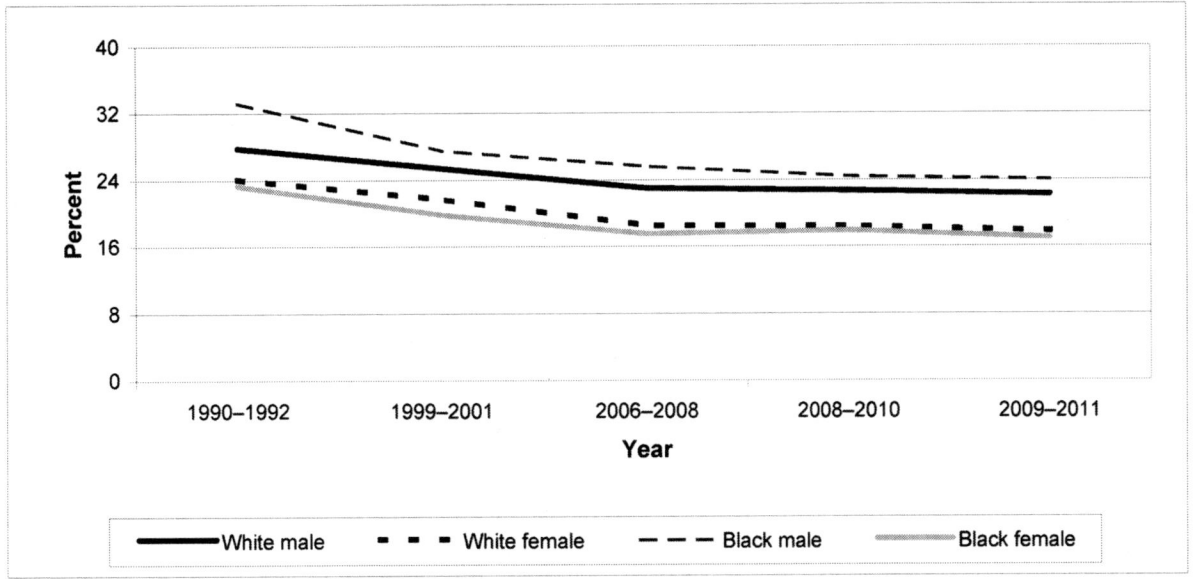

Table 3-27A. Use of Selected Substances in the Past Month Among Persons 12 Years of Age and Over, by Age, Sex, Race, and Hispanic Origin, Selected Years, 2002–2009

(Percent.)

Age, sex, race, and Hispanic origin	Any illicit drug[1]			Marijuana			Nonmedical use of any psychotherapeutic drug[2]		
	2002	2008	2009	2002	2008	2009	2002	2008	2009
Total, 12 Years and Over	8.3	8.0	8.7	6.2	6.1	6.6	2.7	2.5	2.8
Age									
12 to 13 years	4.2	3.3	3.6	1.4	1.0	0.8	1.7	1.5	1.6
14 to 15 years	11.2	8.6	9.0	7.6	5.7	6.3	4.0	3.0	3.3
16 to 17 years	19.8	15.2	16.7	15.7	12.7	14.0	6.3	4.0	4.3
18 to 25 years	20.2	19.6	21.2	17.3	16.5	18.1	5.5	5.9	6.3
26 to 34 years	10.5	11.2	12.3	7.7	8.8	9.6	3.7	3.2	3.8
35 years and over	4.6	4.7	4.9	3.1	3.2	3.4	1.6	1.6	1.7
Sex									
Male	10.3	9.9	10.8	8.1	7.9	8.6	2.8	2.6	3.1
Female	6.4	6.3	6.6	4.4	4.4	4.8	2.6	2.4	2.4
Age and Sex									
12 to 17 years	11.6	9.3	10.0	8.2	6.7	7.3	4.0	2.9	3.1
Male	12.3	9.5	10.6	9.1	7.3	8.3	3.6	2.5	2.8
Female	10.9	9.1	9.4	7.2	6.0	6.3	4.4	3.3	3.5
Hispanic Origin and Race[3]									
Not Hispanic or Latino									
White only	8.5	8.2	8.8	6.5	6.2	6.8	2.8	2.8	3.0
Black or African American only	9.7	10.1	9.6	7.4	8.3	7.8	2.0	1.8	2.0
American Indian or Alaska Native only	10.1	9.5	18.3	6.7	8.2	10.6	3.2	3.0	6.2
Native Hawaiian or Other Pacific Islander only	7.9	7.3	*	4.4	5.5	4.3	3.8	1.7	*
Asian only	3.5	3.6	3.7	1.8	2.0	2.4	0.7	1.0	1.4
Two or more races	11.4	14.7	14.3	9.0	13.1	12.2	3.5	2.7	3.4
Hispanic or Latino	7.2	6.2	7.9	4.3	4.2	5.8	2.9	1.8	2.4

* = Figure does not meet standards of reliability or precision. Data not shown if the relative standard error is greater than 17.5 percent of the log transformation of the proportion, the minimum effective sample size is less than 68, the minimum nominal sample size is less than 100, or the prevalence is close to 0 percent or 100 percent.   [1]Any illicit drug includes marijuana/hashish, cocaine (including crack), heroin, hallucinogens (including LSD and PCP), inhalants, or any prescription-type psychotherapeutic drug used nonmedically.   [2]Nonmedical use of prescription-type psychotherapeutic drugs includes the nonmedical use of pain relievers, tranquilizers, stimulants, or sedatives and does not include over-the-counter drugs.   [3]Persons of Hispanic origin may be of any race.

Table 3-27B. Use of Selected Substances in the Past Month Among Persons 12 Years of Age and Over, by Age, Sex, Race, and Hispanic Origin, Selected Years, 2002–2009

(Percent.)

Age, sex, race, and Hispanic origin	Alcohol use			Binge alcohol use[1]			Heavy alcohol use[2]		
	2002	2008	2009	2002	2008	2009	2002	2008	2009
Total, 12 Years and Over	51.0	51.6	51.9	22.9	23.3	23.7	6.7	6.9	6.8
Age									
12 to 13 years	4.3	3.4	3.5	1.8	1.5	1.6	0.3	0.2	0.2
14 to 15 years	16.6	13.1	13.0	9.2	6.9	7.0	1.9	1.1	1.4
16 to 17 years	32.6	26.2	26.3	21.4	17.2	17.0	5.6	4.4	4.5
18 to 25 years	60.5	61.2	61.8	40.9	41.0	41.7	14.9	14.5	13.7
26 to 34 years	61.4	63.5	64.3	33.1	36.4	36.3	9.0	10.6	10.1
35 years and over	52.1	52.8	52.7	18.6	18.8	19.2	5.2	5.3	5.3
Sex									
Male	57.4	57.7	57.6	31.2	31.6	31.6	10.8	10.6	10.3
Female	44.9	45.9	46.5	15.1	15.4	16.1	3.0	3.4	3.5
Age and Sex									
12 to 17 years	17.6	14.6	14.7	10.7	8.8	8.8	2.5	2.0	2.1
Male	17.4	14.2	15.1	11.4	8.9	9.6	3.1	2.3	2.3
Female	17.9	15.0	14.3	9.9	8.7	8.0	1.9	1.6	1.9
Hispanic Origin and Race [3]									
Not Hispanic or Latino									
White only	55.0	56.2	56.7	23.4	24.0	24.8	7.5	7.7	7.9
Black or African American only	39.9	41.9	42.8	21.0	20.4	19.8	4.4	5.6	4.5
American Indian or Alaska Native only	44.7	43.3	37.1	27.9	24.4	22.2	8.7	5.7	8.3
Native Hawaiian or Other Pacific Islander only	*	*	*	25.2	*	*	8.3	3.5	3.6
Asian only	37.1	37.0	37.6	12.4	11.9	11.1	2.6	2.4	1.5
Two or more races	49.9	47.5	47.6	19.8	22.0	24.1	7.5	7.4	6.4
Hispanic or Latino	42.8	43.2	41.7	24.8	25.6	25.0	5.9	5.7	5.2

* = Figure does not meet standards of reliability or precision. Data not shown if the relative standard error is greater than 17.5 percent of the log transformation of the proportion, the minimum effective sample size is less than 68, the minimum nominal sample size is less than 100, or the prevalence is close to 0 percent or 100 percent.   [1]Binge alcohol use is defined as drinking five or more drinks on the same occasion on at least 1 day in the past 30 days. Occasion is defined as at the same time or within a couple of hours of each other.   [2]Heavy alcohol use is defined as drinking five or more drinks on the same occasion on each of 5 or more days in the past 30 days. By definition, all heavy alcohol users are also binge alcohol users.   [3]Persons of Hispanic origin may be of any race.

Table 3-27C. Use of Selected Substances in the Past Month Among Persons 12 Years of Age and Over, by Age, Sex, Race, and Hispanic Origin, Selected Years, 2002–2009

(Percent.)

Age, sex, race, and Hispanic origin	Any tobacco[1]			Cigarettes			Cigars		
	2002	2008	2009	2002	2008	2009	2002	2008	2009
Total, 12 Years and Over	30.4	28.4	27.7	26.0	23.9	23.3	5.4	5.3	5.3
Age									
12 to 13 years	3.8	2.5	2.3	3.2	2.1	1.4	0.7	0.6	0.7
14 to 15 years	13.4	9.7	9.8	11.2	7.6	7.5	3.8	3.1	3.1
16 to 17 years	29.0	21.1	21.6	24.9	16.8	16.9	9.3	7.3	7.7
18 to 25 years	45.3	41.4	41.6	40.8	35.7	35.8	11.0	11.3	11.4
26 to 34 years	38.2	38.3	39.6	32.7	33.6	34.0	6.6	7.2	7.4
35 years and over	27.9	26.1	24.5	23.4	21.6	20.4	4.1	3.8	3.7
Sex									
Male	37.0	34.5	33.5	28.7	26.3	25.3	9.4	9.0	8.7
Female	24.3	22.5	22.2	23.4	21.7	21.4	1.7	1.7	2.0
Age and Sex									
12 to 17 years	15.2	11.4	11.6	13.0	9.1	8.9	4.5	3.8	4.0
Male	16.0	12.6	13.6	12.3	9.0	9.2	6.2	5.3	5.2
Female	14.4	10.2	9.5	13.6	9.2	8.6	2.7	2.2	2.7
Hispanic Origin and Race [2]									
Not Hispanic or Latino									
White only	32.0	30.4	29.6	26.9	25.2	24.5	5.5	5.3	5.2
Black or African American only	28.8	28.6	26.5	25.3	24.8	22.8	6.8	7.0	7.2
American Indian or Alaska Native only	44.3	48.7	41.8	37.1	44.1	33.0	5.2	5.6	6.9
Native Hawaiian or Other Pacific Islander only	28.8	*	*	*	*	15.4	4.1	2.2	*
Asian only	18.6	13.9	11.9	17.7	11.9	10.9	1.1	1.2	1.5
Two or more races	38.1	37.3	36.6	35.0	32.2	30.7	5.5	7.2	7.7
Hispanic or Latino	25.2	21.3	23.2	23.0	19.4	21.2	5.0	4.5	4.7

* = Figure does not meet standards of reliability or precision. Data not shown if the relative standard error is greater than 17.5 percent of the log transformation of the proportion, the minimum effective sample size is less than 68, the minimum nominal sample size is less than 100, or the prevalence is close to 0 percent or 100 percent. [1]Any tobacco product includes cigarettes, smokeless tobacco (i.e., chewing tobacco or snuff), cigars, or pipe tobacco. [2]Persons of Hispanic origin may be of any race.

Table 3-28. Heavier Drinking and Drinking Five or More Drinks in a Day Among Adults 18 Years of Age and Over, by Selected Characteristics, Selected Years, 1997–2011

(Percent.)

Characteristic	Heavier drinker[1]				Five or more drinks in a day on at least 1 day in the past year[1]				Five or more drinks in a day on at least 12 days in the past year[1]			
	1997	2000	2010	2011	1997	2000	2010	2011	1997	2000	2010	2011
BOTH SEXES												
18 years and over, age-adjusted[2]	4.9	4.3	5.2	4.8	21.1	19.2	23.8	23.1	9.7	8.7	10.1	9.4
18 years and over, crude	5.0	4.3	5.2	4.8	21.5	19.3	23.2	22.4	9.8	8.7	9.9	9.2
Age												
All persons												
18 to 44 years	5.2	4.7	5.7	4.9	29.2	26.9	32.5	31.6	13.2	12.2	13.7	13.1
18 to 24 years	5.3	5.8	6.2	5.2	31.8	30.3	34.0	31.7	15.2	15.5	16.2	15.1
25 to 44 years	5.2	4.3	5.5	4.8	28.5	25.8	31.9	31.5	12.6	11.1	12.7	12.3
45 to 64 years	5.5	4.6	5.4	5.5	15.9	14.4	19.0	18.1	7.6	6.4	8.1	7.2
45 to 54 years	5.5	4.4	5.9	5.6	19.0	16.4	22.9	21.4	8.7	7.0	9.3	8.3
55 to 64 years	5.4	5.0	4.7	5.3	11.1	11.3	14.1	14.2	5.8	5.4	6.7	5.9
65 years and over	3.1	2.6	3.7	3.4	4.9	3.8	5.5	5.5	2.2	1.8	2.6	2.4
65 to 74 years	3.9	3.1	4.4	4.2	6.7	5.2	7.9	7.7	3.0	2.5	3.5	3.3
75 years and over	2.1	2.0	2.8	2.4	2.4	2.1	2.7	2.7	1.1	*0.9	*1.4	1.3
Race [2,3]												
White only	5.2	4.5	5.6	5.2	22.9	20.8	26.3	25.2	10.3	9.2	11.1	10.3
Black or African American only	4.0	3.5	4.1	3.3	11.7	11.6	14.0	14.2	6.5	6.5	6.1	6.3
American Indian or Alaska Native only	*	*	*	*7.9	29.2	23.7	15.3	26.4	17.4	*12.1	*9.5	15.4
Asian only	*1.9	*2.3	*1.3	*1.7	11.4	8.8	12.1	13.3	*4.8	3.6	4.3	4.7
Native Hawaiian or Other Pacific Islander only	NA	*	*	*	NA	*	*	*	NA	*	*	*
Two or more races	NA	*7.5	*5.9	5.8	NA	28.0	25.7	25.9	NA	15.9	12.5	8.4
Hispanic Origin and Race [2,3]												
Hispanic or Latino	3.9	3.2	2.8	3.1	20.4	17.3	19.7	21.2	11.2	9.0	9.2	9.0
Mexican	4.4	3.8	3.1	3.9	21.2	19.9	21.4	23.8	12.6	10.8	10.1	10.4
Not Hispanic or Latino	5.1	4.5	5.6	5.1	21.3	19.7	24.7	23.6	9.5	8.8	10.3	9.6
White only	5.4	4.7	6.2	5.6	23.5	21.5	27.9	26.2	10.3	9.3	11.5	10.6
Black or African American only	3.9	3.4	4.2	3.3	11.6	11.5	13.9	14.1	6.5	6.5	6.1	6.2
Percent of Poverty Level [2,4]												
Below 100 percent	4.8	4.3	4.7	4.5	17.3	15.0	17.6	18.9	9.7	8.6	8.5	8.9
100 percent to 199 percent	4.9	4.2	4.9	4.8	18.4	15.7	20.9	20.1	9.8	8.0	9.8	9.3
200 percent to 399 percent	4.9	4.2	4.8	4.6	21.0	18.7	23.3	22.7	9.8	8.9	10.1	9.4
400 percent or more	5.1	4.4	6.0	5.0	24.3	22.1	28.1	26.4	9.7	8.9	10.9	9.9
Disability Measure [2,5]												
Any basic actions difficulty or complex activity limitation	5.7	5.2	5.5	5.0	20.2	18.8	21.9	21.2	10.2	9.3	9.5	9.0
Any basic actions difficulty	5.8	5.3	5.5	5.2	20.6	19.1	22.3	21.6	10.5	9.4	9.7	9.3
Any complex activity limitation	4.5	4.3	5.5	3.9	16.4	14.3	16.2	16.7	8.8	7.3	7.8	7.6
No disability	4.9	4.1	5.3	4.9	21.8	19.7	25.0	24.1	9.6	8.7	10.4	9.6
MALE												
18 years and over, age-adjusted[2]	6.1	5.1	5.7	5.3	30.7	28.3	32.4	32.0	15.8	14.4	15.6	15.0
18 years and over, crude	6.1	5.2	5.7	5.4	31.7	29.0	32.2	31.5	16.3	14.7	15.6	14.8
Age												
All persons												
18 to 44 years	6.5	5.6	6.1	5.6	40.6	37.8	42.5	42.3	21.1	19.6	20.6	20.5
18 to 24 years	6.0	6.3	6.0	6.0	40.6	38.0	39.9	41.0	22.9	22.9	21.5	22.9
25 to 44 years	6.6	5.3	6.2	5.4	40.6	37.7	43.5	42.8	20.6	18.5	20.2	19.6
45 to 64 years	6.6	5.5	5.8	6.0	25.3	23.5	27.3	26.1	12.7	11.3	13.2	11.3
45 to 54 years	6.6	5.7	5.9	6.1	29.4	26.3	32.0	29.7	14.5	12.3	14.5	12.5
55 to 64 years	6.6	5.4	5.7	5.9	18.9	19.0	21.4	21.8	10.0	9.8	11.6	9.8
65 years and over	3.7	3.1	4.0	3.3	9.3	7.4	9.8	9.9	4.7	3.7	4.7	4.5
65 to 74 years	4.8	3.9	4.4	4.3	12.2	9.5	13.5	13.2	6.1	4.9	6.3	6.1
75 years and over	*2.1	*2.0	*3.5	*2.1	5.1	4.4	4.6	5.2	*2.5	*2.0	*2.5	2.4
Race [2,3]												
White only	6.3	5.1	6.1	5.6	32.8	29.9	35.3	34.4	16.7	14.9	17.1	16.1
Black or African American only	5.3	5.4	4.6	4.5	18.4	19.8	20.2	22.2	11.0	12.4	9.8	10.7
American Indian or Alaska Native only	*	*	*	*9.4	45.7	29.2	*20.5	32.8	30.4	*14.0	*15.7	20.7
Asian only	*2.3	*3.5	*1.4	*1.6	17.8	14.1	17.2	18.7	*7.5	*5.9	6.8	7.7
Native Hawaiian or Other Pacific Islander only	NA	*	*	*	NA	*	*	*	NA	*	*	*
Two or more races	NA	*12.1	*8.4	*6.4	NA	39.2	37.6	31.6	NA	23.7	20.3	12.9
Hispanic Origin and Race [2,3]												
Hispanic or Latino	5.7	5.2	3.9	4.2	30.9	27.9	28.8	31.8	18.8	15.9	14.6	14.9
Mexican	6.9	6.6	4.4	5.4	34.2	32.2	32.2	34.8	21.9	19.1	16.3	16.6
Not Hispanic or Latino	6.1	5.2	6.0	5.5	30.7	28.6	33.3	32.3	15.5	14.3	15.9	15.1
White only	6.4	5.2	6.5	5.9	33.3	30.6	36.9	35.3	16.6	15.0	17.6	16.5
Black or African American only	5.3	5.4	4.7	4.5	18.4	19.7	20.3	22.0	11.1	12.3	9.9	10.5
Percent of Poverty Level [2,4]												
Below 100 percent	6.8	6.4	6.5	6.3	26.9	24.8	26.0	28.7	16.5	15.7	14.1	15.0
100 percent to 199 percent	7.1	5.8	5.8	6.4	27.3	23.6	29.1	28.8	16.4	13.3	14.8	15.5
200 percent to 399 percent	6.6	5.3	5.8	5.0	30.4	27.4	31.8	30.6	16.0	14.7	16.4	14.5
400 percent or more	5.0	4.4	5.4	4.7	33.6	31.3	36.4	35.3	15.4	14.4	15.8	15.2
Disability Measure [2,5]												
Any basic actions difficulty or complex activity limitation	7.2	6.8	6.6	6.1	29.4	28.9	30.6	29.0	17.0	16.5	14.8	14.3
Any basic actions difficulty	7.5	6.8	6.7	6.2	30.4	29.8	31.8	29.8	17.7	16.8	15.5	14.7
Any complex activity limitation	5.4	5.8	6.6	4.7	23.1	20.5	21.1	21.5	14.2	11.9	11.3	11.0
No disability	5.8	4.8	5.4	5.0	31.5	28.5	33.5	33.0	15.6	14.1	15.9	15.1

Table 3-28. Heavier Drinking and Drinking Five or More Drinks in a Day Among Adults 18 Years of Age and Over, by Selected Characteristics, Selected Years, 1997–2011—Continued

(Percent.)

Characteristic	Heavier drinker[1]				Five or more drinks in a day on at least 1 day in the past year[1]				Five or more drinks in a day on at least 12 days in the past year[1]			
	1997	2000	2010	2011	1997	2000	2010	2011	1997	2000	2010	2011
FEMALE												
18 years and over, age-adjusted[2]	3.9	3.5	4.8	4.3	12.2	10.8	15.6	14.6	3.9	3.4	4.8	4.1
18 years and over, crude	3.9	3.5	4.8	4.4	12.1	10.6	14.9	13.8	3.9	3.3	4.6	3.9
Age												
All persons												
18 to 44 years	4.0	3.8	5.2	4.2	18.3	16.5	22.6	21.0	5.5	5.2	6.9	5.7
18 to 24 years	4.5	5.2	6.4	4.4	23.0	22.8	28.1	22.2	7.6	8.3	10.9	7.1
25 to 44 years	3.9	3.4	4.8	4.1	16.9	14.5	20.6	20.5	4.9	4.2	5.4	5.2
45 to 64 years	4.4	3.8	4.9	5.0	7.2	6.0	11.1	10.6	2.9	1.9	3.4	3.3
45 to 54 years	4.5	3.2	5.9	5.2	9.2	7.1	14.3	13.6	3.3	2.1	4.3	4.2
55 to 64 years	4.4	4.6	3.8	4.9	4.1	4.4	7.3	7.1	2.1	1.5	2.3	2.3
65 years and over	2.6	2.2	3.4	3.4	1.6	1.2	2.3	2.1	*0.4	*0.4	*	*0.7
65 to 74 years	3.1	2.5	4.5	4.2	2.3	1.7	*3.1	3.0	*	*	*	*0.8
75 years and over	2.0	1.9	2.3	2.6	*0.7	*	*1.4	*1.0	*	*	*	*
Race [2,3]												
White only	4.2	4.0	5.2	4.8	13.5	12.1	17.4	16.2	4.2	3.7	5.2	4.5
Black or African American only	2.9	2.0	3.8	2.3	6.5	5.2	9.0	7.6	2.9	1.9	3.1	2.6
American Indian or Alaska Native only	*	*	*	*	18.1	*19.0	*11.7	19.2	*	*	*	*
Asian only	*	*	*	*	*5.2	*3.7	7.3	8.5	*	*	*	*2.0
Native Hawaiian or Other Pacific Islander only	NA	*	*	*	NA	*	*	*	NA	*	*	*
Two or more races	NA	*	*	*4.8	NA	17.0	16.4	20.5	NA	*8.2	*6.3	*4.1
Hispanic Origin and Race [2,3]												
Hispanic or Latina	2.2	1.2	1.7	1.9	9.7	6.8	10.3	10.2	3.5	2.1	3.6	2.9
Mexican	*1.9	*1.1	*1.7	2.1	8.2	7.1	10.4	11.6	3.2	*2.2	3.7	3.4
Not Hispanic or Latina	4.1	3.8	5.3	4.7	12.6	11.5	16.6	15.5	4.0	3.6	5.0	4.4
White only	4.4	4.3	5.9	5.3	14.2	13.0	19.1	17.5	4.3	4.0	5.6	4.9
Black or African American only	2.9	2.0	3.8	2.3	6.2	5.2	8.9	7.6	2.9	1.9	3.0	2.5
Percent of Poverty Level [2,4]												
Below 100 percent	3.6	2.8	3.4	3.2	10.8	8.2	11.3	11.9	5.1	3.6	4.2	4.4
100 percent to 199 percent	3.1	2.9	4.1	3.3	10.5	9.0	13.5	12.3	4.0	3.5	5.1	3.8
200 percent to 399 percent	3.3	3.2	3.9	4.2	12.1	10.7	15.3	14.6	4.0	3.5	4.2	4.2
400 percent or more	5.2	4.5	6.7	5.3	14.2	12.6	19.2	16.8	3.4	3.3	5.6	4.0
Disability Measure [2,5]												
Any basic actions difficulty or complex activity limitation	4.5	4.1	4.7	4.2	13.1	11.3	15.2	15.2	5.0	4.1	5.4	5.1
Any basic actions difficulty	4.5	4.2	4.7	4.3	13.2	11.6	15.4	15.6	5.1	4.1	5.4	5.3
Any complex activity limitation	3.7	*3.2	4.6	3.2	10.8	9.1	12.3	12.6	4.2	*3.1	5.0	4.6
No disability	3.9	3.5	5.1	4.7	12.0	10.9	16.1	14.8	3.6	3.3	4.7	3.9

NA = Not available.   * = Figure does not meet standards of reliability or precision. Data preceded by an asterisk have a relative standard error (RSE) of 20 percent to 30 percent. Data not shown have an RSE of greater than 30 percent.   [1]Heavier drinking is based on self-reported responses to questions about average alcohol consumption and is defined as more than 14 drinks per week for men and more than seven drinks per week for women on average. Respondents were also asked, "In the past year, on how many days did you have five or more drinks of any alcoholic beverage?"   [2]Estimates are age adjusted to the year 2000 standard population using four age groups: 18 to 24 years, 25 to 44 years, 45 to 64 years, and 65 years and over. Age-adjusted estimates in this table may differ from other age-adjusted estimates based on the same data and presented elsewhere if different age groups are used in the adjustment procedure.   [3]The race groups White, Black, American Indian or Alaska Native, Asian, Native Hawaiian or Other Pacific Islander, and two or more races, include persons of Hispanic and non-Hispanic origin. Persons of Hispanic origin may be of any race.   [4]Percent of poverty level is based on family income and family size and composition using U.S. Census Bureau poverty thresholds. Missing family income data were imputed for 1997 and beyond.   [5]Any basic actions difficulty or complex activity limitation is defined as having one or more of the following limitations or difficulties: movement difficulty, emotional difficulty, sensory (seeing or hearing) difficulty, cognitive difficulty, self-care (activities of daily living or instrumental activities of daily living) limitation, social limitation, or work limitation.

Table 3-29. Age-Adjusted Prevalence of Current Cigarette Smoking[1] Among Adults 25 Years of Age and Over, by Sex, Race, and Education Level, Selected Years, 1974–2011

(Percent.)

Sex, race, and education level	1974[2]	1979[2]	1985[2]	1990[2]	1995[2]	2000	2005	2006	2007	2008	2009	2010	2011
25 YEARS AND OVER, AGE-ADJUSTED [3]													
All Persons [4]	36.9	33.1	30.0	25.4	24.5	22.6	20.3	20.3	19.3	20.5	20.4	19.2	19.0
No high school diploma or GED	43.7	40.7	40.8	36.7	35.6	31.6	28.2	28.8	26.9	29.8	28.9	26.9	27.2
High school diploma or GED	36.2	33.6	32.0	29.1	29.1	29.2	27.0	26.5	26.6	28.1	28.7	27.0	27.4
Some college, no bachelor's degree	35.9	33.2	29.5	23.4	22.6	21.7	21.8	22.1	20.1	22.1	21.4	21.3	20.7
Bachelor's degree or higher	27.2	22.6	18.5	13.9	13.6	10.9	9.1	8.2	9.0	8.5	9.0	8.3	7.5
All Males [4]	42.9	37.3	32.8	28.2	26.4	24.7	22.7	22.9	21.4	22.6	22.4	21.0	21.2
No high school diploma or GED	52.3	47.6	45.7	42.0	39.7	36.0	31.7	31.6	30.8	32.5	32.3	29.7	31.6
High school diploma or GED	42.4	38.9	35.5	33.1	32.7	32.1	29.9	29.7	29.4	31.4	31.4	29.3	29.8
Some college, no bachelor's degree	41.8	36.5	32.9	25.9	23.7	23.3	24.9	25.2	21.6	24.3	23.0	23.2	22.6
Bachelor's degree or higher	28.3	22.7	19.6	14.5	13.8	11.6	9.7	9.2	10.4	9.1	9.6	8.7	7.9
White Males [4,5]	41.9	36.7	31.7	27.6	25.9	24.7	22.4	22.7	21.6	22.6	22.7	21.0	21.3
No high school diploma or GED	51.5	47.6	45.0	41.8	38.7	38.2	31.6	31.4	30.8	33.1	32.2	29.4	32.0
High school diploma or GED	42.0	38.5	34.8	32.9	32.9	32.4	30.0	29.2	29.9	31.9	32.4	29.6	29.9
Some college, no bachelor's degree	41.6	36.4	32.2	25.4	23.3	23.5	24.5	25.8	21.8	23.7	22.4	23.4	22.4
Bachelor's degree or higher	27.8	22.5	19.1	14.4	13.4	11.3	9.3	8.9	10.5	9.1	9.6	8.8	7.9
Black or African American Males [4,5]	53.4	44.4	42.1	34.5	31.6	26.4	26.5	25.4	23.7	25.9	23.7	23.9	23.9
No high school diploma or GED	58.1	49.7	50.5	41.6	41.9	38.2	35.9	35.2	30.4	35.0	39.1	34.4	32.3
High school diploma or GED	*50.7	48.6	41.8	37.4	36.6	29.0	30.1	31.3	29.6	28.3	26.0	28.8	29.4
Some college, no bachelor's degree	*45.3	39.2	41.8	28.1	26.4	19.9	27.4	21.0	23.6	29.5	26.5	24.2	24.7
Bachelor's degree or higher	*41.4	*36.8	*32.0	*20.8	*17.3	14.6	10.0	12.9	*13.5	*10.0	9.9	8.1	7.9
All Females [4]	32.0	29.5	27.5	22.9	22.9	20.5	18.0	17.9	17.2	18.4	18.5	17.5	16.8
No high school diploma or GED	36.6	34.8	36.5	31.8	31.7	27.1	24.6	26.0	22.7	27.0	24.8	23.7	22.7
High school diploma or GED	32.2	29.8	29.5	26.1	26.4	26.6	24.1	23.4	23.8	25.0	26.1	24.9	24.7
Some college, no bachelor's degree	30.1	30.0	26.3	21.0	21.6	20.4	19.1	19.6	18.9	20.1	20.0	19.6	19.0
Bachelor's degree or higher	25.9	22.5	17.1	13.3	13.3	10.1	8.5	7.2	7.7	8.1	8.4	7.9	7.1
White Females [4,5]	31.7	29.7	27.3	23.3	23.1	21.0	18.6	18.5	18.0	19.4	19.0	18.3	17.6
No high school diploma or GED	36.8	35.8	36.7	33.4	32.4	28.4	24.6	25.9	23.8	28.4	24.4	24.0	22.7
High school diploma or GED	31.9	29.9	29.4	26.5	26.8	27.8	25.9	24.6	25.2	27.1	26.5	25.8	26.8
Some college, no bachelor's degree	30.4	30.7	26.7	21.2	22.2	21.1	19.5	20.5	19.6	21.6	21.2	21.0	20.0
Bachelor's degree or higher	25.5	21.9	16.5	13.4	13.5	10.2	9.1	7.7	8.2	8.5	9.1	8.7	7.5
Black or African American Females [4,5]	35.6	30.3	32.0	22.4	25.7	21.6	17.5	19.1	16.6	17.5	19.3	17.0	16.1
No high school diploma or GED	36.1	31.6	39.4	26.3	32.3	31.1	27.8	31.2	23.1	28.9	31.0	25.8	29.6
High school diploma or GED	40.9	32.6	32.1	24.1	27.8	25.4	18.2	18.6	19.8	20.0	27.3	22.9	16.9
Some college, no bachelor's degree	32.3	*28.9	23.9	22.7	20.8	20.4	17.5	18.9	17.2	15.9	16.2	15.0	15.0
Bachelor's degree or higher	*36.3	*43.3	26.6	17.0	17.3	10.8	*6.6	*8.5	*6.0	*9.3	*7.3	*6.6	7.2

* = Figure does not meet standards of reliability or precision. Data preceded by an asterisk have a relative standard error of 20 percent to 30 percent. [1]Starting with 1993 data (shown in spreadsheet version), current cigarette smokers were defined as ever smoking 100 cigarettes in their lifetime and smoking now every day or some days. [2]Data prior to 1997 are not strictly comparable with data for later years due to the 1997 questionnaire redesign. [3]Estimates are age adjusted to the year 2000 standard population using four age groups: 25 to 34 years, 35 to 44 years, 45 to 64 years, and 65 years and over. [4]Includes unknown education level. Education categories shown are for 1997 and subsequent years. GED is General Educational Development high school equivalency diploma. [5]The race groups White and Black include persons of Hispanic and non-Hispanic origin.

Table 3-30. Current Cigarette Smoking[1] Among Adults, by Sex, Race, Hispanic Origin, Age, and Education Level, Average Annual, Selected Years, 1990–1992 Through 2009–2011

(Percent.)

Characteristic	Male					Female				
	1990–1992[2]	1999–2001	2006–2008	2008–2010	2009–2011	1990–1992[2]	1999–2001	2006–2008	2008–2010	2009–2011
18 Years and Over, Age-Adjusted [3]										
All persons[4]	27.9	25.0	22.8	22.4	21.9	23.7	21.1	18.0	18.0	17.4
Race [5]										
White only	27.4	25.1	22.9	22.6	22.1	24.3	22.2	18.9	18.8	18.3
Black or African American only	33.9	27.2	24.8	23.7	23.2	23.1	19.7	17.2	17.5	16.8
American Indian or Alaska Native only	34.2	30.3	31.5	25.1	23.7	36.7	34.7	22.2	21.0	23.6
Asian only	24.8	20.3	15.6	15.3	15.0	6.3	6.7	4.4	5.5	5.7
Native Hawaiian or Other Pacific Islander only	NA	*	*	*	*	NA	*	*	*	*
2 or more races	NA	34.4	25.1	27.7	26.9	NA	30.7	24.6	20.9	22.5
American Indian or Alaska Native; White	NA	38.7	34.6	34.6	31.2	NA	38.9	28.6	26.5	29.8
Hispanic Origin and Race [5]										
Hispanic or Latino	25.7	22.2	18.6	17.3	16.4	15.8	12.1	9.5	9.6	9.0
Mexican	26.2	21.9	18.7	17.5	16.9	14.8	10.6	8.8	8.4	7.9
Not Hispanic or Latino	28.1	25.5	23.7	23.4	23.0	24.4	22.3	19.4	19.5	18.9
White only	27.7	25.5	24.0	23.9	23.5	25.2	23.5	20.9	20.9	20.3
Black or African American only	33.9	27.2	25.1	24.0	23.5	23.2	19.7	17.2	17.7	17.0
18 Years and Over, Crude										
All persons[4]	28.4	25.5	23.1	22.7	22.2	23.6	21.0	17.9	17.8	17.3
Race [5]										
White only	27.8	25.4	23.0	22.7	22.2	24.1	21.7	18.5	18.4	17.8
Black or African American only	33.2	27.5	25.6	24.4	24.0	23.3	19.8	17.5	17.9	17.0
American Indian or Alaska Native only	35.5	31.8	30.7	25.6	24.1	37.3	36.9	23.0	21.6	24.5
Asian only	24.9	21.4	16.5	15.7	15.6	6.3	6.9	4.6	5.6	5.9
Native Hawaiian or Other Pacific Islander only	NA	*	*	*	*	NA	*	*	*	*
2 or more races	NA	35.9	27.0	29.2	28.4	NA	31.5	25.3	21.9	23.0
American Indian or Alaska Native; White	NA	41.1	33.5	33.9	31.6	NA	40.1	30.0	27.5	29.9
Hispanic Origin and Race [5]										
Hispanic or Latino	26.5	23.2	19.6	18.4	17.2	16.6	12.6	9.7	9.8	9.1
Mexican	27.1	22.8	19.4	18.6	17.7	15.0	11.0	8.8	8.5	8.1
Not Hispanic or Latino	28.5	25.8	23.7	23.4	23.0	24.2	21.9	19.1	19.0	18.5
White only	28.0	25.5	23.7	23.6	23.2	24.8	22.7	20.1	20.0	19.4
Black or African American only	33.3	27.5	26.0	24.7	24.3	23.3	19.8	17.6	18.0	17.3
Age and Hispanic Origin and Race [5]										
18 to 24 Years										
Hispanic or Latino	19.3	22.6	18.4	19.3	16.4	12.8	12.9	8.0	8.0	7.7
Not Hispanic or Latino										
White only	28.9	32.7	29.1	28.2	27.9	28.7	30.8	24.1	21.2	20.5
Black or African American only	17.7	21.9	23.6	18.4	18.6	10.8	13.0	13.5	14.9	12.6
25 to 34 Years										
Hispanic or Latino	29.9	23.2	20.4	20.1	18.6	19.2	12.5	9.5	9.6	9.0
Not Hispanic or Latino										
White only	32.7	30.8	31.6	30.8	30.9	30.9	27.4	26.7	26.5	25.5
Black or African American only	34.6	23.3	28.5	25.7	25.5	29.2	16.9	16.2	19.1	19.0
35 to 44 Years										
Hispanic or Latino	32.1	25.3	20.5	18.2	18.1	19.9	14.1	10.2	10.4	9.7
Not Hispanic or Latino										
White only	32.3	29.6	25.9	26.5	25.0	27.3	28.3	24.1	24.7	24.5
Black or African American only	44.1	32.0	20.9	23.2	24.3	31.3	27.5	19.4	19.0	18.5
45 to 64 Years										
Hispanic or Latino	26.6	24.7	21.4	19.2	18.0	17.1	13.5	12.5	12.2	11.0
Not Hispanic or Latino										
White only	28.4	25.1	23.5	24.1	24.3	26.1	22.1	20.7	21.0	20.4
Black or African American only	38.0	34.0	31.8	31.7	30.1	26.1	23.6	23.2	21.6	20.5
65 Years and Over										
Hispanic or Latino	16.1	12.6	9.4	8.2	9.1	6.6	5.9	4.7	5.5	5.3
Not Hispanic or Latino										
White only	14.2	10.0	10.5	9.8	9.2	12.3	9.8	8.6	9.5	9.0
Black or African American only	25.2	17.6	16.3	13.7	12.6	10.7	11.0	7.8	9.8	10.2
Percent of Poverty Level [2,6]										
Below 100 percent	40.5	36.5	32.1	32.5	33.2	30.7	29.1	28.1	28.6	26.7
100 percent to 199 percent	35.0	32.8	29.4	29.3	28.4	26.9	25.6	22.4	22.8	22.3
200 percent to 399 percent	26.5	27.3	24.8	24.3	23.6	22.6	22.3	18.5	18.5	18.1
400 percent or more	22.5	18.8	17.0	16.0	15.1	19.0	15.9	12.5	11.8	10.9
Hispanic Origin and Race and Percent of Poverty Level [2,4,6]										
Hispanic or Latino										
Below 100 percent	29.2	25.3	20.8	20.2	20.8	16.3	14.4	11.9	11.4	10.6
100 percent to 199 percent	29.5	22.0	18.4	17.8	17.0	16.0	11.8	8.3	8.7	8.4
200 percent to 399 percent	23.7	23.6	19.7	16.6	15.4	15.9	12.0	8.6	10.2	9.6
400 percent or more	19.7	18.1	15.7	15.1	13.3	13.6	9.4	9.9	7.9	6.2
Not Hispanic or Latino										
White only										
Below 100 percent	44.2	40.7	38.6	40.6	41.1	37.8	38.3	38.0	39.4	38.1
100 percent to 199 percent	36.3	37.5	35.0	35.3	34.5	31.1	32.0	30.7	30.7	30.1
200 percent to 399 percent	26.4	28.5	27.0	27.4	26.7	23.7	24.8	22.1	21.9	21.4
400 percent or more	22.5	19.1	17.4	16.3	15.8	19.5	17.1	13.6	13.1	12.2
Black or African American only										
Below 100 percent	43.5	40.6	38.2	36.5	36.5	28.9	27.7	27.0	29.1	27.1
100 percent to 199 percent	36.0	33.9	30.9	30.4	30.3	20.3	21.3	18.6	19.6	18.6
200 percent to 399 percent	31.4	24.9	21.8	20.7	20.5	21.4	17.3	13.5	13.2	13.3
400 percent or more	24.3	17.9	18.4	15.6	13.4	19.2	12.6	10.3	8.2	7.4
Disability Measure [7]										
Any basic actions difficulty or complex activity limitation	NA	33.1	32.1	30.3	29.9	NA	28.1	26.8	26.8	26.4
Any basic actions difficulty	NA	33.2	32.5	30.5	30.3	NA	28.2	27.0	27.0	26.7
Any complex activity limitation	NA	37.6	34.2	33.2	33.0	NA	30.6	31.8	31.5	31.5
No disability	NA	22.8	20.1	19.8	19.2	NA	18.8	14.9	14.6	14.1

Table 3-30. Current Cigarette Smoking[1] Among Adults, by Sex, Race, Hispanic Origin, Age, and Education Level, Average Annual, Selected Years, 1990–1992 Through 2009–2011—Continued

(Percent.)

Characteristic	Male					Female				
	1990–1992[2]	1999–2001	2006–2008	2008–2010	2009–2011	1990–1992[2]	1999–2001	2006–2008	2008–2010	2009–2011
Education, Hispanic Origin, and Race [5,8] 25 years and over, age-adjusted[9]										
No high school diploma or GED Hispanic or Latino	30.2	24.3	19.5	18.5	17.5	15.8	12.1	8.6	8.6	7.9
Not Hispanic or Latino										
White only	46.1	43.5	42.0	45.1	46.7	40.4	39.3	42.9	44.0	42.0
Black or African American only	45.4	40.0	35.9	37.2	37.2	31.3	29.4	28.7	29.9	30.4
High school diploma or GED Hispanic or Latino	29.6	24.1	21.7	20.3	21.0	18.4	12.5	10.7	11.4	11.0
Not Hispanic or Latino										
White only	32.9	31.8	32.7	34.4	33.3	28.4	29.2	28.8	30.3	30.6
Black or African American only	38.2	31.4	29.5	27.8	28.3	25.4	23.0	19.8	23.7	22.5
Some college or more Hispanic or Latino	20.4	17.1	15.8	12.9	11.5	14.3	11.1	10.3	9.9	9.0
Not Hispanic or Latino										
White only	19.3	17.6	16.2	15.9	15.8	18.1	16.7	14.7	15.5	15.1
Black or African American only	25.6	19.2	19.3	19.8	18.6	22.8	16.9	13.7	12.7	12.3

NA = Not available.   * = Figure does not meet standards of reliability or precision. Data preceded by an asterisk have a relative standard error (RSE) of 20 percent to 30 percent. Data not shown have an RSE of greater than 30 percent.   [1]Starting with 1993 data, current cigarette smokers were defined as ever smoking 100 cigarettes in their lifetime and smoking now every day or some days.   [2]Data prior to 1997 are not strictly comparable with data for later years due to the 1997 questionnaire redesign.   [3]Estimates are age adjusted to the year 2000 standard population using five age groups: 18 to 24 years, 25 to 34 years, 35 to 44 years, 45 to 64 years, and 65 years and over. For age groups where smoking is 0 percent or 100 percent, the age-adjustment procedure was modified to substitute the percentage smoking from the previous 3-year period.   [4]Includes all other races not shown separately, unknown education level, and unknown disability measure.   [5]The race groups White, Black, American Indian or Alaska Native, Asian, Native Hawaiian or Other Pacific Islander, and two or more races include persons of Hispanic and non–Hispanic origin. Persons of Hispanic origin may be of any race.   [6]Percent of poverty level is based on family income and family size and composition using U.S. Census Bureau poverty thresholds. Missing family income data were imputed for 1990 and beyond.   [7]Any basic actions difficulty or complex activity limitation is defined as having one or more of the following limitations or difficulties: movement difficulty, emotional difficulty, sensory (seeing or hearing) difficulty, cognitive difficulty, self–care (activities of daily living or instrumental activities of daily living) limitation, social limitation, or work limitation.   [8]Education categories shown are for 1997 and subsequent years. GED is General Educational Development high school equivalency diploma.   [9]Estimates are age adjusted to the year 2000 standard using four age groups: 25 to 34 years, 35 to 44 years, 45 to 64 years, and 65 years and over.

Table 3-31. Current Cigarette Smoking[1] Among Adults 18 Years of Age and Over, by Sex, Race, and Age, Selected Years, 1965–2011

(Percent.)

Sex, race, and age	1965[2]	1974[2]	1983[2]	1985[2]	1990[2]	1995[2]	2000	2005	2006	2007	2008	2009	2010	2011
18 Years and Over, Age-Adjusted[3]														
All persons	41.9	37.0	31.9	29.9	25.3	24.6	23.1	20.8	20.8	19.7	20.6	20.6	19.3	19.0
Male	51.2	42.8	34.8	32.2	28.0	26.5	25.2	23.4	23.6	22.0	22.8	23.2	21.2	21.2
Female	33.7	32.2	29.4	27.9	22.9	22.7	21.1	18.3	18.1	17.5	18.5	18.1	17.5	16.8
White male[4]	50.4	41.7	34.2	31.3	27.6	26.2	25.4	23.3	23.5	22.2	23.0	23.6	21.4	21.4
Black or African American male[4]	58.8	53.6	41.7	40.2	32.8	29.4	25.7	25.9	26.1	23.4	24.7	23.1	23.3	23.2
White female[4]	33.9	32.0	29.6	27.9	23.5	23.4	22.0	19.1	18.8	18.5	19.5	18.7	18.3	17.7
Black or African American female[4]	31.8	35.6	31.3	30.9	20.8	23.5	20.7	17.1	18.5	15.6	17.4	18.5	16.6	15.2
18 Years and Over, Crude														
All persons	42.4	37.1	32.1	30.1	25.5	24.7	23.2	20.9	20.8	19.8	20.6	20.6	19.3	19.0
Male	51.9	43.1	35.1	32.6	28.4	27.0	25.6	23.9	23.9	22.3	23.1	23.5	21.5	21.6
Female	33.9	32.1	29.5	27.9	22.8	22.6	20.9	18.1	18.0	17.4	18.3	17.9	17.3	16.5
White male[4]	51.1	41.9	34.5	31.7	28.0	26.6	25.7	23.6	23.6	22.3	23.1	23.6	21.4	21.6
Black or African American male[4]	60.4	54.3	40.6	39.9	32.5	28.5	26.2	26.5	27.0	24.6	25.3	23.7	24.3	23.8
White female[4]	34.0	31.7	29.4	27.7	23.4	23.1	21.4	18.7	18.4	18.1	19.1	18.3	17.9	17.2
Black or African American female[4]	33.7	36.4	32.2	31.0	21.2	23.5	20.8	17.3	18.8	15.9	17.8	18.8	17.0	15.3
All Males														
18 to 44 years	57.9	47.9	37.7	35.2	31.4	29.9	29.2	27.1	26.7	25.8	25.6	26.9	23.9	23.6
18 to 24 years	54.1	42.1	32.9	28.0	26.6	27.8	28.1	28.0	28.5	25.4	23.6	28.0	22.8	21.3
25 to 34 years	60.7	50.5	38.8	38.2	31.6	29.5	28.9	27.7	27.4	28.8	28.5	27.6	26.1	27.5
35 to 44 years	58.2	51.0	41.0	37.6	34.5	31.5	30.2	26.0	24.8	23.2	24.3	25.4	22.5	21.2
45 to 64 years	51.9	42.6	35.9	33.4	29.3	27.1	26.4	25.2	24.5	22.6	24.8	24.5	23.2	24.4
45 to 54 years	55.9	46.8	39.0	34.9	32.1	27.2	28.8	28.1	26.6	24.8	26.4	27.3	25.2	27.0
55 to 64 years	46.6	37.7	32.6	31.9	25.9	26.9	22.6	21.1	21.5	19.6	22.6	20.8	20.7	21.4
65 years and over	28.5	24.8	22.0	19.6	14.6	14.9	10.2	8.9	12.6	9.3	10.5	9.5	9.7	8.9
White Male [4]														
18 to 44 years	57.1	46.8	37.5	34.6	31.3	30.1	30.2	27.7	27.1	26.6	26.7	28.1	24.6	24.3
18 to 24 years	53.0	40.8	32.5	28.4	27.4	28.4	30.4	29.7	28.9	26.5	25.2	30.0	23.8	22.1
25 to 34 years	60.1	49.5	38.6	37.3	31.6	29.9	29.7	27.7	27.9	29.0	29.5	28.4	26.6	28.6
35 to 44 years	57.3	50.1	40.8	36.6	33.5	31.2	30.6	26.3	25.3	24.4	24.9	26.3	23.1	21.4
45 to 64 years	51.3	41.2	35.0	32.1	28.7	26.3	25.8	24.5	23.4	22.1	24.0	24.0	22.5	24.0
45 to 54 years	55.3	45.0	38.0	33.7	31.3	25.9	28.0	27.4	25.7	24.4	26.1	27.1	24.5	26.6
55 to 64 years	46.1	36.6	31.9	30.5	25.6	27.0	22.5	20.4	20.4	19.1	21.2	20.1	20.1	20.8
65 years and over	27.7	24.3	20.6	18.9	13.7	14.1	9.8	7.9	12.6	8.9	9.9	9.3	9.6	8.6
Black or African American Male [4]														
18 to 44 years	66.3	58.1	39.4	39.6	32.9	26.4	25.5	25.1	26.2	24.2	22.0	22.5	22.6	22.7
18 to 24 years	62.8	54.9	34.2	27.2	21.3	*	20.9	21.6	31.2	21.4	*17.0	18.9	18.8	18.4
25 to 34 years	68.4	58.5	39.9	45.6	33.8	25.1	23.2	29.8	26.3	32.3	25.9	24.1	25.7	25.0
35 to 44 years	67.3	61.5	45.5	45.0	42.0	36.3	30.7	23.3	22.2	17.4	21.8	24.0	22.6	24.3
45 to 64 years	57.9	57.8	44.8	46.1	36.7	33.9	32.2	32.4	32.6	28.3	33.6	28.9	31.8	28.9
45 to 54 years	62.4	63.6	47.8	47.7	42.0	36.9	35.6	33.9	32.0	29.3	31.7	28.1	33.2	29.2
55 to 64 years	51.8	50.1	41.1	44.4	30.2	29.1	26.3	29.8	33.5	26.8	36.6	30.1	29.6	28.4
65 years and over	36.4	29.7	38.9	27.7	21.5	28.5	14.2	16.8	16.0	14.3	17.5	14.0	10.0	13.7
All Females														
18 to 44 years	42.1	37.5	33.8	31.4	25.6	25.6	24.5	21.2	20.6	19.5	20.6	20.0	19.1	18.8
18 to 24 years	38.1	34.1	35.5	30.4	22.5	21.8	24.9	20.7	19.3	19.1	19.0	15.6	17.4	16.4
25 to 34 years	43.7	38.8	32.6	32.0	28.2	26.4	22.3	21.5	21.5	19.6	21.4	21.8	20.6	19.5
35 to 44 years	43.7	39.8	33.8	31.5	24.8	27.1	26.2	21.3	20.6	19.6	20.9	21.2	19.0	19.9
45 to 64 years	32.0	33.4	31.0	29.9	24.8	24.0	21.7	18.8	19.3	19.5	20.5	19.5	19.1	18.5
45 to 54 years	37.5	36.0	34.1	32.4	28.5	24.3	22.2	20.9	22.5	22.1	23.7	22.3	21.3	21.6
55 to 64 years	25.0	30.4	28.0	27.4	20.5	23.7	20.9	16.1	14.9	16.2	16.3	16.1	16.5	15.0
65 years and over	9.6	12.0	13.1	13.5	11.5	11.5	9.3	8.3	8.3	7.6	8.3	9.5	9.3	7.1
White Female [4]														
18 to 44 years	42.2	37.3	34.2	31.6	26.5	26.6	26.5	22.6	22.2	21.2	22.1	21.2	20.5	20.3
18 to 24 years	38.4	34.0	36.5	31.8	25.4	24.9	28.5	22.6	20.7	21.6	20.1	16.7	18.4	18.4
25 to 34 years	43.4	38.6	32.2	32.0	28.5	27.3	24.9	23.1	23.7	21.4	23.1	22.7	22.0	20.6
35 to 44 years	43.9	39.3	34.8	31.0	25.0	27.0	26.6	22.2	21.7	20.7	22.6	22.9	20.5	21.5
45 to 64 years	32.7	33.0	30.6	29.7	25.4	24.3	21.4	18.9	18.8	19.6	20.9	19.4	19.5	19.0
45 to 54 years	38.2	34.9	33.3	32.4	29.1	24.6	21.9	21.0	22.1	22.2	24.2	22.4	22.4	22.5
55 to 64 years	25.7	30.6	28.1	27.2	21.2	23.8	20.6	16.2	14.4	16.2	16.8	15.8	15.9	15.1
65 years and over	9.8	12.3	13.2	13.3	11.5	11.7	9.1	8.4	8.4	8.0	8.6	9.6	9.4	7.0
Black or African American Female [4]														
18 to 44 years	42.9	41.1	34.6	33.5	22.8	24.0	20.8	16.9	17.3	14.2	18.0	18.3	17.1	15.0
18 to 24 years	37.1	35.6	32.0	23.7	10.0	*8.8	14.2	14.2	14.8	*8.7	16.6	13.3	14.2	9.1
25 to 34 years	47.8	42.2	38.0	36.2	29.1	26.7	15.5	16.9	15.4	14.9	17.6	20.1	19.3	17.5
35 to 44 years	42.8	46.4	32.7	40.2	25.5	31.9	30.2	19.0	21.0	17.7	19.6	20.0	17.2	17.4
45 to 64 years	25.7	38.9	36.3	33.4	22.6	27.5	25.6	21.0	25.5	22.6	21.3	22.7	19.8	18.3
45 to 54 years	32.3	46.2	43.6	36.4	26.5	28.3	26.5	22.2	29.3	26.3	24.9	23.5	20.4	20.1
55 to 64 years	16.5	29.3	28.0	29.8	17.6	26.3	24.2	19.1	19.5	17.0	15.9	21.4	18.9	16.0
65 years and over	7.1	*8.9	*13.1	14.5	11.1	13.3	10.2	10.0	9.3	6.4	8.1	11.5	9.4	9.1

* = Figure does not meet standards of reliability or precision. Data preceded by an asterisk have a relative standard error (RSE) of 20 percent to 30 percent. Data not shown have an RSE of greater than 30 percent.   [1]Starting with 1993 data, current cigarette smokers were defined as ever smoking 100 cigarettes in their lifetime and smoking now every day or some days.   [2]Data prior to 1997 are not strictly comparable with data for later years due to the 1997 questionnaire redesign.   [3]Estimates are age adjusted to the year 2000 standard population using five age groups: 18 to 24 years, 25 to 34 years, 35 to 44 years, 45 to 64 years, and 65 years and over. For age groups where smoking is 0 percent or 100 percent, the age-adjustment procedure was modified to substitute the percentage smoking from the previous 3-year period.   [4]The race groups White, Black, American Indian or Alaska Native, Asian, Native Hawaiian or Other Pacific Islander, and two or more races include persons of Hispanic and non-Hispanic origin. Persons of Hispanic origin may be of any race.

Table 3-32. Use of Selected Substances Among High School Seniors, 10th Graders, and 8th Graders, by Sex and Race, Selected Years, 1980–2010

(Percent.)

Substance, grade in school, sex, and race	1980	1985	1990	1995	2000	2005	2006	2007	2008	2009	2010
Cigarettes											
All high school seniors	30.5	30.1	29.4	33.5	31.4	23.2	21.6	21.6	20.4	20.1	19.2
Male	26.8	28.2	29.1	34.5	32.8	24.8	22.4	23.1	21.5	22.1	21.9
Female	33.4	31.4	29.2	32.0	29.7	20.7	20.1	19.6	19.1	17.6	15.7
White	31.0	31.7	32.5	37.3	36.6	27.0	24.7	25.2	24.1	23.7	22.2
Black or African American	25.2	18.7	12.0	15.0	13.6	10.0	11.0	10.6	10.1	9.3	10.7
All 10th graders	NA	NA	NA	27.9	23.9	14.9	14.5	14.0	12.3	13.1	13.6
Male	NA	NA	NA	27.7	23.8	14.5	13.4	14.6	12.7	13.7	15.0
Female	NA	NA	NA	27.9	23.6	15.1	15.5	13.3	11.9	12.5	12.1
White	NA	NA	NA	31.2	27.3	17.0	16.3	16.1	14.1	14.6	14.8
Black or African American	NA	NA	NA	12.2	11.3	7.7	8.5	5.8	7.1	6.4	7.0
All 8th graders	NA	NA	NA	19.1	14.6	9.3	8.7	7.1	6.8	6.5	7.1
Male	NA	NA	NA	18.8	14.3	8.7	8.1	7.5	6.7	6.7	7.4
Female	NA	NA	NA	19.0	14.7	9.7	8.9	6.4	6.7	6.0	6.8
White	NA	NA	NA	21.7	16.4	9.5	9.1	7.1	7.3	7.3	7.9
Black or African American	NA	NA	NA	8.2	8.4	6.7	5.4	4.8	4.4	4.5	4.0
Marijuana											
All high school seniors	33.7	25.7	14.0	21.2	21.6	19.8	18.3	18.8	19.4	20.6	21.4
Male	37.8	28.7	16.1	24.6	24.7	23.6	19.7	22.3	22.2	24.3	25.2
Female	29.1	22.4	11.5	17.2	18.3	15.8	16.4	15.0	16.2	16.8	16.9
White	34.2	26.4	15.6	21.5	22.0	21.7	19.2	19.9	20.4	21.2	21.6
Black or African American	26.5	21.7	5.2	17.8	17.5	15.1	16.7	15.4	17.1	20.6	19.7
All 10th graders	NA	NA	NA	17.2	19.7	15.2	14.2	14.2	13.8	15.9	16.7
Male	NA	NA	NA	19.2	23.3	16.7	15.7	15.8	15.2	18.7	20.1
Female	NA	NA	NA	15.0	16.2	13.4	12.6	12.5	12.3	13.2	13.3
White	NA	NA	NA	17.7	20.1	15.7	14.7	14.8	13.5	15.6	15.9
Black or African American	NA	NA	NA	15.1	17.0	13.5	14.2	11.0	12.3	15.1	15.9
All 8th graders	NA	NA	NA	9.1	9.1	6.6	6.5	5.7	5.8	6.5	8.0
Male	NA	NA	NA	9.8	10.2	7.6	6.7	6.2	6.6	7.5	9.2
Female	NA	NA	NA	8.2	7.8	5.7	6.0	4.9	4.8	5.3	6.8
White	NA	NA	NA	9.0	8.3	6.0	5.7	5.1	4.9	5.9	7.1
Black or African American	NA	NA	NA	7.0	8.5	8.2	6.7	6.0	6.2	7.2	8.2
Cocaine											
All high school seniors	5.2	6.7	1.9	1.8	2.1	2.3	2.5	2.0	1.9	1.3	1.3
Male	6.0	7.7	2.3	2.2	2.7	2.6	3.0	2.4	2.3	1.5	1.9
Female	4.3	5.6	1.3	1.3	1.6	1.8	2.1	1.5	1.3	0.9	0.7
White	5.4	7.0	1.8	1.7	2.2	2.3	2.6	2.3	2.0	1.2	1.2
Black or African American	2.0	2.7	0.5	0.4	1.0	0.5	1.0	0.5	0.5	0.2	0.9
All 10th graders	NA	NA	NA	1.7	1.8	1.5	1.5	1.3	1.2	0.9	0.9
Male	NA	NA	NA	1.8	2.1	1.9	1.6	1.4	1.4	1.0	1.1
Female	NA	NA	NA	1.5	1.4	1.2	1.3	1.1	1.0	0.8	0.5
White	NA	NA	NA	1.7	1.7	1.5	1.5	1.2	1.0	0.7	0.7
Black or African American	NA	NA	NA	0.4	0.4	0.8	0.7	0.4	0.7	0.5	0.6
All 8th graders	NA	NA	NA	1.2	1.2	1.0	1.0	0.9	0.8	0.8	0.6
Male	NA	NA	NA	1.1	1.3	0.9	1.0	0.7	0.9	0.8	0.6
Female	NA	NA	NA	1.2	1.1	1.0	0.9	1.0	0.7	0.7	0.6
White	NA	NA	NA	1.0	1.1	0.9	0.8	0.6	0.6	0.6	0.5
Black or African American	NA	NA	NA	0.4	0.5	0.3	0.4	0.6	0.4	0.7	0.3
Inhalants											
All high school seniors	1.4	2.2	2.7	3.2	2.2	2.0	1.5	1.2	1.4	1.2	1.4
Male	1.8	2.8	3.5	3.9	2.9	2.4	1.5	1.5	1.6	1.2	2.1
Female	1.0	1.7	2.0	2.5	1.7	1.6	1.4	0.9	1.2	1.0	0.7
White	1.4	2.4	3.0	3.7	2.1	2.1	1.5	1.2	1.5	1.1	1.1
Black or African American	1.0	0.8	1.5	1.1	2.1	1.4	1.2	0.9	1.0	1.1	1.5
All 10th graders	NA	NA	NA	3.5	2.6	2.2	2.3	2.5	2.1	2.2	2.0
Male	NA	NA	NA	3.8	3.0	1.9	2.2	2.7	1.9	1.8	1.6
Female	NA	NA	NA	3.2	2.2	2.5	2.4	2.4	2.3	2.6	2.4
White	NA	NA	NA	3.9	2.8	2.2	2.4	2.6	1.6	1.9	1.7
Black or African American	NA	NA	NA	1.2	1.5	1.4	1.8	1.5	1.9	1.3	1.8
All 8th graders	NA	NA	NA	6.1	4.5	4.2	4.1	3.9	4.1	3.8	3.6
Male	NA	NA	NA	5.6	4.1	3.1	3.6	3.4	2.9	3.3	2.8
Female	NA	NA	NA	6.6	4.8	5.3	4.7	4.3	5.3	4.3	4.4
White	NA	NA	NA	7.0	4.8	4.0	4.2	3.6	3.8	3.7	3.2
Black or African American	NA	NA	NA	2.3	2.3	2.9	2.7	2.8	2.8	3.4	2.2
MDMA (Ecstasy)											
All high school seniors	NA	NA	NA	NA	3.6	1.0	1.3	1.6	1.8	1.8	1.4
Male	NA	NA	NA	NA	4.1	1.0	1.5	1.5	2.3	2.4	1.5
Female	NA	NA	NA	NA	3.1	1.0	1.1	1.6	1.2	1.2	1.2
White	NA	NA	NA	NA	3.9	1.0	1.4	1.7	1.7	1.7	0.9
Black or African American	NA	NA	NA	NA	1.9	0.9	0.6	0.8	1.1	1.8	1.1
All 10th graders	NA	NA	NA	NA	2.6	1.0	1.2	1.2	1.1	1.3	1.9
Male	NA	NA	NA	NA	2.5	1.0	1.5	1.3	1.6	1.6	2.3
Female	NA	NA	NA	NA	2.5	0.9	0.8	1.1	0.7	1.0	1.5
White	NA	NA	NA	NA	2.5	1.0	1.3	1.4	1.0	1.0	1.5
Black or African American	NA	NA	NA	NA	1.8	0.3	1.0	0.4	0.1	0.6	1.1
All 8th graders	NA	NA	NA	NA	1.4	0.6	0.7	0.6	0.8	0.6	1.1
Male	NA	NA	NA	NA	1.6	0.8	0.5	0.7	0.7	0.5	1.2
Female	NA	NA	NA	NA	1.2	0.4	0.8	0.6	0.9	0.6	1.1
White	NA	NA	NA	NA	1.4	0.6	0.5	0.5	0.7	0.6	1.0
Black or African American	NA	NA	NA	NA	0.8	0.9	0.7	0.8	0.3	0.1	0.5
Alcohol [1]											
All high school seniors	72.0	65.9	57.1	51.3	50.0	47.0	45.3	44.4	43.1	43.5	41.2
Male	77.4	69.8	61.3	55.7	54.0	50.7	47.3	47.1	45.8	47.8	44.2
Female	66.8	62.1	52.3	47.0	46.1	43.3	43.0	41.4	40.9	38.9	37.9
White	75.8	70.2	62.2	54.8	55.3	52.2	49.1	49.4	47.8	46.6	44.1
Black or African American	47.7	43.6	32.9	37.4	29.3	28.8	29.5	27.9	29.3	32.2	30.8

Table 3-32. Use of Selected Substances Among High School Seniors, 10th Graders, and 8th Graders, by Sex and Race, Selected Years, 1980–2010—*Continued*

(Percent.)

Substance, grade in school, sex, and race	1980	1985	1990	1995	2000	2005	2006	2007	2008	2009	2010
All 10th graders	NA	NA	NA	38.8	41.0	33.2	33.8	33.4	28.8	30.4	28.9
Male	NA	NA	NA	39.7	43.3	32.8	33.8	33.4	28.6	31.0	30.1
Female	NA	NA	NA	37.8	38.6	33.6	33.8	33.3	29.0	29.8	27.7
White	NA	NA	NA	41.3	44.3	36.7	36.0	35.7	30.5	32.4	29.2
Black or African American	NA	NA	NA	24.9	24.7	20.8	22.4	21.0	20.4	20.1	21.3
All 8th graders	NA	NA	NA	24.6	22.4	17.1	17.2	15.9	15.9	14.9	13.8
Male	NA	NA	NA	25.0	22.5	16.2	16.3	15.6	15.4	14.7	13.2
Female	NA	NA	NA	24.0	22.0	17.9	17.6	16.0	16.4	14.9	14.3
White	NA	NA	NA	25.4	23.9	17.3	16.5	14.7	15.8	15.1	12.8
Black or African American	NA	NA	NA	17.3	15.1	13.9	12.4	12.3	13.5	11.1	12.7
Binge Drinking [2]											
All high school seniors	41.2	36.7	32.2	29.8	30.0	27.1	25.4	25.9	24.6	25.2	23.2
Male	52.1	45.3	39.1	36.9	36.7	32.6	28.9	30.7	28.4	30.5	28.0
Female	30.5	28.2	24.4	23.0	23.5	21.6	21.5	21.5	21.3	20.2	18.4
White	44.6	40.1	36.2	32.9	34.4	31.8	28.9	30.5	29.3	28.7	26.5
Black or African American	17.0	16.7	11.6	15.5	11.0	10.9	11.9	11.0	10.8	13.7	12.6
All 10th graders	NA	NA	NA	22.0	24.1	19.0	19.9	19.6	16.0	17.5	16.3
Male	NA	NA	NA	24.1	27.6	19.9	21.0	20.9	16.6	18.8	17.9
Female	NA	NA	NA	19.7	20.6	17.9	18.9	18.3	15.4	16.1	14.6
White	NA	NA	NA	24.1	26.6	21.5	21.8	21.7	17.4	18.4	16.0
Black or African American	NA	NA	NA	9.6	10.6	8.4	9.9	10.0	9.6	10.0	11.5
All 8th graders	NA	NA	NA	12.3	11.7	8.4	8.7	8.3	8.1	7.8	7.2
Male	NA	NA	NA	12.5	11.7	8.2	8.6	8.2	8.1	7.8	6.5
Female	NA	NA	NA	12.1	11.3	8.6	8.5	8.2	8.0	7.7	7.8
White	NA	NA	NA	12.6	12.5	8.4	8.4	7.7	8.0	7.4	6.7
Black or African American	NA	NA	NA	7.8	6.2	5.8	5.5	5.7	5.7	4.8	5.9

NA = Not available.   [1]In 1993, the alcohol question was changed to indicate that a drink meant more than a few sips.   [2]Five or more alcoholic drinks in a row at least once in the prior 2-week period.

AMBULATORY CARE

Figure 3-8. Influenza Vaccination Among Adults Age 18 Years and Over, by Age, 2000–2011

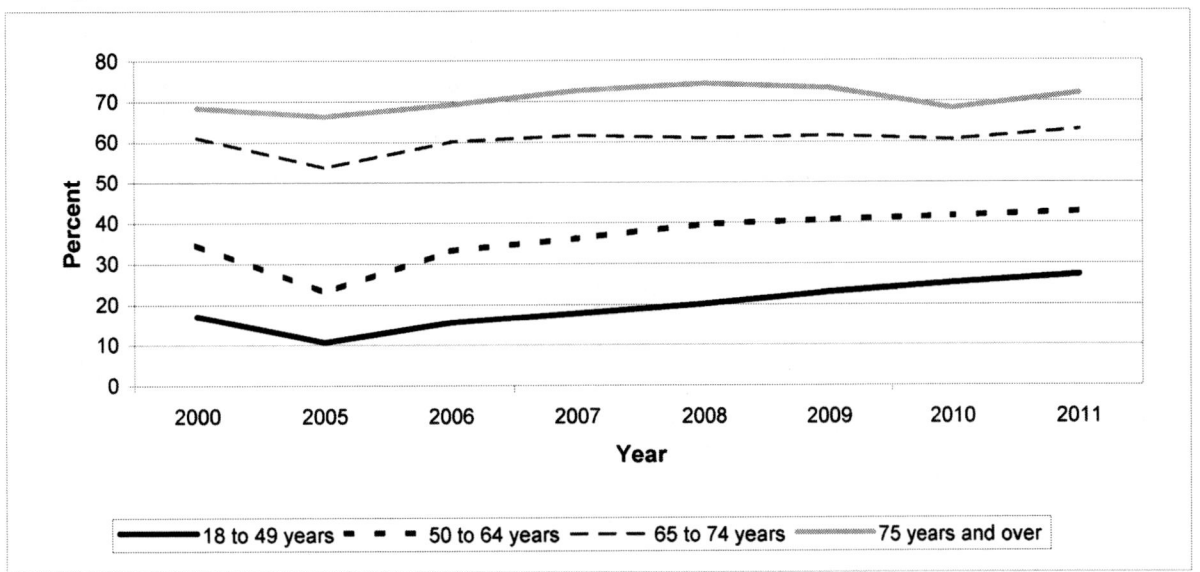

Figure 3-9. Percent of People Who Delayed or Did Not Get Medical Care Due to Cost, Highest and Lowest Among States with the 25 Largest Populations, 2010–2011

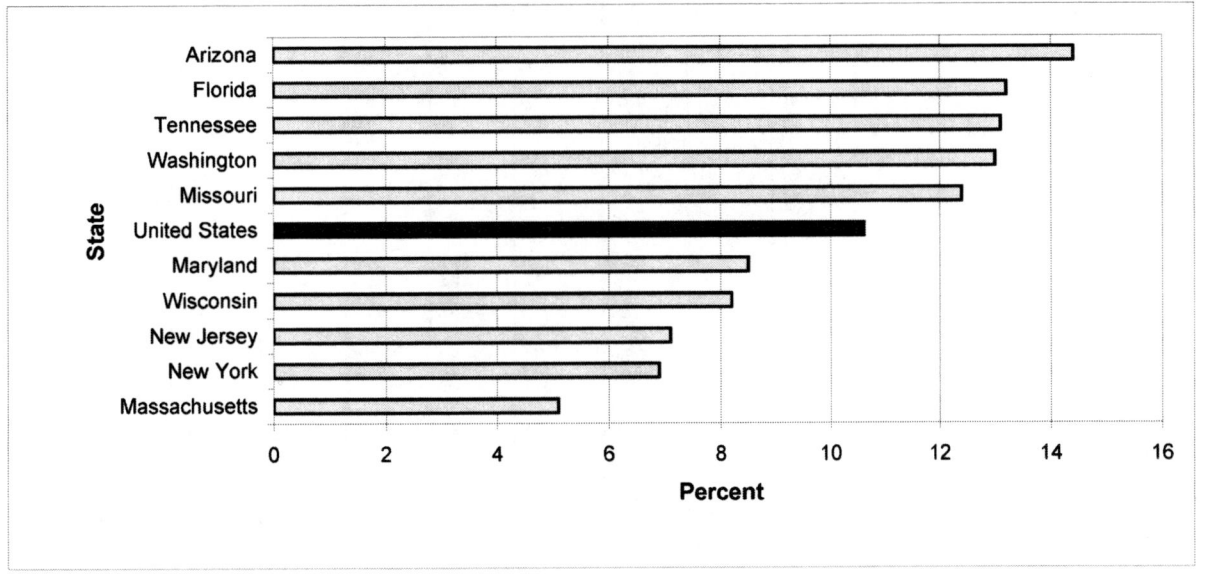

Table 3-33. No Usual Source of Health Care Among Children Under 18 Years of Age, by Selected Characteristics, Annual Average, Selected Years, 1993–1994 Through 2010–2011

(Percent.)

Characteristic	Under 18 years				Under 6 years				6 to 17 years			
	1993–1994[1]	1999–2000	2009–2010	2010–2011	1993–1994[1]	1999–2000	2009–2010	2010–2011	1993–1994[1]	1999–2000	2009–2010	2010–2011
Percent of Children without a Usual Source of Health Care[2]												
All Children[3]	7.7	6.9	5.4	4.7	5.2	4.6	4.1	3.0	9.0	8.0	6.2	5.6
Sex												
Male	8.1	6.7	5.5	4.6	5.3	4.5	4.2	2.9	9.6	7.8	6.1	5.6
Female	7.3	7.1	5.4	4.8	5.0	4.7	4.0	3.2	8.5	8.2	6.2	5.6
Race[4]												
White only	7.0	6.3	5.3	4.5	4.7	4.4	3.8	2.6	8.3	7.2	6.1	5.4
Black or African American only	10.3	7.7	5.6	5.3	7.6	4.4	4.3	4.5	11.9	9.1	6.3	5.8
American Indian or Alaska Native only	*9.3	*9.4	*	*7.0	*	*	*	*	*8.7	*9.4	*9.2	*9.6
Asian only	9.7	10.0	6.1	5.8	*3.4	*5.8	*3.9	*2.7	13.5	12.2	7.3	7.5
Native Hawaiian or Other Pacific Islander only	NA	*	*	*	NA	*	*	*	NA	*	*	*
Two or more races	NA	*4.9	4.6	4.8	NA	*	*4.2	*4.7	NA	*7.2	*4.9	4.8
Hispanic Origin and Race[4]												
Hispanic or Latino	14.3	14.2	9.5	7.9	9.3	9.0	5.8	4.3	17.7	17.2	11.8	10.2
Not Hispanic or Latino	6.7	5.5	4.3	3.7	4.4	3.6	3.5	2.6	7.8	6.3	4.7	4.3
White only	5.7	4.7	3.8	3.1	3.7	3.3	2.9	2.0	6.7	5.4	4.1	3.6
Black or African American only	10.2	7.6	5.4	5.4	7.7	4.5	4.3	4.5	11.6	9.0	6.0	5.8
Percent of Poverty Level[5]												
Below 100 percent	13.9	13.1	8.3	6.8	9.4	7.6	6.6	4.3	16.8	16.2	9.3	8.4
100 percent to 199 percent	9.8	10.6	7.5	7.1	6.7	7.5	4.8	4.3	11.6	12.2	9.0	8.6
200 percent to 399 percent	3.7	4.8	4.7	3.9	1.9	3.2	*3.1	2.2	4.5	5.6	5.5	4.8
400 percent or more	3.7	2.6	2.1	1.7	*1.6	1.5	*1.9	*1.3	5.0	3.0	2.2	1.8
Hispanic Origin and Race and Percent of Poverty Level[4,5]												
Hispanic or Latino												
Below 100 percent	19.6	19.4	10.7	8.0	12.7	11.6	7.1	*3.7	24.8	24.5	13.4	11.1
100 percent to 199 percent	15.3	17.1	10.6	9.6	9.9	11.3	6.3	5.5	18.9	20.4	13.2	12.1
200 percent to 399 percent	5.2	8.3	8.5	7.3	*	*5.0	*4.1	*4.1	6.7	10.1	10.9	9.2
400 percent or more	*	*3.8	*3.6	*3.1	*	*	*	*	*	*5.0	*4.1	*3.3
Not Hispanic or Latino												
White only												
Below 100 percent	10.2	10.7	6.1	4.8	6.5	*6.3	*5.0	*	12.7	13.1	*6.8	5.9
100 percent to 199 percent	8.7	7.8	5.7	5.4	6.3	5.7	*4.0	*3.9	10.1	8.8	6.6	6.2
200 percent to 399 percent	3.3	4.0	3.7	2.9	1.6	2.7	*	*1.3	4.0	4.6	4.2	3.7
400 percent or more	4.0	2.3	2.1	1.4	*1.7	*1.5	*1.9	*	5.4	2.6	2.1	1.6
Black or African American only												
Below 100 percent	13.7	9.4	6.3	6.6	10.9	*4.7	*6.2	*6.0	15.5	11.8	6.4	7.0
100 percent to 199 percent	9.1	9.7	6.2	6.7	*6.0	*6.4	*	*	10.8	11.2	8.1	8.0
200 percent to 399 percent	5.0	5.0	5.1	3.5	*	*	*	*	6.2	5.7	5.4	3.4
400 percent or more	*	*3.5	*	*	*	*	*	*	*	*4.0	*	*
Health Insurance Status at the Time of Interview[6]												
Insured	5.0	3.9	3.4	2.8	3.3	2.6	2.8	2.0	5.9	4.5	3.7	3.2
Private	3.8	3.4	2.6	2.1	1.9	2.2	1.7	1.3	4.6	3.9	3.0	2.5
Medicaid	8.9	5.3	4.4	3.7	6.4	3.5	3.7	2.7	11.3	6.7	4.9	4.4
Uninsured	23.5	29.3	28.8	28.4	18.0	20.8	21.4	19.5	26.0	32.9	31.5	31.5
Health Insurance Status Prior to Interview[6]												
Insured continuously all 12 months	4.6	3.6	3.2	2.6	3.1	2.3	2.7	1.9	5.5	4.2	3.4	3.0
Uninsured for any period up to 12 months	15.3	15.0	11.7	12.8	10.9	12.5	10.4	9.2	18.1	16.4	12.4	14.6
Uninsured more than 12 months	27.6	35.8	36.2	36.2	21.4	26.8	27.5	29.5	30.0	39.1	38.5	37.7
Geographic Region												
Northeast	4.1	2.8	2.7	2.2	2.9	2.3	*2.6	*1.8	4.8	3.0	2.7	2.4
Midwest	5.2	5.3	4.3	3.8	4.1	3.7	3.6	2.3	5.9	6.0	4.6	4.5
South	10.9	8.5	6.2	5.5	7.3	5.8	4.4	3.7	12.7	9.8	7.1	6.5
West	8.6	9.7	7.4	6.0	5.3	5.7	4.9	3.5	10.6	11.7	8.7	7.4
Location of Residence												
Within MSA[7]	7.7	6.8	5.5	4.9	5.0	4.7	4.2	3.2	9.2	7.8	6.2	5.8
Outside MSA[7]	7.8	7.4	5.0	3.8	6.0	4.2	3.3	*2.3	8.7	8.7	5.8	4.6

NA = Not available.   * = Figure does not meet standards of reliability or precision. Data preceded by an asterisk have a relative standard error (RSE) of 20 percent to 30 percent. Data not shown have an RSE of greater than 30 percent.   [1]Data prior to 1997 are not strictly comparable with data for later years due to the 1997 questionnaire redesign.   [2]Persons who report the emergency department as their usual source of care are defined as having no usual source of care.   [3]Includes all other races not shown separately and unknown health insurance status.   [4]The race groups White, Black, American Indian or Alaska Native, Asian, Native Hawaiian or Other Pacific Islander, and two or more races include persons of Hispanic and non-Hispanic origin. Persons of Hispanic origin may be of any race.   [5]Percent of poverty level is based on family income and family size and composition using U.S. Census Bureau poverty thresholds. Missing family income data were imputed starting in 1993.   [6]Health insurance categories are mutually exclusive. Persons who reported both Medicaid and private coverage are classified as having private coverage. Medicaid includes other public assistance through 1996. Starting with 1997 data, state-sponsored health plan coverage is included as Medicaid coverage. Starting with 1999 data, coverage by the Children's Health Insurance Program (CHIP) is included with Medicaid coverage. Persons not covered by private insurance, Medicaid, CHIP, public assistance (through 1996), state-sponsored or other government-sponsored health plans (starting in 1997), Medicare, or military plans are considered to have no health insurance coverage. Persons with only Indian Health Service coverage are considered to have no health insurance coverage. Health insurance status was unknown for 8 to 9 percent of children in 1993–1996 and about 1 percent in 1997–2011.   [7]MSA = metropolitan statistical area.

Table 3-34. No Usual Source of Health Care Among Adults 18 to 64 Years of Age, by Selected Characteristics, Annual Average, Selected Years, 1993–1994 Through 2010–2011

(Percent.)

Characteristic	1993–1994[1]	1995–1996[1]	1997–1998	1999–2000	2001–2002	2003–2004	2004–2005	2005–2006	2006–2007	2007–2008	2008–2009	2009–2010	2010–2011
PERCENT OF ADULTS WITHOUT A USUAL SOURCE OF HEALTH CARE[2]													
Total, 18 to 64 Years[3]	18.9	16.9	17.7	17.8	16.4	17.3	18.0	18.4	18.5	18.5	19.5	20.3	19.6
Age													
18 to 44 years	21.7	19.6	21.1	21.6	20.6	21.7	22.8	23.5	23.5	23.6	25.0	26.0	25.2
18 to 24 years	26.6	22.6	27.0	27.2	27.2	28.0	29.9	29.8	28.7	28.6	29.6	29.8	28.1
25 to 44 years	20.3	18.8	19.3	19.9	18.5	19.5	20.3	21.3	21.8	21.8	23.4	24.7	24.1
45 to 64 years	12.8	11.3	11.2	10.9	9.2	10.4	10.6	10.7	11.2	11.0	11.6	12.3	11.8
45 to 54 years	14.1	12.2	12.6	12.0	10.3	11.7	11.9	12.3	13.3	13.1	13.6	14.7	14.0
55 to 64 years	11.1	9.8	9.0	9.2	7.6	8.7	8.8	8.4	8.3	8.3	9.0	9.3	9.0
Sex													
Male	23.9	21.4	23.6	24.1	21.6	22.5	23.3	23.9	23.9	23.9	25.3	25.9	24.6
Female	14.1	12.6	12.0	11.8	11.4	12.4	12.9	13.0	13.3	13.1	13.8	14.8	14.7
Race[3]													
White only	18.4	16.5	17.0	16.7	15.4	17.0	17.7	18.1	18.3	18.0	18.9	19.7	18.9
Black or African American only	20.0	18.3	19.4	19.2	16.9	18.4	19.3	19.8	19.8	20.5	21.5	22.4	22.5
American Indian or Alaska Native only	19.7	16.5	21.3	19.2	16.3	21.5	22.8	21.9	24.4	24.4	24.8	26.7	22.4
Asian only	24.8	21.5	21.7	22.1	20.1	19.3	18.8	17.9	17.3	17.8	19.4	20.8	20.8
Native Hawaiian or Other Pacific Islander only	NA	NA	NA	*	*	*	*	*	*	*	*	*	*
Two or more races	NA	NA	NA	21.0	20.1	18.4	18.1	20.9	20.4	21.4	26.1	27.5	24.4
American Indian or Alaska Native; White	NA	NA	NA	25.8	18.1	17.8	19.1	21.4	19.3	20.9	25.9	27.1	23.9
Hispanic Origin and Race[4]													
Hispanic or Latino	30.3	27.4	30.4	32.6	32.5	32.9	34.0	35.1	34.3	32.5	32.8	33.3	33.3
Mexican	32.4	29.8	35.9	36.5	36.5	36.4	37.8	39.3	39.0	36.6	36.1	35.7	35.2
Not Hispanic or Latino	17.7	15.7	16.2	15.8	14.0	14.9	15.4	15.6	15.9	16.0	17.1	17.9	17.0
White only	17.1	15.0	15.4	14.9	13.1	14.0	14.6	14.8	15.2	15.1	16.0	16.8	15.8
Black or African American only	19.7	18.1	19.3	19.2	16.8	18.1	19.0	19.2	18.9	20.2	21.4	22.2	22.1
Percent of Poverty Level[5]													
Below 100 percent	29.5	26.1	29.1	29.6	29.3	28.9	31.8	32.1	30.6	30.4	32.7	33.8	32.8
100 percent to 199 percent	25.4	22.9	25.6	27.1	25.6	26.6	27.1	27.8	28.6	29.1	30.3	30.5	30.4
200 percent to 399 percent	15.6	13.4	16.6	17.2	16.0	17.3	17.9	17.8	18.5	18.9	19.7	20.5	19.3
400 percent or more	13.4	13.8	11.6	11.6	9.6	10.1	10.3	10.4	10.4	10.2	10.6	10.8	9.7
Hispanic Origin and Race and Percent of Poverty Level[4,5]													
Hispanic or Latino													
Below 100 percent	40.0	34.3	42.8	44.4	46.3	42.8	44.5	46.7	46.7	43.7	44.1	45.5	44.3
100 percent to 199 percent	36.9	32.9	35.4	40.6	40.0	39.7	40.7	41.8	42.1	40.6	40.7	39.7	40.4
200 percent to 399 percent	20.7	19.5	23.6	26.9	27.9	28.2	30.1	31.2	29.5	28.0	27.9	29.1	28.9
400 percent or more	13.8	16.3	14.4	16.1	13.7	16.4	16.2	16.4	15.9	16.9	16.6	14.0	13.4
Not Hispanic or Latino													
White only													
Below 100 percent	28.2	23.6	25.0	24.2	23.4	23.0	26.8	26.2	25.0	25.2	27.8	28.8	27.5
100 percent to 199 percent	23.3	20.7	22.4	23.0	20.7	22.0	22.8	23.5	24.5	24.9	26.0	26.6	26.0
200 percent to 399 percent	14.8	12.5	15.4	15.3	13.6	15.4	15.6	15.3	16.2	16.7	17.7	18.6	17.2
400 percent or more	13.4	13.7	11.3	11.2	9.1	9.4	9.6	9.8	10.0	9.5	9.9	10.3	9.1
Black or African American only													
Below 100 percent	24.7	21.9	23.9	23.7	22.8	24.3	28.3	29.5	26.5	27.1	29.4	30.1	30.3
100 percent to 199 percent	22.3	22.1	25.3	24.4	20.4	22.8	22.1	22.6	23.4	25.7	27.6	28.5	29.6
200 percent to 399 percent	16.5	14.5	17.6	18.2	16.2	16.3	16.6	16.2	18.0	19.7	19.9	20.1	18.1
400 percent or more	11.7	12.6	11.2	12.0	9.6	11.3	11.3	10.3	9.1	10.2	11.2	10.5	10.6
Health Insurance Status at the Time of Interview[6]													
Insured	13.3	11.4	11.4	10.9	9.1	9.4	9.7	9.7	9.9	10.1	10.4	10.6	10.2
Private	13.1	11.3	11.5	11.1	9.0	9.5	9.5	9.6	9.8	10.0	10.3	10.6	10.1
Medicaid	16.3	13.0	10.3	9.9	11.1	9.9	12.1	11.6	11.5	11.7	12.1	12.5	12.3
Uninsured	43.1	41.8	46.7	49.2	49.1	50.2	52.5	53.0	52.8	52.1	54.1	55.6	54.2
Health Insurance Status Prior to Interview[6]													
Insured continuously all 12 months	12.7	10.8	10.6	10.3	8.3	8.7	8.9	8.9	9.0	9.1	9.5	9.8	9.3
Uninsured for any period up to 12 months	30.9	29.6	30.7	31.2	33.3	32.1	34.0	33.4	33.6	35.1	36.7	36.5	33.6
Uninsured more than 12 months	46.9	44.8	51.4	54.8	54.6	55.0	57.4	58.0	57.9	56.1	57.2	59.5	58.3
Disability Measure[7]													
Any basic actions difficulty or complex activity limitation	NA	NA	15.5	14.1	13.2	14.3	15.0	15.2	15.7	16.6	17.1	16.8	16.2
Any basic actions difficulty	NA	NA	15.7	14.1	13.1	14.5	15.2	15.4	15.8	16.5	17.1	16.6	16.2
Any complex activity limitation	NA	NA	13.1	11.6	10.4	10.7	11.5	11.1	12.6	13.6	13.8	13.5	13.1
No disability	NA	NA	18.2	18.8	17.5	18.2	18.8	19.4	19.5	19.1	20.3	21.5	20.7
Geographic Region													
Northeast	14.7	13.4	13.3	12.8	11.9	12.1	11.7	12.2	13.1	12.5	12.9	14.0	13.9
Midwest	16.2	14.7	15.1	17.0	14.1	14.7	15.4	15.8	16.2	16.6	17.3	17.5	16.7
South	21.8	18.7	20.7	19.7	18.3	19.7	21.0	21.4	21.4	21.4	22.5	23.5	22.3
West	21.1	19.9	20.2	20.1	19.9	21.0	21.2	21.1	20.5	20.0	21.8	22.9	22.4
Location of Residence													
Within MSA[8]	19.3	17.3	17.9	18.1	16.6	17.6	18.3	18.7	18.9	18.7	19.5	20.3	19.8
Outside MSA[8]	17.5	15.4	17.0	16.8	15.4	16.2	16.6	16.7	16.5	16.9	19.4	20.4	18.4

NA = Not available.   * = Figure does not meet standards of reliability or precision. Data not shown have an RSE of greater than 30 percent.   [1]Data prior to 1997 are not strictly comparable with data for later years due to the 1997 questionnaire redesign.   [2]Persons who report the emergency department as their usual source of care are defined as having no usual source of care.   [3]Includes all other races not shown separately, unknown health insurance status, and unknown disability status.   [4]The race groups White, Black, American Indian or Alaska Native, Asian, Native Hawaiian or Other Pacific Islander, and two or more races include persons of Hispanic and non-Hispanic origin. Persons of Hispanic origin may be of any race.   [5]Percent of poverty level is based on family income and family size and composition using U.S. Census Bureau poverty thresholds. Missing family income data were imputed starting in 1993.   [6]Health insurance categories are mutually exclusive. Persons who reported both Medicaid and private coverage are classified as having private coverage. Medicaid includes other public assistance through 1996. Starting with 1997 data, state-sponsored health plan coverage is included as Medicaid coverage. Starting with 1999 data, coverage by the Children's Health Insurance Program (CHIP) is included with Medicaid coverage. Persons not covered by private insurance, Medicaid, CHIP, public assistance (through 1996), state-sponsored or other government-sponsored health plans (starting in 1997), Medicare, or military plans are considered to have no health insurance coverage. Persons with only Indian Health Service coverage are considered to have no health insurance coverage. Health insurance status was unknown for 8 to 9 percent of children in 1993-1996 and about 1 percent in 1997-2011.   [7]Any basic actions difficulty or complex activity limitation is defined as having one or more of the following limitations or difficulties: movement difficulty, emotional difficulty, sensory (seeing or hearing) difficulty, cognitive difficulty, self-care (activities of daily living or instrumental activities of daily living) limitation, social limitation, or work limitation.   [8]MSA = metropolitan statistical area.

Table 3-35. Reduced Access to Medical Care, Dental Care, and Prescription Drugs During the Past 12 Months Due to Cost, by Selected Characteristics, Selected Years, 1997–2011

(Percent.)

Characteristic	Did not get or delayed medical care due to cost[1]				Did not get prescription drugs due to cost[2]				Did not get dental care due to cost[3]			
	1997	2005	2010	2011	1997	2005	2010	2011	1997	2005	2010	2011
TOTAL [4]	8.3	8.5	10.9	10.3	4.8	7.2	8.3	7.7	8.6	10.7	13.5	12.9
Age												
Under 19 years	4.5	4.3	4.5	4.0	2.1	3.0	2.8	2.4	6.0	7.3	6.6	6.2
Under 18 years	4.4	4.2	4.4	3.8	2.2	2.9	2.7	2.3	6.0	7.3	6.6	6.1
Under 6 years	3.3	3.3	3.7	2.9	1.6	2.5	2.5	1.4	3.9	3.7	3.9	3.9
6 to 17 years	4.9	4.7	4.8	4.2	2.4	3.1	2.8	2.7	6.8	8.4	7.5	6.9
18 to 64 years	10.7	11.0	14.7	14.0	6.3	9.4	11.2	10.5	10.6	13.0	17.3	16.4
18 to 44 years	11.0	11.3	14.5	13.6	6.9	9.8	11.2	10.3	11.7	14.1	17.9	16.7
18 to 24 years	10.2	11.3	13.5	11.8	6.7	9.6	9.7	7.6	11.6	13.7	17.4	13.3
25 to 34 years	11.4	11.8	15.3	15.1	6.9	10.2	12.0	11.7	12.3	15.1	18.3	18.5
35 to 44 years	11.0	10.8	14.4	13.5	7.1	9.6	11.3	10.9	11.2	13.3	17.8	17.3
19 to 25 years	11.1	12.5	14.8	13.2	7.7	10.3	10.9	8.3	13.1	14.8	18.9	14.7
45 to 64 years	10.1	10.6	14.9	14.4	5.1	8.7	11.3	10.8	8.4	11.5	16.5	16.1
45 to 54 years	10.6	10.8	15.0	15.6	5.6	9.2	11.5	11.6	9.4	12.1	17.8	17.4
55 to 64 years	9.3	10.4	14.6	13.1	4.2	8.0	11.0	9.8	7.0	10.7	14.9	14.6
65 years and over	4.6	4.6	5.0	4.6	2.8	5.1	4.7	4.3	3.5	5.2	6.9	7.0
65 to 74 years	5.0	5.4	6.3	5.8	3.4	6.4	6.3	5.7	4.2	6.2	9.0	9.0
75 years and over	4.1	3.7	3.4	3.1	2.0	3.6	2.8	2.6	2.6	4.0	4.3	4.5
18 TO 64 YEARS												
Sex												
Male	9.3	10.0	13.5	12.9	5.1	7.2	8.8	8.7	8.8	10.8	15.2	14.5
Female	12.0	12.1	15.7	15.0	7.4	11.4	13.5	12.3	12.4	15.2	19.4	18.3
Race [5]												
White only	10.8	11.1	14.5	13.9	5.9	9.1	10.8	10.2	10.6	12.8	17.1	16.4
Black or African American only	10.8	12.0	17.4	15.4	9.5	11.6	15.6	13.7	10.8	15.2	20.7	18.3
American Indian or Alaska Native only	14.5	13.2	*15.7	16.4	*10.1	*14.1	18.6	11.0	18.8	19.2	23.1	17.2
Asian only	6.3	5.0	8.0	8.9	*2.8	*3.5	4.2	5.1	7.8	6.8	8.7	9.9
Native Hawaiian or Other Pacific Islander only	NA	*	*	*	NA	*	*	*	NA	*	*	*
Two or more races	NA	19.9	24.0	20.0	NA	22.9	16.6	14.7	NA	23.0	25.6	22.5
Hispanic Origin and Race [5]												
Hispanic or Latino	10.5	11.5	15.4	15.8	6.7	11.2	13.0	12.5	11.5	15.5	21.6	21.1
Mexican	9.7	11.4	15.6	15.4	6.5	12.0	13.5	12.1	11.3	16.3	22.0	21.6
Not Hispanic or Latino	10.7	11.0	14.5	13.6	6.3	9.0	10.9	10.1	10.5	12.6	16.6	15.6
White only	10.9	11.1	14.3	13.6	5.9	8.7	10.3	9.7	10.5	12.3	16.2	15.4
Black or African American only	10.8	12.0	17.5	15.3	9.5	11.4	15.6	13.8	10.8	15.3	20.8	18.2
Education [6]												
No high school diploma or GED	16.2	16.2	20.6	20.2	11.5	16.4	18.1	18.3	14.5	20.3	26.3	26.2
High school diploma or GED	11.1	11.7	16.1	16.4	7.0	10.5	13.8	13.1	11.4	14.6	20.1	19.8
Some college or more	9.2	9.8	13.4	12.5	4.3	7.1	9.2	8.8	8.8	10.4	14.4	14.0
Percent of Poverty Level [7]												
Below 100 percent	19.6	20.0	23.4	24.1	14.8	19.5	21.5	20.2	19.4	24.4	30.4	29.4
100 percent to 199 percent	17.9	18.9	24.0	23.5	11.6	16.3	18.4	17.9	18.3	21.0	29.2	28.6
200 percent to 399 percent	10.5	11.8	15.2	14.2	5.5	9.5	11.4	10.6	10.2	13.7	17.3	15.8
400 percent or more	4.6	5.0	6.8	5.5	1.7	3.3	3.9	3.2	4.5	5.9	7.0	6.2
Hispanic Origin and Race and Percent of Poverty Level [5,7]												
Hispanic or Latino												
Below 100 percent	14.6	14.8	19.0	22.3	10.6	17.3	18.9	18.0	16.1	23.5	30.5	32.2
100 percent to 199 percent	12.2	14.5	18.6	18.3	8.1	13.0	14.7	14.6	13.5	18.2	25.2	27.7
200 percent to 399 percent	8.0	9.6	13.9	13.4	4.4	9.1	11.5	11.3	9.2	12.5	18.1	13.6
400 percent or more	5.1	6.2	7.7	6.2	*	*4.2	4.6	*3.1	4.5	5.8	9.1	6.3
Not Hispanic or Latino												
White only												
Below 100 percent	24.3	23.6	26.1	27.2	17.3	20.5	24.6	21.4	23.4	25.1	31.8	29.5
100 percent to 199 percent	20.9	21.8	27.6	27.6	12.4	18.2	19.9	20.1	20.6	22.9	31.7	31.3
200 percent to 399 percent	11.4	13.1	16.0	14.7	5.4	10.0	11.3	10.6	10.6	14.4	18.0	16.9
400 percent or more	4.6	5.0	6.9	5.5	1.7	3.2	3.8	3.3	4.5	5.9	6.9	6.3
Black or African American only												
Below 100 percent	16.1	20.1	24.4	22.6	14.9	21.7	21.1	22.6	14.8	25.5	29.7	28.8
100 percent to 199 percent	14.3	16.2	22.9	20.7	13.9	14.3	21.3	17.2	16.4	19.0	28.2	24.4
200 percent to 399 percent	8.8	9.2	14.6	12.8	7.0	7.9	13.7	11.6	8.6	12.0	16.1	14.3
400 percent or more	4.6	5.5	8.1	5.4	*2.9	*4.1	5.6	*3.9	4.3	*7.0	9.1	5.8
Health Insurance Status at the Time of Interview												
Insured	6.8	6.8	9.1	8.5	3.7	6.0	7.3	6.9	7.2	8.7	11.8	11.1
Private	6.0	5.9	8.2	7.4	2.9	4.7	6.0	5.3	6.2	6.7	9.2	8.3
Medicaid	11.9	12.0	12.5	12.7	11.1	14.0	13.5	13.7	14.8	21.8	24.2	22.8
Uninsured	27.6	29.5	34.5	34.8	18.0	23.1	25.7	24.2	26.1	30.7	37.7	36.6
Health Insurance Status Prior to Interview												
Insured continuously all 12 months	5.5	5.5	7.6	6.9	2.8	5.0	6.2	5.9	6.0	7.5	10.5	10.0
Uninsured for any period up to 12 months	28.7	31.7	35.1	34.4	17.7	23.5	25.1	23.0	25.2	30.3	33.6	31.5
Uninsured more than 12 months	30.6	31.1	35.9	36.2	18.9	24.5	26.2	24.7	28.0	32.1	39.4	37.8

Table 3-35. Reduced Access to Medical Care, Dental Care, and Prescription Drugs During the Past 12 Months Due to Cost, by Selected Characteristics, Selected Years, 1997–2011—*Continued*

(Percent.)

Characteristic	Did not get or delayed medical care due to cost[1]				Did not get prescription drugs due to cost[2]				Did not get dental care due to cost[3]			
	1997	2005	2010	2011	1997	2005	2010	2011	1997	2005	2010	2011
Disability Measure [8]												
Any basic actions difficulty or complex activity limitation	23.3	24.8	28.9	28.5	14.8	20.0	22.6	22.6	19.8	23.8	28.8	29.6
Any basic actions difficulty	24.2	26.1	28.9	30.1	15.3	20.5	23.3	23.2	20.1	24.4	29.2	30.2
Any complex activity limitation	25.7	26.9	30.8	29.4	19.4	25.3	27.3	27.8	23.2	27.3	33.7	34.5
No disability	9.0	9.8	13.2	12.3	3.4	5.7	7.0	6.0	7.5	9.4	13.1	11.5
Geographic Region												
Northeast	8.8	8.7	10.2	9.9	4.9	7.2	7.7	7.9	8.9	10.6	12.9	11.8
Midwest	10.5	10.6	14.8	13.7	5.9	9.0	11.6	9.5	9.7	11.9	16.0	14.3
South	11.8	12.6	16.5	15.3	7.3	11.3	13.5	12.2	10.9	14.7	19.6	17.9
West	10.8	11.1	15.1	15.3	6.3	8.2	10.0	10.8	13.1	13.6	18.4	19.7
Location of Residence												
Within MSA[9]	10.2	10.6	14.2	13.7	5.9	8.8	10.8	10.2	10.0	12.7	17.0	16.3
Outside MSA[9]	12.5	12.8	17.4	15.6	7.9	11.8	13.6	12.3	12.9	14.6	19.1	17.4

NA = Not available.   * = Figure does not meet standards of reliability or precision. Data preceded by an asterisk have a relative standard error (RSE) of 20 percent to 30 percent. Data not shown have an RSE of greater than 30 percent.   NA = Data not available.   [1]Based on persons responding to the question, "During the past 12 months was there any time when person needed medical care but did not get it because person couldn't afford it?" and "During the past 12 months has medical care been delayed because of worry about the cost?"   [2]Based on persons responding to the question, "During the past 12 months was there any time when person needed prescription medicine but didn't get it because person couldn't afford it?"   [3]Based on persons responding to the question, "During the past 12 months was there any time when person needed dental care (including checkups) but didn't get it because person couldn't afford it?"   [4]Includes all other races not shown separately, unknown health insurance status, unknown education level, and unknown disability status.   [5]The race groups White, Black, American Indian or Alaska Native, Asian, Native Hawaiian or Other Pacific Islander, and two or more races include persons of Hispanic and non-Hispanic origin. Persons of Hispanic origin may be of any race.   [6]Estimates are for persons 25 to 64 years of age.   [7]Percent of poverty level is based on family income and family size and composition using U.S. Census Bureau poverty thresholds. Missing family income data were imputed for 1997 and beyond.   [8]Any basic actions difficulty or complex activity limitation is defined as having one or more of the following limitations or difficulties: movement difficulty, emotional difficulty, sensory (seeing or hearing) difficulty, cognitive difficulty, self-care (activities of daily living or instrumental activities of daily living) limitation, social limitation, or work limitation.   [9]MSA = metropolitan statistical area.

Table 3-36. Reduced Access to Medical Care During the Past 12 Months Due to Cost, 25 Largest States, Selected Annual Averages, 1997–1998 Through 2010–2011

(Percent for the 25 states with the largest populations in 2010–2011.)

State	Did not get or delayed medical care due to cost[1]			Did not get prescription drugs due to cost[2]			Did not get dental care[3]		
	1997–1998	2000–2001	2010–2011	1997–1998	2000–2001	2010–2011	1997–1998	2000–2001	2010–2011
United States	7.9	7.5	10.6	4.5	5.3	8.0	8.1	8.4	13.2
Alabama	7.6	7.7	11.9	6.8	8.3	12.3	8.7	10.3	15.0
Arizona	8.0	7.4	14.4	4.1	4.6	11.1	9.4	8.4	20.6
California	6.8	6.6	10.4	3.9	4.7	7.2	8.3	8.1	15.0
Colorado	6.4	8.1	12.2	3.1	5.5	6.9	8.9	11.5	13.5
Florida	9.8	9.6	13.2	4.8	5.8	10.1	7.2	8.4	17.4
Georgia	8.0	7.7	12.1	4.2	4.0	9.7	5.8	5.3	13.8
Illinois	6.1	6.5	8.7	3.0	4.2	6.0	5.7	6.8	9.9
Indiana	9.0	8.6	12.0	5.1	6.8	11.9	7.2	6.9	12.2
Louisiana	9.8	11.1	11.4	8.7	9.8	12.0	11.3	16.4	18.0
Maryland	8.0	7.4	8.5	5.8	5.2	5.7	9.8	7.8	9.1
Massachusetts	5.1	4.3	5.1	*1.7	4.2	4.7	5.0	5.2	7.9
Michigan	7.2	7.0	11.4	3.8	5.1	9.8	7.5	7.9	15.9
Minnesota	8.1	7.0	10.3	3.6	3.9	6.0	8.7	8.3	10.7
Missouri	7.1	6.4	12.4	4.3	5.2	8.4	7.3	7.1	14.7
New Jersey	7.2	6.1	7.1	3.8	3.5	4.7	7.3	5.9	9.9
New York	6.4	5.8	6.9	2.8	3.8	5.4	5.6	7.5	7.8
North Carolina	7.8	7.9	11.3	4.0	5.8	7.9	8.2	7.9	12.4
Ohio	9.2	7.6	10.5	5.0	5.1	8.1	8.8	8.1	10.5
Pennsylvania	5.9	5.9	9.1	4.3	3.5	7.0	7.4	6.0	11.4
South Carolina	7.6	6.3	11.2	5.2	4.4	8.4	5.7	5.2	11.3
Tennessee	10.0	8.6	13.1	8.0	8.5	10.7	10.5	10.4	15.3
Texas	7.9	8.1	12.0	4.7	6.6	9.9	8.8	10.4	16.4
Virginia	6.2	7.2	9.3	4.1	5.2	6.9	8.3	7.4	9.6
Washington	8.6	9.2	13.0	4.8	6.8	8.3	11.6	11.9	17.6
Wisconsin	6.5	5.9	8.2	3.0	4.0	5.0	5.5	6.6	10.6

* = Figure does not meet standards of reliability or precision. Data preceded by an asterisk have a relative standard error (RSE) of 20 percent to 30 percent.   [1]Based on persons responding to the question, "During the past 12 months was there any time when person needed medical care but did not get it because person couldn't afford it?" and "During the past 12 months has medical care been delayed because of worry about the cost?" [2]Based on persons responding to the question, "During the past 12 months was there any time when you needed prescription medicine but didn't get it because you couldn't afford it?" [3]Based on persons responding to the question, "During the past 12 months was there any time when you needed dental care (including check ups) but didn't get it because you couldn't afford it?"

Table 3-37. No Health Care Visits[1] to an Office or Clinic Within the Past 12 Months Among Children Under 18 Years of Age, by Selected Characteristics, Selected Annual Averages, 1997–1998 Through 2010–2011

(Percent.)

Characteristic	Under 18 years				Under 6 years				6 to 17 years			
	1997–1998	2005–2006	2009–2010	2010–2011	1997–1998	2005–2006	2009–2010	2010–2011	1997–1998	2005–2006	2009–2010	2010–2011
ALL CHILDREN [2]	12.8	11.7	9.6	9.1	5.7	6.1	4.9	4.8	16.3	14.4	12.1	11.3
Sex												
Male	12.9	12.0	9.8	9.3	4.9	6.2	5.0	5.3	16.8	14.7	12.4	11.4
Female	12.7	11.4	9.4	8.9	6.5	6.1	4.8	4.3	15.8	14.0	11.8	11.3
Race [3]												
White only	12.2	11.3	9.4	8.8	5.5	6.3	4.5	4.4	15.5	13.8	11.8	11.0
Black or African American only	14.3	11.7	10.1	9.3	6.5	4.6	6.4	6.1	18.1	15.1	12.1	11.0
American Indian or Alaska Native only	13.8	*15.7	*12.4	13.3	*	*	*	*	*17.6	*17.7	*14.7	16.7
Asian only	16.3	17.5	12.7	12.6	*5.6	10.5	*4.8	*6.1	22.1	20.8	17.0	16.1
Native Hawaiian or Other Pacific Islander only	NA	*	*	*	NA	*	*	*	NA	*	*	*
Two or more races	NA	10.4	8.3	8.5	NA	*	*5.7	*5.7	NA	14.8	10.1	10.5
Hispanic Origin and Race [3]												
Hispanic or Latino	19.3	17.4	13.5	12.6	9.7	9.6	7.7	6.7	25.3	21.9	17.2	16.4
Not Hispanic or Latino	11.6	10.3	8.5	8.0	4.8	5.1	4.0	4.2	14.9	12.6	10.7	9.9
White only	10.7	9.4	7.7	7.2	4.3	5.0	3.1	3.5	13.7	11.4	9.8	9.0
Black or African American only	14.5	11.7	10.3	9.3	6.5	*4.4	6.4	5.9	18.3	15.1	12.4	11.1
Percent of Poverty Level [4]												
Below 100 percent	17.6	14.2	12.4	11.3	8.1	7.7	6.9	6.1	23.6	18.2	16.0	14.7
100 percent to 199 percent	16.2	14.9	12.7	12.3	7.2	8.4	6.4	6.6	20.8	18.2	16.2	15.5
200 percent to 399 percent	11.7	11.1	9.0	8.5	4.9	6.1	4.2	4.4	14.8	13.4	11.4	10.5
400 percent or more	7.4	7.8	5.3	5.0	3.0	2.8	*2.3	2.1	9.5	10.0	6.7	6.2
Health Insurance Status at the Time of Interview [5]												
Insured	10.4	9.5	7.7	7.6	4.5	4.9	4.3	4.3	13.4	11.9	9.6	9.3
Private	10.4	9.4	7.0	6.8	4.3	4.4	3.5	3.2	13.1	11.6	8.6	8.4
Medicaid	10.1	9.5	8.8	8.7	5.0	5.8	5.3	5.5	14.4	12.2	11.1	10.9
Uninsured	28.8	31.7	31.0	27.8	14.6	20.6	14.4	14.1	34.9	35.6	37.3	32.6
Health Insurance Status Prior to Interview [5]												
Insured continuously all 12 months	10.3	9.5	7.4	7.4	4.4	4.9	4.1	4.1	13.2	11.9	9.2	9.1
Uninsured for any period up to 12 months	15.9	15.8	16.3	14.3	7.7	9.3	7.7	8.8	20.9	18.8	20.9	17.2
Uninsured more than 12 months	34.9	39.0	38.6	36.5	19.9	28.0	22.8	21.4	40.2	42.2	42.9	40.0
Geographic Region												
Northeast	7.0	6.8	5.6	5.7	3.1	4.0	3.3	4.4	8.9	8.1	6.7	6.4
Midwest	12.2	9.8	8.6	7.7	5.9	5.2	3.5	3.5	15.3	12.0	11.2	9.8
South	14.3	12.4	9.9	9.0	5.6	6.2	5.2	4.7	18.5	15.5	12.4	11.3
West	16.3	16.5	12.9	12.8	7.9	8.8	6.9	6.6	20.7	20.3	16.1	16.1
Location of Residence												
Within MSA[6]	12.3	11.4	9.4	9.0	5.4	5.9	4.7	4.9	15.9	14.1	11.9	11.2
Outside MSA[6]	14.6	12.9	10.8	9.5	6.9	7.4	6.0	4.3	17.9	15.4	13.1	12.2

NA = Not available.   * = Figure does not meet standards of reliability or precision. Data preceded by an asterisk have a relative standard error (RSE) of 20 percent to 30 percent. Data not shown have an RSE of greater than 30 percent.   [1]Respondents were asked how many times a doctor or other health care professional was seen in the past 12 months at a doctor's office, clinic, or some other place. Excluded are visits to emergency rooms, hospitalizations, home visits, and telephone calls. Starting with 2000 data, dental visits were also excluded.   [2]Includes all other races not shown separately and unknown health insurance status.   [3]The race groups White, Black, American Indian or Alaska Native, Asian, Native Hawaiian or Other Pacific Islander, and two or more races include persons of Hispanic and non-Hispanic origin. Persons of Hispanic origin may be of any race.   [4]Percent of poverty level is based on family income and family size and composition using U.S. Census Bureau poverty thresholds. Missing family income data were imputed starting in 1993.   [5]Health insurance categories are mutually exclusive. Persons who reported both Medicaid and private coverage are classified as having private coverage. Medicaid includes other public assistance through 1996. Starting with 1997 data, state-sponsored health plan coverage is included as Medicaid coverage. Starting with 1999 data, coverage by the Children's Health Insurance Program (CHIP) is included with Medicaid coverage. Persons not covered by private insurance, Medicaid, CHIP, public assistance (through 1996), state-sponsored or other government-sponsored health plans (starting in 1997), Medicare, or military plans are considered to have no health insurance coverage. Persons with only Indian Health Service coverage are considered to have no health insurance coverage. Health insurance status was unknown for 8 to 9 percent of children in 1993–1996 and about 1 percent in 1997–2011.   [6]MSA = metropolitan statistical area.

Table 3-38. Health Care Visits to Doctors' Offices, Emergency Departments, and Home Visits within the Past 12 Months, by Selected Characteristics, Selected Years, 2000–2011

(Percent distribution of health care visits to doctors' offices, emergency departments, and home visits during a 12-month period.)

Characteristic	None				1 to 3 visits				4 to 9 visits				10 or more visits			
	2000	2005	2010	2011	2000	2005	2010	2011	2000	2005	2010	2011	2000	2005	2010	2011
Total, age-adjusted[1,2]	16.6	15.5	15.6	15.5	45.1	45.9	45.4	46.8	25.1	25.1	25.8	13.0	13.2	13.6	13.2	13.0
Total, crude[1]	16.7	15.4	15.4	15.2	45.2	45.9	45.2	46.5	25.0	25.1	26.0	13.2	13.1	13.6	13.5	13.2
Age																
Under 18 years	12.3	10.2	8.1	8.3	53.5	56.0	55.6	57.3	26.7	26.5	28.2	7.4	7.6	7.4	8.2	7.4
Under 6 years	6.2	5.1	3.7	4.5	44.0	47.4	48.9	50.1	38.7	38.0	36.8	9.1	11.0	9.5	10.6	9.1
6 to 17 years	15.1	12.6	10.4	10.3	57.9	60.1	59.1	61.0	21.0	20.9	23.6	6.5	5.9	6.3	6.9	6.5
18 to 44 years	23.4	22.9	24.2	23.7	44.9	45.8	43.9	45.5	19.6	19.2	20.6	11.6	12.1	12.0	11.3	11.6
18 to 24 years	24.5	24.2	25.9	25.3	45.0	44.4	43.4	46.1	19.4	19.6	21.1	10.1	11.1	11.8	9.6	10.1
25 to 44 years	23.0	22.5	23.6	23.2	44.9	46.3	44.1	45.4	19.6	19.1	20.5	12.1	12.5	12.1	11.9	12.1
45 to 64 years	14.9	14.0	14.8	14.6	43.1	42.9	42.8	44.0	26.2	26.8	26.1	15.3	15.8	16.3	16.4	15.3
45 to 54 years	16.3	15.8	17.6	16.8	44.9	44.8	43.5	45.2	24.3	24.3	23.9	13.9	14.5	15.0	15.0	13.9
55 to 64 years	12.7	11.4	11.1	12.0	40.4	40.2	41.9	42.7	29.2	30.3	28.8	17.0	17.7	18.2	18.2	17.0
65 years and over	7.4	5.6	5.3	5.5	31.8	30.7	33.8	34.0	37.3	37.5	36.7	24.7	23.5	26.2	24.2	24.7
65 to 74 years	8.9	5.9	6.3	6.2	34.2	34.4	36.1	36.0	35.1	35.8	35.7	22.9	21.9	23.9	21.9	22.9
75 years and over	5.7	5.2	4.1	4.7	29.0	26.4	31.0	31.5	39.9	39.5	38.0	26.8	25.5	28.8	27.0	26.8
Sex [2]																
Male	21.6	20.4	20.4	20.0	45.7	46.7	46.4	47.8	22.7	22.2	22.7	10.3	10.0	10.7	10.5	10.3
Female	11.8	10.7	10.9	11.0	44.4	45.1	44.4	45.9	27.5	27.9	28.8	15.5	16.2	16.3	15.9	15.5
Race [2,3]																
White only	16.0	15.1	15.3	15.2	44.8	45.6	44.9	46.4	25.7	25.4	26.1	13.2	13.6	13.9	13.7	13.2
Black or African American only	17.1	15.9	15.7	15.0	46.4	47.4	47.2	47.6	24.0	23.8	24.7	13.1	12.5	12.9	12.4	13.1
American Indian or Alaska Native only	21.2	20.4	19.4	18.6	42.8	36.4	40.3	47.5	20.3	29.8	28.1	11.7	15.7	13.4	12.2	11.7
Asian only	20.2	21.5	20.4	20.4	49.0	49.3	49.9	49.8	21.1	20.8	22.1	7.8	9.7	8.4	7.6	7.8
Native Hawaiian and Other Pacific Islander only	*	*	*	*	*	*	*	*	*	*	*	*	*	*	*	*
Two or more races	12.0	15.4	13.9	14.0	41.4	37.3	42.3	45.7	28.8	27.6	25.2	15.9	17.9	19.7	18.6	15.9
Hispanic Origin and Race [2,3]																
Hispanic or Latino	26.7	23.9	23.5	23.3	41.5	42.1	43.2	43.7	20.2	22.2	22.6	10.4	11.5	11.8	10.7	10.4
Mexican	30.9	26.6	25.2	25.6	40.6	41.5	43.3	42.8	18.2	20.8	21.4	9.9	10.3	11.1	10.1	9.9
Not Hispanic or Latino	15.1	13.9	14.0	13.9	45.6	46.5	45.8	47.4	25.8	25.7	26.5	13.4	13.6	13.9	13.7	13.4
White only	14.4	13.0	13.2	13.1	45.1	46.4	45.3	47.1	26.5	26.2	27.1	13.9	14.0	14.5	14.4	13.9
Black or African American only	17.0	15.9	15.6	14.8	46.5	47.4	47.3	47.9	24.0	23.8	24.9	13.0	12.5	12.9	12.2	13.0
Percent of Poverty Level [2,4]																
Below 100 percent	21.9	20.7	20.4	18.9	37.3	37.3	37.5	39.5	23.4	24.7	25.1	16.9	17.4	17.3	17.0	16.9
100 percent to 199 percent	21.6	20.2	20.8	21.1	42.3	42.0	42.1	42.7	22.1	23.4	23.1	13.5	14.1	14.4	13.9	13.5
200 percent to 399 percent	16.9	15.9	16.2	15.7	45.3	47.3	46.3	48.1	25.0	24.0	25.4	12.4	12.8	12.8	12.1	12.4
400 percent or more	12.3	11.0	10.2	10.5	48.1	49.2	49.4	51.0	27.3	27.0	27.6	11.7	12.4	12.8	12.7	11.7
Hispanic Origin and Race and Percent of Poverty Level [2,3,4]																
Hispanic or Latino																
Below 100 percent	32.3	27.9	28.7	26.4	33.3	37.2	36.5	38.6	19.2	20.2	22.5	13.2	15.1	14.6	12.3	13.2
100 percent to 199 percent	30.5	27.6	27.7	29.2	40.6	38.8	42.7	41.4	17.6	22.6	19.9	9.3	11.3	11.1	9.8	9.3
200 percent to 399 percent	24.2	22.7	21.6	19.6	45.5	44.9	45.0	45.9	19.9	23.1	23.1	10.3	10.3	9.2	10.3	10.3
400 percent or more	17.0	13.4	11.3	14.1	47.2	50.4	51.1	52.1	26.3	23.0	26.1	9.5	9.5	13.2	11.5	9.5
Not Hispanic or Latino																
White only																
Below 100 percent	18.0	16.4	15.0	15.6	36.9	36.1	37.0	38.8	25.3	28.0	27.4	19.2	19.8	19.5	20.6	19.2
100 percent to 199 percent	18.5	17.5	18.4	17.9	41.5	41.8	40.4	42.8	24.1	24.0	24.7	15.7	15.9	16.8	16.5	15.7
200 percent to 399 percent	15.3	13.8	14.7	14.4	44.6	47.3	46.0	47.7	26.1	24.7	26.3	13.7	13.9	14.2	13.0	13.7
400 percent or more	11.8	10.3	9.9	9.8	47.8	48.9	48.2	50.2	27.6	27.6	28.4	12.2	12.8	13.1	13.5	12.2
Black or African American only																
Below 100 percent	18.3	17.8	18.4	15.2	40.0	40.1	39.8	40.2	24.9	24.8	25.0	18.2	16.7	17.3	16.8	18.2
100 percent to 199 percent	20.8	16.1	17.6	17.2	44.2	47.0	45.7	45.5	20.7	24.3	24.3	13.0	14.3	12.6	12.5	13.0
200 percent to 399 percent	17.1	17.2	15.1	15.7	48.5	49.0	49.0	51.4	24.4	22.9	25.7	9.8	10.1	10.9	10.2	9.8
400 percent or more	11.3	12.1	10.0	10.4	52.2	52.0	58.2	54.7	24.8	24.7	22.5	11.6	11.7	11.2	9.3	11.6
Health Insurance Status at the Time of Interview [5,6]																
Under 65 years																
Insured	14.0	12.4	12.3	12.4	48.2	49.6	48.5	50.3	25.1	25.0	26.1	12.4	12.7	13.0	13.1	12.4
Private	14.3	12.8	12.4	12.7	49.9	51.5	51.0	53.1	24.8	24.5	25.5	9.9	11.0	11.2	11.1	9.9
Medicaid	10.4	9.9	10.9	10.6	32.4	37.8	38.2	40.0	27.6	26.8	28.0	23.0	29.6	25.5	23.0	23.0
Uninsured	36.8	37.5	37.2	37.1	41.9	42.0	42.2	43.5	14.1	14.7	15.2	5.5	7.2	5.8	5.4	5.5
Health Insurance Status Prior to Interview [5,6]																
Under 65 years																
Insured continuously all 12 months	13.9	12.3	12.1	12.2	48.5	49.8	48.6	50.5	25.1	25.0	26.2	12.3	12.6	12.9	13.0	12.3
Uninsured for any period up to 12 months	20.4	18.9	18.5	19.0	44.1	44.9	47.8	47.3	21.5	22.5	22.0	12.2	13.9	13.7	11.6	12.2
Uninsured more than 12 months	43.1	43.5	43.8	43.0	39.5	40.0	39.7	41.7	12.3	12.3	12.6	4.1	5.1	4.2	3.9	4.1
Respondent-Assessed Health Status [2]																
Fair or poor	8.9	9.0	8.4	10.3	21.7	21.5	24.0	23.0	28.2	28.1	30.2	38.7	41.2	41.3	37.3	38.7
Good to excellent	17.2	16.1	16.3	16.2	47.3	48.2	47.5	49.2	25.0	24.8	25.5	10.3	10.5	10.8	10.7	10.3

Table 3-38. Health Care Visits to Doctors' Offices, Emergency Departments, and Home Visits within the Past 12 Months, by Selected Characteristics, Selected Years, 2000–2011—*Continued*

(Percent distribution of health care visits to doctors' offices, emergency departments, and home visits during a 12-month period.)

Characteristic	None				1 to 3 visits				4 to 9 visits				10 or more visits			
	2000	2005	2010	2011	2000	2005	2010	2011	2000	2005	2010	2011	2000	2005	2010	2011
Disability Measure Among Adults 18 Years of Age and Over [2,7]																
Any basic actions difficulty or complex activity limitation	10.8	9.6	11.5	10.3	28.0	29.7	30.9	30.1	30.1	29.6	29.3	30.0	31.1	31.1	28.3	30.0
Any basic actions difficulty	10.7	9.7	11.5	10.1	28.0	29.4	30.3	30.1	30.2	29.6	29.2	30.0	31.1	31.3	29.0	30.0
Any complex activity limitation	7.1	5.9	6.9	6.9	19.5	21.1	23.0	21.5	27.5	27.8	29.1	44.3	45.9	45.2	41.0	44.3
No disability	20.5	19.8	20.5	20.6	48.2	48.8	47.5	49.7	22.9	22.7	23.4	7.8	8.4	8.6	8.5	7.8
Geographic Region [2]																
Northeast	12.4	11.3	12.6	13.0	45.9	46.8	46.3	47.0	27.8	27.0	26.4	13.8	13.9	14.9	14.7	13.8
Midwest	14.3	13.8	13.4	13.6	45.8	47.2	46.8	49.2	26.1	25.2	26.4	13.0	13.8	13.9	13.3	13.0
South	18.4	16.0	16.1	15.4	44.4	45.7	44.2	45.5	24.5	25.1	26.6	13.4	12.8	13.3	13.2	13.4
West	20.2	20.0	19.1	19.3	44.6	44.2	45.2	46.5	22.5	23.3	23.5	11.5	12.7	12.5	12.2	11.5
Location of Residence [2]																
Within MSA[8]	16.6	15.5	15.6	15.4	45.5	46.2	45.8	47.4	24.9	24.9	25.6	12.7	13.0	13.3	13.0	12.7
Outside MSA[8]	16.7	15.3	15.9	15.7	43.3	44.5	42.7	43.6	26.0	25.6	27.0	14.5	14.1	14.6	14.4	14.5

* = Figure does not meet standards of reliability or precision. Data preceded by an asterisk have a relative standard error (RSE) of 20 percent to 30 percent. Data not shown have an RSE of greater than 30 percent. [1]Includes all other races not shown separately, unknown health insurance status, and unknown disability status. [2]Estimates are age adjusted to the year 2000 standard population using six age groups: under 18 years, 18 to 44 years, 45 to 54 years, 55 to 64 years, 65 to 74 years, and 75 years and over. [3]The race groups White, Black, American Indian or Alaska Native, Asian, Native Hawaiian or Other Pacific Islander, and 2 or more races, include persons of Hispanic and non-Hispanic origin. Persons of Hispanic origin may be of any race. [4]Percent of poverty level is based on family income and family size and composition. Missing family income data were imputed for 1997 and beyond. [5]Estimates for persons under 65 years of age are age adjusted to the year 2000 standard population using four age groups: under 18 years, 18 to 44 years, 45 to 54 years, and 55 to 64 years. [6]Health insurance categories are mutually exclusive. Persons who reported both Medicaid and private coverage are classified as having private coverage. Medicaid includes other public assistance through 1996. Starting with 1997 data, state-sponsored health plan coverage is included as Medicaid coverage. Starting with 1999 data, coverage by the Children's Health Insurance Program (CHIP) is included with Medicaid coverage. Persons not covered by private insurance, Medicaid, CHIP, public assistance (through 1996), state-sponsored or other government-sponsored health plans (starting in 1997), Medicare, or military plans are considered to have no health insurance coverage. Persons with only Indian Health Service coverage are considered to have no health insurance coverage. Health insurance status was unknown for 8 to 9 percent of children in 1993–1996 and about 1 percent in 1997–2011. [7]Any basic actions difficulty or complex activity limitation is defined as having one or more of the following limitations or difficulties: movement difficulty, emotional difficulty, sensory (seeing or hearing) difficulty, cognitive difficulty, self-care (activities of daily living or instrumental activities of daily living) limitation, social limitation, or work limitation. [8]MSA = metropolitan statistical area.

Table 3-39A. Vaccination Coverage Among Children 19 to 35 Months of Age for Selected Diseases, by Race, Hispanic Origin, Poverty Level, and Location of Residence in Metropolitan Statistical Area, Selected Years, 1995–2011

(Percent.)

| Vaccination and year | Race and Hispanic origin[1] | | | | | | | Hispanic or Latino | Poverty level | | Location of residence | | |
| | All | Not Hispanic or Latino | | | | | | | Below poverty level | At or above poverty level | Inside MSA[2] | | Outside MSA |
		White	Black or African American	American Indian or Alaska Native	Asian[3]	Native Hawaiian or Other Pacific Islander[3]	Two or more races				Central city	Remaining area	
Combined Series (4:3:1:3*:3:1:4)[4]													
2009	44	45	40	*	39	*	41	46	41	46	45	45	42
2010	57	57	55	64	59	*	61	56	53	59	57	57	55
2011	69	69	64	66	71	*	71	70	64	72	70	68	67
DTP/DT/DTaP (4 Doses or More)[5]													
1995	78	80	74	71	84	*	NA	75	71	81	77	79	78
1996	81	83	79	85	85	*	NA	77	74	84	79	83	81
1997	82	84	77	80	80	*	NA	78	76	84	80	83	81
1998	84	87	77	83	89	*	NA	81	80	86	82	85	85
1999	83	86	79	80	87	*	NA	80	79	85	82	84	83
2000	82	84	76	75	85	*	NA	79	76	84	80	83	83
2001	82	84	76	77	84	*	NA	83	77	84	81	83	82
2002	82	84	76	*	88	*	78	79	75	84	79	84	80
2003	85	88	80	80	89	*	84	82	80	87	84	86	83
2004	86	88	80	77	90	*	86	84	81	87	84	87	85
2005	86	87	84	*	89	*	86	84	82	87	85	87	85
2006	85	87	81	83	86	*	84	85	81	87	84	86	85
2007	85	85	82	86	88	*	84	84	81	86	85	85	83
2008	85	85	80	82	92	*	88	85	80	87	85	85	82
2009	84	86	79	82	87	93	82	83	80	86	84	84	84
2010	84	85	84	82	88	*	83	84	81	86	84	85	84
2011	85	85	81	73	92	93	87	84	81	87	86	84	82
Polio (3 Doses or More)													
1995	88	89	84	86	90	*	NA	87	85	89	87	88	89
1996	91	92	90	90	90	*	NA	89	88	92	89	92	92
1997	91	92	89	90	89	*	NA	90	89	92	90	91	92
1998	91	92	88	85	93	*	NA	89	90	92	89	91	93
1999	90	90	87	88	90	*	NA	89	87	91	89	90	90
2000	90	91	87	90	93	*	NA	88	87	90	88	90	91
2001	89	90	85	88	90	*	NA	91	87	90	88	90	91
2002	90	91	87	*	92	95	87	90	88	91	89	91	90
2003	92	93	89	91	91	90	91	90	89	93	91	92	92
2004	92	92	90	87	93	*	92	91	90	92	91	92	92
2005	92	91	91	*	93	*	94	92	90	92	91	93	92
2006	93	93	90	91	92	96	92	93	92	93	93	93	93
2007	93	93	91	95	95	87	92	93	92	93	92	93	94
2008	94	94	92	91	97	*	94	94	92	94	94	94	93
2009	93	93	91	92	94	97	93	93	92	93	94	92	92
2010	93	93	94	95	93	95	90	94	92	94	93	94	93
2011	94	94	94	88	97	97	94	94	94	94	94	93	94
Measles, Mumps, Rubella													
1995	90	91	87	88	95	*	NA	88	86	91	90	90	89
1996	91	91	90	89	93	*	NA	88	87	92	90	91	91
1997	90	91	89	92	90	*	NA	88	86	92	90	91	91
1998	92	93	89	91	92	*	NA	91	90	93	92	92	93
1999	92	92	90	92	93	*	NA	90	90	92	91	92	90
2000	91	92	88	87	90	*	NA	90	89	91	90	91	91
2001	91	92	89	94	90	*	NA	92	89	92	91	92	91
2002	92	93	90	84	95	94	89	91	90	92	90	93	90
2003	93	93	92	92	96	*	94	93	92	93	93	93	92
2004	93	94	91	89	94	*	94	93	91	94	93	94	92
2005	92	91	92	90	92	90	94	91	89	92	92	92	90
2006	92	93	91	89	95	94	91	92	91	93	93	93	92
2007	92	92	92	96	94	88	95	93	91	93	92	93	92
2008	92	91	92	96	95	97	94	93	92	92	93	92	90
2009	90	91	88	95	91	97	89	89	89	91	91	89	89
2010	92	91	92	93	92	97	90	93	91	91	92	91	91
2011	92	91	91	95	94	99	91	92	91	92	92	91	92
Hib (Full Series)[6]													
2009	55	55	51	*	55	*	54	55	51	57	56	55	53
2010	67	68	65	77	70	*	70	65	61	70	67	68	63
2011	80	81	75	74	84	*	82	82	76	83	81	80	78
Hepatitis A (2 Doses or More)													
2008	40	NA	NA	NA	NA	NA	NA	NA	NA	NA	NA	NA	NA
2009	47	46	41	33	51	*	48	49	47	46	48	47	47
2010	50	46	49	*	51	*	50	57	51	49	52	49	45
2011	52	50	51	*	57	*	50	56	51	53	55	51	48
Hepatitis B (3 Doses or More)													
1995	68	68	66	52	80	*	NA	70	65	69	69	71	59
1996	82	82	82	79	85	*	NA	81	78	83	81	83	81
1997	84	85	82	83	88	*	NA	81	81	85	82	85	85
1998	87	88	84	82	89	*	NA	86	85	88	85	88	87
1999	88	89	87	*	88	*	NA	87	87	89	87	89	88
2000	90	91	89	91	91	*	NA	88	87	91	89	90	92
2001	89	90	85	86	90	*	NA	90	87	90	88	90	89
2002	90	91	88	*	94	94	84	90	88	90	89	91	90
2003	92	93	92	90	94	*	93	91	91	93	92	93	93
2004	92	93	91	91	93	*	94	92	91	93	92	93	93
2005	93	93	93	90	93	*	94	93	91	94	92	94	93
2006	93	94	92	95	92	97	92	94	93	94	93	94	93
2007	93	93	91	97	94	*	92	94	92	93	92	93	94
2008	94	93	92	92	98	*	95	94	91	94	93	94	93
2009	92	92	92	93	93	96	93	93	92	93	93	92	92

Table 3-39A. Vaccination Coverage Among Children 19 to 35 Months of Age for Selected Diseases, by Race, Hispanic Origin, Poverty Level, and Location of Residence in Metropolitan Statistical Area, Selected Years, 1995–2011—Continued

(Percent.)

Vaccination and year	All	Race and Hispanic origin[1]								Poverty level		Location of residence		
		Not Hispanic or Latino						Hispanic or Latino	Below poverty level	At or above poverty level	Inside MSA[2]		Outside MSA
		White	Black or African American	American Indian or Alaska Native	Asian[3]	Native Hawaiian or Other Pacific Islander[3]	Two or more races					Central city	Remaining area	
2010	92	91	92	97	92	97	90	93	92	92	91	92	93
2011	91	90	92	93	96	91	91	92	92	91	91	91	93
Varicella [7]													
1997	26	28	21	20	36	*	NA	22	17	29	26	29	17
1998	43	42	42	28	53	*	NA	47	41	44	45	45	34
1999	58	56	58	*	64	*	NA	61	55	58	59	61	47
2000	68	66	67	62	77	*	NA	70	64	69	69	70	60
2001	76	75	75	69	82	*	NA	80	74	77	78	78	68
2002	81	79	83	71	87	*	79	82	79	81	81	83	75
2003	85	84	85	81	91	*	86	86	84	85	86	86	80
2004	88	87	86	84	91	*	89	89	86	88	88	89	85
2005	88	86	91	82	92	*	90	89	87	88	88	88	86
2006	89	89	89	85	93	90	91	90	88	90	90	90	86
2007	90	89	90	95	94	89	92	91	89	90	90	90	89
2008	91	90	90	94	94	92	91	92	90	91	92	90	88
2009	90	89	88	89	90	98	91	91	89	90	91	89	89
2010	90	89	92	96	93	93	89	92	90	91	91	90	90
2011	91	90	91	90	94	99	92	92	90	91	91	91	90
PCV (4 doses or more) [8]													
2005	54	57	46	*	56	*	54	51	45	57	52	58	48
2006	68	71	61	63	65	*	71	67	62	71	69	71	62
2007	75	77	70	80	75	*	74	75	73	76	75	77	71
2008	80	81	76	71	82	*	85	79	74	83	81	81	75
2009	80	83	73	76	73	*	73	81	75	83	80	82	82
2010	83	84	80	85	79	*	83	84	79	86	83	84	83
2011	84	85	81	75	85	93	84	85	81	87	85	85	82
Rotavirus vaccine [9]													
2009	44	46	38	*	42	*	38	44	38	47	45	47	36
2010	59	60	53	*	63	*	58	61	52	63	59	62	52
2011	67	68	63	58	67	*	68	68	61	71	69	67	63

NOTE: Final estimates from the National Immunization Survey include an adjustment for children with missing immunization provider data. Poverty level is based on family income and family size using U.S. Census Bureau poverty thresholds. In 2011, 5.9 percent of all 19,144 children with provider-reported vaccination history data, 9.5 percent of Hispanic, 3.6 percent of non-Hispanic White, and 6.5% of non-Hispanic Black children were missing information about poverty level and were omitted from the estimates of vaccination coverage by poverty level.

NA = Not available.   * = Estimates are considered unreliable. For data prior to 2007, percents not shown if the unweighted sample size for the numerator was less than 30, or the confidence interval half-width divided by the estimate was greater than 50 percent, or the confidence interval half-width was greater than 10. Starting with 2007 data, percents not shown if the unweighted sample size for the denominator was less than 30, or the confidence interval half-width divided by the estimate was greater than 60 percent, or the confidence interval half-width was greater than 10.   [1]Persons of Hispanic origin may be of any race.   [2]MSA = metropolitan statistical area.   [3]Prior to data year 2002, the category Asian included Native Hawaiian and Other Pacific Islander.   [4]The 4:3:1:3:3:1:4 combined series consists of 4 or more doses of diphtheria and tetanus toxoids and pertussis vaccine (DTP), diphtheria and tetanus toxoids (DT), or diphtheria and tetanus toxoids and acellular pertussis vaccine (DTaP);3 or more doses of any poliovirus vaccine; 1 or more doses of a measles-containing vaccine (MCV); 3 or more doses of Haemophilus influenzae type b vaccine (Hib); 3 or more doses of hepatitis B vaccine; 1 or more doses of varicella vaccine; and 4 or more doses of pneumococcal conjugate vaccine (PCV).   [5]Diphtheria and tetanus toxoids and pertussis vaccine (DTP), diphtheria and tetanus toxoids (DT), and diphtheria and tetanus toxoids and acellular pertussis vaccine (DTaP).   [6]Haemophilus influenzae type b vaccine (Hib) full series includes primary series plus the booster dose. Before January 2009, NIS did not distinguish between Hib vaccine product types; therefore, children who received 3 doses of a vaccine product that requires 4 doses were misclassified as fully vaccinated. In addition, there was a Hib vaccine shortage during December 2007-September 2009.   [7]Recommended in 1996. Data collection for varicella began in July 1996.   [8]PCV is pneumococcal conjugate vaccine. Recommended in 2000.   [9]Rotavirus vaccine includes 2 or more or 3 or more doses, depending on the product type received.

Table 3-39B. Vaccination Coverage Among Children 19 to 35 Months of Age for Selected Diseases, by Race, Hispanic Origin, Poverty Level, and Location of Residence in Metropolitan Statistical Area, 2009–2011

(Percent.)

Vaccination and year	Not Hispanic or Latino				Hispanic or Latino[1]	
	White		Black or African American		Below poverty level	At or above poverty level
	Below poverty level	At or above poverty level	Below poverty level	At or above poverty level		
Combined Series (4:3:1:3*:3:1:4) [2]						
2009	43	46	38	44	44	49
2010	49	59	53	56	55	55
2011	60	72	61	68	68	71

NOTE: Final estimates from the National Immunization Survey include an adjustment for children with missing immunization provider data. Poverty level is based on family income and family size using U.S. Census Bureau poverty thresholds. In 2011, 5.9 percent of all 19,144 children with provider-reported vaccination history data, 9.5 percent of Hispanic, 3.6 percent of non-Hispanic White, and 6.5% of non-Hispanic Black children were missing information about poverty level and were omitted from the estimates of vaccination coverage by poverty level.

NA = Not available.   * = Estimates are considered unreliable. For data prior to 2007, percents not shown if the unweighted sample size for the numerator was less than 30, or the confidence interval half-width divided by the estimate was greater than 50 percent, or the confidence interval half-width was greater than 10. Starting with 2007 data, percents not shown if the unweighted sample size for the denominator was less than 30, or the confidence interval half-width divided by the estimate was greater than 60 percent, or the confidence interval half-width was greater than 10.   [1]Persons of Hispanic origin may be of any race.   [2]The 4:3:1:3:3:1:4 combined series consists of 4 or more doses of diphtheria and tetanus toxoids and pertussis vaccine (DTP), diphtheria and tetanus toxoids (DT), or diphtheria and tetanus toxoids and acellular pertussis vaccine (DTaP);3 or more doses of any poliovirus vaccine; 1 or more doses of a measles-containing vaccine (MCV); 3 or more doses of Haemophilus influenzae type b vaccine (Hib); 3 or more doses of hepatitis B vaccine; 1 or more doses of varicella vaccine; and 4 or more doses of pneumococcal conjugate vaccine (PCV).

Table 3-40A. Vaccination Coverage Among Children 19 to 35 Months of Age, by State and Selected Urban Area, Selected Years, 2002–2009

(Percent.)

State and selected urban area	2002	2003	2004	2005	2006	2007	2008	2009
Percent of Children 19 to 35 Months of Age with 4:3:1:3:3:1 Combined Series [1]								
United States	66	73	76	76	77	77	76	70
Alabama	73	79	80	82	79	78	75	73
Jefferson County (Birmingham)	74	79	81	85	NA	NA	NA	NA
Alaska	56	73	66	68	67	70	69	64
Arizona	59	68	73	75	71	75	76	70
Maricopa County (Phoenix)	62	69	72	76	68	NA	NA	NA
Arkansas	68	75	81	64	73	72	76	63
California	67	76	79	74	79	77	79	75
Alameda County	NA	NA	NA	71	NA	76	NA	NA
Fresno County	NA	NA	NA	NA	73	NA	NA	NA
Los Angeles County (Los Angeles)	72	79	77	78	79	78	76	78
Northern California	NA	NA	NA	NA	71	NA	69	NA
Santa Clara County (Santa Clara)	75	77	80	NA	78	NA	81	NA
Santa Bernadino County	NA	NA	NA	63	NA	70	NA	NA
San Diego County (San Diego)	71	75	74	NA	80	NA	NA	NA
Colorado	56	63	73	79	76	78	79	65
Denver	NA	NA	NA	79	NA	NA	NA	NA
Connecticut	73	89	85	82	82	87	70	47
Delaware	70	66	80	82	80	80	72	65
District of Columbia	68	72	80	72	79	82	78	75
Florida	66	74	85	78	79	80	80	75
Dade County (Miami)	60	73	73	NA	80	76	78	NA
Duval County (Jacksonville)	70	75	69	77	76	NA	NA	NA
Orange County	NA	NA	NA	NA	NA	NA	79	NA
Georgia	77	75	82	82	81	80	72	69
Fulton/DeKalb Counties (Atlanta)	75	71	81	72	75	NA	NA	NA
Hawaii	69	79	80	78	79	88	77	67
Idaho	53	61	70	68	68	66	60	52
Illinois	58	69	74	77	74	74	75	73
Chicago	58	71	71	70	77	71	78	72
Madison/St Clair County	NA	NA	NA	NA	NA	NA	75	NA
Indiana	59	62	68	70	76	74	76	66
Lake County	NA	NA	NA	NA	NA	NA	NA	65
Marion County (Indianapolis)	62	66	74	NA	77	71	NA	72
Iowa	58	63	76	76	79	76	75	66
Kansas	55	63	66	72	70	76	77	77
Eastern Kansas	NA	NA	NA	NA	74	NA	NA	NA
Kentucky	64	79	77	71	80	78	74	66
Louisiana	62	65	70	74	70	77	82	77
Orleans Parish (New Orleans)	53	68	68	NA	NA	NA	NA	NA
Maine	62	69	74	76	76	73	74	53
Maryland	71	77	76	79	78	91	80	80
Baltimore City	69	74	80	77	72	NA	75	63
Massachusetts	78	83	84	91	84	78	82	81
Boston	71	86	79	NA	82	NA	NA	NA
Michigan	72	79	79	81	78	79	75	71
Detroit	60	64	66	71	65	NA	NA	NA
Minnesota	62	71	78	78	78	81	75	58
Twin Cities	NA	NA	NA	NA	NA	NA	75	NA
Mississippi	64	78	80	79	73	77	76	73
Missouri	60	74	75	73	81	76	73	61
St. Louis County	NA	NA	NA	74	NA	NA	NA	NA
Montana	49	65	65	65	66	65	59	55
Nebraska	64	68	73	84	75	83	72	60
Nevada	65	66	65	63	60	63	68	59
Clark County	NA	NA	NA	59	NA	NA	NA	NA
New Hampshire	66	76	78	77	76	91	81	79
New Jersey	66	64	74	72	76	81	69	67
Newark	50	64	64	67	68	NA	NA	NA
New Mexico	59	71	79	75	72	76	77	68
New York	67	73	78	74	77	78	73	69
New York City	71	69	77	71	72	76	75	72
North Carolina	70	77	78	82	82	77	71	56
North Dakota	56	63	71	79	80	77	70	56
Ohio	64	71	71	78	75	78	82	74
Cuyahoga County (Cleveland)	65	66	78	77	77	NA	NA	NA
Franklin County (Columbus)	69	71	79	81	NA	NA	NA	NA
Oklahoma	60	67	71	72	78	79	72	70
Oregon	60	70	74	65	74	71	71	65
Pennsylvania	68	79	82	77	79	79	78	69
Allegheny County	NA	NA	NA	NA	74	NA	NA	NA
Philadelphia	68	75	75	77	80	82	80	74
Rhode Island	81	80	82	80	81	76	78	51
South Carolina	74	80	77	76	81	80	78	67

Table 3-40A. Vaccination Coverage Among Children 19 to 35 Months of Age, by State and Selected Urban Area, Selected Years, 2002–2009—*Continued*

(Percent.)

State and selected urban area	2002	2003	2004	2005	2006	2007	2008	2009
South Dakota	62	60	73	80	74	77	77	75
Tennessee	67	74	79	80	77	79	81	74
Davidson County (Nashville)	67	76	88	81	NA	NA	NA	NA
Shelby County (Memphis)	61	69	71	74	73	NA	NA	NA
Texas	65	70	69	77	75	77	78	74
Bexar County (San Antonio)	72	75	73	71	75	80	76	71
Dallas County (Dallas)	68	67	67	73	73	72	74	74
El Paso County (El Paso)	61	72	64	69	69	77	75	71
Houston	56	63	62	77	70	73	72	70
Utah	61	70	68	68	78	74	77	70
Vermont	58	65	67	63	75	67	65	65
Virginia	65	80	74	82	77	76	73	70
Washington	52	56	67	66	71	69	74	70
Eastern Washington	NA	NA	NA	NA	72	NA	NA	NA
Eastern/Western Washington	NA	NA	NA	NA	NA	NA	76	67
King County (Seattle)	56	61	74	69	71	NA	NA	NA
Western Washington	NA	NA	NA	NA	NA	71	NA	NA
West Virginia	66	63	76	68	68	76	77	65
Wisconsin	68	73	78	77	81	77	80	59
Milwaukee County (Milwaukee)	60	71	73	74	78	NA	NA	NA
Wyoming	54	57	64	67	63	70	65	62

NA = Not available.   [1]The 4:3:1:3:3:1 combined series consists of 4 or more doses of diphtheria and tetanus toxoids and pertussis vaccine (DTP), diphtheria and tetanus toxoids (DT), or diphtheria and tetanus toxoids and acellular pertussis vaccine (DTaP); 3 or more doses of any poliovirus vaccine; 1 or more doses of a measles-containing vaccine (MCV); 3 or more doses of Haemophilus influenzae type b vaccine (Hib) regardless of vaccine brand type; 3 or more doses of hepatitis B vaccine; and 1 or more doses of varicella vaccine. This series is the most complete series for which long-term state trend data are currently available.

Table 3-40B. Vaccination Coverage Among Children 19 to 35 Months of Age for Selected Diseases, by Race, Hispanic Origin, Poverty Level, and Location of Residence in Metropolitan Statistical Area, 2009–2011

(Percent.)

Vaccination and year	Not Hispanic or Latino				Hispanic or Latino[1]	
	White		Black or African American		Below poverty level	At or above poverty level
	Below poverty level	At or above poverty level	Below poverty level	At or above poverty level		
Combined Series (4:3:1:3*:3:1:4) [2]						
2009	43	46	38	44	44	49
2010	49	59	53	56	55	55
2011	60	72	61	68	68	71

NOTE: Final estimates from the National Immunization Survey include an adjustment for children with missing immunization provider data. Poverty level is based on family income and family size using U.S. Census Bureau poverty thresholds. In 2011, 5.9 percent of all 19,144 children with provider-reported vaccination history data, 9.5 percent of Hispanic, 3.6 percent of non-Hispanic White, and 6.5% of non-Hispanic Black children were missing information about poverty level and were omitted from the estimates of vaccination coverage by poverty level.

NA = Not available.   * = Estimates are considered unreliable. For data prior to 2007, percents not shown if the unweighted sample size for the numerator was less than 30, or the confidence interval half-width divided by the estimate was greater than 50 percent, or the confidence interval half-width was greater than 10. Starting with 2007 data, percents not shown if the unweighted sample size for the denominator was less than 30, or the confidence interval half-width divided by the estimate was greater than 60 percent, or the confidence interval half-width was greater than 10.   [1]Persons of Hispanic origin may be of any race.   [2]The 4:3:1:3:3:1:4 combined series consists of 4 or more doses of diphtheria and tetanus toxoids and pertussis vaccine (DTP), diphtheria and tetanus toxoids (DT), or diphtheria and tetanus toxoids and acellular pertussis vaccine (DTaP);3 or more doses of any poliovirus vaccine; 1 or more doses of a measles-containing vaccine (MCV); 3 or more doses of Haemophilus influenzae type b vaccine (Hib); 3 or more doses of hepatitis B vaccine; 1 or more doses of varicella vaccine; and 4 or more doses of pneumococcal conjugate vaccine (PCV).

Table 3-41A. Vaccination Coverage Among Adolescents 13 to 17 Years of Age for Selected Diseases, by Selected Characteristics, 2006–2011

(Percent.)

Vaccination coverage	2006[1]	2007[1]	2008	2009	2010	2011
Percent of Adolescents, 13 to 17 Years						
Measles, mumps, rubella (2 doses or more)	86.9	88.9	89.3	89.1	90.5	91.1
Hepatitis B (3 doses or more)	81.3	87.6	87.9	89.9	91.6	92.3
History of varicella or received varicella vaccine (2 doses or more)[2]	NA	NA	73.5	75.7	76.8	79.9
Td or Tdap (1 dose or more)[3]	60.1	72.3	72.2	76.2	81.2	85.3
Tdap (1 dose or more)[3]	10.8	30.4	40.8	55.6	68.7	78.2
Meningococcal conjugate vaccine (MenACWY) (1 dose or more)[4]	11.7	32.4	41.8	53.6	62.7	70.5
Human papillomavirus (HPV) (1 dose or more among females)	NA	25.1	37.2	44.3	48.7	53.0
Human papillomavirus (HPV) (3 doses or more among females)	NA	NA	17.9	26.7	32.0	34.8
Human papillomavirus (HPV) (1 dose or more among males)	X	X	X	X	X	8.3
Human papillomavirus (HPV) (3 doses or more among males)	X	X	X	X	X	1.3

NA = Not available.   X = Not applicable.   * = Estimates are not reliable and not shown if the unweighted sample size for the denominator is less than 30 or the confidence interval half-width divided by the estimate is greater than 0.588.   [1]For 2006 and 2007, data were only collected in the 4th quarter of the year. Starting with 2008, data were collected for the entire year. [2]Varicella is chickenpox. [3]Td or Tdap refers to tetanus toxoid-diphtheria vaccine (Td) or tetanus toxoid, reduced diphtheria toxoid, and acellular pertussis vaccine (Tdap) received since the age of 10 years. [4]Includes persons receiving MenACWY or meningococcal-unknown type vaccine.

Table 3-41B. Vaccination Coverage Among Adolescents 13 to 17 Years of Age for Selected Diseases, by Selected Characteristics, 2006–2011

(Percent.)

Vaccination coverage, 2011	Race and Hispanic origin[1]					Poverty level[2]		Location of residence		
	Not Hispanic or Latino				Hispanic or Latino	Below poverty level	At or above poverty level	Inside MSA		Outside MSA[3]
	White	Black or African American	American Indian or Alaska Native	Asian				Remaining area	Central city	
Percent of Adolescents, 13 to 17 Years										
Measles, mumps, rubella (2 doses or more)	91.4	90.6	81.1	94.6	90.6	90.3	91.4	90.5	91.7	91.1
Hepatitis B (3 doses or more)	92.8	91.7	89.1	91.9	91.7	91.4	92.6	91.3	93.3	91.9
History of varicella or received varicella vaccine (2 doses or more)[4]	67.3	65.3	61.8	74.8	71.4	67.2	68.4	70.9	69.0	58.0
Td or Tdap (1 dose or more)[5]	85.1	83.1	80.8	89.6	86.7	81.5	86.5	87.3	86.2	77.7
Tdap (1 dose or more)[5]	78.6	75.7	72.3	83.8	78.4	74.0	79.5	80.2	78.7	71.6
Meningococcal conjugate vaccine (MenACWY) (1 dose or more)[6]	68.4	72.1	64.4	76.0	75.3	69.0	70.7	73.9	72.5	56.1
Human papillomavirus (HPV) (1 dose or more among females)	47.5	56.0	59.4	55.8	65.0	62.1	50.1	56.9	53.1	43.1
Human papillomavirus (HPV) (3 doses or more among females)	33.0	31.7	37.8	35.0	41.6	39.0	33.4	37.1	35.4	27.3
Human papillomavirus (HPV) (1 dose or more among males)	5.6	10.6	*	*	14.9	14.1	6.7	10.3	7.2	6.4
Human papillomavirus (HPV) (3 doses or more among males)	0.8	*	*	*	2.7	2.5	1.1	1.8	1.1	1.0

NA = Not available.   X = Not applicable.   * = Estimates are not reliable and not shown if the unweighted sample size for the denominator is less than 30 or the confidence interval half-width divided by the estimate is greater than 0.588.   [1]Persons of Hispanic origin may be of any race.   [2]Poverty level is based on family income and family size using U.S. Census Bureau poverty thresholds. In 2011, less than 4 percent (unweighted) of adolescents with provider-reported vaccination data were missing information about poverty level and were not included in the estimates of vaccination coverage by poverty level.   [3]MSA = metropolitan statistical area.   [4]Varicella is chickenpox.   [5]Td or Tdap refers to tetanus toxoid-diphtheria vaccine (Td) or tetanus toxoid, reduced diphtheria toxoid, and acellular pertussis vaccine (Tdap) received since the age of 10 years.   [6]Includes persons receiving MenACWY or meningococcal-unknown type vaccine.

Table 3-42. Influenza Vaccination[1] Among Adults 18 Years of Age and Over, by Selected Characteristics, Selected Years, 1989–2011

(Percent.)

Characteristic	1989	1995	2000	2005	2006	2007	2008	2009	2010	2011
18 years and over, age-adjusted[2,3]	9.6	23.7	28.7	21.6	27.4	29.9	32.1	34.1	35.1	37.1
18 years and over, crude[3]	9.1	23.0	28.4	21.4	27.6	30.1	32.6	34.7	35.8	37.9
Age										
18 to 49 years	3.4	13.1	17.1	10.7	15.6	17.8	20.1	23.0	25.2	27.2
50 years and over	19.9	41.9	47.9	38.1	45.9	48.5	50.7	51.1	50.5	52.4
50 to 64 years	10.6	27.0	34.6	23.0	33.2	36.2	39.6	40.7	41.6	42.7
65 years and over	30.4	58.2	64.4	59.7	64.3	66.7	67.2	66.8	63.9	66.9
65 to 74 years	28.0	54.9	61.1	53.7	60.1	61.6	60.9	61.5	60.5	63.0
75 years and over	34.2	63.0	68.4	66.3	69.2	72.6	74.3	73.2	68.2	71.9
50 YEARS AND OVER										
Sex										
Male	19.2	40.2	45.9	34.7	43.2	45.6	47.6	49.2	47.4	49.3
Female	20.6	43.4	49.5	40.9	48.3	51.0	53.5	52.8	53.2	55.1
Race [4]										
White only	20.9	43.6	49.8	39.7	47.2	49.9	52.1	52.4	51.5	53.8
Black or African American only	12.5	28.2	33.2	26.9	34.9	38.2	41.1	41.7	40.4	40.8
American Indian or Alaska Native only	26.2	*	43.6	*22.9	56.3	45.8	49.3	42.8	54.7	51.2
Asian only	*9.2	35.6	43.3	30.6	44.8	45.3	47.1	50.4	55.9	53.4
Native Hawaiian or Other Pacific Islander only	NA	NA	*	*	*	*	*	*	*	*
Two or more races	NA	NA	50.7	30.4	40.2	44.8	46.3	47.7	49.8	47.7
Hispanic Origin and Race [4]										
Hispanic or Latino	13.2	33.8	34.4	24.7	31.7	35.5	38.0	40.3	40.6	43.2
Mexican	13.0	35.4	33.0	26.1	33.5	36.1	36.5	40.4	41.3	44.9
Not Hispanic or Latino	20.3	42.4	48.8	39.1	47.1	49.6	51.9	52.1	51.5	53.3
White only	21.3	44.3	50.6	41.0	48.6	51.3	53.6	53.7	52.7	54.9
Black or African American only	12.4	28.5	33.2	26.9	35.1	38.1	41.0	41.7	40.0	41.0
Percent of Poverty Level [5]										
Below 100 percent	19.6	39.7	44.1	35.8	42.1	44.8	44.4	45.2	37.5	42.8
100 percent to 199 percent	24.0	43.2	50.7	41.2	47.5	47.9	52.0	49.4	47.6	50.4
200 percent to 399 percent	20.5	43.7	51.5	42.1	48.0	50.7	51.8	52.6	51.2	53.9
400 percent or more	17.5	39.3	44.3	33.9	44.4	48.0	50.8	52.0	54.3	54.5
Hispanic Origin and Race and Percent of Poverty Level [4,5]										
Hispanic or Latino										
Below 100 percent	12.7	29.7	35.8	22.3	30.9	41.1	37.0	42.2	36.3	37.9
100 percent to 199 percent	20.4	34.7	35.6	27.5	32.0	42.7	41.3	32.4	36.6	43.2
200 percent to 399 percent	12.7	34.2	33.7	22.3	33.8	31.3	34.5	41.1	41.8	43.7
400 percent or more	*9.8	39.1	32.2	26.6	29.5	28.9	39.9	48.7	47.7	47.8
Not Hispanic or Latino										
White only										
Below 100 percent	22.5	44.4	48.6	42.2	47.8	47.4	49.3	49.8	38.7	46.1
100 percent to 199 percent	26.1	46.7	54.8	46.1	51.7	50.8	57.0	54.3	51.1	53.0
200 percent to 399 percent	21.6	45.4	54.6	46.4	50.8	54.3	54.6	55.0	53.4	56.4
400 percent or more	18.1	40.8	46.0	35.1	45.9	50.2	52.3	53.3	54.9	56.0
Black or African American only										
Below 100 percent	14.6	31.8	35.5	28.9	34.8	38.9	36.7	37.8	32.4	36.4
100 percent to 199 percent	12.0	28.3	37.9	27.4	35.0	35.6	38.4	41.8	39.2	42.3
200 percent to 399 percent	14.1	29.0	31.0	25.7	36.2	41.2	44.1	45.1	42.6	43.5
400 percent or more	*8.8	*20.0	28.7	26.2	34.6	36.2	42.9	41.0	44.4	40.6
Disability Measure [6]										
Any basic actions difficulty or complex activity limitation	NA	NA	55.2	46.5	53.4	55.8	57.2	56.9	54.5	58.6
Any basic actions difficulty	NA	NA	55.3	46.7	53.7	56.0	57.6	57.1	54.8	59.0
Any complex activity limitation	NA	NA	57.1	50.3	56.0	56.8	58.9	58.8	55.3	60.3
No disability	NA	NA	41.3	29.7	38.4	41.6	44.8	46.0	47.0	46.7
Geographic Region										
Northeast	17.9	39.7	45.9	38.4	44.1	49.0	52.7	52.0	52.4	54.0
Midwest	20.0	43.2	49.3	39.9	49.4	51.4	53.7	52.9	51.8	51.7
South	20.2	41.4	46.8	37.3	43.9	47.2	49.4	50.9	49.3	52.7
West	21.8	43.8	50.1	36.8	47.3	46.9	48.1	48.8	49.5	51.2
Location of Residence										
Within MSA[7]	18.9	41.6	47.1	37.2	44.9	47.1	50.2	51.0	50.8	52.3
Outside MSA[7]	23.3	42.9	50.2	41.0	49.7	53.7	53.0	51.6	49.3	52.7

NA = Not available.　* = Figure does not meet standards of reliability or precision.　NA = Data not available.　[1]Questions concerning use of influenza vaccination differed slightly on the National Health Interview Survey across the years for which data are shown.　[2]Estimates are age adjusted to the year 2000 standard population using four age groups: 18 to 49 years, 50 to 64 years, 65 to 74 years, and 75 years and over.　[3]Includes all other races not shown separately, unknown disability status, and unknown poverty level in 1989.　[4]The race groups White, Black, American Indian or Alaska Native, Asian, Native Hawaiian or Other Pacific Islander, and two or more races, include persons of Hispanic and non-Hispanic origin. Persons of Hispanic origin may be of any race.　[5]Percent of poverty level is based on family income and family size and composition using U.S. Census Bureau poverty thresholds. Poverty level was unknown for 11 percent of persons 18 years of age and over in 1989. Missing family income data were imputed for 1991 and beyond.　[6]Any basic actions difficulty or complex activity limitation is defined as having one or more of the following limitations or difficulties: movement difficulty, emotional difficulty, sensory (seeing or hearing) difficulty, cognitive difficulty, self-care (activities of daily living or instrumental activities of daily living) limitation, social limitation, or work limitation.　[7]MSA = metropolitan statistical area.

Table 3-43. Pneumococcal Vaccination[1] Among Adults 18 Years of Age and Over, by Selected Characteristics, Selected Years, 1989–2011

(Percent.)

Characteristic	1989	1995	2000	2005	2006	2007	2008	2009	2010	2011
18 years and over, age-adjusted[2,3]	4.6	12.0	15.4	16.7	17.0	16.7	18.3	19.0	19.0	20.4
18 years and over, crude[3]	4.4	11.7	15.1	16.5	17.0	16.7	18.5	19.3	19.6	21.1
Age										
18 to 49 years	2.1	6.5	5.4	5.8	5.7	5.3	6.8	7.5	7.3	8.8
50 to 64 years	4.4	10.0	14.7	17.1	18.2	17.3	18.5	19.2	21.0	20.9
65 years and over	14.1	34.0	53.1	56.2	57.1	57.7	60.0	60.6	59.7	62.3
65 to 74 years	13.1	31.4	48.2	49.4	52.0	51.8	52.5	54.6	54.6	56.0
75 years and over	15.7	37.8	59.1	63.9	63.0	64.4	68.7	68.0	66.0	70.0
High-Risk Group [4]										
Total, 18 to 64 years	NA	NA	18.3	22.6	23.1	24.4	24.9	17.4	18.3	20.0
18 to 49 years	NA	NA	12.2	15.0	13.5	16.0	16.0	11.2	10.6	13.6
50 to 64 years	NA	NA	26.0	30.6	32.5	32.2	33.9	28.2	30.8	30.1
65 YEARS AND OVER										
Sex										
Male	13.9	34.6	52.1	53.4	54.3	55.1	56.4	59.2	57.6	59.5
Female	14.3	33.6	53.9	58.4	59.2	59.6	62.8	61.7	61.3	64.5
Race [5]										
White only	14.8	35.3	55.6	58.4	60.0	60.1	62.5	63.1	61.6	64.7
Black or African American only	6.4	21.9	30.6	40.2	35.5	43.7	44.1	44.2	45.5	47.5
American Indian or Alaska Native only	31.2	*	70.1	*	*57.5	*	66.9	*	*48.5	53.0
Asian only	*	*23.4	40.9	35.0	35.6	33.4	45.7	44.8	47.9	40.3
Native Hawaiian or Other Pacific Islander only	NA	NA	*	*	*	*	*	*	*	*
Two or more races	NA	NA	55.6	64.8	63.6	55.8	*35.9	67.9	65.5	77.1
Hispanic Origin and Race [5]										
Hispanic or Latino	9.8	23.2	30.4	27.5	33.3	31.8	36.4	40.1	39.0	43.1
Mexican	12.9	*18.8	32.0	31.3	29.3	34.3	39.5	42.8	41.4	47.1
Not Hispanic or Latino	14.3	34.5	54.4	58.1	58.7	59.6	61.8	62.2	61.3	63.8
White only	15.0	35.9	56.8	60.6	62.0	62.2	64.5	64.8	63.5	66.5
Black or African American only	6.2	21.8	30.6	40.4	35.6	44.0	44.5	44.7	46.2	47.6
Percent of Poverty Level [6]										
Below 100 percent	11.2	28.7	40.6	46.7	45.4	48.7	46.5	48.5	42.6	49.6
100 percent to 199 percent	15.1	30.7	51.4	54.5	55.8	55.6	59.5	60.6	57.2	60.3
200 percent to 399 percent	15.1	36.1	55.8	60.8	59.9	59.8	61.4	62.9	62.2	63.4
400 percent or more	15.5	39.5	56.9	55.3	59.3	59.8	62.8	61.5	64.0	66.4
Hispanic Origin and Race and Percent of Poverty Level [5,6]										
Hispanic or Latino										
Below 100 percent	*	*14.1	23.8	20.9	24.5	*22.4	*25.7	32.6	30.2	34.8
100 percent to 199 percent	*11.0	*15.6	32.3	26.9	30.9	37.9	32.9	41.8	36.9	49.3
200 percent to 399 percent	*11.1	*34.4	37.6	35.2	42.3	29.6	44.8	40.0	45.8	39.2
400 percent or more	*	*55.1	*26.4	*25.2	*38.2	*33.7	42.4	49.1	43.0	49.1
Not Hispanic or Latino										
White only										
Below 100 percent	13.3	32.5	47.9	55.6	56.0	59.7	60.4	61.0	51.1	60.3
100 percent to 199 percent	16.0	33.5	56.1	60.5	61.6	60.8	66.3	66.3	61.3	64.6
200 percent to 399 percent	15.7	37.1	57.6	64.1	62.6	63.4	64.5	66.3	64.9	66.9
400 percent or more	15.9	39.3	59.5	57.4	63.0	62.4	64.1	62.9	66.0	68.6
Black or African American only										
Below 100 percent	*5.0	*22.6	28.8	42.3	38.4	40.7	37.6	33.8	34.9	39.5
100 percent to 199 percent	7.8	*20.9	28.1	36.6	36.2	41.9	43.5	46.9	46.4	45.6
200 percent to 399 percent	*5.9	*21.7	35.5	41.6	40.0	48.7	44.5	49.3	51.8	54.2
400 percent or more	*	*	*32.6	44.6	*24.7	43.6	56.5	45.8	50.1	49.1
Any Basic Actions Difficulty or Complex Activity Limitation [7]										
Any basic actions difficulty or complex activity limitation	NA	NA	56.6	61.6	61.4	64.2	64.9	65.9	63.9	67.0
Any basic actions difficulty	NA	NA	56.8	61.6	61.6	64.4	65.1	66.0	64.2	67.3
Any complex activity limitation	NA	NA	58.0	63.3	61.6	63.9	67.0	67.8	65.2	66.7
No disability	NA	NA	48.0	47.8	50.0	47.0	53.4	53.1	53.3	55.6
Geographic Region										
Northeast	10.4	28.2	51.2	55.8	53.7	54.6	60.9	58.5	56.7	60.0
Midwest	13.7	31.0	52.6	58.5	61.5	60.6	63.8	58.4	61.2	65.6
South	14.9	35.9	51.3	57.4	55.7	58.5	59.8	61.9	60.9	63.2
West	17.9	41.1	59.7	51.4	57.2	55.6	55.4	63.0	58.9	59.5
Location of Residence										
Within MSA[8]	13.1	33.8	52.4	55.1	56.6	56.5	59.1	60.0	58.8	61.7
Outside MSA[8]	17.1	34.8	55.4	59.8	58.9	61.7	63.2	62.9	63.3	64.6

NA = Not available.   * = Estimates are considered unreliable. Data preceded by an asterisk have a relative standard error (RSE) of 20 percent to 30 percent. Data not shown have an RSE of greater than 30 percent.   [1]Respondents were asked, "Have you ever had a pneumonia shot? This shot is usually given only once or twice in a person's lifetime and is different from the flu shot. It is also called the pneumococcal vaccine."   [2]Estimates are age adjusted to the year 2000 standard population using four age groups: 18 to 49 years, 50 to 64 years, 65 to 74 years, and 75 years and over.   [3]Includes all other races not shown separately, unknown poverty level in 1989, and unknown disability status.   [4]High-risk group membership is based on recommendations of the Advisory Committee on Immunization Practices (ACIP). The high-risk group includes persons who reported diabetes, cancer, heart, lung, liver, or kidney disease. Starting in 2009, this group also includes persons who reported asthma or cigarette smoking, to be consistent with the revised ACIP recommendation.   [5]The race groups White, Black, American Indian or Alaska Native, Asian, Native Hawaiian or Other Pacific Islander, and two or more races, include persons of Hispanic and non-Hispanic origin. Persons of Hispanic origin may be of any race.   [6]Percent of poverty level is based on family income and family size and composition using U.S. Census Bureau poverty thresholds. Poverty level was unknown for 11 percent of persons 18 years of age and over in 1989. Missing family income data were imputed for 1991 and beyond.   [7]Any basic actions difficulty or complex activity limitation is defined as having one or more of the following limitations or difficulties: movement difficulty, emotional difficulty, sensory (seeing or hearing) difficulty, cognitive difficulty, self-care (activities of daily living or instrumental activities of daily living) limitation, social limitation, or work limitation.   [8]MSA = metropolitan statistical area.

Table 3-44. Use of Mammography[1] Among Women 40 Years of Age and Over, by Selected Characteristics, Selected Years, 1987–2010

(Percent.)

Characteristic	1987	1990	1991	1993	1994	1998	1999	2000	2003	2005	2008	2010
40 years and over, age-adjusted[2,3]	29.0	51.7	54.7	59.7	61.0	67.0	70.3	70.4	69.5	66.6	67.1	66.5
40 years and over, crude[2]	28.7	51.4	54.6	59.7	60.9	66.9	70.3	70.4	69.7	66.8	67.6	67.1
50 years and over, age-adjusted[2,3]	27.3	49.8	54.3	59.7	60.9	69.0	72.1	73.7	72.4	68.2	70.3	68.8
50 years and over, crude[2]	27.4	49.7	54.1	59.7	60.6	68.9	71.9	73.6	72.4	68.4	70.5	69.2
Age												
40 to 49 years	31.9	55.1	55.6	59.9	61.3	63.4	67.2	64.3	64.4	63.5	61.5	62.3
50 to 64 years	31.7	56.0	60.3	65.1	66.5	73.7	76.5	78.7	76.2	71.8	74.2	72.6
65 years and over	22.8	43.4	48.1	54.2	55.0	63.8	66.8	67.9	67.7	63.8	65.5	64.4
65 to 74 years	26.6	48.7	55.7	64.2	63.0	69.4	73.9	74.0	74.6	72.5	72.6	71.9
75 years and over	17.3	35.8	37.8	41.0	44.6	57.2	58.9	61.3	60.6	54.7	57.9	55.7
Race [4]												
40 years and over, crude												
White only	29.6	52.2	55.6	60.0	60.6	67.4	70.6	71.4	70.1	67.4	67.9	67.4
Black or African American only	24.0	46.4	48.0	59.1	64.3	66.0	71.0	67.8	70.4	64.9	68.0	67.9
American Indian or Alaska Native only	*	43.2	54.5	49.8	65.8	45.2	63.0	47.4	63.1	72.8	62.7	71.2
Asian only	*	46.0	45.9	55.1	55.8	60.2	58.3	53.5	57.6	54.6	66.1	62.4
Native Hawaiian or Other Pacific Islander only	NA	NA	NA	NA	NA	NA	*	*	*	*	*	*
Two or more races	NA	NA	NA	NA	NA	NA	70.2	69.2	65.3	63.7	55.2	51.4
Hispanic Origin and Race [4]												
40 years and over, crude												
Hispanic or Latina	18.3	45.2	49.2	50.9	51.9	60.2	65.7	61.2	65.0	58.8	61.2	64.2
Not Hispanic or Latina	29.4	51.8	54.9	60.3	61.5	67.5	70.7	71.1	70.1	67.5	68.3	67.4
White only	30.3	52.7	56.0	60.6	61.3	68.0	71.1	72.2	70.5	68.3	68.7	67.8
Black or African American only	23.8	46.0	47.7	59.2	64.4	66.0	71.0	67.9	70.5	65.2	68.3	67.4
Age, Hispanic Origin, and Race [4]												
40 to 49 years												
Hispanic or Latina	*15.3	45.1	44.0	52.6	47.5	55.2	61.6	54.1	59.4	54.2	54.1	59.8
Not Hispanic or Latina												
White only	34.3	57.0	58.1	61.6	62.0	64.4	68.3	67.2	65.2	65.5	64.1	62.6
Black or African American only	27.8	48.4	48.0	55.6	67.2	65.0	69.2	60.9	68.2	62.1	59.5	63.5
50 to 64 years												
Hispanic or Latina	23.0	47.5	61.7	59.2	60.1	67.2	69.7	66.5	69.4	61.5	71.3	68.6
Not Hispanic or Latina												
White only	33.6	58.1	61.5	66.2	67.5	75.3	77.9	80.6	77.2	73.5	74.1	73.5
Black or African American only	26.4	48.4	52.4	65.5	63.6	71.2	75.0	77.7	76.2	71.6	76.7	74.0
65 years and over												
Hispanic or Latina	*	41.1	40.9	*35.7	48.0	59.0	67.2	68.3	69.5	63.8	59.0	65.2
Not Hispanic or Latina												
White only	24.0	43.8	49.1	54.7	54.9	64.3	66.8	68.3	68.1	64.7	66.1	65.0
Black or African American only	14.1	39.7	41.6	56.3	61.0	60.6	68.1	65.5	65.4	60.5	66.4	60.9
Age and Percent of Poverty Level [5]												
40 years and over, crude												
Below 100 percent	14.6	30.8	35.2	41.1	44.2	50.1	57.4	54.8	55.4	48.5	51.4	51.4
100 percent to 199 percent	20.9	39.1	44.4	47.5	48.6	56.1	59.5	58.1	60.8	55.3	55.8	53.8
200 percent to 399 percent	29.7	53.3	57.5	63.2	65.0	67.4	69.1	68.8	69.9	67.2	64.4	66.2
400 percent or more	42.9	68.7	69.8	74.1	74.1	76.8	79.8	81.5	77.7	76.6	79.0	78.1
40 to 49 years												
Below 100 percent	18.6	32.2	33.0	36.1	43.0	44.8	51.3	47.4	50.6	42.5	46.6	48.1
100 percent to 199 percent	18.4	39.0	43.8	47.8	47.6	46.9	52.8	43.6	54.0	49.8	46.5	46.2
200 percent to 399 percent	31.2	55.2	56.3	63.0	64.5	61.8	63.0	60.2	63.0	61.8	56.8	59.2
400 percent or more	44.1	68.9	69.6	69.6	69.9	72.7	77.4	75.8	71.6	73.6	72.5	73.6
50 to 64 years												
Below 100 percent	14.6	29.9	37.3	47.3	46.2	52.7	63.3	61.7	58.3	50.4	57.5	54.7
100 percent to 199 percent	24.2	39.8	50.2	47.0	49.0	61.8	64.9	68.3	64.0	58.8	58.9	57.3
200 percent to 399 percent	29.7	56.2	60.2	66.1	69.6	71.1	74.8	75.1	74.1	70.7	69.8	70.7
400 percent or more	44.7	71.6	72.6	78.7	78.0	83.4	83.4	86.9	84.9	80.6	84.3	82.8
65 years and over												
Below 100 percent	13.1	30.8	35.2	40.4	43.9	51.9	57.6	54.8	57.0	52.3	49.1	50.6
100 percent to 199 percent	19.9	38.6	41.8	47.6	48.8	57.8	60.2	60.3	62.8	56.1	59.4	55.5
200 percent to 399 percent	27.7	47.4	55.9	60.3	61.0	69.5	70.0	71.1	72.3	68.6	65.0	67.2
400 percent or more	34.7	61.2	63.0	71.3	73.0	71.1	76.7	81.9	73.0	72.6	78.3	74.5
Health Insurance Status at the Time of Interview [6]												
40 to 64 years												
Insured	NA	NA	NA	66.2	68.3	72.3	75.5	76.0	75.1	72.5	73.4	74.1
Private	NA	NA	NA	67.1	69.4	73.4	76.3	77.1	76.3	74.5	74.2	75.6
Medicaid	NA	NA	NA	51.9	54.5	59.7	62.5	61.7	63.5	55.6	64.2	64.4
Uninsured	NA	NA	NA	36.0	34.0	40.1	44.8	40.7	41.5	38.1	39.7	36.0
Health Insurance Status Prior to Interview [6]												
40 to 64 years												
Insured continuously all 12 months	NA	NA	NA	66.6	68.6	73.0	76.1	76.8	75.6	73.1	74.1	74.7
Uninsured for any period up to 12 months	NA	NA	NA	49.4	49.9	47.6	57.1	53.0	56.0	51.3	55.3	57.3
Uninsured more than 12 months	NA	NA	NA	28.4	26.6	36.3	38.9	34.0	37.0	32.9	34.6	30.0

Table 3-44. Use of Mammography[1] Among Women 40 Years of Age and Over, by Selected Characteristics, Selected Years, 1987–2010—*Continued*

(Percent.)

Characteristic	1987	1990	1991	1993	1994	1998	1999	2000	2003	2005	2008	2010
Age and Education [7]												
40 years and over, crude												
No high school diploma or GED	17.8	36.4	40.0	46.4	48.2	54.5	56.7	57.7	58.1	52.8	53.8	53.0
High school diploma or GED	31.3	52.7	55.8	59.0	61.0	66.7	69.2	69.7	67.8	64.9	65.2	64.4
Some college or more	37.7	62.8	65.2	69.5	69.7	72.8	77.3	76.2	75.1	72.7	73.4	72.1
40 to 49 years												
No high school diploma or GED	15.1	38.5	40.8	43.6	50.4	47.3	48.8	46.8	53.3	51.2	46.9	44.9
High school diploma or GED	32.6	53.1	52.0	56.6	55.8	59.1	60.8	59.0	60.8	58.8	57.2	58.4
Some college or more	39.2	62.3	63.7	66.1	68.7	68.3	74.4	70.6	68.1	68.3	66.3	66.5
50 to 64 years												
No high school diploma or GED	21.2	41.0	43.6	51.4	51.6	58.8	62.3	66.5	63.4	56.9	64.9	56.7
High school diploma or GED	33.8	56.5	60.8	62.4	67.8	73.3	77.2	76.6	71.8	70.1	70.4	69.9
Some college or more	40.5	68.0	72.7	78.5	74.7	79.8	81.2	84.2	82.7	77.0	78.5	77.0
65 years and over												
No high school diploma or GED	16.5	33.0	37.7	44.2	45.6	54.7	56.6	57.4	56.9	50.7	49.2	54.1
High school diploma or GED	25.9	47.5	54.0	57.4	59.1	66.8	68.4	71.8	69.7	64.3	65.7	62.5
Some college or more	32.3	56.7	57.9	64.8	64.3	71.3	77.1	74.1	75.1	73.0	75.6	70.9
Disability Measure [8]												
40 years and over, crude												
Any basic actions difficulty or complex activity limitation	NA	NA	NA	NA	NA	65.8	67.6	67.8	67.2	63.5	63.9	63.3
Any basic actions difficulty	NA	NA	NA	NA	NA	65.9	67.1	67.9	67.3	63.5	63.9	63.3
Any complex activity limitation	NA	NA	NA	NA	NA	61.8	64.8	64.1	62.3	59.9	60.2	58.2
No disability	NA	NA	NA	NA	NA	68.2	72.3	72.6	71.8	69.8	71.1	70.8

NA = Not available.   * = Estimates are considered unreliable. Data preceded by an asterisk have a relative standard error (RSE) of 20 percent to 30 percent. Data not shown have an RSE of greater than 30 percent.   [1]Questions concerning use of mammography differed slightly on the National Health Interview Survey across the years for which data are shown.   [2]Includes all other races not shown separately, unknown poverty level in 1987, unknown health insurance status, unknown education level, and unknown disability status.   [3]Estimates for women 40 years of age and over are age-adjusted to the year 2000 standard population using four age groups: 40 to 49 years, 50 to 64 years, 65 to 74 years, and 75 years and over. Estimates for women 50 years of age and over are age-adjusted using three age groups.   [4]The race groups White, Black, American Indian or Alaska Native, Asian, Native Hawaiian or Other Pacific Islander, and two or more races, include persons of Hispanic and non-Hispanic origin. Persons of Hispanic origin may be of any race.   [5]Percent of poverty level is based on family income and family size and composition using U.S. Census Bureau poverty thresholds. Poverty level was unknown for 11 percent of women 40 years of age and over in 1987. Missing family income data were imputed for 1997 and beyond.   [6]Health insurance categories are mutually exclusive. Persons who reported both Medicaid and private coverage are classified as having private coverage. Medicaid includes other public assistance through 1996. Starting with 1997 data, state-sponsored health plan coverage is included as Medicaid coverage. Starting with 1999 data, coverage by the Children's Health Insurance Program (CHIP) is included with Medicaid coverage. Persons not covered by private insurance, Medicaid, CHIP, public assistance (through 1996), state-sponsored or other government-sponsored health plans (starting in 1997), Medicare, or military plans are considered to have no health insurance coverage. Persons with only Indian Health Service coverage are considered to have no health insurance coverage. Health insurance status was unknown for 8 to 9 percent of children in 1993-1996 and about 1 percent in 1997-2011.   [7]Education categories shown are for 1998 and subsequent years. GED is General Educational Development high school equivalency diploma. In years prior to 1998, the following categories based on number of years in school completed were used: less than 12 years, 12 years, and 13 years or more.   [8]Any basic actions difficulty or complex activity limitation is defined as having one or more of the following limitations or difficulties: movement difficulty, emotional difficulty, sensory (seeing or hearing) difficulty, cognitive difficulty, self-care (activities of daily living or instrumental activities of daily living) limitation, social limitation, or work limitation.

Table 3-45. Percent of Women 18 Years of Age and Over Who Have Had a Pap Smear[1] Within the Last Three Years, by Selected Characteristics, Selected Years, 1987–2010

(Percent.)

Characteristic	1987	1993	1994	1998	1999	2000	2003	2005	2008	2010
18 years and over, age-adjusted[2,3]	74.1	77.7	76.8	79.3	80.8	81.3	79.2	77.9	75.6	73.7
18 years and over, crude[2]	74.4	77.7	76.8	79.1	80.8	81.2	79.0	77.7	75.1	73.2
Age										
18 to 44 years	83.3	84.6	82.8	84.4	86.8	84.9	83.9	83.6	81.8	80.4
18 to 24 years	74.8	78.8	76.6	73.6	76.8	73.5	75.1	74.5	70.5	69.0
25 to 44 years	86.3	86.3	84.6	87.6	89.9	88.5	86.8	86.8	85.7	84.6
45 to 64 years	70.5	77.2	77.4	81.4	81.7	84.6	81.3	80.6	78.8	76.9
45 to 54 years	75.7	82.1	81.9	83.7	83.8	86.3	83.6	83.4	81.0	79.9
55 to 64 years	65.2	70.6	71.0	78.0	78.4	82.0	77.8	76.8	76.0	73.2
65 years and over	50.8	57.6	57.3	59.8	61.0	64.5	60.8	54.9	50.0	47.1
65 to 74 years	57.9	64.7	64.9	67.0	70.0	71.6	70.1	66.3	61.6	58.0
75 years and over	40.4	48.0	47.3	51.2	50.8	56.7	51.1	42.7	37.5	34.6
Race[4]										
18 years and over, crude										
White only	74.1	77.3	76.2	78.9	80.6	81.3	78.7	77.7	74.9	72.8
Black or African American only	80.7	82.7	83.5	84.2	85.7	85.1	84.0	81.1	80.1	77.9
American Indian or Alaska Native only	85.4	78.1	73.5	74.6	92.2	76.8	84.8	75.2	69.4	73.4
Asian only	51.9	68.8	66.4	68.5	64.4	66.4	68.3	64.1	65.1	68.0
Native Hawaiian or Other Pacific Islander only	NA	NA	NA	NA	*	*	*	*	*	*
Two or more races	NA	NA	NA	NA	86.9	80.0	81.6	86.2	77.1	70.8
Hispanic Origin and Race[4]										
18 years and over, crude										
Hispanic or Latina	67.6	77.2	74.4	75.2	76.3	77.0	75.4	75.5	75.4	73.6
Not Hispanic or Latina	74.9	77.8	77.0	79.6	81.3	81.7	79.5	78.0	75.1	73.1
White only	74.7	77.3	76.5	79.3	81.0	81.8	79.3	78.1	74.9	72.8
Black or African American only	80.9	82.7	83.8	84.2	86.0	85.1	83.8	81.2	80.0	77.4
Age, Hispanic Origin, and Race[4]										
18 to 44 years										
Hispanic or Latina	73.9	80.9	80.6	76.4	77.0	78.1	75.9	76.5	77.9	75.9
Not Hispanic or Latina										
White only	84.5	85.3	82.9	85.7	88.7	86.6	85.8	85.8	83.8	82.1
Black or African American only	89.1	88.0	89.1	88.9	90.8	88.5	88.6	86.4	83.5	84.2
45 to 64 years										
Hispanic or Latina	57.7	75.8	70.1	78.3	79.5	77.8	77.9	78.4	78.2	75.4
Not Hispanic or Latina										
White only	71.2	77.2	77.5	81.7	81.9	85.9	81.4	81.4	79.0	77.2
Black or African American only	76.2	80.3	82.2	84.1	84.6	85.7	84.7	80.5	82.1	78.2
65 years and over										
Hispanic or Latina	41.7	57.1	43.8	59.8	63.7	66.8	64.6	60.0	52.6	54.2
Not Hispanic or Latina										
White only	51.8	57.1	58.2	59.7	60.5	64.2	60.7	54.1	49.0	46.5
Black or African American only	44.8	61.2	59.5	61.7	64.5	67.2	59.6	60.1	58.7	48.0
Age and Percent of Poverty Level[5]										
18 years and over, crude										
Below 100 percent	64.3	70.3	68.8	69.8	73.6	72.0	70.5	68.7	68.9	65.1
100 percent to 199 percent	68.2	71.2	68.8	70.6	72.5	73.4	71.4	69.0	65.0	64.3
200 percent to 399 percent	77.6	80.6	80.1	79.7	80.6	80.2	78.6	77.9	72.5	71.3
400 percent or more	83.6	85.1	85.4	87.0	87.6	89.1	86.6	85.7	84.4	83.1
18 to 44 years										
Below 100 percent	77.1	77.0	78.9	77.1	79.7	77.1	77.1	76.2	76.5	73.0
100 percent to 199 percent	80.4	81.9	78.2	79.2	84.0	79.4	79.5	78.1	75.5	75.7
200 percent to 399 percent	84.8	86.6	84.5	85.3	86.7	86.1	84.0	85.5	82.6	79.8
400 percent or more	88.9	91.3	88.7	89.8	91.1	89.8	89.5	88.7	87.0	88.9
45 to 64 years										
Below 100 percent	53.6	66.5	62.0	67.6	73.1	73.6	66.0	65.9	66.2	61.7
100 percent to 199 percent	60.4	64.8	66.2	69.9	70.4	76.1	71.4	69.6	65.6	63.2
200 percent to 399 percent	71.0	79.5	80.3	79.7	79.9	80.0	80.8	79.3	75.3	75.2
400 percent or more	79.1	83.9	84.0	88.2	87.4	91.5	87.5	87.4	87.1	85.7
65 years and over										
Below 100 percent	33.2	47.4	44.0	48.2	51.9	53.7	52.6	44.4	41.6	35.1
100 percent to 199 percent	50.4	55.7	51.5	55.1	54.7	61.0	55.4	49.5	43.5	40.7
200 percent to 399 percent	58.0	59.7	63.7	64.2	64.0	65.1	62.4	56.8	45.8	47.1
400 percent or more	65.2	67.5	76.2	67.5	70.4	75.4	70.2	64.6	65.7	57.7
Health Insurance Status at the Time of Interview[6]										
18 to 64 years, crude										
Insured	NA	84.7	83.8	86.0	87.2	87.8	86.4	85.6	83.4	82.8
Private	NA	84.8	83.6	86.5	87.5	88.0	87.0	86.5	84.2	84.2
Medicaid	NA	82.7	86.2	83.0	84.2	85.8	82.8	80.9	80.3	78.0
Uninsured	NA	69.4	68.6	69.6	73.3	70.4	66.6	67.7	67.1	61.9
Health Insurance Status Prior to Interview[6]										
18 to 64 years, crude										
Insured continuously all 12 months	NA	84.8	83.7	86.3	87.3	88.0	86.6	85.8	83.7	83.2
Uninsured for any period up to 12 months	NA	81.8	83.4	81.7	83.5	83.7	81.8	81.3	78.9	78.3
Uninsured more than 12 months	NA	65.1	63.6	64.0	68.8	65.1	60.2	62.0	62.1	55.2

Table 3-45. Percent of Women 18 Years of Age and Over Who Have Had a Pap Smear[1] Within the Last Three Years, by Selected Characteristics, Selected Years, 1987–2010—*Continued*

(Percent.)

Characteristic	1987	1993	1994	1998	1999	2000	2003	2005	2008	2010
Age and Education [7]										
25 years and over, crude										
No high school diploma or GED	57.1	61.9	60.9	65.0	66.1	69.9	64.9	64.1	60.6	56.7
High school diploma or GED	76.4	78.2	76.0	77.4	79.3	79.8	75.9	73.8	69.5	66.8
Some college or more	84.0	84.4	85.2	86.9	87.8	88.0	86.2	84.6	82.6	80.7
25 to 44 years										
No high school diploma or GED	75.1	73.6	73.6	76.8	79.0	79.6	71.7	75.5	76.2	69.1
High school diploma or GED	85.6	85.4	82.4	83.9	87.6	86.2	84.3	83.1	80.0	79.0
Some college or more	90.1	89.8	89.1	91.5	93.0	91.4	90.8	90.5	89.3	89.0
45 to 64 years										
No high school diploma or GED	58.0	65.6	66.1	69.2	71.6	75.7	71.4	69.7	70.4	63.4
High school diploma or GED	72.3	77.6	75.9	81.0	79.8	81.8	77.6	79.0	73.9	72.4
Some college or more	80.1	83.0	84.7	85.5	85.7	89.1	86.2	84.1	83.0	81.5
65 years and over										
No high school diploma or GED	44.0	50.7	47.7	52.4	51.8	56.6	52.5	46.0	36.7	37.7
High school diploma or GED	55.4	61.6	61.2	60.7	63.7	66.9	61.2	52.5	49.3	42.6
Some college or more	59.4	62.3	66.5	67.9	68.8	69.8	67.8	63.8	59.0	54.9
Disability measure [8]										
18 years and over, crude										
Any basic actions difficulty or complex activity limitation	NA	NA	NA	72.7	74.4	75.4	72.7	69.1	66.1	63.8
Any basic actions difficulty	NA	NA	NA	72.4	74.3	75.1	72.6	69.1	66.2	63.6
Any complex activity limitation	NA	NA	NA	67.9	69.3	71.0	67.6	62.2	60.1	58.5
No disability	NA	NA	NA	82.5	83.8	84.1	82.5	82.6	80.4	78.9

NA = Not available.   * = Figure does not meet standards of reliability or precision. Data not shown have an RSE of greater than 30 percent.   [1]Questions concerning use of Pap smears differed slightly on the National Health Interview Survey across the years for which data are shown.   [2]Includes all other races not shown separately, unknown poverty level in 1987, unknown health insurance status, unknown education level, and unknown disability status.   [3]Estimates are age adjusted to the year 2000 standard population using five age groups: 18 to 44 years, 45 to 54 years, 55 to 64 years, 65 to 74 years, and 75 years and over.   [4]The race groups White, Black, American Indian or Alaska Native, Asian, Native Hawaiian or Other Pacific Islander, and two or more races, include persons of Hispanic and non-Hispanic origin. Persons of Hispanic origin may be of any race.   [5]Percent of poverty level is based on family income and family size and composition. Missing family income data were imputed for 1993 and beyond.   [6]Health insurance categories are mutually exclusive. Persons who reported both Medicaid and private coverage are classified as having private coverage. Medicaid includes other public assistance through 1996. Starting with 1997 data, state-sponsored health plan coverage is included as Medicaid coverage. Starting with 1999 data, coverage by the Children's Health Insurance Program (CHIP) is included with Medicaid coverage. Persons not covered by private insurance, Medicaid, CHIP, public assistance (through 1996), state-sponsored or other government-sponsored health plans (starting in 1997), Medicare, or military plans are considered to have no health insurance coverage. Persons with only Indian Health Service coverage are considered to have no health insurance coverage. Health insurance status was unknown for 8 to 9 percent of children in 1993–1996 and about 1 percent in 1997–2011.   [7]Education categories shown are for 1998 and subsequent years. GED is General Educational Development high school equivalency diploma. In years prior to 1998, the following categories based on number of years in school completed were used: less than 12 years, 12 years, and 13 years or more.   [8]Any basic actions difficulty or complex activity limitation is defined as having one or more of the following limitations or difficulties: movement difficulty, emotional difficulty, sensory (seeing or hearing) difficulty, cognitive difficulty, self-care (activities of daily living or instrumental activities of daily living) limitation, social limitation, or work limitation.

Table 3-46. Use of Colorectal Tests or Procedures Among Adults 50 to 75 Years of Age, by Selected Characteristics, Selected Years, 2000–2010

(Percent.)

Characteristic	Any colorectal test or procedure[1,2]					Colonoscopy[2,3]				
	2000	2003	2005	2008	2010	2000	2003	2005	2008	2010
All Adults, 50 to 75 Years [4]	33.9	39.1	44.3	51.6	58.7	19.1	29.2	37.6	46.7	54.9
Sex										
Male	33.1	40.1	44.4	51.4	58.5	19.5	30.2	37.9	46.9	54.7
Female	34.5	38.1	44.2	51.9	58.8	18.8	28.4	37.4	46.6	55.1
Race [5]										
White only	34.9	39.8	45.6	52.8	59.8	19.7	30.0	38.9	47.8	56.0
Black or African American only	29.6	35.2	38.1	46.9	55.2	17.4	24.8	32.2	43.1	51.8
American Indian or Alaska Native only	*35.2	*37.9	*33.9	28.5	48.9	*	*	*	*26.7	46.7
Asian only	20.4	26.7	30.8	47.1	47.1	*8.6	20.0	24.4	39.3	43.6
Native Hawaiian and Other Pacific Islander only	*	*	*	*	*	*	*	*	*	*
Two or more races	37.5	40.7	33.8	38.4	51.9	*25.1	29.7	29.6	37.4	48.4
Hispanic Origin and Race [5]										
Hispanic or Latino	21.7	27.2	28.5	34.0	46.5	13.3	19.8	23.1	29.3	43.9
Mexican	19.3	22.4	24.6	27.5	44.6	11.2	14.2	18.2	21.2	41.3
Not Hispanic or Latino	34.7	40.0	45.6	53.3	59.9	19.5	30.0	38.9	48.4	56.0
White only	35.7	41.0	47.4	54.8	61.3	20.0	30.9	40.5	49.8	57.3
Black or African American only	29.7	35.3	38.0	47.4	55.3	17.5	25.0	32.0	43.5	52.0
Percent of Poverty Level [6]										
Below 100 percent	26.5	29.7	28.7	33.9	37.9	16.3	22.0	23.6	28.5	34.8
100 percent to 199 percent	29.4	31.9	38.4	42.7	47.9	17.7	23.3	31.5	38.0	43.3
200 percent to 399 percent	33.7	38.8	43.6	49.9	58.0	18.6	29.4	37.0	44.3	54.6
400 percent or more	37.1	43.8	49.6	58.9	67.3	20.5	32.7	42.8	54.5	63.6
Hispanic Origin and Race and Percent of Poverty Level [5,6]										
Hispanic or Latino										
Below 100 percent	15.3	21.4	19.3	21.1	33.7	*9.3	15.2	13.1	17.9	32.1
100 percent to 199 percent	16.8	20.5	24.6	27.7	39.6	8.6	16.0	19.4	24.4	36.3
200 percent to 399 percent	23.6	29.0	28.3	39.3	47.5	*13.7	20.7	21.6	33.8	46.0
400 percent or more	31.1	37.9	42.1	43.9	63.3	22.4	27.1	39.3	37.6	59.5
Not Hispanic or Latino										
White only										
Below 100 percent	29.6	33.9	30.6	39.8	40.4	19.3	26.8	26.8	33.2	36.4
100 percent to 199 percent	32.1	34.7	42.4	46.0	50.0	19.7	25.7	35.0	40.7	44.5
200 percent to 399 percent	35.2	40.3	47.3	51.6	59.7	19.3	31.0	40.2	45.8	56.3
400 percent or more	37.9	44.3	50.6	60.5	68.0	20.7	32.9	43.8	56.3	64.3
Black or African American only										
Below 100 percent	27.5	27.4	29.0	35.1	39.2	14.5	17.6	23.5	30.1	36.4
100 percent to 199 percent	28.7	30.0	36.2	46.7	49.0	17.2	20.0	30.3	43.2	46.5
200 percent to 399 percent	27.7	36.8	35.8	48.5	60.5	16.5	25.6	31.8	44.7	56.2
400 percent or more	33.9	43.5	48.9	54.3	68.1	20.7	33.3	40.2	50.6	64.6
Education [7]										
No high school diploma or GED	25.9	28.9	34.5	36.2	44.6	14.9	21.2	29.0	31.8	41.5
High school diploma or GED	33.1	38.3	42.1	48.5	53.7	19.0	29.3	35.7	44.6	50.8
Some college or more	37.8	43.3	48.7	57.5	64.7	20.9	32.1	41.6	52.1	60.4
Disability Measure [8]										
Any basic actions difficulty or complex activity limitation	37.8	42.0	47.7	54.2	59.5	22.1	31.9	40.1	48.5	55.5
Any basic actions difficulty	38.1	41.9	47.9	54.6	59.7	22.5	31.9	40.6	48.9	55.8
Any complex activity limitation	37.4	41.5	48.1	52.4	59.4	22.6	31.3	39.7	46.7	55.1
No disability	30.9	36.9	41.6	50.0	58.5	16.6	27.1	35.6	45.8	54.9
Geographic Region										
Northeast	34.4	43.5	50.9	54.7	64.3	19.1	33.1	44.8	51.0	61.7
Midwest	35.2	40.4	43.5	52.5	58.4	19.8	30.6	36.6	47.8	55.2
South	32.5	36.7	43.9	51.6	57.4	20.0	28.5	38.1	47.4	54.4
West	34.1	37.0	39.6	48.2	56.3	16.3	24.3	31.3	41.1	49.7
Location of Residence										
Within MSA[9]	34.1	40.3	44.7	52.4	59.6	19.0	29.9	37.9	47.6	55.8
Outside MSA[9]	33.2	34.8	42.7	48.5	54.4	19.6	26.8	36.7	43.3	50.9

* = Figure does not meet standards of reliability or precision. Data preceded by an asterisk have a relative standard error (RSE) of 20 percent to 30 percent. Data not shown have an RSE of greater than 30 percent. [1]Includes reports of home fecal occult blood test (FOBT) in the past year, sigmoidoscopy procedure in the past 5 years with FOBT in the past 3 years, or colonoscopy in the past 10 years. Colorectal procedures are performed for diagnostic and screening purposes. [2]Questions differed slightly on the National Health Interview Survey across the years for which data are shown. [3]Includes any colonoscopy in the past 10 years. [4]Includes all other races not shown separately, unknown disability status, and unknown education level. [5]The race groups White, Black, American Indian or Alaska Native, Asian, Native Hawaiian or Other Pacific Islander, and two or more races include persons of Hispanic and non-Hispanic origin. Persons of Hispanic origin may be of any race. [6]Based on family income and family size and composition using U.S. Census Bureau poverty thresholds. Missing family income data were imputed. [7]GED is General Educational Development high school equivalency diploma. [8]Any basic actions difficulty or complex activity limitation is defined as having one or more of the following limitations or difficulties: movement difficulty, emotional difficulty, sensory (seeing or hearing) difficulty, cognitive difficulty, self-care (activities of daily living or instrumental activities of daily living) limitation, social limitation, or work limitation. [9]MSA = metropolitan statistical area.

Table 3-47. Emergency Department Visits Within the Past 12 Months Among Children Under 18 Years of Age, by Selected Characteristics, Selected Years, 1997–2011

(Percent.)

Characteristic	Under 18 years					Under 6 years					6 to 17 years				
	1997	2000	2005	2010	2011	1997	2000	2005	2010	2011	1997	2000	2005	2010	2011
PERCENT OF CHILDREN WITH ONE OR MORE EMERGENCY DEPARTMENT VISITS															
All Children [1]	19.9	20.3	20.5	22.1	18.5	24.3	25.7	26.8	27.8	24.2	17.7	17.6	17.4	19.1	15.6
Sex															
Male	21.5	21.5	21.7	23.3	18.9	25.2	27.7	27.6	29.3	25.1	19.6	18.6	18.8	20.1	15.7
Female	18.3	19.0	19.2	20.9	18.1	23.3	23.7	25.9	26.3	23.3	15.7	16.6	15.9	18.2	15.4
Race [2]															
White only	19.4	19.9	19.8	21.2	17.9	22.6	24.8	25.3	26.6	22.7	17.8	17.6	17.1	18.4	15.5
Black or African American only	24.0	22.7	23.8	27.6	22.6	33.1	30.8	31.6	34.0	30.7	19.4	19.0	20.0	24.2	18.2
American Indian or Alaska Native only	*24.1	38.0	*32.1	20.9	21.9	*24.3	*	67.1	*35.4	*33.7	*24.0	*39.0	*	*	*16.8
Asian only	12.6	12.3	14.6	15.0	9.3	20.8	*16.7	20.2	18.4	17.7	8.6	9.8	12.3	13.3	4.7
Native Hawaiian and Other Pacific Islander only	NA	*	*	*	*	NA	*	*	*	*	NA	*	*	*	*
Two or more races	NA	24.2	24.8	27.2	24.1	NA	31.7	38.3	34.9	31.7	NA	18.3	17.1	21.6	19.0
Hispanic Origin and Race [2]															
Hispanic or Latino	21.1	18.6	19.5	23.6	19.2	25.7	23.9	28.0	30.2	25.3	18.1	15.6	14.5	19.4	15.5
Not Hispanic or Latino	19.7	20.6	20.7	21.7	18.3	24.0	26.2	26.5	27.0	23.8	17.6	18.0	18.0	19.0	15.6
White only	19.2	20.2	19.9	20.4	17.6	22.2	25.1	24.5	25.1	21.7	17.7	17.9	17.9	18.2	15.7
Black or African American only	23.6	22.7	23.8	27.2	22.8	32.7	30.9	31.8	34.4	31.2	19.2	19.0	20.0	23.3	18.3
Percent of Poverty Level [3]															
Below 100 percent	25.1	25.0	27.3	30.6	24.9	29.5	30.7	33.5	35.4	30.0	22.2	21.7	23.5	27.6	21.4
100 percent to 199 percent	22.0	22.4	21.8	25.7	19.8	28.0	27.4	30.8	31.6	27.4	19.0	19.9	17.4	22.3	15.9
200 percent to 399 percent	18.0	19.0	18.9	18.4	15.9	21.4	25.7	25.9	22.7	20.5	16.4	15.9	15.7	16.4	13.6
400 percent or more	16.3	17.0	16.8	15.9	14.6	19.1	20.3	19.1	21.7	18.5	15.1	15.6	15.8	13.3	12.9
Hispanic Origin and Race and Percent of Poverty Level [2,3]															
Hispanic or Latino															
Below 100 percent	21.9	19.9	21.8	27.0	21.5	25.0	25.7	28.4	32.0	26.5	19.6	16.4	17.4	23.4	18.0
100 percent to 199 percent	20.8	18.2	17.8	23.3	18.8	28.8	20.8	26.1	31.6	27.3	15.6	16.6	13.1	18.0	13.9
200 percent to 399 percent	21.4	17.9	20.2	19.5	17.7	24.6	26.1	31.7	25.2	22.5	19.6	13.3	14.3	16.1	14.9
400 percent or more	17.7	17.6	15.3	21.4	15.4	*20.2	*22.9	23.3	28.6	*18.9	16.4	15.4	*11.5	18.0	14.0
Not Hispanic or Latino															
White only															
Below 100 percent	25.5	26.5	34.1	33.7	27.8	27.2	35.6	37.3	37.4	30.9	24.4	21.2	32.2	31.6	25.8
100 percent to 199 percent	22.3	24.7	22.8	26.3	20.4	25.8	29.2	30.7	29.2	25.3	20.7	22.7	19.1	24.7	18.0
200 percent to 399 percent	17.8	19.5	17.9	17.6	15.1	20.9	26.0	22.9	21.2	18.0	16.3	16.6	15.7	15.9	13.7
400 percent or more	16.5	16.9	16.8	15.5	14.6	19.0	18.5	18.7	21.0	18.6	15.4	16.2	16.0	13.2	13.0
Black or African American only															
Below 100 percent	29.3	27.8	27.1	32.4	27.1	39.5	28.9	34.8	41.6	31.3	23.0	27.3	22.6	26.6	23.9
100 percent to 199 percent	22.5	20.8	24.1	27.5	22.2	31.7	35.3	33.3	34.5	34.2	18.5	13.8	20.3	23.7	17.4
200 percent to 399 percent	18.5	19.6	22.6	22.3	19.9	23.9	28.3	33.3	24.6	32.9	16.3	16.2	17.8	21.4	14.4
400 percent or more	16.1	19.3	16.9	18.9	15.2	*18.8	32.8	*	*24.1	*19.6	15.2	*13.9	17.4	16.1	13.5
Health Insurance Status at the Time of Interview [4]	19.8	20.7	20.7	22.3	18.8	24.4	25.8	26.8	28.1	24.4	17.5	18.2	17.7	19.2	15.9
Insured	17.5	18.4	17.4	17.1	14.9	20.9	22.8	21.7	21.8	18.8	15.9	16.5	15.5	14.9	13.2
Private	28.2	28.6	28.5	30.0	24.4	33.0	33.2	35.5	35.5	30.2	24.1	25.5	23.6	26.4	20.2
Medicaid	20.2	17.2	18.4	19.4	13.8	23.0	24.5	26.6	24.0	20.1	18.9	13.9	15.4	17.6	12.0
Uninsured															
Health Insurance Status Prior to Interview [4]															
Insured continuously all 12 months	19.6	20.2	20.5	22.2	18.6	24.1	25.3	26.7	28.1	23.9	17.3	17.8	17.3	19.1	15.7
Uninsured for any period up to 12 months	24.0	25.9	26.0	23.7	22.9	27.1	33.9	34.4	28.0	32.1	21.9	21.7	22.4	21.3	18.3
Uninsured more than 12 months	18.4	14.7	14.4	17.6	9.2	19.3	19.1	*15.7	*21.3	*	18.1	13.1	14.0	16.7	9.0
Geographic Region															
Northeast	18.5	19.7	20.9	22.3	19.1	20.7	21.6	26.3	27.8	23.8	17.4	18.8	18.5	19.6	16.8
Midwest	19.5	20.3	21.8	23.3	19.0	26.0	25.6	30.1	28.8	24.5	16.4	17.8	17.8	20.7	16.1
South	21.8	21.9	21.7	23.4	19.8	25.6	28.6	27.1	30.4	25.5	19.9	18.7	18.8	19.5	16.8
West	18.5	18.0	16.7	19.1	15.7	23.5	24.7	22.9	23.3	22.2	15.9	14.7	13.8	16.8	12.3
Location of Residence															
Within MSA[5]	19.7	19.9	20.0	21.8	17.9	23.9	24.5	25.7	27.7	23.9	17.4	17.6	17.2	18.6	14.8
Outside MSA[5]	20.8	21.9	22.4	24.2	21.9	26.2	31.3	31.8	28.6	25.8	18.6	17.8	18.2	22.1	19.8
PERCENT OF CHILDREN WITH TWO OR MORE EMERGENCY DEPARTMENT VISITS															
All Children [1]	7.1	7.0	6.8	8.4	5.9	9.6	10.0	9.8	10.8	8.6	5.8	5.6	5.4	7.2	4.5
Sex															
Male	7.3	7.3	7.2	8.5	5.4	9.9	10.3	10.7	11.3	8.8	6.0	5.8	5.4	7.0	3.6
Female	6.9	6.7	6.5	8.3	6.4	9.4	9.6	8.9	10.3	8.3	5.7	5.3	5.3	7.3	5.4
Race															
White only	6.6	6.4	6.3	7.6	5.3	8.4	8.7	9.1	10.1	7.6	5.7	5.4	4.9	6.3	4.2
Black or African American only	9.6	10.5	9.2	12.6	8.4	14.9	16.2	12.7	15.7	12.9	6.9	7.9	7.5	11.0	6.0
American Indian or Alaska Native only	*	*	*	*	*8.6	*	*	*	*	*	*	*	*	*	*8.3
Asian only	*5.7	*3.1	*4.6	7.3	*2.9	*12.9	*	*	*	*5.8	*	*	*3.9	*7.1	*
Native Hawaiian and Other Pacific Islander only	NA	*	*	*	*	NA	*	*	*	*	NA	*	*	*	*
Two or more races	NA	*8.7	*8.6	10.3	9.1	NA	*14.3	*13.2	*11.7	12.2	NA	*	*	*9.2	*7.0
Hispanic Origin and Race [2]															
Hispanic or Latino	8.9	7.0	7.7	8.6	6.5	11.8	9.4	12.1	11.7	9.5	7.0	5.6	5.2	6.6	4.7
Not Hispanic or Latino	6.8	7.0	6.6	8.4	5.7	9.2	10.1	9.2	10.5	8.2	5.7	5.6	5.4	7.3	4.4
White only	6.2	6.3	5.9	7.4	5.1	7.8	8.6	8.2	9.3	6.9	5.5	5.2	4.9	6.4	4.2
Black or African American only	9.3	10.6	9.1	12.3	8.4	14.6	16.6	12.4	15.8	13.2	6.8	7.9	7.5	10.4	5.9
Percent of Poverty Level [3]															
Below 100 percent	11.1	11.9	11.2	13.4	10.3	14.5	16.4	15.9	15.3	13.7	8.9	9.4	8.4	12.1	7.9
100 percent to 199 percent	8.3	8.0	7.9	10.3	6.3	12.2	11.8	12.7	13.4	9.5	6.3	6.1	5.5	8.4	4.7
200 percent to 399 percent	6.2	5.6	5.7	6.3	4.5	7.4	8.0	7.6	7.3	6.9	5.6	4.5	4.8	5.9	3.3
400 percent or more	4.0	4.7	4.4	5.0	3.1	5.0	5.8	5.1	7.3	3.4	3.6	4.2	4.0	3.9	2.9
Hispanic Origin and Race and Percent of Poverty Level [2,3]															
Hispanic or Latino															
Below 100 percent	10.4	8.2	10.0	9.9	7.8	13.9	10.9	13.8	10.9	9.8	8.0	6.6	7.4	9.2	6.4
100 percent to 199 percent	8.2	7.4	6.1	9.4	6.0	12.0	8.5	*8.7	15.4	10.2	5.7	6.7	*4.7	5.5	*3.6
200 percent to 399 percent	8.5	6.2	7.7	5.9	5.9	10.0	9.2	14.2	*8.0	*9.1	*7.6	*4.5	*4.4	*4.6	*3.9
400 percent or more	*5.0	*4.0	*5.4	*6.5	*4.6	*	*	*	*	*	*	*	*	*5.2	*

Table 3-47. Emergency Department Visits Within the Past 12 Months Among Children Under 18 Years of Age, by Selected Characteristics, Selected Years, 1997–2011—*Continued*

(Percent.)

Characteristic	Under 18 years					Under 6 years					6 to 17 years				
	1997	2000	2005	2010	2011	1997	2000	2005	2010	2011	1997	2000	2005	2010	2011
Not Hispanic or Latino															
White only															
Below 100 percent	10.7	12.8	13.5	14.0	11.8	12.2	18.4	18.6	15.5	15.5	9.8	*9.5	10.4	13.1	9.5
100 percent to 199 percent	8.0	8.0	8.2	10.4	6.2	11.2	11.8	13.7	12.3	*8.1	6.4	6.3	*5.5	9.4	5.3
200 percent to 399 percent	6.0	5.4	5.1	5.7	4.1	6.7	7.7	6.1	*6.5	5.4	5.6	4.4	4.6	5.4	3.4
400 percent or more	3.7	4.5	3.7	5.0	2.9	4.6	4.5	4.1	7.6	*3.4	3.3	4.5	3.5	3.9	2.7
Black or African American only															
Below 100 percent	12.7	14.7	11.4	16.1	13.1	19.1	18.5	16.2	22.1	17.1	8.8	12.8	8.6	12.4	9.9
100 percent to 199 percent	9.2	8.9	8.4	12.4	7.7	*13.5	17.5	*13.3	*14.6	*12.6	*7.2	*4.8	*6.5	11.1	*5.7
200 percent to 399 percent	5.8	7.8	*7.6	9.9	*4.6	*8.9	*12.5	*	*10.2	*	*4.5	*6.0	*7.5	*9.8	*3.0
400 percent or more	*	*8.9	*7.2	*3.7	*	*	*17.8	*	*	*	*	*	*	*	*
Health Insurance Status at the Time of Interview [4]															
Insured	7.0	7.0	6.8	8.5	6.0	9.6	9.6	9.7	11.0	8.7	5.7	5.7	5.3	7.1	4.5
Private	5.2	5.2	5.0	5.5	3.5	6.8	7.1	6.2	7.4	5.0	4.5	4.5	4.4	4.6	2.9
Medicaid	13.1	13.1	11.1	12.8	9.6	16.2	15.9	15.8	15.3	12.7	10.4	11.2	7.7	11.2	7.4
Uninsured	7.7	6.6	7.0	8.0	4.2	9.8	11.3	11.5	*8.5	*	6.8	4.5	5.4	7.8	*3.7
Health Insurance Status Prior to Interview [4]															
Insured continuously all 12 months	6.9	6.7	6.7	8.4	5.8	9.4	9.2	9.7	10.8	8.3	5.7	5.5	5.2	7.1	4.4
Uninsured for any period up to 12 months	8.5	10.6	8.9	10.1	9.0	11.5	16.0	13.6	13.3	13.1	6.6	7.7	6.9	8.4	7.0
Uninsured more than 12 months	6.8	5.8	5.5	7.8	*	*8.6	8.9	*	*	*	6.2	4.7	5.3	*7.9	*
Geographic Region															
Northeast	6.2	6.4	6.2	7.8	6.7	7.6	7.9	8.9	10.3	8.1	5.4	5.6	5.0	6.6	6.0
Midwest	6.6	6.6	6.9	9.1	5.9	10.4	9.0	9.6	11.4	8.9	4.8	5.5	5.5	8.0	4.4
South	8.0	8.5	7.9	9.1	6.1	10.1	12.6	10.8	12.9	9.1	6.9	6.6	6.3	7.1	4.5
West	7.1	5.4	5.5	7.2	4.9	10.0	8.5	9.1	7.6	7.7	5.6	3.9	3.9	7.0	3.4
Location of Residence															
Within MSA [5]	7.2	6.6	6.7	8.3	5.6	9.6	8.9	9.5	10.6	8.4	5.9	5.5	5.2	7.0	4.1
Outside MSA [5]	6.8	8.6	7.5	9.3	7.3	9.7	15.0	11.2	12.2	9.2	5.6	5.8	5.9	7.9	6.3

NA = Not available.   * = Figure does not meet standards of reliability or precision. Data preceded by an asterisk have a relative standard error (RSE) of 20 percent to 30 percent. Data not shown have an RSE of greater than 30 percent.   [1]Includes all other races not shown separately and unknown health insurance status.   [2]The race groups, White, Black, American Indian or Alaska Native, Asian, Native Hawaiian or Other Pacific Islander, and 2 or more races, include persons of Hispanic and non-Hispanic origin. Persons of Hispanic origin may be of any race.   [3]Percent of poverty level is based on family income and family size and composition using U.S. Census Bureau poverty thresholds. Missing family data were imputed for 1997 and beyond.   [4]Health insurance categories are mutually exclusive. Persons who reported both Medicaid and private coverage are classified as having private coverage. Medicaid includes other public assistance through 1996. Starting with 1997 data, state-sponsored health plan coverage is included as Medicaid coverage. Starting with 1999 data, coverage by the Children's Health Insurance Program (CHIP) is included with Medicaid coverage. Persons not covered by private insurance, Medicaid, CHIP, public assistance (through 1996), state-sponsored or other government-sponsored health plans (starting in 1997), Medicare, or military plans are considered to have no health insurance coverage. Persons with only Indian Health Service coverage are considered to have no health insurance coverage. Health insurance status was unknown for 8 to 9 percent of children in 1993–1996 and about 1 percent in 1997–2011.   [5]MSA = metropolitan statistical area.

Table 3-48. Emergency Department Visits Within the Past 12 Months Among Adults 18 Years of Age and Over, by Selected Characteristics, Selected Years, 1997–2011

(Percent.)

Characteristic	One or more emergency department visits					Two or more emergency department visits				
	1997	2000	2005	2010	2011	1997	2000	2005	2010	2011
18 years and over, age-adjusted[1,2]	19.6	20.2	20.5	21.4	20.4	6.7	6.9	7.1	7.8	7.4
18 years and over, crude[1]	19.6	20.1	20.4	21.3	20.3	6.7	6.8	7.0	7.7	7.3
Age										
18 to 44 years	20.7	20.5	20.8	22.0	20.6	6.8	7.0	7.1	8.4	7.7
18 to 24 years	26.3	25.7	25.3	25.4	23.8	9.1	8.8	8.9	9.6	9.0
25 to 44 years	19.0	18.8	19.2	20.7	19.5	6.2	6.4	6.5	8.0	7.2
45 to 64 years	16.2	17.6	18.2	19.2	18.2	5.6	5.6	6.4	6.7	6.6
45 to 54 years	15.7	17.9	17.6	18.6	18.0	5.5	5.8	6.1	6.6	6.6
55 to 64 years	16.9	17.0	19.0	19.8	18.5	5.7	5.3	6.8	6.8	6.6
65 years and over	22.0	23.7	23.7	23.7	23.3	8.1	8.6	8.2	7.7	7.8
65 to 74 years	20.3	21.6	20.8	20.7	20.4	7.1	7.4	7.4	6.4	6.7
75 years and over	24.3	26.2	27.1	27.4	27.0	9.3	10.0	9.1	9.4	9.3
Sex [2]										
Male	19.1	18.7	18.6	18.5	18.0	5.9	5.7	5.9	6.0	5.9
Female	20.2	21.6	22.3	24.3	22.7	7.5	7.9	8.2	9.6	8.8
Race [2,3]										
White only	19.0	19.4	19.8	20.7	19.8	6.2	6.4	6.5	7.2	6.8
Black or African American only	25.9	26.5	26.3	28.6	28.0	11.1	10.8	11.9	12.6	12.3
American Indian or Alaska Native only	24.8	30.3	31.0	22.6	27.3	13.1	*12.6	*11.1	*11.8	12.7
Asian only	11.6	13.6	15.4	13.3	9.9	*2.9	*3.8	*3.8	3.3	2.3
Native Hawaiian and Other Pacific Islander only	NA	*	*	*	*	NA	*	*	*	*
Two or more races	NA	32.5	25.7	29.7	24.3	NA	11.3	12.8	11.1	12.7
American Indian or Alaska Native; White	NA	33.9	29.3	31.1	26.1	NA	*9.4	*15.3	*15.2	*17.2
Hispanic Origin and Race [2,3]										
Hispanic or Latino	19.2	18.3	20.1	19.8	18.9	7.4	7.0	7.1	6.9	7.0
Mexican	17.8	17.4	17.2	18.1	17.4	6.4	7.1	5.8	6.1	6.4
Not Hispanic or Latino	19.7	20.6	20.7	21.9	20.7	6.7	6.9	7.1	8.1	7.5
White only	19.1	19.8	20.1	21.1	20.1	6.2	6.4	6.4	7.4	6.9
Black or African American only	25.9	26.5	26.2	29.0	27.9	11.0	10.8	11.9	12.7	12.5
Percent of Poverty Level [2,4]										
Below 100 percent	28.1	29.0	29.8	30.6	30.5	12.8	13.3	13.7	14.9	14.5
100 percent to 199 percent	23.8	23.9	23.2	25.6	24.1	9.3	9.6	9.6	10.5	10.0
200 percent to 399 percent	18.3	19.8	20.2	20.4	18.8	5.9	6.3	6.5	6.8	6.5
400 percent or more	15.9	16.8	16.9	17.0	16.1	3.9	4.5	4.5	4.7	4.0
Hispanic Origin and Race and Percent of Poverty Level [2,3,4]										
Hispanic or Latino										
Below 100 percent	22.1	22.4	24.0	23.6	22.6	9.8	9.7	9.2	11.5	10.0
100 percent to 199 percent	19.2	18.1	18.7	19.9	19.1	8.1	6.7	7.1	6.3	7.3
200 percent to 399 percent	18.5	17.3	18.9	18.1	17.2	6.0	7.4	5.9	5.2	6.3
400 percent or more	14.6	16.4	20.9	18.8	15.6	*3.8	*4.3	*6.9	*5.5	*2.9
Not Hispanic or Latino										
White only										
Below 100 percent	29.5	30.1	30.8	33.3	31.6	13.0	13.9	13.7	15.5	14.8
100 percent to 199 percent	24.3	25.5	24.3	26.8	25.4	9.1	10.4	9.8	11.2	10.8
200 percent to 399 percent	18.1	20.1	20.7	20.3	19.1	5.8	6.3	6.4	6.5	6.4
400 percent or more	15.8	16.3	16.2	16.9	16.4	3.8	4.1	4.0	4.9	3.9
Black or African American only										
Below 100 percent	34.6	35.4	35.4	36.9	41.1	17.5	17.4	18.3	20.2	22.1
100 percent to 199 percent	29.2	28.5	28.9	33.5	31.6	12.8	12.2	14.2	15.9	13.0
200 percent to 399 percent	20.8	23.2	21.5	25.7	21.3	8.1	8.0	8.7	10.2	8.4
400 percent or more	18.2	22.6	22.6	18.8	18.6	5.9	8.8	*9.2	*4.0	6.9
Health Insurance Status at the Time of Interview [5,6]										
18 to 64 years										
Insured	18.8	19.5	20.0	20.8	19.4	6.1	6.4	6.6	7.5	6.9
Private	16.9	17.6	17.3	17.4	15.7	4.7	5.1	4.8	5.2	4.3
Medicaid	37.6	42.2	40.1	40.2	37.6	19.7	21.0	20.1	21.1	19.7
Uninsured	20.0	19.3	19.5	21.3	21.0	7.5	6.9	8.0	8.9	8.7
Health Insurance Status Prior to Interview [5,6]										
18 to 64 years										
Insured continuously all 12 months	18.3	19.0	19.4	20.2	18.7	5.8	6.1	6.3	7.1	6.5
Uninsured for any period up to 12 months	25.5	28.2	28.0	26.0	28.3	9.4	10.3	12.4	12.5	11.0
Uninsured more than 12 months	18.9	17.3	18.0	20.6	19.4	7.1	6.4	7.0	8.1	8.1

Table 3-48. Emergency Department Visits Within the Past 12 Months Among Adults 18 Years of Age and Over, by Selected Characteristics, Selected Years, 1997–2011—*Continued*

(Percent.)

Characteristic	One or more emergency department visits					Two or more emergency department visits				
	1997	2000	2005	2010	2011	1997	2000	2005	2010	2011
Percent of Poverty Level and Health Insurance Status Prior to Interview [4,5,6]										
18 to 64 years										
Below 100 percent										
Insured continuously all 12 months	30.2	31.6	33.6	35.2	32.4	14.7	15.4	15.3	18.3	16.6
Uninsured for any period up to 12 months	34.1	43.7	39.1	34.2	39.3	16.1	18.1	21.5	16.5	17.4
Uninsured more than 12 months	20.8	20.5	20.5	23.4	25.7	8.1	9.1	8.5	11.7	12.2
100 percent to 199 percent										
Insured continuously all 12 months	24.5	25.5	23.7	26.1	25.5	8.9	10.2	9.8	10.8	10.8
Uninsured for any period up to 12 months	28.7	27.7	28.4	29.7	30.5	12.3	11.7	12.7	15.6	12.5
Uninsured more than 12 months	19.0	17.4	18.5	21.2	17.5	8.3	6.4	7.7	7.8	7.6
200 to 399 percent										
Insured continuously all 12 months	17.5	19.5	19.7	19.6	17.3	5.3	6.3	6.4	6.0	6.0
Uninsured for any period up to 12 months	21.6	24.6	26.8	25.4	22.8	6.6	7.3	10.6	12.2	7.8
Uninsured more than 12 months	16.8	15.6	14.7	17.6	17.0	5.9	4.5	4.5	5.7	5.3
400 percent or more										
Insured continuously all 12 months	14.9	15.5	15.6	15.9	14.5	3.7	3.7	3.6	4.5	3.3
Uninsured for any period up to 12 months	18.0	20.1	20.2	12.5	22.0	*3.1	6.4	7.2	*	*5.6
Uninsured more than 12 months	19.1	15.8	17.9	19.4	13.0	*	*5.2	*7.4	*	*
Disability Measure [2,7]										
Any basic actions difficulty or complex activity limitation	30.8	32.0	34.4	34.9	34.7	13.5	14.6	15.6	16.8	17.3
Any basic actions difficulty	30.5	32.4	34.9	35.0	35.3	13.5	14.9	15.8	17.2	17.7
Any complex activity limitation	39.7	41.5	42.3	43.8	42.9	19.9	21.2	22.4	24.5	23.9
No disability	14.5	15.3	14.9	16.1	14.2	3.7	3.9	3.9	4.4	3.6
Geographic Region [2]										
Northeast	19.5	20.0	21.6	22.6	20.8	6.9	6.2	7.2	8.4	6.9
Midwest	19.3	20.1	21.6	22.3	20.9	6.2	6.9	7.2	8.2	7.9
South	20.9	21.2	20.7	22.1	21.6	7.3	7.6	7.6	8.0	8.2
West	17.7	18.6	17.8	18.9	17.8	6.0	6.3	6.0	6.7	6.0
Location of Residence [2]										
Within MSA [8]	19.1	19.6	20.1	20.8	20.0	6.4	6.6	6.8	7.5	7.1
Outside MSA [8]	21.5	22.5	22.3	25.5	23.0	7.8	7.8	8.1	9.8	9.2

NA = Not available.   * = Figure does not meet standards of reliability or precision. Data preceded by an asterisk have a relative standard error (RSE) of 20 percent to 30 percent. Data not shown have an RSE of greater than 30 percent.   [1]Includes all other races not shown separately, unknown health insurance status, and unknown disability status.   [2]Estimates are for persons 18 years of age and over and are age adjusted to the year 2000 standard population using five age groups: 18 to 44 years, 45 to 54 years, 55 to 64 years, 65 to 74 years, and 75 years and over.   [3]The race groups White, Black, American Indian or Alaska Native, Asian, Native Hawaiian or Other Pacific Islander, and two or more races include persons of Hispanic and non-Hispanic origin. Persons of Hispanic origin may be of any race.   [4]Percent of poverty level is based on family income and family size and composition using U.S. Census Bureau poverty thresholds. Missing family income data were imputed for 1997 and beyond.   [5]Estimates for persons 18 to 64 years of age are age adjusted to the year 2000 standard population using three age groups: 18 to 44 years, 45 to 54 years, and 55 to 64 years.   [6]Health insurance categories are mutually exclusive. Persons who reported both Medicaid and private coverage are classified as having private coverage. Medicaid includes other public assistance through 1996. Starting with 1997 data, state-sponsored health plan coverage is included as Medicaid coverage. Starting with 1999 data, coverage by the Children's Health Insurance Program (CHIP) is included with Medicaid coverage. Persons not covered by private insurance, Medicaid, CHIP, public assistance (through 1996), state-sponsored or other government-sponsored health plans (starting in 1997), Medicare, or military plans are considered to have no health insurance coverage. Persons with only Indian Health Service coverage are considered to have no health insurance coverage. Health insurance status was unknown for 8 to 9 percent of children in 1993–1996 and about 1 percent in 1997–2011.   [7]Any basic actions difficulty or complex activity limitation is defined as having one or more of the following limitations or difficulties: movement difficulty, emotional difficulty, sensory (seeing or hearing) difficulty, cognitive difficulty, self-care (activities of daily living or instrumental activities of daily living) limitation, social limitation, or work limitation.   [8]MSA = metropolitan statistical area.

Table 3-49. Initial Injury-Related Visits to Hospital Emergency Departments, by Sex, Age, and Intent and Mechanism of Injury, Selected Annual Averages, 2005–2006 Through 2009–2010

(Numbers in thousands; rate per 10,000 population.)

Sex, age, and intent and mechanism of injury[1]	Initial injury-related visits in thousands				Initial injury-related visits per 10,000 persons			
	2005–2006	2007–2008[2]	2008–2009	2009–2010	2005–2006	2007–2008[2]	2008–2009	2009–2010
Both Sexes								
All ages, age-adjusted[2,3]	31,706	28,699	31,328	32,204	1,076.4	960.9	1,040.8	1,063.2
All ages, crude[2]	31,706	28,699	31,328	32,204	1,068.6	951.3	1,029.4	1,049.7
Unintentional injuries[4]	25,658	23,670	25,725	26,523	864.7	784.6	845.3	864.5
Falls	8,100	8,144	8,900	9,393	273.0	270.0	292.4	306.2
Struck by or against objects or persons	2,935	2,746	2,916	3,055	98.9	91.0	95.8	99.6
Motor vehicle traffic	3,714	3,387	3,508	3,622	125.2	112.3	115.3	118.1
Cut or pierce	2,145	1,944	2,008	1,829	72.3	64.4	66.0	59.6
Intentional injuries	1,977	1,888	2,313	2,418	66.6	62.6	76.0	78.8
Male								
All ages, age-adjusted[2,3]	16,966	15,332	16,640	17,124	1,166.1	1,039.7	1,118.0	1,143.0
All ages, crude[2]	16,966	15,332	16,640	17,124	1,164.2	1,033.8	1,111.8	1,133.8
Unintentional injuries[4]	13,736	12,611	13,590	14,083	942.5	850.3	908.0	932.4
Falls	3,685	3,581	3,944	4,285	252.9	241.4	263.5	283.7
Struck by or against objects or persons	1,833	1,771	1,863	1,931	125.8	119.4	124.4	127.8
Motor vehicle traffic	1,733	1,693	1,734	1,762	118.9	114.2	115.8	116.7
Cut or pierce	1,392	1,270	1,263	1,183	95.5	85.7	84.4	78.3
Intentional injuries	1,135	1,020	1,266	1,348	77.8	68.8	84.6	89.3
Under 18 years[2]	5,072	4,602	5,132	5,403	1,346.6	1,216.8	1,351.1	1,416.3
Unintentional injuries[4]	4,391	3,995	4,509	4,817	1,165.8	1,056.0	1,187.1	1,262.9
Falls	1,362	1,305	1,512	1,647	361.5	345.0	398.1	431.8
Struck by or against objects or persons	816	850	909	1,022	216.6	224.6	239.2	267.9
Motor vehicle traffic	357	265	305	309	94.8	70.0	80.3	81.0
Cut or pierce	291	264	284	248	77.3	69.8	74.8	64.9
Intentional injuries	190	198	194	173	50.4	52.2	51.1	45.3
18 to 24 years[2]	2,552	2,305	2,562	2,516	1,729.5	1,547.4	1,695.5	1,630.1
Unintentional injuries[4]	1,985	1,788	1,947	1,878	1,345.4	1,200.6	1,288.6	1,216.7
Falls	318	309	366	375	215.2	207.7	242.4	243.0
Struck by or against objects or persons	290	280	283	216	196.9	188.0	187.4	140.2
Motor vehicle traffic	386	366	373	406	261.6	245.8	247.0	263.2
Cut or pierce	265	190	215	187	179.5	127.8	142.6	121.4
Intentional injuries	273	308	381	389	185.2	206.9	252.2	252.2
25 to 44 years[2]	5,199	4,471	4,611	4,719	1,243.6	1,072.7	1,109.5	1,140.9
Unintentional injuries[4]	4,001	3,531	3,540	3,577	957.1	847.0	851.8	864.8
Falls	763	677	703	739	182.4	162.5	169.2	178.7
Struck by or against objects or persons	472	384	401	400	112.9	92.1	96.4	96.8
Motor vehicle traffic	629	638	578	585	150.5	153.0	139.1	141.5
Cut or pierce	480	426	401	380	114.8	102.2	96.5	91.9
Intentional injuries	436	350	495	586	104.4	83.9	119.2	141.6
45 to 64 years[2]	2,842	2,707	2,996	3,071	790.0	718.3	780.7	788.7
Unintentional injuries[4]	2,275	2,223	2,437	2,531	632.5	590.0	635.1	649.9
Falls	599	651	669	775	166.6	172.8	174.2	199.0
Struck by or against objects or persons	208	205	216	208	57.9	54.3	56.4	53.3
Motor vehicle traffic	262	331	375	334	72.9	87.9	97.7	85.9
Cut or pierce	285	309	306	297	79.2	81.9	79.7	76.2
Intentional injuries	205	145	168	180	57.1	38.4	43.9	46.2
65 years and over[2]	1,301	1,247	1,340	1,415	837.5	768.6	805.1	824.7
Unintentional injuries[4]	1,082	1,073	1,157	1,280	696.8	661.7	695.2	746.1
Falls	644	638	694	749	414.5	393.2	416.7	436.3
Struck by or against objects or persons	46	*52	*54	84	29.8	*32.3	*32.2	49.1
Motor vehicle traffic	98	93	103	127	63.4	57.4	61.7	74.1
Cut or pierce	70	81	*57	71	45.3	50.0	*34.0	41.1
Intentional injuries	*	*	*	*	*	*	*	*

Table 3-49. Initial Injury-Related Visits to Hospital Emergency Departments, by Sex, Age, and Intent and Mechanism of Injury, Selected Annual Averages, 2005–2006 Through 2009–2010—*Continued*

(Numbers in thousands; rate per 10,000 population.)

Sex, age, and intent and mechanism of injury[1]	Initial injury-related visits in thousands				Initial injury-related visits per 10,000 persons			
	2005–2006	2007–2008[2]	2008–2009	2009–2010	2005–2006	2007–2008[2]	2008–2009	2009–2010
Female								
All ages, age-adjusted[2,3]	14,740	13,367	14,688	15,080	980.5	874.2	955.6	976.8
All ages, crude[2]	14,740	13,367	14,688	15,080	976.3	871.6	949.7	968.2
Unintentional injuries[4]	11,922	11,060	12,134	12,439	789.7	721.1	784.6	798.6
Falls	4,415	4,564	4,956	5,109	292.4	297.6	320.4	328.0
Struck by or against objects or persons	1,102	976	1,053	1,124	73.0	63.6	68.1	72.2
Motor vehicle traffic	1,981	1,695	1,774	1,860	131.2	110.5	114.7	119.4
Cut or pierce	753	673	745	646	49.9	43.9	48.2	41.5
Intentional injuries	843	867	1,048	1,070	55.8	56.5	67.7	68.7
Under 18 years[2]	3,625	3,062	3,508	3,645	1,008.7	848.2	967.5	1,001.6
Unintentional injuries[4]	3,058	2,690	3,008	3,115	851.1	745.3	829.5	855.9
Falls	1,039	1,014	1,096	1,144	289.1	280.9	302.3	314.3
Struck by or against objects or persons	419	391	439	454	116.7	108.3	121.1	124.7
Motor vehicle traffic	367	282	249	285	102.1	78.2	68.6	78.3
Cut or pierce	160	145	154	139	44.4	40.1	42.4	38.2
Intentional injuries	188	163	222	207	52.3	45.1	61.4	56.8
18 to 24 years[2]	1,882	1,698	1,736	1,854	1,329.3	1,186.5	1,194.5	1,259.9
Unintentional injuries[4]	1,431	1,318	1,325	1,437	1,010.5	921.0	911.7	976.4
Falls	290	301	307	299	205.0	210.5	210.9	203.5
Struck by or against objects or persons	146	106	110	135	103.4	74.0	75.4	91.6
Motor vehicle traffic	397	378	360	426	280.6	264.5	247.5	289.8
Cut or pierce	116	89	77	*81	82.2	61.9	53.2	*55.1
Intentional injuries	176	209	232	262	124.2	145.8	159.7	177.9
25 to 44 years[2]	4,173	3,733	4,087	4,152	1,004.2	905.4	996.6	1,016.6
Unintentional injuries[4]	3,266	2,865	3,179	3,244	785.8	694.7	775.1	794.2
Falls	873	900	1,004	986	210.1	218.2	244.7	241.4
Struck by or against objects or persons	309	216	198	250	74.3	52.4	48.3	61.2
Motor vehicle traffic	719	572	621	612	173.1	138.8	151.3	149.9
Cut or pierce	269	214	270	230	64.7	51.8	65.9	56.4
Intentional injuries	313	345	396	396	75.4	83.6	96.5	96.9
45 to 64 years[2]	2,904	2,681	3,061	3,106	767.8	677.5	760.0	759.3
Unintentional injuries[4]	2,278	2,209	2,539	2,536	602.2	558.3	630.4	619.9
Falls	865	886	1,012	1,067	228.7	223.9	251.2	260.8
Struck by or against objects or persons	160	171	216	205	42.2	43.2	53.5	50.0
Motor vehicle traffic	359	345	399	403	94.8	87.3	99.0	98.4
Cut or pierce	158	163	190	159	41.7	41.1	47.2	38.8
Intentional injuries	149	130	161	184	39.4	32.9	39.9	45.0
65 years and over[2]	2,155	2,193	2,294	2,322	1,002.9	989.9	1,016.3	1,014.2
Unintentional injuries[4]	1,889	1,978	2,083	2,108	879.1	892.5	922.8	920.4
Falls	1,347	1,463	1,538	1,612	626.9	660.1	681.2	704.1
Struck by or against objects or persons	69	91	91	81	31.9	41.2	40.4	35.5
Motor vehicle traffic	139	116	146	134	64.5	52.5	64.7	58.3
Cut or pierce	*50	*64	*54	*37	*23.3	*28.8	*23.9	*16.3
Intentional injuries	*	*	*	*	*	*	*	*

NOTE: An emergency department visit was considered injury related if the first-listed diagnosis was injury related (ICD-9-CM 800-909.2, 909.4, 909.9-994.9, 995.50-995.59, and 995.80-995.85) or the first-listed external cause code (E code) was injury related (ICD-9-CM E800-E869, E880-E929, and E950-E999).

* = Figure does not meet standards of reliability or precision. Data preceded by an asterisk have a relative standard error (RSE) of 20 percent to 30 percent. Data not shown have an RSE greater than 30 percent.   [1]Intent and mechanism of injury are based on the first-listed external cause of injury code (E code). Intentional injuries include suicide attempts and assaults.   [2]Includes all injury-related visits not shown separately in table, including those with undetermined intent (2 percent in 2009 to 2010) and insufficient or no information to code cause of injury (9 percent in 2009 to 2010).   [3]Rates are age adjusted to the year 2000 standard population using six age groups: under 18 years, 18 to 24 years, 25 to 44 years, 45 to 64 years, 65 to 74 years, and 75 years and over.   [4]Includes unintentional injury-related visits with mechanism of injury not shown in table.

Table 3-50A. Visits to Physician Offices, by Age, Sex, and Race, Selected Years, 1995–2010

(Number; rate.)

Age, sex, and race	All places[1]				Physician offices			
	1995	2000	2009	2010	1995	2000	2009	2010
Number of Visits in Thousands								
Age								
Total	860,859	1,014,848	1,270,001	1,239,387	697,082	823,542	1,037,796	1,008,802
Under 18 years	194,644	212,165	239,590	246,228	150,351	163,459	183,999	191,500
18 to 44 years	285,184	315,774	341,209	342,797	219,065	243,011	257,890	261,941
45 to 64 years	188,320	255,894	374,775	352,001	159,531	216,783	316,395	296,385
45 to 54 years	104,891	142,233	190,701	171,039	88,266	119,474	158,120	140,819
55 to 64 years	83,429	113,661	184,074	180,962	71,264	97,309	158,275	155,566
65 years and over	192,712	231,014	314,428	298,362	168,135	200,289	279,514	258,976
65 to 74 years	102,605	116,505	153,884	151,075	90,544	102,447	137,452	132,201
75 years and over	90,106	114,510	160,544	147,287	77,591	97,842	142,062	126,775
Number of Visits per 100 Persons								
Total, age-adjusted[2]	334	374	414	401	271	304	337	325
Total, crude	329	370	421	408	266	300	344	332
Under 18 years	275	293	322	331	213	226	247	257
18 to 44 years	264	291	309	310	203	224	234	237
45 to 64 years	364	422	475	441	309	358	401	371
45 to 54 years	339	385	431	388	286	323	358	320
55 to 64 years	401	481	532	505	343	412	457	434
65 years and over	612	706	829	767	534	612	737	666
65 to 74 years	560	656	749	713	494	577	669	624
75 years and over	683	766	923	831	588	654	817	715
Sex and Age								
Male, age-adjusted[2]	290	325	358	350	232	261	290	283
Male, crude	277	314	356	350	220	251	289	283
Under 18 years	273	302	334	340	209	231	257	262
18 to 44 years	190	203	201	205	139	148	145	151
45 to 54 years	275	316	361	324	229	260	296	265
55 to 64 years	351	428	473	460	300	367	403	396
65 to 74 years	508	614	731	680	445	539	654	597
75 years and over	711	771	907	871	616	670	807	760
Female, age-adjusted[2]	377	420	469	452	309	345	383	367
Female, crude	378	424	483	464	310	348	397	379
Under 18 years	277	285	310	322	217	221	237	252
18 to 44 years	336	377	416	415	265	298	322	323
45 to 54 years	400	451	499	450	339	384	417	372
55 to 64 years	446	529	586	546	382	453	507	469
65 to 74 years	603	692	764	741	534	609	681	647
75 years and over	666	763	934	804	571	645	823	685
Race and Age [3]								
White, age-adjusted[2]	339	380	421	408	282	315	351	336
White, crude	338	381	434	421	281	316	365	349
Under 18 years	295	306	339	341	237	243	269	270
18 to 44 years	267	301	312	319	211	239	244	249
45 to 54 years	334	386	432	389	286	330	369	326
55 to 64 years	397	480	531	505	345	416	466	440
65 to 74 years	557	641	752	727	496	568	678	642
75 years and over	689	764	936	838	598	658	835	723
Black or African American, age-adjusted[2]	309	353	459	439	204	239	314	316
Black or African American, crude	281	324	438	425	178	214	296	303
Under 18 years	193	264	315	351	100	167	198	241
18 to 44 years	260	257	373	339	158	149	228	222
45 to 54 years	387	383	486	466	281	269	329	339
55 to 64 years	414	495	645	617	294	373	478	481
65 to 74 years	553	656	821	715	429	512	667	565
75 years and over	534	745	908	845	395	568	718	682

* = Estimates are considered unreliable. Data preceded by an asterisk have a relative standard error (RSE) of 20 percent to 30 percent. Data not shown have an RSE greater than 30 percent.   [1]All places includes visits to physician offices and hospital outpatient and emergency departments.   [2]Estimates are age adjusted to the year 2000 standard population using six age groups: under 18 years, 18 to 44 years, 45 to 54 years, 55 to 64 years, 65 to 74 years, and 75 years and over.   [3]Estimates by racial group should be used with caution because information on race was collected from medical records. In 2010, race data were missing and imputed for 23 percent of visits to physician offices, 14 percent of visits to hospital outpatient departments, and 11 percent of visits to hospital emergency departments.

Table 3-50B. Visits to Hospital Outpatient Departments and Hospital Emergency Departments, by Age, Sex, and Race, Selected Years, 1995–2010

(Number; rate.)

Age, sex, and race	Hospital outpatient departments				Hospital emergency departments			
	1995	2000	2009	2010	1995	2000	2009	2010
Number of Visits in Thousands								
Age								
Total	67,232	83,289	96,132	100,742	96,545	108,017	136,072	129,843
Under 18 years	17,636	21,076	22,418	24,913	26,657	27,630	33,173	29,815
18 to 44 years	24,299	26,947	29,535	28,159	41,820	45,816	53,784	52,697
45 to 64 years	14,811	20,772	29,083	27,739	13,978	18,339	29,297	27,877
45 to 54 years	8,029	11,558	15,310	13,639	8,595	11,201	17,271	16,581
55 to 64 years	6,782	9,214	13,774	14,100	5,383	7,138	12,026	11,296
65 years and over	10,486	14,494	15,096	19,932	14,090	16,232	19,818	19,454
65 to 74 years	6,004	7,515	8,036	10,675	6,057	6,543	8,396	8,199
75 years and over	4,482	6,979	7,060	9,257	8,033	9,690	11,423	11,255
Number of Visits per 100 Persons								
Total, age-adjusted[1]	26	31	31	33	37	40	46	43
Total, crude	26	30	32	33	37	39	45	43
Under 18 years	25	29	30	33	38	38	45	40
18 to 44 years	22	25	27	25	39	42	49	48
45 to 64 years	29	34	37	35	27	30	37	35
45 to 54 years	26	31	35	31	28	30	39	38
55 to 64 years	33	39	40	39	26	30	35	32
65 years and over	33	44	40	51	45	50	52	50
65 to 74 years	33	42	39	50	33	37	41	39
75 years and over	34	47	41	52	61	65	66	64
Sex and Age								
Male, age-adjusted[1]	21	26	25	27	37	38	42	40
Male, crude	21	25	26	27	36	38	42	39
Under 18 years	25	29	30	34	40	41	46	43
18 to 44 years	14	17	16	16	37	38	40	38
45 to 54 years	20	26	28	24	26	30	36	35
55 to 64 years	26	32	35	32	25	30	34	32
65 to 74 years	29	38	37	47	34	36	40	37
75 years and over	34	42	37	50	61	59	63	60
Female, age-adjusted[1]	31	35	37	38	37	41	49	47
Female, crude	31	35	38	39	37	41	48	46
Under 18 years	25	29	30	33	35	35	43	37
18 to 44 years	31	33	38	35	40	46	57	57
45 to 54 years	32	36	41	37	29	31	42	40
55 to 64 years	38	45	44	46	26	31	35	31
65 to 74 years	36	46	41	54	32	37	42	40
75 years and over	34	49	43	53	61	69	68	66
Race and Age[2]								
White, age-adjusted[1]	23	28	29	31	34	37	41	41
White, crude	23	28	29	32	34	37	41	40
Under 18 years	23	27	29	33	35	36	40	39
18 to 44 years	20	23	24	25	36	39	43	45
45 to 54 years	23	28	30	28	25	28	34	34
55 to 64 years	28	36	34	36	24	28	30	29
65 to 74 years	29	38	35	48	32	35	38	37
75 years and over	31	44	36	52	60	63	64	62
Black or African American, age-adjusted[1]	48	51	59	51	58	62	85	73
Black or African American, crude	45	48	58	50	58	62	84	72
Under 18 years	39	40	42	48	53	57	75	62
18 to 44 years	38	40	50	37	64	68	94	81
45 to 54 years	55	61	74	54	51	53	83	73
55 to 64 years	73	70	91	73	47	52	76	62
65 to 74 years	*77	85	*81	*85	47	59	73	66
75 years and over	66	85	*	*74	73	92	95	89

* = Estimates are considered unreliable. Data preceded by an asterisk have a relative standard error (RSE) of 20 percent to 30 percent. Data not shown have an RSE greater than 30 percent. [1]Estimates are age adjusted to the year 2000 standard population using six age groups: under 18 years, 18 to 44 years, 45 to 54 years, 55 to 64 years, 65 to 74 years, and 75 years and over. [2]Estimates by racial group should be used with caution because information on race was collected from medical records. In 2010, race data were missing and imputed for 23 percent of visits to physician offices, 14 percent of visits to hospital outpatient departments, and 11 percent of visits to hospital emergency departments.

Table 3-51A. Visits to Primary Care Generalist and Specialist Physicians, by Selected Characteristics and Type of Physician, Selected Years, 1980–2010

(Percent.)

| Age, sex, and race | Type of primary care generalist physician[1] | | | | | | | | | | | | | | |
| | All primary care generalists | | | | | General and family practice | | | | | Internal medicine | | | | |
	1980	1990	2000	2009	2010	1980	1990	2000	2009	2010	1980	1990	2000	2009	2010
Age															
Total	66.2	63.6	58.9	55.9	55.2	33.5	29.9	24.1	23.1	21.1	12.1	13.8	15.3	14.8	13.9
Under 18 years	77.8	79.5	79.7	78.8	80.9	26.1	26.5	19.9	16.3	15.3	2.0	2.9	*	*	*
18 to 44 years	65.3	65.2	62.1	61.5	62.7	34.3	31.9	28.2	29.7	27.8	8.6	11.8	12.7	11.0	11.6
45 to 64 years	60.2	55.5	51.2	48.6	46.7	36.3	32.1	26.4	25.5	23.1	19.5	18.6	20.1	18.0	18.5
45 to 54 years	60.2	55.6	52.3	50.9	48.7	37.4	32.0	27.8	27.5	26.2	17.1	17.1	18.7	17.1	15.7
55 to 64 years	60.2	55.5	49.9	46.4	44.8	35.4	32.1	24.7	23.5	20.4	21.8	20.0	21.7	19.0	21.0
65 years and over	61.6	52.6	46.5	43.9	38.3	37.5	28.1	20.2	18.8	16.4	22.7	23.3	24.5	23.5	20.5
65 to 74 years	61.2	52.7	46.6	41.9	37.3	37.4	28.1	19.7	19.9	17.5	22.1	23.0	24.5	20.0	18.2
75 years and over	62.3	52.4	46.4	45.9	39.2	37.6	28.0	20.8	17.7	15.4	23.5	23.7	24.5	26.9	22.8
Sex and Age															
Male															
Under 18 years	77.3	78.1	77.7	77.6	80.1	25.6	24.1	18.3	15.2	15.7	2.0	3.0	*	*	*
18 to 44 years	50.8	51.8	51.5	52.4	51.7	38.0	35.9	34.2	36.6	33.7	11.5	15.0	14.4	14.1	16.4
45 to 64 years	55.6	50.6	49.4	45.2	43.7	34.4	31.0	28.7	26.4	24.4	20.5	19.2	19.8	18.7	19.1
65 years and over	58.2	51.2	43.1	38.6	36.6	35.6	27.7	19.3	18.3	16.2	22.3	23.3	23.8	20.1	20.3
Female															
Under 18 years	78.5	81.1	82.0	80.2	81.7	26.6	29.1	21.7	17.6	14.9	2.0	2.8	*	*	*
18 to 44 years	72.1	71.3	67.2	65.6	67.9	32.5	30.0	25.3	26.6	25.0	7.3	10.3	11.9	9.6	9.4
45 to 64 years	63.4	58.8	52.5	51.1	48.9	37.7	32.8	24.9	24.9	22.2	18.9	18.2	20.2	17.6	18.1
65 years and over	63.9	53.5	48.9	47.8	39.6	38.7	28.3	20.9	19.2	16.7	22.9	23.3	25.0	26.0	20.5
Race and Age[2]															
White															
Under 18 years	77.6	79.2	78.5	78.1	79.6	26.4	27.1	21.2	16.3	15.6	2.0	2.3	*	*	*
18 to 44 years	64.8	64.4	61.4	60.4	61.2	34.5	31.9	29.2	30.3	27.9	8.6	10.6	11.0	10.1	11.1
45 to 64 years	59.6	54.2	49.3	47.6	45.2	36.0	31.5	27.3	25.9	22.8	19.2	17.6	17.1	17.0	17.5
65 years and over	61.4	51.9	45.1	43.2	37.6	36.6	27.5	20.3	18.7	16.6	23.3	23.1	23.0	22.9	19.7
Black or African American															
Under 18 years	79.9	85.5	87.3	80.8	88.0	23.7	20.2	*	*15.5	*16.5	*2.2	9.8	*	*	*
18 to 44 years	68.5	68.3	65.0	64.4	72.6	31.7	31.9	22.0	26.6	29.4	9.0	18.1	20.9	*15.2	*14.0
45 to 64 years	66.1	61.6	61.7	50.0	57.0	38.6	31.2	23.3	23.4	26.7	22.6	26.9	35.9	*21.4	24.5
65 years and over	64.6	58.6	52.8	45.7	45.2	49.0	28.9	*18.5	*15.8	*18.6	14.2	28.7	33.4	*28.6	*25.4

NOTE: This table presents data on visits to physician offices and excludes visits to other sites, such as hospital outpatient and emergency departments.

X = Not applicable.   * = Figure does not meet standards of reliability or precision. Data preceded by an asterisk have a relative standard error (RSE) of 20 percent to 30 percent. Data not shown have a RSE greater than 30 percent. [1]Type of physician is based on physician's self-designated primary area of practice. Primary care generalist physicians are defined as practitioners in the fields of general and family practice, general internal medicine, general obstetrics and gynecology, and general pediatrics and exclude primary care specialists. Primary care generalists in general and family practice exclude primary care specialties, such as sports medicine and geriatrics. Primary care internal medicine physicians exclude internal medicine specialists, such as allergists, cardiologists, and endocrinologists. Primary care obstetrics and gynecology physicians exclude obstetrics and gynecology specialties, such as gynecological oncology, maternal and fetal medicine, obstetrics and gynecology critical care medicine, and reproductive endocrinology. Primary care pediatricians exclude pediatric specialists, such as adolescent medicine specialists, neonatologists, pediatric allergists, and pediatric cardiologists. [2]Estimates by racial group should be used with caution because information on race was collected from medical records. In 2010, race data were missing and imputed for 23 percent of visits.

Table 3-51B. Visits to Primary Care Generalist and Specialist Physicians, by Selected Characteristics and Type of Physician, Selected Years, 1980–2010

(Percent.)

Age, sex, and race	Type of primary care generalist physician[1]										Specialty care physicians				
	Obstetrics and gynecology					Pediatrics									
	1980	1990	2000	2009	2010	1980	1990	2000	2009	2010	1980	1990	2000	2009	2010
Age															
Total	9.6	8.7	7.8	7.0	7.8	10.9	11.2	11.7	11.1	12.4	33.8	36.4	41.1	44.1	44.8
Under 18 years	1.3	1.2	*1.1	0.8	*1.3	48.5	48.9	57.3	60.5	63.4	22.2	20.5	20.3	21.2	19.1
18 to 44 years	21.7	20.8	20.4	19.8	22.3	0.7	0.7	*0.9	*1.1	1.0	34.7	34.8	37.9	38.5	37.3
45 to 64 years	4.2	4.6	4.5	4.9	4.9	*	*	*	*	*	39.8	44.5	48.8	51.4	53.3
45 to 54 years	5.6	6.3	5.6	6.0	6.7	*	*	*	*	*	39.8	44.4	47.7	49.1	51.3
55 to 64 years	2.9	3.1	3.3	3.8	3.3	*	*	*	*	*	39.8	44.5	50.1	53.6	55.2
65 years and over	1.4	1.1	1.5	*1.5	1.3	*	*	*	*	*	38.4	47.4	53.5	56.1	61.7
65 to 74 years	1.7	1.6	2.0	*1.8	1.7	*	*	*	*	*	38.8	47.3	53.4	58.1	62.7
75 years and over	1.0	*0.6	*1.0	*1.1	*1.0	*	*	*	*	*	37.7	47.6	53.6	54.1	60.8
Sex and Age															
Male															
Under 18 years	X	X	X	X	X	49.4	50.7	58.0	61.2	63.7	22.7	21.9	22.3	22.4	19.9
18 to 44 years	X	X	X	X	X	1.0	0.7	*1.7	*1.8	*1.4	49.2	48.2	48.5	47.6	48.3
45 to 64 years	X	X	X	X	X	*	*	*	*	*	44.4	49.4	50.6	54.8	56.3
65 years and over	X	X	X	X	X	*	*	*	*	*	41.8	48.8	56.9	61.4	63.4
Female															
Under 18 years	2.5	2.3	2.1	1.7	*2.8	47.4	46.9	56.5	59.8	63.1	21.5	18.9	18.0	19.8	18.3
18 to 44 years	31.7	30.4	29.6	28.7	32.5	0.6	0.7	*	*	*0.9	27.9	28.7	32.8	34.4	32.1
45 to 64 years	6.7	7.7	7.3	8.4	8.5	*	*	*	*	*	36.6	41.2	47.5	48.9	51.1
65 years and over	2.1	1.8	2.6	*2.5	2.4	*	*	*	*	*	36.1	46.5	51.1	52.2	60.4
Race and Age[2]															
White															
Under 18 years	1.1	1.0	*1.2	*0.7	*1.3	48.2	48.8	54.7	60.1	61.7	22.4	20.8	21.5	21.9	20.4
18 to 44 years	21.0	21.1	20.4	18.8	21.1	0.7	0.7	*0.8	*1.2	*1.1	35.2	35.6	38.6	39.6	38.8
45 to 64 years	4.1	4.8	4.7	4.5	4.7	*	*	*	*	*	40.4	45.8	50.7	52.4	54.8
65 years and over	1.4	1.2	1.5	*1.4	*1.3	*	*	*	*	*	38.6	48.1	54.9	56.8	62.4
Black or African American															
Under 18 years	2.8	*3.4	*	*	*	51.2	52.1	75.0	62.7	70.2	20.1	14.5	*12.7	*19.2	*12.0
18 to 44 years	27.1	17.9	20.7	22.1	28.4	*	*	*	*	*	31.5	31.7	35.0	35.6	27.4
45 to 64 years	4.8	3.5	*2.4	*5.1	*5.6	*	*	*	*	*	33.9	38.4	38.3	50.0	43.0
65 years and over	*	*	*	*	*1.2	*	*	*	*	*	35.4	41.4	47.2	54.3	54.8

NOTE: This table presents data on visits to physician offices and excludes visits to other sites, such as hospital outpatient and emergency departments.

X = Not applicable.   * = Figure does not meet standards of reliability or precision. Data preceded by an asterisk have a relative standard error (RSE) of 20 percent to 30 percent. Data not shown have a RSE greater than 30 percent.   [1]Type of physician is based on physician's self-designated primary area of practice. Primary care generalist physicians are defined as practitioners in the fields of general and family practice, general internal medicine, general obstetrics and gynecology, and general pediatrics and exclude primary care specialists. Primary care generalists in general and family practice exclude primary care specialties, such as sports medicine and geriatrics. Primary care internal medicine physicians exclude internal medicine specialists, such as allergists, cardiologists, and endocrinologists. Primary care obstetrics and gynecology physicians exclude obstetrics and gynecology specialties, such as gynecological oncology, maternal and fetal medicine, obstetrics and gynecology critical care medicine, and reproductive endocrinology. Primary care pediatricians exclude pediatric specialists, such as adolescent medicine specialists, neonatologists, pediatric allergists, and pediatric cardiologists.   [2]Estimates by racial group should be used with caution because information on race was collected from medical records. In 2010, race data were missing and imputed for 23 percent of visits.

Table 3-52. Dental Visits in the Past Year, by Selected Characteristics, Selected Years, 1997–2011

(Percent.)

Characteristic	2 years and over				2 to 17 years				18 to 64 years				65 years and over[1]			
	1997	2000	2010	2011	1997	2000	2010	2011	1997	2000	2010	2011	1997	2000	2010	2011
Total with Dental Visit [2,3]	65.1	66.2	64.7	66.0	72.7	74.1	78.9	81.4	64.1	65.1	61.1	61.6	54.8	56.6	57.7	61.2
Sex																
Male	62.9	63.5	61.7	63.5	72.3	73.7	78.3	81.4	60.4	60.7	56.8	57.5	55.4	56.1	56.2	61.2
Female	67.1	68.8	67.5	68.3	73.0	74.6	79.6	81.4	67.7	69.4	65.4	65.5	54.4	56.9	58.9	61.2
Race [3]																
White only	66.4	67.9	65.6	66.7	74.0	75.8	79.2	81.8	65.7	67.2	62.4	62.6	56.8	58.4	59.3	63.1
Black or African American only	58.9	59.5	58.8	61.4	68.8	70.0	79.0	81.3	57.0	57.1	53.1	55.5	35.4	38.2	40.6	44.9
American Indian or Alaska Native only	55.1	58.6	57.4	61.6	66.8	71.3	73.2	86.9	49.9	55.0	49.8	53.0	*	*	72.2	46.7
Asian only	62.5	67.1	66.5	66.3	69.9	72.8	74.8	76.0	60.3	65.6	64.6	63.9	53.9	60.6	61.9	61.7
Native Hawaiian and Other Pacific Islander only	NA	*	*	*	NA	*	*	*	NA	*	*	*	NA	*	*	*
Two or more races	NA	65.1	65.2	66.5	NA	71.4	77.9	80.5	NA	60.5	54.7	56.6	NA	57.4	48.1	50.0
Black or African American; White	NA	63.5	72.5	71.9	NA	65.7	78.4	81.3	NA	60.7	62.1	56.1	NA	*	*	*
American Indian or Alaska Native; White	NA	61.7	54.7	56.3	NA	63.4	70.0	72.2	NA	61.6	49.0	52.3	NA	*57.8	*54.5	48.6
Hispanic Origin and Race [4]																
Hispanic or Latino	54.0	52.3	56.5	57.2	61.0	60.6	74.8	79.7	50.8	48.6	48.5	46.5	47.8	44.5	42.1	46.6
Not Hispanic or Latino	66.4	68.2	66.2	67.6	74.7	76.8	80.1	81.9	65.7	67.5	63.4	64.3	55.2	57.2	59.0	62.4
White only	68.0	69.9	67.6	69.0	76.4	78.9	80.9	82.6	67.5	69.4	65.4	66.1	57.2	59.1	60.9	64.4
Black or African American only	58.8	59.4	58.7	61.4	68.8	70.0	79.2	81.4	56.9	57.2	53.1	55.7	35.3	38.0	40.5	45.4
Percent of Poverty Level [5]																
Below 100 percent	50.5	50.4	50.6	51.7	62.0	62.4	73.2	75.5	46.9	46.8	41.0	41.3	31.5	33.3	32.8	36.7
100 percent to 199 percent	50.8	52.2	51.6	52.3	62.5	66.1	73.4	77.9	48.3	48.4	44.1	43.0	40.8	43.0	43.8	44.2
200 percent to 399 percent	66.2	65.6	63.5	65.2	76.1	75.5	79.0	81.4	63.4	62.2	59.6	60.4	60.7	62.8	57.9	62.1
400 percent or more	78.9	79.5	79.3	80.9	85.7	85.9	88.0	89.6	77.7	78.5	77.5	78.9	74.7	73.8	77.2	80.5
Hispanic Origin and Race and Percent of Poverty Level [4,5]																
Hispanic or Latino																
Below 100 percent	45.7	43.4	50.8	52.4	55.9	54.2	74.3	79.0	39.2	36.8	34.7	33.6	33.6	31.3	32.4	36.3
100 percent to 199 percent	47.2	45.5	50.8	51.8	53.8	56.9	71.1	78.5	43.5	39.2	40.2	37.5	47.9	42.9	39.5	40.7
200 percent to 399 percent	61.2	57.2	59.1	59.6	70.5	65.6	76.5	77.6	57.5	53.7	54.1	53.6	57.0	54.8	46.0	49.9
400 percent or more	73.0	70.0	73.3	73.3	82.4	78.4	84.2	90.3	70.8	68.7	71.6	68.4	64.9	53.4	54.3	72.1
Not Hispanic or Latino																
White only																
Below 100 percent	51.7	53.6	49.3	49.8	64.4	65.0	69.1	70.9	50.6	53.3	44.4	44.4	32.0	37.2	36.4	37.5
100 percent to 199 percent	52.4	53.8	52.7	51.0	66.1	69.7	75.3	75.5	50.4	51.7	47.2	43.8	42.3	43.4	45.4	45.4
200 percent to 399 percent	67.5	67.6	64.7	66.4	77.1	78.3	79.6	82.7	65.0	64.4	61.4	61.9	61.9	63.9	59.8	63.8
400 percent or more	79.7	80.8	79.8	82.4	86.8	87.5	88.6	90.4	78.5	79.7	77.9	80.6	75.5	76.1	78.8	82.2
Black or African American only																
Below 100 percent	52.8	51.8	52.0	54.3	66.1	67.1	78.0	77.2	46.2	44.4	39.7	43.4	27.7	21.7	20.9	30.9
100 percent to 199 percent	48.7	52.4	50.0	55.1	61.2	67.3	75.9	83.3	46.3	48.0	41.5	45.9	26.9	35.2	33.6	33.4
200 percent to 399 percent	63.3	62.3	61.2	64.3	75.0	74.0	81.2	83.7	60.7	58.4	57.2	60.0	41.5	48.4	45.3	50.5
400 percent or more	74.6	72.8	77.2	74.8	81.8	74.2	87.2	86.0	73.4	73.3	75.9	73.1	66.1	60.5	69.8	70.6
Disability Measure [6]																
Any basic actions difficulty or complex activity limitation	X	X	X	X	X	X	X	X	55.1	57.3	53.5	52.2	49.0	50.7	50.7	54.7
Any basic actions difficulty	X	X	X	X	X	X	X	X	54.7	57.0	53.2	51.9	48.7	50.7	50.5	54.5
Any complex activity limitation	X	X	X	X	X	X	X	X	51.0	52.5	47.4	48.2	44.6	44.4	43.1	48.5
No disability	X	X	X	X	X	X	X	X	67.4	67.7	64.2	65.1	64.2	65.7	68.8	72.2
Geographic Region																
Northeast	69.6	72.3	70.1	71.5	77.5	81.1	83.8	84.2	69.6	72.1	67.9	69.2	55.5	58.1	61.5	63.6
Midwest	68.4	69.9	67.3	67.6	76.4	77.2	80.8	80.6	67.4	69.2	64.3	64.2	57.8	58.6	58.2	61.5
South	60.2	61.0	60.9	62.6	68.0	69.5	77.4	81.2	59.4	59.8	56.5	56.9	49.0	50.8	54.1	58.7
West	65.0	65.3	63.9	65.2	71.5	72.0	76.1	80.5	62.9	63.0	60.2	60.3	61.9	63.1	59.8	63.0
Location of Residence																
Within MSA[7]	66.7	67.5	65.9	67.1	73.6	74.3	79.3	81.9	65.7	66.5	62.4	62.6	57.6	58.9	59.4	63.9
Outside MSA[7]	59.1	61.2	58.4	60.0	69.3	73.3	76.4	78.6	58.0	59.7	53.8	55.9	46.1	49.3	51.3	50.9

NA = Not available.   X = Not applicable.   * = Estimates do not meet the standards of reliability and precision.   [1]Based on the 1997-2011 National Health Interview Surveys, about 23 to 30 percent of persons 65 years and over were edentulous (having lost all their natural teeth). In 1997-2011, about 69 to 73 percent of older dentate persons, compared with 17 to 23 percent of older edentate persons, had a dental visit in the past year.   [2]Respondents were asked, "About how long has it been since you last saw or talked to a dentist?"   [3]Includes all other races not shown separately and unknown disability status.   [4]The race groups White, Black, American Indian or Alaska Native, Asian, Native Hawaiian or Other Pacific Islander, and two or more races include persons of Hispanic and non-Hispanic origin. Persons of Hispanic origin may be of any race.   [5]Percent of poverty level is based on family income and family size and composition using U.S. Census Bureau poverty thresholds. Missing family income data were imputed for 1997 and beyond.   [6]Any basic actions difficulty or complex activity limitation is defined as having one or more of the following limitations or difficulties: movement difficulty, emotional difficulty, sensory (seeing or hearing) difficulty, cognitive difficulty, self-care (activities of daily living or instrumental activities of daily living) limitation, social limitation, or work limitation.   [7]MSA = metropolitan statistical area.

Table 3-53A. Prescription Drug Use in the Past 30 Days, by Sex, Age, and Race, Selected Years, 1988–1994 Through 2007–2010

(Percent.)

Sex and age	All persons[1]				White only			
	1988–1994	2001–2004	2005–2008	2007–2010	1988–1994	2001–2004	2005–2008	2007–2010
PERCENT OF POPULATION WITH AT LEAST ONE PRESCRIPTION DRUG IN PAST 30 DAYS								
Both Sexes, Age-Adjusted[2]	39.1	46.7	47.2	47.5	41.1	50.6	52.0	52.8
Male	32.7	41.6	41.8	42.8	34.2	45.0	46.1	47.5
Female	45.0	51.5	52.4	52.0	47.6	56.0	57.9	57.9
Both Sexes, Crude	37.8	46.5	47.9	48.5	41.4	52.6	55.0	56.2
Male	30.6	40.5	41.7	43.0	33.5	46.0	48.4	50.3
Female	44.6	52.2	53.9	53.8	48.9	59.0	61.5	61.8
Under 18 years	20.5	23.9	25.3	24.0	22.9	27.3	29.9	28.1
18 to 44 years	31.3	37.7	37.8	38.7	34.3	43.5	45.1	47.5
45 to 64 years	54.8	66.2	64.8	66.2	55.5	68.6	67.7	69.7
65 years and over	73.6	87.3	90.1	89.7	74.0	88.3	91.1	90.2
Male								
Under 18 years	20.4	25.3	25.3	24.5	22.3	29.4	29.2	27.4
18 to 44 years	21.5	29.2	27.5	29.5	23.5	33.4	33.3	37.1
45 to 64 years	47.2	58.7	59.3	61.3	48.1	60.8	62.3	5.2
65 years and over	67.2	83.6	89.7	88.8	67.4	84.8	91.6	90.1
Female								
Under 18 years	20.6	22.4	25.2	23.5	23.6	25.1	30.7	28.8
18 to 44 years	40.7	45.9	47.9	47.6	44.7	53.5	56.6	57.6
45 to 64 years	62.0	73.4	70.2	70.8	62.6	76.3	73.0	74.1
65 years and over	78.3	90.1	90.5	90.4	78.8	91.0	90.7	90.2
PERCENT OF POPULATION WITH THREE OR MORE PRESCRIPTION DRUGS IN PAST 30 DAYS								
Both Sexes, Age-Adjusted[2]	11.8	20.2	20.8	20.8	12.4	21.8	22.3	22.4
Male	9.4	17.3	18.3	19.1	9.9	18.7	19.5	20.6
Female	13.9	22.8	23.2	22.5	14.6	24.8	25.1	24.3
Both Sexes, Crude	11.0	19.9	21.4	21.7	12.5	23.6	25.3	25.8
Male	8.3	16.4	17.8	19.0	9.5	19.5	21.3	22.9
Female	13.6	23.4	24.8	24.2	15.4	27.6	29.1	28.6
Under 18 years	2.4	4.0	4.4	3.8	3.2	5.0	5.3	4.0
18 to 44 years	5.7	10.2	9.8	9.7	6.3	12.2	12.1	12.3
45 to 64 years	20.0	34.2	34.1	34.4	20.9	35.6	35.6	36.6
65 years and over	35.3	59.8	65.0	66.6	35.0	62.0	65.7	66.8
Male								
Under 18 years	2.6	4.1	5.0	4.4	3.3	4.9	5.7	4.5
18 to 44 years	3.6	8.0	6.2	7.1	4.1	9.8	8.0	9.1
45 to 64 years	15.1	28.3	28.6	30.4	15.8	29.1	29.4	32.7
65 years and over	31.3	54.2	64.6	66.8	30.9	56.4	66.3	67.8
Female								
Under 18 years	2.3	3.9	3.8	3.1	3.0	5.2	4.8	3.6
18 to 44 years	7.6	12.3	13.3	12.2	8.5	14.7	16.1	15.3
45 to 64 years	24.7	39.9	39.4	38.1	25.8	41.9	41.8	40.4
65 years and over	38.2	64.0	65.3	66.4	38.0	66.2	65.3	66.1
PERCENT OF POPULATION WITH FIVE OR MORE PRESCRIPTION DRUGS IN PAST 30 DAYS								
Both Sexes, Age-Adjusted[2]	4.0	9.2	10.2	10.1	4.2	9.8	10.7	10.7
Male	2.9	7.9	8.9	9.2	3.1	8.4	9.3	9.8
Female	4.9	10.4	11.5	11.0	5.1	11.1	12.1	11.6
Both Sexes, Crude	3.6	9.0	10.5	10.6	4.2	10.8	12.4	12.6
Male	2.5	7.3	8.6	9.1	2.9	8.8	10.3	11.0
Female	4.7	10.7	12.4	12.1	5.4	12.8	14.5	14.2
Under 18 years	*	0.8	1.0	0.8	*	*0.9	1.2	0.9
18 to 44 years	1.2	3.3	3.4	3.1	1.4	3.8	4.2	3.9
45 to 64 years	7.4	15.7	17.0	16.8	7.8	16.3	17.4	17.7
65 years and over	13.8	33.3	38.3	39.7	13.9	35.4	38.6	39.4
Male								
Under 18 years	*	*0.8	*1.1	0.8	*	*	*	*
18 to 44 years	*0.8	2.6	*1.8	2.1	*	2.9	*2.4	*2.8
45 to 64 years	4.8	12.5	13.7	14.4	5.0	13.2	13.8	15.2
65 years and over	11.3	30.6	38.4	39.5	11.6	31.9	39.2	39.9
Female								
Under 18 years	*	*0.7	*0.8	*0.7	*	*0.9	*	*
18 to 44 years	1.7	3.9	5.0	4.0	1.8	4.6	6.0	4.9
45 to 64 years	9.7	18.8	20.2	19.1	10.3	19.4	20.9	20.2
65 years and over	15.6	35.4	38.3	39.8	15.7	38.0	38.2	39.0

* = Figure does not meet standards of reliability or precision. Data preceded by an asterisk have a relative standard error (RSE) of 20 to 30 percent. Data not shown have an RSE of greater than 30 percent. [1]Includes persons of all races and Hispanic origins, not just those shown separately. [2]Age adjusted to the 2000 standard population using four age groups: under 18 years, 18 to 44 years, 45 to 64 years, and 65 years and over.

Table 3-53B. Prescription Drug Use in the Past 30 Days, by Sex, Age, Race and Hispanic Origin, Selected Years, 1988–1994 Through 2007–2010

(Percent.)

Sex and age	Black or African American only				Mexican[1]			
	1988–1994	2001–2004	2005–2008	2007–2010	1988–1994	2001–2004	2005–2008	2007–2010
PERCENT OF POPULATION WITH AT LEAST ONE PRESCRIPTION DRUG IN PAST 30 DAYS								
Both Sexes, Age-Adjusted [2]	36.9	40.5	42.1	33.9	31.7	34.5	32.2	33.9
Male	31.1	36.2	37.2	31.0	27.5	28.8	28.8	31.0
Female	41.4	43.8	46.0	37.0	36.0	40.5	35.6	37.0
Both Sexes, Crude	31.2	36.5	39.5	26.4	24.0	25.4	24.5	26.4
Male	25.5	31.6	33.9	23.7	20.1	20.6	21.4	23.7
Female	36.2	40.7	44.4	29.4	28.1	30.6	27.9	29.4
Under 18 years	14.8	18.0	20.8	16.8	16.1	16.3	17.0	16.8
18 to 44 years	27.8	29.4	29.4	19.4	21.1	20.9	17.7	19.4
45 to 64 years	57.5	63.4	62.6	49.7	48.1	53.8	50.1	49.7
65 years and over	74.5	80.8	89.1	86.2	67.7	79.6	76.7	86.2
Male								
Under 18 years	15.5	18.8	23.4	17.6	16.3	16.9	17.3	17.6
18 to 44 years	21.1	22.6	20.9	16.7	14.9	14.1	14.2	16.7
45 to 64 years	48.2	58.0	54.7	43.9	43.8	42.7	46.0	43.9
65 years and over	64.4	75.9	85.1	80.2	61.3	74.4	67.8	80.2
Female								
Under 18 years	14.2	17.1	18.1	16.0	16.0	15.7	16.7	16.0
18 to 44 years	33.4	35.0	36.6	22.8	28.1	28.6	22.0	22.8
45 to 64 years	64.4	67.7	69.1	55.7	52.2	65.8	54.1	55.7
65 years and over	81.3	84.0	91.7	91.1	73.0	83.9	83.9	91.1
PERCENT OF POPULATION WITH THREE OR MORE PRESCRIPTION DRUGS IN PAST 30 DAYS								
Both Sexes, Age-Adjusted [2]	12.6	17.7	20.0	15.0	9.0	14.4	13.8	15.0
Male	10.2	15.1	17.5	13.4	7.0	12.1	11.6	13.4
Female	14.3	19.7	21.8	16.6	11.0	16.7	15.9	16.6
Both Sexes, Crude	9.2	14.7	17.5	9.0	4.8	7.9	7.8	9.0
Male	7.0	11.9	14.4	7.6	3.4	6.2	6.1	7.6
Female	11.1	17.1	20.2	10.6	6.4	9.8	9.7	10.6
Under 18 years	1.5	2.8	3.6	2.6	*1.2	2.0	2.7	2.6
18 to 44 years	5.4	8.1	7.3	*3.0	3.0	4.3	2.7	*3.0
45 to 64 years	21.9	33.7	34.5	24.1	16.0	27.5	24.5	24.1
65 years and over	41.2	50.1	67.0	61.6	31.3	47.8	52.5	61.6
Male								
Under 18 years	1.7	3.4	5.3	3.1	*0.9	*1.7	3.5	3.1
18 to 44 years	4.2	6.1	*4.9	2.6	*1.8	2.6	*1.5	2.6
45 to 64 years	18.7	28.2	29.0	19.7	11.6	23.8	19.7	19.7
65 years and over	31.7	44.0	61.5	56.6	27.6	42.0	45.0	56.6
Female								
Under 18 years	*1.2	2.1	*1.9	2.1	*1.5	2.4	1.8	2.1
18 to 44 years	6.4	9.7	9.4	*3.5	4.3	*6.2	4.1	*3.5
45 to 64 years	24.3	38.1	39.1	28.5	20.3	31.4	29.0	28.5
65 years and over	47.7	54.2	70.6	65.7	34.5	52.7	58.6	65.7
PERCENT OF POPULATION WITH FIVE OR MORE PRESCRIPTION DRUGS IN PAST 30 DAYS								
Both Sexes, Age-Adjusted [2]	3.8	8.7	11.2	7.9	2.9	6.1	6.9	7.9
Male	2.9	7.6	9.4	7.2	2.0	4.8	5.9	7.2
Female	4.5	9.5	12.6	8.7	3.7	7.6	7.9	8.7
Both Sexes, Crude	2.6	7.1	9.6	4.1	1.4	2.9	3.4	4.1
Male	1.8	5.9	7.6	3.4	0.9	2.1	2.6	3.4
Female	3.3	8.2	11.4	4.9	1.9	3.8	4.4	4.9
Under 18 years	*	*0.7	*0.9	*	*	*	*0.5	*
18 to 44 years	1.0	4.1	2.8	*	*	*	*	*
45 to 64 years	7.1	16.8	20.6	12.1	5.4	12.4	11.5	21.1
65 years and over	14.3	25.4	42.0	39.4	11.6	23.4	31.1	39.4
Male								
Under 18 years	*	*	*	*	*	*	*	*
18 to 44 years	*	*3.2	*	*	*	*	*	*
45 to 64 years	5.9	15.0	17.5	10.4	*3.5	*7.8	8.7	10.4
65 years and over	9.9	22.3	35.3	36.3	*8.7	20.7	28.9	36.3
Female								
Under 18 years	*	*	*	*	*	*	*	*
18 to 44 years	1.2	4.7	3.6	*	*0.6	*	*	*
45 to 64 years	8.0	18.2	23.2	13.9	*7.2	17.2	14.2	13.9
65 years and over	17.4	27.5	46.4	41.9	14.0	25.6	32.9	41.9

* = Figure does not meet standards of reliability or precision. Data preceded by an asterisk have a relative standard error (RSE) of 20 to 30 percent. Data not shown have an RSE of greater than 30 percent. [1]Persons of Mexican origin may be of any race. [2]Age adjusted to the 2000 standard population using four age groups: under 18 years, 18 to 44 years, 45 to 64 years, and 65 years and over.

Table 3-54. Selected Prescription Drug Classes Used in the Past 30 Days, by Sex and Age, Selected Years, 1988–1994 Through 2005–2008

(Percent.)

Age group and Multum Lexicon Plus therapeutic class[1] (primary indications for use)	Total			Male			Female		
	1988–1994	2001–2004	2005–2008	1988–1994	2001–2004	2005–2008	1988–1994	2001–2004	2005–2008
All Ages									
Antihyperlipidemic agents (high cholesterol)	1.7	7.8	11.4	1.5	8.7	12.0	1.8	7.0	10.8
Analgesics (pain relief)	7.2	11.1	9.0	5.4	8.8	7.7	9.0	13.3	10.2
Antidepressants (depression and related disorders)	1.8	7.8	8.9	1.2	5.4	5.0	2.3	10.0	12.7
Beta-adrenergic blocking agents (high blood pressure, heart disease)	3.1	5.4	7.3	2.7	5.2	6.8	3.5	5.5	7.6
Proton pump inhibitors (gastrointestinal reflux, ulcers)	*	5.0	6.3	*	4.6	5.6	*	5.4	6.9
ACE inhibitors (high blood pressure, heart disease)	2.4	5.2	5.9	2.4	5.4	6.3	2.4	5.1	5.6
Sex hormones (contraceptives, menopause, hot flashes)	X	X	X	X	X	X	9.9	13.3	9.7
Diuretics (high blood pressure, heart disease, kidney disease)	3.4	4.6	5.3	2.3	3.3	4.5	4.4	5.8	6.1
Thyroid drugs (hyper- and hypothyroidism)	2.3	4.5	5.2	0.8	1.7	1.7	3.7	7.1	8.5
Antidiabetic agents (diabetes)	2.6	4.3	5.2	2.5	4.1	4.8	2.6	4.4	5.5
Bronchodilators (asthma, breathing)	2.6	3.7	4.9	2.5	3.5	4.5	2.7	4.0	5.2
Anxiolytics, sedatives, and hypnotics (generalized anxiety and related disorders)	2.8	3.8	4.5	1.9	2.8	3.2	3.6	4.8	5.7
Antihypertensive combinations (high blood pressure)	2.4	3.5	4.1	1.4	2.8	3.0	3.3	4.1	5.1
Calcium channel blocking agents (high blood pressure, heart disease)	3.6	3.8	4.0	3.4	3.4	3.6	3.8	4.2	4.4
Antihistamines (allergies)	2.7	4.4	3.8	2.2	3.8	2.9	3.2	4.9	4.6
Under 18 Years									
Bronchodilators (asthma, breathing)	3.0	4.3	5.4	3.3	4.5	6.0	2.7	4.0	4.7
Penicillins (bacterial infections)	6.1	4.1	3.8	5.9	3.9	3.4	6.4	4.3	4.2
CNS stimulants (attention deficit disorder, hyperactivity)	*0.8	3.1	3.7	*1.2	4.8	4.8	*	1.3	2.6
Antihistamines (allergies)	2.0	4.0	2.9	2.1	4.1	3.0	1.9	4.0	2.7
Leukotriene modifiers (asthma, allergies)	X	1.1	2.9	X	1.2	3.3	X	*1.0	*2.4
Upper respiratory combinations (cough and cold, congestion)	2.3	2.6	1.8	2.6	2.7	1.6	2.0	2.4	1.9
Respiratory inhalant products (asthma, chronic obstructive pulmonary disease, and related disorders)	*0.7	1.3	1.8	*	1.3	2.4	*	1.3	1.3
Adrenal cortical steroids (anti-inflammatory)	*0.5	0.9	1.6	*	*0.9	2.1	*0.5	0.8	1.1
Antidepressants (depression and related disorders)	*	1.6	1.5	*	1.8	*1.5	*	*1.4	*1.6
Analgesics (pain relief)	1.2	1.7	1.4	*1.2	1.6	1.0	1.4	1.8	2.0
Cephalosporins (bacterial infections)	1.8	1.4	1.1	1.8	*1.7	1.1	1.8	*1.1	*1.2
Macrolide derivatives (bacterial infections)	1.0	1.1	*0.9	*0.7	1.3	*1.1	*1.3	*0.9	
18 to 44 Years									
Antidepressants (depression and related disorders)	1.6	7.3	7.8	*1.0	4.1	3.6	2.3	10.4	11.9
Analgesics (pain relief)	7.2	10.0	7.7	5.1	7.5	6.5	9.1	12.5	8.9
Sex hormones (contraceptives, menopause, hot flashes)	X	X	X	X	X	X	11.7	13.8	15.7
Proton pump inhibitors (gastrointestinal reflux, ulcers)	*	3.3	3.5	*	3.0	2.8	*	3.7	4.2
Bronchodilators (asthma, breathing)	1.4	2.4	3.3	*1.1	2.2	2.3	*1.8	2.6	4.2
Antihistamines (allergies)	2.5	4.0	3.2	1.8	3.9	*1.7	3.2	4.1	4.6
Anxiolytics, sedatives, and hypnotics (generalized anxiety and related disorders)	1.4	2.9	3.2	*1.0	2.2	2.1	1.9	3.7	4.3
Anticonvulsants (epilepsy, seizure, and related disorders)	0.8	2.2	2.9	*0.6	1.9	*2.0	1.0	2.5	3.8
Thyroid drugs (hyper- and hypothyroidism)	1.4	2.3	2.8	*	*	*	2.1	4.1	4.9
Antihyperlipidemic agents (high cholesterol)	*0.4	1.8	2.5	*	2.5	3.1	*	*1.2	*2.0
Antidiabetic agents (diabetes)	*1.0	1.8	2.1	*	1.6	1.7	*1.0	2.0	2.4
ACE inhibitors (high blood pressure, heart disease)	0.7	1.6	1.9	*0.9	2.1	1.7	*0.6	*1.2	2.0
Penicillins (bacterial infections)	3.1	2.1	1.8	2.3	*1.6	*1.1	3.8	2.7	2.5
Muscle relaxants (muscle spasm and related disorders)	1.0	1.7	1.6	*1.3	*1.5	*1.1	*0.7	1.9	2.0
Beta-adrenergic blocking agents (high blood pressure, heart disease)	1.1	1.4	1.4	*0.9	*1.5	*1.2	1.3	1.2	1.5
45 to 64 Years									
Antihyperlipidemic agents (high cholesterol)	4.3	15.3	19.6	4.4	18.7	21.2	4.2	12.1	18.0
Antidepressants (depression and related disorders)	3.5	14.1	15.3	*2.3	10.7	8.5	4.6	17.3	21.9
Analgesics (pain relief)	11.9	18.6	14.0	9.2	16.0	12.3	14.3	21.1	15.7
Beta-adrenergic blocking agents (high blood pressure, heart disease)	6.6	9.8	11.0	7.0	9.7	10.5	6.2	9.9	11.6
Proton pump inhibitors (gastrointestinal reflux, ulcers)	*	9.0	10.9	*	8.4	10.6	*	9.5	11.2
ACE inhibitors (high blood pressure, heart disease)	5.2	9.8	10.3	5.7	10.5	11.4	4.6	9.2	9.3
Antidiabetic agents (diabetes)	5.5	7.8	9.4	5.9	8.4	9.5	5.1	7.2	9.3
Thyroid drugs (hyper- and hypothyroidism)	4.7	8.2	8.5	*1.2	*3.1	*2.9	8.1	12.9	13.9
Sex hormones (contraceptives, menopause, hot flashes)	X	X	X	X	X	X	19.9	23.9	11.2
Antihypertensive combinations (high blood pressure)	5.3	6.9	8.1	3.3	6.6	6.3	7.1	7.3	9.7
Anxiolytics, sedatives, and hypnotics (generalized anxiety and related disorders)	6.0	6.8	7.8	4.3	*5.3	6.2	7.5	8.3	9.3
Diuretics (high blood pressure, heart disease, kidney disease)	6.1	7.2	6.7	4.8	4.8	6.0	7.3	9.6	7.5
Calcium channel blocking agents (high blood pressure, heart disease)	7.0	5.7	6.1	8.2	5.6	5.3	5.9	5.8	6.9
Anticonvulsants (epilepsy, seizure, and related disorders)	2.7	5.3	6.0	*2.5	4.5	5.0	2.9	6.0	7.0
65 Years and Over									
Antihyperlipidemic agents (high cholesterol)	5.9	30.2	44.5	5.3	32.8	50.6	6.4	28.3	40.0
Beta-adrenergic blocking agents (high blood pressure, heart disease)	11.8	21.5	32.0	10.4	22.4	34.8	12.8	20.9	29.9
Diuretics (high blood pressure, heart disease, kidney disease)	16.2	21.4	24.5	12.2	18.3	24.6	19.1	23.7	24.4
ACE inhibitors (high blood pressure, heart disease)	9.5	19.7	21.0	9.8	21.1	25.1	9.3	18.6	18.1
Analgesics (pain relief)	13.8	20.8	18.1	11.4	16.8	17.8	15.6	23.7	18.3
Calcium channel blocking agents (high blood pressure, heart disease)	16.1	18.7	17.1	14.5	17.1	17.3	17.3	19.9	17.0
Proton pump inhibitors (gastrointestinal reflux, ulcers)	*	13.3	17.0	*	13.7	16.9	*	13.0	17.1
Antidiabetic agents (diabetes)	9.0	14.5	16.0	9.0	14.9	15.9	9.0	14.2	16.1
Thyroid drugs (hyper- and hypothyroidism)	7.1	14.5	15.5	3.5	8.2	6.2	9.8	19.2	22.4
Antidepressants (depression and related disorders)	3.0	10.4	14.2	*2.3	8.3	10.0	3.5	11.9	17.3
Antihypertensive combinations (high blood pressure)	9.6	11.9	13.2	6.0	8.6	9.6	12.2	14.4	15.8
Angiotensin II inhibitors (high blood pressure, heart disease)	X	7.5	10.7	X	6.6	9.7	X	8.2	11.5
Anxiolytics, sedatives, and hypnotics (generalized anxiety and related disorders)	7.8	8.6	9.8	6.1	5.9	7.1	9.1	10.5	11.8
Bisphosphonates (osteoporosis and related disorders)	*	7.1	8.4	*	*1.4	*	*	11.3	13.8
Antiadrenergic agents, peripherally acting (prostate conditions)[2]	X	X	X	2.8	14.4	15.9	X	X	X

Table 3-54. Selected Prescription Drug Classes Used in the Past 30 Days, by Sex and Age, Selected Years, 1988–1994 Through 2005–2008—Continued

(Percent.)

Age group and Multum Lexicon Plus therapeutic class[1] (primary indications for use)	Total			Male			Female		
	1988–1994	2001–2004	2005–2008	1988–1994	2001–2004	2005–2008	1988–1994	2001–2004	2005–2008
65 to 74 Years									
Antihyperlipidemic agents (high cholesterol)	7.3	33.5	44.3	6.2	36.2	52.1	8.1	31.1	38.2
Beta-adrenergic blocking agents (high blood pressure, heart disease)	11.3	20.9	29.0	10.6	22.7	32.2	11.9	19.3	26.4
Diuretics (high blood pressure, heart disease, kidney disease)	14.2	16.8	21.0	10.8	15.0	19.6	17.0	18.3	22.1
ACE inhibitors (high blood pressure, heart disease)	9.6	19.6	19.5	10.6	22.4	24.2	8.9	17.2	15.8
Analgesics (pain relief)	13.0	21.8	18.6	10.5	17.8	16.5	15.0	25.3	20.3
Antidiabetic agents (diabetes)	8.8	16.0	17.8	8.0	16.6	18.2	9.4	15.4	17.5
Proton pump inhibitors (gastrointestinal reflux, ulcers)	*	13.6	16.9	*	14.2	17.0	*	13.0	16.8
Antidepressants (depression and related disorders)	2.8	10.4	15.0	*2.3	7.1	9.6	3.1	13.2	19.3
Calcium channel blocking agents (high blood pressure, heart disease)	15.0	16.7	14.0	14.0	16.5	15.5	15.8	16.8	12.9
Antihypertensive combinations (high blood pressure)	8.1	11.5	13.7	4.8	8.1	11.0	10.8	14.4	15.8
Thyroid drugs (hyper- and hypothyroidism)	6.6	12.9	13.1	*3.8	7.0	4.3	8.9	18.0	19.9
Angiotensin II inhibitors (high blood pressure, heart disease)	X	6.9	9.7	X	6.0	9.2	X	7.7	10.1
Anxiolytics, sedatives, and hypnotics (generalized anxiety and related disorders)	6.9	8.4	9.4	6.0	*5.7	6.8	7.6	10.7	11.4
Antiadrenergic agents, peripherally acting (prostate conditions)[2]	X	X	X	*2.6	14.9	13.1	X	X	X
Bisphosphonates (osteoporosis and related disorders)	*	6.2	7.2	*	*	*	*	10.8	12.5
Anticonvulsants (epilepsy, seizure, and related disorders)	3.0	6.0	7.1	*2.7	4.1	5.7	3.2	*7.6	8.2
75 Years and Over									
Antihyperlipidemic agents (high cholesterol)	3.8	26.5	44.8	*3.5	28.2	48.7	4.0	25.4	42.0
Beta-adrenergic blocking agents (high blood pressure, heart disease)	12.5	22.3	35.6	9.8	22.0	38.1	14.1	22.5	33.8
Diuretics (high blood pressure, heart disease, kidney disease)	19.2	26.7	28.7	14.7	22.9	31.1	21.9	29.1	27.0
ACE inhibitors (high blood pressure, heart disease)	9.3	19.8	22.9	8.5	19.3	26.2	9.8	20.1	20.6
Calcium channel blocking agents (high blood pressure, heart disease)	17.8	21.0	20.8	15.3	17.9	19.6	19.2	22.9	21.6
Thyroid drugs (hyper- and hypothyroidism)	8.0	16.4	18.5	3.0	9.9	8.7	10.9	20.5	25.2
Analgesics (pain relief)	15.1	19.5	17.5	13.0	15.3	19.5	16.3	22.2	16.1
Proton pump inhibitors (gastrointestinal reflux, ulcers)	*	13.0	17.3	*	13.0	16.8	*	12.9	17.6
Antidiabetic agents (diabetes)	9.3	12.8	13.9	10.7	12.4	12.9	8.5	13.0	14.5
Antidepressants (depression and related disorders)	3.4	10.4	13.3	*2.3	10.0	10.6	4.0	10.6	15.1
Antihypertensive combinations (high blood pressure)	11.9	12.4	12.6	8.3	9.2	7.8	14.0	14.4	15.9
Antiplatelet agents (blood thinning, reduce or prevent blood clots)	4.4	6.7	11.7	*4.2	9.1	14.6	4.6	5.2	9.7
Angiotensin II inhibitors (high blood pressure, heart disease)	X	8.2	11.9	X	7.4	10.2	X	8.7	13.0
Anticoagulants (blood thinning, reduce or prevent blood clots)	2.9	8.8	10.4	3.7	10.6	14.3	*2.4	7.7	7.7
Anxiolytics, sedatives, and hypnotics (generalized anxiety and related disorders)	9.2	8.8	10.3	6.3	6.2	7.5	10.9	10.3	12.3
Bisphosphonates (osteoporosis and related disorders)	*	8.1	10.0	*	*	*	*	11.8	15.4
Minerals and electrolytes mineral deficiencies)	7.5	9.2	8.4	5.6	8.4	6.8	8.7	9.8	9.6
Antiadrenergic agents, peripherally acting (prostate conditions)[2]	X	X	X	*3.1	13.7	19.5	X	X	X

X = Not applicable.   * = Figure does not meet standards of reliability or precision. Data preceded by an asterisk have a relative standard error (RSE) of 20 to 30 percent. Data not shown have an RSE of greater than 30 percent.   [1]The drug therapeutic class is based on Lexicon Plus, a proprietary database of Cerner Multum, Inc. Lexicon Plus is a comprehensive database of all prescription and some nonprescription drug products available in the U.S. drug market. Data on prescription drug use are collected by the National Health and Nutrition Examination Survey. Respondents were asked if they had taken a prescription drug in the past 30 days. Those who answered "yes" were asked to show the interviewer the medication containers for all prescriptions. If no container was available, the respondent was asked to verbally report the name of the medication. Each drug's complete name was recorded and classified. Data presented are based on the second level classification of prescription drugs. Up to four classes are assigned to each drug. Drugs classified into more than one class were counted in each class. Some drug classes were not available for 1988–1994.   [2]Although some antiadrenergic agents are used to treat high blood pressure, they are generally used currently to treat prostate hyperplasia and related conditions.

Table 3-55. Dietary Supplement Use Among Persons 20 Years of Age and Over, by Selected Characteristics, Selected Years, 1988–1994 Through 2005–2008

(Percent.)

Sex, age, race and Hispanic origin[1], and percent of poverty level	Any supplement use in past 30 days[2]			Any vitamin D supplement use in past 30 days[3]			Any folic acid supplement use in past 30 days[4]		
	1988–1994	2001–2004	2005–2008	1988–1994	2001–2004	2005–2008	1988–1994	2001–2004	2005–2008
20 YEARS AND OVER, AGE-ADJUSTED [5]									
Sex									
Both sexes[6]	42.1	53.1	50.9	28.4	38.8	38.0	30.3	38.6	37.5
Male	35.7	47.0	44.4	24.3	33.3	32.2	26.2	34.7	32.9
Female	47.8	58.7	56.9	32.2	43.8	43.4	34.2	42.3	42.0
Race									
Not Hispanic or Latino									
White only, male	37.5	51.4	48.7	26.1	36.8	35.8	28.2	38.4	36.6
White only, female	50.9	64.5	61.3	35.4	49.9	47.7	37.7	48.5	46.1
Black or African American only, male	29.5	32.3	31.0	18.5	20.3	22.6	18.2	22.1	23.0
Black or African American only, female	38.2	38.3	43.0	22.7	25.2	30.5	23.7	25.2	30.3
Mexican male	28.9	31.9	30.0	17.1	20.9	19.6	18.6	21.1	19.2
Mexican female	36.8	43.8	41.5	21.9	30.8	28.1	23.3	28.0	26.5
Percent of Poverty Level [7]									
Below 199 percent	30.0	37.1	33.5	16.8	24.2	23.2	18.3	23.4	21.7
100 percent to 199 percent	36.0	45.9	43.9	23.3	30.1	30.3	24.1	29.3	30.4
200 percent to 399 percent	44.0	52.5	52.5	30.2	39.8	39.4	32.5	39.1	38.8
400 percent or more	51.0	63.9	60.8	35.8	48.8	47.7	38.5	49.3	47.3
20 YEARS AND OVER, CRUDE									
Sex									
Both sexes[6]	41.8	52.7	51.3	28.4	38.6	38.3	30.3	38.4	37.8
Male	35.3	46.2	44.2	24.2	32.8	32.1	26.0	34.1	32.8
Female	47.7	58.8	57.8	32.2	43.9	44.1	34.3	42.4	42.5
Race									
Not Hispanic or Latino									
White only, male	37.4	51.5	49.7	26.0	37.0	36.4	28.1	38.6	37.3
White only, female	51.1	65.5	63.3	35.4	50.5	49.1	37.7	48.9	47.2
Black or African American only, male	28.9	31.0	30.3	18.8	19.4	22.6	18.5	21.0	22.7
Black or African American only, female	37.0	37.6	42.4	22.9	24.7	30.4	23.9	24.8	30.1
Mexican male	25.6	26.6	24.1	15.5	17.3	16.0	17.1	17.3	15.7
Mexican female	34.9	39.1	37.6	21.9	27.1	26.5	23.1	25.8	25.8
Percent of Poverty Level [7]									
Below 199 percent	29.4	34.9	31.9	17.1	23.2	22.4	18.4	22.5	21.2
100 percent to 199 percent	36.8	46.7	45.2	24.0	30.6	31.3	24.9	29.9	31.1
200 percent to 399 percent	43.6	52.2	53.1	30.4	39.6	39.9	32.7	38.9	39.1
400 percent or more	50.8	63.7	61.0	36.0	48.6	47.6	38.7	49.1	47.3
Male									
20 to 34 years	31.0	34.7	31.2	21.9	24.2	22.9	23.5	24.9	23.0
35 to 44 years	36.8	43.2	38.4	26.3	31.1	29.2	28.5	32.5	29.6
45 to 54 years	32.8	47.9	47.0	23.6	35.3	32.4	25.3	36.1	33.9
55 to 64 years	42.9	55.9	56.6	28.1	41.5	42.1	30.2	43.2	43.0
65 to 74 years	39.4	64.4	60.0	24.4	43.8	43.7	26.3	46.6	44.3
75 years and over	40.9	64.0	64.0	23.0	41.7	44.7	24.1	44.4	45.1
Female									
20 to 34 years	43.6	47.9	44.4	33.1	36.3	35.6	35.5	37.1	35.6
35 to 44 years	46.5	52.0	49.7	32.2	38.7	37.9	34.8	37.9	38.2
45 to 54 years	47.8	62.7	60.3	32.3	45.6	44.9	33.7	44.5	43.2
55 to 64 years	52.3	72.6	70.2	33.4	55.7	53.8	35.8	51.3	52.0
65 to 74 years	52.9	69.3	75.5	30.0	51.6	57.7	31.2	46.8	52.1
75 years and over	54.0	72.2	71.1	29.8	53.1	50.6	30.7	48.6	44.8

[1]Persons of Hispanic origin may be of any race.   [2]Respondents were asked "Have you used or taken any vitamins, minerals, herbals, or other dietary supplements in the past 30 days? Include prescription and non-prescription supplements." To facilitate their response, respondents were shown a card with some examples of different types of dietary supplements. The question wording differs slightly on the earlier, 1988–1994, survey.   [3]Includes supplements with vitamin D, cholecalciferol, calciferol, ergocalciferol, or calcitriol as an ingredient.   [4]Includes supplements with folic acid as an ingredient.   [5]Age adjusted to the 2000 standard population using five age groups: 20 to 34 years, 35 to 44 years, 45 to 54 years, 55 to 64 years, and 65 years and over.   [6]Includes persons of all races and Hispanic origins, not just those shown separately.   [7]Percent of poverty level is based on family income and family size. Persons with unknown percent of poverty level are excluded (5 percent in 2005–2008).

INPATIENT CARE

Figure 3-10. Percent of Persons with a Hospital Stay in the Past Year, by Age, 2011

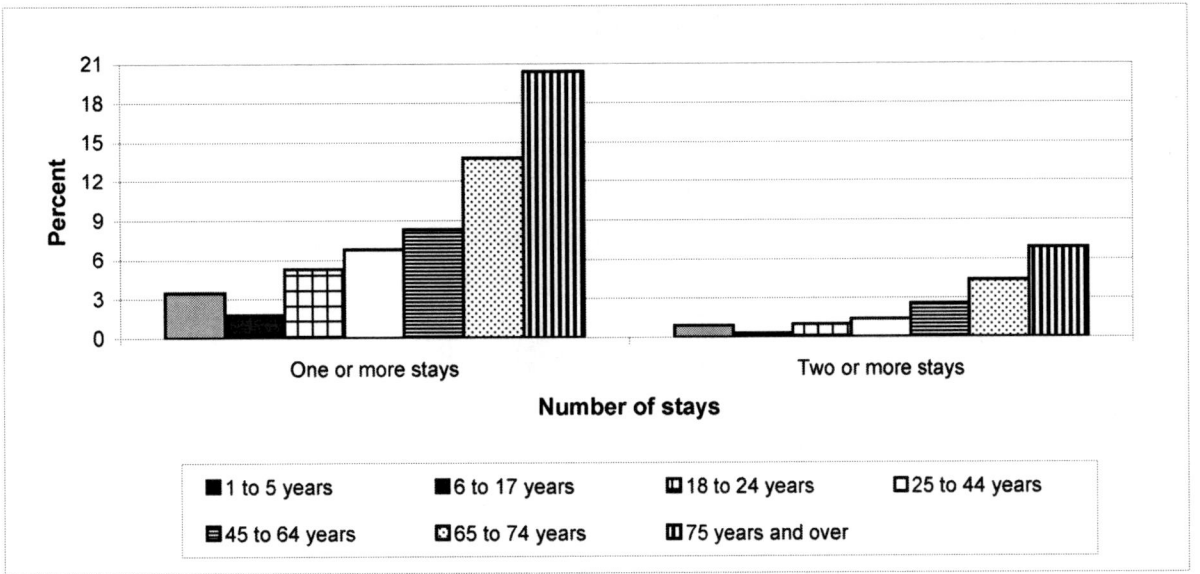

Figure 3-11. Average Length of Stay in Non-Federal, Short-Stay Hospitals, by Sex, Selected Years, 1990–2009

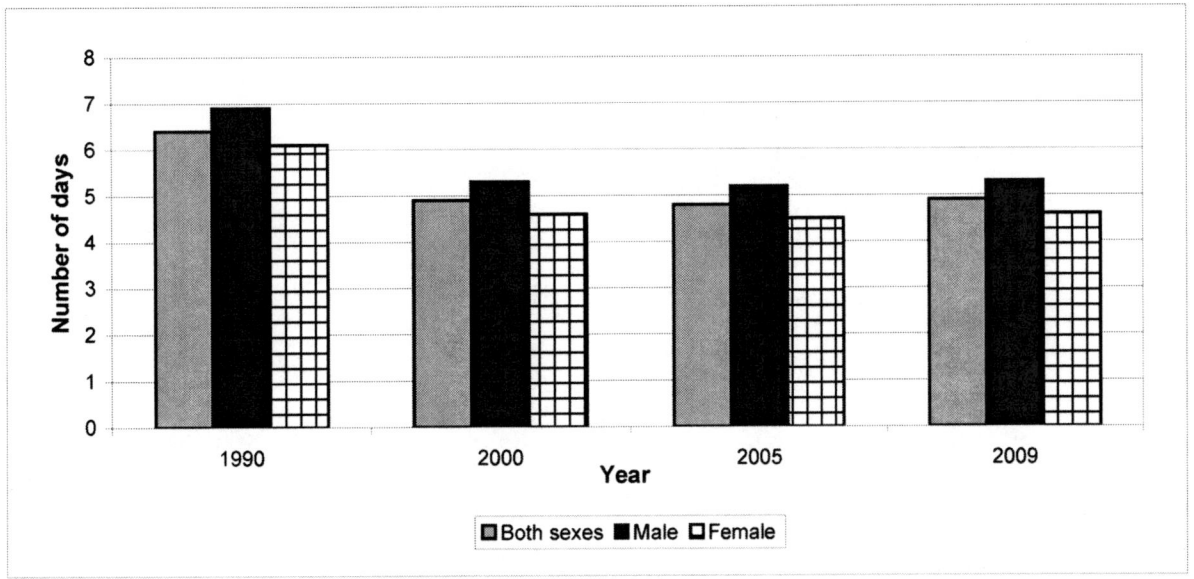

Table 3-56. Persons with Hospital Stays in the Past Year, by Selected Characteristics, Selected Years, 1997–2011

(Percent.)

Characteristic	One or more hospital stays[1]					Two or more hospital stays[1]				
	1997	2000	2005	2010	2011	1997	2000	2005	2010	2011
1 year and over, age-adjusted[2,3]	7.8	7.6	7.4	7.0	7.1	1.8	1.8	1.7	1.8	1.9
1 year and over, crude[2]	7.7	7.5	7.4	7.2	7.3	1.7	1.8	1.8	1.9	2.0
Age										
1 to 17 years	2.8	2.5	2.5	2.4	2.3	0.5	0.4	0.4	0.5	0.5
1 to 5 years	3.9	3.8	3.7	3.4	3.5	0.7	0.7	0.8	0.6	0.9
6 to 17 years	2.3	1.9	2.0	1.9	1.8	0.4	0.3	0.3	0.5	0.3
18 to 44 years	7.4	7.0	6.7	6.3	6.4	1.2	1.1	1.1	1.3	1.3
18 to 24 years	7.9	7.0	6.3	5.7	5.3	1.3	1.1	1.0	1.1	1.0
25 to 44 years	7.3	7.0	6.9	6.6	6.8	1.2	1.2	1.2	1.3	1.4
45 to 64 years	8.2	8.4	8.2	8.3	8.3	2.2	2.2	2.2	2.5	2.6
45 to 54 years	6.9	7.3	7.1	7.3	6.6	1.7	1.8	1.8	2.1	2.0
55 to 64 years	10.2	10.0	9.8	9.5	10.2	2.9	2.8	2.9	2.9	3.3
65 years and over	18.0	18.2	17.8	16.1	16.7	5.4	5.8	5.4	4.9	5.5
65 to 74 years	16.1	16.1	14.5	13.6	13.8	4.8	4.9	4.5	3.8	4.4
75 years and over	20.4	20.7	21.4	19.0	20.4	6.2	6.8	6.4	6.2	6.9
75 to 84 years	19.8	20.1	19.9	18.3	19.6	6.1	6.2	6.1	6.1	6.4
85 years and over	22.8	23.4	26.6	20.8	22.5	6.2	9.0	7.4	6.6	8.0
1 to 64 Years										
Total, 1 to 64 years[2,4]	6.3	6.1	5.9	5.7	5.7	1.3	1.2	1.2	1.3	1.4
Sex										
Male, crude	4.4	4.2	4.5	4.2	4.2	0.9	1.0	1.1	1.1	1.2
1 to 17 years	2.9	2.4	2.8	2.4	2.3	0.6	0.4	0.5	0.5	0.5
18 to 44 years	3.6	3.1	3.2	2.9	3.1	0.6	0.6	0.7	0.7	0.7
45 to 64 years	6.0	7.0	6.6	6.4	5.5	1.4	1.8	1.9	1.9	1.7
65 years and over	11.1	10.2	10.3	9.3	10.1	3.0	3.0	3.4	2.8	3.4
Female, crude	8.0	7.9	7.5	7.6	7.5	1.6	1.5	1.4	1.7	1.7
1 to 17 years	2.6	2.5	2.2	2.3	2.3	0.5	0.4	0.4	0.5	0.5
18 to 44 years	11.2	10.8	10.2	9.8	9.7	1.8	1.7	1.6	1.9	1.8
45 to 64 years	7.6	7.6	7.6	8.3	7.6	2.0	1.9	1.7	2.3	2.3
65 years and over	9.4	9.8	9.3	9.7	10.4	2.9	2.7	2.4	2.9	3.2
Race [4,5]										
White only	6.2	5.9	5.9	5.6	5.6	1.2	1.1	1.1	1.3	1.3
Black or African American only	7.6	7.4	6.6	6.7	6.8	1.9	1.9	1.8	1.9	2.3
American Indian or Alaska Native only	7.6	7.0	6.9	*7.6	4.9	*	*	*2.5	*2.4	*1.5
Asian only	3.9	3.9	3.9	3.6	3.4	*0.5	*0.6	*0.5	*0.4	0.6
Native Hawaiian and Other Pacific Islander only	NA	*	*	*	*	NA	*	*	*	*
Two or more races	NA	8.8	6.0	7.7	6.9	NA	*1.6	*1.9	*2.4	2.2
Hispanic Origin and Race [4,5]										
Hispanic or Latino	6.8	5.5	5.4	5.2	4.9	1.3	0.9	1.2	1.1	1.3
Not Hispanic or Latino	6.2	6.1	6.0	5.8	5.8	1.3	1.3	1.2	1.4	1.4
White only	6.1	6.0	6.0	5.7	5.8	1.2	1.2	1.1	1.3	1.3
Black or African American only	7.5	7.4	6.6	6.7	6.8	1.9	1.9	1.7	1.9	2.2
Percent of Poverty Level [4,6]										
Below 100 percent	10.3	9.1	8.8	8.3	8.5	2.8	2.6	2.5	2.7	2.9
100 percent to 199 percent	7.3	7.3	7.4	7.0	6.6	1.7	1.9	1.9	1.9	1.8
200 percent to 399 percent	6.0	6.0	5.4	5.2	5.3	1.2	1.1	1.1	1.1	1.2
400 percent or more	4.7	5.0	4.8	4.5	4.4	0.7	0.8	0.8	0.8	0.8
Hispanic Origin and Race and Percent of Poverty Level [4,5,6]										
Hispanic or Latino										
Below 100 percent	9.1	7.4	7.6	7.3	7.1	2.0	1.6	2.0	2.0	2.1
100 percent to 199 percent	5.9	5.4	5.9	4.8	4.7	1.0	0.8	1.4	1.1	1.3
200 percent to 399 percent	5.9	4.6	4.4	4.3	4.2	1.1	0.7	0.8	0.7	0.9
400 percent or more	5.5	4.7	3.8	4.4	3.5	*1.1	*0.6	*0.6	*0.8	*0.8
Not Hispanic or Latino										
White only										
Below 100 percent	10.7	9.6	9.3	8.8	9.3	3.2	2.7	2.5	2.9	3.2
100 percent to 199 percent	7.7	7.8	8.2	7.8	7.5	1.8	2.2	2.0	2.2	2.0
200 percent to 399 percent	6.1	6.1	5.8	5.5	5.7	1.2	1.1	1.1	1.2	1.1
400 percent or more	4.7	5.0	4.9	4.6	4.5	0.7	0.8	0.7	0.8	0.8
Black or African American only										
Below 100 percent	11.4	10.8	9.4	9.4	10.1	3.3	3.4	3.1	3.1	3.9
100 percent to 199 percent	8.0	8.5	7.7	7.7	7.0	2.1	2.3	2.0	2.3	2.1
200 percent to 399 percent	6.2	6.1	5.2	5.3	5.6	1.5	1.3	1.3	1.4	1.8
400 percent or more	4.7	5.8	5.1	4.5	4.4	*0.9	*1.3	*1.2	*1.0	1.3
Health Insurance Status at the Time of Interview [4,7]										
Insured	6.6	6.4	6.3	6.2	6.1	1.3	1.3	1.3	1.4	1.5
Private	5.6	5.5	5.2	5.0	4.8	1.0	1.0	0.9	0.9	0.9
Medicaid	16.1	15.9	14.6	12.7	12.1	4.9	4.7	4.1	4.5	4.6
Uninsured	4.8	4.5	4.4	4.0	4.1	1.0	0.9	0.9	0.9	1.0
Health Insurance Status Prior to Interview [4,7]										
Insured continuously all 12 months	6.5	6.3	6.1	6.0	5.9	1.3	1.2	1.2	1.4	1.4
Uninsured for any period up to 12 months	8.5	8.4	9.0	7.9	8.1	1.8	1.9	2.4	1.9	2.1
Uninsured more than 12 months	3.8	3.5	3.2	3.0	3.1	0.8	0.8	0.6	0.8	0.8
Disability Measure Among Adults 18 to 64 Years [4,8]										
Any basic actions difficulty or complex activity limitation	14.1	15.1	15.2	14.3	14.7	4.1	4.4	4.9	5.2	5.6
Any basic actions difficulty	13.9	15.1	15.1	14.2	14.9	4.1	4.4	4.9	5.1	5.8
Any complex activity limitation	21.5	22.6	23.2	21.2	20.8	7.7	8.8	8.6	8.6	9.5
No disability	5.8	5.6	5.4	5.4	4.9	0.6	0.7	0.6	0.8	0.6
Geographic Region [4]										
Northeast	6.0	5.5	5.8	5.2	5.2	1.2	1.0	1.1	1.2	1.4
Midwest	6.5	6.3	6.3	6.3	6.3	1.5	1.3	1.3	1.5	1.5
South	6.8	6.6	6.3	6.0	6.1	1.4	1.5	1.4	1.5	1.5
West	5.4	5.2	4.8	4.9	4.7	0.8	0.9	0.8	1.1	1.1
Location of Residence [4]										
Within MSA[9]	6.1	5.8	5.7	5.5	5.5	1.2	1.1	1.2	1.3	1.3
Outside MSA[9]	7.0	6.9	6.8	6.9	6.5	1.6	1.5	1.4	1.6	1.7

Table 3-56. Persons with Hospital Stays in the Past Year, by Selected Characteristics, Selected Years, 1997–2011—*Continued*

(Percent.)

Characteristic	One or more hospital stays[1]					Two or more hospital stays[1]				
	1997	2000	2005	2010	2011	1997	2000	2005	2010	2011
65 Years and Over										
Total, 65 years and over[2,10]	18.1	18.3	17.8	16.2	16.9	5.4	5.8	5.4	4.9	5.5
65 to 74 years	16.1	16.1	14.5	13.6	13.8	4.8	4.9	4.5	3.8	4.4
75 years and over	20.4	20.7	21.4	19.0	20.4	6.2	6.8	6.4	6.2	6.9
Sex [10]										
Male	19.0	19.5	18.6	16.2	16.8	5.8	5.8	6.0	5.4	5.0
Female	17.5	17.4	17.3	16.2	17.0	5.1	5.7	4.9	4.6	6.0
Hispanic Origin and Race [5,10]										
Hispanic or Latino	17.3	16.6	17.7	13.9	16.5	6.2	6.4	5.7	5.0	5.3
Not Hispanic or Latino	18.2	18.4	17.9	16.4	16.9	5.4	5.8	5.4	4.9	5.6
White only	18.3	18.4	17.9	16.5	16.8	5.4	5.7	5.4	4.9	5.4
Black or African American only	18.9	19.8	19.0	16.9	20.5	5.5	7.5	6.3	5.5	8.2
Percent of Poverty Level [6,10]										
Below 100 percent	20.9	20.9	22.1	18.8	20.6	6.4	7.5	7.9	5.1	7.8
100 percent to 199 percent	19.6	19.2	19.2	17.2	18.8	6.5	6.6	5.9	5.2	6.3
200 percent to 399 percent	17.3	18.1	17.2	16.0	16.5	4.9	5.8	4.8	5.5	5.6
400 percent or more	16.6	16.0	16.1	15.0	15.2	4.7	4.2	5.1	4.1	4.4
Disability Measure [8,10]										
Any basic actions difficulty or complex activity limitation	22.6	24.7	24.1	20.2	23.1	7.2	8.6	8.3	6.4	8.1
Any basic actions difficulty	22.7	24.7	24.2	20.4	23.3	7.2	8.7	8.5	6.6	8.3
Any complex activity limitation	29.0	31.5	29.3	25.4	29.5	10.8	12.2	11.1	9.2	11.5
No disability	7.8	9.7	8.3	10.6	9.1	1.1	1.9	*1.6	*1.6	*1.7
Geographic Region [10]										
Northeast	17.2	16.6	16.1	16.5	18.4	5.1	4.5	4.5	6.1	6.4
Midwest	18.2	19.5	18.9	16.4	17.1	5.6	7.2	5.8	4.7	5.4
South	19.4	19.5	19.7	16.4	17.4	6.1	6.3	6.3	4.7	5.8
West	16.5	16.4	15.0	15.3	14.7	4.4	4.4	4.3	4.5	4.5
Location of Residence [10]										
Within MSA[9]	17.8	17.8	17.4	15.9	17.1	5.2	5.4	5.2	4.8	5.7
Outside MSA[9]	19.1	19.6	19.2	17.3	16.3	6.3	6.9	6.2	5.6	5.1

NA = Not available.   * = Figure does not meet standards of reliability or precision. Data preceded by an asterisk have a relative standard error (RSE) of 20 to 30 percent. Data not shown have an RSE of greater than 30 percent.   [1]These estimates exclude hospitalizations for institutionalized persons and those who died while hospitalized.   [2]Includes all other races not shown separately, unknown health insurance status, and unknown disability status.   [3]Estimates are for persons 1 year of age and over and are age adjusted to the year 2000 standard population using six age groups: 1 to 17 years, 18 to 44 years, 45 to 54 years, 55 to 64 years, 65 to 74 years, and 75 years and over.   [4]Estimates are for persons 1 to 64 years of age and are age adjusted to the year 2000 standard population using four age groups: 1 to 17 years, 18 to 44 years, 45 to 54 years, and 55 to 64 years. The disability measure is age adjusted using the three adult age groups.   [5]The race groups White, Black, American Indian or Alaska Native, Asian, Native Hawaiian or Other Pacific Islander, and two or more races include persons of Hispanic and non-Hispanic origin. Persons of Hispanic origin may be of any race.   [6]Percent of poverty level is based on family income and family size and composition using U.S. Census Bureau poverty thresholds. Missing family data were imputed for 1997 and beyond.   [7]Health insurance categories are mutually exclusive. Persons who reported both Medicaid and private coverage are classified as having private coverage. Medicaid includes other public assistance through 1996. Starting with 1997 data, state-sponsored health plan coverage is included as Medicaid coverage. Starting with 1999 data, coverage by the Children's Health Insurance Program (CHIP) is included with Medicaid coverage. Persons not covered by private insurance, Medicaid, CHIP, public assistance (through 1996), state-sponsored or other government-sponsored health plans (starting in 1997), Medicare, or military plans are considered to have no health insurance coverage. Persons with only Indian Health Service coverage are considered to have no health insurance coverage. Health insurance status was unknown for 8 to 9 percent of children in 1993–1996 and about 1 percent in 1997–2011.   [8]Any basic actions difficulty or complex activity limitation is defined as having one or more of the following limitations or difficulties: movement difficulty, emotional difficulty, sensory (seeing or hearing) difficulty, cognitive difficulty, self-care (activities of daily living or instrumental activities of daily living) limitation, social limitation, or work limitation.   [9]MSA = metropolitan statistical area.   [10]Estimates are for persons 65 years of age and over and are age adjusted to the standard population using two age groups: 65 to 74 years and 75 years and over.

Table 3-57. Discharges, Days of Care, and Average Length of Stay in Nonfederal Short-Stay Hospitals, by Selected Characteristics, Selected Years, 1980 Through 2009–2010

(Rate per 10,000 population, number.)

Characteristic	1980[1]	1985[1]	1990	1995	2000	2005	2006	2007	2008[2]	2009[2]	2009–2010[2]
DISCHARGES PER 10,000 POPULATION											
Total, age-adjusted[3]	1,744.5	1,522.3	1,252.4	1,180.2	1,132.8	1,162.4	1,153.1	1,124.0	1,150.3	1,149.3	1,125.1
Total, crude	1,676.8	1,484.1	1,222.7	1,157.4	1,128.3	1,174.4	1,168.7	1,143.9	1,178.6	1,181.2	1,160.3
Age											
Under 18 years	756.5	614.0	463.5	423.7	402.6	411.0	393.9	376.7	343.3	340.2	336.2
Under 1 year	2,317.6	2,137.9	1,915.3	1,977.6	2,027.6	1,949.3	1,818.4	1,639.3	1,657.5	1,550.7	1,542.6
1 to 4 years	864.6	650.2	466.9	457.1	458.0	429.7	418.8	389.9	337.1	335.2	340.8
5 to 17 years	609.3	477.4	334.1	290.2	268.6	286.5	276.0	271.5	238.2	244.9	239.5
18 to 44 years	1,578.8	1,301.2	1,026.6	914.3	849.4	898.0	906.7	888.8	884.6	886.7	867.3
18 to 24 years	1,570.3	1,297.8	1,065.3	928.9	854.1	862.4	870.4	846.1	817.0	811.8	789.0
25 to 44 years	1,582.8	1,302.5	1,013.8	909.9	847.9	910.3	919.3	903.8	908.6	914.0	896.0
25 to 34 years	1,682.9	1,416.9	1,140.3	1,015.0	942.5	1,007.8	1,011.2	1,003.5	1,003.8	998.1	981.9
35 to 44 years	1,438.3	1,153.1	868.8	808.0	764.8	821.5	834.6	810.4	817.4	830.2	809.3
45 to 64 years	1,947.6	1,707.8	1,354.5	1,185.4	1,114.2	1,147.0	1,161.2	1,143.9	1,197.6	1,221.3	1,200.5
45 to 54 years	1,750.2	1,470.7	1,123.9	984.7	920.8	964.3	970.5	959.3	1,033.3	1,021.8	999.3
55 to 64 years	2,153.6	1,948.0	1,632.6	1,483.4	1,415.0	1,402.4	1,422.1	1,391.2	1,413.8	1,476.6	1,453.1
65 years and over	3,836.9	3,698.0	3,341.2	3,477.4	3,533.6	3,595.6	3,507.9	3,395.1	3,576.5	3,521.5	3,436.1
65 to 74 years	3,158.4	2,972.6	2,616.3	2,600.0	2,546.0	2,628.9	2,533.6	2,439.9	2,531.3	2,554.9	2,487.1
75 years and over	4,893.0	4,756.1	4,340.3	4,590.7	4,619.6	4,588.4	4,512.6	4,392.4	4,698.4	4,591.7	4,493.8
75 to 84 years	4,638.6	4,464.2	3,957.0	4,155.7	4,124.4	4,131.7	4,025.9	3,983.3	4,213.1	4,068.0	3,982.8
85 years and over	5,764.6	5,728.9	5,606.3	5,925.1	6,050.9	5,758.1	5,711.4	5,358.9	5,803.2	5,814.6	5,667.7
Sex[3]											
Male	1,543.9	1,382.5	1,130.0	1,048.5	990.8	1,013.0	1,000.5	973.8	997.3	1,004.3	975.3
Female	1,951.9	1,675.6	1,389.5	1,317.3	1,277.3	1,319.6	1,312.3	1,280.6	1,311.8	1,303.4	1,283.5
Sex and Age											
Male, all ages	1,390.4	1,240.2	1,002.2	941.7	910.6	959.0	954.9	936.7	964.9	978.8	957.4
Under 18 years	762.6	626.4	463.1	431.3	408.6	412.2	401.5	385.6	353.1	348.0	343.1
18 to 44 years	950.9	776.9	579.2	507.2	450.0	471.1	476.8	460.8	439.3	456.0	434.0
45 to 64 years	1,953.1	1,775.6	1,402.7	1,212.0	1,127.4	1,148.8	1,175.7	1,156.6	1,214.1	1,235.4	1,209.8
65 to 74 years	3,474.1	3,255.2	2,877.6	2,762.2	2,649.1	2,742.6	2,584.3	2,559.3	2,601.6	2,678.2	2,598.5
75 to 84 years	5,093.5	5,031.8	4,417.3	4,361.1	4,294.1	4,388.1	4,220.3	4,162.6	4,498.4	4,242.3	4,137.3
85 years and over	6,372.3	6,406.9	6,420.9	6,387.9	6,166.6	5,984.1	5,983.5	5,440.6	6,003.9	6,425.5	6,193.4
Female, all ages	1,944.0	1,712.2	1,431.7	1,362.9	1,336.6	1,382.2	1,375.3	1,344.0	1,385.2	1,377.2	1,357.1
Under 18 years	750.2	601.0	464.1	415.7	396.2	409.8	385.9	367.3	333.1	332.0	329.0
18 to 44 years	2,180.2	1,808.3	1,468.0	1,318.0	1,248.1	1,330.9	1,343.5	1,324.5	1,338.7	1,326.4	1,310.2
45 to 64 years	1,942.5	1,645.9	1,309.7	1,160.5	1,101.7	1,145.3	1,147.3	1,131.7	1,182.0	1,207.8	1,191.6
65 to 74 years	2,916.6	2,754.8	2,411.2	2,469.4	2,461.0	2,533.1	2,490.7	2,338.4	2,471.3	2,449.3	2,391.0
75 to 84 years	4,370.4	4,130.4	3,678.9	4,024.1	4,013.5	3,957.7	3,893.0	3,859.8	4,015.1	3,944.7	3,871.9
85 years and over	5,500.3	5,458.0	5,289.6	5,743.7	6,003.3	5,654.4	5,584.1	5,320.0	5,706.2	5,531.7	5,415.6
Geographic Region[3]											
Northeast	1,622.9	1,428.7	1,332.2	1,335.3	1,274.8	1,245.9	1,261.4	1,274.6	1,283.7	1,361.0	1,299.6
Midwest	1,925.2	1,584.7	1,287.5	1,132.8	1,109.2	1,174.9	1,168.0	1,125.5	1,172.1	1,153.7	1,146.8
South	1,814.1	1,569.4	1,325.0	1,252.4	1,209.2	1,202.5	1,198.8	1,139.9	1,179.0	1,149.3	1,136.1
West	1,519.7	1,469.6	1,006.6	967.4	894.0	1,005.9	964.1	966.0	960.2	959.2	932.7
DAYS OF CARE PER 10,000 POPULATION											
Total, age-adjusted[3]	13,027.0	10,017.9	8,189.3	6,386.2	5,576.8	5,541.7	5,474.7	5,404.1	5,577.2	5,536.3	5,369.2
Total, crude	12,166.8	9,576.6	7,840.5	6,201.7	5,546.5	5,620.9	5,577.8	5,539.4	5,773.9	5,748.1	5,598.7
Age											
Under 18 years	3,415.1	2,812.3	2,263.1	1,846.7	1,789.7	1,918.3	1,857.6	1,785.0	1,482.8	1,491.6	1,479.5
Under 1 year	13,213.9	14,141.2	11,484.7	10,834.5	11,524.0	12,131.6	11,624.2	8,466.7	9,401.0	9,277.7	9,170.4
1 to 4 years	3,333.5	2,280.4	1,700.1	1,525.6	1,482.2	1,355.3	1,405.4	1,280.3	1,018.8	1,041.0	1,111.0
5 to 17 years	2,698.5	2,049.8	1,633.2	1,240.3	1,172.1	1,300.9	1,239.1	1,406.4	984.0	1,012.6	990.5
18 to 44 years	8,323.6	6,294.7	4,676.7	3,517.2	3,093.8	3,305.0	3,360.6	3,258.0	3,180.3	3,268.3	3,147.4
18 to 24 years	7,174.6	5,287.2	4,015.9	2,987.4	2,679.5	2,819.9	2,889.4	2,738.7	2,606.0	2,755.3	2,687.1
25 to 44 years	8,861.4	6,685.2	4,895.5	3,676.4	3,225.5	3,472.8	3,524.5	3,439.7	3,383.8	3,454.9	3,316.3
25 to 34 years	8,497.5	6,688.9	4,939.7	3,536.1	3,161.7	3,434.3	3,462.2	3,423.1	3,462.0	3,482.0	3,342.6
35 to 44 years	9,386.6	6,680.4	4,844.8	3,812.3	3,281.5	3,507.9	3,581.9	3,455.2	3,308.9	3,428.0	3,289.7
45 to 64 years	15,969.5	12,015.9	9,139.3	6,574.5	5,515.4	5,717.3	5,793.0	5,868.2	6,284.3	6,184.5	6,058.0
45 to 54 years	13,167.2	9,692.8	6,996.6	5,162.0	4,374.2	4,711.2	4,667.4	4,745.9	5,185.7	4,772.0	4,719.7
55 to 64 years	18,895.4	14,369.5	11,722.6	8,671.6	7,290.8	7,124.0	7,333.6	7,371.8	7,729.7	7,993.0	7,739.0
65 years and over	40,983.5	32,279.7	28,956.1	23,736.5	21,118.9	19,882.8	19,197.5	18,951.7	20,391.2	19,933.0	19,225.8
65 to 74 years	31,470.3	24,373.3	20,878.2	16,847.0	14,389.7	13,985.3	13,170.2	13,274.8	13,911.2	13,888.2	13,504.6
75 years and over	55,788.2	43,812.7	40,090.8	32,478.1	28,518.6	25,939.4	25,413.1	24,878.5	27,347.0	26,625.9	25,602.5
75 to 84 years	51,836.2	40,521.6	35,995.1	28,947.5	25,397.8	23,155.3	22,671.7	22,658.1	24,400.0	23,644.1	22,884.1
85 years and over	69,332.0	54,782.4	53,616.9	43,305.9	37,537.8	33,071.5	32,165.5	30,124.5	34,055.6	33,588.7	31,848.6
Sex[3]											
Male	12,475.8	9,792.1	8,057.8	6,239.0	5,358.8	5,301.3	5,208.8	5,157.4	5,376.4	5,342.4	5,158.3
Female	13,662.9	10,340.4	8,404.5	6,548.8	5,809.7	5,828.7	5,764.2	5,685.1	5,832.4	5,784.1	5,630.6
Sex and Age											
Male, all ages	10,674.1	8,518.8	6,943.0	5,507.5	4,860.8	4,979.7	4,947.3	4,937.6	5,176.0	5,178.1	5,043.5
Under 18 years	3,473.1	2,942.7	2,335.7	1,998.0	1,955.7	2,006.2	1,968.0	1,858.1	1,646.9	1,526.4	1,555.6
18 to 44 years	6,102.4	4,746.6	3,517.4	2,729.7	2,175.0	2,282.7	2,375.6	2,241.8	2,045.7	2,203.9	2,036.6
45 to 64 years	15,894.9	12,290.1	9,434.2	6,822.7	5,704.4	5,773.5	6,004.3	6,103.5	6,553.3	6,443.8	6,327.1
65 to 74 years	33,697.6	26,220.5	22,515.5	17,697.4	14,897.4	14,502.6	13,262.1	13,666.7	14,473.2	14,915.8	14,462.9
75 to 84 years	54,723.3	44,087.4	38,257.8	29,642.6	26,616.7	25,106.9	23,972.7	23,894.6	26,208.6	24,959.5	24,184.6
85 years and over	77,013.1	58,609.5	60,347.3	45,263.6	37,765.3	35,179.0	32,604.0	31,480.6	37,292.7	37,649.7	35,211.1
Female, all ages	13,560.1	10,566.3	8,691.1	6,863.4	6,202.7	6,239.5	6,186.8	6,121.1	6,352.3	6,300.0	6,137.1
Under 18 years	3,354.5	2,675.5	2,186.8	1,687.9	1,615.1	1,826.1	1,741.8	1,708.3	1,310.9	1,455.1	1,399.7
18 to 44 years	10,450.7	7,792.0	5,820.3	4,297.9	4,010.8	4,341.8	4,361.5	4,292.3	4,337.0	4,354.8	4,283.0
45 to 64 years	16,037.1	11,765.5	8,865.1	6,341.7	5,336.4	5,663.9	5,592.2	5,644.3	6,028.1	5,937.5	5,801.9
65 to 74 years	29,764.7	22,949.2	19,592.7	16,162.0	13,971.3	13,549.0	13,092.4	12,942.1	13,431.6	13,007.9	12,678.4
75 to 84 years	50,133.3	38,424.7	34,628.3	28,502.5	24,601.0	21,830.1	21,782.1	21,806.2	23,144.7	22,713.5	21,949.6
85 years and over	65,990.5	53,253.6	51,000.5	42,538.6	37,444.4	32,103.5	31,960.3	29,479.5	32,492.0	31,707.4	30,236.0
Geographic Region[3]											
Northeast	14,024.4	11,143.1	10,266.8	8,389.7	7,185.9	6,636.5	6,608.5	7,284.4	7,055.4	7,512.7	7,072.6
Midwest	14,871.9	10,803.6	8,306.5	5,908.8	5,005.3	4,954.3	4,893.5	4,775.3	5,176.9	4,990.1	4,932.7
South	12,713.5	9,642.6	8,204.1	6,659.9	5,925.1	5,830.4	5,844.8	5,555.7	5,667.9	5,610.4	5,514.2
West	9,635.2	8,300.7	5,755.1	4,510.6	4,082.0	4,690.3	4,451.6	4,184.5	4,528.7	4,241.2	4,084.4

Table 3-57. Discharges, Days of Care, and Average Length of Stay in Nonfederal Short-Stay Hospitals, by Selected Characteristics, Selected Years, 1980 Through 2009–2010—*Continued*

(Rate per 10,000 population, number.)

Characteristic	1980[1]	1985[1]	1990	1995	2000	2005	2006	2007	2008[2]	2009[2]	2009–2010[2]
AVERAGE LENGTH OF STAY IN DAYS											
Total, age-adjusted[3]	7.5	6.6	6.5	5.4	4.9	4.8	4.7	4.8	4.8	4.8	4.8
Total, crude	7.3	6.5	6.4	5.4	4.9	4.8	4.8	4.8	4.9	4.9	4.8
Age											
Under 18 years	4.5	4.6	4.9	4.4	4.4	4.7	4.7	4.7	4.3	4.4	4.4
Under 1 year	5.7	6.6	6.0	5.5	5.7	6.2	6.4	5.2	5.7	6.0	5.9
1 to 4 years	3.9	3.5	3.6	3.3	3.2	3.2	3.4	3.3	3.0	3.1	3.3
5 to 17 years	4.4	4.3	4.9	4.3	4.4	4.5	4.5	5.2	4.1	4.1	4.1
18 to 44 years	5.3	4.8	4.6	3.8	3.6	3.7	3.7	3.7	3.6	3.7	3.6
18 to 24 years	4.6	4.1	3.8	3.2	3.1	3.3	3.3	3.2	3.2	3.4	3.4
25 to 44 years	5.6	5.1	4.8	4.0	3.8	3.8	3.8	3.8	3.7	3.8	3.7
25 to 34 years	5.0	4.7	4.3	3.5	3.4	3.4	3.4	3.4	3.4	3.5	3.4
35 to 44 years	6.5	5.8	5.6	4.7	4.3	4.3	4.3	4.3	4.0	4.1	4.1
45 to 64 years	8.2	7.0	6.7	5.5	5.0	5.0	5.0	5.1	5.2	5.1	5.0
45 to 54 years	7.5	6.6	6.2	5.2	4.8	4.9	4.8	4.9	5.0	4.7	4.7
55 to 64 years	8.8	7.4	7.2	5.8	5.2	5.1	5.2	5.3	5.5	5.4	5.3
65 years and over	10.7	8.7	8.7	6.8	6.0	5.5	5.5	5.6	5.7	5.7	5.6
65 to 74 years	10.0	8.2	8.0	6.5	5.7	5.3	5.2	5.4	5.5	5.4	5.4
75 years and over	11.4	9.2	9.2	7.1	6.2	5.7	5.6	5.7	5.8	5.8	5.7
75 to 84 years	11.2	9.1	9.1	7.0	6.2	5.6	5.6	5.7	5.8	5.8	5.7
85 years and over	12.0	9.6	9.6	7.3	6.2	5.7	5.6	5.6	5.9	5.8	5.6
Sex[3]											
Male	8.1	7.1	7.1	6.0	5.4	5.2	5.2	5.3	5.4	5.3	5.3
Female	7.0	6.2	6.0	5.0	4.5	4.4	4.4	4.4	4.4	4.4	4.4
Sex and Age											
Male, all ages	7.7	6.9	6.9	5.8	5.3	5.2	5.2	5.3	5.4	5.3	5.3
Under 18 years	4.6	4.7	5.0	4.6	4.8	4.9	4.9	4.8	4.7	4.4	4.5
18 to 44 years	6.4	6.1	6.1	5.4	4.8	4.8	5.0	4.9	4.7	4.8	4.7
45 to 64 years	8.1	6.9	6.7	5.6	5.1	5.0	5.1	5.3	5.4	5.2	5.2
65 to 74 years	9.7	8.1	7.8	6.4	5.6	5.3	5.1	5.3	5.6	5.6	5.6
75 to 84 years	10.7	8.8	8.7	6.8	6.2	5.7	5.7	5.7	5.8	5.9	5.8
85 years and over	12.1	9.1	9.4	7.1	6.1	5.9	5.4	5.8	6.2	5.9	5.7
Female, all ages	7.0	6.2	6.1	5.0	4.6	4.5	4.5	4.6	4.6	4.6	4.5
Under 18 years	4.5	4.5	4.7	4.1	4.1	4.5	4.5	4.7	3.9	4.4	4.3
18 to 44 years	4.8	4.3	4.0	3.3	3.2	3.3	3.2	3.2	3.2	3.3	3.3
45 to 64 years	8.3	7.1	6.8	5.5	4.8	4.9	4.9	5.0	5.1	4.9	4.9
65 to 74 years	10.2	8.3	8.1	6.5	5.7	5.3	5.3	5.5	5.4	5.3	5.3
75 to 84 years	11.5	9.3	9.4	7.1	6.1	5.5	5.6	5.6	5.8	5.8	5.7
85 years and over	12.0	9.8	9.6	7.4	6.2	5.7	5.7	5.5	5.7	5.7	5.6
Geographic Region[3]											
Northeast	8.6	7.8	7.7	6.3	5.6	5.3	5.2	5.7	5.5	5.5	5.4
Midwest	7.7	6.8	6.5	5.2	4.5	4.2	4.2	4.2	4.4	4.3	4.3
South	7.0	6.1	6.2	5.3	4.9	4.8	4.9	4.9	4.8	4.9	4.9
West	6.3	5.6	5.7	4.7	4.6	4.7	4.6	4.3	4.7	4.4	4.4

[1]Comparisons of data from 1980–1985 with data from subsequent years should be made with caution because estimates of change may reflect improvements in the survey design rather than true changes in hospital use.   [2]Starting with 2008 data, the sample of nonfederal short-stay hospitals was cut in half. This smaller sample size has increased standard errors. Therefore, caution should be exercised in interpreting trends in these data.   [3]Estimates are age adjusted to the year 2000 standard population using six age groups: under 18 years, 18 to 44 years, 45 to 54 years, 55 to 64 years, 65 to 74 years, and 75 years and over.

Table 3-58. Discharges in Nonfederal Short-Stay Hospitals, by Sex, Age, and Selected First-Listed Diagnosis, Selected Years, 1990 Through 2009–2010

(Numbers in thousands.)

Age and first-listed diagnosis	Both sexes				Male				Female			
	1990	1995	2009[1]	2009–2010[1]	1990	1995	2009[1]	2009–2010[1]	1990	1995	2009[1]	2009–2010[1]
ALL AGES [2]	30,788	30,722	36,120	35,599	12,280	12,198	14,721	14,461	18,508	18,525	21,398	21,139
Under 18 Years [2]	3,072	3,002	*2,536	*2,506	1,572	1,565	*1,327	*1,309	1,500	1,437	*1,209	*1,197
Dehydration	63	106	*73	*64	32	59	*39	*35	31	47	*34	*29
Acute bronchitis and bronchiolitis	114	170	*109	*119	67	109	*70	*73	47	61	*40	*46
Pneumonia	221	250	170	*167	126	143	*86	*84	95	107	*84	*83
Asthma	182	227	*143	*140	111	137	*92	*88	71	90	*50	*52
Appendicitis	83	69	*76	*72	50	41	*47	*45	34	28	29	*26
Injury	329	286	161	*173	210	171	*96	*104	119	115	*65	*69
Fracture	117	102	*67	*76	76	66	*42	*48	42	36	*25	*28
Complications of care and adverse effects	41	46	*43	*39	22	25	*23	*21	19	*21	*20	*18
18 to 44 Years [2]	11,138	9,996	9,963	9,746	3,120	2,761	2,588	2,465	8,018	7,235	7,375	7,280
HIV/AIDS	*20	88	23	24	*15	66	*17	17	*	22	*6	*7
Cancer, all	181	150	113	114	64	47	*35	40	116	102	77	74
Childbirth	X	X	X	X	X	X	X	X	3,815	3,574	3,862	3,851
Uterine fibroids	X	X	X	X	X	X	X	X	110	115	81	84
Diabetes	105	102	159	159	61	52	79	79	44	50	80	81
Alcohol and drug	284	363	224	215	199	255	152	147	84	107	71	69
Schizophrenia, mood disorders, delusional disorders, nonorganic psychoses	384	551	544	541	184	262	268	271	200	289	276	271
Schizophrenia	145	*181	148	140	88	*118	88	84	57	63	*61	56
Mood disorders	211	324	359	368	83	121	160	166	128	203	199	202
Heart disease	236	265	239	228	163	157	144	140	73	108	95	88
Ischemic heart disease	129	130	72	68	95	90	48	47	34	39	*25	21
Pneumonia	136	149	126	107	69	74	59	51	67	75	67	56
Asthma	106	119	90	85	27	30	*28	26	79	89	62	59
Intervertebral disc disorders	222	157	105	96	138	94	53	49	84	62	52	47
Injury	935	688	555	503	641	465	359	316	294	223	196	187
Fracture	302	250	221	203	217	176	162	142	85	74	59	61
Poisoning and toxic effects	124	118	134	125	54	59	58	55	70	59	76	70
Complications of care and adverse effects	135	146	195	187	63	64	81	74	72	82	114	113
45 to 64 Years [2]	6,244	6,168	9,686	9,585	3,115	3,053	4,781	4,710	3,129	3,115	4,906	4,874
HIV/AIDS	*3	20	*16	16	*3	15	*12	12	*	*5	*4	*4
Cancer, all	545	461	525	497	236	193	255	244	309	268	269	253
Colorectal cancer	59	29	66	60	33	17	32	30	26	13	34	29
Lung/bronchus/tracheal cancer	101	76	68	62	60	37	31	28	41	39	*37	34
Breast cancer[3]	X	X	X	X	X	X	X	X	69	61	48	47
Prostate cancer	X	X	X	X	19	32	*57	*53	X	X	X	X
Uterine fibroids	X	X	X	X	X	X	X	X	70	74	93	95
Diabetes	134	172	256	255	65	86	124	128	70	86	132	127
Alcohol and drug	100	128	191	194	77	100	138	142	23	28	53	52
Schizophrenia, mood disorders, delusional disorders, nonorganic psychoses	152	194	384	379	56	75	177	169	95	118	207	210
Schizophrenia	47	*67	119	115	19	*	*66	61	28	36	54	54
Mood disorders	91	112	241	242	32	37	98	97	58	74	142	146
Heart disease	1,100	1,152	1,204	1,162	704	749	756	730	397	403	448	432
Ischemic heart disease	739	762	579	544	502	537	393	371	237	225	187	173
Heart attack	233	256	205	210	165	188	144	147	68	68	61	63
Arrhythmias	131	131	186	197	79	75	115	121	53	56	71	76
Heart failure	122	143	271	254	68	75	161	145	54	68	111	109
Hypertension	75	82	155	143	38	37	76	69	37	45	80	74
Stroke	162	182	275	288	91	96	149	160	72	86	126	127
Pneumonia	154	163	264	261	76	75	141	135	79	88	122	126
Chronic obstructive pulmonary disease	73	154	236	231	39	72	95	94	34	82	141	137
Asthma	86	87	132	125	26	21	40	34	59	66	93	92
Osteoarthritis	87	110	476	491	36	47	211	211	51	64	265	280
Intervertebral disc disorders	145	115	167	162	82	65	85	82	63	51	81	79
Injury	334	296	441	450	178	165	229	242	157	131	211	208
Fracture	149	147	211	233	74	74	109	122	75	72	102	111
Poisoning and toxic effects	29	30	101	95	10	13	44	43	19	17	57	52
Internal organ injury	36	38	64	56	23	27	36	35	14	11	*28	*21
Complications of care and adverse effects	148	186	402	398	79	92	204	199	69	94	198	199
65 to 74 Years [2]	4,689	4,832	5,312	5,251	2,268	2,290	2,569	2,540	2,421	2,542	2,743	2,711
Septicemia	49	65	139	150	27	27	67	76	21	38	72	74
Cancer, all	436	416	326	311	222	203	178	171	214	212	147	140
Colorectal cancer	48	46	43	35	24	22	*23	20	24	24	*20	15
Lung/bronchus/tracheal cancer	77	73	61	58	50	44	*34	33	26	29	27	25
Breast cancer[3]	X	X	X	X	X	X	X	X	42	35	*21	19
Prostate cancer	X	X	X	X	40	41	*34	29	X	X	X	X
Diabetes	93	93	107	96	34	44	45	45	59	49	61	51
Schizophrenia, mood disorders, delusional disorders, nonorganic psychoses	59	80	*65	*62	20	20	*26	*21	39	60	*38	*41
Dementia and Alzheimer's disease	10	18	*14	*18	4	11	*	*	*6	7	*	*9
Heart disease	1,000	1,115	888	860	547	618	514	498	453	497	375	363
Ischemic heart disease	576	614	389	359	331	365	241	229	245	250	148	131
Heart attack	185	210	138	131	110	129	83	81	75	82	54	50
Arrhythmias	124	153	176	180	67	74	97	97	57	79	79	82
Heart failure	188	233	209	198	93	126	114	110	95	107	95	88
Hypertension	39	42	*77	61	13	14	*32	*24	26	28	*45	38
Stroke	222	250	225	231	108	141	125	124	114	109	100	107
Pneumonia	176	214	174	177	90	105	79	85	86	109	95	92
Chronic obstructive pulmonary disease	81	191	211	208	41	83	96	91	40	107	115	117
Gallstones	79	78	49	47	30	31	25	23	49	46	23	24
Kidney disease	18	31	121	121	9	16	65	70	9	15	56	51
Urinary tract infection	54	50	82	80	17	20	29	25	37	30	53	56
Hyperplasia of the prostate	X	X	X	X	113	62	*23	21	X	X	X	X
Osteoarthritis	122	154	308	339	44	53	115	133	78	101	193	206
Injury	193	176	201	203	71	67	80	75	122	109	121	128
Fracture	120	109	121	126	36	36	37	37	85	72	84	88
Hip fracture	48	44	40	39	12	15	12	12	36	29	*28	27
Complications of care and adverse effects	125	144	204	203	68	66	107	102	57	78	97	101

Table 3-58. Discharges in Nonfederal Short-Stay Hospitals, by Sex, Age, and Selected First-Listed Diagnosis, Selected Years, 1990 Through 2009–2010—Continued

(Numbers in thousands.)

Age and first-listed diagnosis	Both sexes				Male				Female			
	1990	1995	2009[1]	2009–2010[1]	1990	1995	2009[1]	2009–2010[1]	1990	1995	2009[1]	2009–2010[1]
75 to 84 Years [2]	3,949	4,590	5,349	5,257	1,660	1,880	2,311	2,283	2,289	2,710	3,038	2,973
Septicemia	54	87	171	183	24	38	81	84	30	50	90	99
Cancer, all	300	281	236	227	158	131	108	109	142	150	128	119
Colorectal cancer	50	46	39	39	20	22	*15	17	29	24	24	22
Lung/bronchus/tracheal cancer	36	32	44	44	22	17	*21	22	*15	15	23	22
Breast cancer[3]	X	X	X	X	X	X	X	X	24	24	*10	13
Prostate cancer	X	X	X	X	37	18	*5	*6	X	X	X	X
Diabetes	44	73	100	88	17	30	39	37	27	43	*60	51
Schizophrenia, mood disorders, delusional disorders, nonorganic psychoses	39	44	*	*	*10	10	*	*	28	35	*23	*24
Dementia and Alzheimer's disease	20	46	53	58	9	19	*29	26	11	26	*25	33
Heart disease	865	1,057	1,025	976	377	471	480	466	488	585	545	510
Ischemic heart disease	382	479	358	328	177	228	189	173	205	251	169	156
Heart attack	156	188	165	149	83	91	79	70	73	97	86	78
Arrhythmias	133	175	241	223	58	83	99	92	76	92	143	131
Heart failure	261	290	296	291	108	116	132	137	153	174	164	154
Hypertension	23	31	64	50	*	*11	*21	*17	19	20	43	33
Stroke	258	297	258	260	104	129	123	116	154	169	135	144
Pneumonia	224	282	234	237	112	142	109	107	112	140	124	130
Chronic obstructive pulmonary disease	55	143	181	173	34	63	86	83	22	80	94	91
Gallstones	48	55	51	52	20	22	20	22	28	33	*31	30
Kidney disease	24	28	143	145	10	17	70	68	*14	12	73	77
Urinary tract infection	86	99	158	162	25	35	46	48	61	64	112	114
Hyperplasia of the prostate	X	X	X	X	69	41	*21	21	X	X	X	X
Osteoarthritis	69	115	205	213	25	34	80	84	44	80	125	129
Injury	259	270	306	313	58	77	104	104	201	193	202	208
Fracture	195	208	211	219	35	53	60	62	161	154	151	158
Hip fracture	115	122	83	92	20	29	20	25	95	93	63	66
Complications of care and adverse effects	81	108	159	162	38	40	81	83	43	68	78	79
85 Years and Over [2]	1,694	2,134	3,274	3,256	543	648	1,145	1,153	1,151	1,486	2,129	2,102
Septicemia	41	57	134	150	12	17	52	60	29	40	82	90
Cancer, all	77	77	94	83	31	32	43	39	45	45	51	44
Colorectal cancer	14	17	*12	10	*5	*	*	*4	9	11	*7	*6
Lung/bronchus/tracheal cancer	*6	*4	*13	*14	*	*2	*	*	*	*	*	*6
Breast cancer[3]	X	X	X	X	X	X	X	X	*9	8	*	*5
Prostate cancer	X	X	X	X	*7	*	*	*4	X	X	X	X
Diabetes	16	22	*34	34	*5	*	*13	13	11	15	*21	*21
Schizophrenia, mood disorders, delusional disorders, nonorganic psychoses	*8	16	*	*	*	*	*	*8	*7	*12	*	*
Dementia and Alzheimer's disease	15	28	42	44	*2	*6	16	18	13	22	26	26
Heart disease	335	446	611	606	112	135	236	228	223	311	376	378
Ischemic heart disease	128	144	139	142	49	48	62	60	79	96	76	82
Heart attack	60	73	88	92	23	28	37	37	37	44	51	56
Arrhythmias	51	72	127	122	16	20	37	40	35	51	90	82
Heart failure	126	181	263	259	39	52	101	98	87	129	162	161
Hypertension	*5	8	37	28	*	*	*12	*9	*4	*6	*25	19
Stroke	129	156	162	163	35	42	48	52	95	114	114	111
Pneumonia	151	194	207	204	64	73	74	80	88	121	134	124
Chronic obstructive pulmonary disease	13	39	81	83	*6	18	*28	32	*7	21	53	50
Gallstones	18	21	*24	23	*6	*7	*7	*8	13	15	*17	15
Kidney disease	14	16	90	96	8	*8	36	43	*6	*9	54	53
Urinary tract infection	65	74	195	185	20	*18	46	40	45	56	149	144
Hyperplasia of the prostate	X	X	X	X	13	9	*6	*6	X	X	X	X
Osteoarthritis	13	20	36	40	*	*6	*10	*10	8	14	26	30
Injury	164	216	300	302	37	47	78	80	127	169	223	222
Fracture	133	172	227	228	28	32	54	51	104	140	173	177
Hip fracture	82	108	123	122	19	19	29	29	63	88	94	93
Complications of care and adverse effects	29	29	75	73	11	*10	*27	30	18	19	48	43

X = Not applicable. * = Figure does not meet standards of reliability or precision. Data preceded by an asterisk have a relative standard error (RSE) of 20 to 30 percent. Data not shown have an RSE of greater than 30 percent. [1]Starting with 2008 data, the sample of nonfederal short-stay hospitals was cut in half. This smaller sample size has increased standard errors. Therefore, caution should be exercised in interpreting trends in these data. [2]Includes discharges with first-listed diagnoses not shown in table. [3]Shown for women only.

Table 3-59. Discharge Rate in Nonfederal Short-Stay Hospitals, by Sex, Age, and Selected First-Listed Diagnosis, Selected Years, 1990 Through 2009–2010

(Number per 10,000 population.)

Age and first-listed diagnosis	Both sexes				Male				Female			
	1990	2000	2009[1]	2009–2010[1]	1990	2000	2009[1]	2009–2010[1]	1990	2000	2009[1]	2009–2010[1]
All Ages, Age-Adjusted [2,3]	1,252.4	1,132.8	1,149.3	1,125.1	1,130.0	990.8	1,004.3	975.3	1,389.5	1,277.3	1,303.4	1,283.5
All Ages, Crude [3]	1,222.7	1,128.3	1,181.2	1,160.3	1,002.2	910.6	978.8	957.4	1,431.7	1,336.6	1,377.2	1,357.1
Under 18 Years [3]	463.5	402.6	*340.2	*336.2	463.1	408.6	*348.0	*343.1	464.1	396.2	*332.0	*329.0
Dehydration	9.5	15.7	*9.8	*8.6	9.4	17.2	*10.4	*9.1	9.7	14.2	*9.2	*8.0
Acute bronchitis and bronchiolitis	17.2	27.8	*14.7	*16.0	19.6	31.4	*18.3	*19.1	14.6	24.1	*10.9	*12.7
Pneumonia	33.3	25.2	22.7	*22.4	37.0	25.7	*22.5	*22.0	29.5	24.6	*23.0	*22.7
Asthma	27.5	29.6	*19.1	*18.7	32.7	34.8	*24.2	*23.1	22.0	24.0	*13.8	*14.2
Appendicitis	12.6	11.9	*10.2	*9.6	14.6	13.0	*12.2	*11.9	10.5	10.8	8.1	*7.2
Injury	49.7	33.6	21.6	*23.2	62.0	42.0	*25.1	*27.2	36.8	24.8	*17.9	*19.1
Fracture	17.7	13.8	*8.9	*10.2	22.3	18.3	*10.9	*12.6	12.9	9.0	*6.9	*7.8
Complications of care and adverse effects	6.2	*7.3	*5.8	*5.2	6.5	*7.9	*6.0	*5.5	5.9	*6.6	*5.5	*4.9
18 to 44 Years [3]	1,026.6	849.4	886.7	867.3	579.2	450.0	456.0	434.0	1,468.0	1,248.1	1,326.4	1,310.2
HIV/AIDS	*1.8	4.3	2.1	2.2	*2.8	5.8	*3.0	3.1	*	2.8	*1.1	*1.2
Cancer, all	16.6	10.5	10.0	10.1	11.9	7.3	*6.2	7.0	21.3	13.7	13.9	13.3
Childbirth	X	X	X	X	X	X	X	X	698.6	645.2	694.5	693.1
Uterine fibroids	X	X	X	X	X	X	X	X	20.2	21.7	14.6	15.2
Diabetes	9.7	11.5	14.1	14.2	11.3	13.0	13.9	13.9	8.1	9.9	14.4	14.5
Alcohol and drug	26.2	29.7	19.9	19.2	37.0	39.1	26.9	25.8	15.5	*20.2	12.8	12.4
Schizophrenia, mood disorders, delusional disorders, nonorganic psychoses	35.4	*53.6	48.5	48.2	34.1	*53.2	47.3	47.6	36.7	*53.9	49.7	48.7
Schizophrenia	13.4	*14.4	13.2	12.4	16.4	*18.6	15.5	14.8	10.5	*10.1	*10.9	10.0
Mood disorders	19.4	*35.9	31.9	32.8	15.4	*31.0	28.2	29.3	23.4	*40.9	35.8	36.3
Heart disease	21.7	21.8	21.3	20.3	30.2	26.6	25.4	24.6	13.4	17.0	17.1	15.8
Ischemic heart disease	11.9	9.9	6.4	6.0	17.7	14.2	8.4	8.3	6.3	5.6	*4.5	3.7
Pneumonia	12.5	10.9	11.2	9.5	12.8	10.0	10.4	8.9	12.2	11.9	12.0	10.1
Asthma	9.8	9.0	8.0	7.6	5.1	5.4	*4.9	4.6	14.4	12.6	11.1	10.7
Intervertebral disc disorders	20.5	12.5	9.3	8.5	25.6	14.5	9.4	8.6	15.4	10.4	9.3	8.4
Injury	86.2	45.8	49.4	44.8	119.0	62.3	63.2	55.7	53.8	29.4	35.3	33.6
Fracture	27.8	17.8	19.7	18.1	40.2	25.4	28.5	25.0	15.5	10.2	10.6	11.0
Poisoning and toxic effects	11.4	8.5	11.9	11.2	10.0	6.7	10.2	9.7	12.7	10.3	13.7	12.6
Complications of care and adverse effects	12.5	12.2	17.4	16.6	11.7	11.2	14.3	13.1	13.3	13.1	20.5	20.3
45 to 64 Years [3]	1,354.5	1,114.2	1,221.3	1,200.5	1,402.7	1,127.4	1,235.4	1,209.8	1,309.7	1,101.7	1,207.8	1,191.6
HIV/AIDS	*0.6	*3.2	*2.0	2.0	*1.2	*4.9	*3.0	3.0	*	*	*1.0	*1.1
Cancer, all	118.3	62.9	66.1	62.2	106.3	62.1	65.9	62.6	129.5	63.6	66.3	61.8
Colorectal cancer	12.7	7.9	8.3	7.5	14.8	8.9	8.2	7.8	10.8	6.9	8.3	7.2
Lung/bronchus/tracheal cancer	21.8	6.9	8.6	7.8	26.8	8.6	8.1	7.2	17.2	5.2	*9.2	8.3
Breast cancer[4]	X	X	X	X	X	X	X	X	29.0	14.2	11.8	11.5
Prostate cancer	X	X	X	X	8.5	9.6	*14.6	*13.5	X	X	X	X
Uterine fibroids	X	X	X	X	X	X	X	X	29.3	35.6	22.9	23.3
Diabetes	29.1	33.1	32.3	32.0	29.1	37.4	32.0	32.9	29.2	29.0	32.6	31.1
Alcohol and drug	21.7	23.3	24.1	24.2	34.6	33.5	35.6	36.4	9.6	13.7	13.0	12.7
Schizophrenia, mood disorders, delusional disorders, nonorganic psychoses	32.9	42.7	48.4	47.5	25.4	*39.6	45.7	43.5	39.8	45.6	50.9	51.3
Schizophrenia	10.1	12.8	15.1	14.4	8.4	*14.4	*17.0	15.7	11.7	11.3	13.2	13.2
Mood disorders	19.6	*26.9	30.3	30.4	14.5	*21.6	25.4	24.9	24.4	*32.0	35.1	35.6
Heart disease	238.7	203.6	151.8	145.6	316.8	264.0	195.3	187.5	166.1	146.4	110.3	105.6
Ischemic heart disease	160.3	126.4	73.1	68.2	226.1	177.3	101.4	95.4	99.2	78.2	46.0	42.3
Heart attack	50.6	38.8	25.9	26.4	74.4	58.7	37.3	37.8	28.4	19.9	15.0	15.4
Arrhythmias	28.5	25.1	23.5	24.7	35.5	31.8	29.8	31.1	22.1	18.7	17.5	18.6
Heart failure	26.4	31.4	34.2	31.8	30.7	33.5	41.5	37.3	22.4	29.3	27.3	26.6
Hypertension	16.3	19.0	19.6	17.9	16.9	17.6	19.6	17.6	15.6	20.3	19.6	18.2
Stroke	35.2	36.7	34.7	36.0	40.8	38.3	38.6	41.2	30.1	35.2	31.0	31.1
Pneumonia	33.5	35.3	33.2	32.6	34.0	34.2	36.5	34.7	33.0	36.4	30.2	30.7
Chronic obstructive pulmonary disease	15.8	30.8	29.7	28.9	17.4	30.8	24.5	24.1	14.3	30.8	34.8	33.5
Asthma	18.6	13.4	16.7	15.7	11.8	6.2	10.3	8.7	24.9	20.2	22.8	22.4
Osteoarthritis	18.9	24.0	60.0	61.5	16.3	20.8	54.6	54.1	21.2	27.0	65.1	68.4
Intervertebral disc disorders	31.5	21.2	21.0	20.3	36.8	22.5	22.1	21.2	26.5	20.0	20.0	19.4
Injury	72.5	47.9	55.6	56.4	79.9	51.2	59.3	62.2	65.6	44.7	52.0	50.8
Fracture	32.4	26.2	26.6	29.2	33.4	25.3	28.2	31.3	31.5	27.0	25.0	27.2
Poisoning and toxic effects	6.3	6.3	12.7	11.9	4.5	5.5	11.3	11.0	8.0	7.1	14.1	12.7
Internal organ injury	7.9	4.5	8.1	7.1	10.2	5.9	9.3	9.1	5.7	3.2	*6.8	*5.1
Complications of care and adverse effects	32.0	34.5	50.7	49.8	35.6	36.3	52.8	51.0	28.7	32.7	48.8	48.7
65 to 74 Years [3]	2,616.3	2,546.0	2,554.9	2,487.1	2,877.6	2,649.1	2,678.2	2,598.5	2,411.2	2,461.0	2,449.3	2,391.0
Septicemia	27.2	35.6	66.9	71.3	34.9	40.1	69.7	77.9	21.2	32.0	64.5	65.5
Cancer, all	243.1	159.0	156.6	147.5	281.4	176.4	186.0	175.3	213.0	144.7	131.4	123.6
Colorectal cancer	27.0	22.8	20.5	16.6	30.6	29.9	*24.1	20.1	24.1	16.9	*17.4	13.5
Lung/bronchus/tracheal cancer	42.9	26.1	29.2	27.3	63.9	28.2	*35.2	33.6	26.4	24.5	24.0	21.9
Breast cancer[4]	X	X	X	X	X	X	X	X	42.3	31.2	*18.8	16.7
Prostate cancer	X	X	X	X	50.6	37.1	*35.9	30.1	X	X	X	X
Diabetes	51.8	46.4	51.3	45.4	43.6	46.8	47.1	45.7	58.3	46.2	54.9	45.2
Schizophrenia, mood disorders, delusional disorders, nonorganic psychoses	32.7	37.1	*31.0	*29.2	25.3	*34.2	*27.5	*21.6	38.6	39.6	*34.0	*35.7
Dementia and Alzheimer's disease	5.6	*11.2	*6.9	*8.3	4.9	*16.2	*	*	*6.1	*7.0	*	*7.6
Heart disease	558.1	604.8	427.2	407.4	694.2	706.4	535.4	509.0	451.3	521.0	334.4	319.8
Ischemic heart disease	321.3	307.0	187.0	170.2	419.9	396.5	251.4	233.9	243.9	233.2	131.8	115.2
Heart attack	103.3	100.3	66.3	62.0	139.8	124.7	86.9	82.8	74.6	80.2	48.6	44.1
Arrhythmias	69.1	102.6	84.6	85.1	84.7	108.3	101.4	99.4	56.9	97.9	70.2	72.7
Heart failure	105.2	131.6	100.6	93.9	118.0	136.4	119.3	112.3	95.1	127.6	84.6	78.0
Hypertension	21.8	21.5	*37.0	29.1	16.2	16.5	*33.0	*24.3	26.2	25.5	*40.4	33.2
Stroke	123.9	127.1	108.1	109.5	137.5	131.8	129.9	126.6	113.1	123.2	89.4	94.7
Pneumonia	98.1	121.3	83.5	83.8	113.6	127.7	81.9	86.8	85.9	116.1	84.9	81.2
Chronic obstructive pulmonary disease	45.3	102.3	101.5	98.5	52.6	102.6	100.1	92.8	39.6	102.0	102.7	103.4
Gallstones	44.2	33.4	23.4	22.2	38.2	30.2	26.4	23.6	48.9	36.0	20.9	21.1
Kidney disease	9.9	19.1	58.2	57.1	11.0	21.0	67.9	71.3	9.0	17.5	49.9	44.9
Urinary tract infection	30.2	25.5	39.4	38.0	21.7	19.7	29.8	25.4	36.9	30.3	47.6	49.0
Hyperplasia of the prostate	X	X	X	X	143.5	53.6	*23.7	21.6	X	X	X	X
Osteoarthritis	68.0	101.4	148.0	160.7	55.2	103.1	119.9	136.4	78.0	100.1	172.0	181.7
Injury	107.7	101.5	96.8	96.4	90.7	83.8	83.4	77.1	121.1	116.2	108.3	112.9
Fracture	67.2	63.3	58.2	59.5	45.2	46.8	38.8	38.0	84.4	76.9	74.8	77.9
Hip fracture	26.7	26.4	19.2	18.3	15.3	*20.0	12.4	12.2	35.7	31.7	*25.0	23.6
Complications of care and adverse effects	69.7	80.0	98.3	96.3	85.7	95.7	112.0	104.5	57.2	67.1	86.4	89.3

Table 3-59. Discharge Rate in Nonfederal Short-Stay Hospitals, by Sex, Age, and Selected First-Listed Diagnosis, Selected Years, 1990 Through 2009–2010—*Continued*

(Number per 10,000 population.)

Age and first-listed diagnosis	Both sexes				Male				Female			
	1990	2000	2009[1]	2009–2010[1]	1990	2000	2009[1]	2009–2010[1]	1990	2000	2009[1]	2009–2010[1]
75 to 84 Years[3]	3,957.0	4,124.4	4,068.0	3,982.8	4,417.3	4,294.1	4,242.3	4,137.3	3,678.9	4,013.5	3,944.7	3,871.9
Septicemia	53.9	68.3	129.9	138.7	63.8	78.1	148.5	151.6	47.9	61.9	116.7	129.3
Cancer, all	300.3	194.0	179.8	172.3	420.8	211.0	198.9	197.3	227.6	182.9	166.3	154.3
Colorectal cancer	49.8	33.0	29.8	29.8	54.0	37.5	*27.4	30.8	47.3	30.1	31.4	29.1
Lung/bronchus/tracheal cancer	36.5	27.0	33.4	33.5	57.2	32.2	*38.4	40.5	*24.0	23.6	29.8	28.5
Breast cancer[4]	X	X	X	X	X	X	X	X	38.7	30.8	*12.5	16.5
Prostate cancer	X	X	X	X	99.2	27.4	*9.4	*11.1	X	X	X	X
Diabetes	44.3	63.4	75.7	66.9	44.8	68.1	72.0	67.5	44.0	60.3	*78.3	66.5
Schizophrenia, mood disorders, delusional disorders, nonorganic psychoses	38.8	41.4	*	*	*27.3	*30.6	*	*	45.7	48.5	*29.7	*31.3
Dementia and Alzheimer's disease	20.0	36.5	40.7	44.0	22.8	36.8	*52.4	46.2	18.3	36.3	*32.4	42.3
Heart disease	866.6	954.8	779.8	739.5	1,003.8	1,062.5	881.6	844.7	783.7	884.3	707.7	663.8
Ischemic heart disease	382.4	416.7	272.1	248.7	470.5	528.5	346.4	312.9	329.1	343.6	219.5	202.7
Heart attack	155.9	166.9	125.5	112.8	220.9	212.8	144.2	127.7	116.7	136.9	112.2	102.2
Arrhythmias	133.4	176.8	183.6	168.7	153.3	174.4	181.6	165.9	121.4	178.3	185.1	170.7
Heart failure	261.4	263.1	225.1	220.7	286.2	271.1	242.9	248.3	246.4	257.9	212.5	200.9
Hypertension	22.6	39.7	48.9	38.0	*	*28.4	*38.9	*31.7	30.7	47.1	56.0	42.5
Stroke	259.0	255.5	196.5	196.9	277.7	278.4	225.7	210.6	247.7	240.6	175.8	187.1
Pneumonia	224.6	263.5	177.7	179.3	297.8	310.8	201.0	193.3	180.4	232.6	161.3	169.3
Chronic obstructive pulmonary disease	55.4	146.2	137.5	131.4	89.4	179.6	158.7	149.9	34.8	124.3	122.5	118.0
Gallstones	47.6	39.6	38.7	39.1	51.9	41.4	36.5	39.0	45.0	38.5	*40.2	39.1
Kidney disease	24.5	37.6	108.9	110.2	27.6	48.7	129.1	123.9	*22.6	30.4	94.6	100.3
Urinary tract infection	86.0	85.6	120.1	123.0	66.6	72.5	84.6	87.6	97.8	94.2	145.2	148.5
Hyperplasia of the prostate	X	X	X	X	183.3	67.2	*39.1	38.5	X	X	X	X
Osteoarthritis	68.6	100.6	156.0	161.4	65.2	76.5	147.5	152.6	70.7	116.4	162.1	167.8
Injury	259.1	229.1	232.8	237.0	153.4	171.7	190.3	189.0	323.0	266.6	262.9	271.5
Fracture	195.8	170.2	160.4	166.2	92.6	116.4	110.4	111.8	258.1	205.4	195.7	205.3
Hip fracture	115.2	99.0	63.2	69.4	53.7	68.6	36.0	45.6	152.4	118.8	82.3	86.5
Complications of care and adverse effects	81.5	101.4	121.1	123.1	101.4	136.0	149.4	150.8	69.4	78.8	101.1	103.2
85 Years and Over[3]	5,606.3	6,050.9	5,814.6	5,667.7	6,420.9	6,166.6	6,425.5	6,193.4	5,289.6	6,003.3	5,531.7	5,415.6
Septicemia	135.6	153.9	237.5	261.4	139.0	207.3	292.9	320.8	134.3	131.9	211.8	232.8
Cancer, all	254.0	194.5	167.7	144.0	370.6	250.5	241.0	209.0	208.7	171.5	133.7	112.8
Colorectal cancer	47.6	49.7	*21.8	17.0	*59.1	*58.8	*	*20.7	43.2	45.9	*18.3	*15.2
Lung/bronchus/tracheal cancer	*19.1	12.1	*23.1	*25.0	*	*20.9	*	*	*	*8.5	*	*15.2
Breast cancer[4]	X	X	X	X	X	X	X	X	*41.7	*20.5	*	*12.0
Prostate cancer	X	X	X	X	*87.8	*49.3	*	*20.0	X	X	X	X
Diabetes	53.0	65.6	*59.8	58.7	*53.5	*54.2	*70.1	69.4	52.8	70.3	*55.1	*53.6
Schizophrenia, mood disorders, delusional disorders, nonorganic psychoses	*27.9	*37.3	*	*	*	*	*	*40.6	*30.7	*43.0	*	*
Dementia and Alzheimer's disease	49.7	107.0	73.8	77.2	*28.9	94.3	88.7	96.2	57.7	112.2	66.9	68.0
Heart disease	1,107.0	1,298.2	1,085.8	1,054.7	1,320.3	1,407.4	1,323.1	1,224.2	1,024.1	1,253.4	975.9	973.4
Ischemic heart disease	423.0	427.2	246.1	246.9	581.6	534.4	349.8	323.5	361.3	383.2	198.1	210.2
Heart attack	199.8	251.1	155.6	161.0	274.2	296.0	205.0	197.1	170.9	232.7	132.7	143.6
Arrhythmias	167.2	232.4	225.0	212.3	189.6	247.1	207.0	213.2	158.5	226.4	233.3	211.9
Heart failure	416.7	480.4	466.6	451.7	460.5	455.7	565.1	528.8	399.7	490.5	421.0	414.7
Hypertension	*17.9	41.1	66.2	49.1	*	*18.3	*69.3	*47.6	*19.3	50.4	*64.8	49.8
Stroke	427.2	373.8	288.3	284.1	408.2	396.7	270.7	278.5	434.6	364.3	296.4	286.8
Pneumonia	501.0	514.9	367.9	355.3	753.7	607.8	412.7	429.2	402.8	476.8	347.1	319.9
Chronic obstructive pulmonary disease	44.1	130.9	144.3	144.0	*72.9	150.4	*157.2	173.4	*32.9	123.0	138.4	129.8
Gallstones	60.7	39.2	*42.4	39.7	*68.2	*29.7	*40.4	*40.6	57.8	*43.1	*43.3	39.3
Kidney disease	47.1	49.5	160.2	167.4	92.4	*68.1	202.1	230.5	*29.4	*41.9	140.8	137.1
Urinary tract infection	216.5	191.5	346.0	321.9	239.3	153.1	259.5	217.0	207.6	207.2	386.1	372.1
Hyperplasia of the prostate	X	X	X	X	158.6	*69.9	*33.5	*31.8	X	X	X	X
Osteoarthritis	44.5	56.0	64.5	70.2	*	*	*57.3	*54.9	35.8	57.3	67.8	77.6
Injury	542.0	545.5	533.3	525.3	435.4	355.6	435.1	428.4	583.4	623.5	578.9	571.7
Fracture	439.0	450.9	403.5	396.6	335.7	252.4	302.1	275.7	479.2	532.4	450.4	454.6
Hip fracture	272.3	275.1	218.2	211.6	224.4	146.5	160.6	155.4	291.0	327.9	244.9	238.6
Complications of care and adverse effects	96.6	79.1	132.8	127.1	132.3	90.5	*151.7	160.0	82.7	74.4	124.1	111.4

X = Not applicable.   * = Figure does not meet standards of reliability or precision. Data preceded by an asterisk have a relative standard error (RSE) of 20 to 30 percent. Data not shown have an RSE of greater than 30 percent.   [1]Starting with 2008 data, the sample of nonfederal short-stay hospitals was cut in half. This smaller sample size has increased standard errors. Therefore, caution should be exercised in interpreting trends in these data.   [2]Estimates are age adjusted to the year 2000 standard population using six age groups: under 18 years, 18 to 44 years, 45 to 54 years, 55 to 64 years, 65 to 74 years, and 75 years and over.   [3]Includes discharges with first-listed diagnoses not shown in table.   [4]Shown for women only.

Table 3-60. Average Length of Stay[1] in Nonfederal Short-Stay Hospitals, by Sex, Age, and Selected First-Listed Diagnosis, Selected Years, 1990 Through 2009–2010

(Number of days.)

Age and first-listed diagnosis	Both sexes					Male					Female				
	1990	2000	2005	2009[2]	2009–2010[2]	1990	2000	2005	2009[2]	2009–2010[2]	1990	2000	2005	2009[2]	2009–2010[2]
All Ages, Crude [3]	6.4	4.9	4.8	4.9	4.8	6.9	5.3	5.2	5.3	5.3	6.1	4.6	4.5	4.6	4.5
Under 18 Years [3]	4.9	4.4	4.7	4.4	4.4	5.0	4.8	4.9	4.4	4.5	4.7	4.1	4.5	4.4	4.3
Dehydration	3.0	2.2	2.0	2.1	2.1	2.9	2.2	2.1	2.0	2.0	3.0	2.1	2.0	2.3	2.2
Acute bronchitis and bronchiolitis	3.7	3.1	2.9	3.4	3.2	3.6	3.0	3.0	3.4	3.3	3.8	*3.3	2.9	3.3	3.0
Pneumonia	4.6	3.6	3.2	3.4	3.5	4.6	3.4	3.1	3.5	3.7	4.7	3.9	3.3	3.4	3.3
Asthma	2.9	2.2	2.3	2.5	2.5	2.8	2.1	2.3	2.3	2.3	3.1	2.3	2.2	2.7	2.8
Appendicitis	4.0	3.2	3.4	3.1	3.2	3.9	2.9	3.6	3.1	3.3	4.0	3.5	*3.1	3.2	2.9
Injury	4.1	3.8	*4.2	3.2	3.3	4.2	4.1	*4.8	2.9	3.3	3.8	*3.2	3.0	3.6	3.2
Fracture	4.5	3.5	3.5	3.1	3.4	4.2	3.9	*3.8	2.9	3.4	5.0	2.5	3.0	3.3	3.4
Complications of care and adverse effects	*5.3	*5.7	5.9	5.9	5.6	*6.0	*5.5	5.5	*7.1	6.4	*4.5	*5.9	*6.1	*4.7	4.6
18 to 44 Years [3]	4.6	3.6	3.7	3.7	3.6	6.1	4.8	4.8	4.8	4.7	4.0	3.2	3.3	3.3	3.3
HIV/AIDS	*10.7	*8.8	*8.8	8.5	7.9	*10.6	*9.4	7.5	8.9	8.5	*	*7.5	*	7.4	6.4
Cancer, all	7.8	6.3	6.9	6.6	6.3	8.4	7.9	7.5	*9.4	7.9	7.5	5.4	*6.6	5.4	5.4
Childbirth	X	X	X	X	X	X	X	X	X	X	2.8	2.5	2.6	2.7	2.7
Uterine fibroids	X	X	X	X	X	X	X	X	X	X	4.2	2.5	2.7	2.4	2.2
Diabetes	5.8	3.9	3.8	3.7	3.3	6.2	3.7	3.7	3.7	3.3	5.2	4.3	3.9	3.6	3.3
Alcohol and drug	9.0	*5.0	4.8	3.5	3.7	8.9	4.8	4.6	3.6	3.8	9.1	*5.3	*5.1	3.4	3.3
Schizophrenia, mood disorders, delusional disorders, nonorganic psychoses	14.3	*7.9	*7.4	7.7	7.1	13.8	*8.2	*8.3	7.8	7.3	14.8	*7.6	*6.7	7.5	6.9
Schizophrenia	15.4	*11.0	*10.2	10.7	9.9	15.3	*10.6	*10.7	10.0	9.4	15.6	*11.9	9.4	11.8	10.7
Mood disorders	14.3	*6.6	*6.3	6.4	6.0	*13.2	*6.6	*6.7	6.9	6.3	15.0	*6.5	*6.0	6.0	5.8
Heart disease	5.4	3.6	4.0	4.2	4.0	5.4	3.5	3.8	3.9	3.6	5.4	3.7	4.4	4.7	4.7
Ischemic heart disease	4.6	3.0	3.1	3.4	3.2	4.8	2.8	3.3	3.8	3.3	4.1	3.6	2.8	2.7	3.1
Pneumonia	6.9	5.1	5.0	4.1	4.3	7.8	5.0	5.7	4.4	4.5	6.0	5.2	4.5	3.9	4.1
Asthma	4.4	2.9	2.7	3.8	3.4	3.8	2.5	2.4	2.2	2.3	4.6	3.1	2.8	*4.5	3.9
Intervertebral disc disorders	4.4	2.3	2.3	2.5	2.5	4.2	2.2	2.3	2.1	2.2	4.7	2.3	2.2	3.0	2.7
Injury	5.1	4.3	4.3	4.2	4.2	5.0	4.5	4.4	4.6	4.6	5.3	4.1	4.1	3.4	3.6
Fracture	6.0	4.9	5.1	4.5	4.8	5.6	5.0	5.0	4.4	4.9	6.9	4.4	5.4	4.5	4.6
Poisoning and toxic effects	2.7	2.5	2.9	2.5	2.6	2.7	2.8	3.5	2.6	3.0	2.7	2.4	2.3	2.4	2.3
Complications of care and adverse effects	5.6	4.7	5.1	5.2	5.1	5.3	4.9	5.4	5.8	5.5	*5.9	4.6	4.9	4.8	4.8
45 to 64 Years [3]	6.7	5.0	5.0	5.1	5.0	6.7	5.1	5.0	5.2	5.2	6.8	4.8	4.9	4.9	4.9
HIV/AIDS	*	*	*9.9	8.6	8.2	*	*	10.4	8.3	8.7	*	*	*	*9.5	*7.0
Cancer, all	8.8	6.2	6.4	5.9	6.1	9.3	6.8	6.6	6.0	6.1	8.4	5.6	6.1	5.7	6.1
Colorectal cancer	13.3	7.4	7.3	7.5	7.6	*13.0	7.4	7.9	7.7	7.9	*13.6	7.4	6.7	7.3	7.2
Lung/bronchus/tracheal cancer	7.7	6.2	6.8	6.5	6.8	7.1	6.0	7.3	6.6	7.1	8.6	6.4	6.3	6.5	6.6
Breast cancer[4]	X	X	X	X	X	X	X	X	X	X	4.3	2.0	2.5	2.3	2.4
Prostate cancer	X	X	X	X	X	7.3	3.2	3.1	1.4	1.7	X	X	X	X	X
Uterine fibroids	X	X	X	X	X	X	X	X	X	X	4.5	2.8	3.0	2.2	2.2
Diabetes	8.1	5.6	5.1	5.8	5.2	7.3	6.0	5.3	6.8	5.7	8.9	5.2	4.9	4.8	4.8
Alcohol and drug	8.5	4.8	4.7	4.7	4.6	8.6	4.6	4.8	5.0	4.8	8.3	*5.0	4.4	4.1	4.2
Schizophrenia, mood disorders, delusional disorders, nonorganic psychoses	14.3	*7.9	*7.4	7.7	8.1	13.8	*8.2	*8.3	7.8	7.9	14.8	*7.6	*6.7	7.5	8.3
Schizophrenia	15.6	*11.9	10.9	11.0	10.8	14.2	*11.4	10.1	11.0	9.9	16.5	*12.5	11.6	11.0	11.7
Mood disorders	14.7	*7.9	7.8	7.2	6.9	13.4	*7.3	8.1	7.0	6.7	15.4	*8.3	7.6	7.3	7.1
Heart disease	5.9	3.9	4.1	4.1	4.2	5.8	3.8	3.8	3.8	4.0	6.1	4.1	4.7	4.5	4.6
Ischemic heart disease	5.7	3.7	3.8	3.7	3.9	5.7	3.6	3.5	3.4	3.7	5.8	3.8	*4.5	4.2	4.3
Heart attack	7.5	4.8	4.9	4.6	4.8	7.5	4.7	4.6	4.5	4.6	7.6	5.0	5.6	5.0	5.3
Arrhythmias	4.6	2.9	2.9	3.0	3.3	4.6	2.8	2.7	3.2	3.3	4.6	2.9	3.2	2.8	3.3
Heart failure	7.0	4.9	5.2	5.0	5.0	6.9	5.2	4.9	4.9	4.7	7.3	4.7	5.6	5.1	5.4
Hypertension	3.9	2.2	2.1	2.2	2.2	*4.3	2.0	2.1	2.1	2.3	3.8	2.4	2.0	2.2	2.2
Stroke	10.3	5.3	5.6	4.6	5.2	10.0	5.2	5.9	4.5	5.2	10.7	5.5	5.4	4.8	5.3
Pneumonia	8.0	5.8	5.5	4.9	5.2	8.0	6.0	5.7	4.9	5.3	7.9	5.7	5.3	5.0	5.1
Chronic obstructive pulmonary disease	6.5	4.7	4.1	5.7	4.9	6.8	5.0	3.6	4.3	4.1	6.2	4.4	4.5	*6.7	5.5
Asthma	5.2	3.9	3.9	4.1	4.1	5.3	*3.2	3.4	*4.5	3.9	5.2	4.0	4.1	4.0	4.2
Osteoarthritis	7.4	3.9	3.5	3.4	3.3	7.1	3.6	3.4	3.2	3.1	7.5	4.1	3.6	3.6	3.4
Intervertebral disc disorders	5.2	2.8	2.9	3.5	3.3	5.0	2.6	2.5	*3.8	*3.5	5.4	3.1	3.2	3.1	3.0
Injury	6.5	5.1	5.0	4.8	5.7	6.6	5.5	5.0	4.7	*6.4	6.4	4.6	4.9	4.9	4.8
Fracture	7.6	5.6	5.3	5.4	*7.1	7.2	6.4	5.6	5.2	*	7.9	4.9	5.0	5.6	5.4
Poisoning and toxic effects	4.9	3.0	3.4	3.3	3.3	*	*2.9	3.4	2.8	3.0	4.3	3.1	3.3	3.6	3.6
Internal organ injury	*8.3	7.6	6.7	5.9	5.8	*	8.3	7.3	5.9	5.9	*8.1	*	*5.6	6.1	5.6
Complications of care and adverse effects	7.9	6.1	6.0	6.1	6.0	8.4	5.9	6.2	6.2	6.1	7.4	6.4	5.8	6.0	6.0
65 to 74 Years [3]	8.0	5.7	5.3	5.4	5.4	7.8	5.6	5.3	5.6	5.6	8.1	5.7	5.3	5.3	5.3
Septicemia	*15.9	8.6	8.1	8.7	9.3	*	8.5	8.1	7.9	9.7	14.4	8.8	8.1	9.5	9.0
Cancer, all	9.4	7.0	6.7	6.7	6.4	9.9	6.9	6.8	6.8	6.8	9.0	7.1	6.5	6.5	5.9
Colorectal cancer	12.9	9.1	7.7	7.2	7.0	11.3	9.2	7.9	8.1	7.4	14.5	9.0	7.5	6.1	6.5
Lung/bronchus/tracheal cancer	9.2	7.0	7.3	6.1	5.9	8.7	6.8	7.6	6.3	6.0	10.2	*7.1	7.1	5.9	5.7
Breast cancer[4]	X	X	X	X	X	X	X	X	X	X	4.4	*	*3.2	2.0	2.1
Prostate cancer	X	X	X	X	X	6.5	3.8	*3.3	2.0	2.2	X	X	X	X	X
Diabetes	8.4	5.9	5.2	4.9	5.4	9.1	6.2	5.6	5.0	5.8	8.0	5.6	4.8	4.8	5.2
Schizophrenia, mood disorders, delusional disorders, nonorganic psychoses	16.6	11.7	10.7	11.9	12.8	17.4	*11.7	10.0	12.8	13.0	16.3	11.7	11.1	11.3	12.7
Dementia and Alzheimer's disease	*12.6	*9.3	*8.4	*7.8	8.5	*10.4	*9.6	*8.1	*8.6	*8.4	*14.0	*8.9	*8.6	*7.1	8.7
Heart disease	7.0	4.8	4.4	4.7	4.7	7.0	4.7	4.4	4.5	4.6	7.0	4.9	4.4	4.9	4.7
Ischemic heart disease	6.6	4.6	4.2	4.1	4.2	6.8	4.3	4.3	4.0	4.2	6.3	4.9	4.0	4.3	4.3
Heart attack	8.4	5.9	5.8	4.9	5.2	8.8	5.3	6.1	4.7	5.1	7.8	6.6	5.3	5.1	5.3
Arrhythmias	5.7	3.8	3.3	3.5	3.6	5.6	3.8	3.4	3.1	3.4	5.8	3.7	3.2	4.1	3.8
Heart failure	8.4	5.5	4.9	5.4	5.0	7.9	5.7	4.9	5.1	4.9	8.8	5.4	4.9	5.7	5.2
Hypertension	4.3	2.6	2.3	2.1	2.1	*4.6	*2.7	2.4	2.0	2.1	4.1	2.4	2.3	2.2	2.1
Stroke	8.4	4.7	4.5	4.9	5.1	8.3	4.5	4.6	4.6	4.7	8.5	4.8	4.3	5.3	5.7
Pneumonia	9.5	6.4	5.3	5.6	5.7	9.5	6.4	5.1	5.7	5.8	9.5	6.3	5.6	5.5	5.6
Chronic obstructive pulmonary disease	8.2	4.8	4.8	4.4	4.6	8.6	4.5	4.8	4.2	4.4	7.7	5.0	4.8	4.6	4.7
Gallstones	6.6	4.4	4.2	5.4	5.0	6.9	*5.2	4.3	5.1	4.9	6.5	3.9	4.2	5.8	5.1
Kidney disease	10.4	7.6	6.9	6.5	6.2	8.4	6.9	7.2	6.8	5.9	*12.4	8.2	6.6	6.1	6.6
Urinary tract infection	8.0	4.8	4.4	4.4	4.0	7.2	5.1	5.1	4.6	4.2	8.4	4.7	4.1	4.2	3.9
Hyperplasia of the prostate	X	X	X	X	X	4.5	2.8	2.4	2.1	2.0	X	X	X	X	X
Osteoarthritis	9.3	4.7	3.8	3.5	3.5	8.8	4.7	3.8	3.4	3.4	9.5	4.7	3.8	3.6	3.6
Injury	9.2	5.6	5.8	6.0	5.6	8.4	5.7	6.4	6.9	6.3	9.7	5.6	5.4	5.4	5.2
Fracture	11.1	5.9	5.5	6.4	5.8	10.2	6.4	5.6	*7.8	7.2	11.5	5.7	5.5	5.7	5.2
Hip fracture	*15.5	7.1	7.1	*7.6	6.7	*11.8	*7.9	*7.2	*	*8.9	*16.7	6.7	7.0	5.9	5.7
Complications of care and adverse effects	7.8	6.4	6.5	5.6	5.8	7.3	6.1	6.0	5.7	6.0	8.5	6.8	7.1	5.4	5.6

Table 3-60. Average Length of Stay[1] in Nonfederal Short-Stay Hospitals, by Sex, Age, and Selected First-Listed Diagnosis, Selected Years, 1990 Through 2009–2010—*Continued*

(Number of days.)

Age and first-listed diagnosis	Both sexes					Male					Female				
	1990	2000	2005	2009[2]	2009–2010[2]	1990	2000	2005	2009[2]	2009–2010[2]	1990	2000	2005	2009[2]	2009–2010[2]
75 to 84 Years [3]	9.1	6.2	5.6	5.8	5.7	8.7	6.2	5.7	5.9	5.8	9.4	6.1	5.5	5.8	5.7
Septicemia	12.1	7.9	8.0	8.8	8.6	12.9	7.4	8.1	9.1	9.0	11.5	8.4	7.8	8.6	8.3
Cancer, all	10.4	7.2	7.3	6.3	6.5	9.3	7.2	7.2	6.4	6.5	11.7	7.2	7.4	6.2	6.5
Colorectal cancer	12.9	9.0	9.3	7.8	8.1	12.5	*9.3	9.1	8.3	8.3	13.2	8.8	9.4	7.4	8.0
Lung/bronchus/tracheal cancer	9.5	6.5	6.9	6.4	6.2	9.6	6.2	6.9	6.7	6.1	*9.4	6.9	6.9	6.2	6.2
Breast cancer[4]	X	X	X	X	X	X	X	X	X	X	5.7	*3.2	*	2.1	*2.6
Prostate cancer	X	X	X	X	X	6.6	*5.1	*5.7	2.9	*4.7	X	X	X	X	X
Diabetes	12.5	6.0	5.6	*6.3	5.9	11.7	6.4	7.1	*6.3	6.5	13.1	5.6	4.6	*6.2	5.5
Schizophrenia, mood disorders, delusional disorders, nonorganic psychoses	15.8	10.8	9.3	*11.7	12.5	*15.7	*11.6	*9.7	*11.6	*11.8	15.8	10.4	9.1	11.7	12.8
Dementia and Alzheimer's disease	*15.3	8.2	8.5	8.8	8.7	*12.8	7.6	7.2	6.8	7.7	*	8.6	*9.2	11.0	9.4
Heart disease	8.0	5.3	4.7	5.1	5.0	8.1	5.4	4.7	5.2	5.0	7.8	5.3	4.7	5.0	4.9
Ischemic heart disease	7.9	5.1	4.6	4.8	4.8	8.5	5.2	4.8	5.2	4.9	7.4	5.1	4.4	4.4	4.5
Heart attack	9.7	6.2	6.2	5.6	5.7	10.1	5.8	6.6	6.0	5.8	9.3	6.6	5.8	5.3	5.7
Arrhythmias	6.6	4.2	3.4	4.8	4.5	6.5	4.3	3.2	5.2	4.5	6.7	4.1	3.6	4.6	4.5
Heart failure	8.0	5.9	5.1	5.3	5.3	7.7	6.1	5.1	4.9	5.2	8.2	5.8	5.1	5.6	5.3
Hypertension	6.0	2.6	2.7	3.1	2.7	*	*2.1	2.7	2.3	2.0	*5.6	2.8	2.6	*3.5	3.0
Stroke	10.4	5.9	5.1	4.6	5.4	10.0	5.7	5.6	4.6	5.5	10.6	6.0	4.7	4.6	5.3
Pneumonia	10.4	6.3	5.9	6.1	5.7	9.8	6.4	5.8	6.5	5.7	11.0	6.3	5.9	5.8	5.8
Chronic obstructive pulmonary disease	8.0	4.9	5.4	4.7	4.7	6.6	4.8	*5.9	4.6	4.7	*10.1	4.9	4.9	4.7	4.7
Gallstones	8.5	5.3	4.9	5.0	5.6	8.0	5.6	4.5	5.6	6.2	8.8	5.1	5.3	4.6	5.1
Kidney disease	10.5	7.4	6.7	6.3	6.2	11.0	8.2	6.6	5.7	5.6	*10.1	6.6	6.8	6.9	6.7
Urinary tract infection	11.0	5.2	4.6	5.2	4.9	8.1	5.5	5.2	5.2	5.3	12.3	5.1	4.4	5.2	4.8
Hyperplasia of the prostate	X	X	X	X	X	6.0	3.1	*3.0	*	*	X	X	X	X	X
Osteoarthritis	10.1	4.6	3.9	3.7	3.7	9.9	4.4	3.8	3.4	3.6	10.2	4.7	3.9	3.9	3.8
Injury	10.1	6.8	5.5	6.0	6.1	8.9	*8.2	6.3	7.7	7.1	10.4	6.3	5.2	5.2	5.5
Fracture	11.0	7.4	5.7	6.0	6.1	10.0	*	6.8	7.6	7.1	11.2	6.7	5.4	5.4	5.7
Hip fracture	12.1	7.7	6.7	6.3	6.2	10.4	7.8	7.7	7.4	6.9	12.5	7.6	6.3	6.0	5.9
Complications of care and adverse effects	12.5	7.1	6.1	6.1	6.2	14.0	8.1	5.9	6.2	6.5	11.2	6.0	6.4	6.1	5.9
85 Years and Over [3]	9.6	6.2	5.7	5.8	5.6	9.4	6.1	5.9	5.9	5.7	9.6	6.2	5.7	5.7	5.6
Septicemia	12.6	6.9	7.1	8.5	7.9	*11.8	6.7	7.7	10.2	8.6	12.9	6.9	6.8	7.4	7.4
Cancer, all	12.1	7.5	6.8	6.6	6.7	13.4	8.6	6.6	6.0	5.9	11.3	6.8	6.9	7.0	7.5
Colorectal cancer	22.4	*10.1	9.4	8.7	9.7	*	*	*	8.0	8.4	*21.1	8.2	8.9	9.2	10.5
Lung/bronchus/tracheal cancer	*	*8.0	7.0	5.3	5.0	*	*5.9	*	3.2	3.8	*5.3	*	*6.8	6.7	6.6
Breast cancer[4]	X	X	X	X	X	X	X	X	X	X	*	*	*	*2.4	2.5
Prostate cancer	X	X	X	X	X	*7.5	*	*	*5.5	5.3	X	X	X	X	X
Diabetes	9.1	6.0	5.4	4.9	5.2	*	*	*5.3	*6.9	5.8	9.2	4.9	*5.5	3.8	4.9
Schizophrenia, mood disorders, delusional disorders, nonorganic psychoses	*	*10.5	*11.4	*9.5	*10.6	*	*	*	8.4	*8.4	*	*10.8	*12.0	*10.5	*12.2
Dementia and Alzheimer's disease	11.4	7.9	*7.6	6.5	6.8	*	*8.8	*7.3	5.7	7.3	*11.0	*7.6	*7.7	7.0	6.5
Heart disease	8.1	5.2	4.9	5.0	4.9	7.8	5.1	4.9	5.3	5.2	8.2	5.3	4.9	4.8	4.8
Ischemic heart disease	7.5	5.4	4.9	4.6	4.9	6.8	5.4	5.2	5.2	4.9	7.9	5.4	4.6	4.2	4.8
Heart attack	9.8	6.7	5.8	5.5	5.7	8.9	6.4	6.4	6.6	5.9	10.3	6.9	5.5	4.7	5.6
Arrhythmias	8.3	4.4	4.2	4.4	4.3	*9.6	4.3	3.7	5.0	4.4	7.7	4.4	4.4	4.2	4.2
Heart failure	8.6	5.3	5.3	5.4	5.2	8.0	4.9	5.0	5.6	5.7	8.8	5.5	5.4	5.2	4.9
Hypertension	*	*4.2	2.8	2.8	2.9	*	*	*	2.9	2.8	*	*	2.6	2.8	2.9
Stroke	9.6	5.3	5.3	*	*7.4	9.6	5.6	5.1	6.3	5.5	9.5	5.1	5.5	*	*8.4
Pneumonia	10.9	7.0	5.9	6.2	5.9	11.1	6.1	6.0	5.6	5.3	10.7	7.5	5.9	6.5	6.3
Chronic obstructive pulmonary disease	*9.0	5.7	5.0	4.7	4.6	*7.8	5.5	4.7	5.3	4.5	*	5.7	5.3	4.4	4.6
Gallstones	10.3	5.8	6.1	5.6	5.5	*9.3	*5.6	*	5.7	6.4	10.7	*5.9	6.4	5.6	5.1
Kidney disease	*12.6	8.5	5.7	6.3	5.7	*	*9.0	*6.1	5.8	5.3	*13.8	*8.2	5.5	6.6	5.9
Urinary tract infection	10.2	5.6	5.0	4.9	4.5	9.3	5.7	4.7	5.5	4.8	10.7	5.5	5.1	4.7	4.4
Hyperplasia of the prostate	X	X	X	X	X	6.6	*3.7	*4.3	3.8	3.2	X	X	X	X	X
Osteoarthritis	10.5	4.7	4.2	3.7	3.9	*	*	*4.0	3.4	3.7	*9.6	4.4	4.3	3.9	4.0
Injury	10.5	5.9	5.5	5.2	5.2	11.0	6.4	6.2	5.8	5.7	10.3	5.8	5.3	5.0	5.0
Fracture	11.1	6.1	5.7	5.3	5.3	11.2	6.4	*6.9	5.7	5.8	11.1	6.0	5.4	5.2	5.2
Hip fracture	12.7	6.5	5.8	5.8	5.8	12.6	6.8	6.1	5.8	5.8	12.7	6.5	5.7	5.7	5.8
Complications of care and adverse effects	*11.7	*8.2	6.1	6.1	5.9	*10.7	*6.4	*6.2	7.0	6.3	*12.3	*9.1	6.0	5.6	5.5

X = Not applicable.   * = Figure does not meet standards of reliability or precision. Data preceded by an asterisk have a relative standard error (RSE) of 20 to 30 percent. Data not shown have an RSE of greater than 30 percent.   [1]Average length of stay is calculated by dividing days of care by number of discharges.   [2]Starting with 2008 data, the sample of nonfederal short-stay hospitals was cut in half. This smaller sample size has increased standard errors. Therefore, caution should be exercised in interpreting trends in these data.   [3]Includes discharges with first-listed diagnoses not shown in table.   [4]Shown for women only.

Table 3-61. Discharges with at Least One Procedure in Nonfederal Short-Stay Hospitals, by Sex, Age, and Selected Procedures, Selected Years, 1990 Through 2009–2010

(Percent; rate per 10,000 population.)

Age and procedure (any listed)	Both sexes					Male					Female				
	1990	2000	2005	2009[1]	2009-2010[1]	1990	2000	2005	2009[1]	2009-2010[1]	1990	2000	2005	2009[1]	2009-2010[1]
18 Years and Over															
Hospital discharges with at least one procedure, crude (percent)[2]	67.4	62.1	62.6	63.3	63.2	65.2	59.2	59.4	60.0	59.9	68.7	63.9	64.7	65.5	65.3
Hospital discharges with at least one procedure, age-adjusted[2,3]	1,020.1	859.9	893.5	908.8	900.0	882.2	701.4	722.0	733.7	697.8	1,176.4	1,026.2	1,078.1	1,098.0	1,091.3
Hospital discharges with at least one procedure, crude[2]	1,006.4	856.8	893.8	920.0		788.1	648.4	683.9	716.3		1,205.9	1,049.8	1,090.9	1,112.3	
Operations on vessels of heart	28.3	41.2	41.2	36.0	33.1	41.9	56.9	58.5	50.2	46.7	15.8	26.7	25.0	22.6	20.2
Coronary angioplasty or arthrectomy	14.0	26.2	28.5	25.6	23.2	20.5	34.9	40.5	34.8	31.7	8.0	18.1	17.3	17.0	15.1
Coronary artery stent insertion	X	21.7	27.0	22.6	20.5	X	28.7	38.5	30.4	28.0	X	15.3	16.2	15.2	13.5
Drug-eluting stent insertion	X	X	23.9	15.8	15.0	X	X	34.1	21.0	20.4	X	X	14.4	10.9	9.9
Coronary artery bypass graft (CABG)	14.1	15.0	11.8	10.5	9.9	21.2	21.8	16.6	15.6	15.0	7.7	8.7	7.2	5.7	5.1
Cardiac catheterization	52.1	57.8	53.9	46.1	43.1	68.3	72.1	68.5	55.1	53.0	37.4	44.6	40.2	37.5	33.7
Pacemaker	8.6	8.5	9.6	9.2	8.7	10.1	8.5	10.5	9.0	9.0	7.1	8.5	8.8	9.4	8.4
Carotid (neck arteries) endarterectomy	3.6	5.9	4.6	4.0	4.1	4.1	6.6	5.7	4.6	4.7	3.1	5.3	3.6	3.5	3.5
Endoscopy of small intestine	40.8	42.5	45.8	45.7	44.6	38.6	39.1	42.3	42.3	40.7	42.8	45.6	49.1	48.9	48.3
Endoscopy of large intestine	27.9	25.0	24.0	21.9	20.6	22.5	20.2	19.7	19.1	18.0	32.8	29.4	28.0	24.4	23.1
Gall bladder removal	27.9	19.6	17.7	18.4	18.2	16.5	13.3	13.2	14.5	13.1	38.2	25.5	21.9	22.2	23.0
Laparoscopic gall bladder removal	X	14.8	13.5	14.7	14.8	X	9.2	8.8	10.4	9.6	X	20.1	17.9	18.7	19.7
Treatment of intra-abdominal scar tissue	17.0	14.4	15.3	15.1	14.7	6.5	5.7	6.5	7.8	7.8	26.6	22.4	23.5	22.0	21.3
Reduction of fracture	27.6	24.9	23.2	22.8	23.2	27.3	22.0	21.1	20.5	20.0	27.8	27.7	25.2	25.0	26.3
Excision of intervertebral disc and spinal fusion	18.7	18.2	18.4	22.3	21.8	22.3	20.0	18.8	22.5	21.4	15.4	16.4	18.0	22.2	22.1
Total hip replacement	6.4	7.3	10.5	13.8	13.9	5.4	6.8	10.1	14.0	13.6	7.3	7.7	10.9	13.5	14.1
Partial hip replacement	4.8	5.0	10.2	13.3	13.1	2.0	2.3	7.8	*11.3	10.9	7.3	7.6	12.3	15.2	15.1
Total knee replacement	6.7	13.8	23.1	28.0	28.8	4.9	11.0	16.4	20.2	21.6	8.4	16.4	29.3	35.4	35.6
CT scan	68.4	29.2	27.9	*17.1	*17.0	68.6	27.4	26.1	16.0	15.7	68.2	30.9	29.7	*18.1	*18.2
Arteriography and angiocardiography with contrast	59.7	63.0	59.9	56.4	53.8	75.6	76.2	72.1	64.9	63.4	45.2	50.7	48.5	48.3	44.8
Diagnostic ultrasound	72.3	36.9	36.0	34.7	34.9	62.1	33.1	35.2	34.0	33.9	81.7	40.4	36.7	35.4	35.9
Magnetic resonance imaging	9.5	9.2	11.2	*10.1	9.8	9.4	8.2	10.3	*9.4	9.0	9.6	10.2	12.1	*10.7	*10.6
Mechanical ventilation	17.6	23.0	27.0	32.9	32.4	18.8	23.9	29.5	34.9	34.0	16.4	22.1	24.7	31.1	30.9
18 to 44 Years															
Hospital discharges with at least one procedure, crude (percent)[2]	73.0	71.7	71.7	71.9	72.4	62.6	55.9	54.0	53.6	53.7	77.0	77.4	78.1	78.4	78.7
Hospital discharges with at least one procedure[2]	749.3	609.1	644.0	638.0	627.6	362.8	251.6	254.4	244.3	233.3	1,130.6	965.9	1,039.0	1,039.7	1,030.6
Operations on vessels of heart	3.0	3.9	4.1	*3.1	2.8	4.9	5.5	5.7	4.5	4.1	*1.2	2.3	2.4	*	*1.5
Coronary angioplasty or arthrectomy	1.9	3.0	3.0	*2.5	*2.3	3.0	4.3	4.3	*3.5	3.4	*0.8	1.6	*1.7	*	*1.2
Coronary artery stent insertion	X	2.5	3.1	*2.3	*2.0	X	3.6	4.3	*3.1	*2.9	X	1.4	*1.8	*	*1.1
Drug-eluting stent insertion	X	X	2.6	*	*1.5	X	X	3.4	*	*2.1	X	X	*1.8	*	*
Coronary artery bypass graft (CABG)	1.0	0.9	0.8	*	*0.5	*1.8	1.1	*1.1	*	*0.8	*	*0.7	*	*	*
Cardiac catheterization	9.0	8.5	7.6	7.1	6.3	12.5	11.0	9.6	8.7	8.3	5.5	5.9	5.6	5.5	4.3
Endoscopy of small intestine	13.1	10.3	13.3	15.7	14.7	13.2	10.4	11.7	12.2	11.4	13.0	10.2	14.9	19.3	18.0
Endoscopy of large intestine	6.9	5.5	6.5	7.2	6.2	5.6	4.7	5.5	*6.2	5.3	8.1	6.3	7.5	8.3	7.0
Gall bladder removal	18.7	11.9	11.5	13.5	12.8	6.2	4.3	5.1	6.5	5.1	31.0	19.4	17.9	20.6	20.7
Laparoscopic gall bladder removal	X	9.9	9.9	11.0	11.0	X	3.0	4.1	4.5	3.7	X	16.8	15.8	17.7	18.4
Treatment of intra-abdominal scar tissue	14.1	10.8	11.7	11.1	10.5	2.0	1.5	*1.8	*2.9	*2.5	26.0	20.1	21.7	19.4	18.6
Hysterectomy	X	X	X	X	X	X	X	X	X	X	63.3	55.7	51.2	37.4	38.0
Abdominal hysterectomy	X	X	X	X	X	X	X	X	X	X	47.1	34.6	31.5	22.8	21.3
Vaginal hysterectomy	X	X	X	X	X	X	X	X	X	X	15.8	19.1	15.6	*10.6	*12.3
Forceps, vacuum, and breech delivery	X	X	X	X	X	X	X	X	X	X	77.5	59.9	51.1	*45.0	*43.9
Episiotomy	X	X	X	X	X	X	X	X	X	X	293.3	160.8	90.9	52.3	53.6
Other procedures inducing or assisting delivery	X	X	X	X	X	X	X	X	X	X	387.9	384.2	396.7	418.5	422.6
Medical induction of labor	X	X	X	X	X	X	X	X	X	X	41.1	77.7	107.5	120.5	125.9
Cesarean section	X	X	X	X	X	X	X	X	X	X	167.1	149.5	220.7	232.5	233.5
Reduction of fracture	19.1	13.7	13.2	12.0	11.6	27.9	19.0	18.9	17.2	15.3	10.4	8.4	7.5	6.8	7.9
Excision of intervertebral disc and spinal fusion	17.0	14.1	11.7	11.9	10.7	21.5	16.2	13.1	11.7	10.3	12.6	12.1	10.3	12.1	11.0
CT scan	27.5	10.6	12.6	*6.5	*6.6	32.3	11.0	12.3	5.8	*6.1	22.7	10.3	12.8	*7.2	*7.1
Arteriography and angiocardiography with contrast	12.5	10.3	10.5	9.7	9.1	17.4	12.9	12.2	9.7	9.9	7.6	7.7	8.7	9.7	8.2
Diagnostic ultrasound	34.2	11.6	12.3	9.8	10.0	19.3	8.3	9.5	*7.3	7.2	48.9	14.9	15.1	12.3	12.8
Magnetic resonance imaging	4.9	3.8	4.3	*4.4	*4.1	4.9	3.6	3.8	*	*2.9	4.9	*4.0	4.8	*5.6	*5.4
Mechanical ventilation	4.6	7.0	8.8	11.0	9.9	5.4	8.2	10.1	11.9	11.2	3.8	5.8	7.5	10.1	8.6
45 to 64 Years															
Hospital discharges with at least one procedure, crude (percent)[2]	68.2	62.3	62.6	63.2	63.0	68.9	63.4	63.3	63.5	63.3	67.6	61.3	61.8	62.9	62.8
Hospital discharges with at least one procedure[2]	924.2	694.6	717.4	771.7	756.7	965.9	714.4	727.3	784.1	766.2	885.4	675.9	708.1	759.9	747.7
Operations on vessels of heart	53.0	57.7	53.5	42.5	40.0	83.2	88.5	83.5	62.8	59.5	24.8	28.4	24.9	23.1	21.4
Coronary angioplasty or arthrectomy	29.4	37.5	38.4	31.2	28.9	45.3	55.9	59.4	46.1	42.7	14.5	20.0	18.3	17.1	15.8
Coronary artery stent insertion	X	31.1	36.7	26.9	25.4	X	46.5	57.7	39.9	37.5	X	16.5	16.7	14.6	13.8
Drug-eluting stent insertion	X	X	33.0	18.7	18.7	X	X	51.8	28.1	27.5	X	X	15.1	9.8	10.2
Coronary artery bypass graft (CABG)	23.4	20.3	14.0	11.5	11.1	37.5	32.5	21.9	17.1	16.9	10.3	8.6	6.4	*6.1	*5.5
Cardiac catheterization	98.2	83.0	69.7	56.6	54.4	136.8	113.9	95.6	75.7	72.3	62.3	53.7	45.1	38.4	37.2
Pacemaker	7.8	4.0	3.9	3.2	3.2	10.9	5.2	4.6	*4.5	4.2	*4.9	2.8	3.2	*2.0	*2.3
Carotid (neck arteries) endarterectomy	4.0	5.2	2.9	2.6	3.1	5.2	5.2	3.7	*3.1	3.6	3.0	*5.2	2.2	*2.1	*2.7
Endoscopy of small intestine	45.0	36.4	42.5	43.5	43.2	46.3	40.7	44.7	45.3	42.2	43.8	32.3	40.3	41.9	44.2
Endoscopy of large intestine	28.5	19.3	19.4	18.9	18.0	25.4	18.1	17.4	16.7	15.9	31.4	20.4	21.2	21.0	20.0
Gall bladder removal	36.4	20.6	17.6	18.4	18.0	22.3	16.3	14.0	15.6	13.8	49.5	24.6	20.9	21.0	21.9
Laparoscopic gall bladder removal	X	15.3	13.0	15.0	14.6	X	12.1	9.0	11.8	10.6	X	18.5	16.8	18.0	18.5
Treatment of intra-abdominal scar tissue	17.1	15.0	15.6	14.6	13.8	9.5	7.0	6.2	8.5	8.2	24.2	22.6	24.5	20.4	19.1

Table 3-61. Discharges with at Least One Procedure in Nonfederal Short-Stay Hospitals, by Sex, Age, and Selected Procedures, Selected Years, 1990 Through 2009–2010—Continued

(Percent; rate per 10,000 population.)

Age and procedure (any listed)	Both sexes					Male					Female				
	1990	2000	2005	2009[1]	2009-2010[1]	1990	2000	2005	2009[1]	2009-2010[1]	1990	2000	2005	2009[1]	2009-2010[1]
Removal of prostate	X	X	X	X	X	35.8	15.6	14.4	*17.9	16.9	X	X	X	X	X
Transurethral prostatectomy	X	X	X	X	X	30.4	7.0	4.6	*2.7	3.3	X	X	X	X	X
Hysterectomy	X	X	X	X	X	X	X	X	X	X	76.4	78.2	63.8	54.5	54.1
Abdominal hysterectomy	X	X	X	X	X	X	X	X	X	X	58.4	53.2	39.7	33.9	32.1
Vaginal hysterectomy	X	X	X	X	X	X	X	X	X	X	17.6	21.6	19.3	14.4	15.4
Reduction of fracture	20.3	18.5	16.5	17.0	18.2	19.5	17.6	17.9	16.7	18.1	21.0	19.3	15.3	17.3	18.3
Excision of intervertebral disc and spinal fusion	26.1	25.7	26.9	31.1	30.8	29.4	27.1	27.0	30.6	31.3	23.1	24.4	26.8	31.7	30.2
Total hip replacement	6.2	8.1	10.9	18.3	18.0	5.7	9.1	12.3	20.8	19.0	6.5	7.2	9.6	15.8	17.1
Partial hip replacement	*	*1.3	9.1	*14.0	*13.8	*	*0.8	8.8	*14.1	*13.7	*	*1.7	9.5	*13.9	*13.8
Total knee replacement	6.7	12.7	25.4	36.5	37.1	5.8	8.7	17.7	27.0	27.8	*7.4	16.4	32.7	45.5	46.0
Mastectomy	X	X	X	X	.	X	X	X	X	X	21.2	10.6	8.1	8.5	9.3
CT scan	65.4	25.2	26.1	17.0	*17.1	69.9	25.9	26.7	18.0	17.4	61.2	24.5	25.5	*16.1	*16.9
Arteriography and angiocardiography with contrast	105.4	85.3	73.2	66.3	64.3	138.5	111.4	94.6	86.7	83.3	74.6	60.7	52.8	46.9	46.3
Diagnostic ultrasound	69.5	34.3	33.5	30.9	31.8	73.8	38.0	39.4	35.9	36.3	65.5	30.9	27.9	26.2	27.5
Magnetic resonance imaging	10.9	8.9	11.6	8.9	9.2	10.7	9.4	12.4	9.2	9.2	11.0	8.4	11.0	*8.6	9.2
Mechanical ventilation	17.6	21.2	24.7	32.2	32.9	18.6	22.9	28.0	33.5	34.4	16.7	19.6	21.6	30.8	31.5
65 to 74 Years															
Hospital discharges with at least one procedure, crude (percent)[2]	66.5	61.3	62.9	63.9	63.2	69.3	63.9	65.0	64.4	64.6	63.8	58.9	60.9	63.4	62.0
Hospital discharges with at least one procedure[2]	1,739.4	1,559.8	1,653.0	1,632.6	1,573.0	1,994.1	1,692.3	1,783.2	1,725.0	1,678.0	1,539.4	1,450.6	1,543.1	1,553.5	1,482.5
Operations on vessels of heart	97.0	139.8	142.1	117.4	104.2	148.9	195.3	211.0	165.8	152.6	56.3	94.1	84.0	75.9	62.4
Coronary angioplasty or arthrectomy	44.1	86.3	91.2	83.2	69.4	64.9	116.0	138.2	113.2	96.6	27.8	61.9	51.5	57.4	45.9
Coronary artery stent insertion	X	71.7	92.6	73.6	61.1	X	94.9	129.4	97.3	83.3	X	52.5	49.8	53.2	42.0
Drug-eluting stent insertion	X	X	76.8	53.5	46.1	X	X	115.7	69.1	62.5	X	X	44.0	*40.2	32.1
Coronary artery bypass graft (CABG)	52.1	53.9	47.4	34.4	34.7	83.1	79.7	68.1	52.9	55.9	27.7	32.6	30.0	*18.6	16.5
Cardiac catheterization	164.0	174.2	170.3	130.9	120.4	213.8	222.7	230.4	159.3	153.7	124.9	134.2	119.6	106.6	91.7
Pacemaker	24.6	22.5	23.7	19.6	18.6	32.1	22.8	29.0	*17.3	18.1	18.7	22.3	19.1	*21.5	19.0
Carotid (neck arteries) endarterectomy	14.6	24.1	24.0	*17.8	15.6	18.0	29.5	31.2	*21.8	21.8	11.9	19.6	18.0	*14.3	*10.3
Endoscopy of small intestine	92.8	106.6	102.5	99.4	93.2	91.5	102.4	102.6	106.7	99.0	93.7	110.0	102.4	93.2	88.2
Endoscopy of large intestine	70.3	64.8	58.3	45.7	44.3	62.5	59.7	52.1	44.9	41.6	76.5	69.0	63.6	46.4	46.7
Gall bladder removal	45.0	42.1	34.4	31.3	30.0	42.0	37.9	34.0	33.7	31.9	47.4	45.5	34.8	29.3	28.3
Laparoscopic gall bladder removal	X	29.5	23.6	21.9	22.0	X	24.4	22.4	*20.3	21.2	X	33.7	24.6	23.2	22.6
Treatment of intra-abdominal scar tissue	23.1	21.4	23.5	27.4	29.0	17.1	14.5	19.6	*20.5	24.3	27.7	27.1	26.8	*33.2	33.0
Removal of prostate	X	X	X	X	X	201.1	83.7	65.3	56.9	50.8	X	X	X	X	X
Transurethral prostatectomy	X	X	X	X	X	180.9	59.4	39.5	*23.7	24.1	X	X	X	X	X
Hysterectomy	X	X	X	X	X	X	X	X	X	X	37.4	35.9	28.0	*29.3	30.2
Abdominal hysterectomy	X	X	X	X	X	X	X	X	X	X	20.8	20.5	12.8	*12.2	15.0
Vaginal hysterectomy	X	X	X	X	X	X	X	X	X	X	16.5	14.7	14.1	*15.0	*14.1
Reduction of fracture	36.2	36.4	38.0	34.8	32.9	24.3	26.2	25.8	19.0	18.4	45.5	44.8	48.3	48.3	45.5
Excision of intervertebral disc and spinal fusion	16.3	21.1	31.1	41.7	42.1	14.2	22.5	27.6	*45.9	39.2	18.0	20.0	34.1	*38.0	*44.5
Total hip replacement	24.0	25.4	36.6	37.4	39.3	23.0	26.4	36.2	34.6	37.1	24.9	24.5	37.0	39.9	41.2
Partial hip replacement	8.9	7.6	20.1	*24.7	*25.3	*4.0	.	15.4	*20.8	*19.1	*12.7	10.5	24.1	*27.9	*30.7
Total knee replacement	33.2	65.4	99.5	104.6	108.3	26.4	64.5	71.8	76.2	84.0	38.6	66.0	122.8	128.9	129.3
Mastectomy	X	X	X	X	X	X	X	X	X	X	30.7	22.7	*11.5	*15.5	*12.9
CT scan	153.7	64.3	53.8	*30.9	*29.4	163.4	65.7	53.6	*32.6	*31.1	146.1	63.1	53.7	*29.5	*27.9
Arteriography and angiocardiography with contrast	184.5	186.2	180.8	153.6	146.5	239.0	231.9	233.2	191.5	186.7	141.7	148.5	136.6	121.2	111.9
Diagnostic ultrasound	155.2	92.7	80.9	82.7	79.8	165.2	94.1	87.0	*93.0	85.6	147.4	91.6	75.8	73.9	74.8
Magnetic resonance imaging	20.6	17.2	24.4	*18.1	*18.3	19.2	*14.6	19.9	*19.2	18.9	21.7	*19.3	28.3	*	*17.8
Mechanical ventilation	48.6	60.0	70.1	79.5	79.9	58.7	70.3	83.0	86.0	90.7	40.6	51.6	59.3	73.9	70.7
75 to 84 Years															
Hospital discharges with at least one procedure, crude (percent)[2]	59.0	53.6	54.9	57.1	56.4	61.7	56.3	58.1	59.6	59.0	57.0	51.8	52.5	55.2	54.5
Hospital discharges with at least one procedure[2]	2,332.9	2,212.3	2,269.1	2,322.2	2,247.8	2,723.9	2,416.5	2,549.4	2,528.1	2,441.4	2,096.7	2,078.8	2,078.7	2,176.6	2,108.7
Operations on vessels of heart	69.1	143.2	142.3	138.6	126.0	107.6	202.5	199.6	208.3	189.8	45.8	104.5	103.4	89.2	80.2
Coronary angioplasty or arthrectomy	22.4	84.7	97.3	87.3	82.7	33.7	109.3	134.8	121.2	116.8	15.7	68.7	71.9	63.3	58.2
Coronary artery stent insertion	X	69.8	88.2	79.6	75.3	X	86.5	122.2	111.4	107.5	X	58.8	65.2	57.1	52.2
Drug-eluting stent insertion	X	X	75.5	55.6	54.7	X	X	104.9	77.5	77.5	X	X	55.6	*40.2	38.2
Coronary artery bypass graft (CABG)	47.0	57.7	44.4	*50.7	42.7	74.7	90.5	62.6	*86.2	*72.3	30.3	36.2	32.0	*25.7	*21.5
Cardiac catheterization	116.6	190.2	183.9	159.3	149.3	166.0	236.9	238.1	179.6	179.9	86.8	159.6	147.1	144.8	127.4
Pacemaker	50.8	58.1	67.9	59.9	60.0	70.6	72.2	91.0	79.6	84.9	38.8	48.9	52.2	46.0	42.1
Carotid (neck arteries) endarterectomy	19.8	32.8	24.4	23.3	23.7	24.2	45.5	34.1	31.6	29.6	*17.1	24.5	17.7	*17.5	19.5
Endoscopy of small intestine	171.4	189.7	182.2	167.4	166.0	188.9	193.8	202.0	162.5	164.2	160.8	187.0	168.7	170.9	167.3
Endoscopy of large intestine	131.1	123.7	106.4	93.7	87.9	126.1	113.8	109.3	89.5	83.9	134.1	130.1	104.3	96.7	90.7
Gall bladder removal	51.8	43.4	43.3	38.2	43.6	64.4	46.7	48.9	50.7	50.5	44.2	41.3	39.4	29.3	38.7
Laparoscopic gall bladder removal	X	28.9	30.5	32.3	35.9	X	29.6	30.4	40.7	39.2	X	28.5	30.5	26.4	33.6
Treatment of intra-abdominal scar tissue	34.0	28.6	27.9	28.1	30.2	28.2	26.3	*34.5	*30.0	28.7	37.5	30.2	23.4	26.7	31.3
Removal of prostate	X	X	X	X	X	273.5	98.0	65.4	*47.0	41.2	X	X	X	X	X
Transurethral prostatectomy	X	X	X	X	X	257.5	89.0	58.6	*44.0	36.6	X	X	X	X	X
Hysterectomy	X	X	X	X	X	X	X	X	X	X	28.5	25.5	16.1	*23.2	18.5
Abdominal hysterectomy	X	X	X	X	X	X	X	X	X	X	18.8	16.2	8.6	*14.7	*11.1
Vaginal hysterectomy	X	X	X	X	X	X	X	X	X	X	*9.4	8.1	7.1	*	*5.6
Reduction of fracture	86.2	80.1	70.7	61.9	68.1	43.4	57.2	41.5	*41.9	46.0	112.1	95.0	90.6	76.0	84.0
Excision of intervertebral disc and spinal fusion	12.0	17.4	16.4	36.1	36.5	*13.2	*20.4	14.3	*42.8	*39.9	11.3	15.3	17.8	31.3	34.0
Total hip replacement	30.7	26.3	44.4	47.3	49.4	*26.9	*21.3	36.6	*44.4	47.2	33.1	29.6	49.7	49.4	51.1
Partial hip replacement	43.6	36.6	39.9	41.2	37.9	*14.3	20.0	27.4	*29.9	*29.9	61.2	47.5	48.3	49.1	43.7
Total knee replacement	28.4	59.3	90.4	89.8	86.2	*19.5	48.7	83.6	80.4	80.4	34.3	66.4	95.0	96.0	90.1
Mastectomy	X	X	X	X	X	X	X	X	X	X	29.2	22.0	16.2	*8.7	*11.3
CT scan	279.7	119.2	95.8	*56.8	*55.2	307.2	127.9	92.3	*58.3	*51.0	263.0	113.5	98.1	*55.8	*58.3
Arteriography and angiocardiography with contrast	141.0	219.2	212.4	198.1	187.8	192.3	287.9	269.9	219.0	223.3	109.9	174.3	173.3	183.4	162.2
Diagnostic ultrasound	273.5	134.1	133.0	122.4	122.0	315.7	142.8	148.3	135.8	137.7	248.0	128.4	122.6	113.0	110.8
Magnetic resonance imaging	30.5	*37.3	38.4	*38.5	*37.6	43.0	*33.6	41.3	*47.9	*44.0	*23.0	*39.8	36.5	*31.9	*33.0
Mechanical ventilation	79.8	91.1	102.6	105.3	102.0	110.3	106.5	119.4	139.7	119.5	61.3	80.9	91.1	81.1	89.5

Table 3-61. Discharges with at Least One Procedure in Nonfederal Short-Stay Hospitals, by Sex, Age, and Selected Procedures, Selected Years, 1990 Through 2009–2010—*Continued*

(Percent; rate per 10,000 population.)

Age and procedure (any listed)	Both sexes					Male					Female				
	1990	2000	2005	2009[1]	2009-2010[1]	1990	2000	2005	2009[1]	2009-2010[1]	1990	2000	2005	2009[1]	2009-2010[1]
85 Years and Over															
Hospital discharges with at least one procedure, crude (percent)[2]	49.3	44.6	45.4	47.0	46.8	52.4	45.4	47.7	51.4	50.5	47.8	44.3	44.2	44.6	44.7
Hospital discharges with at least one procedure[2]	2,762.1	2,700.5	2,612.5	2,731.1	2,650.6	3,367.3	2,797.9	2,857.1	3,301.9	3,125.0	2,526.8	2,660.6	2,500.2	2,466.7	2,423.0
Operations on vessels of heart	*14.0	51.1	53.9	60.9	55.5	*	83.0	86.2	*124.2	98.6	*	38.0	39.1	*31.6	34.8
Coronary angioplasty or arthrectomy	*	36.3	45.0	*51.7	44.6	*	*52.9	*64.6	*101.8	74.6	*	29.5	35.9	*28.4	*30.2
Coronary artery stent insertion	X	31.6	43.2	45.5	40.0	X	*48.9	*62.3	*83.9	66.6	X	*24.4	34.4	*27.7	*27.2
Drug-eluting stent insertion	X	X	38.4	*27.2	22.7	X	X	*55.8	*	*36.9	X	X	30.4	*19.6	*15.8
Coronary artery bypass graft (CABG)	*	*15.1	*	*	*10.1	*	*30.1	*	*	*22.5	*	*9.0	*3.0	*	*4.2
Cardiac catheterization	*23.7	87.7	88.8	*96.7	78.5	*	122.8	122.5	*145.1	111.7	*19.0	73.2	73.3	*74.4	62.6
Pacemaker	79.5	82.9	92.7	105.3	89.3	120.4	104.3	122.7	*121.0	100.6	63.5	74.2	78.9	*98.0	84.0
Carotid (neck arteries) endarterectomy	*	*12.0	*9.2	*	*	*	*	*	*	*7.1	*	*4.8	*	*	*
Endoscopy of small intestine	228.8	262.4	251.8	192.1	192.2	288.7	245.1	217.8	224.3	228.5	205.5	269.5	267.3	177.2	174.7
Endoscopy of large intestine	180.8	158.1	139.4	99.2	98.1	188.0	133.3	104.3	131.1	128.9	178.0	168.3	155.6	84.4	83.4
Gall bladder removal	46.4	40.9	29.1	*24.7	23.0	*68.4	*42.9	*48.4	*	*30.2	37.8	*40.1	20.3	*22.7	*19.5
Laparoscopic gall bladder removal	X	*30.4	18.6	*15.6	15.4	X	*	*28.2	*	*	X	*30.5	*14.2	*13.5	*14.0
Treatment of intra-abdominal scar tissue	29.6	24.3	29.0	*28.9	23.0	*	*16.4	*20.6	*	*13.9	33.7	*27.5	*32.8	*35.2	*27.4
Removal of prostate	X	X	X	X	X	257.2	*113.0	73.0	*39.7	42.7	X	X	X	X	X
Transurethral prostatectomy	X	X	X	X	X	247.1	*110.0	67.1	*39.7	41.8	X	X	X	X	X
Hysterectomy	X	X	X	X	X	X	X	X	X	X	*	*	*	*	*
Abdominal hysterectomy	X	X	X	X	X	X	X	X	X	X	*	*	*5.9	*	*
Vaginal hysterectomy	X	X	X	X	X	X	X	X	X	X	*	*	*4.3	*	*
Reduction of fracture	196.2	200.5	160.6	182.9	180.3	150.6	93.8	75.4	147.5	132.8	213.9	244.3	199.7	199.4	203.0
Excision of intervertebral disc and spinal fusion	*	*2.3	*	*	*6.2	*	*	*	*	*	*	*	*	*	*
Total hip replacement	*27.8	*20.7	*24.8	*31.6	*25.5	*	*	*	*	*	*23.2	*26.3	*23.6	*	*21.6
Partial hip replacement	67.4	82.2	71.2	78.1	77.1	*52.9	*44.1	56.4	67.0	66.2	73.1	97.9	78.0	83.3	82.3
Total knee replacement	*12.4	*22.9	*30.2	*26.7	34.0	*	*	*27.0	*	*31.3	*	*16.2	*31.7	*31.1	35.3
Mastectomy	X	X	X	X	X	X	X	X	X	X	*28.9	*15.7	*	*	*
CT scan	378.4	158.7	123.7	*86.2	*84.9	401.2	141.4	*131.8	*79.2	*84.8	369.5	165.9	119.9	*	*85.0
Arteriography and angiocardiography with contrast	50.6	120.8	126.6	156.8	135.6	*87.6	164.4	175.2	197.2	161.9	36.2	102.8	104.3	138.2	123.0
Diagnostic ultrasound	327.7	208.5	179.3	203.3	200.6	394.5	181.4	200.7	215.6	216.3	301.7	219.6	169.6	*197.6	193.1
Magnetic resonance imaging	*18.5	*40.4	40.5	*	*35.7	*	*	*40.8	*	*35.9	*16.2	*40.5	*	*	*
Mechanical ventilation	91.5	106.0	110.0	139.1	130.3	97.9	116.5	166.1	199.1	172.2	89.1	101.7	84.3	111.3	110.2

X = Not applicable.   * = Figure does not meet standards of reliability or precision. Data preceded by an asterisk have a relative standard error (RSE) of 20 to 30 percent. Data not shown have an RSE of greater than 30 percent.   [1]Starting with 2008 data, the sample of nonfederal short-stay hospitals was cut in half. This smaller sample size has increased standard errors. Therefore, caution should be exercised in interpreting trends in these data.   [2]Includes discharges for procedures not shown separately.

Table 3-62A. Certified Intermediate Care Facilities and Specialty Hospitals, Number of Facilities and Beds, by State, Selected Years, 1995–2010

(Number.)

State	ICF/MR[1] Long-term		Hospitals Psychiatric		Rehabilitation		Children's		CAH[2]			
	1995	2010	1995	2010	1995	2010	1995	2010	1995	2010	1995	2010
United States	7,106	6,424	175	438	689	508	190	233	70	76	X	1,325
Alabama	8	5	2	7	10	11	5	7	1	2	X	3
Alaska	6	0	0	1	3	2	0	0	0	0	X	13
Arizona	12	12	3	8	11	8	4	7	1	2	X	14
Arkansas	40	40	0	8	9	9	6	8	1	1	X	29
California	687	1,164	8	20	64	32	12	5	7	10	X	31
Colorado	7	16	5	8	9	9	5	3	2	1	X	29
Connecticut	145	115	5	3	10	6	1	1	1	1	X	0
Delaware	6	2	0	1	3	4	1	0	1	1	X	0
District of Columbia	122	81	0	2	2	3	1	1	1	1	X	0
Florida	110	101	10	19	43	25	13	13	2	2	X	13
Georgia	12	9	5	15	28	15	2	3	1	2	X	34
Hawaii	15	18	1	1	1	1	1	1	1	1	X	9
Idaho	48	67	0	3	6	5	1	1	0	0	X	27
Illinois	315	309	4	6	19	14	3	4	2	2	X	51
Indiana	578	529	5	14	30	23	6	6	0	0	X	35
Iowa	116	141	0	2	4	4	0	0	0	0	X	82
Kansas	47	32	2	5	10	4	4	4	0	1	X	83
Kentucky	9	14	0	6	13	11	4	5	0	0	X	30
Louisiana	454	534	13	39	40	39	9	21	1	1	X	27
Maine	42	17	0	0	4	4	1	1	0	0	X	16
Maryland	5	3	4	4	14	9	3	2	2	2	X	0
Massachusetts	8	6	21	16	18	14	5	8	2	1	X	3
Michigan	503	1	2	19	15	11	4	4	1	1	X	36
Minnesota	348	215	1	2	6	8	0	0	3	3	X	79
Mississippi	12	14	1	10	4	5	1	0	0	0	X	28
Missouri	26	17	3	12	17	13	2	5	3	3	X	36
Montana	3	1	0	1	2	2	0	0	0	0	X	48
Nebraska	4	3	1	2	5	3	1	1	2	2	X	65
Nevada	14	9	2	6	5	7	2	3	0	0	X	11
New Hampshire	7	1	0	0	3	2	2	2	0	0	X	13
New Jersey	10	8	3	7	14	17	8	8	1	2	X	0
New Mexico	32	42	2	3	6	2	5	5	1	0	X	7
New York	892	569	7	4	35	28	4	0	2	1	X	13
North Carolina	320	332	2	9	15	10	1	2	0	0	X	23
North Dakota	65	66	1	2	1	3	1	0	0	0	X	36
Ohio	416	429	5	25	19	14	0	3	8	6	X	34
Oklahoma	37	86	4	13	18	10	3	2	2	2	X	34
Oregon	2	1	0	1	4	3	0	0	0	0	X	25
Pennsylvania	252	199	5	23	31	24	17	16	5	5	X	13
Rhode Island	55	5	2	1	3	2	1	1	0	0	X	0
South Carolina	174	85	1	6	9	8	3	6	0	0	X	5
South Dakota	10	1	0	1	2	1	0	0	0	1	X	38
Tennessee	74	113	2	9	16	11	5	6	3	2	X	17
Texas	879	860	35	77	52	37	28	49	7	8	X	78
Utah	14	15	1	3	7	3	1	1	1	1	X	11
Vermont	6	1	0	0	2	1	0	0	0	0	X	8
Virginia	20	41	3	5	19	9	4	9	2	3	X	7
Washington	28	14	2	2	4	5	1	1	2	2	X	38
West Virginia	63	66	0	2	5	4	6	5	0	0	X	18
Wisconsin	44	14	1	5	17	11	2	2	1	2	X	59
Wyoming	4	1	1	0	2	2	1	1	0	0	X	16

X = Not applicable. [1]ICF/MR is intermediate care facilities for persons with mental retardation. [2]CAH is critical access hospital. CAHs were created as part of the Balanced Budget Act of 1997.

Table 3-62B. Certified Intermediate Care Facilities and Specialty Hospitals, Number of Facilities and Beds, by State, Selected Years, 1995–2010

(Number.)

State	ICF/MR[1] Long-term		Beds — Hospitals Psychiatric		Rehabilitation		Children's		CAH[2]			
	1995	2010	1995	2010	1995	2010	1995	2010	1995	2010	1995	2010
United States	159,557	108,427	21,373	29,388	105,165	68,531	13,731	14,999	12,719	13,204	X	32,844
Alabama	981	281	341	429	1,760	1,056	289	392	225	434	X	75
Alaska	121	0	0	60	244	205	0	0	0	0	X	217
Arizona	690	242	203	557	955	874	211	396	15	250	X	299
Arkansas	1,802	1,590	0	283	730	919	446	463	280	280	X	763
California	14,334	10,998	1,477	1,825	7,737	4,922	838	367	1,346	1,980	X	1,054
Colorado	382	188	1,264	430	1,375	943	271	226	378	253	X	600
Connecticut	1,350	1,134	796	715	1,990	1,032	60	60	98	129	X	0
Delaware	405	170	0	35	514	483	60	0	97	180	X	0
District of Columbia	797	492	0	171	583	800	160	160	279	279	X	0
Florida	3,495	2,955	745	1,119	5,385	2,925	833	1,042	376	467	X	344
Georgia	2,240	1,647	372	713	4,103	2,797	108	168	235	483	X	857
Hawaii	207	91	13	9	88	88	100	100	232	207	X	88
Idaho	541	555	0	140	221	263	54	56	0	0	X	555
Illinois	13,001	10,413	1,385	805	3,172	2,321	371	448	351	339	X	1,190
Indiana	7,387	4,129	265	649	2,213	1,555	388	316	0	0	X	946
Iowa	3,679	3,127	0	74	522	287	0	0	0	0	X	2,401
Kansas	2,233	994	54	167	1,717	718	217	257	0	34	X	1,928
Kentucky	1,203	930	0	546	2,086	1,695	225	288	0	0	X	737
Louisiana	6,847	6,347	797	1,852	3,868	2,098	435	549	188	201	X	685
Maine	555	192	0	0	551	392	80	100	0	0	X	398
Maryland	1,042	238	465	465	3,846	1,788	352	131	165	150	X	0
Massachusetts	2,707	1,674	4,218	3,561	2,137	1,449	636	1,064	458	421	X	69
Michigan	3,556	272	249	1,012	3,280	1,308	340	240	260	228	X	836
Minnesota	5,162	1,871	264	356	1,432	458	0	0	329	339	X	2,190
Mississippi	2,131	2,739	25	393	316	1,741	110	0	0	0	X	800
Missouri	1,659	1,020	317	675	1,969	1,792	120	297	592	432	X	867
Montana	188	56	0	40	54	194	0	0	0	0	X	998
Nebraska	761	261	192	148	767	488	60	72	142	200	X	1,418
Nevada	229	121	79	413	407	644	122	189	0	0	X	231
New Hampshire	78	25	0	0	423	341	152	152	0	0	X	316
New Jersey	4,637	3,622	476	442	3,486	3,249	848	783	60	120	X	0
New Mexico	604	272	86	106	397	124	194	212	37	0	X	174
New York	15,379	8,860	1,351	1,010	14,199	6,327	428	0	404	92	X	301
North Carolina	5,294	5,173	182	490	2,941	3,435	80	213	0	0	X	775
North Dakota	721	635	68	72	328	303	88	0	0	0	X	795
Ohio	8,936	7,268	683	1,693	3,079	1,448	0	199	2,535	1,356	X	840
Oklahoma	3,132	2,078	194	636	1,726	638	219	107	168	160	X	777
Oregon	546	76	0	28	670	742	0	0	0	0	X	830
Pennsylvania	7,412	4,536	369	1,355	7,334	3,472	1,574	1,395	721	1,103	X	337
Rhode Island	297	51	1,062	495	371	177	82	82	0	0	X	0
South Carolina	3,550	1,828	166	308	1,089	1,093	213	355	0	0	X	125
South Dakota	558	240	0	24	145	320	0	0	0	114	X	766
Tennessee	2,590	1,247	125	335	1,721	1,215	350	370	395	200	X	395
Texas	15,868	12,659	1,803	4,068	6,561	4,299	1,838	2,769	1,447	1,631	X	1,746
Utah	965	855	34	111	741	486	50	84	194	232	X	236
Vermont	36	6	0	0	164	149	0	0	0	0	X	194
Virginia	2,758	1,715	892	236	1,677	1,345	231	353	250	296	X	175
Washington	1,482	940	97	73	1,541	1,417	102	102	276	276	X	1,130
West Virginia	782	511	0	60	564	485	246	280	0	0	X	722
Wisconsin	4,083	961	34	204	1,720	1,133	135	121	186	338	X	1,321
Wyoming	164	142	230	0	266	98	15	41	0	0	X	343

X = Not applicable.   [1]ICF/MR is intermediate care facilities for persons with mental retardation.   [2]CAH is critical access hospital. CAHs were created as part of the Balanced Budget Act of 1997.

HEALTH PERSONNEL

Figure 3-12. Annual Mean Wages for Selected Occupations in the Health Care Industry, May 2012

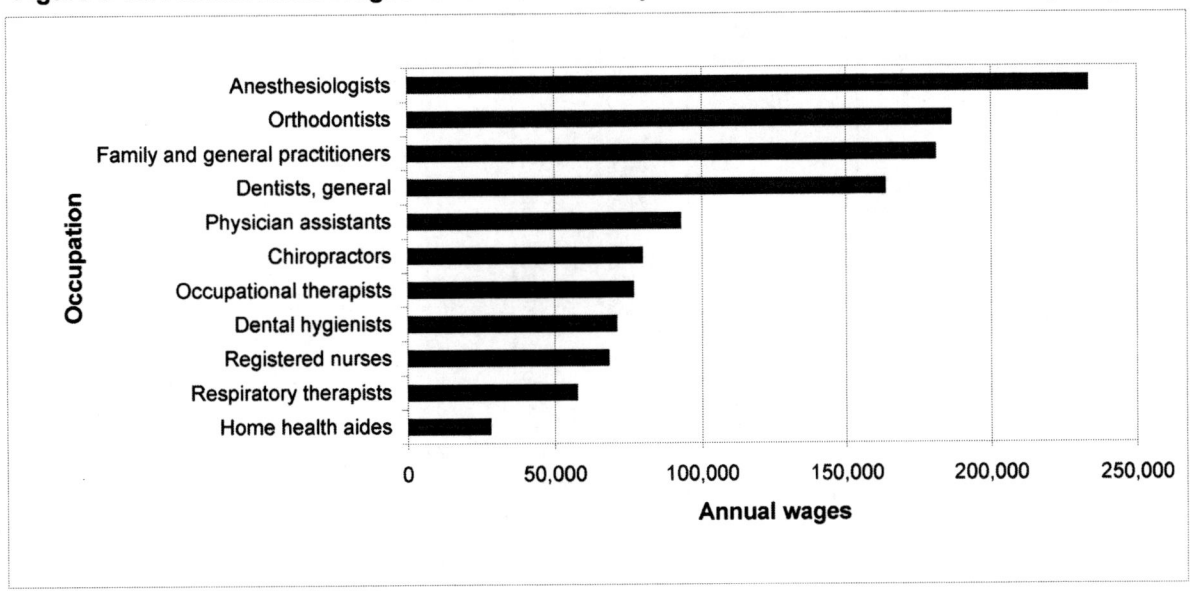

Figure 3-13. Annual Wages for Selected Specialties in Medicine, May 2012

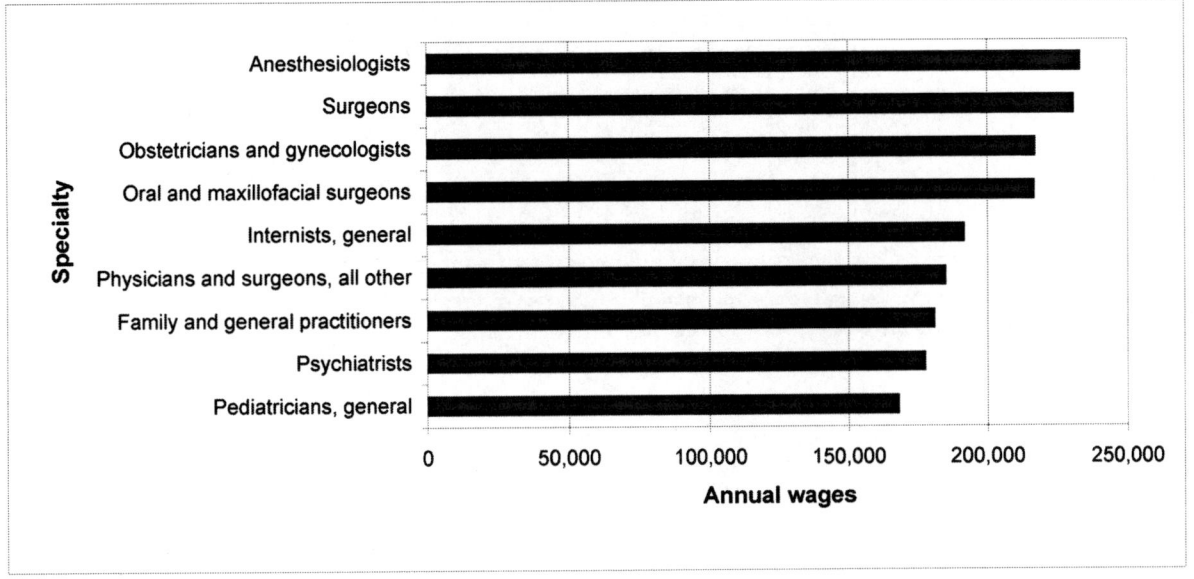

Table 3-63. Health Care Employment and Wages, by Selected Occupations, Selected Years, 2001–2011

(Number; dollars.)

Occupation title	Employment[1]					AAPC[2]	Mean hourly wage (dollars)[3]					AAPC[2]
	2001	2005	2009	2010	2011	2001–2011	2001	2005	2009	2010	2011	2001–2011
Health Care Practitioners and Technical Occupations												
Audiologists	11,040	10,030	12,590	12,860	12,490	1.2	23.89	27.72	32.14	33.58	34.13	3.6
Cardiovascular technologists and technicians	40,990	43,560	48,070	48,720	50,410	2.1	17.55	19.99	23.91	24.38	25.08	3.6
Dental hygienists	149,880	161,140	173,900	177,520	184,110	2.1	27.30	29.15	32.63	33.02	33.54	2.1
Diagnostic medical sonographers	32,990	43,590	51,630	53,010	54,760	5.2	23.08	26.65	30.60	31.20	31.63	3.2
Dietetic technicians	28,940	23,780	24,510	23,890	23,490	-2.1	11.23	12.20	13.72	13.86	14.04	2.3
Dietitians and nutritionists	43,200	48,850	53,220	53,510	56,130	2.7	19.74	22.09	25.59	26.13	26.66	3.1
Emergency medical technicians and paramedics	170,690	196,880	217,920	221,760	229,340	3.0	12.24	13.68	15.88	16.01	16.36	2.9
Licensed practical and licensed vocational nurses	683,790	710,020	728,670	730,290	729,140	0.6	15.14	17.41	19.66	19.88	20.21	2.9
Medical and clinical laboratory technicians	146,920	144,710	152,420	156,480	156,860	0.7	14.52	15.95	18.20	18.36	18.73	2.6
Medical and clinical laboratory technologists	145,400	160,760	166,860	164,430	165,220	1.3	20.70	23.37	26.74	27.34	27.94	3.0
Medical records and health information techni-cians	142,170	164,700	170,580	176,090	180,280	2.4	12.20	13.81	16.29	16.83	17.27	3.5
Nuclear medicine technologists	17,360	18,280	21,670	21,600	21,200	2.0	24.65	29.10	32.91	33.20	33.64	3.2
Occupational therapists	77,080	87,430	97,840	100,300	103,570	3.0	25.10	28.41	33.98	35.28	36.05	3.7
Opticians, dispensing	63,120	70,090	60,840	62,200	60,680	-0.4	13.49	14.80	16.73	16.73	16.70	2.2
Pharmacists	223,630	229,740	267,860	268,030	272,320	2.0	35.02	42.62	51.27	52.59	53.92	4.4
Pharmacy technicians	207,140	266,790	331,890	333,500	343,550	5.2	10.82	12.19	13.92	14.10	14.43	2.9
Physical therapists	126,450	151,280	174,490	180,280	185,440	3.9	28.43	31.42	36.64	37.50	38.38	3.0
Physician assistants	56,200	63,350	76,900	81,420	83,540	4.0	30.00	34.17	40.78	41.89	43.01	3.7
Psychiatric technicians	59,750	62,040	70,730	72,650	69,840	1.6	12.94	14.04	14.77	15.15	15.08	1.5
Radiation therapists	13,460	14,120	15,570	16,590	18,380	3.2	25.71	30.59	37.18	37.64	38.14	4.0
Radiologic technologists and technicians	168,240	184,580	213,560	216,730	220,540	2.7	18.68	22.60	26.05	26.80	27.29	3.9
Recreational therapists	26,830	23,260	21,960	20,830	19,650	-3.1	14.92	16.90	19.84	19.92	20.65	3.3
Registered nurses	2,217,990	2,368,070	2,583,770	2,655,020	2,724,570	2.1	23.19	27.35	31.99	32.56	33.23	3.7
Respiratory therapists	82,930	95,320	107,270	109,270	113,980	3.2	19.17	22.24	26.06	26.54	27.05	3.5
Respiratory therapy technicians	28,700	22,060	15,100	13,570	13,940	-7.0	16.93	18.57	21.96	22.28	22.76	3.0
Speech-language pathologists	83,110	94,660	111,640	112,530	117,210	3.5	24.20	27.89	32.86	33.60	34.61	3.6
Health Care Support Occupations												
Dental assistants	267,840	270,720	294,020	294,030	296,810	1.0	13.29	14.41	16.35	16.41	16.70	2.3
Home health aides	560,190	663,280	955,220	982,840	924,650	5.1	8.90	9.34	10.39	10.46	10.49	1.7
Massage therapists	26,440	37,670	55,920	60,040	63,810	9.2	15.93	19.33	19.13	19.12	19.19	1.9
Medical assistants	345,930	382,720	495,970	523,260	539,220	4.5	11.71	12.58	14.16	14.31	14.51	2.2
Medical equipment preparers	33,540	41,790	47,070	47,310	49,560	4.0	11.29	12.42	14.32	14.59	14.99	2.9
Medical transcriptionists	94,090	90,380	82,810	78,780	76,570	-2.0	12.99	14.36	16.03	16.12	16.37	2.3
Nursing aides, orderlies, and attendants	1,307,600	1,391,430	1,438,010	1,451,090	1,466,700	1.2	9.54	10.67	12.01	12.09	12.22	2.5
Occupational therapy aides	7,560	6,220	8,040	7,180	7,090	-0.6	11.70	13.20	13.89	14.95	15.28	2.7
Occupational therapy assistants	17,520	22,160	26,680	27,720	29,130	5.2	17.39	19.13	24.44	24.66	25.07	3.7
Pharmacy aides	58,130	46,610	52,230	49,580	45,130	-2.5	9.22	9.76	10.74	10.98	11.23	2.0
Physical therapist aides	35,250	41,930	44,160	45,900	47,640	3.1	10.45	11.01	12.01	12.02	12.11	1.5
Physical therapist assistants	47,810	58,670	63,750	65,960	67,550	3.5	17.18	18.98	23.36	23.95	24.57	3.6
Psychiatric aides	59,640	56,150	62,610	64,730	71,570	1.8	11.42	11.47	13.19	12.84	13.11	1.4

NOTE: This table excludes occupations such as dentists, physicians, and chiropractors, which have a large percentage of workers who are self-employed.

[1]Employment is the number of filled positions. This table includes both full-time and part-time wage and salary positions. Estimates do not include business establishments where persons are self-employed, owners and partners in unincorporated firms, household workers, or unpaid family workers and were rounded to the nearest 10. [2]Average annual percent change. [3]The mean hourly wage rate for an occupation is the total wages that all workers in the occupation earn in an hour divided by the total employment of the occupation.

Table 3-64. Employment and Wages in the Health Care Industry, by Occupation, May 2012

(Number; dollars.)

Occupation	Employment	Employment per 1,000 jobs	Median hourly wage (dollars)	Mean hourly wage (dollars)	Annual mean wage (dollars)
Healthcare Practitioners and Technical Occupations	4,680,350	35.923	35.29	44.18	91,890
Chiropractors	27,740	0.213	31.81	38.25	79,550
Dentists, General	93,580	0.718	69.83	78.48	163,240
Oral and Maxillofacial Surgeons	4,990	0.038	(1)	104.06	216,440
Orthodontists	5,530	0.042	(1)	89.58	186,320
Prosthodontists	310	0.002	81.31	80.83	168,120
Dentists, All Other Specialists	5,150	0.04	74.51	79.22	164,780
Dietitians and Nutritionists	58,240	0.447	26.56	27.00	56,170
Optometrists	29,180	0.224	47.03	52.80	109,810
Pharmacists	281,560	2.161	56.09	55.27	114,950
Anesthesiologists	29,930	0.23	(1)	111.94	232,830
Family and General Practitioners	110,050	0.845	82.70	86.95	180,850
Internists, General	45,210	0.347	(1)	92.08	191,520
Obstetricians and Gynecologists	20,880	0.16	(1)	104.21	216,760
Pediatricians, General	30,560	0.235	74.35	80.59	167,640
Psychiatrists	24,210	0.186	83.33	85.35	177,520
Surgeons	42,410	0.325	(1)	110.84	230,540
Physicians and Surgeons, All Other	308,410	2.367	(1)	88.86	184,820
Physician Assistants	83,640	0.642	43.72	44.45	92,460
Podiatrists	9,090	0.07	55.98	63.69	132,470
Registered Nurses	2,633,980	20.217	31.48	32.66	67,930
Occupational Therapists	105,540	0.81	36.25	36.73	76,400
Physical Therapists	191,460	1.47	38.39	38.99	81,110
Radiation Therapists	18,230	0.14	37.29	38.66	80,410
Recreational Therapists	19,180	0.147	20.33	21.29	44,280
Respiratory Therapists	116,960	0.898	26.86	27.50	57,200
Speech-Language Pathologists	121,690	0.934	33.59	34.97	72,730
Therapists, All Other	12,480	0.096	25.58	27.29	56,760
Veterinarians	56,020	0.43	40.61	44.83	93,250
Audiologists	12,060	0.093	33.52	35.04	72,890
Health Diagnosing and Treating Practitioners, All Other	30,590	0.235	34.96	41.22	85,740
Medical and Clinical Laboratory Technicians	160,700	1.233	27.69	28.19	58,640
Dental Hygienists	190,290	1.461	33.75	33.99	70,700
Cardiovascular Technologists and Technicians	50,530	0.388	25.04	25.51	53,050
Diagnostic Medical Sonographers	57,700	0.443	31.66	31.90	66,360
Nuclear Medicine Technologists	20,480	0.157	33.74	34.06	70,840
Radiologic Technologists	194,790	1.495	26.26	27.14	56,450
Emergency Medical Technicians and Paramedics	29,560	0.227	31.42	31.45	65,410
Dietetic Technicians	24,660	0.189	12.62	13.79	28,680
Pharmacy Technicians	353,340	2.712	14.10	14.63	30,430
Psychiatric Technicians	67,760	0.52	14.45	15.93	33,140
Respiratory Therapy Technicians	13,460	0.103	22.48	22.84	47,510
Surgical Technologists	97,150	0.746	20.09	20.91	43,480
Veterinary Technologists and Technicians	83,350	0.64	14.56	15.13	31,470
Licensed Practical and Licensed Vocational Nurses	718,800	5.517	19.97	20.39	42,400
Medical Records and Health Information Technicians	182,370	1.4	16.42	17.68	36,770
Opticians, Dispensing	64,930	0.498	16.03	16.83	35,010
Orthotists and Prosthetists	7,890	0.061	30.13	33.64	69,960
Hearing Aid Specialists	4,980	0.038	19.92	22.49	46,780
Health Technologists and Technicians, All Other	84,510	0.649	19.57	21.35	44,400
Occupational Health and Safety Specialists	59,610	0.458	32.11	32.67	67,960
Occupational Health and Safety Technicians	11,890	0.091	22.81	24.11	50,150
Athletic Trainers	20,780	0.159	(2)	(2)	44,010
Genetic Counselors	2,000	0.015	27.31	26.84	55,820
Healthcare Practitioners and Technical Workers, All Other	48,130	0.369	22.20	25.78	53,610
Healthcare Support Occupations	3,915,460	30.052	12.28	13.36	27,780
Home Health Aides	839,930	6.447	10.01	10.49	21,830
Nursing Assistants	1,420,020	10.899	11.74	12.32	25,620
Psychiatric Aides	77,880	0.598	11.82	12.83	26,680
Occupational Therapy Assistants	29,500	0.226	25.60	25.52	53,090
Occupational Therapy Aides	7,950	0.061	12.91	14.36	29,870
Physical Therapist Assistants	69,810	0.536	25.08	25.15	52,320
Physical Therapist Aides	48,700	0.374	11.48	12.22	25,410
Massage Therapists	71,040	0.545	17.29	19.40	40,350
Dental Assistants	300,160	2.304	16.59	16.86	35,080
Medical Assistants	553,140	4.246	14.12	14.69	30,550
Medical Equipment Preparers	50,230	0.386	14.82	15.51	32,260
Medical Transcriptionists	74,810	0.574	16.36	16.66	34,650
Pharmacy Aides	42,600	0.327	10.51	11.28	23,460
Veterinary Assistants and Laboratory Animal Caretakers	71,500	0.549	11.12	11.90	24,740
Phlebotomists	100,380	0.77	14.29	14.86	30,910
Healthcare Support Workers, All Other	103,890	0.797	15.77	16.29	33,880

[1]This wage is equal to or greater than $90.00 per hour or $187,199 per year.   [2]Wages for some occupations that do not generally work year-round, full time, are reported either as hourly wages or annual salaries depending on how they are typically paid.

Table 3-65. Employment and Wages for the Highest- and Lowest-Paying Detailed Health Sector Occupations, May 2012

(Dollars; number.)

Occupation title	Median hourly wage (dollars)[1]	Annual mean wage (dollars)	Employment
Highest-Paying Positions			
Anesthesiologists	(2)	232,830	29,930
Surgeons	(2)	230,540	42,410
Obstetricians and Gynecologists	(2)	216,760	20,880
Oral and Maxillofacial Surgeons	(2)	216,440	4,990
Internists, General	(2)	191,520	45,210
Orthodontists	(2)	186,320	5,530
Physicians and Surgeons, All Other	(2)	184,820	308,410
Family and General Practitioners	82.70	180,850	110,050
Psychiatrists	83.33	177,520	24,210
Prosthodontists	81.31	168,120	310
Lowest-Paying Positions			
Dietetic Technicians	12.62	28,680	24,660
Pharmacy Technicians	14.10	30,430	353,340
Veterinary Technologists and Technicians	14.56	31,470	83,350
Psychiatric Technicians	14.45	33,140	67,760
Emergency Medical Technicians and Paramedics	14.91	34,370	232,860
Opticians, Dispensing	16.03	35,010	26,570
Ophthalmic Medical Technicians	16.46	35,590	9,210
Medical Records and Health Information Technicians	16.42	36,770	300,830
Medical and Clinical Laboratory Technicians	17.90	39,340	168,410
Licensed Practical and Licensed Vocational Nurses	19.97	42,400	47,510

[1]The median wage is the wage where half the workers in the occupation earn more and half earn less. The OES program does not estimate percentile wages above $187,200.   [2]This wage is equal to or greater than $90.00 per hour or $187,199 per year.

Table 3-66. Industries with the Highest Levels of Employment and Highest Concentration of Employment in Health Care and Practitioner and Technical Occupations, May 2012

(Number; dollars.)

Industry	Employment[1]	Percent of industry employment	Hourly mean wage (dollars)	Annual mean wage (dollars)[2]
Industries with the Highest Levels of Employment in Health Care and Practitioner and Technical Occupations				
General Medical and Surgical Hospitals	2,863,320	54.68	32.93	68,490
Offices of Physicians	994,810	41.87	55.33	115,080
Nursing Care Facilities (Skilled Nursing Facilities)	418,310	25.16	25.12	52,240
Health and Personal Care Stores	348,470	34.80	29.93	62,250
Home Health Care Services	297,820	25.28	30.33	63,080
Industries with the Highest Concentration of Employment in Health Care and Practitioner and Technical Occupations				
Other Ambulatory Health Care Services	145,660	55.34	17.80	37,030
General Medical and Surgical Hospitals	2,863,320	54.68	32.93	68,490
Specialty (Except Psychiatric and Substance Abuse) Hospitals	113,570	49.29	34.64	72,060
Offices of Physicians	994,810	41.87	55.33	115,080
Medical and Diagnostic Laboratories	97,550	41.46	30.51	63,460

[1]Estimates for detailed occupations do not sum to the totals because the totals include occupations not shown separately. Estimates do not include self-employed workers. [2]Annual wages have been calculated by multiplying the hourly mean wage by a "year-round, full-time" hours figure of 2,080 hours; for those occupations where there is not an hourly mean wage published, the annual wage has been directly calculated from the reported survey data.

Table 3-67. States with the Highest Level of Employment and Highest Concentration of Jobs in Health Care Practitioner and Technical Occupations, May 2012

(Number, dollar.)

State	Employment[1]	Employment per thousand jobs	Location quotient[2]	Hourly mean wage (dollars)	Annual mean wage (dollars)[3]
States with the Highest Employment Level in This Occupation					
California	721,930	50.47	0.86	42.60	88,610
Texas	567,220	53.62	0.91	33.83	70,370
New York	494,330	57.87	0.99	39.22	81,580
Florida	459,410	63.16	1.08	33.71	70,110
Pennsylvania	351,870	62.87	1.07	34.08	70,900
States with the Highest Concentration of Jobs and Location Quotients in This Occupation					
West Virginia	52,670	74.06	1.26	29.49	61,340
Massachusetts	227,840	71.15	1.21	38.84	80,780
South Dakota	27,650	69.36	1.18	30.48	63,400
Mississippi	74,920	69.34	1.18	28.61	59,510
Maine	40,270	69.30	1.18	35.95	74,770

[1]Estimates for detailed occupations do not sum to the totals because the totals include occupations not shown separately. Estimates do not include self-employed workers.   [2]The location quotient is the ratio of the area concentration of occupational employment to the national average concentration. A location quotient greater than one indicates the occupation has a higher share of employment than average, and a location quotient less than one indicates the occupation is less prevalent in the area than average.   [3]Annual wages have been calculated by multiplying the hourly mean wage by a "year-round, full-time" hours figure of 2,080 hours; for those occupations where there is not an hourly mean wage published, the annual wage has been directly calculated from the reported survey data.

Table 3-68. Top Paying Metropolitan Area for Health Care Practitioner and Technical Occupations, May 2012

(Number, dollar.)

Metropolitan area	Employment[1]	Employment per thousand jobs	Location quotient[2]	Hourly mean wage (dollars)	Annual mean wage (dollars)[3]
San Jose-Sunnyvale-Santa Clara, CA	36,380	40.48	0.69	51.12	106,330
Oakland-Fremont-Hayward, CA Metropolitan Division	53,380	54.96	0.94	49.39	102,730
San Francisco-San Mateo-Redwood City, CA Metropolitan Division	42,730	42.71	0.73	48.36	100,590
Vallejo-Fairfield, CA	8,230	68.34	1.16	47.11	97,980
Sacramento–Arden-Arcade–Roseville, CA	43,730	53.50	0.91	47.04	97,840
Bethesda-Rockville-Frederick, MD Metropolitan Division	37,960	67.78	1.15	45.60	94,860
Napa, CA	4,240	67.64	1.15	45.02	93,460
Modesto, CA	9,760	63.73	1.09	44.47	92,500
Salinas, CA	6,090	39.10	0.67	44.31	92,170
Nassau-Suffolk, NY Metropolitan Division	77,330	63.22	1.08	43.86	91,230

[1]Estimates for detailed occupations do not sum to the totals because the totals include occupations not shown separately. Estimates do not include self-employed workers.   [2]The location quotient is the ratio of the area concentration of occupational employment to the national average concentration. A location quotient greater than one indicates the occupation has a higher share of employment than average, and a location quotient less than one indicates the occupation is less prevalent in the area than average.   [3]Annual wages have been calculated by multiplying the hourly mean wage by a "year-round, full-time" hours figure of 2,080 hours; for those occupations where there is not an hourly mean wage published, the annual wage has been directly calculated from the reported survey data.

Table 3-69. Employers' Costs Per Employee Hour Worked for Total Compensation, Wages and Salaries, and Health Insurance, by Selected Characteristics, Selected Years, 1991–2012

(Dollars; percent.)

Characteristic	1991	1995	2000	2005	2006	2007	2008	2009	2010	2011	2012
TOTAL COMPENSATION PER EMPLOYEE-HOUR WORKED											
State and local government	22.31	24.86	29.05	35.50	36.96	38.66	37.84	39.51	39.81	40.54	41.16
Total private industry	15.40	17.10	19.85	24.17	25.09	25.91	26.76	27.46	27.73	28.10	28.78
Industry											
Goods producing	18.48	20.75	23.55	28.48	29.36	30.12	31.38	32.29	32.42	32.91	33.76
Service providing	14.31	15.88	18.72	23.11	24.05	24.84	25.63	26.37	26.77	27.11	27.78
Occupational Group [1]											
White collar	18.15	20.50	24.19	NA	NA	NA	NA	NA	NA	NA	NA
Blue collar	15.15	16.69	18.73	NA	NA	NA	NA	NA	NA	NA	NA
Service	7.82	8.39	9.72	NA	NA	NA	NA	NA	NA	NA	NA
Management, professional, and related	NA	NA	NA	42.09	44.32	46.05	47.55	48.82	48.80	50.08	50.88
Sales and office	NA	NA	NA	19.30	19.93	20.55	21.15	21.40	21.77	22.02	22.60
Service	NA	NA	NA	12.07	12.30	12.87	13.27	13.53	13.71	13.98	14.03
Natural resources, construction, and maintenance	NA	NA	NA	27.26	28.07	28.96	30.13	30.97	31.10	30.93	31.46
Production, transportation, and material moving	NA	NA	NA	20.82	21.19	22.22	23.07	23.28	23.72	23.70	24.08
Census Region											
Northeast	17.56	20.09	22.67	27.09	28.75	29.56	30.56	31.73	32.13	32.16	32.99
Midwest	15.05	15.89	19.22	24.23	24.65	25.16	25.98	26.44	26.75	27.47	27.92
South	13.68	15.31	17.81	21.36	22.35	23.17	23.90	24.45	24.72	24.93	26.16
West	15.97	18.35	20.88	25.98	26.56	27.77	28.70	29.53	29.52	29.95	30.03
Union Status											
Union	19.76	22.40	25.88	33.17	34.07	35.27	36.28	36.59	37.16	37.68	38.41
Nonunion	14.56	16.26	19.07	23.09	24.03	24.82	25.64	26.39	26.67	27.08	27.80
Establishment Employment Size											
1 to 99 employees	13.38	14.58	17.16	20.22	20.43	21.29	22.23	22.56	22.84	23.21	23.84
100 or more employees	17.34	19.44	22.81	28.94	30.34	30.86	31.68	32.83	33.33	33.69	34.65
100 to 499 employees	14.31	16.30	19.30	24.44	25.91	26.31	26.80	28.19	28.55	28.69	29.15
500 or more employees	20.60	22.85	26.93	34.59	35.94	36.48	37.60	38.71	39.76	40.53	42.33
WAGES AND SALARIES AS A PERCENT OF TOTAL COMPENSATION											
State and local government	69.6	69.6	70.8	68.3	67.6	67.0	65.9	65.7	65.9	65.5	65.2
Total private industry	72.3	71.6	73.0	71.0	70.7	70.8	70.6	70.8	70.6	70.7	70.4
Industry											
Goods producing	68.7	67.3	69.0	65.5	66.2	66.8	66.7	66.9	66.7	66.5	66.7
Service providing	74.0	73.5	74.5	72.6	72.0	72.0	71.8	71.9	71.6	71.7	71.3
Occupational Group [1]											
White collar	73.8	73.0	74.0	NA	NA	NA	NA	NA	NA	NA	NA
Blue collar	68.4	67.6	69.4	NA	NA	NA	NA	NA	NA	NA	NA
Service	76.3	75.7	77.9	NA	NA	NA	NA	NA	NA	NA	NA
Management, professional, and related	NA	NA	NA	71.5	70.9	71.1	71.0	71.1	70.7	70.8	70.3
Sales and office	NA	NA	NA	72.6	72.2	72.1	72.0	71.8	71.6	71.6	71.4
Service	NA	NA	NA	75.7	75.3	75.0	74.8	75.3	75.4	75.4	75.2
Natural resources, construction, and maintenance	NA	NA	NA	68.0	68.0	68.3	68.3	68.2	68.0	68.3	67.8
Production, transportation, and material moving	NA	NA	NA	66.2	66.7	66.8	66.6	67.0	66.8	66.7	66.8
Census Region											
Northeast	72.1	70.9	72.2	70.4	70.0	69.7	69.8	69.6	69.0	69.5	69.2
Midwest	71.1	70.8	72.4	70.1	69.4	69.9	69.8	70.3	70.0	69.8	69.5
South	73.3	72.1	73.5	72.1	72.1	72.0	71.8	71.9	71.8	71.9	71.5
West	72.8	73.0	74.0	70.9	71.0	71.0	70.8	71.1	71.1	71.0	70.8
Union Status											
Union	65.9	64.3	65.2	62.6	62.3	62.2	61.9	62.2	61.6	61.1	60.3
Nonunion	74.0	73.2	74.4	72.4	72.1	72.2	72.1	72.2	72.0	72.1	71.8
Establishment Employment Size											
1 to 99 employees	74.7	74.1	75.5	73.9	73.7	73.8	73.8	74.0	73.6	74.0	73.7
100 or more employees	70.5	69.9	71.0	68.5	68.4	68.5	68.2	68.4	68.2	68.0	67.6
100 to 499 employees	72.1	71.3	72.8	70.2	70.0	70.1	69.8	70.0	70.0	69.9	69.7
500 or more employees	69.3	68.8	69.4	67.0	66.9	67.1	66.9	67.0	66.5	66.2	65.6

Table 3-69. Employers' Costs Per Employee Hour Worked for Total Compensation, Wages and Salaries, and Health Insurance, by Selected Characteristics, Selected Years, 1991–2012—Continued

(Dollars; percent.)

Characteristic	1991	1995	2000	2005	2006	2007	2008	2009	2010	2011	2012
HEALTH INSURANCE AS A PERCENT OF TOTAL COMPENSATION											
State and local government	6.9	7.8	7.8	10.2	10.6	10.9	11.0	10.9	11.4	11.7	11.6
Total private industry	6.0	6.2	5.5	6.8	6.9	7.1	7.2	7.3	7.5	7.5	7.7
Industry											
Goods producing	6.9	7.4	6.9	8.0	8.4	8.4	8.5	8.7	8.9	8.9	8.9
Service providing	5.5	5.7	4.9	6.4	6.4	6.7	6.8	6.9	7.2	7.2	7.4
Occupational Group [1]											
White collar	5.6	5.7	5.0	NA	NA	NA	NA	NA	NA	NA	NA
Blue collar	7.0	7.5	6.8	NA	NA	NA	NA	NA	NA	NA	NA
Service	4.6	5.1	4.3	NA	NA	NA	NA	NA	NA	NA	NA
Management, professional, and related	NA	NA	NA	5.5	5.6	5.8	5.8	6.0	6.2	6.3	6.5
Sales and office	NA	NA	NA	7.5	7.5	7.8	7.9	8.3	8.6	8.6	8.9
Service	NA	NA	NA	6.1	6.2	6.7	6.8	6.7	6.7	6.5	6.5
Natural resources, construction, and maintenance	NA	NA	NA	7.5	7.7	7.6	7.6	7.9	8.0	8.0	8.2
Production, transportation, and material moving	NA	NA	NA	8.9	9.0	9.3	9.6	9.7	9.9	10.1	9.9
Census Region											
Northeast	6.2	6.4	5.6	6.8	6.7	6.9	6.9	7.2	7.5	7.8	7.9
Midwest	6.3	6.7	5.8	7.3	7.6	7.8	7.9	8.1	8.3	8.3	2.4
South	5.5	6.0	5.4	6.6	6.7	6.9	6.9	7.0	7.2	7.2	7.1
West	5.8	5.6	5.0	6.3	6.4	6.7	6.9	6.9	7.1	7.1	7.3
Union Status											
Union	8.2	9.3	8.4	10.3	10.3	10.8	10.9	11.4	11.8	12.3	12.9
Nonunion	5.4	5.5	5.0	6.2	6.3	6.4	6.5	6.6	6.8	6.8	6.9
Establishment Employment Size											
1 to 99 employees	5.1	5.3	4.8	5.9	6.0	6.1	6.1	6.3	6.4	6.3	6.4
100 or more employees	6.6	6.9	6.0	7.5	7.5	7.8	8.0	8.1	8.4	8.6	8.7
100 to 499 employees	6.3	6.5	5.6	7.5	7.4	7.7	7.9	7.9	8.3	8.4	8.5
500 or more employees	6.8	7.2	6.4	7.6	7.6	7.9	8.0	8.2	8.5	8.7	8.9

NOTE: Total compensation includes wages and salaries and benefits.

NA =Data not available. [1]Starting with 2004 data, sample establishments were classified by industry categories based on the North American Industry Classification System (NAICS), as defined by the U.S. Office of Management and Budget. Within a sample establishment, specific job categories were selected and classified into about 840 occupational classifications according to the 2000 Standard Occupational Classification (SOC) system. Individual occupations were combined to represent one of five higher-level aggregations, such as management, professional, and related occupations. NAICS and SOC have replaced the 1987 Standard Industrial Classification System and the Occupational Classification System.

HEALTH EXPENDITURES

Figure 3-14. Consumer Price Index (CPI), All Items and Medical Care, 2000–2011

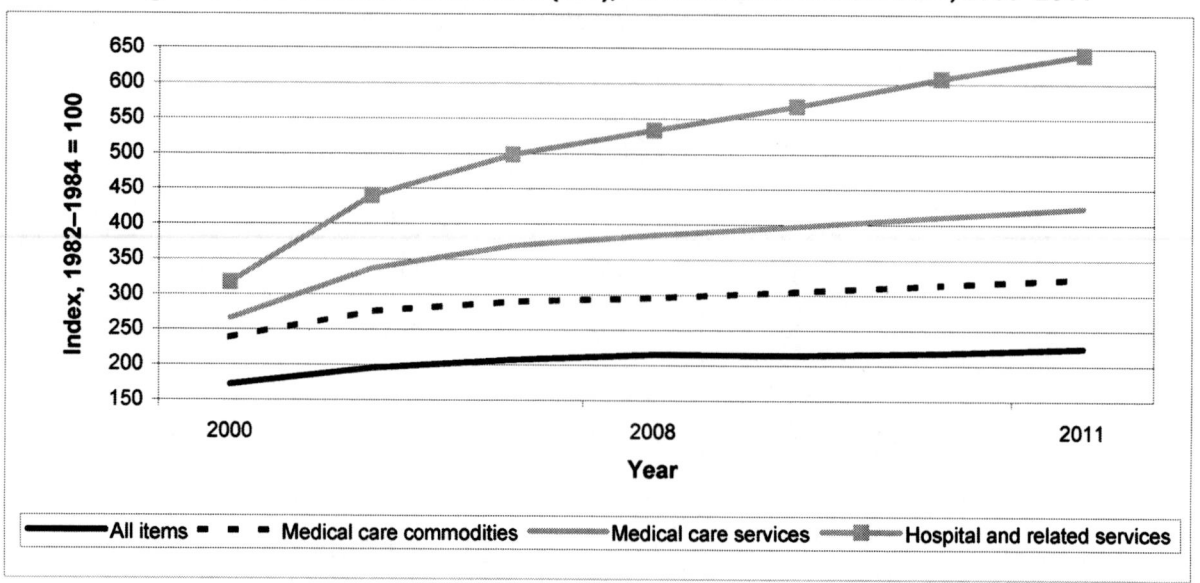

Figure 3-15. Percent Distribution of Personal Health Care Expenditures, by Type, 2010

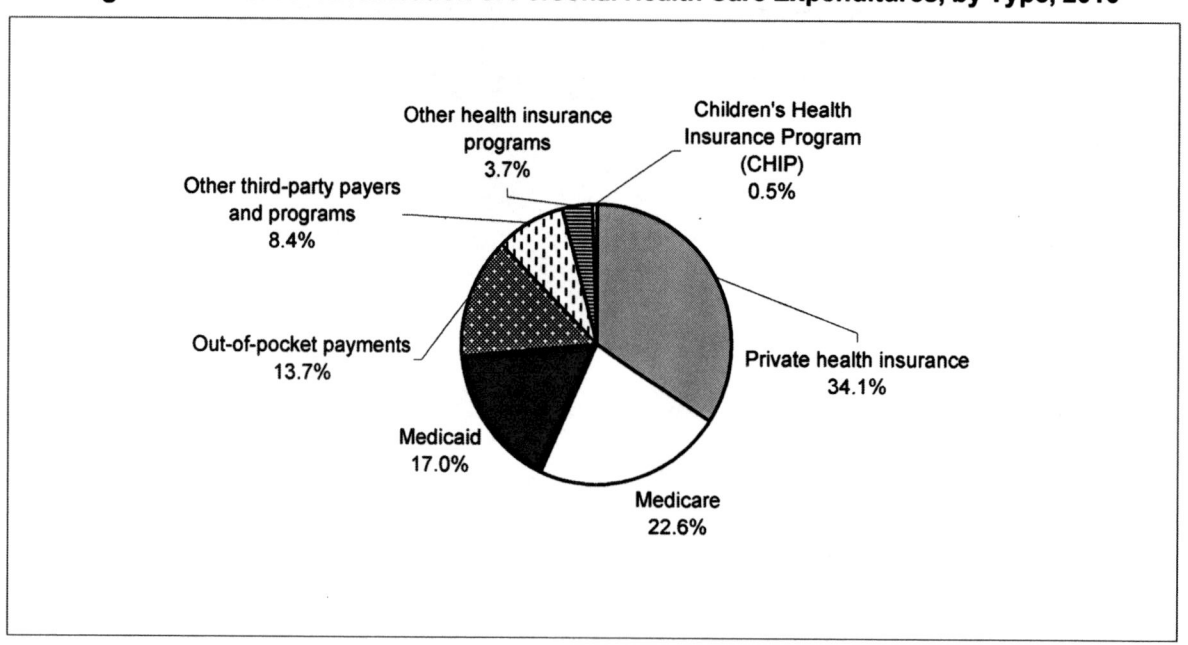

Table 3-70. Gross Domestic Product, National Health Expenditures, Per Capita Amounts, Percent Distribution, and Average Annual Percent Change, Selected Years, 1960–2010

(Number; dollars.)

Gross domestic product and national health expenditures	1960	1970	1980	1990	2000	2005	2008	2009	2010
Gross domestic product (GDP)	526	1,038	2,788	5,801	9,952	12,623	14,292	13,939	14,527
Implicit price deflator for GDP[1] (2005 = 1000)	18.6	24.3	47.8	72.3	88.7	100.0	108.6	109.7	111.0
Amount (in Billions)									
National health expenditures	27.4	74.9	255.8	724.3	1,377.2	2,029.1	2,403.9	2,495.8	2,593.6
Health consumption expenditures	24.8	67.1	235.7	675.6	1,289.6	1,902.6	2,250.1	2,349.5	2,444.6
Personal health care	23.4	63.1	217.2	616.8	1,165.4	1,697.2	2,010.2	2,109.0	2,186.0
Administration and net cost of private health insurance	1.1	2.6	12.0	38.8	81.2	149.2	167.2	164.3	176.1
Public health	0.4	1.4	6.4	20.0	43.0	56.2	72.7	76.2	82.5
Investment[2]	2.6	7.8	20.1	48.7	87.5	126.5	153.8	146.3	149.0
Per Capita Amount (in Dollars)									
National health expenditures	147	356	1,110	2,854	4,878	6,868	7,911	8,149	8,402
Health consumption expenditures	133	319	1,023	2,662	4,568	6,440	7,405	7,671	7,919
Personal health care	125	300	943	2,430	4,128	5,745	6,615	6,886	7,082
Administration and net cost of private health insurance	6	12	52	153	288	505	550	536	570
Public health	2	6	28	79	152	190	239	249	267
Investment[2]	14	37	87	192	310	428	506	478	483
Percent									
National health expenditures as percent of GDP	5.2	7.2	9.2	12.5	13.8	16.1	16.8	17.9	17.9
Percent Distribution									
National health expenditures	100.0	100.0	100.0	100.0	100.0	100.0	100.0	100.0	100.0
Health consumption expenditures	90.6	89.6	92.1	93.3	93.6	93.8	93.6	94.1	94.3
Personal health care	85.4	84.3	84.9	85.2	84.6	83.6	83.6	84.5	84.3
Administration and net cost of private health insurance	3.9	3.5	4.7	5.4	5.9	7.4	7.0	6.6	6.8
Public health	1.4	1.8	2.5	2.8	3.1	2.8	3.0	3.1	3.2
Investment[2]	9.4	10.4	7.9	6.7	6.4	6.2	6.4	5.9	5.7
Average Annual Percent Change from Previous Year Shown									
GDP	X	7.0	10.4	7.6	5.5	4.9	4.2	-2.5	4.2
National health expenditures	X	10.6	13.1	11.0	6.6	8.1	5.8	3.8	3.9
Health consumption expenditures	X	10.5	13.4	11.1	6.7	8.1	5.8	4.4	4.0
Personal health care	X	10.4	13.2	11.0	6.6	7.8	5.8	4.9	3.7
Administration and net cost of private health insurance	X	9.0	16.5	12.5	7.7	12.9	3.9	-1.7	7.2
Public health	X	13.3	16.4	12.1	8.0	5.5	9.0	4.8	8.3
Investment[2]	X	11.6	9.9	9.3	6.0	7.7	6.7	-4.9	1.8
National health expenditures	X	9.2	12.0	9.9	5.5	7.1	4.8	3.0	3.1
Health consumption expenditures	X	9.1	12.4	10.0	5.5	7.1	4.8	3.6	3.2
Personal health care	X	9.1	12.1	9.9	5.4	6.8	4.8	4.1	2.8
Administration and net cost of private health insurance	X	7.2	15.8	11.4	6.5	11.9	2.9	-2.5	6.3
Public health	X	11.6	16.7	10.9	6.8	4.6	7.9	4.2	7.2
Investment[2]	X	10.2	8.9	8.2	4.9	6.7	5.7	-5.5	1.0

NOTE: Dollar amounts are in current dollars. The data reflect preliminary annual estimates of the resident population for the United States, as of July 1, 2010, excluding the Armed Forces overseas.

X = Not applicable.   [1]Year 2005 = 100.   [2]Investment consists of research and structures and equipment.

Table 3-71. Consumer Price Index and Average Annual Percent Change for All Items, Selected Items and Medical Care Components, Selected Years, 1960–2011

(Number; percent change.)

Items and medical care components	1960	1970	1980	1990	1995	2000	2005	2007	2008	2009	2010	2011
Consumer Price Index (CPI)												
All items	29.6	38.8	82.4	130.7	152.4	172.2	195.3	207.3	215.3	214.5	218.1	224.9
All items less medical care	30.2	39.2	82.8	128.8	148.6	167.3	188.7	200.1	207.8	206.6	209.7	216.4
Services	24.1	35.0	77.9	139.2	168.7	195.3	230.1	246.8	255.5	259.2	261.3	265.8
Food	30.0	39.2	86.8	132.4	148.4	167.8	190.7	202.9	214.1	218.0	219.6	227.8
Apparel	45.7	59.2	90.9	124.1	132.0	129.6	119.5	119.0	118.9	120.1	119.5	122.1
Housing	NA	36.4	81.1	128.5	148.5	169.6	195.7	209.6	216.3	217.1	216.3	219.1
Energy	22.4	25.5	86.0	102.1	105.2	124.6	177.1	207.7	236.7	193.1	211.4	243.9
Medical care	22.3	34.0	74.9	162.8	220.5	260.8	323.2	351.1	364.1	375.6	388.4	400.3
Components of Medical Care												
Medical care services	19.5	32.3	74.8	162.7	224.2	266.0	336.7	369.3	384.9	397.3	411.2	423.8
Professional services	NA	37.0	77.9	156.1	201.0	237.7	281.7	300.8	311.0	319.4	328.2	335.7
Physicians' services	21.9	34.5	76.5	160.8	208.8	244.7	287.5	303.2	311.3	320.8	331.3	340.3
Dental services	27.0	39.2	78.9	155.8	206.8	258.5	324.0	358.4	376.9	388.1	398.8	408.0
Eyeglasses and eye care[1]	NA	NA	NA	117.3	137.0	149.7	163.2	171.6	174.1	175.5	176.7	178.3
Services by other medical professionals[1]	NA	NA	NA	120.2	143.9	161.9	186.8	197.4	205.5	209.8	214.4	217.4
Hospital and related services	NA	NA	69.2	178.0	257.8	317.3	439.9	498.9	534.0	567.9	607.7	641.5
Hospital services[2]	NA	NA	NA	NA	NA	115.9	161.6	183.6	197.2	210.7	227.2	241.2
Inpatient hospital services[2,3]	NA	NA	NA	NA	NA	113.8	156.6	178.1	190.8	203.6	221.5	236.6
Outpatient hospital services[1,3]	NA	NA	NA	138.7	204.6	263.8	373.0	424.2	456.8	490.6	520.6	546.9
Hospital rooms	9.3	23.6	68.0	175.4	251.2	NA	NA	NA	NA	NA	NA	NA
Other inpatient services[1]	NA	NA	NA	142.7	206.8	NA	NA	NA	NA	NA	NA	NA
Nursing homes and adult day care[2]	NA	NA	NA	NA	NA	117.0	145.0	159.6	165.3	171.6	177.0	182.2
Health insurance[4]	NA	NA	NA	NA	NA	NA	NA	113.5	114.2	110.5	106.6	105.5
Medical care commodities	46.9	46.5	75.4	163.4	204.5	238.1	276.0	290.0	296.0	305.1	314.7	324.1
Medicinal drugs[5]	NA	NA	NA	NA	NA	NA	NA	NA	NA	NA	102.3	105.5
Prescription drugs[6]	54.0	47.4	72.5	181.7	235.0	285.4	349.0	369.2	378.3	391.1	407.8	425.0
Nonprescription drugs[5]	NA	NA	NA	NA	NA	NA	NA	NA	NA	NA	100.0	98.6
Medical equipment and supplies[5]	NA	NA	NA	NA	NA	NA	NA	NA	NA	NA	99.1	99.3
Nonprescription drugs and medical supplies[1,7]	NA	NA	NA	120.6	140.5	149.5	151.7	156.8	158.3	161.4	NA	NA
Internal and respiratory over-the-counter drugs[8]	NA	42.3	74.9	145.9	167.0	176.9	179.7	186.4	188.7	193.0	NA	NA
Nonprescription medical equipment and supplies[9]	NA	NA	79.2	138.0	166.3	178.1	180.6	185.1	185.6	188.2	NA	NA
Average Annual Percent Change from Previous Year Shown												
All items	X	2.7	7.8	4.7	3.1	2.5	2.5	3.0	3.8	2.4	1.6	3.2
All items less medical care	X	2.6	7.8	4.5	2.9	2.4	2.4	3.0	3.8	2.3	1.5	3.2
Services	X	3.8	8.3	6.0	3.9	3.0	3.3	3.6	3.5	3.0	0.8	1.7
Food	X	2.7	8.3	4.3	2.3	2.5	2.6	3.1	5.5	3.4	0.8	3.7
Apparel	X	2.6	4.4	3.2	1.2	-0.4	-1.6	-0.2	-0.1	0.1	-0.5	2.2
Housing	X	NA	8.3	4.7	2.9	2.7	2.9	3.5	3.2	2.6	-0.4	1.3
Energy	X	1.3	12.9	1.7	0.6	3.4	7.3	8.3	13.9	2.2	9.5	15.4
Medical care	X	4.3	8.2	8.1	6.3	3.4	4.4	4.2	3.7	3.8	3.4	3.0
Components of Medical Care												
Medical care services	X	5.2	8.8	8.1	6.6	3.5	4.8	4.7	4.2	4.2	3.5	3.1
Professional services	X	NA	7.7	7.2	5.2	3.4	3.5	3.3	3.4	3.2	2.8	2.3
Physicians' services	X	4.6	8.3	7.7	5.4	3.2	3.3	2.7	2.7	2.8	3.3	2.7
Dental services	X	3.8	7.2	7.0	5.8	4.6	4.6	5.2	5.1	4.6	2.7	2.3
Eyeglasses and eye care[1]	X	NA	NA	NA	3.2	1.8	1.7	2.5	1.4	1.8	0.7	0.9
Services by other medical professionals[1]	X	NA	NA	NA	3.7	2.4	2.9	2.8	4.1	2.9	2.2	1.4
Hospital and related services	X	NA	NA	9.9	7.7	4.2	6.8	6.5	7.0	6.6	7.0	5.6
Hospital services[2]	X	NA	NA	NA	NA	NA	6.9	6.6	7.4	6.9	7.8	6.2
Inpatient hospital services[2,3]	X	NA	NA	NA	NA	NA	6.6	6.6	6.6	6.8	8.8	6.8
Outpatient hospital services[1,3]	X	NA	NA	NA	8.1	5.2	7.2	6.6	7.7	7.1	6.1	5.1
Hospital rooms	X	9.8	11.2	9.9	7.4	NA	NA	NA	NA	NA	NA	NA
Other inpatient services[1]	X	NA	NA	NA	7.7	NA	NA	NA	NA	NA	NA	NA
Nursing homes and adult day care[2]	X	NA	NA	NA	NA	NA	4.4	4.9	3.6	4.3	3.1	2.9
Health insurance[4]	X	NA	NA	NA	NA	NA	NA	NA	0.6	NA	-3.5	-1.1
Medical care commodities	X	-0.1	5.0	8.0	4.6	3.1	3.0	2.5	2.1	2.5	3.1	3.0
Medicinal drugs[5]	X	NA	NA	NA	NA	NA	NA	NA	NA	NA	X	3.1
Prescription drugs[6]	X	-1.3	4.3	9.6	5.3	4.0	4.1	2.9	2.5	2.9	4.3	4.2
Nonprescription drugs[5]	X	NA	NA	NA	NA	NA	NA	NA	NA	NA	X	-1.3
Medical equipment and supplies[5]	X	NA	NA	NA	NA	NA	NA	NA	NA	NA	X	0.3
Nonprescription drugs and medical supplies[1,7]	X	NA	NA	NA	3.1	1.2	0.3	1.7	0.9	1.6	NA	NA
Internal and respiratory over-the-counter drugs[8]	X	NA	5.9	6.9	2.7	1.2	0.3	1.8	1.2	1.8	NA	NA
Nonprescription medical equipment and supplies[9]	X	NA	NA	5.7	3.8	1.4	0.3	1.2	0.3	1.0	NA	NA

NOTE: CPI for all urban consumers (CPI-U) U.S. city average, detailed expenditure categories. 1982-1984 = 100, except where noted. Data are not seasonally adjusted.

NA = Not available.   X = Not applicable.   [1]December 1986 = 100.   [2]December 1996 = 100.   [3]Special index based on a substantially smaller sample.   [4]December 2005 = 100.   [5]December 2009 = 100.   [6]Prior to 2006, this category included medical supplies.   [7]Starting with 2010 updates, this index series will no longer be published.   [8]Starting with 2010 updates, replaced by the series, nonprescription drugs.   [9]Starting with 2010 updates, replaced by the series, medical equipment and supplies.

Table 3-72. Growth in Personal Health Care Expenditures and Percent Distribution of Factors Affecting Growth, 1960–2009

(Percent.)

Period	Average annual percent increase	Factors affecting personal health care expenditure growth				Intensity growth[4]
		All factors	Inflation[1]		Population growth	
			Economy-wide inflation[2]	Excess medical price inflation[3]		
		Percent distribution of factors affecting growth[5]				
1960–2009	9.6	100	39	13	11	36
1960–1965	8.3	100	17	9	18	56
1965–1970	12.7	100	33	11	8	47
1970–1975	12.4	100	55	0	8	37
1975–1980	13.9	100	54	12	7	27
1980–1985	11.7	100	46	30	9	15
1985–1990	10.4	100	32	21	10	37
1990–1995	7.2	100	35	17	16	32
1995–2000	5.9	100	29	10	17	43
1995–1996	5.6	100	35	5	18	42
1996–1997	5.7	100	31	1	19	49
1997–1998	5.5	100	21	17	19	43
1998–1999	5.9	100	26	17	17	40
1999–2000	6.9	100	32	11	14	43
2000–2005	7.8	100	32	11	13	44
2000–2001	8.6	100	27	17	12	44
2001–2002	8.5	100	20	17	12	52
2002–2003	7.8	100	28	11	12	49
2003–2004	7.2	100	40	10	14	36
2004–2005	6.8	100	50	-4	14	40
2005–2006	6.3	100	53	-3	16	34
2006–2007	5.9	100	51	7	18	24
2007–2008	4.9	100	45	9	19	26
2008–2009	4.6	100	20	40	19	21

NOTE: The inflation rates used to calculate the factors affecting growth have a base year of 2005.

[1]Two measures of inflation are presented: economy-wide and excess medical inflation (changes in medical-specific prices in excess of those included in economy-wide inflation).   [2]Economy-wide inflation is calculated using the implicit price deflator (IDP) for gross domestic product (GDP). The IDP is a broad measure of the prices of the goods and services that the U.S. produces.   [3]Excess medical price inflation is the measured amount of medical price growth above general economy-wide price growth. This excess rate captures if medical prices have tended to rise more or less quickly than general economy-wide prices.   [4]Intensity is the residual percentage of growth that cannot be attributed to inflation or population growth. It includes changes in the use or kinds of services and supplies, and it captures any errors in measuring prices or total spending.   [5]Percents may not sum to 100 due to rounding.

Table 3-73. National Health Expenditures, Average Annual Percent Change and Percent Distribution, by Type of Expenditure, Selected Years, 1960–2010

(Dollars; percent.)

Type of national health expenditure	1960	1970	1980	1990	2000	2005	2008	2009	2010
Amount (in Billions of Dollars)									
National health expenditures	27.4	74.9	255.8	724.3	1,377.2	2,029.1	2,403.9	2,495.8	2,593.6
Health consumption expenditures	24.8	67.1	235.7	675.6	1,289.6	1,902.6	2,250.1	2,349.5	2,444.6
Personal health care	23.4	63.1	217.2	616.8	1,165.4	1,697.2	2,010.2	2,109.0	2,186.0
Hospital care	9.0	27.2	100.5	250.4	415.5	609.4	729.3	776.1	814.0
Professional services	8.0	19.8	64.6	208.1	390.2	557.0	652.6	671.2	688.6
Physician and clinical services	5.6	14.3	47.7	158.9	290.9	416.9	486.6	502.7	515.5
Other professional services	0.4	0.7	3.5	17.4	37.0	53.0	63.6	66.0	68.4
Dental services	2.0	4.7	13.4	31.7	62.3	87.0	102.4	102.5	104.8
Other health, residential, and personal care	0.5	1.3	8.5	24.3	64.6	96.5	113.3	122.0	128.5
Home health care[1]	0.1	0.2	2.4	12.6	32.4	48.7	61.5	66.1	70.2
Nursing care facilities and continuing care retirement communities[1]	0.8	4.0	15.3	44.9	85.1	112.5	132.7	138.7	143.1
Retail outlet sales of medical products	5.0	10.6	25.9	76.5	177.6	273.2	321.0	334.9	341.6
Prescription drugs	2.7	5.5	12.0	40.3	120.9	204.8	243.6	256.1	259.1
Durable medical equipment	0.7	1.7	4.1	13.8	25.1	31.2	34.9	35.2	37.7
Other nondurable medical products	1.6	3.3	9.8	22.4	31.6	37.2	42.5	43.6	44.8
Government administration[2]	0.1	0.7	2.8	7.2	17.1	28.0	29.5	29.6	30.1
Net cost of health insurance[3]	1.0	1.9	9.3	31.6	64.2	121.2	137.8	134.7	146.0
Government public health activities[4]	0.4	1.4	6.4	20.0	43.0	56.2	72.7	76.2	82.5
Investment	2.6	7.8	20.1	48.7	87.5	126.5	153.8	146.3	149.0
Research[5]	0.7	2.0	5.4	12.7	25.5	40.3	43.4	45.7	49.3
Structures and equipment	1.9	5.8	14.7	36.0	62.1	86.2	110.4	100.6	99.8
Average Annual Percent Change from Previous Year Shown									
National health expenditures	X	10.6	13.1	11.0	6.6	8.1	5.8	3.8	3.9
Health consumption expenditures	X	10.5	13.4	11.1	6.7	8.1	5.8	4.4	4.0
Personal health care	X	10.4	13.2	11.0	6.6	7.8	5.8	4.9	3.7
Hospital care	X	11.7	14.0	9.6	5.2	8.0	6.2	6.4	4.9
Professional services	X	9.5	12.6	12.4	6.5	7.4	5.4	2.9	2.6
Physician and clinical services	X	9.8	12.8	12.8	6.2	7.5	5.3	3.3	2.5
Other professional services	X	5.8	17.5	17.4	7.8	7.5	6.3	3.8	3.6
Dental services	X	8.9	11.0	9.0	7.0	6.9	5.6	0.1	2.2
Other health, residential, and personal care	X	10.0	20.7	11.1	10.3	8.4	5.5	7.7	5.3
Home health care[1]	X	7.2	28.2	18.0	9.9	8.5	8.1	7.5	6.2
Nursing care facilities and continuing care retirement communities[1]	X	17.5	14.4	11.4	6.6	5.7	5.7	4.5	3.2
Retail outlet sales of medical products	X	7.7	9.4	11.4	8.8	9.0	5.5	4.3	2.0
Prescription drugs	X	7.4	8.1	12.9	11.6	11.1	6.0	5.1	1.2
Durable medical equipment	X	9.3	9.2	12.9	6.2	4.4	3.8	0.9	7.1
Other nondurable medical products	X	7.5	11.5	8.6	3.5	3.3	4.5	2.6	2.8
Government administration[2]	X	30.0	14.1	10.0	9.1	10.4	1.6	0.4	1.7
Net cost of health insurance[3]	X	6.4	17.3	13.1	7.3	13.6	4.4	-2.2	8.4
Government public health activities[4]	X	13.8	16.9	12.0	8.0	5.5	9.0	4.9	8.2
Investment	X	11.7	10.0	9.2	6.0	7.6	6.7	-4.9	1.9
Research[5]	X	10.9	10.8	8.9	7.2	9.6	2.5	5.3	7.9
Structures and equipment	X	12.0	9.7	9.4	5.6	6.8	8.6	-8.9	-0.8
Percent Distribution									
National health expenditures	100.0	100.0	100.0	100.0	100.0	100.0	100.0	100.0	100.0
Health consumption expenditures	90.6	89.6	92.1	93.3	93.6	93.8	93.6	94.1	94.3
Personal health care	85.4	84.3	84.9	85.2	84.6	83.6	83.6	84.5	84.3
Hospital care	32.8	36.3	39.3	34.6	30.2	30.0	30.3	31.1	31.4
Professional services	29.3	26.4	25.3	28.7	28.3	27.4	27.1	26.9	26.6
Physician and clinical services	20.6	19.1	18.7	21.9	21.1	20.5	20.2	20.1	19.9
Other professional services	1.4	1.0	1.4	2.4	2.7	2.6	2.6	2.6	2.6
Dental services	7.3	6.3	5.2	4.4	4.5	4.3	4.3	4.1	4.0
Other health, residential, and personal care	1.6	1.8	3.3	3.4	4.7	4.8	4.7	4.9	5.0
Home health care[1]	0.2	0.3	0.9	1.7	2.4	2.4	2.6	2.6	2.7
Nursing care facilities and continuing care retirement communities[1]	3.0	5.4	6.0	6.2	6.2	5.5	5.5	5.6	5.5
Retail outlet sales of medical products	18.4	14.1	10.1	10.6	12.9	13.5	13.4	13.4	13.2
Prescription drugs	9.8	7.3	4.7	5.6	8.8	10.1	10.1	10.3	10.0
Durable medical equipment	2.7	2.3	1.6	1.9	1.8	1.5	1.5	1.4	1.5
Other nondurable medical products	5.9	4.4	3.8	3.1	2.3	1.8	1.8	1.7	1.7
Government administration[2]	0.2	1.0	1.1	1.0	1.2	1.4	1.2	1.2	1.2
Net cost of health insurance[3]	3.7	2.5	3.6	4.4	4.7	6.0	5.7	5.4	5.6
Government public health activities[4]	1.4	1.8	2.5	2.8	3.1	2.8	3.0	3.1	3.2
Investment	9.4	10.4	7.9	6.7	6.4	6.2	6.4	5.9	5.7
Research[5]	2.5	2.6	2.1	1.8	1.8	2.0	1.8	1.8	1.9
Structures and equipment	6.8	7.8	5.7	5.0	4.5	4.2	4.6	4.0	3.8

X = Not applicable. [1]Includes expenditures for care in freestanding facilities only. Additional services of this type are provided in hospital-based facilities and are considered hospital care. [2]Includes all administrative costs (federal and state and local employees' salaries, contracted employees including fiscal intermediaries, rent and building costs, computer systems and programs, other materials and supplies, and other miscellaneous expenses) associated with insuring individuals enrolled in the following health insurance programs: Medicare, Medicaid, Children's Health Insurance Program, Department of Defense, Department of Veterans Affairs, Indian Health Service, workers' compensation, maternal and child health, vocational rehabilitation, Substance Abuse and Mental Health Services Administration, and other federal programs. [3]Net cost of health insurance is calculated as the difference between calendar year incurred premiums earned and benefits paid for private health insurance. This includes administrative costs, and in some cases, additions to reserves, rate credits and dividends, premium taxes, and plan profits or losses. Also included in this category is the difference between premiums earned and benefits paid for the private health insurance companies that insure the enrollees of the following programs: Medicare, Medicaid, Children's Health Insurance Program, and workers' compensation (health portion only). [4]Includes personal care services delivered by government public health agencies. [5]Research and development expenditures of drug companies and other manufacturers and providers of medical equipment and supplies are excluded. They are included in the expenditure class in which the product falls because such expenditures are covered by the payment received for that product.

Table 3-74. Personal Health Care Expenditures, by Source of Funds and Type of Expenditure, Selected Years, 1960–2010

(Number; percent.)

Type of personal health care expenditures and source of funds	1960	1970	1980	1990	2000	2005	2008	2009	2010
Amount in Billions									
Per capita	125.0	300.0	943.0	2,430.0	4,128.0	5,745.0	6,615.0	6,886.0	7,082.0
Amount in Billions									
All personal health care expenditures[1]	23.4	63.1	217.2	616.8	1,165.4	1,697.2	2,010.2	2,109.0	2,186.0
Out-of-pocket payments	13.1	25.0	58.4	138.7	201.8	263.4	294.0	294.4	299.7
Health insurance	6.6	29.6	132.0	403.3	844.8	1,281.4	1,544.9	1,637.1	1,703.0
Private health insurance	4.9	14.0	61.4	205.1	407.1	607.7	707.5	734.0	746.0
Medicare	X	7.3	36.3	107.3	215.8	325.3	442.0	471.2	493.8
Medicaid	X	5.0	24.7	69.7	186.9	287.7	317.1	345.9	371.6
Federal	X	2.7	13.7	40.3	109.3	165.5	187.8	230.5	251.5
State and local	X	2.3	11.0	29.4	77.6	122.2	129.3	115.4	120.1
CHIP[2]	X	X	X	X	2.5	6.4	8.7	9.6	10.0
Federal	X	X	X	X	1.8	4.5	6.1	6.7	7.0
State and local	X	X	X	X	0.8	2.0	2.6	2.8	3.0
Other health insurance programs[3]	1.7	3.3	9.6	21.2	32.4	54.3	69.6	76.5	81.6
Other third-party payers and programs[4]	3.7	8.5	26.8	74.9	118.8	152.5	171.4	177.4	183.3
Amount in Billions									
Personal health care implicit price deflator[5] (2005 = 100.0)	10.1	14.7	31.4	63.1	85.0	100.0	109.3	112.3	115.3
Percent Distribution									
All sources of funds	100.0	100.0	100.0	100.0	100.0	100.0	100.0	100.0	100.0
Out-of-pocket payments	55.9	39.6	26.9	22.5	17.3	15.5	14.6	14.0	13.7
Health insurance	28.3	46.9	60.8	65.4	72.5	75.5	76.8	77.6	77.9
Private health insurance	21.1	22.2	28.3	33.3	34.9	35.8	35.2	34.8	34.1
Medicare	X	11.5	16.7	17.4	18.5	19.2	22.0	22.3	22.6
Medicaid	X	8.0	11.4	11.3	16.0	17.0	15.8	16.4	17.0
Federal	X	4.3	6.3	6.5	9.4	9.8	9.3	10.9	11.5
State and local	X	3.7	5.1	4.8	6.7	7.2	6.4	5.5	5.5
CHIP[2]	X	X	X	X	0.2	0.4	0.4	0.5	0.5
Federal	X	X	X	X	0.2	0.3	0.3	0.3	0.3
State and local	X	X	X	X	0.1	0.1	0.1	0.1	0.1
Other health insurance programs[3]	7.2	5.2	4.4	3.4	2.8	3.2	3.5	3.6	3.7
Other third-party payers and programs[4]	15.8	13.5	12.3	12.1	10.2	9.0	8.5	8.4	8.4
Amount in Billions									
Hospital expenditures[6]	9.0	27.2	100.5	250.4	415.5	609.4	729.3	776.1	814.0
Percent Distribution									
All sources of funds	100.0	100.0	100.0	100.0	100.0	100.0	100.0	100.0	100.0
Out-of-pocket payments	20.6	9.0	5.4	4.5	3.3	3.2	3.2	3.2	3.2
Health insurance	50.7	71.4	79.6	82.6	86.1	87.4	87.7	87.6	87.8
Private health insurance	35.6	32.5	36.7	38.7	34.2	35.8	36.6	36.0	35.1
Medicare	X	19.7	26.1	26.9	29.6	28.8	28.2	27.9	27.8
Medicaid	X	9.7	9.2	10.6	17.1	17.2	17.0	17.7	18.7
Federal	X	5.2	5.0	6.3	10.3	10.0	10.1	11.7	12.6
State and local	X	4.5	4.2	4.3	6.8	7.2	6.9	6.0	6.1
CHIP[2]	X	X	X	X	0.2	0.4	0.4	0.4	0.4
Federal	X	X	X	X	0.2	0.3	0.3	0.3	0.3
State and local	X	X	X	X	0.1	0.1	0.1	0.1	0.1
Other health insurance programs[3]	15.1	9.5	7.7	6.3	5.0	5.1	5.5	5.6	5.7
Other third-party payers and programs[4]	28.7	19.5	15.0	13.0	10.6	9.4	9.1	9.2	9.1
Amount in Billions									
Physician and clinical expenditures	5.6	14.3	47.7	158.9	290.9	416.9	486.6	502.7	515.5
Percent Distribution									
All sources of funds	100.0	100.0	100.0	100.0	100.0	100.0	100.0	100.0	100.0
Out-of-pocket payments	60.1	45.1	29.9	18.9	11.2	10.2	10.0	9.5	9.6
Health insurance	32.6	48.8	59.9	67.8	76.6	79.2	80.3	81.3	81.2
Private health insurance	28.3	29.4	34.9	42.2	47.5	48.4	47.9	47.2	46.4
Medicare	X	11.5	17.4	19.2	20.2	20.6	21.3	22.2	22.2
Medicaid	X	4.5	5.1	4.4	6.6	7.2	7.3	8.0	8.3
Federal	X	2.4	2.9	2.6	3.9	4.3	4.5	5.5	5.8
State and local	X	2.1	2.2	1.8	2.7	2.9	2.8	2.5	2.5
CHIP[2]	X	X	X	X	0.3	0.4	0.6	0.6	0.6
Federal	X	X	X	X	0.2	0.3	0.4	0.4	0.4
State and local	X	X	X	X	0.1	0.1	0.2	0.2	0.2
Other health insurance programs[3]	4.3	3.4	2.4	2.1	2.1	2.6	3.2	3.5	3.6
Other third-party payers and programs[4]	7.3	6.1	10.2	13.2	12.2	10.6	9.7	9.2	9.2
Amount in Billions									
Nursing care facilities and continuing care retirement communities expenditures[7]	0.8	4.0	15.3	44.9	85.1	112.5	132.7	138.7	143.1
Percent Distribution									
All sources of funds	100.0	100.0	100.0	100.0	100.0	100.0	100.0	100.0	100.0
Out-of-pocket payments	74.8	49.5	40.7	40.3	31.9	28.9	29.1	28.5	28.3
Health insurance	0.0	28.5	51.9	48.8	61.1	64.7	64.7	65.3	65.5
Private health insurance	0.0	0.2	1.3	6.2	8.8	7.4	8.2	8.5	8.9
Medicare	X	3.5	2.0	3.8	12.7	18.3	20.8	21.6	22.3
Medicaid	X	23.3	46.2	36.6	37.4	36.6	33.0	32.4	31.5
Federal	X	12.5	26.1	20.6	21.7	20.6	19.3	21.6	21.4
State and local	X	10.8	20.1	16.0	15.7	15.9	13.7	10.8	10.1
CHIP[2]	X	X	X	X	0.0	0.0	0.0	0.0	0.0
Federal	X	X	X	X	0.0	0.0	0.0	0.0	0.0
State and local	X	X	X	X	0.0	0.0	0.0	0.0	0.0
Other health insurance programs[3]	0.0	1.5	2.4	2.2	2.2	2.5	2.8	2.9	2.8
Other third-party payers and programs[4]	25.2	21.9	7.4	10.9	6.9	6.4	6.2	6.2	6.3

Table 3-74. Personal Health Care Expenditures, by Source of Funds and Type of Expenditure, Selected Years, 1960–2010—*Continued*

(Number; percent.)

Type of personal health care expenditures and source of funds	1960	1970	1980	1990	2000	2005	2008	2009	2010
Amount in Billions									
Home health care expenditures	0.1	0.2	2.4	12.6	32.4	48.7	61.5	66.1	70.2
Percent Distribution									
All sources of funds	100.0	100.0	100.0	100.0	100.0	100.0	100.0	100.0	100.0
Out-of-pocket payments	12.5	9.4	15.2	17.9	19.6	12.8	8.2	7.2	7.1
Health insurance	5.6	37.9	53.7	66.2	71.4	81.5	88.1	89.6	89.8
Private health insurance	2.5	3.0	14.7	22.9	23.8	12.6	7.3	6.7	6.4
Medicare	X	26.7	26.8	26.0	26.4	37.4	43.8	45.3	44.9
Medicaid	X	6.7	11.7	17.1	20.9	31.0	36.2	36.8	37.3
Federal	X	3.3	6.2	9.1	11.3	16.8	20.5	23.9	24.6
State and local	X	3.4	5.4	7.9	9.6	14.3	15.7	12.9	12.7
CHIP[2]	X	X	X	X	0.0	0.0	0.0	0.0	0.0
Federal	X	X	X	X	0.0	0.0	0.0	0.0	0.0
State and local	X	X	X	X	0.0	0.0	0.0	0.0	0.0
Other health insurance programs[3]	3.1	1.4	0.5	0.3	0.3	0.5	0.7	0.9	1.2
Other third-party payers and programs[4]	81.9	52.7	31.1	16.0	9.0	5.6	3.7	3.2	3.1
Amount in Billions									
Prescription drug expenditures	2.7	5.5	12.0	40.3	120.9	204.8	243.6	256.1	259.1
Percent Distribution									
All sources of funds	100.0	100.0	100.0	100.0	100.0	100.0	100.0	100.0	100.0
Out-of-pocket payments	96.0	82.4	71.3	56.8	28.1	25.2	21.0	19.9	18.8
Health insurance	1.5	16.5	26.9	40.3	70.0	72.9	77.6	78.8	79.9
Private health insurance	1.3	8.8	15.0	27.0	50.2	49.6	45.2	45.8	45.2
Medicare	X	X	X	0.5	1.7	1.9	20.8	21.3	23.0
Medicaid	X	7.6	11.7	12.6	16.3	17.7	7.8	7.8	7.8
Federal	X	4.1	6.8	7.2	9.3	10.1	4.6	5.2	5.3
State and local	X	3.5	4.9	5.4	7.0	7.6	3.2	2.6	2.5
CHIP[2]	X	X	X	X	0.3	0.5	0.5	0.6	0.6
Federal	X	X	X	X	0.2	0.4	0.4	0.4	0.4
State and local	X	X	X	X	0.1	0.2	0.2	0.2	0.2
Other health insurance programs[3]	0.1	0.1	0.2	0.2	1.5	3.1	3.2	3.3	3.3
Other third-party payers and programs[4]	2.5	1.1	1.8	3.0	1.9	1.9	1.5	1.4	1.3
Amount in Billions									
Dental services expenditures	2.0	4.7	13.4	31.7	62.3	87.0	102.4	102.5	104.8
Percent Distribution									
All sources of funds	100.0	100.0	100.0	100.0	100.0	100.0	100.0	100.0	100.0
Out-of-pocket payments	96.0	90.0	65.8	48.1	44.4	44.0	44.4	42.0	41.3
Health insurance	3.2	9.5	33.3	51.3	55.0	55.6	55.2	57.5	58.2
Private health insurance	1.9	4.5	28.4	48.1	50.2	49.3	47.9	48.7	48.7
Medicare	X	X	X	0.0	0.1	0.1	0.2	0.3	0.2
Medicaid	X	3.4	3.7	2.4	3.7	4.8	5.4	6.6	7.1
Federal	X	1.8	2.0	1.3	2.1	2.7	3.2	4.5	4.9
State and local	X	1.6	1.7	1.0	1.6	2.0	2.1	2.1	2.2
CHIP[2]	X	X	X	X	0.4	0.5	0.7	0.7	1.0
Federal	X	X	X	X	0.3	0.4	0.5	0.5	0.7
State and local	X	X	X	X	0.1	0.2	0.2	0.2	0.3
Other health insurance programs[3]	1.3	1.6	1.2	0.9	0.6	0.9	1.0	1.1	1.2
Other third-party payers and programs[4]	0.8	0.4	0.8	0.6	0.6	0.4	0.4	0.5	0.5
Amount in Billions									
All other personal health care expenditures[8]	3.2	7.1	25.8	77.9	158.3	218.0	254.3	266.8	279.4
Percent Distribution									
All sources of funds	100.0	100.0	100.0	100.0	100.0	100.0	100.0	100.0	100.0
Out-of-pocket payments	84.8	74.5	57.2	49.9	38.3	33.3	32.1	31.3	31.2
Health insurance	3.4	8.3	25.0	33.2	44.2	49.9	50.7	51.6	52.0
Private health insurance	2.0	3.4	6.7	12.0	12.6	13.0	13.0	12.7	12.7
Medicare	X	1.0	2.8	5.5	8.0	9.7	10.7	10.7	10.6
Medicaid	X	2.9	14.7	14.9	22.6	25.9	26.2	27.3	27.6
Federal	X	1.6	8.1	8.5	12.9	14.7	15.5	18.1	18.7
State and local	X	1.4	6.7	6.4	9.7	11.2	10.8	9.2	8.9
CHIP[2]	X	X	X	X	0.2	0.3	0.4	0.4	0.4
Federal	X	X	X	X	0.1	0.2	0.3	0.3	0.3
State and local	X	X	X	X	0.1	0.1	0.1	0.1	0.1
Other health insurance programs[3]	1.4	0.9	0.8	0.9	0.8	1.0	0.4	0.5	0.7
Other third-party payers and programs[4]	11.7	17.2	17.9	16.9	17.5	16.8	17.1	17.0	16.8

X = Not applicable.   0.0 = Quantity more than zero but less than 0.05.   [1]Includes all expenditures for specified health services and supplies other than expenses for government administration, net cost of health insurance, public health activities, research, and structures and equipment.   [2]Children's Health Insurance Program (CHIP). Medicaid CHIP expansions are included.   [3]Includes Department of Defense and Department of Veterans Affairs.   [4]Includes worksite health care, other private revenues, Indian Health Service, workers' compensation, general assistance, maternal and child health, vocational rehabilitation, other federal programs, Substance Abuse and Mental Health Services Administration, other state and local programs, and school health.   [5]Constructed from the Producer Price Indexes for hospitals, offices of physicians, medical and diagnostic laboratories, home health care services, and nursing care facilities; and Consumer Price Indices specific to each of the remaining personal health care components.   [6]Includes expenditures for hospital-based nursing home and home health agency care.   [7]Includes expenditures for care in freestanding nursing homes. Expenditures for care in hospital-based nursing homes are included with hospital care.   [8]Includes expenditures for other professional services, other nondurable medical products, durable medical equipment, and other health, residential, and personal care, not shown separately.

Table 3-75. Cost of Hospital Discharges with Common Hospital Operating Room Procedures in Nonfederal Community Hospitals, by Age and Selected Principal Procedure, Selected Years, 2000–2010

(Dollars.)

Age and principal operating room procedure[1]	Mean inflation-adjusted cost per hospitalization: 2010 dollars[2]			Number of discharges with operating room principal procedure			Total inflation-adjusted national costs: 2010 dollars (in millions of dollars)		
	2000	2005	2010	2000	2005	2010	2000	2005	2010
All Ages									
Hospital discharges with an operating room principal procedure[3]	12,994	15,551	17,922	9,022,288	10,285,810	10,049,810	116,513	160,101	179,935
Laminectomy (back surgery)	7,999	9,025	11,089	294,345	255,955	213,277	2,365	2,312	2,364
Heart valve procedures	42,003	51,340	52,442	82,826	96,715	102,543	3,473	4,985	5,383
Coronary artery bypass graft (CABG)	30,615	37,191	38,895	349,967	227,774	173,074	10,754	8,485	6,734
Percutaneous coronary angioplasty (PTCA) (balloon angioplasty of heart)	14,665	18,030	19,498	601,832	749,572	511,109	8,828	13,521	9,968
Insertion, revision, replacement, removal of cardiac pacemaker or cardioverter/defibrillator	27,106	34,553	35,311	68,723	165,619	128,664	1,878	5,715	4,539
Colorectal resection (removal of part of the bowel)	19,069	22,122	23,788	261,519	283,453	272,865	5,089	6,278	6,488
Appendectomy	7,175	8,298	9,242	277,029	308,634	284,039	1,965	2,561	2,625
Cholecystectomy (gall bladder removal)	10,185	11,808	12,822	400,818	388,252	394,304	4,047	4,585	5,060
Hysterectomy	6,400	7,097	8,941	596,889	567,964	368,471	3,792	4,038	3,298
Cesarean section	5,323	5,349	5,874	927,397	1,301,770	1,275,164	4,820	6,966	7,498
Treatment, fracture or dislocation of hip and femur	12,322	14,913	17,549	244,706	259,071	258,181	3,066	3,861	4,528
Arthroplasty knee (knee replacement)	13,517	15,240	16,348	328,118	549,867	721,443	4,409	8,384	11,799
Hip replacement	14,661	16,682	17,510	304,709	381,318	453,621	4,523	6,355	7,940
Spinal fusion	17,068	24,214	28,665	210,677	331,912	463,470	3,512	8,045	13,290
Under 18 Years									
Hospital discharges with an operating room principal procedure[3]	13,029	18,858	19,655	394,504	551,952	431,421	4,969	10,366	8,496
Incision and excision of CNS (a type of brain surgery)	28,254	34,200	41,131	6,581	11,786	9,308	179	404	383
Tonsillectomy and/or adenoidectomy	4,312	5,580	5,992	12,524	16,842	13,571	56	94	83
Small bowel resection (removal of part of the small bowel)	35,453	49,331	41,795	1,769	3,075	2,811	61	150	117
Appendectomy	5,909	5,615	6,252	24,419	29,549	23,501	130	167	147
Cesarean section	28,651	44,961	52,211	7,704	13,305	11,087	218	593	578
Spinal fusion	8,587	9,683	11,735	2,894,835	3,202,648	2,960,738	24,325	31,043	34,745
18 to 44 Years									
Hospital discharges with an operating room principal procedure[3]	24,939	29,799	36,389	20,221	18,779	23,874	485	563	875
Incision and excision of CNS (a type of brain surgery)	7,197	8,405	10,427	98,649	69,320	46,309	714	584	484
Laminectomy	6,609	7,552	8,476	137,667	140,028	120,890	897	1,058	1,025
Appendectomy	8,343	9,187	10,191	136,587	133,060	144,351	1,095	1,223	1,473
Cholecystectomy	6,218	7,216	8,919	39,388	34,430	33,422	248	249	298
Oophorectomy (removal of one or both ovaries)	4,605	4,442	5,157	77,428	77,073	47,276	337	343	244
Ligation of fallopian tubes ("tying" of fallopian tubes)	5,933	6,444	8,116	299,858	262,861	155,684	1,754	1,696	1,265
Hysterectomy	5,306	5,338	5,862	900,964	1,267,786	1,246,610	4,678	6,772	7,315
Cesarean section	9,143	11,556	14,101	70,112	61,369	62,138	629	708	875
Treatment, fracture or dislocation of lower extremity (other than hip or femur)	16,042	22,414	26,903	75,502	89,893	93,911	1,171	2,016	2,527
Spinal fusion	14,212	17,052	20,079	2,513,848	3,001,674	3,220,135	35,570	51,255	64,557
45 to 64 Years									
Hospital discharges with an operating room principal procedure[3]	8,068	8,909	11,447	111,022	98,847	83,913	897	881	959
Laminectomy	39,460	47,027	50,688	23,731	27,467	29,926	931	1,299	1,518
Heart valve procedures	28,601	34,059	37,437	144,812	97,449	77,190	4,162	3,327	2,891
Coronary artery bypass graft (CABG)	14,193	17,408	19,125	261,110	328,248	234,877	3,699	5,719	4,493
Percutaneous coronary angioplasty (PTCA)	33,171	37,492	37,210	16,558	45,357	38,159	545	1,699	1,419
Insertion, revision, replacement, removal of cardiac pacemaker or cardioverter/defibrillator	17,156	19,705	21,872	78,937	98,142	104,318	1,381	1,937	2,284
Colorectal resection	9,604	11,366	12,904	120,985	121,446	125,138	1,162	1,383	1,615
Cholecystectomy	7,449	8,484	9,994	21,888	23,172	38,646	163	196	386
Oophorectomy	6,529	7,237	9,060	238,417	249,676	170,718	1,554	1,810	1,548
Hysterectomy	13,828	15,294	16,382	98,691	205,869	303,860	1,357	3,149	4,979
Arthroplasty knee (knee replacement)	15,233	16,920	17,182	67,121	108,449	155,998	1,030	1,832	2,679
Hip replacement	16,382	22,501	27,364	90,101	154,618	227,953	1,437	3,482	6,240
Spinal fusion									
65 to 74 Years									
Hospital discharges with an operating room principal procedure[3]	15,924	18,985	21,245	1,559,874	1,653,945	1,720,707	24,970	31,451	36,493
Laminectomy	8,456	8,997	10,675	47,332	47,031	45,588	400	423	486
Heart valve procedures	42,981	52,231	52,757	24,127	25,535	27,262	1,028	1,338	1,440
Coronary artery bypass graft (CABG)	31,155	37,932	38,996	116,648	72,447	56,415	3,633	2,751	2,200
Percutaneous coronary angioplasty (PTCA)	14,602	17,861	19,577	172,403	202,718	130,974	2,513	3,623	2,564
Insertion, revision, replacement, removal of cardiac pacemaker or cardioverter/defibrillator	29,608	35,659	36,741	19,805	46,292	34,225	589	1,648	1,256
Endarterectomy (plaque removal from artery lining of brain, head, neck)	8,517	9,106	10,070	52,875	41,903	36,037	462	383	363
Colorectal resection	19,168	22,404	24,319	65,640	64,326	61,732	1,296	1,444	1,497
Cholecystectomy	11,260	13,479	14,878	67,897	57,382	54,433	777	774	809
Arthroplasty knee	13,769	15,195	16,208	114,150	182,838	241,232	1,556	2,781	3,913
Hip replacement	14,605	16,409	17,235	74,103	89,657	110,806	1,098	1,471	1,909
Spinal fusion	18,050	26,008	30,017	24,143	48,299	88,132	434	1,257	2,646
75 to 84 Years									
Hospital discharges with an operating room principal procedure[3]	16,165	19,633	21,373	1,263,420	1,405,406	1,240,660	20,720	27,626	26,466
Laminectomy	9,127	9,876	10,854	31,988	32,853	29,357	295	324	319
Heart valve procedures	44,332	55,018	54,089	21,844	25,893	27,829	980	1,431	1,506
Coronary artery bypass graft (CABG)	33,778	42,167	41,615	71,235	46,557	31,244	2,426	1,965	1,301
Percutaneous coronary angioplasty (PTCA)	15,458	19,091	20,196	115,128	149,285	91,574	1,792	2,850	1,850
Insertion, revision, replacement, removal of cardiac pacemaker or cardioverter/defibrillator	24,296	33,516	34,303	20,711	50,092	34,900	513	1,676	1,196
Endarterectomy (plaque removal from artery lining of brain, head, neck)	8,846	9,445	10,242	46,719	39,208	29,200	427	372	299
Colorectal resection	20,905	24,856	26,236	63,982	63,255	50,875	1,374	1,573	1,332
Cholecystectomy	12,890	15,883	16,880	54,014	51,443	44,590	711	816	753
Treatment, fracture or dislocation of hip and femur	11,601	13,897	16,204	75,452	75,221	68,395	901	1,047	1,109
Arthroplasty knee	13,762	15,290	16,285	81,404	125,729	138,682	1,122	1,923	2,260
Hip replacement	14,429	16,553	17,831	95,401	108,919	106,315	1,399	1,802	1,895
Spinal fusion	18,796	27,133	30,514	12,139	23,530	37,687	226	638	1,150

Table 3-75. Cost of Hospital Discharges with Common Hospital Operating Room Procedures in Nonfederal Community Hospitals, by Age and Selected Principal Procedure, Selected Years, 2000–2010—*Continued*

(Dollars.)

Age and principal operating room procedure[1]	Mean inflation-adjusted cost per hospitalization: 2010 dollars[2]			Number of discharges with operating room principal procedure			Total inflation-adjusted national costs: 2010 dollars (in millions of dollars)		
	2000	2005	2010	2000	2005	2010	2000	2005	2010
85 Years and Over									
Hospital discharges with an operating room principal procedure[3]	14,823	18,085	19,456	394,256	450,122	464,057	5,935	8,149	9,028
Heart valve procedures	46,636	59,001	49,030	3,114	4,088	5,887	145	241	289
Coronary artery bypass graft (CABG)	38,005	48,587	48,466	5,483	4,315	3,079	206	211	149
Percutaneous coronary angioplasty (PTCA)	17,554	21,291	20,852	17,268	29,810	24,543	300	634	512
Insertion, revision, replacement, removal of cardiac pacemaker or cardioverter/defibrillator	14,425	24,432	26,701	7,301	14,121	12,167	108	344	324
Colorectal resection	22,602	26,607	28,673	21,347	21,140	19,145	493	563	549
Cholecystectomy	15,705	17,645	18,382	16,163	17,286	17,157	256	304	315
Treatment, fracture or dislocation of hip and femur	11,295	13,347	15,432	79,202	80,284	79,568	921	1,073	1,230
Arthroplasty knee	13,956	16,059	17,237	10,414	16,274	19,466	146	261	335
Hip replacement	14,038	16,620	18,142	51,469	55,699	59,894	734	925	1,087
Amputation of lower extremity (amputation of leg, foot or toe)	12,961	16,793	17,366	13,260	10,403	8,768	175	175	153

[1]Data are based on valid operating room procedures. Operating room procedures were identified using the Centers for Medicare & Medicaid Services' Diagnosis Related Groups (DRGs). For DRGs, physician panels identified International Classification of Diseases (ICD-9-CM) procedure codes, which would be performed in operating rooms in most hospitals. Operating room procedures, as defined by DRGs, are classified by the Clinical Classifications Software (CCS) into 1 of 231 clinically meaningful categories. Mean costs per hospitalization are based on the principal procedure as determined by the CCS. The number of discharges is based on the first-listed (principal) major procedure.   [2]Charges (the amount billed by the hospital) were converted to costs using cost-charge ratios from the Centers for Medicare & Medicaid Services. Costs are for the entire hospitalization including the principal procedure. Costs were adjusted to 2010 dollars for inflation using the gross domestic product deflator.   [3]Includes discharges for operating room principal procedures not shown separately.

Table 3-76. Expenses[1] for Health Care by Selected Population Characteristics, Selected Years, 1987–2008

(Number, percent, dollars.)

Characteristic	Population in millions[2]				Percent of persons with expense				Mean annual expense per person with expense(dollars)[3]			
	1997	2000	2005	2008	1987	2000	2005	2008	1987	2000	2005	2008
All Ages	271.3	278.4	296.2	304.4	84.5	83.5	84.7	84.4	2,960	3,376	4,500	4,470
Under 65 Years												
Total	237.1	243.6	258.7	264.6	83.2	81.8	82.9	82.6	2,305	2,659	3,571	3,571
Under 6 years	23.8	24.1	23.8	24.7	88.9	86.7	88.9	88.8	1,958	1,405	1,711	2,049
6 to 17 years	48.1	48.4	49.7	49.6	80.2	80.0	83.0	82.5	1,291	1,397	1,807	1,699
18 to 44 years	108.9	109.0	111.1	111.0	81.5	77.7	77.1	76.5	2,026	2,382	3,175	2,974
45 to 64 years	56.3	62.1	74.1	79.4	87.0	88.5	89.7	89.1	3,923	4,454	5,769	5,843
Sex												
Male	118.0	120.9	129.2	132.2	78.8	76.6	77.5	77.5	2,174	2,546	3,225	3,299
Female	119.1	122.7	129.6	132.4	87.5	87.0	88.4	87.6	2,416	2,758	3,874	3,811
Hispanic Origin and Race [4]												
Hispanic or Latino	29.4	32.0	41.1	45.0	71.0	69.0	69.3	69.9	1,838	1,812	2,425	2,472
Not Hispanic or Latino												
White	166.2	169.2	166.5	167.3	86.9	86.6	88.1	87.6	2,312	2,782	3,873	3,936
Black or African American	31.3	32.1	32.8	33.5	72.2	71.3	76.4	75.7	2,788	2,824	3,637	3,268
Asian[5]	X	X	11.3	11.7	X	X	75.5	78.1	X	X	2,205	1,871
American Indian, Alaska Native, Native Hawaiian, Other Pacific Islander, and multiple race[5]	10.2	10.2	7.0	7.1	72.8	76.0	82.0	83.7	1,529	2,267	3,291	4,312
Insurance Status [6]												
Any private insurance	174.0	181.6	180.1	178.2	86.5	85.9	87.9	88.1	2,210	2,533	3,597	3,613
Public insurance only	29.8	29.7	42.2	45.8	82.4	83.6	84.2	85.0	3,707	4,037	4,342	4,391
Uninsured all year	33.3	32.3	36.4	40.7	61.8	57.3	56.8	55.7	1,440	1,875	2,046	1,870
65 Years and Over												
Total	34.2	34.8	37.5	39.7	93.7	95.5	96.7	96.6	7,312	7,677	10,003	9,585
Sex												
Male	14.6	15.0	16.0	17.2	92.0	93.4	95.9	95.7	7,482	8,232	9,788	9,433
Female	19.6	19.8	21.5	22.6	94.9	97.1	97.2	97.3	7,192	7,273	10,161	9,698
Hispanic Origin and Race [4]												
Hispanic or Latino	1.7	1.9	2.4	2.8	82.5	92.5	92.0	93.3	6,963	6,889	8,659	9,437
Not Hispanic or Latino												
White	28.8	28.9	30.0	31.5	94.9	95.9	97.3	97.5	7,198	7,793	10,118	9,603
Black or African American	2.8	2.9	3.1	3.5	88.5	94.0	94.9	93.8	8,813	7,383	11,985	10,414
Asian[5]	X	X	1.3	1.3	X	X	94.4	94.9	X	X	5,875	6,037
American Indian, Alaska Native, Native Hawaiian, Other Pacific Islander, and multiple race[5]	*	*	*	*	*	*	*	*	*	*	*	*
Insurance Status [7]												
Medicare only	8.8	12.0	10.9	15.8	85.9	94.8	96.2	95.8	5,760	6,592	9,673	8,886
Medicare and private insurance	21.7	19.2	20.7	18.6	95.4	96.0	97.8	98.2	7,234	7,872	9,610	9,425
Medicare and other public coverage	3.2	3.2	5.5	4.8	94.4	96.3	95.5	96.4	11,235	10,534	12,290	12,486

X = Not applicable.   * = Figure does not meet standards of reliability or precision. Data preceded by an asterisk have a relative standard error equal to or greater than 30 percent. Data not shown if based on fewer than 100 sample cases.   [1]Includes expenses for inpatient hospital and physician services, ambulatory physician and nonphysician services, prescribed medicines, home health services, dental services, and other medical equipment, supplies, and services that were purchased or rented during the year. Excludes expenses for over-the-counter medications, phone contacts with health providers, and premiums for health insurance.   [2]Includes persons in the civilian noninstitutionalized population for all or part of the year. Expenditures for persons in this population for only part of the year are restricted to those incurred during periods of eligibility (e.g., expenses incurred during periods of institutionalization and military service are not included in estimates).   [3]Estimates of expenses were converted to 2008 dollars using the Consumer Price Index (all items).   [4]Persons of Hispanic origin may be of any race.   [5]Starting with 2002 data, MEPS respondents were allowed to report as non-Hispanic Asian-only. Prior to 2002, Asian respondents were reported with the American Indian, Alaska Native, Native Hawaiian, Other Pacific Islander, and multiple race category.   [6]Any private insurance includes individuals with insurance that provided coverage for hospital and physician care at any time during the year, other than Medicare, Medicaid, or other public coverage for hospital or physician services. Public insurance only includes individuals who were not covered by private insurance at any time during the year but were covered by Medicare, Medicaid, other public coverage for hospital or physician services, and/or CHAMPUS/CHAMPVA (TRICARE) at any point during the year. Uninsured includes persons not covered by either private or public insurance throughout the entire year or period of eligibility for the survey. Individuals with Indian Health Service coverage only are considered uninsured.   [7]Populations do not add to total because uninsured persons and persons with unknown insurance status were excluded.

Table 3-77. Out-of-Pocket Health Care Expenses Among Persons with Medical Expenses, by Age, Selected Years, 1987–2008

(Percent.)

Age and year	Percent of persons with expenses	Amount paid out of pocket among persons with expenses[1]						
		Total	$0	$1 to 99	$100 to 499	$500 to 999	$1,000 to 1,999	$2,000+
All Ages								
1987	84.5	100.0	10.4	19.9	36.6	15.3	10.0	7.7
1997	84.1	100.0	8.5	26.1	35.1	14.3	9.4	6.6
1998	83.8	100.0	7.7	26.6	35.6	14.0	9.5	6.5
1999	84.3	100.0	7.4	27.1	34.2	14.5	9.5	7.3
2000	83.5	100.0	6.9	26.6	34.4	14.4	9.8	7.8
2001	85.4	100.0	7.1	24.6	33.8	14.6	11.0	8.8
2002	85.2	100.0	7.8	23.4	32.5	15.1	11.9	9.4
2003	85.6	100.0	7.6	21.9	32.1	15.8	12.1	10.4
2004	84.7	100.0	8.8	22.1	31.2	14.9	12.0	11.1
2005	84.7	100.0	8.7	21.2	31.5	15.8	11.9	10.8
2006	84.6	100.0	8.7	21.4	31.6	15.8	12.2	10.2
2007	84.9	100.0	9.8	22.6	31.6	15.3	11.5	9.2
2008	84.4	100.0	9.9	22.9	32.1	14.8	11.2	9.1
Under 6 Years								
1987	88.9	100.0	19.2	28.0	39.8	8.5	2.5	2.0
1997	88.0	100.0	20.0	44.5	28.7	4.0	2.2	0.7
1998	87.6	100.0	17.4	48.0	28.7	4.0	1.5	0.3
1999	87.9	100.0	17.7	50.7	26.0	4.2	0.7	0.7
2000	86.7	100.0	16.7	51.4	25.9	4.1	1.4	0.5
2001	88.8	100.0	18.5	49.0	27.9	3.0	1.3	0.3
2002	88.8	100.0	21.5	42.8	28.8	4.9	1.4	0.5
2003	91.3	100.0	20.6	42.4	29.6	5.4	1.4	0.6
2004	90.0	100.0	26.0	40.5	26.0	4.8	2.1	0.7
2005	88.9	100.0	27.2	36.6	27.5	6.1	1.9	0.7
2006	89.2	100.0	27.1	39.3	26.4	4.3	1.9	1.0
2007	88.7	100.0	30.2	36.5	24.7	5.1	2.0	1.4
2008	88.8	100.0	31.4	36.1	25.9	3.9	1.9	0.8
6 to 17 Years								
1987	80.2	100.0	15.5	27.4	37.4	9.0	5.7	5.0
1997	81.7	100.0	16.5	36.2	32.1	7.5	3.6	4.1
1998	80.6	100.0	16.3	36.3	32.7	7.9	3.9	3.0
1999	81.5	100.0	15.0	38.0	31.6	7.9	3.8	3.8
2000	80.0	100.0	14.7	37.2	33.0	6.5	4.1	4.5
2001	83.2	100.0	15.0	36.5	32.3	7.3	3.8	5.2
2002	83.6	100.0	16.6	35.8	31.8	7.9	3.7	4.3
2003	84.1	100.0	16.1	32.8	33.1	8.9	5.4	3.8
2004	83.9	100.0	18.7	33.8	30.2	8.3	4.7	4.4
2005	83.0	100.0	18.6	32.4	31.1	9.2	4.6	4.0
2006	83.6	100.0	19.2	32.8	29.9	8.7	4.1	5.3
2007	84.0	100.0	21.6	33.0	29.4	7.6	4.2	4.1
2008	82.5	100.0	22.4	33.0	28.3	7.4	4.0	4.9
18 to 44 Years								
1987	81.5	100.0	10.1	22.0	39.4	14.9	8.3	5.4
1997	78.3	100.0	7.3	28.4	39.4	14.0	6.9	3.9
1998	78.0	100.0	6.4	29.1	40.3	13.1	7.0	4.1
1999	78.9	100.0	6.4	29.6	39.2	13.3	7.1	4.4
2000	77.7	100.0	5.8	29.4	39.8	13.8	6.9	4.4
2001	79.3	100.0	6.0	26.4	39.7	15.1	8.4	4.5
2002	78.5	100.0	6.7	26.3	38.3	14.6	8.8	5.3
2003	79.0	100.0	6.4	24.5	38.8	15.4	9.2	5.7
2004	77.0	100.0	7.2	24.8	37.6	14.8	9.4	6.2
2005	77.1	100.0	7.0	24.8	37.9	15.0	9.0	6.2
2006	76.9	100.0	6.8	24.2	38.3	15.2	8.9	6.5
2007	77.3	100.0	7.7	26.7	37.1	14.2	8.8	5.5
2008	76.5	100.0	7.9	27.1	36.6	14.0	8.3	6.1
45 to 64 Years								
1987	87.0	100.0	5.7	12.5	35.7	20.9	14.7	10.5
1997	89.2	100.0	3.4	16.8	36.3	19.6	14.8	9.2
1998	89.2	100.0	2.9	17.2	36.3	19.7	14.5	9.5
1999	88.9	100.0	2.7	16.6	35.9	20.2	14.7	9.9
2000	88.5	100.0	2.6	15.7	35.2	20.4	15.1	11.0
2001	89.9	100.0	2.4	14.3	33.8	19.9	17.2	12.4
2002	90.0	100.0	2.3	14.0	31.2	21.1	18.3	13.1
2003	89.6	100.0	2.4	12.9	29.9	21.2	18.1	15.6
2004	88.9	100.0	2.7	13.1	30.8	20.8	17.3	15.2
2005	89.7	100.0	2.4	12.9	29.5	21.7	18.6	14.8
2006	89.2	100.0	2.7	12.9	30.4	21.1	17.9	15.0
2007	89.2	100.0	2.9	14.3	30.6	21.2	17.0	14.1
2008	89.1	100.0	2.8	15.2	33.2	20.0	16.4	12.3

Table 3-77. Out-of-Pocket Health Care Expenses Among Persons with Medical Expenses, by Age, Selected Years, 1987–2008 —Continued

(Percent.)

Age and year	Percent of persons with expenses	Amount paid out of pocket among persons with expenses[1]						
		Total	$0	$1 to 99	$100 to 499	$500 to 999	$1,000 to 1,999	$2,000+
65 to 74 Years								
1987	92.8	100.0	5.3	10.0	27.3	21.8	19.4	16.2
1997	94.6	100.0	3.2	10.7	31.6	23.6	17.0	14.0
1998	94.3	100.0	2.0	9.8	33.6	21.6	19.5	13.6
1999	95.3	100.0	1.4	10.0	27.4	23.8	19.4	17.9
2000	94.7	100.0	1.5	10.0	27.2	22.1	21.0	18.3
2001	95.6	100.0	1.5	9.9	27.0	21.5	20.6	19.5
2002	96.1	100.0	1.8	6.3	25.4	21.4	24.1	21.1
2003	95.3	100.0	1.7	6.5	21.0	23.8	23.3	23.8
2004	96.6	100.0	1.5	8.0	23.2	19.3	20.6	27.3
2005	95.9	100.0	1.7	6.5	24.8	20.8	21.5	24.6
2006	95.7	100.0	1.7	7.3	23.7	22.0	25.6	19.7
2007	95.8	100.0	2.7	8.8	28.9	23.0	20.8	15.9
2008	95.8	100.0	1.5	9.6	28.8	22.0	20.4	17.7
75 Years and Over								
1987	95.1	100.0	5.6	7.6	24.7	20.0	19.7	22.4
1997	95.8	100.0	2.4	9.8	27.5	19.5	21.2	19.7
1998	96.3	100.0	3.0	9.6	26.6	20.3	21.0	19.4
1999	95.3	100.0	2.7	8.9	26.3	22.4	19.7	20.0
2000	96.5	100.0	2.6	10.0	25.2	21.5	19.8	20.9
2001	97.0	100.0	1.7	7.0	22.1	19.5	23.0	26.7
2002	96.5	100.0	2.2	6.2	20.1	18.5	24.9	28.2
2003	97.5	100.0	1.9	6.2	19.0	19.5	23.5	29.9
2004	97.7	100.0	1.8	6.1	19.2	16.9	24.8	31.1
2005	97.4	100.0	1.6	6.3	21.2	19.7	19.7	31.4
2006	97.6	100.0	1.7	6.8	22.1	22.8	24.0	22.6
2007	97.3	100.0	1.9	8.7	25.9	19.8	21.8	21.9
2008	97.6	100.0	1.9	10.0	25.9	20.5	22.0	19.7

[1]Estimates of expenses were converted to 2008 dollars using the Consumer Price Index (all items).

Table 3-78. Expenditures for Health Services and Supplies and Percent Distribution, by Sponsor, Selected Years, 1987–2010

(Dollars, percent.)

Type of sponsor	1987	1990	1995	2000	2005	2008	2009	2010
NATIONAL HEALTH EXPENDITURES (AMOUNT IN BILLIONS)	519.1	724.3	1,027.5	1,377.2	2,029.1	2,403.9	2,495.8	2,593.6
Business, Households, and Other Private Revenues								
Private business	354.1	488.2	642.3	888.5	1,226.8	1,407.8	1,402.8	1,429.9
Employer contribution to private health insurance premiums[1]	122.3	178.3	243.6	346.3	487.7	531.4	529.8	534.5
Employer contribution to Medicare hospital insurance trust fund	84.4	129.5	176.2	254.9	370.4	404.9	412.0	414.1
Workers compensation and temporary disability insurance and worksite health care	24.6	29.4	43.1	62.3	72.6	82.8	77.7	79.7
Household	13.4	19.3	24.3	29.1	44.7	43.7	40.1	40.7
Employee contribution to private health insurance premiums and individual policy premiums[2]	189.9	253.0	319.0	434.3	596.7	703.1	705.5	725.5
Employee and self-employment contributions and voluntary premiums paid to Medicare hospital insurance trust fund[3]	44.0	68.5	100.3	133.6	207.6	252.5	256.2	263.1
Premiums paid by individuals to Medicare supplementary medical insurance trust fund	29.5	35.6	56.0	82.6	96.5	112.1	108.2	112.2
Out-of-pocket health spending	6.2	10.2	16.4	16.4	29.3	44.6	46.7	50.6
Other private revenues	110.2	138.7	146.4	201.8	263.4	294.0	294.4	299.7
	41.9	56.9	79.7	107.9	142.3	173.4	167.4	169.9
Governments								
Federal government	165.0	236.1	385.1	488.7	802.4	996.1	1,093.1	1,163.7
Employer contributions to private health insurance premiums	86.1	125.3	217.2	261.0	451.8	582.4	684.0	742.7
Employer contributions to Medicare hospital insurance trust fund	4.9	9.9	11.4	14.3	23.1	25.1	26.8	28.5
Adjusted Medicare[4]	1.7	2.0	2.3	2.7	3.3	3.8	3.9	4.0
Health program expenditures (excluding Medicare)	17.4	27.7	57.6	48.8	119.4	198.7	237.4	254.0
Medicaid[5]	62.1	85.7	145.9	195.3	305.9	354.8	415.8	456.2
Other programs[6]	28.2	43.3	87.9	119.3	182.3	209.2	254.8	278.1
State and local government	33.9	42.5	58.1	75.9	123.6	145.7	161.1	178.0
Employer contributions to private health insurance premiums	78.9	110.8	167.9	227.7	350.6	413.6	409.1	421.1
Employer contributions to Medicare hospital insurance trust fund	16.0	26.4	38.9	56.8	101.8	121.4	127.9	134.1
Health expenditures by program	3.1	4.1	5.6	7.5	9.4	11.0	11.3	11.4
Medicaid[5]	22.7	31.5	60.3	85.3	135.4	145.3	130.5	135.9
Other programs[6]	37.1	48.8	63.1	78.0	104.0	136.0	139.4	139.6
PERCENT DISTRIBUTION								
NATIONAL HEALTH EXPENDITURES	100.0	100.0	100.0	100.0	100.0	100.0	100.0	100.0
Business, Households, and Other Private Revenues								
Private business	68	67	63	65	60	59	56	55
Employer contribution to private health insurance premiums[1]	24	25	24	25	24	22	21	21
Employer contribution to Medicare hospital insurance trust fund	69	73	72	74	76	76	78	77
Workers compensation and temporary disability insurance and worksite health care	20	16	18	18	15	16	15	15
Household	11	11	10	8	9	8	8	8
Employee contribution to private health insurance premiums and individual policy premiums[2]	37	35	31	32	29	29	28	28
Employee and self-employment contributions and voluntary premiums paid to Medicare hospital insurance trust fund[3]	23	27	31	31	35	36	36	36
Premiums paid by individuals to Medicare supplementary medical insurance trust fund	16	14	18	19	16	16	15	15
Out-of-pocket health spending	3	4	5	4	5	6	7	7
Other private revenues	58	55	46	46	44	42	42	41
	8	8	8	8	7	7	7	7
Governments								
Federal government	32	33	37	35	40	41	44	45
Employer contributions to private health insurance premiums	17	17	21	19	22	24	27	29
Employer contributions to Medicare hospital insurance trust fund	6	8	5	5	5	4	4	4
Adjusted Medicare[4]	2	2	1	1	1	1	1	1
Health program expenditures (excluding Medicare)	20	22	27	19	26	34	35	34
Medicaid[5]	72	68	67	75	68	61	61	61
Other programs[6]	33	35	40	46	40	36	37	37
State and local government	39	34	27	29	27	25	24	24
Employer contributions to private health insurance premiums	15	15	16	17	17	17	16	16
Employer contributions to Medicare hospital insurance trust fund	20	24	23	25	29	29	31	32
Health expenditures by program	4	4	3	3	3	3	3	3
Medicaid[5]	76	72	73	72	68	68	66	65
Other programs[6]	29	28	36	37	39	35	32	32
	47	44	38	34	30	33	34	33

[1]Estimates for 2006 and beyond exclude Retiree Drug Subsidy (RDS) payments. [2]Estimates for 2009 and beyond exclude subsidized Consolidated Omnibus Budget Reconciliation Act (COBRA) payments. [3]Includes one-half of self-employment contribution to Medicare hospital insurance trust fund and taxation of Social Security benefits. [4]Excludes Medicaid buy-in premiums for Medicare. Estimates for 2006 and beyond and includes RDS payments to private and state and local plans. [5]Includes Medicaid buy-in premiums for Medicare. [6]Includes maternal and child health, vocational rehabilitation, Substance Abuse and Mental Health Services Administration, Indian Health Service, federal workers' miscellaneous general hospital and medical programs, public health activities, Department of Defense, Department of Veterans Affairs, and Children's Health Insurance Program (CHIP), investment (research, structures, and equipment) and COBRA subsidies.

Table 3-79. Department of Veterans Affairs Health Care Expenditures and Use, and Persons Treated, by Selected Characteristics, Selected Fiscal Years, 1970–2011

(Dollars; numbers in thousands; percent.)

Type of expenditure and use	1970	1980	1985	1990	1995	2000	2005[1]	2006[1]	2007[1]	2008[1]	2009[1]	2010[1]	2011[1]
All Expenditures (Amount in Millions)[2]	1,689	5,981	8,936	11,500	16,126	19,327	30,291	31,909	34,025	38,282	42,955	47,280	50,575
Percent Distribution													
All services	100.0	100.0	100.0	100.0	100.0	100.0	100.0	100.0	100.0	100.0	100.0	100.0	100.0
Inpatient hospital	71.3	64.3	60.3	57.5	49.0	37.3	24.3	24.0	24.0	23.5	22.7	21.4	20.6
Outpatient care	14.0	19.1	18.9	25.3	30.2	45.7	53.4	55.2	53.5	53.2	53.5	52.5	52.6
Nursing home care	5.5	7.1	5.4	9.5	10.0	8.2	8.4	8.2	8.3	8.1	7.8	7.4	7.2
All other[3]	9.1	9.6	12.4	7.7	10.8	8.8	13.9	12.6	14.2	15.2	16.0	18.8	19.6
Health Care Use													
Inpatient hospital discharges[4,5]	787	1,248	1,306	1,029	879	579	614	601	607	622	640	656	653
Outpatient visits[6]	7,312	17,971	19,601	22,602	27,527	38,370	57,169	59,132	62,234	66,484	73,969	79,457	83,146
Nursing home discharges[5,7]	47	57	73	75	79	91	61	59	63	64	65	67	63
Inpatients[8]	NA	NA	NA	598	527	417	488	467	477	492	512	532	540
Percent Distribution													
Total	NA	NA	NA	100.0	100.0	100.0	100.0	100.0	100.0	100.0	100.0	100.0	100.0
Veterans with service-connected disability	NA	NA	NA	38.9	39.3	34.4	37.6	38.8	39.9	41.1	42.6	43.5	44.9
Veterans without service-connected disability	NA	NA	NA	60.3	59.9	64.7	61.5	60.2	59.1	58.0	56.4	55.6	54.3
Low income	NA	NA	NA	54.8	56.2	41.7	39.9	37.9	36.9	35.4	34.8	34.6	33.4
Veterans receiving aid and attendance or housebound benefits or who are catastrophically disabled[9]	NA	NA	NA	NA	NA	16.0	12.1	11.6	11.3	11.1	10.5	10.1	9.8
Veterans receiving medical care subject to copayments[10]	NA	NA	NA	2.8	2.8	5.2	8.6	9.7	9.8	10.0	9.5	9.3	9.3
Other and unknown[11]	NA	NA	NA	2.7	0.9	1.8	1.0	1.0	1.0	1.6	1.6	1.6	1.7
Nonveterans	NA	NA	NA	0.8	0.8	0.9	0.9	0.9	0.9	0.9	1.0	0.9	0.9
Outpatients[8]	NA	NA	NA	2,564	2,790	3,657	5,077	5,180	5,221	5,291	5,439	5,631	5,789
Percent Distribution													
Total	NA	NA	NA	100.0	100.0	100.0	100.0	100.0	100.0	100.0	100.0	100.0	100.0
Veterans with service-connected disability	NA	NA	NA	38.3	37.5	30.7	31.6	32.4	33.8	34.7	37.1	38.6	39.8
Veterans without service-connected disability	NA	NA	NA	49.8	50.5	60.8	62.7	62.0	60.8	59.7	57.2	56.4	55.1
Low income	NA	NA	NA	41.1	42.2	37.6	31.8	30.3	28.9	27.2	25.9	25.7	24.9
Veterans receiving aid and attendance or housebound benefits or who are catastrophically disabled[9]	NA	NA	NA	NA	NA	3.8	3.5	3.4	3.5	3.5	3.4	3.4	3.3
Veterans receiving medical care subject to copayments[10]	NA	NA	NA	3.6	4.2	15.4	25.4	25.7	25.5	25.2	23.8	23.0	22.3
Other and unknown[11]	NA	NA	NA	5.1	4.1	4.0	2.0	2.6	3.0	3.8	4.0	4.3	4.6
Nonveterans	NA	NA	NA	11.8	12.0	8.5	5.7	5.6	5.4	5.7	5.7	5.1	5.1

NA = Not available. [1]Starting with FY2005, the cost report data are taken from a different report than earlier years. The major impact of this change was to assign more cost to outpatient care than inpatient hospital. Also in FY2005, the responsibility for residential rehabilitation programs including domiciliary care was reassigned from extended care to mental health care. [2]Health care expenditures exclude construction, medical administration, and miscellaneous operating expenses at Department of Veterans Affairs headquarters. [3]Includes miscellaneous benefits and services, contract hospitals, education and training, subsidies to state veterans hospitals, nursing homes and residential rehabilitation treatment programs (formerly domiciliaries), and the Civilian Health and Medical Program of the Department of Veterans Affairs. [4]Discharges from medicine, surgery, psychiatry, rehabilitation medicine, spinal cord, and neurology units. Starting with FY2005 data, includes domiciliary care. Does not include long-term stays. One-day dialysis patients were included in 1980. Interfacility transfers were included starting in 1990 data. [5]Until FY2004, includes Department of Veterans Affairs nursing home and residential rehabilitation treatment programs (formerly domiciliary) stays, and community nursing home care stays. [6]Hospital outpatient care. Includes the following services: physicians, laboratory tests, home-based primary care, or outpatient fee-basis care. [7]Includes state nursing home veteran patients. [8]Individuals receiving services. Individuals with multiple discharges or visits are only counted once in the inpatient or outpatient category. [9]Includes veterans who are receiving aid and attendance or housebound benefit and veterans who have been determined by the Department of Veterans Affairs to be catastrophically disabled. [10]Includes veterans who receive medical care subject to copayments according to income level, based on financial means testing. [11]Includes expenditures for services for veterans who were prisoners of war, exposed to Agent Orange, and other. Prior to FY1994, veterans who reported exposure to Agent Orange were classified as having a service-connected disability. Beginning in FY1994, those veterans reporting Agent Orange exposure but not treated for it were means tested and placed in the low income or other group depending on income.

HEALTH INSURANCE

Figure 3-16. Number in Millions of Persons with No Health Insurance, Selected Years, 1984–2011

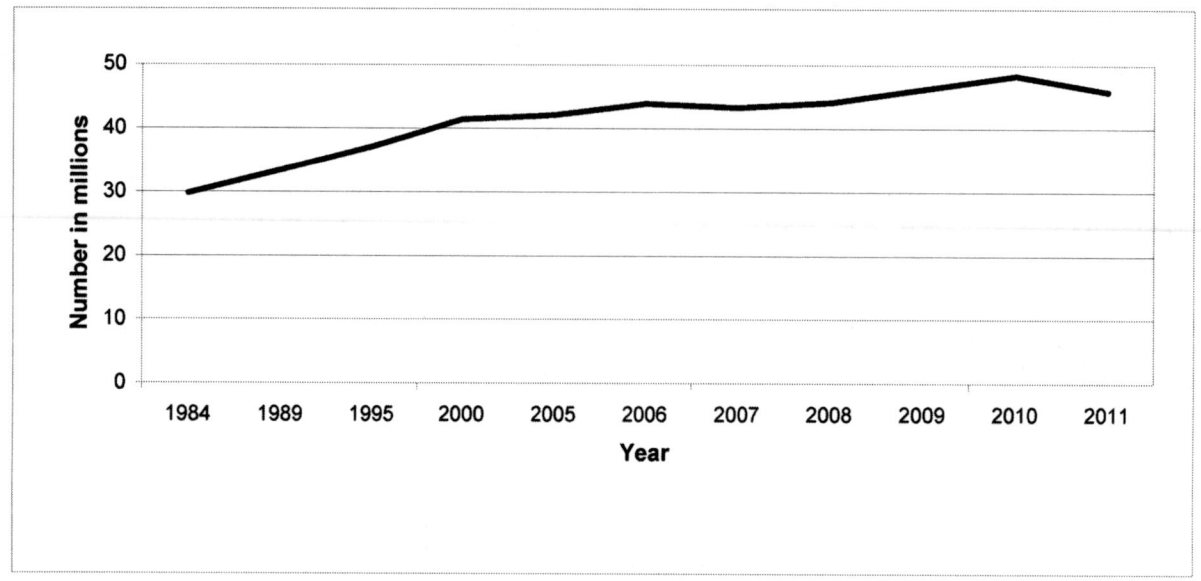

Figure 3-17. Medicaid Coverage Among Persons Age 65 Years and Over, Selected Years, 1984–2011

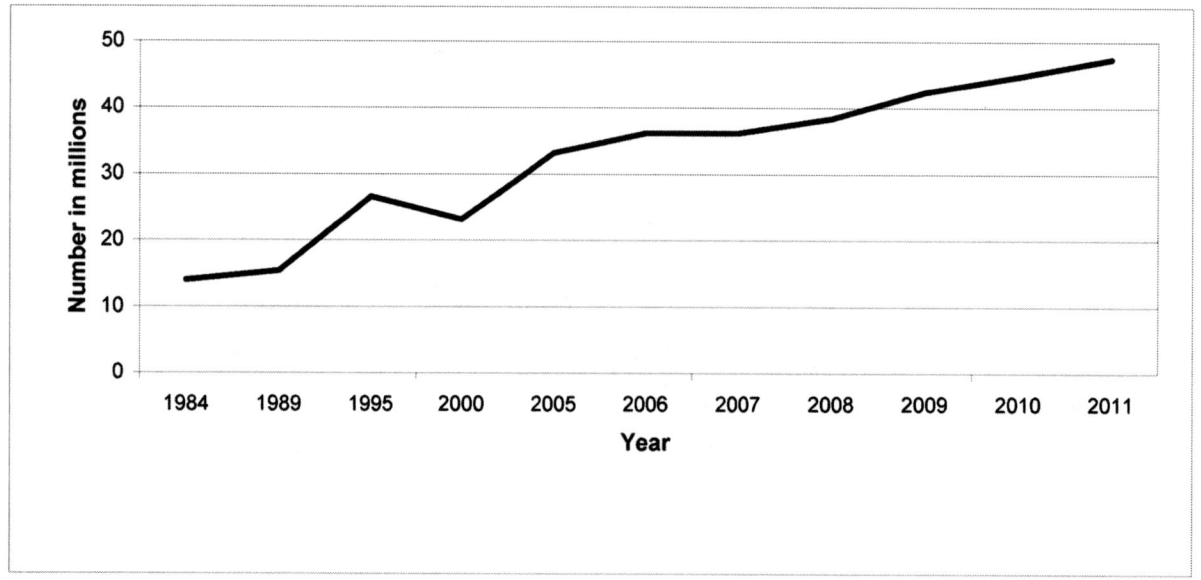

Table 3-80. Private Health Insurance[1] Coverage Among Persons Under 65 Years of Age, by Selected Characteristics, Selected Years, 1984–2011

(Numbers in millions; percent.)

Characteristic	1984[2]	1989[2]	1995[2]	2000[3]	2005	2006	2007	2008	2009	2010	2011
Total (number in millions)[4]	157.5	162.7	164.2	174.0	174.7	171.2	174.1	171.9	166.7	163.9	164.5
Total (percent of population)[4]	76.8	75.9	71.3	71.5	68.2	66.3	66.8	65.6	63.3	61.7	61.8
Age											
Under 19 years	72.6	71.9	65.4	66.7	62.3	59.5	59.9	58.6	56.1	54.3	53.9
Under 6 years	68.1	67.9	59.5	62.7	56.6	54.7	54.1	53.2	50.1	48.3	47.8
6 to 18 years	74.8	73.9	68.3	68.5	64.9	61.7	62.6	61.1	59.0	57.2	56.9
Under 18 years	72.6	71.8	65.2	66.6	62.1	59.4	59.8	58.4	55.8	54.1	53.7
6 to 17 years	74.9	74.0	68.3	68.5	64.7	61.7	62.6	61.1	58.8	57.2	56.7
18 to 64 years	78.6	77.6	73.9	73.5	70.7	69.1	69.5	68.5	66.2	64.7	65.0
18 to 44 years	76.5	75.5	70.9	70.5	66.6	65.0	65.5	64.4	61.7	60.0	60.9
18 to 24 years	67.4	64.5	60.8	60.3	58.0	57.0	59.0	56.2	54.4	52.3	57.2
19 to 25 years	67.4	63.8	60.1	59.1	56.3	56.1	57.9	55.8	53.0	51.8	56.9
25 to 34 years	77.4	75.9	70.1	70.1	65.1	63.0	63.5	62.7	60.0	58.7	58.6
35 to 44 years	83.9	82.7	77.7	77.0	73.7	72.0	71.7	71.7	68.4	66.9	66.0
45 to 64 years	83.3	82.5	80.1	78.7	76.9	75.2	75.5	74.3	72.6	71.3	70.6
45 to 54 years	83.3	83.4	80.9	80.0	77.4	75.1	75.4	74.8	72.6	70.9	70.1
55 to 64 years	83.3	81.6	79.0	76.7	76.2	75.4	75.5	73.6	72.6	71.8	71.2
Sex											
Male	77.3	76.1	71.6	71.6	68.0	65.9	66.4	65.3	62.9	61.1	61.4
Female	76.2	75.7	70.9	71.3	68.4	66.7	67.1	65.9	63.7	62.4	62.2
Sex and Marital Status [5]											
Male											
Married	85.0	84.2	80.2	81.5	79.6	78.1	78.1	77.7	75.8	75.1	74.5
Divorced, separated, widowed	65.5	64.6	62.4	62.2	56.7	55.4	55.8	56.0	52.9	50.6	50.5
Never married	71.3	68.3	65.4	63.8	60.2	57.8	59.8	57.9	54.9	52.5	55.1
Female											
Married	83.8	83.5	79.3	81.0	79.3	78.6	78.4	77.7	76.7	75.6	75.1
Divorced, separated, widowed	63.1	63.6	61.7	63.2	59.9	56.3	57.0	56.3	54.2	53.9	52.6
Never married	72.2	70.0	66.2	64.2	61.5	59.0	60.8	58.8	56.4	54.1	55.9
Race [6]											
White only	79.9	79.1	74.5	75.7	70.9	69.1	69.7	68.5	66.3	64.9	64.9
Black or African American only	58.1	57.7	53.0	55.9	52.9	51.3	51.8	50.0	47.4	44.8	45.9
American Indian or Alaska Native only	49.1	45.5	45.3	43.7	43.0	36.3	36.4	30.7	35.9	31.7	33.7
Asian only	69.9	71.9	68.4	72.1	72.2	72.1	73.2	74.3	71.3	68.1	65.9
Native Hawaiian or Other Pacific Islander only	NA	NA	NA	*	*	*	*	*	*	*	*
Two or more races	NA	NA	NA	61.4	57.6	54.0	52.7	58.0	47.8	52.4	52.3
Hispanic Origin and Race [6]											
Hispanic or Latino	55.7	51.5	46.4	47.8	42.4	40.0	41.7	39.9	37.3	36.8	36.4
Mexican	53.3	46.8	42.6	45.4	39.7	36.5	37.9	36.8	34.7	33.4	33.9
Puerto Rican	48.4	45.6	47.6	51.1	48.5	46.1	54.2	48.2	46.2	46.0	45.5
Cuban	72.5	70.3	63.6	63.9	58.1	63.4	64.8	57.9	54.3	53.8	51.1
Other Hispanic or Latino	61.6	61.0	51.4	50.7	45.6	44.3	44.3	43.5	39.7	40.9	38.1
Not Hispanic or Latino	78.7	78.5	74.4	75.2	73.0	71.3	71.7	70.8	68.6	67.0	67.3
White only	82.4	82.5	78.6	79.5	77.3	75.6	76.2	75.3	73.3	72.0	72.2
Black or African American only	58.2	57.7	53.4	56.0	53.1	52.2	52.3	50.6	48.0	45.1	46.5
Age and Percent of Poverty Level [7]											
Under 65 years											
Below 100 percent	32.2	27.0	22.6	25.2	21.4	21.4	21.4	19.2	15.3	16.0	17.2
100 percent to 199 percent	70.3	64.3	55.3	50.1	44.7	42.8	40.0	38.1	37.4	34.8	35.1
100 percent to 133 percent	59.4	52.8	41.7	39.3	36.0	33.6	29.5	27.3	26.1	24.4	24.1
134 percent to 199 percent	75.2	69.5	62.7	55.3	49.4	47.8	45.4	43.7	43.3	40.3	41.1
200 percent to 399 percent	89.3	89.2	86.4	78.1	74.8	74.9	73.2	72.3	70.6	70.7	71.1
400 percent or more	95.4	94.6	93.2	91.9	90.6	89.8	91.0	90.1	90.2	89.9	90.7
Under 19 years											
Below 100 percent	29.6	24.1	19.0	20.3	15.0	15.0	14.1	12.4	9.7	9.8	10.6
100 percent to 199 percent	73.6	68.5	55.8	49.5	41.6	38.5	35.7	34.1	34.0	31.5	31.2
100 percent to 133 percent	63.8	56.9	42.5	37.1	32.6	29.0	25.4	23.2	21.3	20.1	19.1
134 percent to 199 percent	78.4	74.0	64.4	56.1	47.0	44.6	41.7	40.1	41.3	38.1	38.0
200 percent to 399 percent	91.1	92.1	89.1	80.8	76.6	77.1	75.8	73.7	73.2	72.6	72.4
400 percent or more	96.2	96.2	93.3	93.0	92.5	91.4	93.2	92.0	91.8	91.2	92.7
Under 18 years											
Below 100 percent	28.5	22.3	16.9	19.5	14.2	14.0	12.7	11.3	9.3	9.2	9.7
100 percent to 199 percent	73.9	68.9	56.1	49.4	41.4	38.3	35.6	34.1	34.0	31.5	31.0
100 percent to 133 percent	63.9	57.3	42.3	36.8	32.0	29.0	25.4	23.2	21.1	19.9	19.0
134 percent to 199 percent	78.6	74.5	64.9	56.2	47.0	44.4	41.5	40.1	41.3	38.3	37.7
200 percent to 399 percent	91.3	92.3	89.2	81.1	76.6	77.3	76.0	73.8	73.0	72.6	72.5
400 percent or more	96.1	96.5	93.1	93.1	92.5	91.6	93.4	92.2	91.8	91.4	92.8
18 to 64 years											
Below 100 percent	35.0	30.8	27.0	29.1	25.9	26.1	26.8	24.0	19.2	20.4	21.8
100 percent to 199 percent	68.3	61.5	54.8	50.5	46.5	45.1	42.5	40.2	39.1	36.4	37.2
100 percent to 133 percent	56.6	50.0	41.4	40.9	38.3	36.4	32.1	29.6	28.8	26.9	26.7
134 percent to 199 percent	73.3	66.6	61.5	54.9	50.7	49.4	47.5	45.7	44.3	41.3	42.8
200 percent to 399 percent	88.3	87.6	85.0	76.7	74.0	73.9	72.0	71.7	69.6	70.0	70.5
400 percent or more	95.2	94.4	93.2	91.6	90.1	89.3	90.4	89.6	89.8	89.5	90.2

Table 3-80.   Private Health Insurance[1] Coverage Among Persons Under 65 Years of Age, by Selected Characteristics, Selected Years, 1984–2011—*Continued*

(Numbers in millions; percent.)

Characteristic	1984[2]	1989[2]	1995[2]	2000[3]	2005	2006	2007	2008	2009	2010	2011
Disability Measure among Adults 18 to 64 Years [8]											
Any basic actions difficulty or complex activity limitation	NA	NA	NA	63.1	58.1	56.4	56.4	53.2	51.6	53.0	49.3
Any basic actions difficulty	NA	NA	NA	63.9	58.8	57.1	56.9	54.3	52.3	53.8	49.6
Any complex activity limitation	NA	NA	NA	48.4	44.0	41.7	40.3	37.0	36.0	38.6	35.7
No disability	NA	NA	NA	77.2	73.7	72.5	72.9	73.3	70.4	69.3	70.5
Geographic Region											
Northeast	80.5	82.0	75.4	76.3	74.0	70.8	72.2	71.3	69.7	68.2	66.8
Midwest	80.6	81.5	77.3	78.8	74.6	71.7	72.0	69.9	67.5	66.7	67.9
South	74.3	71.4	66.9	66.8	62.5	61.8	62.6	62.1	59.3	57.5	57.8
West	71.9	71.2	67.5	66.5	65.6	64.6	64.0	62.8	60.6	58.9	58.4
Location of Residence											
Within MSA[9]	77.5	76.5	72.1	72.3	69.0	67.5	67.8	66.5	64.6	62.9	63.2
Outside MSA[9]	75.2	73.8	67.9	67.8	64.6	60.3	61.0	61.1	56.2	55.1	54.1

NA = Not available.   * = Figure does not meet standards of reliability or precision. Data not shown have a relative standard error of greater than 30 percent.   [1]Any private insurance at the time of interview that was originally obtained through a present or former employer or union, or, starting with 1997 data, through the workplace, self-employment, or a professional association; includes those who also had another type of coverage.   [2]Data prior to 1997 are not strictly comparable with data for later years due to the 1997 questionnaire redesign.   [3]Estimates for 2000–2002 were calculated using 2000-based sample weights and may differ from estimates in other reports that used 1990-based sample weights for 2000–2002 estimates.   [4]Includes all other races not shown separately, those with unknown marital status, unknown disability status, and, in 1984 and 1989, persons with unknown poverty level.   [5]Includes persons 14 to 64 years of age.   [6]The race groups White, Black, American Indian or Alaska Native, Asian, Native Hawaiian or Other Pacific Islander, and two or more races include persons of Hispanic and non-Hispanic origin. Persons of Hispanic origin may be of any race.   [7]Percent of poverty level is based on family income and family size and composition using U.S. Census Bureau poverty thresholds. Poverty level was unknown for 10 to 11 percent of persons under 65 years of age in 1984 and 1989. Missing family income data were imputed for 1995 and beyond.   [8]Any basic actions difficulty or complex activity limitation is defined as having one or more of the following limitations or difficulties: movement difficulty, emotional difficulty, sensory (seeing or hearing) difficulty, cognitive difficulty, self-care (activities of daily living or instrumental activities of daily living) limitation, social limitation, or work limitation.   [9]MSA = metropolitan statistical area.

Table 3-81. Private Health Insurance[1] Coverage Obtained Through the Workplace Among Persons Under 65 Years of Age, by Selected Characteristics, Selected Years, 1984–2011

(Numbers in millions; percent.)

Characteristic	1984[2]	1989[2]	1995[2]	2000[3]	2005	2006	2007	2008	2009	2010	2011
Total Population (in Millions)[4]	141.8	146.3	150.7	160.8	160.1	155.8	157.9	155.6	150.2	147.6	146.4
Percent of Population, Total[4]	69.1	68.3	65.4	67.1	63.6	61.5	61.6	60.5	58.0	56.6	56.4
Age											
Under 19 years	66.4	65.6	60.5	63.1	58.7	55.6	55.8	54.5	52.0	50.9	49.9
Under 6 years	62.1	62.3	55.1	58.9	53.4	50.8	50.8	49.6	46.3	44.9	44.3
6 to 18 years	68.4	67.3	63.1	64.9	61.1	57.8	58.1	56.9	54.8	53.8	52.5
Under 18 years	66.5	65.8	60.4	63.0	58.6	55.5	55.8	54.4	51.8	50.7	49.7
6 to 17 years	68.7	67.7	63.3	65.0	61.1	57.8	58.3	56.9	54.7	53.8	52.4
18 to 64 years	70.3	69.4	67.6	68.8	65.7	63.9	63.9	62.9	60.4	58.9	59.1
18 to 44 years	69.6	68.4	65.3	66.5	62.2	60.6	60.3	59.4	56.6	54.6	55.6
18 to 24 years	58.7	55.3	53.5	55.5	52.1	51.7	52.3	49.5	47.4	45.3	51.0
19 to 25 years	59.0	55.0	53.0	54.2	50.6	50.7	51.4	48.9	45.9	44.1	50.5
25 to 34 years	71.2	69.5	65.0	66.4	61.1	59.3	59.0	58.4	55.5	53.3	53.0
35 to 44 years	77.4	76.2	72.7	73.2	69.9	67.5	67.0	67.0	64.3	62.8	61.6
45 to 64 years	71.8	71.6	72.2	72.9	70.9	68.9	69.2	68.0	65.7	64.8	63.9
45 to 54 years	74.6	74.4	74.7	75.6	72.6	70.2	70.4	69.5	67.1	65.9	64.7
55 to 64 years	69.0	68.3	68.4	68.6	68.6	67.2	67.7	66.2	64.0	63.4	63.0
Sex											
Male	69.8	68.7	65.9	67.3	63.6	61.2	61.3	60.3	57.6	56.1	56.1
Female	68.4	67.9	64.9	66.9	63.6	61.8	61.9	60.8	58.4	57.1	56.7
Sex and Marital Status[5]											
Male											
Married	77.9	76.9	74.9	77.5	75.3	73.3	73.3	72.7	70.6	70.1	69.3
Divorced, separated, widowed	58.0	57.3	56.4	57.4	51.9	51.0	50.8	51.0	48.0	45.3	45.0
Never married	61.5	58.8	58.2	58.8	54.9	52.6	53.5	51.9	48.8	46.2	48.4
Female											
Married	76.1	75.5	73.2	76.3	74.2	73.1	72.7	72.2	70.7	69.8	69.2
Divorced, separated, widowed	51.9	54.9	54.6	57.8	54.3	51.5	51.3	51.4	48.6	48.1	46.5
Never married	63.5	60.9	59.2	60.1	56.3	54.2	55.1	53.0	50.6	48.2	50.0
Race[6]											
White only	72.0	71.2	68.4	71.0	66.1	64.0	64.2	63.0	60.6	59.3	59.0
Black or African American only	52.4	52.8	49.3	53.4	50.6	48.5	49.1	47.7	45.3	42.3	43.5
American Indian or Alaska Native only	45.8	40.9	40.2	41.7	39.9	33.7	35.1	29.4	33.6	*29.4	32.4
Asian only	59.0	61.1	59.6	65.8	64.4	64.5	64.6	66.2	62.5	60.6	58.7
Native Hawaiian or Other Pacific Islander only	NA	NA	NA	*	*	*	*	*	*	*	*
Two or more races	NA	NA	NA	59.8	54.8	50.6	49.7	54.3	45.0	49.5	48.3
Hispanic Origin and Race[6]											
Hispanic or Latino	52.0	47.3	43.4	45.3	40.0	37.7	38.8	37.6	34.9	34.6	34.1
Mexican	50.5	44.2	40.9	43.6	37.6	34.9	35.7	35.2	32.6	31.6	32.0
Puerto Rican	45.9	42.3	44.5	49.4	46.2	43.5	51.2	45.9	42.9	43.6	42.8
Cuban	57.4	56.5	54.0	53.6	53.5	56.9	54.7	49.2	46.4	47.4	45.0
Other Hispanic or Latino	57.4	54.7	46.7	47.3	42.6	40.9	40.8	39.8	36.9	37.8	35.1
Not Hispanic or Latino	70.7	70.5	68.2	70.6	68.0	66.0	66.1	65.2	62.8	61.3	61.3
White only	74.0	74.1	72.1	74.5	71.9	69.9	70.2	69.0	66.8	65.7	65.5
Black or African American only	52.5	52.8	49.8	53.6	50.9	49.5	49.5	48.2	45.9	42.6	44.1
Age and Percent of Poverty Level[7]											
Under 65 years											
Below 100 percent	24.1	19.8	17.5	21.0	17.8	17.6	17.4	15.5	11.9	12.4	13.6
100 percent to 199 percent	61.7	56.1	49.3	45.4	40.1	38.3	35.5	33.8	33.3	30.2	30.4
100 percent to 133 percent	50.0	44.3	36.0	35.0	31.3	30.0	25.3	23.8	22.6	20.6	19.7
134 percent to 199 percent	66.9	61.5	56.6	50.5	44.8	42.9	40.7	39.1	39.0	35.3	36.2
200 percent to 399 percent	82.8	82.2	80.5	73.4	69.8	69.7	67.7	66.8	64.7	65.3	65.0
400 percent or more	88.8	87.8	86.7	87.9	86.1	84.7	85.5	84.6	84.1	84.2	85.0
Under 19 years											
Below 100 percent	23.6	18.6	15.1	17.1	13.3	12.7	12.1	11.3	7.9	8.2	9.1
100 percent to 199 percent	67.0	62.1	50.5	45.8	38.3	35.5	32.7	31.4	31.9	28.8	27.9
100 percent to 133 percent	56.1	49.9	37.4	33.6	29.1	27.0	22.4	21.0	19.8	17.9	16.3
134 percent to 199 percent	72.3	67.9	58.8	52.2	43.7	41.0	38.6	37.1	38.9	35.1	34.4
200 percent to 399 percent	85.7	86.0	83.9	76.9	72.4	72.5	71.2	68.3	67.7	68.7	67.0
400 percent or more	90.8	90.3	87.5	89.5	88.3	86.3	87.5	86.9	86.0	86.5	87.5
Under 18 years											
Below 100 percent	23.0	17.5	13.6	16.6	12.5	11.8	11.2	10.3	7.5	7.8	8.4
100 percent to 199 percent	67.5	62.5	50.9	45.8	38.2	35.4	32.7	31.4	32.0	28.8	27.7
100 percent to 133 percent	56.3	50.3	37.2	33.5	28.6	27.1	22.5	21.0	19.8	17.8	16.1
134 percent to 199 percent	72.8	68.4	59.6	52.4	43.9	40.8	38.5	37.1	38.9	35.2	34.1
200 percent to 399 percent	85.9	86.4	84.1	77.1	72.4	72.7	71.5	68.4	67.6	68.7	67.0
400 percent or more	90.7	90.5	87.1	89.7	88.5	86.4	87.7	87.1	86.0	86.6	87.7
18 to 64 years											
Below 100 percent	24.8	21.8	20.5	24.0	21.2	21.3	21.2	18.7	14.8	15.4	16.8
100 percent to 199 percent	58.3	52.3	48.4	45.2	41.1	39.9	37.0	35.1	34.0	30.9	31.8
100 percent to 133 percent	46.0	40.4	35.3	35.9	32.9	31.8	27.0	25.5	24.2	22.1	21.5
134 percent to 199 percent	63.6	57.5	55.0	49.5	45.3	43.9	41.8	40.1	39.0	35.3	37.2
200 percent to 399 percent	81.4	80.2	78.8	71.7	68.7	68.4	66.2	66.1	63.6	63.9	64.3
400 percent or more	88.5	87.5	86.7	87.5	85.4	84.3	84.9	83.9	83.6	83.6	84.2

Table 3-81.   Private Health Insurance[1] Coverage Obtained Through the Workplace Among Persons Under 65 Years of Age, by Selected Characteristics, Selected Years, 1984–2011—*Continued*

(Numbers in millions; percent.)

Characteristic	1984[2]	1989[2]	1995[2]	2000[3]	2005	2006	2007	2008	2009	2010	2011
Disability Measure among Adults 18 to 64 Years [8]											
Any basic actions difficulty or complex activity limitation	NA	NA	NA	58.5	53.3	52.0	51.5	49.1	46.7	48.0	44.4
Any basic actions difficulty	NA	NA	NA	59.1	54.0	52.6	52.1	49.9	47.4	48.9	44.9
Any complex activity limitation	NA	NA	NA	43.5	38.9	37.2	35.4	33.5	31.1	32.8	30.3
No disability	NA	NA	NA	72.5	68.5	67.3	67.1	67.5	64.8	63.5	64.6
Geographic Region											
Northeast	74.0	75.0	69.8	72.5	70.6	67.5	68.2	68.0	65.3	64.4	63.0
Midwest	72.0	73.3	71.2	74.9	70.1	67.0	68.0	64.7	62.0	61.8	62.2
South	66.2	63.6	61.8	62.5	58.0	57.2	57.2	56.7	54.1	52.2	52.3
West	64.7	63.9	60.4	61.1	59.7	58.1	57.3	56.8	54.5	52.7	52.2
Location of Residence											
Within MSA[9]	70.9	69.6	66.6	68.2	64.5	62.7	62.7	61.5	59.3	57.9	57.8
Outside MSA[9]	65.3	63.5	60.7	62.6	59.6	55.4	55.7	55.1	50.8	49.4	48.7

NA = Not available.   * = Figure does not meet standards of reliability or precision. Data not shown have a relative standard error of greater than 30 percent.   [1]Any private insurance at the time of interview that was originally obtained through a present or former employer or union, or, starting with 1997 data, through the workplace, self-employment, or a professional association; includes those who also had another type of coverage.   [2]Data prior to 1997 are not strictly comparable with data for later years due to the 1997 questionnaire redesign.   [3]Estimates for 2000–2002 were calculated using 2000-based sample weights and may differ from estimates in other reports that used 1990-based sample weights for 2000–2002 estimates.   [4]Includes all other races not shown separately, those with unknown marital status, unknown disability status, and, in 1984 and 1989, persons with unknown poverty level.   [5]Includes persons 14 to 64 years of age.   [6]The race groups White, Black, American Indian or Alaska Native, Asian, Native Hawaiian or Other Pacific Islander, and two or more races include persons of Hispanic and non-Hispanic origin. Persons of Hispanic origin may be of any race.   [7]Percent of poverty level is based on family income and family size and composition using U.S. Census Bureau poverty thresholds. Poverty level was unknown for 10 to 11 percent of persons under 65 years of age in 1984 and 1989. Missing family income data were imputed for 1995 and beyond.   [8]Any basic actions difficulty or complex activity limitation is defined as having one or more of the following limitations or difficulties: movement difficulty, emotional difficulty, sensory (seeing or hearing) difficulty, cognitive difficulty, self-care (activities of daily living or instrumental activities of daily living) limitation, social limitation, or work limitation.   [9]MSA = metropolitan statistical area.

Table 3-82. No Health Insurance Coverage Among Persons Under 65 Years of Age, by Selected Characteristics, Selected Years, 1984–2011

(Numbers in millions; percent.)

Characteristic	1984[1]	1989[1]	1995[1]	2000[2]	2005[3]	2006[3]	2007[3]	2008[3]	2009[3]	2010[3]	2011[3]
Total (number in millions)[4]	29.8	33.4	37.1	41.4	42.1	43.9	43.3	44.1	46.2	48.3	45.8
Total (percent of population)[4]	14.5	15.6	16.1	17.0	16.4	17.0	16.6	16.8	17.5	18.2	17.2
Age											
Under 19 years	14.1	15.0	13.7	12.9	9.7	9.8	9.4	9.5	8.5	8.3	7.4
Under 6 years	14.9	15.1	11.8	11.8	7.7	7.5	7.3	7.6	6.6	6.3	5.0
6 to 18 years	13.8	15.0	14.6	13.4	10.6	10.9	10.4	10.5	9.4	9.2	8.5
Under 18 years	13.9	14.7	13.4	12.6	9.3	9.5	9.0	9.0	8.2	7.8	7.0
6 to 17 years	13.4	14.5	14.3	13.0	10.1	10.5	9.9	9.8	9.0	8.6	8.0
18 to 64 years	14.8	16.0	17.3	18.9	19.3	20.0	19.6	19.9	21.2	22.3	21.2
18 to 44 years	17.1	18.4	20.4	22.4	23.5	24.6	23.9	24.4	25.9	27.1	25.4
18 to 24 years	25.0	27.1	28.0	30.4	29.1	29.9	27.9	29.0	29.6	31.4	25.9
19 to 25 years	25.1	27.9	28.8	32.3	31.7	32.4	30.5	31.1	32.8	33.8	27.9
25 to 34 years	16.2	18.3	21.1	23.3	25.6	27.2	26.1	26.6	27.8	28.3	28.1
35 to 44 years	11.2	12.3	15.1	16.9	17.9	18.8	19.1	19.1	21.4	22.6	22.2
45 to 64 years	9.6	10.5	10.9	12.6	12.9	13.2	13.5	13.6	14.6	15.7	15.4
45 to 54 years	10.5	11.0	11.6	12.8	14.2	15.0	14.9	14.9	16.5	17.9	17.4
55 to 64 years	8.7	10.0	9.9	12.4	11.1	10.8	11.6	11.8	12.2	12.8	13.0
Sex											
Male	15.3	16.8	17.4	18.1	17.9	18.8	18.2	18.3	19.4	20.3	18.8
Female	13.8	14.4	14.8	15.9	15.0	15.3	15.1	15.4	15.7	16.1	15.6
Sex and Marital Status [5]											
Male											
Married	11.1	12.5	15.0	14.1	14.4	15.3	15.3	15.4	16.3	17.2	16.5
Divorced, separated, widowed	24.9	25.0	24.0	25.8	28.6	29.1	28.1	27.0	29.8	31.4	30.0
Never married	22.4	25.0	25.6	27.2	27.6	28.6	27.0	27.6	29.4	31.1	28.0
Female											
Married	11.2	11.8	13.6	13.3	13.0	13.5	13.5	13.5	14.2	14.7	14.4
Divorced, separated, widowed	19.2	19.1	18.1	21.3	22.1	23.0	22.6	22.1	22.8	23.6	24.0
Never married	16.3	18.0	17.5	21.1	20.0	20.4	19.5	20.7	21.0	21.9	20.5
Race [6]											
White only	13.6	14.5	15.5	15.4	15.9	16.7	16.3	16.7	17.1	17.6	16.7
Black or African American only	19.9	21.6	18.0	19.5	18.4	18.1	17.0	18.0	18.9	20.6	19.0
American Indian or Alaska Native only	22.5	28.4	34.3	38.4	32.2	38.0	38.8	28.4	32.5	44.0	34.2
Asian only	18.5	16.9	18.6	17.6	17.1	15.0	15.4	13.9	16.2	17.1	16.5
Native Hawaiian or Other Pacific Islander only	NA	NA	NA	*	*	*	*	*	*	*	*
Two or more races	NA	NA	NA	16.8	16.5	18.4	15.0	15.8	18.2	15.8	16.0
Hispanic Origin and Race [6]											
Hispanic or Latino	29.5	33.7	31.4	35.6	33.0	35.0	31.8	33.3	32.9	32.0	31.1
Mexican	33.8	39.9	35.6	39.9	36.0	38.6	34.7	36.1	35.0	34.8	33.0
Puerto Rican	18.3	24.7	17.6	16.4	16.3	16.8	12.8	16.8	17.8	13.7	15.8
Cuban	21.6	20.6	22.3	25.4	23.2	22.8	20.7	28.1	27.8	26.5	28.1
Other Hispanic or Latino	27.4	25.8	30.2	33.4	32.6	33.2	32.7	32.5	33.4	32.4	31.8
Not Hispanic or Latino	13.2	13.7	14.2	14.0	13.4	13.6	13.7	13.5	14.4	15.2	14.2
White only	11.9	12.1	13.0	12.5	12.0	12.5	12.6	12.5	13.2	13.7	12.9
Black or African American only	19.7	21.5	17.9	19.5	18.3	17.5	16.8	17.9	18.8	20.7	18.8
Age and Percent of Poverty Level [7]											
Under 65 years											
Below 100 percent	33.9	35.2	29.6	34.2	30.6	30.2	28.4	29.0	30.4	30.3	28.4
100 percent to 199 percent	21.8	25.6	28.3	31.0	28.6	29.6	30.0	30.6	29.8	32.4	30.0
100 percent to 133 percent	28.8	32.3	34.1	35.7	30.1	31.3	32.0	32.8	30.1	34.9	32.0
134 percent to 199 percent	18.7	22.6	25.1	28.7	27.8	28.7	29.0	29.5	29.6	31.0	28.9
200 percent to 399 percent	7.6	8.3	10.0	15.4	15.7	15.5	16.9	16.6	17.8	17.4	16.5
400 percent or more	3.2	4.2	5.4	5.9	6.3	6.5	5.6	6.2	5.8	5.6	5.2
Under 19 years											
Below 100 percent	29.0	31.7	20.4	22.6	15.2	14.2	12.7	14.0	12.2	11.3	9.4
100 percent to 199 percent	18.0	20.7	22.6	22.1	15.6	16.4	16.4	16.3	13.0	13.5	12.1
100 percent to 133 percent	24.4	27.6	26.4	26.5	15.6	15.6	17.9	17.4	12.9	15.9	12.5
134 percent to 199 percent	14.9	17.4	20.1	19.7	15.6	15.5	15.9	15.8	13.1	12.0	11.9
200 percent to 399 percent	5.1	4.9	6.7	9.6	8.2	7.8	8.5	8.0	8.0	7.4	6.8
400 percent or more	1.8	2.1	4.4	3.5	3.3	3.4	2.3	2.8	2.4	2.3	2.1
Under 18 years											
Below 100 percent	28.9	31.6	20.0	22.0	14.3	13.9	11.9	13.3	11.8	10.6	8.8
100 percent to 199 percent	17.5	20.2	22.0	21.7	15.0	16.0	15.7	15.5	12.3	12.7	11.4
100 percent to 133 percent	24.0	27.1	26.1	26.4	15.1	17.5	16.5	16.4	11.8	15.1	11.5
134 percent to 199 percent	14.4	16.9	19.5	19.1	15.0	15.1	15.3	15.0	12.6	11.3	11.3
200 percent to 399 percent	4.9	4.7	6.6	9.3	7.8	7.4	8.2	7.5	7.8	7.0	6.4
400 percent or more	1.8	1.9	4.6	3.3	3.2	3.1	2.2	2.7	2.3	2.1	2.0
18 to 64 years											
Below 100 percent	37.6	38.2	37.0	42.4	40.9	40.7	38.6	38.6	42.5	42.7	40.4
100 percent to 199 percent	24.4	28.8	32.0	36.4	35.9	36.7	37.9	38.9	38.9	42.1	39.3
100 percent to 133 percent	31.9	35.6	39.7	41.7	38.9	39.8	41.7	42.1	40.4	45.7	42.5
134 percent to 199 percent	21.1	25.9	28.2	34.0	34.4	35.1	36.1	37.3	38.1	40.3	37.6
200 percent to 399 percent	8.9	10.0	11.7	18.2	19.0	18.8	20.5	20.2	21.7	21.3	20.4
400 percent or more	3.4	4.4	5.5	6.6	7.1	7.4	6.5	7.1	6.7	6.5	6.1

Table 3-82. No Health Insurance Coverage Among Persons Under 65 Years of Age, by Selected Characteristics, Selected Years, 1984–2011—Continued

(Numbers in millions; percent.)

Characteristic	1984[1]	1989[1]	1995[1]	2000[2]	2005[3]	2006[3]	2007[3]	2008[3]	2009[3]	2010[3]	2011[3]
Disability Measure among Adults 18 to 64 Years [8]											
Any basic actions difficulty or complex activity limitation	NA	NA	NA	17.6	19.6	20.0	19.6	19.5	21.4	20.8	22.0
Any basic actions difficulty	NA	NA	NA	17.6	19.8	20.0	19.6	19.4	21.2	20.9	22.3
Any complex activity limitation	NA	NA	NA	16.1	16.9	17.3	18.3	15.8	19.2	17.2	18.2
No disability	NA	NA	NA	18.5	19.5	20.5	19.9	19.8	21.2	21.6	20.2
Geographic Region											
Northeast	10.2	10.9	13.3	12.2	11.3	11.2	11.0	11.4	11.4	12.4	11.8
Midwest	11.3	10.7	12.2	12.3	11.9	13.4	13.0	13.9	14.6	14.1	13.4
South	17.7	19.7	19.4	20.5	21.0	21.1	20.1	20.1	21.2	21.9	20.4
West	18.2	18.8	17.9	20.7	18.4	18.8	18.9	18.8	19.4	20.6	20.0
Location of Residence											
Within MSA[9]	13.6	15.2	15.5	16.6	16.1	16.6	16.1	16.4	17.1	17.8	16.7
Outside MSA[9]	16.6	17.0	18.6	18.6	17.8	19.3	19.4	19.1	20.2	20.4	19.8

NA = Not available.   * = Figure does not meet standards of reliability or precision. Data not shown have a relative standard error of greater than 30 percent.   [1]Any private insurance at the time of interview that was originally obtained through a present or former employer or union, or, starting with 1997 data, through the workplace, self-employment, or a professional association; includes those who also had another type of coverage.   [2]Data prior to 1997 are not strictly comparable with data for later years due to the 1997 questionnaire redesign.   [3]Beginning in quarter 3 of the 2004 NHIS, persons under 65 years of age with no reported coverage were asked explicitly about Medicaid coverage. Estimates were calculated without and with the additional information from this question in the columns labeled 2004(1) and 2004(2), respectively, and estimates were calculated with the additional information starting with 2005 data.   [4]Includes all other races not shown separately, those with unknown marital status, unknown disability status, and, in 1984 and 1989, persons with unknown poverty level.   [5]Includes persons 14 to 64 years of age.   [6]The race groups White, Black, American Indian or Alaska Native, Asian, Native Hawaiian or Other Pacific Islander, and two or more races include persons of Hispanic and non-Hispanic origin. Persons of Hispanic origin may be of any race.   [7]Percent of poverty level is based on family income and family size and composition using U.S. Census Bureau poverty thresholds. Poverty level was unknown for 10 to 11 percent of persons under 65 years of age in 1984 and 1989. Missing family income data were imputed for 1995 and beyond.   [8]Any basic actions difficulty or complex activity limitation is defined as having one or more of the following limitations or difficulties: movement difficulty, emotional difficulty, sensory (seeing or hearing) difficulty, cognitive difficulty, self-care (activities of daily living or instrumental activities of daily living) limitation, social limitation, or work limitation.   [9]MSA = metropolitan statistical area.

Table 3-83A. Health Insurance Coverage of Medicare Beneficiaries 65 Years of Age and Over, by Type of Coverage and Selected Characteristics, Selected Years, 1992–2010

(Numbers in millions; percent.)

Characteristic	Medicare Risk Health Maintenance Organization[1]					Medicaid[2]				
	1992	1995	2000	2005	2010	1992	1995	2000	2005	2010
Age										
65 years and over (number in millions)	1.1	2.6	5.9	4.6	10.3	2.7	2.8	2.7	3.2	3.2
65 years and over (percent of population)	3.9	8.9	19.3	14.5	26.7	9.4	9.6	9.0	10.1	8.4
65 to 74 years	4.2	9.5	20.6	13.9	26.9	7.9	8.8	8.5	9.9	7.7
75 to 84 years	3.7	8.3	18.5	15.3	27.6	10.6	9.6	8.9	9.9	9.1
85 years and over	*	7.3	16.3	13.9	23.7	16.6	13.6	11.2	11.9	9.5
Sex										
Male	4.6	9.2	19.3	13.5	25.4	6.3	6.2	6.3	7.2	6.3
Female	3.4	8.6	19.3	15.2	27.8	11.6	12.0	10.9	12.3	10.1
Race and Hispanic Origin										
White, not Hispanic or Latino	3.6	8.4	18.4	13.2	23.9	5.6	5.4	5.1	6.1	5.4
Black, not Hispanic or Latino	*	7.9	20.7	17.1	34.3	28.5	30.3	23.6	23.6	16.8
Hispanic	*	15.5	27.5	27.2	47.2	39.0	40.5	28.7	29.2	18.8
Percent of Poverty Level [3]										
Below 100 percent	3.6	7.7	18.4	NA	NA	22.3	17.2	15.9	NA	NA
100 percent to less than 200 percent	3.7	9.5	23.4	NA	NA	6.7	6.3	8.4	NA	NA
200 percent or more	4.2	10.1	18.0	NA	NA	*	*	*	NA	NA
Marital Status										
Married	4.6	9.5	18.7	13.8	27.1	4.0	4.3	4.3	5.4	3.6
Widowed	2.3	7.7	19.4	15.0	25.4	14.9	15.0	13.6	14.9	12.6
Divorced	*	9.7	24.4	17.1	29.1	23.4	24.5	20.2	20.0	16.9
Never married	*	*	15.8	13.9	23.1	19.2	19.0	17.0	21.3	19.8

NA = Not available.   * = Figure does not meet standards of reliability or precision. Estimates are considered unreliable if the sample cell size is 50 or fewer.   [1]Enrollee has Medicare risk Health Maintenance Organization (HMO) regardless of other insurance.   [2]Enrolled in Medicaid and not enrolled in a Medicare risk HMO.   [3]Percent of poverty level is based on family income and family size and composition using U.S. Census Bureau poverty thresholds.

Table 3-83B. Health Insurance Coverage of Medicare Beneficiaries 65 Years of Age and Over, by Type of Coverage and Selected Characteristics, Selected Years, 1992–2010

(Numbers in millions; percent.)

Characteristic	Employer-sponsored plan[1]					Medigap[2]				
	1992	1995	2000	2005	2010	1992	1995	2000	2005	2010
Age										
65 years and over (number in millions)	12.5	11.3	10.7	11.6	11.9	9.9	9.5	7.6	8.2	7.6
65 years and over (percent of population)	42.8	38.6	35.2	36.4	30.6	33.9	32.5	25.0	25.7	19.6
65 to 74 years	46.9	41.1	36.6	38.1	32.5	31.4	29.9	21.7	23.2	17.4
75 to 84 years	38.2	37.1	35.0	35.5	28.4	37.5	35.2	27.8	27.3	21.3
85 years and over	31.6	30.2	29.4	31.8	28.5	38.3	37.6	31.1	30.8	24.7
Sex										
Male	46.3	42.1	37.7	39.4	32.9	30.6	30.0	23.4	23.8	18.2
Female	40.4	36.0	33.4	34.2	28.9	36.2	34.4	26.2	27.1	20.8
Race and Hispanic Origin										
White, not Hispanic or Latino	45.9	41.3	38.6	39.5	33.5	37.2	36.2	28.3	29.1	23.0
Black, not Hispanic or Latino	25.9	26.7	22.0	27.9	23.7	13.6	10.2	7.5	9.5	6.7
Hispanic	20.7	16.9	15.8	18.6	14.8	15.8	10.1	11.3	11.1	6.4
Percent of Poverty Level [3]										
Below 100 percent	29.0	32.1	28.1	NA	NA	30.8	29.8	22.6	NA	NA
100 percent to less than 200 percent	37.5	32.0	27.0	NA	NA	39.3	39.1	28.4	NA	NA
200 percent or more	58.4	52.8	49.0	NA	NA	32.8	32.2	26.2	NA	NA
Marital Status										
Married	49.9	44.6	41.0	41.7	35.9	33.0	32.6	25.6	27.0	19.6
Widowed	34.1	30.3	28.7	30.4	26.3	37.5	35.2	26.7	26.2	22.0
Divorced	27.3	26.6	22.4	25.1	18.9	27.9	24.1	16.9	19.8	15.3
Never married	38.0	35.1	28.5	29.1	25.2	29.1	26.2	21.9	15.4	17.5

NA = Not available.   * = Figure does not meet standards of reliability or precision. Estimates are considered unreliable if the sample cell size is 50 or fewer.   [1]Private insurance plans purchased through employers (own, current, or former employer, family business, union, or former employer or union of spouse) and not enrolled in a Medicare risk HMO or Medicaid.   [2]Supplemental insurance purchased privately or through organizations such as American Association of Retired Persons or professional organizations, and not enrolled in a Medicare risk HMO, Medicaid, or employer-sponsored plan.   [3]Percent of poverty level is based on family income and family size and composition using U.S. Census Bureau poverty thresholds.

Table 3-83C. Health Insurance Coverage of Medicare Beneficiaries 65 Years of Age and Over, by Type of Coverage and Selected Characteristics, Selected Years, 1992–2010

(Numbers in millions; percent.)

Characteristic	Medicare fee-for-service only or other[1]				
	1992	1995	2000	2005	2010
Age					
65 years and over (number in millions)	2.9	3.1	3.5	4.3	5.7
65 years and over (percent of population)	9.9	10.5	11.5	13.3	14.6
65 to 74 years	9.7	10.7	12.6	14.9	15.5
75 to 84 years	10.1	9.9	9.9	11.9	13.5
85 years and over	10.8	11.3	12.1	11.6	13.6
Sex					
Male	12.2	12.6	13.3	16.2	17.3
Female	8.3	8.9	10.2	11.2	12.5
Race and Hispanic Origin					
White, not Hispanic or Latino	7.7	8.7	9.6	12.2	14.2
Black, not Hispanic or Latino	26.7	25.0	26.1	21.9	18.6
Hispanic	18.3	17.1	16.7	13.9	12.7
Percent of Poverty Level [2]					
Below 100 percent	14.3	13.3	15.1	NA	NA
100 percent to less than 200 percent	12.9	13.1	12.7	NA	NA
200 percent or more	4.0	4.5	6.3	NA	NA
Marital Status					
Married	8.5	9.0	10.5	12.1	13.9
Widowed	11.2	11.9	11.6	13.5	13.7
Divorced	15.7	15.1	16.1	17.9	19.8
Never married	*	13.1	16.8	20.4	14.4

NA = Not available.   * = Figure does not meet standards of reliability or precision. Estimates are considered unreliable if the sample cell size is 50 or fewer.   [1]Medicare fee-for-service only or other public plans (except Medicaid).   [2]Percent of poverty level is based on family income and family size and composition using U.S. Census Bureau poverty thresholds.

Table 3-84. Persons Without Health Insurance Coverage, by State, Average Annual, Selected Years, 1995–1997 Through 2008–2010

(Percent.)

State	1995–1997	1998–2000	2001–2003	2004–2006[1]	2005–2007[1]	2006–2008	2007–2009	2008–2010
United States	15.7	14.4	15.1	15.3	15.4	15.5	15.8	15.8
Alabama	14.0	14.2	13.3	14.1	13.9	13.0	13.6	14.4
Alaska	14.7	18.1	17.8	16.7	17.3	18.2	18.6	18.3
Arizona	23.0	19.5	17.3	19.0	19.6	19.6	19.1	19.1
Arkansas	21.3	15.3	16.6	17.5	17.5	17.6	17.7	18.5
California	20.7	19.2	18.7	18.5	18.6	18.5	18.9	18.9
Colorado	15.5	14.1	16.3	16.6	16.7	16.5	15.9	14.3
Connecticut	10.6	9.5	10.4	10.4	9.9	9.6	10.5	10.5
Delaware	14.1	11.2	10.1	12.5	11.8	11.4	11.8	11.7
District of Columbia	16.1	14.5	13.3	12.4	11.4	10.4	10.6	11.4
Florida	18.9	17.2	17.6	20.3	20.5	20.5	20.9	20.7
Georgia	17.8	15.2	16.4	17.6	17.8	17.7	18.6	19.0
Hawaii	8.3	9.8	9.9	8.6	8.3	8.1	7.8	7.5
Idaho	16.1	16.5	17.5	14.9	14.7	15.0	14.9	16.6
Illinois	11.6	13.3	14.0	13.6	13.7	13.4	13.7	13.8
Indiana	11.5	11.3	12.9	13.1	12.3	11.8	12.6	12.8
Iowa	11.6	8.2	9.5	9.3	9.4	9.8	10.0	10.7
Kansas	11.8	11.0	10.9	11.1	11.8	12.4	12.7	12.5
Kentucky	15.0	13.1	13.3	13.8	13.8	15.0	15.3	15.5
Louisiana	18.8	19.5	19.4	18.5	19.4	20.1	18.2	18.0
Maine	13.5	11.5	10.7	9.5	9.5	9.5	9.8	9.9
Maryland	13.4	11.9	13.2	13.5	13.6	13.2	13.2	12.6
Massachusetts	12.0	9.2	9.6	10.3	8.3	7.1	5.1	5.0
Michigan	10.1	10.6	11.0	10.6	10.8	11.3	12.4	12.5
Minnesota	9.1	8.2	8.2	8.5	8.5	8.7	8.6	8.7
Mississippi	19.4	15.7	17.0	18.1	18.8	19.1	18.1	18.7
Missouri	13.5	9.0	10.9	12.3	12.5	12.8	13.5	13.7
Montana	15.3	18.3	16.1	17.0	16.1	16.3	15.7	16.3
Nebraska	10.4	9.5	10.3	11.1	12.0	12.5	12.2	11.8
Nevada	17.3	17.5	18.3	18.3	17.9	18.5	18.9	20.0
New Hampshire	10.4	8.6	9.9	10.4	10.5	10.7	10.4	10.1
New Jersey	15.8	12.9	13.7	14.6	15.2	15.1	15.2	14.4
New Mexico	23.5	22.6	21.3	21.0	21.9	23.0	22.6	21.8
New York	16.6	15.3	15.5	13.2	13.4	13.8	14.0	14.2
North Carolina	15.3	13.7	16.1	16.0	16.6	16.6	16.6	16.7
North Dakota	11.1	12.1	10.5	11.1	11.1	11.4	10.8	11.7
Ohio	11.6	10.2	11.7	10.7	11.0	11.1	12.5	12.9
Oklahoma	18.0	17.7	18.7	18.7	18.2	16.9	16.6	16.3
Oregon	13.7	13.7	14.8	16.6	16.8	17.0	16.9	16.5
Pennsylvania	9.8	8.3	10.7	10.2	9.8	9.8	10.3	10.5
Rhode Island	11.0	6.9	9.3	10.2	10.3	10.4	11.6	11.5
South Carolina	16.2	13.8	13.1	16.0	16.5	16.1	16.4	17.6
South Dakota	10.2	12.0	11.0	11.6	11.2	11.5	12.0	12.8
Tennessee	14.5	10.8	11.8	13.4	13.9	14.4	14.9	14.7
Texas	24.4	22.2	24.6	24.1	24.4	24.9	25.5	24.8
Utah	12.4	13.2	13.6	15.7	15.6	14.5	13.6	13.2
Vermont	11.3	10.3	9.9	10.8	11.0	10.2	10.1	9.4
Virginia	12.9	12.9	12.5	13.2	13.6	13.5	13.4	12.9
Washington	12.4	12.8	14.3	12.5	12.1	11.8	12.2	12.8
West Virginia	15.8	15.2	14.8	15.5	14.9	14.2	14.4	13.9
Wisconsin	7.9	9.3	9.5	9.4	8.8	8.9	9.1	9.2
Wyoming	15.0	15.1	16.5	14.0	14.3	13.9	14.3	15.3

[1]Data for 2004 and 2005 were revised in March 2007.

Table 3-85. Medicaid Coverage Among Persons Under 65 Years of Age, by Selected Characteristics, Selected Years, 1984–2011

(Percent.)

Characteristic	1984[1]	1989[1]	1995[1]	2000[2]	2005[3]	2006[3]	2007[3]	2008[3]	2009[3]	2010[3]	2011[3]
Total (number in millions)[4]	14.0	15.4	26.6	23.2	33.2	36.2	36.2	38.4	42.4	44.8	47.4
Total (percent of population)[4]	6.8	7.2	11.5	9.5	12.9	14.0	13.9	14.7	16.1	16.9	17.8
Age											
Under 19 years	11.7	12.2	21.1	19.2	26.6	29.4	29.3	30.6	33.9	35.7	37.5
Under 6 years	15.5	15.7	29.3	24.7	34.0	36.6	36.6	38.1	41.4	43.7	46.1
6 to 18 years	9.8	10.5	17.0	16.8	23.3	26.1	25.9	27.1	30.3	31.8	33.4
Under 18 years	11.9	12.6	21.5	19.6	27.2	29.9	29.8	31.3	34.5	36.4	38.2
6 to 17 years	10.1	10.9	17.4	17.2	23.9	26.7	26.4	27.9	30.9	32.5	34.1
18 to 64 years	4.5	4.9	7.1	5.2	7.2	7.7	7.5	8.1	8.9	9.2	9.9
18 to 44 years	5.1	5.2	7.8	5.6	8.3	8.6	8.7	9.2	10.3	10.9	11.6
18 to 24 years	6.4	6.8	10.4	8.1	11.3	11.4	11.4	12.2	14.0	14.5	15.2
19 to 25 years	6.3	6.6	10.2	7.3	10.3	9.7	9.9	10.6	12.2	12.6	13.4
25 to 34 years	5.3	5.2	8.2	5.5	8.0	8.3	8.5	9.3	10.1	11.1	11.5
35 to 44 years	3.5	4.0	5.9	4.3	6.6	7.1	7.0	7.1	7.7	8.1	9.0
45 to 64 years	3.4	4.3	5.6	4.5	5.5	6.3	5.9	6.4	6.9	6.8	7.5
45 to 54 years	3.2	3.8	5.1	4.2	5.2	6.4	6.0	6.2	7.0	7.0	8.0
55 to 64 years	3.6	4.9	6.4	4.9	5.8	6.1	5.7	6.8	6.8	6.6	6.9
Sex											
Male	5.4	5.7	9.6	8.2	11.6	12.6	12.5	13.4	14.4	15.2	16.3
Female	8.1	8.6	13.4	10.8	14.3	15.5	15.2	15.9	17.8	18.5	19.3
Sex and Marital Status [5]											
Male											
Married	1.9	1.8	2.9	2.2	3.5	3.7	3.5	3.6	4.1	4.0	4.9
Divorced, separated, widowed	4.9	5.4	7.7	6.1	7.0	7.9	7.8	8.1	8.3	9.3	9.8
Never married	4.8	5.6	8.1	7.2	10.4	11.6	11.3	12.1	13.1	13.5	14.5
Female											
Married	2.6	3.0	5.2	3.1	4.7	4.6	4.7	5.2	5.3	5.7	6.4
Divorced, separated, widowed	16.0	16.1	19.0	12.7	14.6	16.2	16.3	17.2	18.7	17.6	18.0
Never married	10.7	11.9	16.5	13.2	17.3	19.0	18.1	18.7	20.9	22.2	21.9
Race [6]											
White only	4.6	5.1	8.9	7.1	11.0	11.8	11.4	12.1	13.7	14.5	15.4
Black or African American only	20.5	19.0	28.5	21.2	24.9	26.6	27.7	28.3	29.5	30.4	30.9
American Indian or Alaska Native only	*28.2	29.7	19.0	15.1	24.2	24.3	21.2	37.0	29.7	21.6	29.0
Asian only	*8.7	*8.8	10.5	7.5	8.2	9.7	8.7	9.2	9.9	12.0	14.7
Native Hawaiian or Other Pacific Islander only	NA	NA	NA	*	*	*	*	*	*	*	*
Two or more races	NA	NA	NA	19.1	22.0	24.0	27.9	24.7	30.1	27.4	27.2
Hispanic Origin and Race [6]											
Hispanic or Latino	13.3	13.5	21.9	15.5	22.9	23.1	24.7	24.9	27.6	28.6	30.1
Mexican	12.2	12.4	21.6	14.0	23.0	23.0	25.9	25.4	28.4	29.5	31.0
Puerto Rican	31.5	27.3	33.4	29.4	31.9	35.7	28.0	31.0	32.1	35.7	33.0
Cuban	*4.8	*7.7	13.4	9.2	17.7	*11.3	13.3	13.0	16.7	17.3	20.0
Other Hispanic or Latino	7.9	11.1	18.2	14.5	19.7	20.2	21.4	22.3	24.6	24.5	27.7
Not Hispanic or Latino	6.2	6.5	10.2	8.5	11.1	12.3	11.7	12.6	13.7	14.4	15.2
White only	3.7	4.1	7.1	6.1	8.5	9.5	8.5	9.2	10.4	11.0	11.8
Black or African American only	20.7	19.0	28.1	21.0	24.8	26.2	27.3	27.9	29.1	30.0	30.5
Age and Percent of Poverty Level [7]											
Under 65 years											
Below 100 percent	33.0	37.6	48.4	38.4	45.7	45.8	47.6	49.1	51.2	50.8	51.4
100 percent to 199 percent	5.3	7.5	14.4	16.2	23.4	23.8	26.1	27.4	29.0	28.5	30.6
100 percent to 133 percent	8.7	11.9	23.1	22.4	30.6	30.8	34.8	36.1	39.3	36.3	38.8
134 percent to 199 percent	3.7	5.6	9.7	13.1	19.5	20.0	21.7	22.9	23.6	24.4	26.1
200 percent to 399 percent	0.8	1.3	2.3	4.0	6.6	7.0	6.8	7.8	8.0	8.4	8.9
400 percent or more	0.2	0.5	0.4	0.9	1.5	1.7	1.5	1.6	1.7	2.0	1.7
Under 19 years											
Below 100 percent	42.0	45.8	63.5	56.9	69.4	70.4	72.7	73.4	77.5	78.4	79.9
100 percent to 199 percent	6.5	8.6	21.3	27.8	41.7	44.1	47.2	48.5	52.7	53.5	56.7
100 percent to 133 percent	10.3	13.4	32.4	36.4	51.0	51.3	57.5	60.0	65.6	63.5	69.1
134 percent to 199 percent	4.7	6.3	14.3	23.3	36.2	39.4	41.3	42.3	45.3	47.7	49.9
200 percent to 399 percent	1.0	1.7	3.5	7.6	13.0	13.5	13.3	16.4	16.4	17.7	18.3
400 percent or more	*	*1.2	*	2.1	2.9	3.5	3.0	3.5	3.6	4.3	3.5
Under 18 years											
Below 100 percent	43.3	47.8	66.0	58.5	71.2	72.0	75.0	75.3	78.3	79.8	81.4
100 percent to 199 percent	6.6	8.7	21.6	28.4	42.5	44.7	48.1	49.5	53.5	54.3	57.6
100 percent to 133 percent	10.4	13.5	32.9	36.9	52.0	51.7	58.4	61.1	66.9	64.6	70.1
134 percent to 199 percent	4.8	6.4	14.4	23.8	36.9	40.1	42.2	43.2	45.9	48.2	50.6
200 percent to 399 percent	1.0	1.7	3.5	7.6	13.3	13.8	13.3	16.8	16.8	18.0	18.6
400 percent or more	*	*1.1	*	2.2	2.9	3.4	3.0	3.6	3.7	4.3	3.6
18 to 64 years											
Below 100 percent	25.3	29.1	34.8	24.9	29.6	28.9	30.6	33.0	33.6	32.4	33.0
100 percent to 199 percent	4.5	6.8	10.2	9.1	13.1	13.0	14.0	15.3	16.2	15.7	17.1
100 percent to 133 percent	7.6	10.8	16.3	13.2	17.9	17.8	20.2	21.9	23.7	21.0	22.7
134 percent to 199 percent	3.1	5.1	7.2	7.2	10.7	10.5	11.0	11.8	12.4	13.0	14.1
200 percent to 399 percent	0.7	1.1	1.7	2.4	3.8	4.2	4.0	4.1	4.6	4.8	5.2
400 percent or more	0.2	0.4	0.4	0.6	1.1	1.2	1.1	1.1	1.2	1.3	1.2

Table 3-85. Medicaid Coverage Among Persons Under 65 Years of Age, by Selected Characteristics, Selected Years, 1984–2011 —Continued

(Percent.)

Characteristic	1984[1]	1989[1]	1995[1]	2000[2]	2005[3]	2006[3]	2007[3]	2008[3]	2009[3]	2010[3]	2011[3]
Disability Measure among Adults 18 to 64 Years [8]											
Any basic actions difficulty or complex activity limitation	NA	NA	NA	12.8	16.4	16.2	16.5	18.6	18.2	17.8	19.6
Any basic actions difficulty	NA	NA	NA	12.2	15.5	15.3	15.9	17.7	17.8	16.7	19.1
Any complex activity limitation	NA	NA	NA	23.2	28.5	28.7	28.7	31.0	30.2	30.0	30.8
No disability	NA	NA	NA	3.0	4.9	5.1	5.2	4.9	6.4	6.8	6.9
Geographic Region											
Northeast	8.6	6.6	11.7	10.6	13.3	16.8	15.4	16.1	17.3	17.9	19.6
Midwest	7.4	7.6	10.5	8.0	12.3	13.9	13.7	14.5	16.4	17.3	16.7
South	5.1	6.5	11.3	9.4	12.7	12.9	12.9	13.5	14.8	16.0	17.3
West	7.0	8.5	12.9	10.4	13.8	13.8	14.5	15.7	16.8	17.1	18.4
Location of Residence											
Within MSA[9]	7.1	7.0	11.3	8.9	12.4	13.3	13.3	14.2	15.2	16.1	17.0
Outside MSA[9]	6.1	7.9	12.3	11.9	15.5	17.7	17.1	17.2	20.8	21.4	22.1

NA = Not available.   * = Figure does not meet standards of reliability or precision. Data not shown have a relative standard error of greater than 30 percent.   [1]Any private insurance at the time of interview that was originally obtained through a present or former employer or union, or, starting with 1997 data, through the workplace, self-employment, or a professional association; includes those who also had another type of coverage.   [2]Data prior to 1997 are not strictly comparable with data for later years due to the 1997 questionnaire redesign.   [3]Beginning in quarter 3 of the 2004 NHIS, persons under 65 years of age with no reported coverage were asked explicitly about Medicaid coverage. Estimates were calculated without and with the additional information from this question in the columns labeled 2004(1) and 2004(2), respectively, and estimates were calculated with the additional information starting with 2005 data.   [4]Includes all other races not shown separately, those with unknown marital status, unknown disability status, and, in 1984 and 1989, persons with unknown poverty level.   [5]Includes persons 14 to 64 years of age.   [6]The race groups White, Black, American Indian or Alaska Native, Asian, Native Hawaiian or Other Pacific Islander, and two or more races include persons of Hispanic and non-Hispanic origin. Persons of Hispanic origin may be of any race.   [7]Percent of poverty level is based on family income and family size and composition using U.S. Census Bureau poverty thresholds. Poverty level was unknown for 10 to 11 percent of persons under 65 years of age in 1984 and 1989. Missing family income data were imputed for 1995 and beyond.   [8]Any basic actions difficulty or complex activity limitation is defined as having one or more of the following limitations or difficulties: movement difficulty, emotional difficulty, sensory (seeing or hearing) difficulty, cognitive difficulty, self-care (activities of daily living or instrumental activities of daily living) limitation, social limitation, or work limitation.   [9]MSA = metropolitan statistical area.

Table 3-86. Medicaid Beneficiaries and Payments, by Basis of Eligibility, and Race and Hispanic Origin, Selected Fiscal Years, 1999–2009

(Number, percent, dollar.)

Characteristic	1999	2000	2001	2002	2003	2004	2005	2006	2007	2008	2009
Beneficiaries (Number in Millions) [1]											
All beneficiaries	40.1	42.8	46.2	49.3	52.0	55.6	57.7	57.8	56.8	58.8	56.0
Percent of Beneficiaries											
Basis of eligibility											
Age (65 years and over)	9.4	8.7	8.3	7.9	7.8	7.8	7.6	7.6	7.1	7.1	6.5
Blind and disabled	16.7	16.1	15.4	15.0	14.8	14.6	14.2	14.4	14.8	14.8	14.0
Adults in families with dependent children [2]	18.7	20.5	21.2	22.8	22.5	22.5	21.5	21.9	21.8	21.8	22.6
Children under age 21 [3]	46.9	46.1	45.7	47.1	47.8	47.8	47.5	48.0	48.4	48.0	48.4
Other Title XIX [4]	8.4	8.6	9.4	7.2	7.2	7.3	9.1	8.1	7.8	8.4	8.5
Race and Hispanic Origin [5]											
White	NA	NA	40.1	40.9	41.2	41.1	39.3	39.1	38.6	38.1	36.5
Black or African American	NA	NA	23.0	22.8	22.4	22.1	21.5	21.8	21.6	21.1	21.1
American Indian or Alaska Native	NA	NA	1.3	1.3	1.4	1.3	1.2	1.2	1.2	1.3	1.3
Asian or Pacific Islander	NA	NA	3.3	3.4	3.3	3.3	3.5	3.5	3.5	3.5	3.5
Asian	NA	NA	NA	2.2	2.4	2.4	2.5	2.6	2.6	2.6	2.6
Pacific Islander	NA	NA	NA	1.2	0.9	0.9	0.9	0.9	0.9	0.9	0.8
Hispanic or Latino	NA	NA	17.9	19.0	19.3	19.4	20.6	21.0	21.6	21.7	23.6
Multiple race or unknown	NA	NA	14.5	12.6	12.5	12.7	13.9	13.3	13.5	14.3	14.1
Payments (Billions of Dollars) [6]											
All payments	154	168	187	214	233	258	275	269	276	294	287
Percent Distribution											
Basis of eligibility	100.0	100.0	100.0	100.0	100.0	100.0	100.0	100.0	100.0	100.0	100.0
Age (65 years and over)	27.7	26.4	25.9	24.4	23.7	23.1	23.1	21.6	20.7	20.6	19.2
Blind and disabled	42.9	43.2	43.1	43.3	43.7	43.3	43.4	43.3	43.3	43.5	43.5
Adults in families with dependent children [2]	10.3	10.6	10.8	11.0	11.5	12.0	11.7	12.3	12.4	12.6	13.9
Children under age 21 [3]	15.7	15.9	16.3	16.8	17.1	17.2	17.3	18.8	19.4	19.4	19.9
Other Title XIX [4]	3.4	3.9	3.9	4.5	4.0	4.5	4.6	3.9	4.2	4.0	3.5
Race and Hispanic Origin [5]											
White	NA	NA	54.3	54.1	53.8	53.4	53.0	52.1	50.7	50.2	48.6
Black or African American	NA	NA	19.8	19.6	19.7	19.8	19.8	20.4	20.8	20.6	21.3
American Indian or Alaska Native	NA	NA	1.1	1.1	1.2	1.2	1.2	1.2	1.2	1.3	1.3
Asian or Pacific Islander	NA	NA	2.6	2.8	2.4	2.5	2.7	2.8	2.8	2.9	3.0
Asian	NA	NA	NA	1.5	1.6	1.7	1.9	2.0	2.0	2.1	2.2
Pacific Islander	NA	NA	NA	1.4	0.8	0.8	0.8	0.8	0.8	0.8	0.8
Hispanic or Latino	NA	NA	9.4	9.7	10.6	10.7	12.2	12.8	13.1	13.7	15.2
Multiple race or unknown	NA	NA	12.8	12.6	12.2	12.3	11.1	10.8	11.4	11.4	10.5
Payments per Beneficiary (Dollars) [6]											
All beneficiaries	3,819	3,936	4,049	4,328	4,487	4,639	4,768	4,657	4,862	5,051	5,122
Basis of eligibility											
Age (65 years and over)	11,268	11,929	12,705	13,370	13,677	13,687	14,427	13,276	14,141	14,742	15,141
Blind and disabled	9,832	10,559	11,308	12,470	13,303	13,714	14,531	13,982	14,194	14,843	15,921
Adults in families with dependent children [2]	2,104	2,030	2,057	2,093	2,292	2,471	2,587	2,622	2,753	2,917	3,156
Children under age 21 [3]	1,282	1,358	1,447	1,545	1,606	1,664	1,735	1,825	1,951	2,038	2,107
Other Title XIX [4]	1,532	1,778	1,689	2,718	2,474	2,896	2,380	2,255	2,622	2,407	2,087
Race and Hispanic Origin [5]											
White	NA	NA	5,483	5,721	5,870	6,026	6,422	6,199	6,390	6,657	6,832
Black or African American	NA	NA	3,479	3,733	3,944	4,158	4,397	4,358	4,669	4,928	5,184
American Indian or Alaska Native	NA	NA	3,451	3,774	4,001	4,320	4,626	4,489	4,826	5,218	5,439
Asian or Pacific Islander	NA	NA	3,255	3,562	3,513	3,710	3,696	3,863	4,133	4,445	
Asian	NA	NA	NA	2,836	2,993	3,198	3,624	3,657	3,847	4,123	4,389
Pacific Islander	NA	NA	NA	4,919	4,223	4,366	3,947	3,799	3,907	4,161	4,619
Hispanic or Latino	NA	NA	2,127	2,215	2,463	2,563	2,822	2,831	2,960	3,175	3,298
Multiple race or unknown	NA	NA	3,586	4,338	4,396	4,493	3,816	3,770	4,106	4,014	3,804

NOTE: Data are for fiscal years ending September 30. Hawaii, Massachusetts, Missouri, Pennsylvania, Utah, and Wisconsin did not report 2009 data.

NA = Not available. [1]Beneficiaries include those who received services through Medicaid. [2]Includes adults who meet the requirements for the Aid to Families with Dependent Children (AFDC) program that were in effect in their state on July 16, 1996, or, at state option, more liberal criteria (with some exceptions). Includes adults in the Temporary Assistance for Needy Families (TANF) program. Starting with 2001 data, includes women in the Breast and Cervical Cancer Prevention and Treatment Program and unemployed adults. [3]Includes children (including those in the foster care system) in the TANF program. [4]Includes some participants in the Supplemental Security Income program and other people deemed medically needy in participating states. Prior to 2001, includes unemployed adults. Excludes foster care children and includes unknown eligibility. [5]Race and Hispanic origin are as determined on initial Medicaid application. Categories are mutually exclusive. Starting with 2001 data, the Hispanic category included Hispanic persons, regardless of race. Persons indicating more than one race were included in the multiple race category. [6]Medicaid payments exclude disproportionate share hospital (DSH) payments ($14.7 billion in FY2009) and DSH mental health facility payments ($3.1 billion in FY2009).

Table 3-87. Medicaid Beneficiaries and Payments, by Type of Service, Selected Fiscal Years, 1999–2009

(Number; percent.)

Type of service	1999	2000	2001	2002	2003	2004	2005	2006	2007	2008	2009
Beneficiaries (Number in Millions) [1]											
All beneficiaries	40.2	42.8	46.0	49.3	52.0	55.6	57.7	57.5	56.8	58.8	56.0
Percent											
Inpatient hospital	11.2	11.5	10.6	10.2	10.0	9.8	9.5	10.9	9.0	8.9	9.0
Mental health facility	0.2	0.2	0.2	0.2	0.2	0.2	0.2	0.2	0.2	0.2	0.2
Intermediate care facility for the mentally retarded	0.3	0.3	0.3	0.2	0.2	0.2	0.2	0.2	0.2	0.2	0.2
Nursing facility	4.0	4.0	3.7	3.6	3.3	3.1	3.0	3.0	2.9	2.7	2.6
Physician	45.7	44.7	43.5	44.7	44.0	43.1	42.0	40.2	38.8	36.9	38.2
Dental	14.0	13.8	15.3	16.0	16.4	16.2	16.2	16.4	16.8	16.7	17.8
Other practitioner	9.9	11.1	11.1	11.3	11.1	10.7	10.2	10.1	9.5	8.8	8.9
Outpatient hospital	30.9	30.9	29.8	30.1	29.8	28.7	28.2	27.6	26.2	25.2	27.0
Clinic	16.8	17.9	18.4	19.2	19.6	20.0	20.7	20.5	20.6	20.2	20.3
Laboratory and radiological	25.4	26.6	26.8	28.5	28.3	28.9	27.7	28.0	27.8	26.6	26.4
Home health	2.0	2.3	2.2	2.2	2.3	2.1	2.1	2.1	2.1	1.9	1.8
Prescribed drugs	49.4	48.0	47.6	49.4	50.2	50.3	49.2	47.1	42.1	41.8	43.1
Capitated care	51.5	49.7	50.5	51.7	53.1	54.2	58.1	61.0	64.5	64.9	64.7
Primary care case management	9.7	13.0	13.9	14.6	14.5	15.4	15.1	14.8	12.5	14.9	14.0
Personal support	10.1	10.6	10.8	11.5	11.6	11.3	11.8	11.8	11.6	10.8	11.2
Other care[2]	21.6	21.4	21.5	22.6	23.1	22.9	21.9	21.6	21.5	21.3	21.1
Payments (Billions of Dollars) [3]											
All payments	154	168	186	214	233	258	275	267	276	294	287
Percent Distribution											
Inpatient hospital	100.0	100.0	100.0	100.0	100.0	100.0	100.0	100.0	100.0	100.0	100.0
	14.5	14.4	13.9	13.6	13.5	13.5	12.8	13.5	13.4	12.5	12.4
Mental health facility	1.1	1.1	1.1	1.0	0.9	0.9	0.8	0.9	0.9	0.8	0.8
Intermediate care facility for the mentally retarded	6.1	5.6	5.2	5.0	4.7	4.3	4.3	4.4	4.3	4.2	4.0
Nursing facility	21.7	20.5	20.0	18.4	17.3	16.3	16.3	17.0	16.8	16.1	14.5
Physician	4.3	4.0	4.0	3.9	3.9	4.0	4.1	3.9	3.6	3.5	3.8
Dental	0.8	0.8	1.0	1.1	1.1	1.1	1.1	1.2	1.2	1.3	1.5
Other practitioner	0.3	0.4	0.4	0.4	0.4	0.4	0.4	0.4	0.3	0.3	0.3
Outpatient hospital	4.0	4.2	4.0	4.0	4.0	4.0	3.6	3.8	3.7	3.7	3.8
Clinic	3.8	3.7	3.0	3.1	3.1	3.2	3.2	3.2	3.1	3.1	3.2
Laboratory and radiological	0.8	0.8	0.9	1.0	1.0	1.0	1.1	1.1	1.1	1.0	1.0
Home health	1.9	1.9	1.9	1.8	1.9	1.8	2.0	2.2	2.3	2.2	2.1
Prescribed drugs	10.8	11.9	12.7	13.3	14.5	15.3	15.6	10.4	8.0	7.9	8.0
Capitated care	14.0	14.5	15.7	15.8	16.0	16.5	16.9	18.8	21.2	23.0	23.7
Primary care case management	0.3	0.1	0.1	0.1	0.1	0.2	0.1	0.1	0.1	0.1	0.1
Personal support	6.9	6.9	7.0	7.2	7.4	7.2	7.5	8.0	8.4	8.3	8.6
Other care[2]	8.6	8.8	9.2	10.3	10.2	10.3	10.2	11.1	11.6	12.0	12.2
Payments per Beneficiary (Dollars) [3]											
All beneficiaries	3,819	3,936	4,053	4,328	4,487	4,639	4,768	4,654	4,862	5,051	5,122
Inpatient hospital	4,943	4,919	5,313	5,771	6,047	6,424	6,411	5,781	7,191	7,083	7,047
Mental health facility	18,094	17,800	21,482	21,377	20,503	19,928	19,252	17,156	21,407	21,975	22,172
Intermediate care facility for the mentally retarded	76,443	79,330	83,227	91,588	95,287	97,497	107,028	110,340	113,735	123,053	125,236
Nursing facility	20,568	20,220	21,894	22,326	23,882	24,475	26,185	26,531	28,282	29,533	29,070
Physician	357	356	371	378	403	426	465	456	457	485	506
Dental	214	238	270	293	305	318	326	329	340	389	423
Other practitioner	118	139	149	151	154	160	200	196	170	171	174
Outpatient hospital	491	533	546	571	596	639	617	642	695	736	713
Clinic	860	805	662	706	720	750	749	731	741	772	808
Laboratory and radiological	114	113	131	154	161	168	183	185	185	188	194
Home health	3,571	3,135	3,478	3,689	3,720	3,978	4,487	4,977	5,334	5,789	5,823
Prescribed drugs	837	975	1,083	1,165	1,293	1,411	1,509	1,030	926	957	950
Capitated care	1,040	1,148	1,257	1,318	1,357	1,415	1,386	1,431	1,598	1,786	1,879
Primary care case management	119	30	29	28	28	58	27	29	33	32	41
Personal support	2,583	2,543	2,639	2,704	2,864	2,946	3,035	3,160	3,534	3,852	3,961
Other care[2]	1,508	1,600	1,734	1,963	1,975	2,086	2,228	2,388	2,611	2,856	2,967

[1]Beneficiaries include those who received services through Medicaid.   [2]Unknown services (0.3 percent of beneficiaries and 0.3 percent of payments in 2009) are included with Other Care.   [3]Medicaid payments exclude disproportionate share hospital (DSH) payments ($14.7 billion in FY2009) and DSH mental health facility payments ($3.1 billion in FY2009).

Table 3-88. Medicaid Beneficiaries, Beneficiaries in Managed Care, Payments Per Beneficiary, and Beneficiaries Per 100 Persons Below the Poverty Level, by State, Selected Fiscal Years, 1999–2009

(Number.)

State	Beneficiaries (in thousands)[1]		Percent of beneficiaries in managed care[2]		Payments per beneficiary[3]		Beneficiaries per 100 persons below the poverty level	
	2000	2009	2000	2009	2000	2009	1999–2000	2008–2009
United States	42,763	56,041	56	71	$3,936	$5,122	131	138
Alabama	619	877	60	67	3,860	4,135	88	118
Alaska	96	119	-	-	4,876	8,990	180	175
Arizona	681	1,588	92	90	3,100	5,426	113	117
Arkansas	489	825	57	79	3,086	4,338	113	170
California	7,915	11,519	50	52	2,155	3,058	162	201
Colorado	381	678	90	95	4,747	4,852	107	113
Connecticut	420	558	72	75	6,762	9,475	184	191
Delaware	115	209	79	74	4,584	6,052	147	204
District of Columbia	139	175	66	98	5,715	11,077	179	168
Florida	2,360	3,261	60	66	3,114	4,310	136	122
Georgia	1,290	1,805	96	92	2,774	4,087	136	108
Hawaii	204	NA	74	97	2,626	NA	83	NA
Idaho	131	253	30	84	4,530	5,345	75	123
Illinois	1,516	2,626	10	55	5,150	4,483	115	152
Indiana	705	1,109	67	74	4,224	4,858	148	116
Iowa	314	482	90	83	4,707	5,974	149	162
Kansas	263	355	56	87	4,670	6,528	94	98
Kentucky	771	942	81	83	3,780	5,326	158	126
Louisiana	761	1,184	6	69	3,456	4,585	95	164
Maine	192	315	35	64	6,820	4,704	155	203
Maryland	665	846	81	79	5,396	7,480	170	156
Massachusetts	1,047	NA	64	60	5,153	NA	153	NA
Michigan	1,352	1,890	100	89	3,611	5,381	135	139
Minnesota	559	802	63	63	5,857	8,766	178	145
Mississippi	605	932	39	76	2,987	3,432	139	134
Missouri	890	NA	40	99	3,673	NA	157	NA
Montana	104	113	61	67	4,173	6,344	73	88
Nebraska	229	256	77	84	4,185	6,218	136	139
Nevada	138	281	39	84	3,733	4,259	70	85
New Hampshire	97	141	6	78	6,712	7,037	119	140
New Jersey	822	1,151	59	75	5,724	7,208	128	139
New Mexico	376	562	64	74	3,325	5,185	110	140
New York	3,420	4,985	25	66	7,646	9,004	128	171
North Carolina	1,209	1,782	68	70	3,996	5,423	122	125
North Dakota	61	77	55	68	5,852	7,643	87	106
Ohio	1,305	2,238	21	70	5,434	6,243	103	139
Oklahoma	507	809	69	88	3,163	4,419	106	165
Oregon	542	564	83	88	3,135	4,957	132	115
Pennsylvania	1,492	NA	73	82	4,266	NA	141	NA
Rhode Island	179	203	69	62	5,982	7,654	187	153
South Carolina	685	906	6	100	3,900	5,199	157	143
South Dakota	102	141	93	80	3,935	5,188	155	128
Tennessee	1,568	1,479	100	100	2,226	4,910	211	151
Texas	2,603	4,283	34	65	3,487	4,330	85	102
Utah	224	NA	90	86	4,277	NA	132	NA
Vermont	139	171	47	88	3,451	5,684	208	294
Virginia	627	917	59	64	3,960	6,053	115	108
Washington	895	1,177	100	86	2,717	4,872	155	162
West Virginia	335	386	35	46	4,154	6,699	129	140
Wisconsin	577	NA	44	60	5,039	NA	113	NA
Wyoming	46	72	-	-	4,609	7,635	84	136

NA = Not available.   - = Quantity zero.   [1]Beneficiaries include those who received services through Medicaid.   [2]Medicaid managed care enrollment data include individuals in state health care reform programs that expand eligibility beyond traditional Medicaid eligibility standards. The managed care enrollment data include enrollees receiving comprehensive and limited benefits. Managed care enrollments as of June 30 of year shown. Starting with 2001 data, U.S. total excludes Puerto Rico and the Virgin Islands. Managed care data may change year to year due to a variety of factors, including changes in waiver programs, outreach efforts, and data reporting practices.   [3]Medicaid payments exclude disproportionate share hospital (DSH) payments ($14.7 billion in FY2009) and DSH mental health facility payments ($3.1 billion in FY2009.)

Table 3-89. Medicare Enrollees and Expenditures and Percent Distribution, by Medicare Program and Type of Service, Selected Years, 1970–2010

(Number; dollars; percent.)

Medicare program and type of service	1970	1980	1990	1995	2000	2005	2006	2007	2008	2009[1]	2010[1]
Enrollees (Numbers in Millions)											
Total Medicare[2]	20.4	28.4	34.3	37.6	39.7	42.6	43.4	44.4	45.5	46.6	47.5
Hospital insurance	20.1	28.0	33.7	37.2	39.3	42.2	43.1	44.0	45.1	46.2	47.1
Supplementary medical insurance (SMI)[3]	19.5	27.3	32.6	35.6	37.3	NA	NA	NA	NA	NA	NA
Part B	19.5	27.3	32.6	35.6	37.3	39.8	40.4	41.1	42.0	42.9	43.8
Part D[4]	NA	NA	NA	NA	NA	1.8	30.5	31.2	32.4	33.5	34.5
Expenditures (Dollars in Billions)											
Total Medicare	$7.5	$36.8	$111.0	$184.2	$221.8	$336.4	$408.3	$431.7	$468.1	$509.0	$522.8
Total hospital insurance (HI)	5.3	25.6	67.0	117.6	131.1	182.9	191.9	203.1	235.6	242.5	247.9
HI payments to managed care organizations[5]	NA	0.0	2.7	6.7	21.4	24.9	32.9	39.0	50.6	59.4	60.7
HI payments for fee-for-service utilization	5.1	25.0	63.4	109.5	105.1	156.6	159.6	163.4	172.8	179.5	183.3
Inpatient hospital	4.8	24.1	56.9	82.3	87.1	123.3	124.1	124.1	130.2	134.0	136.1
Skilled nursing facility	0.2	0.4	2.5	9.1	11.1	19.3	20.3	22.6	24.6	26.3	26.9
Home health agency	0.1	0.5	3.7	16.2	4.0	6.0	5.9	6.3	6.7	7.0	7.0
Hospice	NA	NA	0.3	1.9	2.9	8.0	9.3	10.5	11.3	12.2	13.2
Other[6]	NA	NA	NA	NA	NA	NA	NA	NA	NA	NA	0.1
Home health agency transfer[7]	NA	NA	NA	NA	1.7	NA	NA	NA	NA	NA	NA
Medicare Advantage premiums[8]	NA	NA	NA	NA	NA	NA	0.0	0.1	0.1	0.1	0.2
Accounting error (CY 2005-2008)[9]	NA	NA	NA	NA	NA	-1.9	-3.9	-2.7	8.5	NA	NA
Administrative expenses[10]	0.2	0.5	0.9	1.4	2.9	3.3	3.3	3.2	3.6	3.5	3.8
Total supplementary medical insurance (SMI)[3]	2.2	11.2	44.0	66.6	90.7	153.5	216.4	228.6	232.6	266.5	274.9
Total Part B	2.2	11.2	44.0	66.6	90.7	152.4	169.0	178.9	183.3	205.7	212.9
Part B payments to managed care organizations[5]	0.0	0.2	2.8	6.6	18.4	22.0	31.5	38.9	48.1	53.4	55.2
Part B payments for fee-for-service utilization[11]	1.9	10.4	39.6	58.4	72.2	125.0	130.2	134.6	140.5	149.0	154.3
Physician/supplies[12]	1.8	8.2	29.6	NA	NA	NA	NA	NA	NA	NA	NA
Outpatient hospital[13]	0.1	1.9	8.5	NA	NA	NA	NA	NA	NA	NA	NA
Independent laboratory[14]	0.0	0.1	1.5	NA	NA	NA	NA	NA	NA	NA	NA
Physician fee schedule	NA	NA	NA	31.7	37.0	57.7	58.1	58.8	60.6	62.4	64.5
Durable medical equipment	NA	NA	NA	3.7	4.7	8.0	8.3	8.2	8.6	8.0	8.3
Laboratory[15]	NA	NA	NA	4.3	4.0	6.3	6.6	7.1	7.2	8.1	8.4
Other[16]	NA	NA	NA	9.9	13.6	26.7	27.9	28.8	29.6	31.9	32.6
Hospital[17]	NA	NA	NA	8.7	8.4	19.3	21.4	22.6	24.2	27.0	28.4
Home health agency	0.0	0.2	0.1	0.2	4.5	7.1	7.8	9.2	10.3	11.6	12.1
Home health agency transfer[7]	NA	NA	NA	NA	-1.7	NA	NA	NA	NA	NA	NA
Medicare Advantage premiums[8]	NA	NA	NA	NA	NA	NA	0.0	0.1	0.1	0.1	0.2
Accounting error (CY 2005-2008)[9]	NA	NA	NA	NA	NA	1.9	3.9	2.7	-8.5	NA	NA
Administrative expenses[10]	0.2	0.6	1.5	1.6	1.8	2.8	3.1	2.7	3.1	3.2	3.2
Part D start-up costs[18]	NA	NA	NA	NA	NA	0.7	0.2	0.0	0.0	NA	NA
Total Part D[4]	NA	NA	NA	NA	NA	1.1	47.4	49.7	49.3	60.8	62.0
Percent Distribution of Expenditures											
Total hospital insurance (HI)	100.0	100.0	100.0	100.0	100.0	100.0	100.0	100.0	100.0	100.0	100.0
HI payments to managed care organizations[5]	NA	0.0	4.0	5.7	16.3	13.6	17.1	19.2	21.5	24.5	24.5
HI payments for fee-for-service utilization	96.2	97.7	94.6	93.1	80.2	85.6	83.2	80.5	73.3	74.0	73.9
Inpatient hospital	90.6	94.1	84.9	70.0	66.4	67.4	64.7	61.1	55.3	55.3	54.9
Skilled nursing facility	3.8	1.6	3.7	7.7	8.5	10.6	10.6	11.1	10.4	10.8	10.9
Home health agency	1.9	2.0	5.5	13.8	3.1	3.3	3.1	3.1	2.8	2.9	2.8
Hospice	NA	NA	0.4	1.6	2.2	4.4	4.8	5.2	4.8	5.0	5.3
Other[6]	NA	NA	NA	NA	NA	NA	NA	NA	NA	NA	0.0
Home health agency transfer[7]	NA	NA	NA	NA	1.3	NA	NA	NA	NA	NA	NA
Medicare Advantage premiums[8]	NA	NA	NA	NA	NA	NA	0.0	0.0	0.0	0.0	0.1
Accounting error (CY 2005-2008)[9]	NA	NA	NA	NA	NA	-1.0	-2.0	-1.3	3.6	NA	NA
Administrative expenses[10]	3.8	2.0	1.3	1.2	2.2	1.8	1.7	1.6	1.5	1.4	1.5
Total supplementary medical insurance (SMI)[3]	100.0	100.0	100.0	100.0	100.0	100.0	100.0	100.0	100.0	100.0	100.0
Total Part B	100.0	100.0	100.0	100.0	100.0	99.3	78.1	78.3	78.8	77.2	77.4
Part B payments to managed care organizations[5]	1.2	1.8	6.4	9.9	20.2	14.3	14.5	17.0	20.7	20.0	20.1
Part B payments for fee-for-service utilization[11]	88.1	92.8	90.1	87.6	79.6	81.5	60.2	58.9	60.4	55.9	56.1
Physician/supplies[12]	80.9	72.8	67.3	NA	NA	NA	NA	NA	NA	NA	NA
Outpatient hospital[13]	5.2	16.9	19.3	NA	NA	NA	NA	NA	NA	NA	NA
Independent laboratory[14]	0.5	1.0	3.4	NA	NA	NA	NA	NA	NA	NA	NA
Physician fee schedule	NA	NA	NA	47.5	40.8	37.6	26.9	25.7	26.0	23.4	23.5
Durable medical equipment	NA	NA	NA	5.5	5.2	5.2	3.8	3.6	3.7	3.0	3.0
Laboratory[15]	NA	NA	NA	6.4	4.4	4.1	3.1	3.1	3.1	3.0	3.1
Other[16]	NA	NA	NA	14.8	15.0	17.4	12.9	12.6	12.7	12.0	11.8
Hospital[17]	NA	NA	NA	13.0	9.3	12.5	9.9	9.9	10.4	10.1	10.3
Home health agency	1.5	2.1	0.2	0.3	4.9	4.6	3.6	4.0	4.4	4.4	4.4
Home health agency transfer[7]	NA	NA	NA	NA	-1.9	NA	NA	NA	NA	NA	NA
Medicare Advantage premiums[8]	NA	NA	NA	NA	NA	NA	0.0	0.0	0.0	0.0	0.1
Accounting error (CY 2005-2008)[9]	NA	NA	NA	NA	NA	1.2	1.8	1.2	-3.6	NA	NA
Administrative expenses[10]	10.7	5.4	3.5	2.4	2.0	1.8	1.4	1.2	1.3	1.2	1.2
Part D start-up costs[18]	NA	NA	NA	NA	NA	0.4	0.1	0.0	0.0	NA	NA
Total Part D[4]	NA	NA	NA	NA	NA	0.7	21.9	21.7	21.2	22.8	22.6

NA = Not available. 0.0 = Quantity more than zero but less than 0.05. [1]Preliminary estimates. [2]Average number enrolled in the hospital insurance (HI) and/or supplementary medical insurance (SMI) programs for the period. [3]Starting with 2004 data, the SMI trust fund consists of two separate accounts: Part B (which pays for a portion of the costs of physicians' services, outpatient hospital services, and other related medical and health services for voluntarily enrolled individuals) and Part D (Medicare Prescription Drug Account, which pays private plans to provide prescription drug coverage). [4]The Medicare Modernization Act, enacted on December 8, 2003, established within SMI two Part D accounts related to prescription drug benefits: the Medicare Prescription Drug Account and the Transitional Assistance Account. [5]Medicare-approved managed care organizations. [6]Reflects Community Based Care Transition Program ($25 million in 2010) and Electronic Health Records Incentive Program ($113 million in 2010). [7]For 1998 to 2003 data, reflects annual home health HI to SMI transfer amounts. [8]When a beneficiary chooses a Medicare Advantage plan whose monthly premium exceeds the benchmark amount, the additional premiums (that is, amounts beyond those paid by Medicare to the plan) are the responsibility of the beneficiary. [9]Represents misallocation of benefit payments between the HI trust fund and the Part B account of the SMI trust fund from May 2005 to September 2007, and the transfer made in June 2008 to correct the misallocation. [10]Includes expenditures for research, experiments and demonstration projects, peer review activity (performed by Peer Review Organizations from 1983 to 2001 and by Quality Review Organizations from 2002 to present), and to combat and prevent fraud and abuse. [11]Type-of-service reporting categories for fee-for-service reimbursement differ before and after 1991. [12]Includes payment for physicians, practitioners, durable medical equipment, and all suppliers other than independent laboratory through 1990. Starting with 1991 data, physician services subject to the physician fee schedule are shown. Payments for laboratory services paid under the laboratory fee schedule and performed in a physician office are included under Laboratory beginning in 1991. [13]Includes payments for hospital outpatient department services, skilled nursing facility outpatient services, Part B services received as an inpatient in a hospital or skilled nursing facility setting, and other types of outpatient facilities. [14]Starting with 1991 data, those independent laboratory services that were paid under the laboratory fee schedule (most of the independent laboratory category) are included in the Laboratory line; the remaining services are included in the Physician fee schedule and Other lines. [15]Payments for laboratory services paid under the laboratory fee schedule performed in a physician office, independent laboratory, or in a hospital outpatient department. [16]Includes payments for physician-administered drugs; freestanding ambulatory surgical center facility services; ambulance services; supplies; freestanding end-stage renal disease (ESRD) dialysis facility services; rural health clinics; outpatient rehabilitation facilities; psychiatric hospitals; and federally qualified health centers. [17]Includes the hospital facility costs for Medicare Part B services that are predominantly in the outpatient department, with the exception of hospital outpatient laboratory services, which are included on the Laboratory line. Physician reimbursement is included on the Physician fee schedule line. [18]Part D start-up costs were funded through the SMI Part B account in 2004-2008.

Table 3-90. Medicare Enrollees and Program Payments Among Fee-for-Service Medicare Beneficiaries, by Sex and Age, Selected Years, 1994–2010

(Number; percent; dollars.)

Characteristic	1994	1995	2000	2005	2006	2007	2008	2009	2010
Fee-for-Service Enrollees (Numbers in Thousands)									
Total	34,076	34,062	32,740	36,685	35,847	35,490	35,320	35,360	35,910
Sex									
Male	14,533	14,563	14,195	16,251	15,958	15,879	15,890	15,968	16,281
Female	19,543	19,499	18,545	20,433	19,890	19,611	19,430	19,392	19,629
Age									
Under 65 years	4,031	4,239	4,907	6,286	6,225	6,318	6,359	6,435	6,619
65 to 74 years	16,713	16,373	14,230	15,587	15,179	15,041	15,182	15,336	15,648
75 to 84 years	9,845	9,911	9,919	10,689	10,298	9,947	9,592	9,335	9,291
85 years and over	3,486	3,540	3,684	4,123	4,146	4,184	4,187	4,254	4,352
Fee-for-Service Program Payments (Billions of Dollars)									
Total	147	159	174	274	281	289	301	318	331
Sex									
Male	63.9	68.8	76.2	121.0	123.6	126.5	131.5	139.1	145.4
Female	82.6	90.2	98.0	153.2	157.0	162.1	169.7	178.9	185.7
Age									
Under 65 years	18.8	21.0	25.8	46.7	48.4	50.9	54.2	59.7	63.7
65 to 74 years	55.1	58.1	57.5	86.6	87.4	89.1	92.9	98.1	102.5
75 to 84 years	50.7	55.3	62.7	95.2	96.2	96.4	97.9	100.2	101.8
85 years and over	21.8	24.6	28.3	45.6	48.7	52.1	56.1	60.0	63.2
Percent Distribution of Fee-for-Service Program Payments									
Total	100.0	100.0	100.0	100.0	100.0	100.0	100.0	100.0	100.0
Sex									
Male	43.6	43.2	43.7	44.1	44.0	43.8	43.7	43.7	43.9
Female	56.4	56.8	56.3	55.9	56.0	56.2	56.3	56.3	56.1
Age									
Under 65 years	12.9	13.2	14.8	17.0	17.2	17.6	18.0	18.8	19.2
65 to 74 years	37.6	36.5	33.0	31.6	31.1	30.9	30.9	30.9	31.0
75 to 84 years	34.6	34.8	36.0	34.7	34.3	33.4	32.5	31.5	30.7
85 years and over	14.9	15.5	16.2	16.6	17.3	18.0	18.6	18.9	19.1
Average Fee-for-Service Payment Per Enrollee (Dollars) [1]									
Total	4,301	4,667	5,323	7,473	7,830	8,129	8,526	8,993	9,221
Sex									
Male	4,397	4,721	5,370	7,443	7,747	7,964	8,274	8,711	8,931
Female	4,229	4,627	5,286	7,497	7,896	8,263	8,732	9,226	9,461
Age									
Under 65 years	4,673	4,960	5,252	7,435	7,774	8,058	8,530	9,280	9,616
65 to 74 years	3,300	3,548	4,040	5,558	5,756	5,924	6,119	6,398	6,550
75 to 84 years	5,152	5,576	6,320	8,904	9,345	9,696	10,206	10,731	10,953
85 years and over	6,267	6,950	7,684	11,061	11,742	12,440	13,396	14,103	14,527

NOTE: Table includes data for Medicare enrollees residing in Puerto Rico, U.S. Virgin Islands, Guam, other outlying areas, foreign countries, and unknown residence.

[1]Medicare enrollees in managed care plans are not included in the denominator used to calculate average payments.

Table 3-91. Medicare Beneficiaries, by Race, Hispanic Origin, and Selected Characteristics, Selected Years, 1992–2009

(Number; percent; dollars.)

Characteristic	All			White			African American			Hispanic or Latino (of any race)		
	1992	2000	2009	1992	2000	2009	1992	2000	2009	1992	2000	2009
All Medicare beneficiaries (number in millions)	36.8	40.6	47.2	30.9	32.4	36.5	3.3	3.7	4.6	1.9	2.8	3.9
All Medicare beneficiaries (percent distribution)	100.0	100.0	100.0	84.2	80.1	77.3	8.9	9.1	9.8	5.2	7.0	8.2
Medical Care Use												
All Medicare beneficiaries												
Long–term care facility stay	7.7	9.3	8.1	8.0	9.7	8.7	6.2	8.8	8.6	4.2	6.0	4.4
Community-only residents												
Inpatient hospital	17.9	19.2	17.6	18.1	19.2	17.8	18.4	22.8	18.4	16.6	16.2	16.9
Outpatient hospital	57.9	69.8	72.7	57.8	70.7	73.2	61.1	69.0	72.2	53.1	63.7	70.0
Physician/supplier[1]	92.4	94.9	95.9	93.0	95.4	96.3	89.1	92.8	93.4	87.9	92.9	93.3
Dental	40.4	43.5	44.6	43.1	46.9	49.0	23.5	24.1	23.9	29.1	33.9	33.5
Prescription medicine	85.2	91.1	94.3	85.5	91.5	94.4	83.1	89.5	93.0	84.6	90.1	94.6
Expenditures												
All Medicare beneficiaries												
Total health care[2]	6,716	10,490	16,068	6,816	10,475	15,938	7,043	12,328	19,211	5,784	9,089	14,860
Long-term care facility[3]	1,581	2,310	2,438	1,674	2,406	2,533	1,255	2,438	2,598	*758	1,799	1,758
Community-only residents												
Total personal health care	5,054	7,911	12,295	4,988	7,814	12,031	5,530	9,419	14,210	4,938	6,934	12,754
Inpatient hospital	2,098	2,664	2,363	2,058	2,605	2,222	2,493	3,465	3,454	1,999	2,133	2,496
Outpatient hospital	504	875	1,385	478	796	1,312	668	1,523	1,873	511	915	1,414
Physician/supplier[1]	1,524	2,491	3,336	1,525	2,503	3,476	1,398	2,621	2,763	1,587	2,234	2,836
Dental	142	258	408	153	278	460	70	101	204	97	193	220
Prescription medicine	468	1,163	3,013	481	1,182	2,891	417	1,135	3,565	389	1,014	3,316
Long-term care facility residents only												
Long–term care facility[4]	23,054	32,442	42,103	23,177	31,795	41,174	21,272	36,132	44,326	*25,026	*39,057	*50,851
Sex												
Both sexes	100.0	100.0	100.0	100.0	100.0	100.0	100.0	100.0	100.0	100.0	100.0	100.0
Male	42.9	43.4	45.1	42.7	43.3	45.2	42.0	40.0	45.1	46.7	46.9	44.8
Female	57.1	56.6	54.9	57.3	56.7	54.8	58.0	60.0	54.9	53.3	53.1	55.2
Eligibility Criteria and Age												
All Medicare beneficiaries[5]	100.0	100.0	100.0	100.0	100.0	100.0	100.0	100.0	100.0	100.0	100.0	100.0
Disabled	10.2	13.6	16.0	8.6	11.5	13.2	19.1	23.3	31.4	16.5	21.7	23.6
Under 45 years	3.5	3.9	3.7	2.9	3.2	3.0	7.6	7.5	8.0	6.9	5.5	5.6
45 to 64 years	6.5	9.8	12.3	5.8	8.3	10.2	11.5	15.8	23.4	9.6	16.3	18.0
Aged												
65 to 74 years	89.8	86.4	84.0	91.4	88.5	86.9	81.0	76.7	68.5	83.5	78.3	76.4
75 to 84 years	51.5	45.4	45.1	52.0	46.7	45.5	48.0	41.7	39.3	49.4	45.5	47.2
85 years and over	28.8	30.0	26.8	29.5	31.4	28.3	24.0	25.9	20.8	27.1	22.9	21.6
	9.7	10.9	12.1	9.9	11.5	13.2	9.0	9.0	8.4	6.9	9.9	7.6
Living Arrangement												
All living arrangements	100.0	100.0	100.0	100.0	100.0	100.0	100.0	100.0	100.0	100.0	100.0	100.0
Alone	27.0	29.3	29.1	27.5	29.8	30.1	27.7	32.5	31.1	20.2	22.9	21.7
With spouse	51.2	49.0	48.7	53.3	51.0	51.0	33.3	30.0	30.8	50.4	49.2	48.6
With children	9.1	9.5	10.2	7.7	7.6	8.2	16.8	18.6	17.9	16.6	14.8	15.4
With others	7.6	7.1	7.9	6.2	6.2	6.5	18.1	13.7	16.4	10.8	9.9	11.7
Long-term care facility	5.1	5.1	4.1	5.3	5.4	4.3	4.0	5.2	3.8	*2.0	*3.3	*2.7
Age and Limitation of Activity [6]												
Disabled, under age 65 years	100.0	100.0	100.0	100.0	100.0	100.0	100.0	100.0	100.0	100.0	100.0	100.0
None	22.7	27.3	40.9	21.8	25.2	42.8	26.2	35.7	37.5	21.2	30.1	38.3
IADL only	39.0	35.1	32.1	38.9	35.5	31.5	35.8	33.2	36.8	46.1	37.3	28.5
1 or 2 IADL	21.2	21.8	16.8	21.5	23.2	16.6	21.2	17.7	15.0	*20.9	*16.8	*17.9
3 to 5 IADL	17.2	15.9	10.3	17.9	16.1	9.1	*16.8	*13.5	*10.8	*11.9	*15.8	*15.4
65 to 74 years	100.0	100.0	100.0	100.0	100.0	100.0	100.0	100.0	100.0	100.0	100.0	100.0
None	67.0	71.5	72.5	68.7	72.6	74.5	55.1	64.8	68.9	59.2	69.4	61.1
IADL only	17.8	15.4	15.3	17.0	15.1	14.3	22.9	18.0	14.1	*20.9	*13.6	23.0
1 or 2 IADL	10.4	8.6	7.7	9.6	8.2	7.3	14.4	10.8	*9.5	*15.7	*13.2	*10.1
3 to 5 IADL	4.8	4.5	4.5	4.6	4.2	3.9	*7.6	*6.3	*7.5	*4.2	*4.0	*5.8
75 to 84 years	100.0	100.0	100.0	100.0	100.0	100.0	100.0	100.0	100.0	100.0	100.0	100.0
None	46.6	52.2	52.8	47.5	53.1	54.2	42.0	46.2	44.9	44.3	48.3	51.9
IADL only	23.9	23.0	23.1	23.6	22.7	22.9	26.7	20.9	25.7	*27.8	24.9	*20.3
1 or 2 IADL	16.5	14.3	13.6	16.8	13.8	13.5	15.3	17.7	*13.3	*14.9	*18.6	*13.8
3 to 5 IADL	13.0	10.6	10.5	12.2	10.4	9.4	*15.9	15.2	*16.2	*13.0	*8.2	*14.1
85 years and over	100.0	100.0	100.0	100.0	100.0	100.0	100.0	100.0	100.0	100.0	100.0	100.0
None	19.9	24.9	27.0	20.2	25.1	27.7	*19.6	*25.9	*18.0	*19.7	*23.4	*24.7
IADL only	20.9	22.6	26.6	20.2	22.4	26.3	*22.1	*19.7	*33.6	*24.7	24.7	*21.7
1 or 2 IADL	23.5	22.2	19.7	23.5	22.3	20.4	*24.3	*19.3	*12.5	*23.7	*28.1	*16.7
3 to 5 IADL	35.8	30.4	26.8	36.1	30.2	25.6	*34.0	35.1	*35.9	*31.8	*23.8	*37.0

* = Figure does not meet standards of reliability or precision. Estimates are based on 50 persons or fewer or with a relative standard error of 30 percent or higher and are considered unreliable. [1]Physician/supplier services include medical and osteopathic doctor and health practitioner visits, diagnostic laboratory and radiology services, medical and surgical services, and durable medical equipment and nondurable medical supplies. [2]Total health care expenditures by Medicare beneficiaries, including expenses paid by Medicare and all other sources of payment for the following services: inpatient hospital, outpatient hospital, physician/supplier, dental, prescription medicine, home health, and hospice and long-term care facility care. Does not include health insurance premiums. [3]Expenditures for long-term care in facilities for all beneficiaries include facility room and board expenses for beneficiaries who resided in a facility for the full year, for beneficiaries who resided in a facility for part of the year and in the community for part of the year, and expenditures for short-term facility stays for full-year or part-year community residents. [4]Expenditures for facility-based long-term care for facility-based beneficiaries include facility room and board expenses for beneficiaries who resided in a facility for the full year and for beneficiaries who resided in a facility for part of the year and in the community for part of the year. They do not include expenditures for short-term facility stays for full-year community residents. [5]Medicare beneficiaries with end-stage renal disease (ESRD) are included within the subgroups Aged and Disabled. In 2007, less than 1 percent of Medicare beneficiaries qualified because of ESRD. [6]IADL is instrumental activities of daily living; ADL is activities of daily living. Includes data for both community and long-term care facility residents.

Table 3-92. Medicare Enrollees, Enrollees in Managed Care, Payment per Enrollee, and Short-Stay Hospital Utilization, by State, Selected Years, 1994–2010

(Number; percent; dollars; rate per 1,000 enrollees.)

State	Enrollment in thousands[1]		Percent of enrollees in managed care[2]		Payment per fee-for-service enrollee		Discharges per 1,000 enrollees[3]		Average length of stay in days[3]	
	1994	2010	1994	2010	1994	2010	1994	2010	1994	2010
United States [4]	36,190	46,585	7.9	24.3	$4,375	$9,347	345	352	7.5	5.4
Alabama	633	845	0.8	21.4	4,454	8,539	413	385	7.0	5.3
Alaska	33	66	0.6	0.9	3,687	7,492	269	226	6.3	5.2
Arizona	578	930	24.8	36.1	4,442	8,659	292	324	5.9	4.8
Arkansas	416	531	0.2	14.3	3,719	7,849	366	335	7.0	5.2
California	3,582	4,757	30.0	35.4	5,219	9,666	366	318	6.1	5.4
Colorado	413	625	17.2	33.5	3,935	8,234	302	293	6.0	4.7
Connecticut	497	568	2.6	18.3	4,426	10,138	287	359	8.1	5.6
Delaware	99	149	0.2	3.7	4,712	9,207	326	312	8.1	5.8
District of Columbia	80	78	3.9	9.8	5,655	10,428	376	388	10.1	6.1
Florida	2,584	3,375	13.8	30.1	5,027	10,777	326	374	7.1	5.5
Georgia	819	1,236	0.4	21.2	4,402	8,849	378	336	6.9	5.4
Hawaii	146	206	29.8	41.6	3,069	5,960	301	218	9.1	6.6
Idaho	146	230	2.5	29.1	3,045	7,041	274	214	5.2	4.4
Illinois	1,605	1,839	5.5	9.7	4,324	9,691	374	382	7.3	5.2
Indiana	805	1,006	2.6	16.3	3,945	8,900	345	346	6.9	5.2
Iowa	470	517	3.1	13.2	3,080	7,571	322	276	6.6	5.1
Kansas	378	433	3.3	11.0	3,847	8,434	348	303	6.5	5.1
Kentucky	578	760	2.3	16.2	3,862	8,701	396	385	7.2	5.2
Louisiana	572	687	0.4	23.8	5,468	10,757	399	386	7.2	5.6
Maine	198	265	0.1	12.6	3,464	7,249	322	259	7.6	5.1
Maryland	596	785	1.4	8.1	4,997	10,425	362	381	7.5	5.0
Massachusetts	924	1,061	6.1	19.2	5,147	10,282	350	377	7.6	5.2
Michigan	1,331	1,651	0.7	16.3	4,307	10,152	328	391	7.6	5.3
Minnesota	625	786	19.6	41.7	3,394	9,322	334	391	5.7	4.6
Mississippi	391	497	0.1	9.6	4,189	9,879	423	382	7.4	5.8
Missouri	821	1,004	3.4	21.0	4,191	8,651	349	370	7.3	5.2
Montana	128	170	0.4	17.9	3,114	6,838	306	225	5.9	4.7
Nebraska	247	279	2.2	12.0	2,926	8,383	281	292	6.3	5.1
Nevada	187	357	19.0	30.3	4,306	9,069	291	317	7.0	5.5
New Hampshire	152	223	0.2	7.8	3,414	8,260	281	242	7.6	5.2
New Jersey	1,158	1,327	2.6	12.6	4,531	10,569	354	371	10.2	5.9
New Mexico	205	313	13.6	25.1	3,110	6,999	301	268	6.0	5.0
New York	2,601	2,988	6.2	30.2	4,855	10,127	334	402	11.2	6.7
North Carolina	1,001	1,490	0.5	17.8	3,465	8,694	314	333	8.0	5.3
North Dakota	101	109	0.6	8.5	3,218	7,036	327	247	6.3	4.9
Ohio	1,649	1,901	2.4	33.1	3,982	9,600	350	426	7.1	5.1
Oklahoma	481	603	2.5	15.1	4,098	9,097	355	374	7.0	5.2
Oregon	469	621	27.7	41.6	3,285	6,807	305	244	5.2	4.6
Pennsylvania	2,053	2,283	3.3	38.0	5,212	9,419	379	425	8.0	5.6
Rhode Island	166	183	7.0	34.5	4,148	9,108	312	364	8.1	5.9
South Carolina	497	774	0.1	16.0	3,777	8,886	319	330	8.3	5.6
South Dakota	114	137	0.1	8.1	2,952	7,103	356	259	6.1	5.0
Tennessee	754	1,058	0.3	24.5	4,441	8,714	375	373	7.1	5.3
Texas	2,029	3,001	4.1	19.6	4,703	10,694	333	342	7.2	5.4
Utah	182	283	9.4	33.7	3,443	7,667	238	256	5.4	4.4
Vermont	82	112	0.1	4.5	3,182	8,069	283	199	7.6	5.3
Virginia	803	1,141	1.5	14.6	3,748	7,831	348	319	7.3	5.3
Washington	676	972	12.5	25.1	3,401	7,455	269	254	5.3	4.7
West Virginia	326	382	8.3	22.8	3,798	8,213	420	381	7.1	5.6
Wisconsin	752	911	2.0	29.3	3,246	8,056	310	301	6.8	5.0
Wyoming	58	80	3.3	6.8	3,537	7,218	315	236	5.6	4.6

[1]Total persons enrolled in hospital insurance, supplementary medical insurance, or both, as of July 1. Includes fee-for-service and managed care enrollees.   [2]Includes enrollees in Medicare-approved managed care organizations.   [3]Data are for fee-for-service enrollees only.   [4]Includes residents of any of the 50 states and the District of Columbia.

Table 3-93. Medicare-Certified Providers and Suppliers, Selected Years, 1975–2010

(Number of providers or suppliers.)

Providers or suppliers	1975	1980	1985	1990	2000	2005	2006	2007	2008	2009	2010
Skilled nursing facilities	NA	5,052	6,451	8,937	14,841	15,006	15,028	15,054	15,032	15,071	15,084
Home health agencies	2,242	2,924	5,679	5,730	7,857	8,090	8,618	9,024	9,407	10,184	10,914
Clinical Laboratory Improvement Amendments facilities	NA	NA	NA	NA	171,018	196,296	199,817	206,065	210,872	218,139	224,679
End-stage renal disease facilities	NA	999	1,393	1,937	3,787	4,755	4,892	5,095	5,317	5,476	5,631
Outpatient physical therapy	117	419	854	1,195	2,867	2,962	3,009	2,915	2,781	2,640	2,536
Portable X-ray	132	216	308	443	666	553	549	550	547	546	561
Rural health clinics	NA	391	428	551	3,453	3,661	3,723	3,781	3,757	3,752	3,845
Comprehensive outpatient rehabilitation facilities	NA	NA	72	186	522	634	589	539	476	406	354
Ambulatory surgical centers	NA	NA	336	1,197	2,894	4,445	4,707	4,964	5,174	5,260	5,316
Hospices	NA	NA	164	825	2,326	2,872	3,071	3,255	3,346	3,405	3,509
Critical access hospitals	NA	NA	NA	NA	NA	NA	NA	NA	1,302	1,311	1,325

NA = Not available.

NOTES AND DEFINITIONS

SOURCES OF DATA

The principal source for data presented in this part is from *Health, United States, 2011: With Special Feature on Socioeconomic Status and Health,* Hyattsville, MD, 2012, an annual report on trends in health statistics compiled by the National Center of Health Statistics (NCHS), a component of the Centers for Disease Control and Prevention (CDC). Updated tables for this publication can be found at http://www.cdc.gov/nchs/hus/contents2011.htm#023.

The data for Tables 3-63 through 3-69 are from the Bureau of Labor Statistics (BLS), Occupational Employment Statistics. For more detailed information, see Occupational Employment and Wages news release. (USDL-12-0548) OES can be accessed at http://www.bls.gov/oes/.

CONCEPTS AND DEFINITIONS

Age-adjustment—used to compare risks of two or more populations at one point in time or one population at two or more points in time. Age-adjusted rates are computed by the direct method by applying age-specific rates in a population of interest to a standardized age distribution, to eliminate differences in observed rates that result from age differences in population composition. Age-adjusted rates should be viewed as relative indexes rather than actual measures of risk. Age-adjusted estimates from other age-adjusted estimates based on the same data and presented elsewhere if different age groups are used in the adjustment procedure.

Body mass index (BMI)—a measure that adjusts bodyweight for height. It is calculated as weight in kilograms divided by height in meters squared. Overweight for children and adolescents is defined as BMI at or above the sex- and age-specific 95th percentile BMI cut points from the 2000 CDC Growth Charts. Healthy weight for adults is defined as a BMI of 18.5 to less than 25; overweight, as greater than or equal to a BMI of 25; and obesity, as greater than or equal to a BMI of 30.

Cholesterol, serum—a measure of the total blood cholesterol. Elevated total blood cholesterol—a combination of high-density lipoproteins (HDL), low-density lipoproteins (LDL), and very-low density lipoproteins (VLDL)—is a risk factor for cardiovascular disease. According to the National Cholesterol Education Program, high serum cholesterol is defined as greater than or equal to 240 mg/dL (6.20 mmol/L). Borderline high serum cholesterol is defined as greater than or equal to 200 mg/dL and less than 240 mg/dL. Assessments of the components of total cholesterol or lower thresholds for

high total cholesterol may be used for individuals with other risk factors for cardiovascular disease.

Condition—A health condition is a departure from a state of physical or mental well-being. In the National Health interview Survey, each condition reported as a cause of an individual's activity limitation has been classified as chronic, not chronic, or unknown if chronic, based on the nature and duration of the condition.

Consumer Price Index (CPI)—prepared by the U.S. Bureau of Labor Statistics. It is a monthly measure of the average change in the prices paid by urban consumers for a fixed market basket of goods and services. The medical care component of CPI shows trends in medical care prices based on specific indicators of hospital, medical, dental, and drug prices. A revision of the definition of CPI has been in use since January 1988.

Dental caries—evidence of tooth decay on any surface of the tooth. Untreated dental caries are determined by an oral examination conducted by a trained dentist.

Diagnosis—the act or process of identifying or determining the nature and cause of a disease or injury through evaluation of patient history, examination, and review of laboratory data.

Gross domestic product (GDP)—the market value of the goods and services produced by labor and property located in the United States. As long as the labor and property are located in the United States, the suppliers (i.e., the workers and, for property, the owners) may be U.S. residents or residents of other countries.

Health expenditures, national—estimated by the Centers for Medicare & Medicaid Services (CMS) it measures spending for health care in the United States by type of service delivered (e.g., hospital care, physician services, nursing home care) and source of funding for those services (e.g., private health insurance, Medicare, Medicaid, out-of-pocket spending). CMS produces both historical and projected estimates of health expenditures by category.

Health insurance coverage—broadly defined to include both public and private payers who cover medical expenditures incurred by a defined population in a variety of settings.

Health maintenance organization (HMO)—a health care system that assumes or shares both the financial risks and the delivery risks associated with providing comprehensive medical services to a voluntarily enrolled population in a particular geographic area, usually in return for a fixed, prepaid fee. Pure HMO enrollees use only the prepaid capitated health services of the HMO panel of medical care providers. Open-ended HMO enrollees use the prepaid HMO health services but, in addition, may receive medical care from providers who are not part of the HMO panel. There is usually a substantial deductible, co-payment, or co-insurance associated with use of non-panel providers.

Hispanic origin—includes persons of Mexican, Puerto Rican, Cuban, Central and South American, and other or unknown Latin American or Spanish origins. Persons of Hispanic origin may be of any race.

Hypertension—elevated blood pressure or hypertension is defined as having an average systolic blood pressure reading of at least 140mmHg or diastolic pressure of at least 90 mmHg, which is consistent with the Seventh Report of the Joint National Committee on Prevention, Detection, Evaluation, and Treatment of High Blood Pressure. People are also considered to have hypertension if they report that they are taking a prescription medicine for high blood pressure, even if their blood pressure readings are within normal range.

Incidence—the number of cases of disease having their onset during a prescribed period of time. It is often expressed as a rate (e.g., the incidence of measles per 1,000 children 5–15 years of age during a specified year). Incidence is a measure of morbidity or other events that occur within a specified period of time. Measuring incidence may be complicated because the population at risk for the disease may change during the period of interest, for example, due to births, deaths, or migration. In addition, determining that a case is new—that is, that its onset occurred during the prescribed period of time—may be difficult. Because of these difficulties in measuring incidence, many health statistics are measured using prevalence.

Instrumental activities of daily living (IADL)—activities related to independent living and include preparing meals, managing money, shopping for groceries or personal items, performing light or heavy housework, and using a telephone. In the National Health Interview Survey (NHIS) respondents are asked whether they or family members 18 years of age and over need the help of another person for handling routine IADL needs because of a physical, mental, or emotional problem. Persons are considered to have an IADL limitation in the NHIS if any causal condition is chronic.

Limitation of activity—may be defined different ways, depending on the conceptual framework. In the National Health Interview Survey, limitation of activity refers to a long-term reduction in a person's capacity to perform the usual kind or amount of activities associated with his or her age group as a result of a chronic condition. Limitation of activity is assessed by asking persons a series of questions about limitations in their or household members' ability to perform activities usual for their age group because of a

physical, mental, or emotional problem. Persons are asked about limitations in activities of daily living, instrumental activities of daily living, play, school, work, difficulty walking or remembering, and any other activity limitations. For reported limitations, the causal health conditions are determined, and persons are considered limited if one or more of these conditions is chronic. Children under 18 years of age who receive special education or early intervention services are considered to have a limitation of activity.

Mammography—an x-ray image of the breast used to detect irregularities of the breast tissue.

Managed care—a term originally used to refer to the prepaid health care sector (health maintenance organizations or HMOs) where care is provided under a fixed budget and costs are therein capable of being managed. Increasingly, the term is being used to include preferred provider organizations (PPOs) and even forms of indemnity.

Medicare—the federal program which helps pay health care costs for people 65 and older and for certain people under 65 with long-term disabilities.

Medicaid—a program authorized by the Social Security Act in 1965 as a jointly funded cooperative venture between the federal and state governments to assist states in the provision of adequate medical care to eligible needy persons. Families with dependent children, the aged, blind, and disabled who are in financial need are eligible for Medicaid.

Notifiable disease—a disease, that when diagnosed, health providers are required, usually by law, to report to state or local public health officials. Notifiable diseases are those of public interest by reason of their contagiousness, severity, or frequency.

Pap smear—a microscopic examination of cells scraped from the cervix that is used to detect cancerous or precancerous conditions of the cervix or other medical conditions.

Physical activity, leisure-time—starting with 1998 data, leisure-time physical activity is assessed in the National Health Interview Survey by asking adults a series of questions about how often they do vigorous or light/moderate physical activity of at least 10 minutes duration and for about how long these sessions generally last. Vigorous physical activity is described as causing heavy sweating or a large increase in breathing or heart rate and light/moderate as causing light sweating or a slight to moderate increase in breathing or heart rate. Adults classified as inactive did not report any sessions of light/moderate or vigorous leisure-time physical activity of at least 10 minutes duration or reported they were unable to perform leisure-time physical activity. Adults classified with some leisure-time activity reported at least one session of light/moderate or vigorous activity of at least 10 minutes duration but did not meet the requirement for regular leisure-time activity. Adults classified with regular leisure-time activity reported at least three sessions per week of vigorous leisure-time physical activity lasting at least 20 minutes in duration or at least five sessions per week of light/moderate physical activity lasting at least 30 minutes in duration.

Poverty—based on definitions originally developed by the Social Security Administration. These include a set of money income thresholds that vary by family size and composition. Families or individuals with income below their appropriate thresholds are classified as below poverty. These thresholds are updated annually by the U.S. Census Bureau to reflect changes in the Consumer Price Index for all urban consumers (CPI-U). For example, the average poverty threshold for a family of four was $22,314 in 2010, $17,603 in 2000, and $13,359 in 1990.

Preferred provider organization (PPO)—a type of medical plan where coverage is provided to participants through a network of selected health care providers (such as hospitals and physicians). The enrollees may go outside the network, but they would pay a greater percentage of the cost of coverage than within the network.

Prevalence—the number of cases of a disease, infected persons, or persons with some other attribute present during a particular interval of time. It is often expressed as a rate (e.g., the prevalence of diabetes per 1,000 persons during a year).

Short-stay hospital—hospitals that provide general (rather than specialized) care and have an average length of stay of less than 30 days.

Specialty hospital—hospitals that provide a particular type of service to the majority of their patients such as psychiatric, tuberculosis, chronic disease, rehabilitation, maternity, and alcoholic or narcotic.

State Children's Health Insurance Program (SCHIP)—Title XXI of the Social Security Act, known as the State Children's Health Insurance Program (SCHIP), is a program initiated by the Balanced Budget Act of 1997 (BBA). SCHIP provides more federal funds for states to provide health care coverage to low-income, uninsured children. SCHIP gives states broad flexibility in program design while protecting beneficiaries through federal standards. Funds from SCHIP may be used to expand Medicaid or to provide medical assistance to children during a presumptive eligibility period for Medicaid. This is one of several options from which states may select to provide health care coverage for more children, as prescribed within the BBA's Title XXI program.

Substance use—the use of selected substances including alcohol, tobacco products, drugs, inhalants, and other substances that can be consumed, inhaled, injected, or otherwise absorbed into the body with possible detrimental effects.

Suicidal ideation—having thoughts of suicide or of taking action to end one's own life. Suicidal ideation includes all thoughts of suicide, both when the thoughts include a plan to commit suicide and when they do not include a plan. Suicidal ideation is measured in the Youth Risk Behavior Survey by the question "During the past 12 months, did you ever seriously consider attempting suicide?"

Uninsured—in the Current Population Survey (CPS) persons are considered uninsured if they do not have coverage through private health insurance, Medicare, Medicaid, State Children's Health Insurance Program, military or Veterans coverage, another government program, a plan of someone outside the household, or other insurance. Persons with only Indian Health Service coverage are considered uninsured. In addition, if the respondent has missing Medicaid information but has income from certain low-income public programs, then Medicaid coverage is imputed. The questions on health insurance are administered in March and refer to the previous calendar year.

PART D

MARRIAGE

CHAPTER 4: MARRIAGE

Figure 4-1. Marriage and Divorce Rates, United States, Selected States, 2000–2011

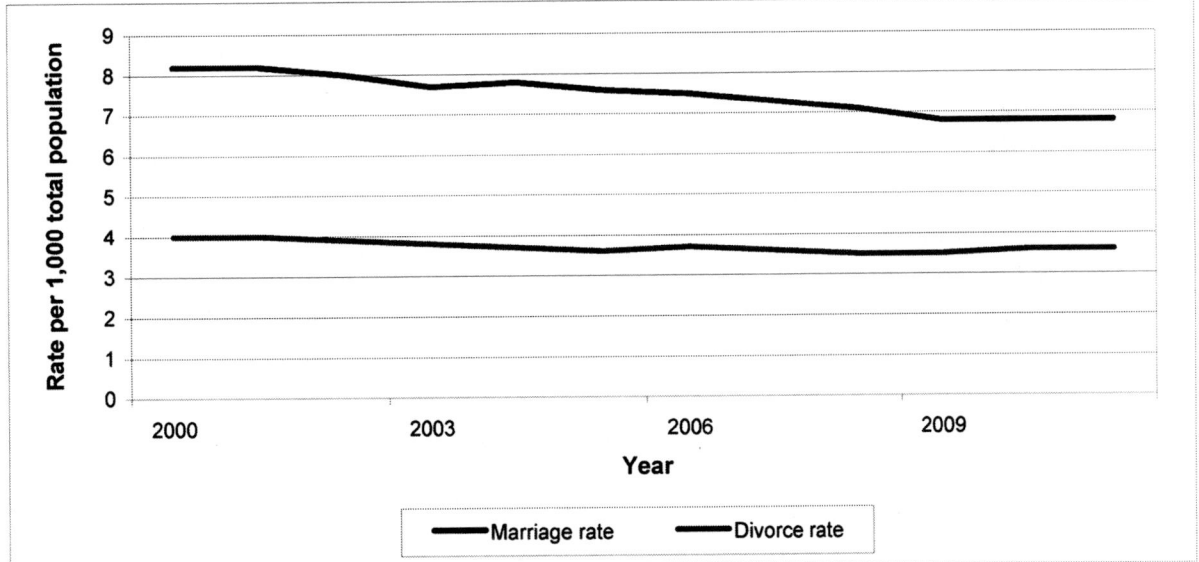

HIGHLIGHTS

- In 2011, Nevada had the highest rate of marriage per 1,000 resident population at 36.9, significantly greater than the next-highest states (Hawaii, 17.6; Arkansas, 10.4; and Tennessee, 9.0). New Jersey had the lowest marriage rate, at 4.8, followed by Mississippi at 4.9, Delaware at 5.2, and Pennsylvania and Wisconsin, each at 5.3. (Table 4-1)

- Among reporting states (California, Georgia, Hawaii, Indiana, Louisiana, and Minnesota did not have available information) in 2011, Iowa had the lowest divorce rate, at 2.4 per 1,000 resident population, followed by Illinois (2.6), Massachusetts and North Dakota (2.7 each), and Pennsylvania (2.8). Nevada, which had the highest marriage rate, also had the highest divorce rate at 5.6, followed by Arkansas (5.3), West Virginia and Oklahoma (5.2 each), and Idaho (4.9). (Table 4-2)

- The median age at first marriage for all races and origins in the United States was 29.1 years for males and 27.1 years for females in 2012. Male median ages ranged from 28.0 for Native Hawaiian and Other Pacific Islanders to 31.0 for Black or African American alone males. Ages for females ranged from 26.5 for Hispanic or Latino origin to 31.0 for Black or African American alone. (Table 4-6)

- In the United States, the median duration of current marriages was 19.3 years in 2012. The District of Columbia had the shortest median duration, at 12.3 years, while South Dakota had the longest median duration, at 22.5 years. (Table 4-10)

Table 4-1. Marriage Rates, by State, Selected Years, 1990–2011

(Rate per 1,000 total population residing in area.)

State	Marriage rate										
	1990	1995	1999	2000	2005	2006	2007	2008	2009	2010	2011
Alabama	10.6	9.8	10.8	10.1	9.2	9.2	8.9	8.6	8.3	8.2	8.4
Alaska	10.2	9.0	8.6	8.9	8.2	8.2	8.5	8.4	7.8	8.0	7.8
Arizona	10.0	8.8	8.2	7.5	6.6	6.5	6.4	6.0	5.6	5.9	5.7
Arkansas	15.3	14.4	14.8	15.4	12.9	12.4	12.0	10.6	10.7	10.8	10.4
California[1]	7.9	6.3	6.4	5.8	6.4	6.3	6.2	6.7	5.8	5.8	5.8
Colorado	9.8	9.0	8.2	8.3	7.6	7.2	7.1	7.4	6.9	6.9	7.0
Connecticut	7.9	6.6	5.8	5.7	5.8	5.5	5.5	5.4	5.9	5.6	5.5
Delaware	8.4	7.3	6.7	6.5	5.9	5.9	5.7	5.5	5.4	5.2	5.2
District of Columbia	8.2	6.1	6.6	4.9	4.1	4.0	4.2	4.1	4.7	7.6	8.7
Florida	10.9	9.9	8.7	8.9	8.9	8.6	8.5	8.0	7.5	7.3	7.4
Georgia	10.3	8.4	7.8	6.8	7.0	7.3	6.8	6.0	6.6	7.3	6.6
Hawaii	16.4	15.7	18.9	20.6	22.6	21.9	20.8	19.1	17.2	17.6	17.6
Idaho	13.9	13.1	12.1	10.8	10.5	10.1	10.0	9.5	8.9	8.8	8.6
Illinois	8.8	6.9	7.0	6.9	5.9	6.2	6.1	5.9	5.7	5.7	5.6
Indiana	9.6	8.6	8.1	7.9	6.9	7.0	7.0	8.0	7.9	6.3	6.8
Iowa	9.0	7.7	7.9	6.9	6.9	6.7	6.6	6.5	7.0	6.9	6.7
Kansas	9.2	8.5	7.1	8.3	6.8	6.8	6.8	6.7	6.4	6.4	6.3
Kentucky	13.5	12.2	10.9	9.8	8.7	8.4	7.8	7.9	7.6	7.4	7.5
Louisiana	9.6	9.3	9.1	9.1	8.0	NA	7.5	6.8	7.1	6.9	6.4
Maine	9.7	8.7	8.6	8.8	8.2	7.8	7.4	7.4	7.1	7.1	7.2
Maryland	9.7	8.4	7.5	7.5	6.9	6.6	6.5	5.9	5.8	5.7	5.8
Massachusetts	7.9	7.1	6.2	5.8	6.2	5.9	5.9	5.7	5.6	5.6	5.5
Michigan	8.2	7.3	6.8	6.7	6.1	5.9	5.7	5.6	5.4	5.5	5.7
Minnesota	7.7	7.0	6.8	6.8	6.0	6.0	5.8	5.4	5.3	5.3	5.6
Mississippi	9.4	7.9	7.8	6.9	5.8	5.7	5.4	5.1	4.8	4.9	4.9
Missouri	9.6	8.3	8.1	7.8	7.0	6.9	6.9	6.8	6.5	6.5	6.6
Montana	8.6	7.6	7.4	7.3	7.4	7.4	7.5	7.6	7.3	7.4	7.8
Nebraska	8.0	7.3	7.5	7.6	7.0	6.8	6.8	6.9	6.6	6.6	6.6
Nevada	99.0	85.2	82.3	72.2	57.4	52.1	48.6	42.3	40.3	38.3	36.9
New Hampshire	9.5	8.3	7.9	9.4	7.3	7.2	7.1	6.8	6.5	7.3	7.1
New Jersey	7.6	6.5	5.9	6.0	5.7	5.5	5.4	5.4	5.0	5.1	4.8
New Mexico	8.8	8.8	8.0	8.0	6.6	6.8	5.6	4.0	5.0	7.7	8.0
New York	8.6	8.0	7.3	7.1	6.8	6.9	6.8	6.6	6.5	6.5	6.9
North Carolina	7.8	8.4	8.5	8.2	7.3	7.3	7.0	6.9	6.6	6.6	6.7
North Dakota	7.5	7.1	6.6	7.2	6.8	6.7	6.6	6.5	6.4	6.5	6.7
Ohio	9.0	8.0	7.8	7.8	6.5	6.3	6.1	6.0	5.8	5.8	5.9
Oklahoma	10.6	8.6	6.8	NA	7.3	7.3	7.3	7.1	6.9	7.2	6.9
Oregon	8.9	8.1	7.6	7.6	7.3	7.3	7.2	6.9	6.6	6.5	6.6
Pennsylvania	7.1	6.2	6.1	6.0	5.8	5.7	5.7	5.5	5.3	5.3	5.3
Rhode Island	8.1	7.3	7.5	7.6	7.0	6.6	6.4	6.1	5.9	5.8	6.0
South Carolina	15.9	11.9	10.2	10.6	8.3	7.8	7.9	7.3	7.3	7.4	7.2
South Dakota	11.1	9.9	9.1	9.4	8.4	8.0	7.8	7.7	7.3	7.3	7.5
Tennessee	13.9	15.5	14.7	15.5	10.9	10.6	10.1	9.4	8.4	8.8	9.0
Texas	10.5	9.9	9.1	9.4	7.8	7.6	7.4	7.3	7.1	7.1	7.1
Utah	11.2	10.7	9.6	10.8	9.8	9.2	9.6	9.0	8.4	8.5	8.6
Vermont	10.9	10.3	10.0	10.0	8.9	8.6	8.5	7.9	8.7	9.3	8.3
Virginia	11.4	10.2	9.2	8.8	8.2	7.8	7.5	7.2	6.9	6.8	6.8
Washington	9.5	7.7	7.2	6.9	6.5	6.5	6.4	6.3	6.0	6.0	6.1
West Virginia	7.2	6.1	7.5	8.7	7.4	7.3	7.3	7.1	6.7	6.7	7.2
Wisconsin	7.9	7.0	6.7	6.7	6.1	6.0	5.7	5.6	5.3	5.3	5.3
Wyoming	10.7	10.6	9.9	10.0	9.3	9.3	9.0	8.6	8.0	7.6	7.8

NA = Not available.   [1]Marriage data includes nonlicensed marriages registered.

Table 4-2. Divorce Rates, by State, Selected Years, 1990–2011

(Rate per 1,000 total population residing in area.)

State	Divorce rate[1]										
	1990	1995	1999	2000	2005	2006	2007	2008	2009	2010	2011
Alabama	6.1	6.0	5.7	5.5	4.9	4.9	4.5	4.3	4.4	4.4	4.3
Alaska	5.5	5.0	5.0	3.9	4.3	4.2	4.3	4.4	4.4	4.7	4.8
Arizona	6.9	6.2	4.6	4.6	4.2	4.0	4.0	3.8	3.6	3.5	3.9
Arkansas	6.9	6.3	6.2	6.4	6.0	5.8	5.9	5.5	5.7	5.7	5.3
California	4.3	NA	NA	NA	NA	NA	NA	NA	NA	NA	NA
Colorado	5.5	NA	4.8	4.7	4.4	4.5	4.4	4.3	4.3	4.3	4.4
Connecticut	3.2	2.9	3.0	3.3	3.0	3.1	3.2	3.4	3.0	2.9	3.1
Delaware	4.4	5.0	4.5	3.9	3.8	3.8	3.7	3.5	3.6	3.5	3.6
District of Columbia	4.5	3.2	3.6	3.2	2.0	2.1	1.7	2.7	2.7	2.8	2.9
Florida	6.3	5.5	5.1	5.1	4.6	4.7	4.6	4.3	4.2	4.4	4.5
Georgia	5.5	5.1	4.1	3.3	NA	NA	NA	NA	NA	NA	NA
Hawaii	4.6	4.6	3.8	3.9	NA	NA	NA	NA	NA	NA	NA
Idaho	6.5	5.8	5.4	5.5	5.0	5.0	4.9	4.8	5.0	5.2	4.9
Illinois	3.8	3.2	3.3	3.2	2.6	2.5	2.6	2.5	2.5	2.6	2.6
Indiana	NA	NA	NA	NA	NA	NA	NA	NA	NA	NA	NA
Iowa	3.9	3.7	3.3	3.3	2.7	2.7	2.5	2.6	2.4	2.4	2.4
Kansas	5.0	4.1	3.4	3.6	3.1	3.1	3.4	3.5	3.6	3.7	3.9
Kentucky	5.8	5.9	5.5	5.1	4.6	5.0	4.6	4.6	4.6	4.5	4.4
Louisiana	NA	NA	NA	NA	NA	NA	NA	NA	NA	NA	NA
Maine	4.3	4.4	5.1	5.0	4.1	4.2	4.2	4.2	4.1	4.2	4.2
Maryland	3.4	3.0	3.2	3.3	3.1	3.0	2.9	2.8	2.8	2.8	2.9
Massachusetts	2.8	2.2	2.5	2.5	2.2	2.3	2.3	2.0	2.2	2.5	2.7
Michigan	4.3	4.1	3.8	3.9	3.4	3.5	3.4	3.4	3.3	3.5	3.4
Minnesota	3.5	3.4	3.2	3.2	NA	NA	NA	NA	NA	NA	NA
Mississippi	5.5	4.8	5.0	5.0	4.4	4.8	4.5	4.3	4.1	4.3	4.0
Missouri	5.1	5.0	4.4	4.5	3.6	3.8	3.8	3.7	3.8	3.9	3.9
Montana	5.1	4.8	2.8	4.2	4.5	4.4	4.0	4.1	4.0	3.9	4.0
Nebraska	4.0	3.8	3.7	3.7	3.3	3.4	3.4	3.3	3.4	3.6	3.5
Nevada	11.4	7.8	7.8	9.9	7.4	6.7	6.4	6.4	6.6	5.9	5.6
New Hampshire	4.7	4.2	5.1	4.8	3.9	4.1	3.8	3.9	3.7	3.8	3.8
New Jersey	3.0	3.0	3.0	3.0	2.9	3.0	3.0	3.0	2.7	3.0	2.9
New Mexico	4.9	6.6	4.6	5.1	4.6	4.3	4.2	4.1	3.9	4.0	3.3
New York	3.2	3.0	3.3	3.0	2.9	3.1	2.9	2.8	2.6	2.9	2.9
North Carolina	5.1	5.0	4.6	4.5	4.1	4.0	4.0	3.8	3.8	3.8	3.7
North Dakota	3.6	3.4	4.4	3.4	2.9	3.0	2.9	2.9	2.8	3.1	2.7
Ohio	4.7	4.3	3.9	4.2	3.5	3.5	3.4	3.3	3.3	3.4	3.4
Oklahoma	7.7	6.6	NA	NA	5.6	5.3	5.2	5.3	4.8	5.2	5.2
Oregon	5.5	4.7	4.6	4.8	4.2	4.0	3.9	3.9	3.9	4.0	3.8
Pennsylvania	3.3	3.2	3.1	3.1	2.3	2.8	2.8	2.7	2.7	2.7	2.8
Rhode Island	3.7	3.6	2.7	2.9	3.0	3.0	2.8	2.7	3.0	3.2	3.2
South Carolina	4.5	3.9	3.8	3.8	2.9	2.9	3.0	2.8	3.0	3.1	3.2
South Dakota	3.7	3.9	3.7	3.5	2.8	3.2	3.1	3.1	3.3	3.4	3.3
Tennessee	6.5	6.2	5.8	5.9	4.6	4.6	4.3	4.2	3.9	4.2	4.3
Texas	5.5	5.2	3.8	4.0	3.3	3.4	3.3	3.3	3.3	3.3	3.2
Utah	5.1	4.4	4.0	4.3	4.1	3.9	3.7	3.8	3.7	3.7	3.7
Vermont	4.5	4.7	4.4	4.1	3.6	3.8	3.6	3.6	3.5	3.8	3.6
Virginia	4.4	4.3	4.4	4.3	4.0	4.0	3.8	3.8	3.7	3.8	3.8
Washington	5.9	5.4	5.0	4.6	4.3	4.1	4.0	3.9	3.9	4.2	4.1
West Virginia	5.3	5.2	4.9	5.1	5.1	5.0	5.1	4.8	5.1	5.1	5.2
Wisconsin	3.6	3.4	3.2	3.2	2.9	3.0	2.9	3.0	2.9	3.0	2.9
Wyoming	6.6	6.6	5.7	5.8	5.2	5.1	4.9	4.9	5.1	5.1	4.8

NA = Not available.   [1]Includes annulments. Includes divorce petitions filed or legal separations for some counties or states.

Table 4-3. Marital Status, United States, 2012 American Community Survey 1-Year Estimates, by Age, Sex, Race and Hispanic Origin, Place of Birth, and Labor Force Status, 2012

(Number; percent.)

Characteristic	Total	Now married (except separated)	Widowed	Divorced	Separated	Never married
Total Population, 15 Years and Over	252,745,149	48.0	5.9	11.1	2.2	32.7
Age and Sex						
Males, 15 years and over	123,174,537	49.8	2.5	9.8	1.9	36.0
15 to 19 years	11,046,052	0.7	0.0	0.0	0.1	99.2
20 to 34 years	32,710,723	27.8	0.1	3.4	1.3	67.4
35 to 44 years	20,268,103	61.0	0.4	11.6	2.8	24.2
45 to 54 years	21,762,309	63.5	1.0	16.3	2.9	16.3
55 to 64 years	18,582,087	68.3	2.5	16.6	2.2	10.3
65 years and over	18,805,263	70.7	12.4	10.8	1.3	4.9
Females, 15 years and over	129,570,612	46.3	9.2	12.4	2.5	29.6
15 to 19 years	10,504,417	1.3	0.0	0.1	0.1	98.5
20 to 34 years	31,853,305	34.7	0.2	4.8	2.3	58.0
35 to 44 years	20,429,983	61.7	1.0	14.3	4.3	18.7
45 to 54 years	22,442,643	61.6	3.0	19.1	3.9	12.4
55 to 64 years	20,005,050	60.5	8.1	20.1	2.7	8.6
65 years and over	24,335,214	42.4	38.2	13.3	1.1	4.9
Race and Hispanic Origin						
One race	247,322,320	48.3	6.0	11.1	2.2	32.3
White	190,522,547	51.4	6.3	11.5	1.8	28.9
Black or African American	30,914,435	28.8	5.8	12.2	4.3	49.0
American Indian and Alaska Native	1,965,345	36.4	5.2	13.3	3.2	41.9
Asian	12,787,170	57.6	4.5	5.2	1.2	31.4
Native Hawaiian and Other Pacific Islander	414,240	47.1	3.7	8.1	2.8	38.2
Some other race	10,718,583	41.5	2.7	7.8	3.8	44.2
Two or more races	5,422,829	33.8	3.5	10.4	2.7	49.6
Hispanic or Latino (of any race)	38,091,097	43.2	3.3	8.5	3.5	41.5
White, not Hispanic or Latino	165,437,009	52.4	6.7	12.0	1.6	27.3
Nativity						
Native born	213,674,013	46.1	6.1	11.7	2.0	34.1
Foreign born	39,071,136	58.6	5.3	7.8	3.1	25.2
Labor Force Participation						
Males, 16 years and over	121,051,882	50.7	2.6	10.0	1.9	34.8
In labor force	83,776,330	54.3	0.9	9.5	1.9	33.4
Females, 16 years and over	127,549,401	47.0	9.3	12.6	2.6	28.5
In labor force	74,952,713	48.1	2.9	14.1	3.0	31.9

Table 4-4. Marital Status, United States, 2012 American Community Survey 1-Year Estimates, by State, 2012

(Number; percent.)

State	Total population, 15 years and over	Now married (except separated)	Widowed	Divorced	Separated	Never married
United States	252,745,149	48.0	5.9	11.1	2.2	32.7
Alabama	3,886,060	48.5	7.0	12.7	2.5	29.3
Alaska	574,398	47.7	3.8	12.4	2.0	34.1
Arizona	5,203,019	47.3	5.5	12.5	2.0	32.7
Arkansas	2,353,968	50.5	6.9	13.3	2.3	26.9
California	30,416,010	46.1	5.1	9.8	2.4	36.6
Colorado	4,152,392	50.6	4.4	12.4	1.7	30.9
Connecticut	2,945,674	48.2	6.0	10.6	1.4	33.8
Delaware	746,748	47.4	6.2	11.8	2.0	32.7
District of Columbia	539,055	26.7	4.5	9.2	2.1	57.5
Florida	16,016,557	46.0	7.1	13.2	2.5	31.1
Georgia	7,830,116	47.1	5.7	11.4	2.6	33.2
Hawaii	1,137,619	49.5	6.2	9.5	1.5	33.4
Idaho	1,239,521	55.0	5.2	12.5	1.3	26.0
Illinois	10,344,646	47.6	5.9	10.0	1.8	34.6
Indiana	5,218,923	49.8	6.0	12.7	1.4	30.0
Iowa	2,472,319	52.7	6.3	11.4	1.3	28.3
Kansas	2,281,272	52.2	5.8	12.2	1.6	28.2
Kentucky	3,530,921	50.1	6.7	13.2	2.2	27.8
Louisiana	3,663,532	43.7	6.6	12.3	2.9	34.5
Maine	1,111,822	50.8	6.4	14.2	1.2	27.4
Maryland	4,773,742	46.7	5.8	10.1	2.6	34.9
Massachusetts	5,498,140	46.1	5.9	10.1	2.0	36.0
Michigan	8,030,918	48.0	6.1	11.8	1.5	32.6
Minnesota	4,315,429	52.4	5.0	10.2	1.1	31.3
Mississippi	2,359,979	44.3	7.2	11.9	3.2	33.4
Missouri	4,856,639	49.1	6.6	12.5	2.0	29.9
Montana	821,687	52.7	6.1	12.3	1.3	27.6
Nebraska	1,465,286	52.8	6.1	10.4	1.2	29.5
Nevada	2,204,567	45.6	5.1	14.6	2.4	32.3
New Hampshire	1,098,030	51.4	5.5	12.3	1.3	29.6
New Jersey	7,196,853	49.2	6.2	8.6	2.0	34.0
New Mexico	1,654,214	46.1	5.8	13.1	1.8	33.1
New York	16,062,969	44.2	6.2	8.8	2.8	38.0
North Carolina	7,840,375	49.1	6.2	10.8	3.2	30.7
North Dakota	569,837	51.9	6.1	9.7	0.9	31.5
Ohio	9,351,828	48.0	6.4	12.5	1.8	31.2
Oklahoma	3,026,600	50.1	6.7	13.5	2.2	27.5
Oregon	3,185,235	49.0	5.5	13.4	1.9	30.2
Pennsylvania	10,519,780	48.1	7.1	9.5	2.2	33.2
Rhode Island	872,769	44.8	6.3	11.5	1.8	35.6
South Carolina	3,818,052	47.3	6.8	10.7	3.4	31.9
South Dakota	662,015	50.9	6.2	11.0	1.3	30.5
Tennessee	5,216,402	49.1	6.4	13.0	2.3	29.2
Texas	20,202,653	49.4	5.1	11.0	2.8	31.6
Utah	2,100,869	55.7	3.7	9.5	1.7	29.5
Vermont	525,211	49.8	5.9	12.1	1.4	30.8
Virginia	6,642,567	50.1	5.5	10.2	2.4	31.8
Washington	5,576,731	50.5	4.9	12.3	1.7	30.7
West Virginia	1,535,612	49.9	7.9	13.3	1.5	27.4
Wisconsin	4,634,334	50.8	5.8	11.0	1.2	31.2
Wyoming	461,254	52.9	5.4	12.8	1.8	27.2

Table 4-5. Median Age at First Marriage, 2012 American Community Survey 1-Year Estimates, by Sex and State, 2012

(Number.)

State	Male median age at first marriage	Female median age at first marriage
United States	29.1	27.1
Alabama	27.7	26.0
Alaska	28.7	25.5
Arizona	28.8	27.3
Arkansas	26.9	25.2
California	30.0	27.9
Colorado	28.1	26.5
Connecticut	30.3	28.7
Delaware	29.7	27.6
District of Columbia	30.2	29.8
Florida	29.9	27.8
Georgia	29.0	26.8
Hawaii	28.4	26.9
Idaho	26.3	24.4
Illinois	29.7	28.2
Indiana	27.8	26.3
Iowa	27.6	26.1
Kansas	27.0	25.7
Kentucky	27.3	25.6
Louisiana	28.9	27.1
Maine	28.7	26.4
Maryland	29.7	28.1
Massachusetts	30.7	29.2
Michigan	29.5	27.5
Minnesota	28.8	26.6
Mississippi	28.4	26.4
Missouri	27.8	26.5
Montana	28.5	26.1
Nebraska	27.3	25.8
Nevada	28.4	26.8
New Hampshire	29.7	27.1
New Jersey	30.6	28.4
New Mexico	26.9	26.3
New York	30.9	29.3
North Carolina	28.3	26.6
North Dakota	27.3	25.8
Ohio	29.0	27.1
Oklahoma	26.6	25.3
Oregon	29.1	27.6
Pennsylvania	29.8	27.7
Rhode Island	31.6	29.5
South Carolina	28.3	26.8
South Dakota	28.3	25.7
Tennessee	27.9	26.1
Texas	27.8	26.1
Utah	26.2	24.1
Vermont	30.6	28.8
Virginia	28.7	26.8
Washington	28.1	26.3
West Virginia	27.1	25.7
Wisconsin	28.6	27.0
Wyoming	26.9	25.0

Table 4-6. Median Age at First Marriage, 2012 American Community Survey 1-Year Estimates, by Sex and Race, United States, 2012

(Number.)

Race and origin	Male median age at first marriage	Female median age at first marriage
Median, Total, United States	29.1	27.1
White alone	28.6	26.7
Black or African American alone	31.0	31.0
American Indian and Alaska Native alone	29.9	27.4
Asian alone	30.1	27.2
Native Hawaiian or Other Pacific Islander alone	28.0	26.9
Some other race alone	29.4	26.7
Two or more races	29.7	28.0
Hispanic or Latino (of any race)	28.8	26.5
White alone, not Hispanic or Latino	28.7	26.8

Table 4-7. Marriages in the Last Year for the Population Age 15 Years and Over, 2012 American Community Survey 1-Year Estimates, by Sex and State, 2012

(Number.)

State	Total, age 15 years and over	Male					Female				
		Total	Never married	Ever married			Total	Never married	Ever Married		
				Total, ever married	Married last year	Not married last year			Total, ever married	Married last year	Not married last year
United States	252,745,149	123,174,537	44,291,637	78,882,900	2,208,051	76,674,849	129,570,612	38,367,449	91,203,163	2,156,833	89,046,330
Alabama	3,886,060	1,858,893	599,765	1,259,128	37,523	1,221,605	2,027,167	537,885	1,489,282	37,737	1,451,545
Alaska	574,398	300,043	117,582	182,461	7,008	175,453	274,355	78,101	196,254	6,757	189,497
Arizona	5,203,019	2,570,325	937,330	1,632,995	45,820	1,587,175	2,632,694	766,043	1,866,651	45,822	1,820,829
Arkansas	2,353,968	1,141,359	346,371	794,988	25,045	769,943	1,212,609	287,878	924,731	24,951	899,780
California	30,416,010	15,018,551	6,049,704	8,968,847	248,942	8,719,905	15,397,459	5,092,645	10,304,814	239,102	10,065,712
Colorado	4,152,392	2,073,202	718,460	1,354,742	45,881	1,308,861	2,079,190	566,395	1,512,795	42,624	1,470,171
Connecticut	2,945,674	1,419,508	525,179	894,329	21,108	873,221	1,526,166	470,937	1,055,229	21,537	1,033,692
Delaware	746,748	357,658	125,252	232,406	5,452	226,954	389,090	118,858	270,232	5,886	264,346
District of Columbia	539,055	251,998	148,943	103,055	5,782	97,273	287,057	160,809	126,248	5,175	121,073
Florida	16,016,557	7,757,505	2,694,915	5,062,590	124,740	4,937,850	8,259,052	2,290,565	5,968,487	119,315	5,849,172
Georgia	7,830,116	3,783,669	1,376,918	2,406,751	79,627	2,327,124	4,046,447	1,226,048	2,820,399	75,360	2,745,039
Hawaii	1,137,619	570,172	215,002	355,170	10,286	344,884	567,447	164,861	402,586	10,321	392,265
Idaho	1,239,521	614,964	178,204	436,760	13,218	423,542	624,557	144,329	480,228	13,933	466,295
Illinois	10,344,646	5,026,063	1,898,189	3,127,874	76,840	3,051,034	5,318,583	1,682,675	3,635,908	76,054	3,559,854
Indiana	5,218,923	2,542,270	843,285	1,698,985	52,902	1,646,083	2,676,653	726,927	1,949,726	51,238	1,898,488
Iowa	2,472,319	1,215,553	382,333	833,220	23,146	810,074	1,256,766	318,365	938,401	22,021	916,380
Kansas	2,281,272	1,127,129	352,894	774,235	25,398	748,837	1,154,143	289,368	864,775	24,382	840,393
Kentucky	3,530,921	1,720,998	539,738	1,181,260	33,599	1,147,661	1,809,923	441,056	1,368,867	34,763	1,334,104
Louisiana	3,663,532	1,771,878	668,775	1,103,103	31,969	1,071,134	1,891,654	594,189	1,297,465	31,961	1,265,504
Maine	1,111,822	538,918	161,676	377,242	8,207	369,035	572,904	142,692	430,212	8,860	421,352
Maryland	4,773,742	2,283,540	849,000	1,434,540	40,222	1,394,318	2,490,202	817,345	1,672,857	39,719	1,633,138
Massachusetts	5,498,140	2,633,255	1,016,940	1,616,315	41,539	1,574,776	2,864,885	960,603	1,904,282	40,910	1,863,372
Michigan	8,030,918	3,903,780	1,397,772	2,506,008	63,050	2,442,958	4,127,138	1,216,379	2,910,759	62,432	2,848,327
Minnesota	4,315,429	2,128,478	730,632	1,397,846	37,936	1,359,910	2,186,951	618,111	1,568,840	37,796	1,531,044
Mississippi	2,359,979	1,126,405	405,014	721,391	19,301	702,090	1,233,574	383,857	849,717	18,861	830,856
Missouri	4,856,639	2,353,637	775,598	1,578,039	48,435	1,529,604	2,503,002	675,076	1,827,926	46,710	1,781,216
Montana	821,687	409,851	129,043	280,808	8,100	272,708	411,836	97,860	313,976	7,917	306,059
Nebraska	1,465,286	723,059	240,484	482,575	12,062	470,513	742,227	192,087	550,140	12,558	537,582
Nevada	2,204,567	1,106,923	398,862	708,061	23,591	684,470	1,097,644	312,613	785,031	23,158	761,873
New Hampshire	1,098,030	536,129	175,494	360,635	8,135	352,500	561,901	149,351	412,550	8,721	403,829
New Jersey	7,196,853	3,470,727	1,297,728	2,172,999	50,601	2,122,398	3,726,126	1,151,256	2,574,870	49,340	2,525,530
New Mexico	1,654,214	813,641	293,989	519,652	15,654	503,998	840,573	253,816	586,757	12,972	573,785
New York	16,062,969	7,693,458	3,159,656	4,533,802	121,945	4,411,857	8,369,511	2,951,737	5,417,774	116,787	5,300,987
North Carolina	7,840,375	3,777,517	1,285,644	2,491,873	69,417	2,422,456	4,062,858	1,123,288	2,939,570	68,943	2,870,627
North Dakota	569,837	290,980	104,080	186,900	5,857	181,043	278,857	75,246	203,611	5,146	198,465
Ohio	9,351,828	4,522,537	1,549,927	2,972,610	74,250	2,898,360	4,829,291	1,369,638	3,459,653	76,355	3,383,298
Oklahoma	3,026,600	1,486,394	460,031	1,026,363	33,303	993,060	1,540,206	372,220	1,167,986	31,607	1,136,379
Oregon	3,185,235	1,564,026	527,989	1,036,037	25,415	1,010,622	1,621,209	434,057	1,187,152	25,860	1,161,292
Pennsylvania	10,519,780	5,081,824	1,846,843	3,234,981	75,192	3,159,789	5,437,956	1,646,017	3,791,939	72,439	3,719,500
Rhode Island	872,769	416,431	163,962	252,469	4,885	247,584	456,338	146,902	309,436	4,561	304,875
South Carolina	3,818,052	1,833,320	634,399	1,198,921	37,350	1,161,571	1,984,732	583,658	1,401,074	36,421	1,364,653
South Dakota	662,015	330,119	112,651	217,468	6,732	210,736	331,896	89,401	242,495	6,999	235,496
Tennessee	5,216,402	2,512,605	808,819	1,703,786	53,883	1,649,903	2,703,797	713,167	1,990,630	52,864	1,937,766
Texas	20,202,653	9,953,055	3,469,917	6,483,138	204,130	6,279,008	10,249,598	2,914,409	7,335,189	198,297	7,136,892
Utah	2,100,869	1,048,088	340,438	707,650	30,116	677,534	1,052,781	279,786	772,995	28,994	744,001
Vermont	525,211	256,714	86,346	170,368	2,727	167,641	268,497	75,169	193,328	2,280	191,048
Virginia	6,642,567	3,227,240	1,122,846	2,104,394	61,226	2,043,168	3,415,327	987,200	2,428,127	61,522	2,366,605
Washington	5,576,731	2,762,858	942,136	1,820,722	55,258	1,765,464	2,813,873	768,444	2,045,429	52,601	1,992,828
West Virginia	1,535,612	749,711	232,165	517,546	13,475	504,071	785,901	188,180	597,721	13,209	584,512
Wisconsin	4,634,334	2,284,469	781,943	1,502,526	35,267	1,467,259	2,349,865	665,400	1,684,465	36,582	1,647,883
Wyoming	461,254	233,110	70,774	162,336	6,504	155,832	228,144	54,550	173,594	6,473	167,121

Table 4-8. Marriages Ending in Widowhood for the Population Age 15 Years and Over, 2012 American Community Survey 1-Year Estimates, by Sex and State, 2012

(Number.)

State	Total, age 15 years and over	Male					Female				
		Total	Never married	Ever married			Total	Never married	Ever married		
				Total, ever married	Widowed last year	Not widowed last year			Total, ever married	Widowed last year	Not widowed last year
United States	252,745,149	123,174,537	44,291,637	78,882,900	439,170	78,443,730	129,570,612	38,367,449	91,203,163	1,002,709	90,200,454
Alabama	3,886,060	1,858,893	599,765	1,259,128	8,869	1,250,259	2,027,167	537,885	1,489,282	20,350	1,468,932
Alaska	574,398	300,043	117,582	182,461	980	181,481	274,355	78,101	196,254	1,001	195,253
Arizona	5,203,019	2,570,325	937,330	1,632,995	7,108	1,625,887	2,632,694	766,043	1,866,651	18,636	1,848,015
Arkansas	2,353,968	1,141,359	346,371	794,988	5,008	789,980	1,212,609	287,878	924,731	9,899	914,832
California	30,416,010	15,018,551	6,049,704	8,968,847	41,805	8,927,042	15,397,459	5,092,645	10,304,814	104,369	10,200,445
Colorado	4,152,392	2,073,202	718,460	1,354,742	5,995	1,348,747	2,079,190	566,395	1,512,795	13,491	1,499,304
Connecticut	2,945,674	1,419,508	525,179	894,329	5,058	889,271	1,526,166	470,937	1,055,229	10,431	1,044,798
Delaware	746,748	357,658	125,252	232,406	1,298	231,108	389,090	118,858	270,232	2,931	267,301
District of Columbia	539,055	251,998	148,943	103,055	178	102,877	287,057	160,809	126,248	1,097	125,151
Florida	16,016,557	7,757,505	2,694,915	5,062,590	32,136	5,030,454	8,259,052	2,290,565	5,968,487	71,741	5,896,746
Georgia	7,830,116	3,783,669	1,376,918	2,406,751	14,772	2,391,979	4,046,447	1,226,048	2,820,399	32,296	2,788,103
Hawaii	1,137,619	570,172	215,002	355,170	1,646	353,524	567,447	164,861	402,586	4,778	397,808
Idaho	1,239,521	614,964	178,204	436,760	1,709	435,051	624,557	144,329	480,228	3,770	476,458
Illinois	10,344,646	5,026,063	1,898,189	3,127,874	17,183	3,110,691	5,318,583	1,682,675	3,635,908	39,726	3,596,182
Indiana	5,218,923	2,542,270	843,285	1,698,985	10,116	1,688,869	2,676,653	726,927	1,949,726	21,976	1,927,750
Iowa	2,472,319	1,215,553	382,333	833,220	5,501	827,719	1,256,766	318,365	938,401	10,732	927,669
Kansas	2,281,272	1,127,129	352,894	774,235	4,053	770,182	1,154,143	289,368	864,775	8,754	856,021
Kentucky	3,530,921	1,720,998	539,738	1,181,260	9,185	1,172,075	1,809,923	441,056	1,368,867	14,721	1,354,146
Louisiana	3,663,532	1,771,878	668,775	1,103,103	6,555	1,096,548	1,891,654	594,189	1,297,465	15,888	1,281,577
Maine	1,111,822	538,918	161,676	377,242	2,947	374,295	572,904	142,692	430,212	2,664	427,548
Maryland	4,773,742	2,283,540	849,000	1,434,540	8,353	1,426,187	2,490,202	817,345	1,672,857	17,722	1,655,135
Massachusetts	5,498,140	2,633,255	1,016,940	1,616,315	6,859	1,609,456	2,864,885	960,603	1,904,282	20,021	1,884,261
Michigan	8,030,918	3,903,780	1,397,772	2,506,008	15,681	2,490,327	4,127,138	1,216,379	2,910,759	34,668	2,876,091
Minnesota	4,315,429	2,128,478	730,632	1,397,846	6,213	1,391,633	2,186,951	618,111	1,568,840	13,499	1,555,341
Mississippi	2,359,979	1,126,405	405,014	721,391	4,725	716,666	1,233,574	383,857	849,717	11,613	838,104
Missouri	4,856,639	2,353,637	775,598	1,578,039	10,661	1,567,378	2,503,002	675,076	1,827,926	21,167	1,806,759
Montana	821,687	409,851	129,043	280,808	1,523	279,285	411,836	97,860	313,976	4,016	309,960
Nebraska	1,465,286	723,059	240,484	482,575	2,950	479,625	742,227	192,087	550,140	6,751	543,389
Nevada	2,204,567	1,106,923	398,862	708,061	3,727	704,334	1,097,644	312,613	785,031	7,643	777,388
New Hampshire	1,098,030	536,129	175,494	360,635	1,794	358,841	561,901	149,351	412,550	4,656	407,894
New Jersey	7,196,853	3,470,727	1,297,728	2,172,999	12,819	2,160,180	3,726,126	1,151,256	2,574,870	27,386	2,547,484
New Mexico	1,654,214	813,641	293,989	519,652	2,788	516,864	840,573	253,816	586,757	6,963	579,794
New York	16,062,969	7,693,458	3,159,656	4,533,802	24,546	4,509,256	8,369,511	2,951,737	5,417,774	63,123	5,354,651
North Carolina	7,840,375	3,777,517	1,285,644	2,491,873	14,275	2,477,598	4,062,858	1,123,288	2,939,570	32,265	2,907,305
North Dakota	569,837	290,980	104,080	186,900	1,029	185,871	278,857	75,246	203,611	2,436	201,175
Ohio	9,351,828	4,522,537	1,549,927	2,972,610	18,191	2,954,419	4,829,291	1,369,638	3,459,653	42,290	3,417,363
Oklahoma	3,026,600	1,486,394	460,031	1,026,363	6,217	1,020,146	1,540,206	372,220	1,167,986	13,642	1,154,344
Oregon	3,185,235	1,564,026	527,989	1,036,037	5,198	1,030,839	1,621,209	434,057	1,187,152	14,670	1,172,482
Pennsylvania	10,519,780	5,081,824	1,846,843	3,234,981	21,670	3,213,311	5,437,956	1,646,017	3,791,939	48,262	3,743,677
Rhode Island	872,769	416,431	163,962	252,469	954	251,515	456,338	146,902	309,436	4,466	304,970
South Carolina	3,818,052	1,833,320	634,399	1,198,921	7,802	1,191,119	1,984,732	583,658	1,401,074	17,951	1,383,123
South Dakota	662,015	330,119	112,651	217,468	893	216,575	331,896	89,401	242,495	2,689	239,806
Tennessee	5,216,402	2,512,605	808,819	1,703,786	10,867	1,692,919	2,703,797	713,167	1,990,630	24,021	1,966,609
Texas	20,202,653	9,953,055	3,469,917	6,483,138	31,774	6,451,364	10,249,598	2,914,409	7,335,189	73,644	7,261,545
Utah	2,100,869	1,048,088	340,438	707,650	2,818	704,832	1,052,781	279,786	772,995	5,250	767,745
Vermont	525,211	256,714	86,346	170,368	632	169,736	268,497	75,169	193,328	1,550	191,778
Virginia	6,642,567	3,227,240	1,122,846	2,104,394	10,757	2,093,637	3,415,327	987,200	2,428,127	26,037	2,402,090
Washington	5,576,731	2,762,858	942,136	1,820,722	9,747	1,810,975	2,813,873	768,444	2,045,429	16,724	2,028,705
West Virginia	1,535,612	749,711	232,165	517,546	3,707	513,839	785,901	188,180	597,721	8,280	589,441
Wisconsin	4,634,334	2,284,469	781,943	1,502,526	6,823	1,495,703	2,349,865	665,400	1,684,465	18,346	1,666,119
Wyoming	461,254	233,110	70,774	162,336	1,075	161,261	228,144	54,550	173,594	1,707	171,887

Table 4-9. Divorces in the Last Year for the Population Age 15 Years and Over, 2012 American Community Survey 1-Year Estimates, by Sex and State, 2012

(Number.)

State	Total, age 15 years and over	Male					Female				
		Total	Never married	Ever married			Total	Never married	Ever married		
				Total, ever married	Divorced last year	Not divorced last year			Total, ever married	Divorced last year	Not divorced last year
United States	252,745,149	123,174,537	44,291,637	78,882,900	1,141,769	77,741,131	129,570,612	38,367,449	91,203,163	1,265,277	89,937,886
Alabama	3,886,060	1,858,893	599,765	1,259,128	20,713	1,238,415	2,027,167	537,885	1,489,282	22,661	1,466,621
Alaska	574,398	300,043	117,582	182,461	2,528	179,933	274,355	78,101	196,254	2,508	193,746
Arizona	5,203,019	2,570,325	937,330	1,632,995	21,785	1,611,210	2,632,694	766,043	1,866,651	26,519	1,840,132
Arkansas	2,353,968	1,141,359	346,371	794,988	14,629	780,359	1,212,609	287,878	924,731	19,307	905,424
California	30,416,010	15,018,551	6,049,704	8,968,847	111,791	8,857,056	15,397,459	5,092,645	10,304,814	121,956	10,182,858
Colorado	4,152,392	2,073,202	718,460	1,354,742	24,525	1,330,217	2,079,190	566,395	1,512,795	24,940	1,487,855
Connecticut	2,945,674	1,419,508	525,179	894,329	12,596	881,733	1,526,166	470,937	1,055,229	14,349	1,040,880
Delaware	746,748	357,658	125,252	232,406	3,141	229,265	389,090	118,858	270,232	4,711	265,521
District of Columbia	539,055	251,998	148,943	103,055	2,002	101,053	287,057	160,809	126,248	1,955	124,293
Florida	16,016,557	7,757,505	2,694,915	5,062,590	73,650	4,988,940	8,259,052	2,290,565	5,968,487	87,158	5,881,329
Georgia	7,830,116	3,783,669	1,376,918	2,406,751	40,144	2,366,607	4,046,447	1,226,048	2,820,399	44,214	2,776,185
Hawaii	1,137,619	570,172	215,002	355,170	3,908	351,262	567,447	164,861	402,586	5,201	397,385
Idaho	1,239,521	614,964	178,204	436,760	8,602	428,158	624,557	144,329	480,228	6,853	473,375
Illinois	10,344,646	5,026,063	1,898,189	3,127,874	39,165	3,088,709	5,318,583	1,682,675	3,635,908	47,968	3,587,940
Indiana	5,218,923	2,542,270	843,285	1,698,985	29,236	1,669,749	2,676,653	726,927	1,949,726	31,940	1,917,786
Iowa	2,472,319	1,215,553	382,333	833,220	12,176	821,044	1,256,766	318,365	938,401	12,297	926,104
Kansas	2,281,272	1,127,129	352,894	774,235	13,844	760,391	1,154,143	289,368	864,775	15,370	849,405
Kentucky	3,530,921	1,720,998	539,738	1,181,260	20,628	1,160,632	1,809,923	441,056	1,368,867	24,102	1,344,765
Louisiana	3,663,532	1,771,878	668,775	1,103,103	14,413	1,088,690	1,891,654	594,189	1,297,465	20,625	1,276,840
Maine	1,111,822	538,918	161,676	377,242	6,766	370,476	572,904	142,692	430,212	4,857	425,355
Maryland	4,773,742	2,283,540	849,000	1,434,540	21,490	1,413,050	2,490,202	817,345	1,672,857	22,685	1,650,172
Massachusetts	5,498,140	2,633,255	1,016,940	1,616,315	19,451	1,596,864	2,864,885	960,603	1,904,282	24,401	1,879,881
Michigan	8,030,918	3,903,780	1,397,772	2,506,008	39,280	2,466,728	4,127,138	1,216,379	2,910,759	39,233	2,871,526
Minnesota	4,315,429	2,128,478	730,632	1,397,846	16,655	1,381,191	2,186,951	618,111	1,568,840	17,815	1,551,025
Mississippi	2,359,979	1,126,405	405,014	721,391	13,158	708,233	1,233,574	383,857	849,717	14,275	835,442
Missouri	4,856,639	2,353,637	775,598	1,578,039	26,057	1,551,982	2,503,002	675,076	1,827,926	26,349	1,801,577
Montana	821,687	409,851	129,043	280,808	4,137	276,671	411,836	97,860	313,976	5,026	308,950
Nebraska	1,465,286	723,059	240,484	482,575	6,464	476,111	742,227	192,087	550,140	6,878	543,262
Nevada	2,204,567	1,106,923	398,862	708,061	13,779	694,282	1,097,644	312,613	785,031	16,144	768,887
New Hampshire	1,098,030	536,129	175,494	360,635	4,925	355,710	561,901	149,351	412,550	5,834	406,716
New Jersey	7,196,853	3,470,727	1,297,728	2,172,999	24,712	2,148,287	3,726,126	1,151,256	2,574,870	24,964	2,549,906
New Mexico	1,654,214	813,641	293,989	519,652	7,796	511,856	840,573	253,816	586,757	8,550	578,207
New York	16,062,969	7,693,458	3,159,656	4,533,802	50,837	4,482,965	8,369,511	2,951,737	5,417,774	66,758	5,351,016
North Carolina	7,840,375	3,777,517	1,285,644	2,491,873	36,019	2,455,854	4,062,858	1,123,288	2,939,570	38,173	2,901,397
North Dakota	569,837	290,980	104,080	186,900	2,682	184,218	278,857	75,246	203,611	2,278	201,333
Ohio	9,351,828	4,522,537	1,549,927	2,972,610	41,775	2,930,835	4,829,291	1,369,638	3,459,653	50,848	3,408,805
Oklahoma	3,026,600	1,486,394	460,031	1,026,363	19,490	1,006,873	1,540,206	372,220	1,167,986	18,790	1,149,196
Oregon	3,185,235	1,564,026	527,989	1,036,037	15,992	1,020,045	1,621,209	434,057	1,187,152	19,068	1,168,084
Pennsylvania	10,519,780	5,081,824	1,846,843	3,234,981	42,160	3,192,821	5,437,956	1,646,017	3,791,939	39,299	3,752,640
Rhode Island	872,769	416,431	163,962	252,469	2,912	249,557	456,338	146,902	309,436	4,196	305,240
South Carolina	3,818,052	1,833,320	634,399	1,198,921	18,362	1,180,559	1,984,732	583,658	1,401,074	18,005	1,383,069
South Dakota	662,015	330,119	112,651	217,468	3,225	214,243	331,896	89,401	242,495	3,125	239,370
Tennessee	5,216,402	2,512,605	808,819	1,703,786	31,692	1,672,094	2,703,797	713,167	1,990,630	28,050	1,962,580
Texas	20,202,653	9,953,055	3,469,917	6,483,138	100,847	6,382,291	10,249,598	2,914,409	7,335,189	113,421	7,221,768
Utah	2,100,869	1,048,088	340,438	707,650	11,722	695,928	1,052,781	279,786	772,995	14,935	758,060
Vermont	525,211	256,714	86,346	170,368	2,098	168,270	268,497	75,169	193,328	2,046	191,282
Virginia	6,642,567	3,227,240	1,122,846	2,104,394	29,053	2,075,341	3,415,327	987,200	2,428,127	31,142	2,396,985
Washington	5,576,731	2,762,858	942,136	1,820,722	26,934	1,793,788	2,813,873	768,444	2,045,429	30,303	2,015,126
West Virginia	1,535,612	749,711	232,165	517,546	9,817	507,729	785,901	188,180	597,721	9,807	587,914
Wisconsin	4,634,334	2,284,469	781,943	1,502,526	19,187	1,483,339	2,349,865	665,400	1,684,465	19,520	1,664,945
Wyoming	461,254	233,110	70,774	162,336	2,819	159,517	228,144	54,550	173,594	3,868	169,726

Table 4-10. Median Duration of Current Marriage in Years for the Population Age 15 Years and Over, 2012 American Community Survey 1-Year Estimates, by Sex, Marital Status, and State, 2012

(Years.)

State	Total, age 15 years and over	Male				Female			
		Total	Married, spouse present	Married, spouse absent	Separated	Total	Married, spouse present	Married, spouse absent	Separated
United States	19.3	19.3	20.0	12.3	14.9	19.4	20.0	12.5	15.2
Alabama	19.8	20.0	20.6	9.9	15.2	19.6	20.7	11.3	13.6
Alaska	16.0	16.2	16.9	9.9	17.6	15.9	16.6	9.8	14.8
Arizona	19.1	19.0	19.6	12.3	15.3	19.2	19.9	11.6	14.2
Arkansas	18.5	18.7	19.4	12.6	13.1	18.3	19.2	11.5	10.4
California	18.2	18.1	18.7	12.0	16.7	18.3	18.8	12.5	17.5
Colorado	17.5	17.5	17.9	11.8	13.0	17.5	18.0	10.7	14.1
Connecticut	20.8	20.6	21.0	12.7	15.6	21.0	21.4	14.1	16.4
Delaware	21.3	21.2	22.1	13.6	11.3	21.3	22.0	8.5	15.1
District of Columbia	12.3	12.3	12.3	7.5	18.7	12.3	11.8	10.6	21.5
Florida	19.9	20.0	20.9	12.8	13.9	19.9	20.9	12.8	14.6
Georgia	17.3	17.2	17.9	10.0	13.1	17.4	17.9	11.2	15.3
Hawaii	19.1	18.7	19.4	11.7	16.9	19.5	19.9	12.3	21.2
Idaho	18.0	18.1	18.6	9.2	11.9	18.0	18.4	8.4	14.3
Illinois	20.0	20.0	20.4	13.3	15.5	20.0	20.4	15.7	16.0
Indiana	19.7	19.7	20.2	12.2	14.5	19.7	20.3	11.9	13.9
Iowa	21.5	21.7	22.1	16.8	11.8	21.4	22.1	11.5	12.1
Kansas	19.6	19.5	19.9	12.1	14.8	19.7	20.3	14.2	12.5
Kentucky	19.6	19.5	20.3	11.6	12.4	19.7	20.5	12.2	12.8
Louisiana	19.1	19.2	20.2	10.0	13.1	19.0	20.1	11.9	12.9
Maine	21.9	21.8	22.0	23.2	12.9	21.9	22.4	11.6	13.4
Maryland	18.7	18.7	19.3	12.0	16.4	18.8	19.3	15.1	16.1
Massachusetts	20.3	20.3	20.7	13.0	18.1	20.3	20.9	12.2	16.4
Michigan	21.3	21.4	21.9	13.2	15.3	21.2	21.7	14.1	15.6
Minnesota	21.1	21.1	21.4	15.0	14.9	21.1	21.5	16.7	15.1
Mississippi	19.1	19.0	20.0	10.8	15.4	19.2	20.3	9.8	15.0
Missouri	20.0	20.0	20.7	12.4	13.6	20.0	20.6	13.5	14.9
Montana	21.2	21.4	21.8	16.4	13.4	21.0	21.8	14.8	13.7
Nebraska	20.8	20.7	21.2	14.2	12.5	20.9	21.3	15.7	12.6
Nevada	16.3	16.4	16.9	11.7	12.3	16.2	16.7	11.8	13.2
New Hampshire	21.8	21.9	22.1	19.3	17.3	21.6	22.1	10.9	17.8
New Jersey	20.1	20.0	20.5	12.5	17.3	20.2	20.7	13.2	17.1
New Mexico	19.6	19.6	20.3	12.4	14.1	19.6	20.3	13.8	14.1
New York	20.0	19.8	20.6	12.3	17.6	20.1	20.7	12.6	18.7
North Carolina	18.9	19.0	19.6	14.0	13.8	18.8	19.7	12.4	14.4
North Dakota	21.9	21.6	21.9	18.2	13.3	22.1	22.4	23.9	14.1
Ohio	20.9	21.0	21.6	14.7	14.4	20.8	21.6	13.1	13.6
Oklahoma	18.2	18.4	19.4	11.0	12.2	18.1	19.3	10.4	11.8
Oregon	19.5	19.5	19.9	14.6	15.4	19.4	20.0	14.9	15.9
Pennsylvania	22.3	22.3	22.8	14.5	16.6	22.3	22.9	18.0	16.0
Rhode Island	20.7	20.7	21.6	10.9	17.1	20.6	21.1	13.3	20.1
South Carolina	19.8	19.7	20.6	11.5	14.9	19.9	20.8	11.0	16.0
South Dakota	22.5	22.6	23.1	22.4	11.6	22.5	23.3	10.1	13.9
Tennessee	18.9	18.8	19.5	10.6	12.9	19.0	19.6	12.0	14.6
Texas	17.2	17.1	17.8	10.7	13.7	17.3	18.0	11.1	13.9
Utah	16.4	16.3	16.7	11.5	10.0	16.5	17.0	10.7	10.9
Vermont	22.1	21.9	22.4	16.1	15.1	22.3	22.8	21.9	15.3
Virginia	18.7	18.7	19.3	11.9	14.7	18.6	19.3	12.4	14.8
Washington	18.5	18.5	18.9	12.5	14.9	18.6	19.1	11.6	14.0
West Virginia	21.5	21.9	22.5	11.7	14.9	21.0	22.1	12.8	12.1
Wisconsin	21.4	21.4	21.7	15.4	15.1	21.5	21.9	17.4	13.4
Wyoming	18.9	19.4	19.6	17.8	15.4	18.6	19.7	11.1	10.7

Table 4-11A. Number of Times Married for the Population Age 15 Years and Over, 2012 American Community Survey 1-Year Estimates, for Males, by Marital Status and State, 2012

(Number.)

State	Total, age 15 years and over	Male					
		Total	Never married	Ever married			
				Total	Once	Twice	Three or more times
United States	252,745,149	123,174,537	44,291,637	78,882,900	59,349,333	15,381,788	4,151,779
Alabama	3,886,060	1,858,893	599,765	1,259,128	861,342	289,556	108,230
Alaska	574,398	300,043	117,582	182,461	130,536	40,483	11,442
Arizona	5,203,019	2,570,325	937,330	1,632,995	1,170,168	355,198	107,629
Arkansas	2,353,968	1,141,359	346,371	794,988	516,362	196,405	82,221
California	30,416,010	15,018,551	6,049,704	8,968,847	7,142,884	1,488,063	337,900
Colorado	4,152,392	2,073,202	718,460	1,354,742	1,008,308	274,037	72,397
Connecticut	2,945,674	1,419,508	525,179	894,329	717,733	152,256	24,340
Delaware	746,748	357,658	125,252	232,406	174,565	47,575	10,266
District of Columbia	539,055	251,998	148,943	103,055	83,498	16,760	2,797
Florida	16,016,557	7,757,505	2,694,915	5,062,590	3,540,339	1,165,296	356,955
Georgia	7,830,116	3,783,669	1,376,918	2,406,751	1,729,189	517,702	159,860
Hawaii	1,137,619	570,172	215,002	355,170	282,236	62,002	10,932
Idaho	1,239,521	614,964	178,204	436,760	304,654	96,740	35,366
Illinois	10,344,646	5,026,063	1,898,189	3,127,874	2,466,594	536,988	124,292
Indiana	5,218,923	2,542,270	843,285	1,698,985	1,205,653	370,025	123,307
Iowa	2,472,319	1,215,553	382,333	833,220	643,897	150,440	38,883
Kansas	2,281,272	1,127,129	352,894	774,235	566,164	157,641	50,430
Kentucky	3,530,921	1,720,998	539,738	1,181,260	822,816	268,349	90,095
Louisiana	3,663,532	1,771,878	668,775	1,103,103	787,816	242,030	73,257
Maine	1,111,822	538,918	161,676	377,242	270,441	85,420	21,381
Maryland	4,773,742	2,283,540	849,000	1,434,540	1,106,369	277,549	50,622
Massachusetts	5,498,140	2,633,255	1,016,940	1,616,315	1,334,045	242,132	40,138
Michigan	8,030,918	3,903,780	1,397,772	2,506,008	1,881,196	504,973	119,839
Minnesota	4,315,429	2,128,478	730,632	1,397,846	1,141,941	215,757	40,148
Mississippi	2,359,979	1,126,405	405,014	721,391	499,951	164,001	57,439
Missouri	4,856,639	2,353,637	775,598	1,578,039	1,107,868	353,101	117,070
Montana	821,687	409,851	129,043	280,808	200,156	61,325	19,327
Nebraska	1,465,286	723,059	240,484	482,575	380,917	81,880	19,778
Nevada	2,204,567	1,106,923	398,862	708,061	484,987	163,844	59,230
New Hampshire	1,098,030	536,129	175,494	360,635	274,413	70,067	16,155
New Jersey	7,196,853	3,470,727	1,297,728	2,172,999	1,803,766	324,907	44,326
New Mexico	1,654,214	813,641	293,989	519,652	380,713	107,944	30,995
New York	16,062,969	7,693,458	3,159,656	4,533,802	3,729,174	696,657	107,971
North Carolina	7,840,375	3,777,517	1,285,644	2,491,873	1,823,136	523,508	145,229
North Dakota	569,837	290,980	104,080	186,900	153,222	28,395	5,283
Ohio	9,351,828	4,522,537	1,549,927	2,972,610	2,187,794	618,153	166,663
Oklahoma	3,026,600	1,486,394	460,031	1,026,363	689,903	239,373	97,087
Oregon	3,185,235	1,564,026	527,989	1,036,037	723,451	233,275	79,311
Pennsylvania	10,519,780	5,081,824	1,846,843	3,234,981	2,579,559	555,864	99,558
Rhode Island	872,769	416,431	163,962	252,469	197,995	46,539	7,935
South Carolina	3,818,052	1,833,320	634,399	1,198,921	858,193	264,006	76,722
South Dakota	662,015	330,119	112,651	217,468	172,982	35,101	9,385
Tennessee	5,216,402	2,512,605	808,819	1,703,786	1,165,152	391,828	146,806
Texas	20,202,653	9,953,055	3,469,917	6,483,138	4,796,443	1,284,003	402,692
Utah	2,100,869	1,048,088	340,438	707,650	543,381	126,300	37,969
Vermont	525,211	256,714	86,346	170,368	127,214	36,806	6,348
Virginia	6,642,567	3,227,240	1,122,846	2,104,394	1,580,363	424,929	99,102
Washington	5,576,731	2,762,858	942,136	1,820,722	1,335,484	373,813	111,425
West Virginia	1,535,612	749,711	232,165	517,546	361,148	119,073	37,325
Wisconsin	4,634,334	2,284,469	781,943	1,502,526	1,189,123	266,534	46,869
Wyoming	461,254	233,110	70,774	162,336	114,099	37,185	11,052

Table 4-11B. Number of Times Married for the Population Age 15 Years and Over, 2012 American Community Survey 1-Year Estimates, for Females, by Marital Status and State, 2012

(Number.)

State	Total, age 15 years and over	Female					
		Total	Never married	Ever married			
				Total	Once	Twice	Three or more times
United States	252,745,149	129,570,612	38,367,449	91,203,163	68,939,223	17,619,555	4,644,385
Alabama	3,886,060	2,027,167	537,885	1,489,282	1,037,888	333,342	118,052
Alaska	574,398	274,355	78,101	196,254	142,649	41,337	12,268
Arizona	5,203,019	2,632,694	766,043	1,866,651	1,342,076	398,629	125,946
Arkansas	2,353,968	1,212,609	287,878	924,731	605,640	225,287	93,804
California	30,416,010	15,397,459	5,092,645	10,304,814	8,221,986	1,710,059	372,769
Colorado	4,152,392	2,079,190	566,395	1,512,795	1,102,481	326,279	84,035
Connecticut	2,945,674	1,526,166	470,937	1,055,229	865,487	165,782	23,960
Delaware	746,748	389,090	118,858	270,232	203,432	54,552	12,248
District of Columbia	539,055	287,057	160,809	126,248	106,218	17,631	2,399
Florida	16,016,557	8,259,052	2,290,565	5,968,487	4,220,477	1,360,033	387,977
Georgia	7,830,116	4,046,447	1,226,048	2,820,399	2,040,104	601,978	178,317
Hawaii	1,137,619	567,447	164,861	402,586	327,313	63,292	11,981
Idaho	1,239,521	624,557	144,329	480,228	329,465	111,043	39,720
Illinois	10,344,646	5,318,583	1,682,675	3,635,908	2,880,472	619,815	135,621
Indiana	5,218,923	2,676,653	726,927	1,949,726	1,385,637	422,718	141,371
Iowa	2,472,319	1,256,766	318,365	938,401	717,058	177,404	43,939
Kansas	2,281,272	1,154,143	289,368	864,775	629,625	177,175	57,975
Kentucky	3,530,921	1,809,923	441,056	1,368,867	950,227	310,089	108,551
Louisiana	3,663,532	1,891,654	594,189	1,297,465	945,623	274,689	77,153
Maine	1,111,822	572,904	142,692	430,212	313,188	93,261	23,763
Maryland	4,773,742	2,490,202	817,345	1,672,857	1,313,653	302,686	56,518
Massachusetts	5,498,140	2,864,885	960,603	1,904,282	1,588,418	280,831	35,033
Michigan	8,030,918	4,127,138	1,216,379	2,910,759	2,205,275	567,257	138,227
Minnesota	4,315,429	2,186,951	618,111	1,568,840	1,274,735	250,583	43,522
Mississippi	2,359,979	1,233,574	383,857	849,717	600,085	187,177	62,455
Missouri	4,856,639	2,503,002	675,076	1,827,926	1,287,158	401,864	138,904
Montana	821,687	411,836	97,860	313,976	223,077	66,482	24,417
Nebraska	1,465,286	742,227	192,087	550,140	429,600	98,345	22,195
Nevada	2,204,567	1,097,644	312,613	785,031	532,996	187,065	64,970
New Hampshire	1,098,030	561,901	149,351	412,550	315,484	81,064	16,002
New Jersey	7,196,853	3,726,126	1,151,256	2,574,870	2,167,820	360,733	46,317
New Mexico	1,654,214	840,573	253,816	586,757	427,556	121,305	37,896
New York	16,062,969	8,369,511	2,951,737	5,417,774	4,524,419	789,899	103,456
North Carolina	7,840,375	4,062,858	1,123,288	2,939,570	2,144,361	634,303	160,906
North Dakota	569,837	278,857	75,246	203,611	164,852	32,889	5,870
Ohio	9,351,828	4,829,291	1,369,638	3,459,653	2,552,900	704,535	202,218
Oklahoma	3,026,600	1,540,206	372,220	1,167,986	775,547	280,889	111,550
Oregon	3,185,235	1,621,209	434,057	1,187,152	822,212	270,207	94,733
Pennsylvania	10,519,780	5,437,956	1,646,017	3,791,939	3,035,654	644,866	111,419
Rhode Island	872,769	456,338	146,902	309,436	251,509	49,855	8,072
South Carolina	3,818,052	1,984,732	583,658	1,401,074	1,019,355	300,589	81,130
South Dakota	662,015	331,896	89,401	242,495	187,925	44,734	9,836
Tennessee	5,216,402	2,703,797	713,167	1,990,630	1,356,356	468,805	165,469
Texas	20,202,653	10,249,598	2,914,409	7,335,189	5,419,969	1,459,737	455,483
Utah	2,100,869	1,052,781	279,786	772,995	591,706	137,703	43,586
Vermont	525,211	268,497	75,169	193,328	148,808	37,912	6,608
Virginia	6,642,567	3,415,327	987,200	2,428,127	1,852,105	470,533	105,489
Washington	5,576,731	2,813,873	768,444	2,045,429	1,485,238	432,011	128,180
West Virginia	1,535,612	785,901	188,180	597,721	420,708	135,777	41,236
Wisconsin	4,634,334	2,349,865	665,400	1,684,465	1,334,260	293,621	56,584
Wyoming	461,254	228,144	54,550	173,594	118,436	40,903	14,255

SOURCES OF DATA

Tables 4-1 and 4-2 are from the Centers for Disease Control and Prevention's National Vital Statistics System. Detailed state tables can be found at http://www.cdc.gov/nchs/mardiv.htm#state_tables.

Tables 4-3 through 4-11 are from the 2012 American Community Survey, which is conducted by the U.S. Census Bureau. Additional information and reports can be found at http://www.census.gov/hhes/socdemo/marriage/data/acs/index.html.

NOTES AND DEFINITIONS

Accuracy of the data—Data are based on a sample and are subject to sampling variability. The degree of uncertainty for an estimate arising from sampling variability is represented through the use of a margin of error. The margin of error can be interpreted roughly as providing a 90 percent probability that the interval defined by the estimate minus the margin of error and the estimate plus the margin of error (the lower and upper confidence bounds) contains the true value. In addition to sampling variability, the ACS estimates are subject to nonsampling error. The effect of nonsampling error is not represented in these tables.

Foreign born—Foreign born excludes people born outside the United States to a parent who is a U.S. citizen.

Population—ACS population comprises individuals age 15 to 54 years.

Widowhood—Widowhood estimates may vary from the mortality data released by the National Center for Health Statistics (NCHS) because of differences in methodology and data collection. NCHS uses information collected on death certificates from each state that record the current marital status of the decedent at the time of death. From these administrative records, NCHS then publishes information about men and women who died in that calendar year by their marital status. By inference, people who were married at their time of death were survived by a widowed spouse. In contrast, the ACS collects survey-based reports from individuals as to whether or not they were widowed in the last 12 months. We recommend using caution when comparing the NCHS estimates to the ACS estimates of widowhood.

INDEX

CPSIA information can be obtained at www.ICGtesting.com
Printed in the USA
BVOW06*1753270714

360527BV00003B/5/P